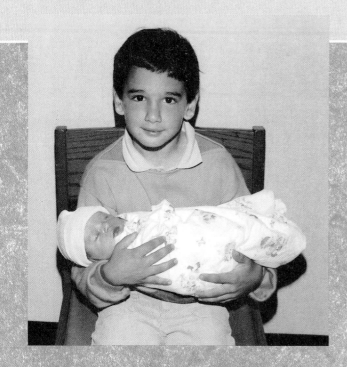

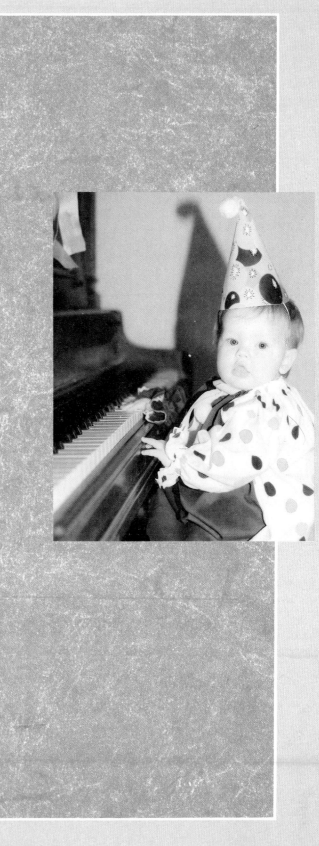

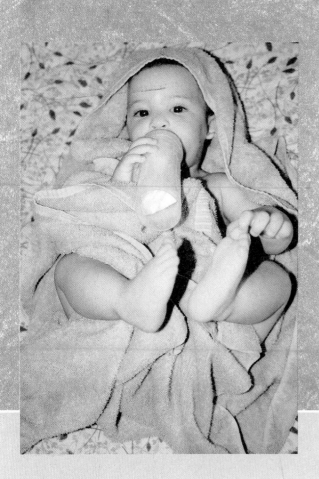

PEDIATRIC NURSING CARE

Gladys M. Scipien, R.N., M.S.
University of Massachusetts
Boston, Harbor Campus
Boston, Massachusetts

Marilyn A. Chard, R.N., Ed.D.
University of Kansas Medical Center
School of Nursing
Kansas City, Kansas

Jeanne Howe, R.N., Ph.D.
Western Carolina University
School of Nursing and Health Sciences
Cullowhee, North Carolina

Martha Underwood Barnard, R.N., Ph.D.
University of Kansas Medical Center
College of Health Sciences and Hospital
Kansas City, Kansas

The C. V. Mosby Company
ST. LOUIS ■ BALTIMORE ■ PHILADELPHIA ■ TORONTO   1990

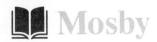

Editor: William Grayson Brottmiller
Senior developmental editor: Sally Adkisson
Design: Liz Fett

This book is dedicated to the memory of Joseph J. Brehm, Jr., a man who by encouraging, supporting, and inspiring us to reach for the seemingly unreachable, played such a significant role in our professional lives. You touched us, Joe.

Printed in the United States of America

The C.V. Mosby Company
11830 Westline Industrial Drive, St. Louis, Missouri 63146

International Standard Book Number 0-8016-6058-0

C/VH/VH   9   8   7   6   5   4   3   2   1

About the Authors

Gladys M. Scipien received a B.S. degree with a major in nursing from Adelphi University and almost immediately began her life-long association with children. For almost twenty years she worked in hospitals, as a staff nurse, head nurse, and supervisor in pediatrics. After receiving an M.S. degree with concentration in Maternal-Child Health from the School of Nursing at Boston University, she assumed a teaching position there, where she remained until its closing in August 1988.

Professor Scipien has published extensively in nursing journals and textbooks. She has served as chief editor of *Comprehensive Pediatric Nursing* through its three editions and is coeditor of *Issues in Comprehensive Pediatric Nursing,* a bimonthly refereed pediatric journal. Her achievements have resulted in alumni awards from Adelphia University and Boston University, the district V MNA Excellence in Nursing Education award, as well as the Mary Ann Garrigan Award for Excellence from the Theta Chapter of Sigma Theta Tau. Professor Scipien, a Fellow in the American Academy of Nursing, currently is Associate Professor at the College of Nursing, Harbor Campus, University of Massachusetts, Boston.

Marilyn A. Chard received a nursing diploma from St. Elizabeth's Hospital in Brighton, a B.S. in nursing from Boston College, an Ed.M. from State College at Worcester, an M.S. in nursing with a major in Maternal Child Nursing from Boston University, and an Ed.D. with a major in Humanistic Behavior and a minor in Adult Education from Boston University. While a doctoral student, she received a certificate as a pediatric nurse practitioner from the University of Kansas. Her thirty-two years of teaching experience include twelve years teaching nursing of children at two diploma schools in Massachusetts; twenty years teaching master's level students in maternal-child nursing at two university schools, one in Massachusetts, and one in Kansas; and five years teaching doctoral level students in nursing in Kansas. From 1975 to 1982, she was program director and teacher in a continuing education nurse practitioner program. Since 1975, she has maintained a part-time collaborative practice as a pediatric nurse practitioner first in Massachusetts and then in Kansas. Dr. Chard has served as coeditor and contributing author for three editions of *Comprehensive Pediatric Nursing.* She has also published several articles in journals and chapters in textbooks.

Jeanne Howe received her B.S.N. degree from the University of Iowa, master's degrees in Pediatric Nursing and Child Development from the University of Pittsburgh, and Ph.D. in Child Development from Florida State University.

Her work has included hospital nursing in pediatric and psychiatric hospitals, hospice home care, editorial freelancing, and twenty years of teaching nursing and related topics at the undergraduate and graduate levels.

She has written and edited seven nursing texts and reference books. The books have received five *American Journal of Nursing* Book of the Year awards and a designation in 1986 as winner of the Second Annual *Pediatric Nursing* Book Awards to recognize excellence in publishing in the child health field.

Dr. Howe resides in Asheville, North Carolina, where she is engaged in private consultation, writing, and the practice of nursing. She directs the Western Carolina University B.S.N. program for registered nurses.

Martha Underwood Barnard is assistant professor of pediatrics at the University of Kansas Medical Center, where she has a joint appointment in the School of Nursing and School of Medicine. She received a B.S. degree in nursing at the University of Missouri, Columbia, and an M.S. degree at the University of Florida with a specialty in Pediatric Nursing. She subsequently joined the nursing faculty at the University of Kansas and received her certificate in the family nurse practitioner program. Because of interests in emotional and compliance problems of children with chronic illnesses, she returned to school to earn an M.S. degree in Child Development and a Ph.D. in Child Psychology, both at the University of Kansas. Dr. Barnard recently completed a post-doctoral program in pediatric psychology at the University of Kansas.

Dr. Barnard has been an editor and author for three editions of *Comprehensive Pediatric Nursing* and coeditor with Gladys Scipien of *Issues in Comprehensive Pediatric Nursing.* She has also edited four other books in pediatric and family nursing and has published extensively in professional journals. Other awards and honors include an outstanding Teaching Award, the American Nurse's Association Certificate of Service, and Outstanding Women of America; and in 1986 she was nominated and appointed to the Nursing Academy of the National Academy of Professionals.

Acknowledgments

Developing a textbook such as this one is an arduous task, made easier by understanding and supportive family members, friends, colleagues, and students as well as conscientious secretaries. There are two professional colleagues who have made significant contributions which deserve special mention. Joyce M. Olson, R.N., M.S.N., a pediatric clinical specialist at the University of Kansas Medical Center, revised and updated Chapters 13, 19, 20, 24, and 27. The editors have appreciated the sharing of her knowledge and expertise as well as her commitment to this project. Tina R. Schwartz, a pediatric clinical nurse specialist at Boston City Hospital, painstakingly prepared all the nursing care plans found in Part III. Her attention to detail and the all-inclusive nature of her efforts enhance the overall quality of that section of the text.

The editors also wish to acknowledge Jacqueline Dowling and Michelle Phillips for preparing the excellent *Instructor's Resource Manual* which accompanies this text. We are confident that this practical manual provides truly creative strategies and support for those teaching pediatric nursing.

We are, in addition, grateful to the following individuals, whose original contributions to our past books have been a source of ideas, idea development, and good teaching sense: Anne Altshuler, R.N., M.S.; Frances J. Anderson, B.S.N., M.A., M.N.; Susan Nelson McCabe, R.N., B.S., M.N., Ph.D.; Eileen Gallagher Nahigian, R.N., B.S.N.E., M.N.; Carolyn Pedigo, R.N., M.S.N.; Barbara Stillman Rothbarth, R.N., M.S.N.; Isobel H. Thorp, R.N., M.A.; June L. Triplett, R.N., Ed.D.

As one might imagine, a project of this proportion requires extensive reviewing and the need for evaluators to expend a considerable amount of time as well as effort in the process. Their comments, suggestions, and recommendations were considered and incorporated within appropriate sections. The editors wish to extend their appreciation to the following nursing colleagues who participated in the review: Nancy Endress, Parkland College; Celia K. Ferguson, San Antonio College; Sharon Ferrante, Middlesex County College; Diane Gallagher, Ohio State University; Ellen Januszkiewicz, Erie Community College; Susan Meehan, Queensborough Community College; Patricia A. Shannon, Phoenix Children's Hospital; Christina D. Slazak, Erie Community College; Sue Ann Symonds, Indiana University at Kokomo; and Edythe Tuchfarber, University of New Mexico.

Lastly, the editors would be remiss in not expressing their gratitude to three publishing colleagues who have been "in the thick of things": Sally Barhydt, Jack Maisel, and Bill Brottmiller.

Gladys M. Scipien
Marilyn A. Chard
Jeanne Howe
Martha Underwood Barnard

Contributors

Kathleen Marie Anderson, R.N., M.S.
Pediatric Nurse Educator
Schneider Children's Hospital
New Hyde Park, New York

Martha Underwood Barnard, R.N., Ph.D.
Faculty and Nurse Clinician
Department of Pediatrics, School of Medicine
School of Nursing
The University of Kansas Medical Center
College of Health Sciences and Hospital
Kansas City, Kansas

Jeanne Quint Benoliel, R.N., D.N.Sc., F.A.A.N.
Professor, Community Health Care Systems
School of Nursing
University of Washington
Seattle, Washington

Laura Maria Bloomquist, R.N., M.N.
Formerly Instructor, Nursing Education Services
Pediatric Staff Development
Dhahran Health Center
Arabian American Oil Company
Dhahran, Saudi Arabia

Marilyn A. Chard, R.N., Ed.D.
Professor, School of Nursing
Assistant Professor, Department of Pediatrics
The University of Kansas Medical Center
College of Health Sciences
Kansas City, Kansas

Teresa Clabots, M.D.
Private Practice
Endocrine Consultants Northwest
Tacoma, Washington

Sherrilyn Passo Coffman, R.N., M.S.
Visiting Assistant Professor
The Division of Nursing
Florida-Atlantic University
Boca Raton, Florida

Mary Jean Denyes, R.N., Ph.D.
Associate Professor, Maternal-Child Health Nursing
Wayne State University,
College of Nursing
Detroit, Michigan

Jacqueline S. Dowling, R.N., M.S.
Director, Nursing Laboratories
Department of Nursing, University of Lowell
Lowell, Massachusetts

Jane Cooper Evans, R.N., Ph.D.
Nurse Researcher and Associate Professor
College of Nursing
Wright State University
Dayton, Ohio

Christina M. Graf, R.N., M.S.
Director, Nursing Management Systems
Massachusetts General Hospital
Boston, Massachusetts

Patricia Ellis Green, R.N., M.S.N., F.A.A.N.
Director of Cancer Nursing
American Cancer Society
New York, New York

Cheryl Hall Harris, R.N., B.S.N.
Instructor, School of Medicine
University of Missouri—Kansas City;
Consultant, Nursing Department
Children's Mercy Hospital
Kansas City, Missouri

Mary Frances Hazinski, R.N., M.S.N.
Clinical Specialist
Pediatric Intensive Care Unit
Vanderbilt University Hospital
Nashville, Tennessee

Jeanne Howe, R.N., Ph.D.
Associate Professor
School of Nursing and Health Sciences
Western Carolina University
Cullowhee, North Carolina

Ann Klingner, R.N., M.S.
Pediatric Clinical Specialist
School of Nursing
University of Texas at Austin
Austin, Texas

Catherine M. Kneut, R.N., M.S.
Pediatric Clinical Nurse Specialist
Rhode Island Hospital
Providence, Rhode Island

Barbara E. Langner, R.N., Ph.D.
Associate Professor
School of Nursing
The University of Kansas Medical Center
College of Health Sciences and Hospital
Kansas City, Kansas

Mira L. Lessick, R.N.
Formerly of the School of Nursing
University of Texas at Austin
Austin, Texas

Sarah Malone, M.S., R.D.
Clinical Nutrition Specialist
The Children's Mercy Hospital
Kansas City, Missouri

Janet A. Marvin, R.N., M.S.N.
Department of Surgery
School of Medicine
University of Washington
Adjunct Assistant Professor
School of Nursing
University of Washington
Seattle, Washington

Janet E. McNally, R.N., M.S.
Nursing Consultant
Handicapped Children Program
Colorado Department of Health
Denver, Colorado

Margaret Shandor Miles, R.N., Ph.D., F.A.A.N.
Professor, School of Nursing
University of North Carolina at Chapel Hill
Chapel Hill, North Carolina

Joyce M. Olson, R.N., M.S.N.
Pediatric Clinical Nurse Specialist
Department of Nursing Services
The University of Kansas Medical Center
College of Health Sciences and Hospital
Kansas City, Kansas

Patricia J. Phillips, R.N., M.N.
Assistant Professor
School of Nursing
Nurse Practitioner, Department of Pediatrics
The University of Kansas Medical Center
College of Health Sciences and Hospital
Kansas City, Kansas

Karen E. Roper, R.N., M.S.N.
Head Nurse in Pediatrics
Delaware County Memorial Hospital
Formerly of the Children's Hospital of Philadelphia,
Pennsylvania

Tina R. Schwartz, R.N., M.S.N.
Clinical Nurse Specialist Nursing of Children
Coordinator Pediatric A.I.D.S. Program
Boston City Hospital
Boston, Massachusetts

Gladys M. Scipien, R.N., M.S., F.A.A.N.
Associate Professor, College of Nursing, Harbor Campus
University of Massachusetts, Boston
Boston, Massachusetts

Marie E. Snyder, R.N., M.S., J.D.
Attorney-at-Law
Boston, Massachusetts

Rachel Spector, R.N., Ph.D.
Associate Professor
Boston College, School of Nursing
Chestnut Hill, Massachusetts

Robin Wheeler, M.S., R.D.
Neonatal Nutritionist
The Children's Mercy Hospital
Kansas City, Missouri

Preface to the Instructor

Basic Pediatric Nursing is designed to present pertinent information for students who are entering their first pediatric clinical and classroom experience. Based on the authors' extensive careers in nursing, both academic and clinical, this text offers students the basic principles on which to build their own professional roles.

The authors recognize the fact that faculty in most undergraduate programs have limited classroom time and clinical hours to convey the essence of pediatric nursing and to help students acquire some mastery of the content. In addition, textbooks have grown to well over 1000 pages, presenting both prerequisite and even graduate-level content. Such a volume of material, although useful in a reference work, may fail to meet the immediate needs of students and may in fact serve only to confuse and discourage them. *Pediatric Nursing Care* has been written in response to survey results that express the need for an undergraduate textbook that goes "back to basics," one which can be carried to and used in the classroom and truly contains only the most pertinent information. To produce such a textbook has been our goal in the development and preparation of this book; we hope that our colleagues will find we have met it.

The chapters in Part I are devoted to introducing the student to the pediatric nursing specialty; discussing factors which influence and promote health; elaborating on the nursing assessment of different age groups; and presenting the ethical and legal issues which are involved in child health. Even though student assignments vary and must take into account the competencies as well as prior experiences of individual students, Chapters 1, 4, 7, and 8 should be required at the start of the course. Growth and development content may be perceived as redundant in curriculums which require a specific course; however, the editors believe its inclusion is essential here. If nurses are to become skillful in recognizing abnormal modes of development, they must be familiar with all aspects of normal development.

The special problems a nurse encounters in pediatrics are found in Part II. Separate chapters cover high-risk neonates and their families and children who are mentally retarded, abused, or chronically or terminally ill. Such elaboration is needed so that students can better understand the ramifications of any one of these problems.

Cases and nursing care plans are included in Part III with the discussion of common but serious disorders which nursing students are most likely to encounter in the basic pediatric course. The editors strongly believe that determining a nursing diagnosis is a critical step in the nursing process and that the process of planning care involves more than simply choosing labels from a list. Students should be encouraged to consider these "generic" care plans as guides to gathering patient data on which care will be based. NANDA-approved diagnoses are used in the care plans, and a complete list of the 1988 NANDA diagnoses is provided in Appendix D at the back of the book.

In Part III, "Nursing Management of Children with Alterations in Body Systems," problems are organized by body system for each age group. Systems are grouped by function. Although this organization may be considered too "medical" an approach, the editors believe it is a real-world format that is more understandable for beginning students.

Study questions and suggestions for classroom and clinical learning activities follow the chapters. Independent learning activities for students are also identified at the ends of chapters. To further aid the instructor, a separate resource manual and test bank is available to adopters.

In a separate Preface for the Student, the editors have suggested one method of using this book efficiently. We have made every effort to provide in this volume the essential content that students will need to pursue the nursing care of children. It is also our hope that we have provided a text and supplementary materials to enhance the enjoyment and professional growth of child health faculty everywhere.

Preface to the Student

Children and adolescents are unique human beings who respond to illness in a highly individualized manner. It is not possible to provide a textbook which allows a student to go to a specific section to acquire all the information necessary to care for that child. Circumstances are different, health needs are different, and, most of all, children are different.

In order to get maximal use of this text, it is essential for students to read portions which are appropriate to the children for whom they have accepted responsibility. Let us say, for example, that you are assigned to care for a hospitalized two-year-old with asthma. It is necessary to read about normal toddler development (Chapter 2), portions of the physical assessment which pertain to the toddler (Chapter 6), this age group's responses to hospitalization (Chapter 9), and then content related to asthma (Chapter 23). This sequence is not all-inclusive because students have different clinical experiences which may require more or less preparation time. It is important for you to identify readings appropriate for your own knowledge needs. Obviously, a child is not cared for in isolation, with a nurse oblivious to the various factors which influence the care provided to that child. Therefore, one cannot simply read the portion of the text which pertains to a health problem requiring hospitalization. It is the constant preparation and reviewing that facilitates the acquisition of an ever-expanding knowledge base. Then and only then is a student prepared to provide safe, effective, quality patient care.

The nursing care plans contained in Part III are generic; they should serve as examples of what needs to be considered in developing plans of care. Children are individuals who function at different developmental levels and are affected by the cultures and families of which they are a part. It is critical to recognize the highly individualized needs of a particular child with a specific health problem because this information must be incorporated into nursing care plans developed by nurses.

When children are stable, nurses also must focus their attention on health promotion activities (Chapter 4), endeavors which maximize wellness. The health patterns of adults can be influenced and affected by the information they acquire in childhood.

The authors have developed this text in the hope that students who begin their work with children will have here the basic information they need in order to work with them effectively. We believe we have provided you with the essential components of pediatric nursing principles. Although we have thoroughly enjoyed and learned a great deal from our professional experiences with children, we have also been challenged and stimulated by our students. We hope that as a result of using this book and working with this population each of you will better understand the remarkable responses of children to illness and appreciate the challenges and rewards they provide the nurses who care for them.

Contents

Appendixes

NURSING CARE PLANS

PART
I

An Introduction to the Nursing Care of Children

1

Nursing of Children: The Development of the Specialty

Objectives

After reading this chapter, the student will be able to:
1. Appreciate the events that influenced the emergence of pediatrics as a specialty.
2. Identify nursing leaders who contributed to improved delivery of health care for children.
3. Discuss variables which affect the delivery of health care for children.
4. Enumerate several challenges pertinent to pediatric nursing in the 1990s.

History of Children in Society

Societal Views of Children

Of what value is a child? In nineteenth-century rural America, the family was a separate economically productive entity with an emphasis on family traditions and continuity. Children were an invaluable part of the work force on a farm. As late as 1880 and 1890, about 20 percent of children died before the second birthday and about 50 percent were not expected to reach the twenty-first birthday; therefore, families were large in an effort to compensate for these expected losses. However, the family unit has been affected by the social and economic forces which gradually transformed this country into an industrial nation.

Today Americans are fearful of the future, of the uncertain economy and spiraling inflation. When one considers that in 1986 it cost a family of average means about $145,000 to raise a child to the age of 18 years, the financial awesomeness of parenting becomes clear. This figure excludes the cost of a college education. The breakdown of categories is as follows: housing, $49,300; food, $36,250; transportation, $24,650; clothing, $11,600; medical care; $7250; education, $2900; other, $15,050 (Daniels, 1986).

The family is being challenged from within and by external factors. There have been breaks in traditional structures, roles, and responsibilities.

Mothers who have returned to the work force have had the greatest impact on the family. The mental stimulation, broadened social horizons, and new economic status have brought independence to women who were previously confined to homes, children, and housework (Nordheimer, 1977). As a result, more and more children are at day care centers or with baby-sitters. Changing attitudes, liberalized divorce laws, and the fact that divorce is now both economically and socially feasible have facilitated the dissolution of unhappy marriages. Divorce rates have more than doubled in the last decade. From November 1, 1984 to October 31, 1985, 1,185,000 divorces were finalized (USDHHS, 1985).

In 1970 there were 3.2 million single-parent families; by 1976 this figure had increased to 4.9 million, all but 500,000 headed by women (Nordheimer, 1977). By 1990, 25 percent of all children in the United States will live in single-parent households (Green, 1986). In 1985 the percentages of mothers employed outside the home were as follows: 70 percent with children 6 years of age and older, 67 percent with children under 3 years of age, and nearly 50 percent with infants under 1 year of age (Crowley, 1986).

After World War II it was thought that indigence was under control in the United States; however, a 1963 study by Harrington revealed that it had reached epidemic proportions, with about 36 million Americans struggling for survival. In 1979 about 8 million (33 percent) of those living at the poverty level were children and youths under 14 years of age (Spector, 1979). By 1982 more than 13 million children in the United States were living in poverty, an increase of 3.1 million since 1979 (Mitchell and Harbin, 1985). While substantial strides have been made to improve the quality of life for children, these efforts must continue because children and adolescents are this country's most valuable resource.

Child-Rearing Practices

Childhood is a fairly recent concept. A glance at medieval art graphically demonstrates the lack of knowledge about children, whose naked bodies are shown with the proportions and musculature of adults rather than the physical characteristics that typify infants and children. Childhood continued to be thought of as an unimportant stage of life until the eighteenth century, when names and birth dates first began to be recorded.

Between 1820 and 1860 Americans began to demonstrate an increasing interest in children and in child-

rearing practices. While it was related to social status, this new interest was associated with the child's being perceived as an extension of parental ambitions. Prior to the Civil War, there was an emerging belief that people had the ability to control their environment and direct their future, which included the molding of a child.

One hundred sixty years ago a mother was considered to be the child's best instructor, the person responsible for developing his character and instituting disciplinary measures. Fathers had very little to do with children, and hence fathering received no attention.

Breast-feeding was common. Babies established their own feeding routines, determining both time and frequency. Weaning occurred in a period of a week or two when the infant was 8 to 12 months old; however, the time at which teeth erupted was an important consideration. Wet nurses, who were frequently unwed mothers, were employed by members of the upper class. Bottle feeding was also prevalent among the more fortunate members of society. Interestingly, supplemental feedings included candy, cake, and some other types of solids. It was not unusual for parents to administer drugs, including laudanum (a form of opium) and alcohol, to crying infants in order to put them to sleep.

For the most part, children after 1820 were loosely dressed and their clothing was light to allow freedom of movement. Since cleanliness was strictly enforced, some infants were not allowed to crawl because they would become dirty in the process. While 10- to 15-month-olds were encouraged to feed themselves in crude high chairs at the supper table, being orderly, neat, and clean in the process of eating met with parental approval (Sunley, 1967).

Religion played a major role in family life during the first half of the nineteenth century. Religious doctrines influenced the moral training of children. For example, the Calvinists extolled the belief that children were totally depraved and doomed unless careful and strict guidance was provided by parents. Hence, total submission and complete obedience were required. As expected, problems arose and resulted in the formation of groups known as the "maternal associations" of the Protestant Calvinist sect, in which mothers met regularly to discuss situations related to child rearing (Sunley, 1967).

Rigid schedules of child rearing continued to be in vogue in the twentieth century. Both children's and parents' roles were defined by the experts. In the late 1940s the emphasis began to shift toward a more relaxed approach and was changed by some parents to a point at which the child seemed to be in command. Some experts believe that this attitude contributed to the rise of the youth counterculture in the 1960s. Also during the 1960s, fathers were encouraged to take a more active role in child rearing. Child-rearing emphasis in the 1970s and 1980s has shifted again but seems to contain a blend of schedules and relaxation. The experts are telling parents that they (the parents) know a great deal about their children and are quite capable of making decisions. The experts may provide guidance, but they no longer claim to hold all knowledge.

Historical Views of the Child

Locke and, later, Rousseau were among the first writers to influence current attitudes toward infants and children. They thought neonates were born without ideas but with natural impulses which their environment taught them to curb. While these men believed it was necessary to "harden" children, they also thought some effort should be directed toward accepting the "naturalness" of childhood behavior (Sunley, 1967). Others believed that children should be treated with consistency, firmness, and understanding and rewarded appropriately. Physical beatings were to be discouraged because children were simply "too tender for such treatment." Horace Bushnell in 1942 proposed that the young were not depraved, nor were they miniature adults; they were individuals who were passing through various stages of development (Whitworth, 1977).

The deleterious effects of prolonged institutionalization of healthy infants were unrecognized until the middle of the twentieth century, when Spitz (1945, 1946) published his results. The infants he studied lived in foundling homes in which one nurse cared for eight infants. A comparison group of infants lived in their parents' homes or in an institution in which they received full-time care from their own mothers or substitute mothers. Spitz discovered that the infants in foundling homes failed to thrive; that is, they were retarded in growth (length and weight) and development. They also were more susceptible to disease than were the infants in the control group.

For some reason, Spitz's findings were not related quickly to the effect of hospitalization on children. Bowlby (1960) made the connection and conducted a study to determine the effects of hospitalization on 15- to 30-month-old toddlers. On the basis of the results, he defined three stages of separation anxiety: protest, despair, and detachment. His studies paved the way for rooming-in. Both Spitz's and Bowlby's data demonstrate the need for consistent mothering in a stimulating environment.

While Spitz was conducting his studies, Spock was writing *The Common Sense Book of Baby and Child Care* at a time when the extended family was being replaced by the nuclear family. This book, retitled *Baby and Child Care* in subsequent editions, has been the "bible" for millions of parents since its publication in 1946. The first edition also emphasized permissiveness. As the youth counterculture emerged in the 1960s, Spock began to think less in prescriptive terms. In the 1976 edition, Spock expressed the belief that parents know more than they think they do and encouraged them to become more independent in their thinking and decision making.

Certainly views of childhood have changed over the years. The child has been thought of as a small adult, as depraved, and finally as a person in his own right. This person has many stages of growth and development to achieve before reaching adulthood.

The Emergence of Pediatrics as a Specialty

Children were not thought to have health needs different from those of adults until 1860, when Dr. Abraham Jacobi, the "father" of American pediatrics and the first chairman of the pediatric section of the American Medical Association, began to lecture to medical students on the special diseases of children treated in a clinic he had established in New York (Rudolph and Oglesby, 1977). Interest in caring for children resulted in the formation of the American Pediatric Society (Rudolph and Ogelsby, 1977), which also incorporated nurses and social workers as well as physicians. The status quo was to remain for some time.

While World War I raged, 1918 was designated as the Children's Year, and the first federally supported health programs for mothers and children were established. Subsequently, the Sheppard-Towner Act of 1921 created a schism in medicine and led to the formation of the American Academy of Pediatrics in 1930. This piece of legislation resulted in the establishment of the first federal grant in the field of health to be specifically aimed at improving the health of mothers and infants. The American Medical Association (AMA) vehemently opposed the bill, and so physicians who were involved in child care broke away from the parent organization. As a result of this legislation, prenatal clinics were established, conferences for expectant mothers were conducted, and many child health centers were created (Grotberg, 1976).

Nursing Leaders in Child Care

Several pediatric and maternity nurses have made important contributions to the nursing care of children, notably Florence Erickson, Florence Blake, Reva Rubin, Ernestine Wiedenbach, Loretta Ford, and Kathryn Barnard. This list is by no means exhaustive.

Erickson (1958) developed the play interview for hospitalized 4-year-old children. The play interview is conducted by offering the child a kit which contains both threatening (e.g., hospital equipment) and nonthreatening (e.g., crayons, toy furniture) materials and dolls representing family members and hospital personnel. The nurse observes and records the child's play with these objects, thereby gaining insight into what the child perceives as traumatic about hospitalization. The combination of both sets of data provides the nurse with a basis to devise a plan of care which will help the child work through his feelings.

Blake (1964) studied eight children (ages 4 to 16 years) who had operable cardiac defects to determine ways in which children and their parents react to and cope with hospitalization, nursing care, and treatment. She provided direct patient care to six of the subjects for periods ranging from 1 to 6 weeks. A detailed report of her experiences with her first subject, 4-year-old Suzie, and her family demonstrated elements of nursing care which can be employed to improve the care given to sick children both preoperatively and postoperatively.

Through this study, Blake demonstrated that nursing

intervention can minimize the child's anxieties, fears, and discomforts and the physical hazards to which he may be subjected.

The progression of maternal touch with the neonate was studied by Rubin (1963). She identified the steps in the touching process as progressing from tentative finger-tip touching to palm to full hand and arm touch as maternal involvement with the neonate increases. Her findings have assumed great significance since Klaus and Kennell's (1970) later work shed more light on the early mother-child relationship. Close body contact during the first few hours after delivery is believed to be important in the development of maternal feelings and behavior.

Family-centered maternity care is another important concept which has been influential in laying the groundwork for parental feelings and behaviors. Wiedenbach (1967), a prime advocate of this concept, was instrumental in bringing the father into the maternity setting and fostered the involvement of both mother and father in the care of the newborn. Family-centered maternity care was a forerunner of what is called rooming-in today.

Ford and Silver (Silver, Ford, and Stearly, 1967) demonstrated the viability of the pediatric nurse's role expansion to include taking a complete health history, performing a thorough physical examination, evaluating the child's developmental level, planning and administering immunizations, advising and counseling parents and youths according to the problems defined, managing common pediatric problems, and collaborating with other health professionals in the provision of primary health care to infants, children, and adolescents. Ford, a pediatric nurse, was a major developer of the nurse practitioner role as it is practiced today not only by pediatric nurse practitioners but also adult, women's, and family nurse practitioners.

Barnard has made many contributions to the nursing care of children. In 1966 she and Paulus designed the "Washington Guide to Promoting Development in the Young Child." This tool was revised in 1969 by Barnard and Erickson (1976). It is widely used by pediatric nurses to evaluate and improve children's developmental levels in a variety of settings. She has been a strong advocate for mentally retarded children and their families (Barnard and Erickson, 1976) and has influenced many nurses, physicians, and legislators in the move to secure the rights and services to which these children and their families are entitled.

The nurses cited in this chapter have had an impact on the care of children from conception through adolescence. They have contributed to the improvement of child health care both in the hospital and in the community.

Variations in Pediatric Nursing Practice

In the 1940s and early 1950s a form of *primary nursing* was practiced on pediatric units. The nurse had responsibility for feeding, bathing, medicating, and performing treatments for each child assigned to her care during an 8-year period. No formal nursing care plans were written, but continuity of care was provided through shift-change reports. At this time nurses were beginning to incorporate the principles of growth and development in pediatric care, but the importance of play as a means of encouraging children to express and work through their feelings was not generally recognized.

In the mid-1950s, *team nursing* emerged and care was fragmented. Children were expected to relate to several people during a single 8-hour period in order to have their needs met. As the importance of play was recognized, yet another person entered the child's milieu, the play therapist. Technology progressed, and varied personnel became involved in child care: the nutritionist, the physical therapist, the respiratory therapist, and the occupational therapist. Care was further fragmented, and efforts toward coordination of care became a nightmare.

A remedy for this dilemma was proposed in the form of *primary nursing.* Although not yet widely adopted, it promulgates continuity of care through making one nurse responsible for the care of several hospitalized children over a 24-hour period. This primary nurse must develop individualized, written care plans for each child. Although the nurse is not physically present 24 hours a day, she is available by phone should the need arise.

In the mid-1960s the role of the *pediatric nurse practitioner* (PNP) was created. PNPs have 24-hour responsibility for a panel of pediatric clients. They (or a designated colleague) are available by telephone evenings, nights, and weekends should an emergency arise. Physicians are available for consultation in medical matters.

The *clinical nurse specialist* was also emerging during the mid-1960s. This role has become highly specialized and requires a master's degree. Clinical specialists in pediatric nursing may be found providing various kinds of nursing care in various settings. For example, they may provide direct care and teaching in the pediatric oncology clinic; on the maternity or pediatric unit or in the clinic they may counsel the parents of infants born with birth defects; in the diabetic clinic or on the pediatric unit they teach diabetic children and their families; and on pediatric units they commonly conduct ward conferences with staff nurses caring for children who have complex problems.

Thus, the nurse can provide services to children and their families through various roles. Service, though, goes beyond direct care. It includes involvement in nursing organizations and other groups that deal with health care issues, e.g., American Nurses' Association (ANA), National League for Nursing (NLN), Association for the Care of Children's Health (ACCH), maternal-child health subgroups, and child advocacy groups; providing information to legislative groups for or against passage of bills related to child health; and community activities such as involvement in youth groups and consultation with other nurses.

Traditionally, nurses have been involved in the teaching of students in the three basic nursing preparation programs, in master's programs, and in doctoral programs. Health teaching to children and their parents through anticipatory guidance, counseling, and the use of audiovisual materials (self-produced or commercially packaged) has been a prime educational role of nursing. Another aspect of teaching involves continuing education (CE) for nurses. Several states now require evidence of CE credits for relicensure, and current trends indicate that several more states will follow this practice.

Another activity which is gaining momentum among pediatric nurses is *scholarly endeavor*. It encompasses the design and implementation of research, the development of teaching materials (e.g., audiovisual aids, textbooks, book chapters, articles, and monographs), and the development of new and innovative educational programs. Through the development of teaching materials and writing, pediatric nurses share the wealth of knowledge they have gained from research and practice.

Variables Affecting Child Care

Infant Mortality

The United States celebrated its hundredth birthday before any efforts were directed toward investigating the cause of death of babies in the first few weeks or months of life. Up to 1897 there were no protests or concern about the conditions under which milk was collected. There was no refrigeration, and consumers frequently purchased sour milk with hundreds of millions of bacteria. Through the efforts of one health officer in Rochester, New York, who had some knowledge of nineteenth-century research regarding the causation of disease, the cleaning of stables, the sterilization of equipment, and the boiling of milk and its eventual distribution to a "milk station" were initiated. At the milk station, infants were weighed and a milk mixture was prescribed according to the baby's body weight (Grotberg, 1976). It was here, too, that mothers had access to a nurse, the health care provider who instructed mothers about fresh air, water, food, sleep, clothing, and the recreational needs of children.

Dr. L. Emmett Holt (of Babies' Hospital in New York City) wrote in 1897 that 20 percent of all infants would die before the end of their second year (Grotberg, 1976). The infant death rate of a country is considered to be an index of the general well-being of its society. In 1900 the U.S. death rate for infants was 100 per 1000 live births (Clemen, Eigsti, and McGuire, 1981); by 1935 it dropped to 55.7 per 1000 live births (Rudolph and Oglesby, 1977). During World War II, between the attack on Pearl Harbor and the end of fighting on V-J day, 281,000 Americans were killed in action. During this same period 430,000 babies died in this country before they were 1 year old, a rather startling comparison (Grotberg, 1976).

By 1950 the mortality rate had dropped to 29.2 per 1000 births (Rudolph and Oglesby, 1977). In 1965 it was 24.7 per 1000 live births, and in 1975 it had dropped to 16.1 per 1000 live births (Pless, 1978). The U.S. infant mortality rate for 1985 was 10.6 per 1000 live births (Smith, 1986). The declines in the death rate after 1955 were due to improved treatment of perinatal illnesses, especially asphyxia, immaturity, and respiratory and gastrointestinal problems.

With the expertise possessed by health care providers and the research capabilities of this country, one would imagine America's infant mortality would be the lowest in the world. In fact, it is higher than that of 15 other countries. Perhaps the unequal distribution of personnel, resources, and access to health care systems has allowed these statistics to prevail.

State and Federal Efforts to Improve Delivery of Care

Efforts to improve the quality of health for children were slow to reach colonial America. By the end of the Civil War, New York had created the Metropolitan Sanitary District and a board of health in order to preserve life and health as well as prevent the spread of disease. In 1869, Massachusetts established a permanent Board of Health and Vital Statistics, which was to provide the most reliable data on infant mortality available before 1900 (Grotberg, 1976). Generally there was little state interest in children or in their specific needs.

Federal involvement followed the first White House Conference on the care of children in 1909. Concern for the plight of children resulted in the establishment of the Children's Bureau in 1912. This federal bureau was charged with investigating all aspects of child care, including infant mortality, the birthrate, conditions in orphanages, desertion of children, and dangerous occupations in which children were participating. It was responsible for compiling and publishing *Infant Care* (1914), the most extensive collection of information ever published on child care, including development (Children's Bureau, 1963).

This federal agency singularly and aggressively directed its efforts to improve the plight of all children in America. Since it was created by Congress, the bureau was able to make proposals for legislation, the most remarkable of which were those authorized by the Social Security Act.

When the Social Security Act of 1935 was signed by President Roosevelt, provisions for the health care of mothers and children were incorporated in Title V and, for the first time, there was recognition of the needs of crippled children (Grotberg, 1976). Both Early and Periodic Screening, Diagnosis, and Treatment (EPSDT) and the Women, Infants, and Children (WIC) programs are examples of the benefits received through this legislation (Grotberg, 1976).

In 1967 the Office of Child Development (OCD) was established; housing both the Children's Bureau and the Bureau of Child Development Services, which operates Head Start and other programs. The secretary of Health and Human Services (HHS) is currently the cabinet officer responsible for the activities of OCD.

In analyzing the progress made in child health and child care, it is apparent that the decade of the 1960s was marked by an increase in access to, and a more equitable distribution of, services. However, in the late 1970s and the 1980s the emphasis was on cost containment. It appears that this issue will continue to be important in the future.

The latest innovation in cost containment is diagnosis-related groupings (DRGs). The National Association of Children's Hospitals and Related Groups has developed 103 children's diagnosis-related groups (CDRGs). Fifty-one of the 103 are from existing DRGs. The CDRGs are to be tested against cost data from several pediatric hospitals ("Trends," 1986). Their advent has great import for nursing practice, education, and research. With early discharge, high-technology care will be provided in the home as well as in the hospital. Professional nurses in the community will need continuing education opportunities to prepare for high-technology home care; educators need to revise their curricula to prepare future practitioners of nursing; and nurse researchers will have an opportunity to study recidivism rates for children who are discharged earlier than had been the practice before the advent of CDRGs.

Violence

The increasing incidence of child abuse, with current annual figures in excess of 2 million cases, has led individual states to enact laws that make abuse reportable; however, the specifics vary greatly from state to state. The definition of abuse and neglect has been expanded to include physical abuse, nutritional deprivation, emotional abuse, medical neglect, and sexual abuse. More recently the use of children in pornography has been revealed. For example, in Los Angeles alone, police estimate that 30,000 children under 5 years of age are used as photography subjects in pornography and that their services are sold by their parents. Initially there was some confusion about what constitutes abuse and when it is reportable, but these points were clarified in 1974, when Congress passed Public Law 93-247.

The incredible acts of violence toward children provided an impetus for analyzing additional acts of physical force which occur within the family. Although exact figures of wife/mother beating and husband/father beating are unknown, witnessing such acts can take its toll on children, potentiating the possibility that the children will become batterers as adults. As a result, Representative Barbara Mikulski of Maryland introduced the Family Violence and Treatment Act in the U.S. House of Representatives in September 1977. This important legislation has been enacted.

Schooling

All states have statutes regarding school programs for children of specific ages. In fact, attendance is mandatory for children and youths between 7 and 16 years of age. However, some states also have exclusion clauses which deny an education to many who have physical, intellectual, or emotional handicaps. The Children's Defense Fund, a large child advocacy organization based in Washington, D.C., estimated that 2 million children between 6 and 17 years were not in classrooms ("Who Speaks?" 1979), and this figure does not include those who are truant, expelled, or suspended. In the annual report of the National Advisory Committee on the Handicapped, 1976 figures showed that 45 percent of handicapped pupils between ages 6 and 19 years and 78 percent of those up to 5 years of age were unserved by any school programs (Keough and Barkett, 1978).

In an effort to improve the situation, "mainstreaming" was started in the 1970s in school systems across the country. Handicapped children began to attend regular classes with nonhandicapped students for part or all of the day. The goal was to allow those with handicaps to function in a society where most individuals did not share their impediments and to enable students without handicaps to gain understanding of what it means to be handicapped.

In the last 10 to 15 years litigation has been a major social force in bringing about a definition of the right to an education. Judicial decisions have also affected "mainstreaming" education; late in 1975 the Education for All Handicapped Children Act became law. This legislation requires that all handicapped children 3 to 21 years of age be given whatever educational services and facilities they need, in the public schools and at no cost. However, implementation has been lagging. The lack of collected evidence to document the social, behavioral, and academic results of mainstreaming endeavors makes it extremely difficult to evaluate the effectiveness and appropriateness of such programs. (See also Chapter 18.)

Child Advocacy

The legal system is based in English law, which always considered children the possessions of their parents. In the absence of a parent, it is incumbent on the state to make decisions based on the child's best interests. It was not until 1948, in *Haley v. Ohio,* that the Supreme Court ruled that the rights guaranteed adults by the Constitution apply to children too. As recently as 1976, in *Planned Parenthood v. Danforth* (abortion for a minor), it was determined that "constitutional rights do not mature and come into being only when one attains the state-defined age" (Stier, 1978, p. 46). However, these precedent-setting decisions have not led to the clarification of other relevant child-focused issues. It appears that legal decisions occur as a result of some overriding social concern rather than out of concern for children themselves. One exception is in the area of juvenile justice, which was settled by the Gault decision of 1967, guaranteeing procedural protection and legal representation for about 100,000 adolescents who were in jail (Reed and Phillips, 1972).

Society is painfully slow in clarifying or extending the rights of children, because of strong, conflicting attitudes regarding children and rights. In spite of the obvious needs of some children for intervention from outside the family, it is widely considered a natural right of parents to control the nurturance of their offspring and, hence, a right that should be preserved at all costs. The caution and hesitation of the courts in these precarious situations have frustrated and discouraged nurses who advocate for children experiencing difficult conditions.

Child advocacy is a term that was first used in 1969, when the Joint Commission on Mental Health of Children recommended the creation of a national system of child advocacy. In 1971 the National Center for Child Advocacy finally was established within the Office of Child Development. It is designed to identify and correct policies and practices which violate basic legal and human rights or are harmful to a child's health or welfare. Prime responsibilities involve organizational or institutional barriers, social or structural impediments, budgetary restrictions, and administrative or statutory constraints which prevent children and families from receiving the assistance they need, whether that assistance pertains to health, education, foster care, handicaps, child development, or day care.

A large private child advocacy group is the Children's Defense Fund (CDF), which was founded about the same time and is based in Washington, D.C. Under the active leadership of Marian Wright Edelman, this organization serves as a congressional watchdog, advising its members through issuing "legislative alerts," publishing a newsletter, and disseminating invaluable relevant information of a national and regional nature.

If overall circumstances are to improve, specific situations need to be challenged, state and federal agencies and personnel should be held accountable, and policies and practices have to be changed so that parents can carry out their responsibilities in preparing their children for the future. Nurses who work with children need to become involved in consumer groups and child advocacy organizations in order to secure the rights and services to which their clients are entitled. They must speak for children who are unable to speak for themselves.

White House Conferences
In 1909 President Theodore Roosevelt convened the first White House Conference as a result of concern regarding the exploitation of children in work settings and their cruel, inhumane treatment in orphanages and foundling homes. This first White House Conference prompted the creation in 1912 of the Children's Bureau, which worked diligently to improve conditions for children but made slow progress.

After the economic crash of 1929 a severe depression paralyzed the country. The White House Conference on Child Health was convened in 1930 to study the health and well-being of children and to determine what ought to be done for them. Nevertheless, by 1932 schoolchildren were suffering from malnutrition, and pellagra was increasing drastically in the south. Despite agendas that included plans for the ill, the handicapped, and the deprived, society's response to the needs of its future citizens has not been as rapid as one might desire.

Since 1930, a White House Conference on Children has been held at the beginning of every decade. Thousands of professionals who work with children, representatives from federal and state agencies, and representatives from national and local voluntary organizations and citizens' groups meet to discuss current issues affecting children. However, the conclusions they draw have little impact, and the recommendations they make are never implemented. There are no permanent members of these conferences, and, more important, the attendees have no power or authority to institute the results of their endeavor. A graphic example is the 1970 White House Conference on Children and Youth. The report from that conference was a scathing indictment of what was being done poorly or not at all. The people at the conference knew the pathetic state of child care in America, yet they were powerless to improve it.

World Health Organization
The United Nations sanctioned the establishment of the World Health Organization (WHO) in 1948. It is headquartered in Geneva, Switzerland, and its primary goal is to improve the health of all people. Although it is the authority where international health issues are concerned, it maintains collaborative relationships with all countries, furnishes health information and a myriad of other services when requested, and promotes programs which will improve the quality of health care for women, infants, and children.

United Nations International Children's Emergency Fund (UNICEF)
The United Nations created UNICEF in 1946 in an effort to meet the emergency needs of children at times of natural disaster (earthquake, famine) or war. While countries voluntarily contribute to this fund, organizations and individuals also support its activities.

In the United States, "Trick or Treat for UNICEF" is an annual occurrence at Halloween as children dressed in costumes collect money to support this international organization. The sale of UNICEF greeting cards and calendars is common in shopping centers and on college campuses as Americans actively support a fund which supplies food and medicines to less fortunate, malnourished, and deprived children around the world.

Challenges for the 1990s

Child health problems have changed dramatically over time. It is important to remember that morbidity and mortality figures were not kept diligently prior to 1900. Although the work of Europeans such as Jenner, Koch, and Pasteur eventually became known in this country, word of their scientific achievements spread slowly. Diarrhea, pneumonia, malnutrition, rickets, scurvy, tuberculosis, beriberi, and the communicable diseases of childhood were common. In the mid-1930s, a U.S. Public Health Service survey revealed that 51 percent of the deaths of children between 1 and 15 years of age were due to infections, parasitic diseases, pneumonia, and diarrhea (Grotberg, 1976). Improved standards of living, clean water, sanitation, and better food production have had a substantial impact on the types of health problems children experience.

Extraordinary progress has occurred in the treatment of a myriad of pathophysiological problems, especially since World War II. Improved technological advancements, the sulfonamides, and penicillin have made it possible to treat previously life-threatening conditions, especially mastoiditis, tuberculosis, meningitis, the pneumonias, and appendicitis. A knowledge of the epidemiology and pathogenesis of streptococcal infections and the prophylactic use of penicillin have drastically affected the occurrence of rheumatic fever and rheumatic heart disease, once major causes of both death and disability. Although millions of children are not immunized properly today, the communicable diseases of childhood can be controlled and complications such as measles encephalitis and the residual effects of poliomyelitis need not occur.

Surgical techniques for many congenital defects and treatments for inborn errors of metabolism have been re-fined to the point where survival has increased dramatically. Biochemical as well as chromosomal studies have enhanced the identification of inherited disorders. Although infant death rates are lower, the causes of death in children have changed significantly. Pneumonia, diarrhea, and infections have been replaced by sudden infant death syndrome, cancer, and accidents. There is a "new morbidity" in pediatrics involving many problems not even mentioned a generation ago. They include learning disorders; allergies; speech, vision, and hearing deficits; behavioral problems; child abuse; and suicide as well as the formerly adult conditions of sexually transmitted disease and substance abuse.

Neonatology, which has emerged as a subspecialty, exemplifies what can be expected in the future. Electronic equipment and vital support systems for sustaining life are complex and costly, necessitating the development of highly specialized regional neonatal centers (Figure 1-1).

Some of the ill newborns who survive live with physical or behavioral handicaps. Chronic disability is one variable which adversely influences child health, and from all indications it appears that chronicity will increase in the future. Developmental disabilities also may increase. In

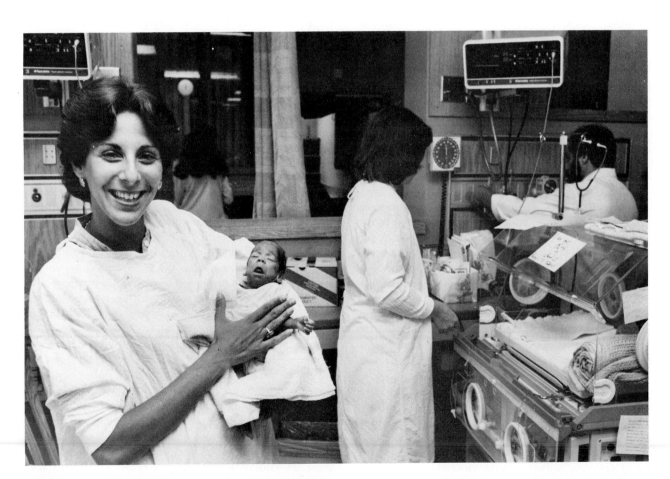

FIGURE 1-1   The highly sophisticated equipment in a neonatal intensive care unit does not overshadow the development of a unique nurse-patient relationship. *(Educational Media Center, New England Medical Center, Boston, Mass. Used with permission.)*

anticipating these possibilities, it is important to design experiences for young people which will help them learn about growth and development before they become parents. Contact with normal and handicapped infants and preschoolers can be instrumental in cultivating positive, accepting attitudes toward both young and handicapped children.

Ethical dilemmas have come to the fore as technology has advanced. The question of who shall live and who shall die involves complicated, frustrating processes. The nurse, who spends the greatest amount of time with these children and their families, is vital in the ethical decision-making process.

The use of CDRGs has placed sophisticated, high-technology care in the home. For example, children are discharged from the hospital on hyperalimentation, ventilators, peritoneal dialysis, and apnea monitors. Parents must be taught how to care for these children. Thus, nurses who work in home health agencies must continue with the education and suppportive help begun by the nurses who cared for these children while hospitalized.

In hospital settings, high-technology care will advance. Robotic devices are already in use in some settings to help deliver medications and serve meals. This technology may "invade" nursing care. Robots will be only as successful as the nurses who program them.

The emphasis in health care has shifted from treating and curing many maladies to preventing them. Screening then becomes an effective strategy; however, getting children into existing screening and treatment programs can pose a substantial logistical problem. The EPSDT program is one example. Implemented in 1972 as an amendment to Title XIX of the Social Security Act, it was to be a highly cost-effective program for individuals under 21 years of age. However, only a small percentage of those eligible have been screened, and less than half with positive findings have been treated (Schoor, 1978). These statistics probably will improve with the development of the Primary Care Network. In this system, families on Aid to Families with Dependent Children (AFDC) must identify a primary physician for their children. If parents choose to have a child seen by another physician (e.g., pediatrician, family practitioner, or specialist) without a referral from the primary physician, AFDC will not pay for the services rendered. Generally, the other physician will not see the child unless an EPSDT examination has been done by the primary physician. In addition, emergency room visits must be authorized by the primary physician. Without referrals and authorizations, families must assume the costs incurred.

Major revisions of AFDC are being debated in Congress. Congressional decisions will have a significant effect on the plight of poor children and families. Issues of concern to pediatric nurses include Medicaid coverage for poor working parents, day care provisions, and promotion of increased parental responsibilities for children.

The problems of any program are not confined to the national level. Bureaucrats at the regional, state, and local levels contribute to the dilemma. The bureaucracy becomes especially evident when one examines the 100 governmental programs which affect maternal and child health. They are administered by 5 cabinet officers, 15 governmental agencies, and 45 separate bureaus (Senator Edward Kennedy, personal communication, Nov. 12, 1980). The sheer numbers of people involved contribute to inadequacy and ineffectiveness.

The size of the pediatric population also strains the resources providing services to children and their families. There were 35 million children in the United States in 1912 and 76 million in 1972 (Reed and Phillips, 1972). These increased numbers complicate the delivery of health care. Admittedly, significant strides were made in the period between 1912 and the decade of the 1980s; however, when one considers the sophisticated technology and the American capacity and potential as a nation, a different, disappointing perspective on progress emerges.

Although pediatric nurses, either singly or collectively, may be unable to cure the ills created by bureaucracy, they can and do have an impact on child health care both in the hospital and in the community. They help prevent disease, injury, and behavior problems in children through planning and administering immunizations and through anticipatory guidance and education in relation to growth and development. Nurses help children achieve and maintain optimum health and development by providing primary, secondary, and tertiary care in conjunction with other members of the health team. Moreover, pediatric nurses assist in restoring health through the care delivered in facilities designed to fill the gap between secondary or tertiary care and home care. Finally, nurses also provide long-term care to children who have chronic problems by helping them reach their potential within the limitations of their disabilities. Nurses who work with children thus are presented with many opportunities to help children attain their potential.

The child's progress from relative fragility and helplessness at birth toward competent functioning as an adult is fraught with many tribulations. The nurse is privileged to observe and guide the child and family and to participate in their delights and struggles. To see a child take his first step, utter his first word, or swim his first stroke allows the adult moments to share in the child's glee that he can do these things and his wonderment that he can now begin to have some control over his own life. These moments multiply as he continues through the various stages of growth and development.

In a wide variety of clinical settings, nurses also have many opportunities to observe and share the joys that children experience. But there are periods of sadness also: the unfavorable prognoses, life-threatening experiences, intrusive procedures, and pain that overshadow happier moments of clinical practice. Unfortunately, these events exist. To endure and to enjoy, a nurse who works with children must recognize and appreciate the uniqueness that each child or adolescent brings to a nurse-patient relationship. It is that characteristic—uniqueness—which needs to be nurtured, understood, respected, and loved.

Study Questions

1. Major factors leading to the creation of the medical specialty of pediatrics include:
   1. Religious views associated with the influence of Christianity in the medieval period.
   2. Nineteenth-century increases in scientific understanding of anatomic and physiological differences between children and adults.
   3. Early twentieth-century governmental programs to promote child health.
   4. Twentieth-century nursing research about anxieties related to hospitalization.

   A. 1 and 2   C. 2 and 3
   B. 2   D. 2, 3, and 4

2. Nurses who are credited with improving health care services for children and families include:
   1. Florence Erickson, who used dolls, toys, and hospital equipment to study children's feelings about hospitalization.
   2. Florence Blake, who showed that nursing intervention can reduce hospitalized children's fear and anxiety.
   3. Loretta Ford, who contributed to the expansion of nurses' roles to include taking a health history, performing a physical examination, and managing common health disorders.
   4. Kathyrn Barnard, who contributed both clinically and politically to the improvement of health services for mentally retarded children.

   A. 1, 2, 3, and 4   C. 3
   B. 1 and 2   D. 3 and 4

3. In 1986 the average cost in U.S. dollars of bringing up a child for the first 18 years of life was approximately:

   A. $52,000.   C. $104,000.
   B. $77,000.   D. $145,000.

4. Diagnosis-related groups (DRGs):
   1. Do not yet apply to children.
   2. Increase the responsibility of nurses to prepare families to care for seriously ill children at home.
   3. Increase Medicare payments to pediatric nurse practitioners.
   4. Lead to earlier discharge from hospitals.

   A. 1   C. 3 and 4
   B. 2, 3, and 4   D. 2 and 4

5. The infant mortality rate in the United States is:
   A. The lowest in the world.
   B. Higher than that of 15 other countries.
   C. The third lowest in the world.
   D. The tenth lowest in the world.

6. Intervening (advocating) on behalf of children whose health or human rights are endangered:
   1. Is taken care of by the police and the court system.
   2. Is the right of the child's parents.
   3. Is taken care of by the World Health Organization.
   4. Is a matter for which nurses share responsibility.

   A. 1 and 2   C. 3
   B. 2   D. 4

References

Barnard, K.E., and M.L. Erickson: *Teaching Children with Developmental Problems,* 2d ed., Mosby, St. Louis, 1976.

Blake, F.G.: *Open Heart Surgery in Children: A Study of Nursing Care,* U.S. Government Printing Office, Washington, D.C., 1964.

Bowlby, J.: "Separation Anxiety," *International Journal of Psychoanalysis,* **41**:81-113, 1960.

Children's Bureau: *Infant Care,* 11th ed., U.S. Government Printing Office, Washington, D.C., 1963.

Clemen, S.A., D.G. Eigsti, and S.L. McGuire: *Comprehensive Family and Community Health Nursing,* McGraw-Hill, New York, 1981.

Crowley, A.: "As I See It. . ." *The American Nurse,* Sept. 1986, pp. 5, 10.

Daniels, D.: "Moneylist: The Cost of Raising a Child," *Kansas City Star,* Oct. 10, 1986, p. IG.

Erickson, F.H.: "Play Interviews for Four-Year-Old Hospitalized Children," *Monographs of the Society for Research in Child Development, Inc.,* **23**(3), ser. no. 69, 1958.

Ginott, H.G.: *Between Parent and Child,* Avon, New York, 1965.

————: *Between Parent and Teenager,* Macmillan, New York, 1969.

Gordon, T.: *P.E.T.: Parent Effectiveness Training,* New American Library, New York, 1970.

Green, M.: "The New American Academy of Pediatrics Health Supervision and Guidelines: Implementation and Evaluation," *Well Child Care,* Ross Laboratories, Columbus, Ohio, 1986.

Grotberg, E.H.: *200 Years of Children,* U.S. Department of Health, Education, and Welfare, Office of Child Development, U.S. Printing Office, Washington, D.C., DHEW(OCD) no. 77-30110, 1976.

Keough, B.K., and C.J. Barkett: "Children's Rights in Assessment and School Placement," *Journal of Social Issues,* **34**(2):87-100, 1978.

Klaus, M., and J. Kennell: "Mothers Separated from Their Newborn Infants," *Pediatric Clinics of North America,* **4**:1020, 1970.

Mitchell, K., and R.E. Harbin: "Our Children: An Economic Priority," *Pediatric Nursing,* **11**(2):82, 1985.

Nordheimer, J.: "The Family in Transition: A Challenge from Within," *The New York Times,* Nov. 27, 1977, pp. 1, 74.

Pless, I.B.: "Current Morbidity and Mortality among the Young," in R.A. Hoekelman et al. (eds.), *Principles of Pediatrics,* McGraw-Hill, New York, 1978, pp. 1873-1891.

Reed, J.H., and M. Phillips: "Child Welfare Since 1912," *Children Today,* **1**(2):13-18, 1972.

Rubin, R.: "Maternal Touch," *Nursing Outlook,* **11**:828-831, 1963.

Rudolph, R.S., and A.C. Oglesby: "The Health Care System," in A.M. Rudolph (ed.), *Pediatrics,* 16th ed., Appleton-Century-Crofts, New York, 1977, pp. 1-8.

Schorr, L.B.: "Social Policy Issues in Improving Child Health Services: A Child Advocate's View," *Pediatrics,* **62**(3):370–376, 1978.

Silver, H.K., L.C. Ford, and S.G. Stearly: "A Program to Increase Health Care for Children: The Pediatric Nurse Practitioner," *Pediatrics,* **39**:756, 1967.

Smith, K.: "Legislative Update," *Pediatric Nursing,* **12**(4); 313, 1986.

Spector, M.: "Poverty: The Barrier to Health Care," in R.E. Spector (ed.), *Cultural Diversity in Health and Illness,* Appleton-Century-Crofts, New York, 1979, pp. 141-163.

Spitz, R.: "Hospitalism: An Inquiry into the Genesis of Psychiatric Conditions in Early Childhood," in D. Fenischel et al. (eds.), *The Psychoanalytic Study of the Child,* vol. I, Int'l. Universities Press, New York, 1945.

————: "Hospitalism: A Follow-up Report," in D. Fenischel et al. (eds.), *The Psychoanalytic Study of the Child,* vol. 2, International Universities Press, New York, 1946.

Spock, B.: *Baby and Child Care,* Pocket Books, New York, 1976.

Steir, S.: "Children's Rights and Society's Duties," *Journal of Social Issues,* **34**(2):46-59, 1978.

Sunley, R.: "Early Nineteenth-Century American Literature in Child-Rearing," in M. Mead and M. Wolfenstein (eds.), *Childhood in Contemporary Cultures,* University of Chicago, 1967.

"Trends," *Nursing 86,* **16**(5), 28, 1986.

U.S. Department of Health and Human Services, "Births, Marriages, Divorces, and Deaths for November 1985," *NCHS Monthly Vital Statistics Report,* **34**(11):1, 1985.

Whitney, L., and K.E. Barnard: "Implication of Operant Learning Theory for Nursing Care of Retarded Children," *Mental Retardation,* **4**:22-29, 1966.

Whitworth, J.M.: "Lost Children," *Journal of the Florida Medical Association,* **64**(7):477-480, 1977.

"Who Speaks for the Child?" *Christian Science Monitor,* Feb. 7, 1979.

Wiedenbach, E.: *Family Centered Maternity Nursing,* 2d ed., Putnam, New York, 1967.

2

Growth and Development in Childhood and Adolescence

Objectives

After reading this chapter, the student will be able to:
1. State four ways in which knowledge about childhood development contributes to the practice of pediatric nursing.
2. State seven principles of child development and give at least one example showing how each principle relates to nursing care.
3. Describe how a nurse can use developmental norms and still design nursing care compatible with the uniqueness of each child and each family.
4. Define *developmental task* and give one example for each childhood age group (newborn, infant, toddler, etc.).
5. Name and describe the specific developmental issue or problem Erikson identified for each of his stages.
6. Name the four developmental stages identified by Piaget and describe the major characteristics of each stage.
7. Record a particular child's weight, height, and head circumference on a growth chart of the type shown in Appendix B.
8. Compare a child of any age with the developmental norms for that age group and identify ways in which the child does and does not conform to the norms.

Why Nurses Need to Understand Child Development

Designing Nursing Care for the Individual

The success of nursing care depends largely on the nurse's accuracy in understanding the client's characteristics and needs. The better the nurse knows "who the client is," the better the nursing plan can be designed to "fit" and the greater the chance that the client will actively participate in the plan and benefit from the nursing intervention. The purpose of this chapter is to help nurses deepen their understanding of what children and adolescents are like, what they need, and why they behave as they do.

Every child is unique, departing in some ways from generalized descriptions of children as a group. There is considerable variation among the babies in a newborn nursery at any one time, for example. Nevertheless, it is helpful to make descriptive statements about newborns as a group so that the novice can have general guidelines about what is usual and normal—what to expect—even though any particular baby probably will not conform in every way to the guidelines.

In human development, similarities are more numerous than differences, and so nursing assessments and interventions can be facilitated by the nurse's knowledge of the principles and theories of child development. It is against the background of these generalizations that the unique qualities of each client care situation can be identified and the nursing approach can be individualized to the client's greatest advantage.

Promoting Each Child's Development

Nursing of children has a larger objective than simply treating illness or even *preventing* and treating illness. Nursing care of children also undertakes to help the growing, changing child reach his individual potential.

Ironically, health care itself, even though intended for the child's good, can impair development. For example, emotional disturbances can result from hospitalization or treatment that otherwise succeeds in correcting a physical disorder. Parents' ability to love and care for a child can be damaged by prolonged separation during the child's hospitalization or by guilt, resentment, or misinformation in regard to the illness.

It is obviously desirable to keep the developmental "costs" of health care at a minimum. Excellence in nursing care is achieved only when, in addition to excellent physical care, all appropriate efforts are made to safeguard the child's progress toward achieving his developmental potential.

Avoiding Problems

As nursing has become increasingly concerned with promoting and maintaining health (in contrast to the traditional emphasis on treating illness), *anticipatory health promotion,* also called *anticipatory guidance,* has become an important part of pediatric nursing. Anticipatory health promotion involves teaching parents (and children, as they become old enough) what is likely to occur in the child's development in the upcoming weeks or months and to assure that the child's well-being will be protected and promoted during that time. Knowledge of developmental expectations *(norms)* is a basic tool for predicting what changes will occur and for making plans to maximize health and safety when the expected changes take place. For example, as an infant gets old enough to crawl from one place to another, it becomes necessary to remove the dangerous objects he will be able to reach.

Increasing the Nurse's Enjoyment

Knowledge about child development is valuable because in helping nurses succeed with their clients, it increases the enjoyment the nurses find in their work. Children, particularly when they are hurt, sick, or scared, can create distress, discouragement, guilt, and anger in the adults who try to provide their care. A crying baby who cannot be comforted, an enraged 4-year-old, or an adolescent who refuses needed medicine can reduce the self-esteem and job satisfaction of a nurse who does not understand the child's actions or know how to respond appropriately.

It is sometimes overlooked that nurses as well as children and parents need and deserve confidence and satisfaction in their work and life situations. Nurses who learn to understand children and contribute to their development make nursing beneficial to themselves as well as to children and their families.

Useful Principles of Child Development

Working effectively with children and enjoying them can be learned. Skill in relating to children and adolescents is not a gift that some people naturally have and others do not. Growth and development, including behavior, follow orderly, predictable patterns. Several principles that provide a framework for understanding children and adolescents are presented below.

Children Are Competent

Children are well endowed with the qualities and abilities needed to ensure their survival and promote their development (Fig. 2-1). Even the rather helpless-appearing newborn is equipped for eating, digesting, breathing, growing, healing, and getting other people to provide food and other necessities. Throughout childhood the fundamental abilities to survive, grow, learn, and develop are repeatedly demonstrated. Children are strong and competent to adapt and thrive if they are given a healthy body and an environment that meets them halfway.

Children Resemble One Another

The characteristics of each age and the changes that occur with increasing age are noticeably similar from child to child. It is usual for children to have physical skills, body measurements such as height and weight, physiological characteristics, and behavior patterns much like those of

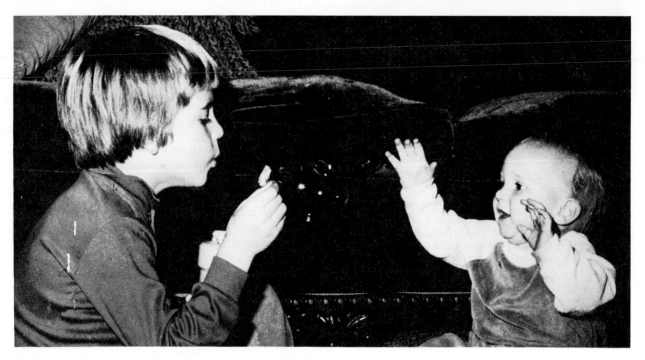

FIGURE 2-1   At each age the healthy child has specific capabilities for interacting with the environment in ways that provide stimulation and promote continuing development. *(Photo by Betsy Smith.)*

age-mates but different from those of children of other ages. This developmental principle has obvious implications for nursing assessment: Comparing a child with the norms for children of that age is a useful and simple preliminary screening technique. For example, by 6 weeks most infants smile when someone smiles at them; if a nurse encounters a baby who at 6 or more weeks does not smile, it is important to recognize this as unusual and find out more about the child's vision, mental development, and social environment.

Each Child Is Unique

Although comparing a child with the norms for his age group is an important screening procedure, norms are averages and must not be accepted as absolute standards. Variations from the norm do not necessarily indicate a problem.

Every child has unique qualities and consequently is likely to differ in several ways from the norms. Even newborns differ from one another and from a hypothetical "average" baby in length and weight, physiological stability, assertiveness, feeding behavior, and so forth. Especially as children grow older and more experienced, they reflect their individual enrichments or deprivations in addition to their unique inborn traits, and considerable difference is to be expected from child to child.

It can be difficult to know how much deviation from the norm is compatible with well-being and at what point differences should arouse professional concern. No general rules are available to show exactly "how much is too much." In the case of a child who differs from expectations in growth, motor ability, language development, social relationships, or some other quality, it is important to include all other relevant considerations in the assessment. Some other points to consider are family patterns; cultural, ethnic, and racial influences; and the child's individuality as shown in his past record. These factors are discussed below.

Family Patterns

The family history may show that siblings or other relatives of the child in question have also been atypical in the same way. If so, this information can help the nurse decide whether intervention is required or whether the long-term outcome may be expected to be satisfactory.

Cultural, Ethnic, and Racial Influences

A child's background may be different from that of the group used for comparison, making assessment difficult. An individual who may appear deviant in terms of the comparison group may not be exceptional in his own group. For example, Asians and blacks are generally smaller at the same age than are children of western European and Scandinavian ancestry, who have predominated in the growth research from which height and weight norms have been developed. Also, language varies widely both among subcultures and regionally so that a child whose speech and language may seem unusual to the nurse may be speaking normally for a child of that age in the family's social group.

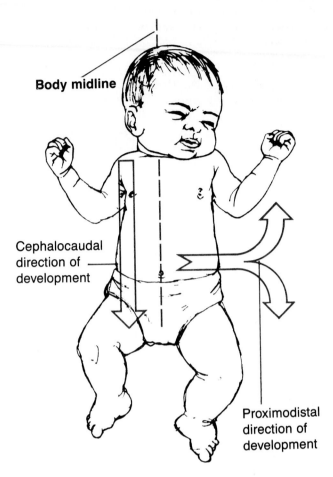

Body midline

Cephalocaudal direction of development

Proximodistal direction of development

FIGURE 2-2 The infant's neuromuscular maturation (e.g., sensory perception and muscle control) is initially more developed in the head and face and gradually progresses downward through the neck and trunk (cephalocaudal direction of development). Similarly, maturation is initially greater near the body midline and slowly extends outward down the arms and legs to include the hands and feet (proximodistal direction of development).

The Child's Own Past History

Since each child grows and develops according to his own pattern, a child's individual history can be used as a standard with which assessment data are compared. Allowing for the occasional spurts and levelings that occur at some points during the maturation process, each child generally follows a consistent pattern with respect to early or late acquisition of new skills, early or late growth, large or small size, etc. For this reason, loss of pace with his own usual pattern may be a more meaningful sign than the way he compares with the norms. Accurate and complete records of a child's growth and development are very valuable in the assessment of current status.

Development Is Directional

The *cephalocaudal, proximodistal,* and *general-to-specific* principles of development can be helpful to nurses. The principle of a cephalocaudal (from head toward tail) development describes the observed fact that

growth, muscle control, and perhaps sensory acuteness are more advanced in the newborn at and near the head and gradually progress downward to the neck, trunk, and extremities (Fig. 2-2). Thus coordination of the mouth for intentional sucking and smiling is achieved very early, and the child gains control of the neck muscles to steady the previously wobbly head before gaining sufficient strength in the trunk muscles to allow sitting.

The word *proximodistal* refers to the fact that the newborn's development is most advanced near the body midline and gradually extends from the central (proximal) part of the body toward the ends (distal parts) of the arms and legs (Fig. 2-2). For example, hip control for sitting precedes leg control for walking. The infant acquires strength and coordination to move the shoulders and arms in order to reach for an object several weeks before becoming able to coordinate the hands to pick it up.

The directional progression of development from head toward buttocks and from the proximal end toward the distal end of the extremities allows the nurse to anticipate, for example, that a baby who is still at the stage of large, uncoordinated arm movements will not need to be restrained from picking at IVs, dressings, or sutures except as required to protect against random arm movements.

Development proceeds also *from the general to the specific,* from the global to the precise. An infant makes varied, random vocal sounds before refining them into speech. Large muscle activities such as throwing precede the fine motor coordination required for fastening buttons or tying shoelaces. Perception and social relationships, as well as these speech and motor examples, seem to develop in accordance with this progression from the more general to the more specific.

Development Is Timely

Sensitive Periods of Development

A *sensitive period,* formerly called a critical period, is a span of time maximally favorable for a new developmental accomplishment. The same developmental progress is more difficult or even impossible for a child to achieve either before or after the sensitive period.

An example of sensitive periods is the last half of the baby's first year, which seems to be a critical time in the infant's development of his special social bond with a parent or another primary caretaker. Early research in orphanages showed that infants deprived of a primary relationship from about age 6 months to 12 months have long-lasting or permanent developmental distortions regardless of the quality of their care before or after that time. The "classic" orphanage babies who lacked a close social tie developed normally for about the first 4 to 6 months of life and then began to show progressive developmental retardation. Those who survived the increased death rates of infancy in institutions often had a long-range inability to form trusting, loving relationships. They also exhibited enuresis (bed-wetting), speech impediments, asocial or delinquent behavior, learning disabilities, and other developmental difficulties that are thought to have been consequences of parenting deprivation during the critical second 6 months.

Developmental Tasks

A *developmental task* may be defined as a skill, a competency, or learning which is necessary for a child to accomplish at a particular time in life. Delay or failure in doing so is said to make subsequent development more difficult.

For example, a developmental task of the newborn is to adapt physiologically to air breathing, maintenance of body temperature, and the other changes required for survival in the extrauterine environment. A task of the school-age child is to become adept at using symbols—numbers and the written word—and at understanding the concepts symbols represent. Among the tasks of late adolescence is mastery of advanced self-care skills and judgments that permit increasing independence from parents.

New Skills Tend to Predominate

Especially in the earlier years of childhood, while the child remains relatively simplistic and incapable of dealing with several things at one time, there is a strong tendency for the current developmental issue to become a preoccupation. The appearance of a new ability is accompanied by a strong drive to practice and perfect that ability.

For example, infants around 9 to 12 months old, which is the usual age to learn to pull from a sitting to a standing position, may be so eager to exercise their new ability that they insist on standing for meals. Even when quite ill, babies this age often stand up in their hospital cribs rather than lie down. Similarly, the application of a plaster cast to one or both legs of a child who has just learned to crawl or walk generally does little to impede practice of the new mobility, as evidenced by the worn-out knees or feet of the cast. A child who has just learned to whistle is not easily stopped from doing so even though his parents may become impatient.

Because of this tendency to attend fully to one aspect of development at a time, any situation in which a child must deal with more than one developmental challenge can be very stressful and probably should not be imposed unnecessarily. For example, a child who is adapting to a recent death or birth of a family member should not be simultaneously subjected to the anxieties of hospitalization if the hospitalization can be postponed. Moreover, hospitalization is not a good time to make changes such as weaning from bottle to cup or discontinuing a "security blanket."

Theories of Child Development

There are many different theories that can help people understand children, although few are widely used in nursing. It is worth noting that none of these theories is completely satisfactory for all purposes or to all who study children. Three approaches to the study and inter-

pretation of children's behavior will be discussed here: Erikson's theory, Piaget's theory, and behaviorism.

Erikson's Theory of Development: The Five Ages of Childhood

Erik Erikson has described the life span from birth through old age as a sequence of eight stages. Each stage is dominated by a major developmental problem that is an either-or situation; that is, for each stage there is a central task or problem that will be resolved either favorably, so that the foundation is well laid for the subsequent stage, or unfavorably, which will make later development more difficult. In none of the stages is the problem resolved totally and forever. Instead, it stands out during the stage it dominates and then becomes less dominant but arises again from time to time to be resolved further.

Infancy: Basic Trust versus Mistrust

During infancy, according to Erikson, the central task is to establish a sense of *basic trust* in predominance to *mistrust*. Infants who find that their needs for food and other kinds of comfort are consistently and effectively met learn that the world is a safe and predictable place and that they can trust others and their own bodies.

In contrast, a sense of mistrust may predominate in babies who do not receive consistent care and those who experience long periods of unrelieved discomfort. Mistrust creates barriers to the formation of interpersonal bonds, since the baby does not consider others trustworthy. Mistrust also interferes with the development of confidence, security, and assertiveness.

Toddlerhood: Autonomy versus Shame and Doubt

The toddler phase is the period during which the child must establish a sense of *autonomy* rather than *shame and doubt*. Toddlers who have learned to trust are developmentally driven to assert their growing awareness that their behavior is under their own control. They can move about and do things, and their will and ability are effective in producing desired outcomes. "I can do it myself, and that delights me" is the earmark of autonomy. Shame ("I can do it, but that isn't nice") and doubt ("I can't do it") are hazards to which toddlers are especially vulnerable if they have carried much mistrust from infancy or if they find that their assertions of independence are unacceptable to others or simply ineffective.

The Preschool Years: Initiative versus Guilt

About the time they become able to walk easily without having to concentrate on coordinating their muscles (Erikson says the child has confidence about "standing on his own feet"), children move into the third developmental stage, in which the central task is to develop a sense of *initiative* in preponderance to a sense of *guilt*. Preschoolers are bent on exploring what they can create and on seeing what they can do with the motor, language, interpersonal, and other skills which are increasing almost daily. The preschooler goes full force into the expanding physical and social worlds. Preschoolers' behavior is characterized by intrusiveness, manifested in endless questions, noises, and physical and intellectual explorations.

Guilt is the major developmental hazard for preschoolers because a good deal of what they try to do is too difficult for them or is unacceptable to the people they wish to please. They are also vulnerable to guilt because the conscience becomes prominent during the preschool years and preschoolers often disapprove of their own actions (or fantasies, which they do not clearly distinguish from reality).

The School-Age Period: Industry versus Inferiority

The preschooler who develops the ability to set acceptable goals and persevere in the attempt to reach them is well prepared for the school-age period, in which the central task as identified by Erikson is to develop a sense of *industry* in predominance to a sense of *inferiority*. The school-age child uses the physical, cognitive (intellectual), and social skills acquired during the preschool phase and turns his attention to learning what he must know in preparation for success in the adult world of facts and tools. There is a lot to learn: mathematics, reading, writing, history, geography, science, the rudiments of religion and politics, social roles, and the social and physical skills required for succeeding in the almost-adult world in which the child operates. Taking on these new situations—dealing with school, making friends outside the family, learning how to get through large parts of the day without direct help from parents or other adults—is what Erikson calls industriousness. Children who have difficulty in school, in interpersonal relationships, and in living up to their own or others' expectations can become discouraged and may come to consider themselves inadequate and inferior. Such a negative self-concept interferes with the developmental tasks of the school-age period.

Adolescence: Identity versus Role Confusion

Erikson characterizes adolescence as centering on the task of developing a sense of *identity*, with the undesirable alternative being *role confusion*. In the quest to find out who one is and who one will be as an adult, the adolescent identifies with and "understudies" a range of people that may include missionaries and mobsters, parents and rock heroes, politicians and artists, and almost anyone else observable. The adolescent's clannishness and intolerance of those who are different are ways of helping to establish who one *is* by separating from and condemning that which one *is not*.

Erikson describes the attainment of identity as a process of young people's coming to feel that who they are is consistent with others' views of them and also with their own views of themselves. The major hazard of adolescence—role confusion—arises from the rapid changes in the experience of self and from the sometimes overwhelming number of possible ways to behave and roles to select. Some young people adopt delinquent or other disapproved "negative" identities as a way of resolving their need for *some* identity rather than continuing to be confused about who they really are.

Piaget's Theory of Intellectual Development

Jean Piaget worked most of his long life to develop a theory of cognitive (intellectual) development. His writings and those of his colleagues and students report thousands of ingenious experiments and describe what they learned about children's intellectual activity and how it changes as children get older.

The First 2 Years: Sensorimotor Thought

Piaget thought that the *way* a child thinks (not just how much he thinks or about what) changes from one period of childhood to another. The earliest kind of thought occurs throughout the first 2 years of life. Piaget called this time span the *sensorimotor period*. The main quality characterizing the sensorimotor period is that thought derives from sensation and movement and so is inseparably linked to (and in fact limited to) the child's motor and sensory experiences. Intellectual experience during the sensorimotor period consists of observing and adaptively manipulating one's body and environment. Beginning with the earliest sensorimotor input revolving around the feeding experience, for example, the infant gradually becomes able to organize information and mentally coordinate the several related components of the experience, such as sucking, feeling, seeing, and tasting.

Object Permanence

Piaget stressed the importance of the infant's learning that objects continue to exist even when they are out of sight. The understanding that an object covered by a blanket continues to exist and can be reclaimed by removing the blanket or reaching under it does not appear to be within a child's grasp until around 8 months of age, when a baby begins to search for an absent object rather than immediately turning attention from it when it disappears. The concept of object permanence is related to the infant's progressing ability to deal with matters of time (continuing existence) and space (existence in other places besides the one currently experienced).

Reaching Goals

Goal-directed behavior appears in infancy and gradually includes alternative ways of achieving a goal. Thus by 12 months an infant not only is able to search for a toy that has rolled under a chair and out of sight, as discussed above, but also can go *around* the chair to repossess the toy rather than having to follow the same path the toy took to end up under the chair. The 12-month-old begins to find a variety of ways to produce an outcome other than the process by which the event has occurred in the child's past experience.

Cause and Effect

During the sensorimotor period the infant gains a primitive grasp of the connection between cause and effect and becomes active in making things happen in accordance with intention. The older infant can carry out a short series of related goal-directed activities, combining behavioral elements into a sequence. Even by the second birthday, however, the child is severely limited in his ability to "think," is bound to the concrete aspects of sensation and activity, and cannot conceptualize or deal abstractly with things beyond the scope of sensorimotor experience.

2 to 7 Years of Age: Preoperational Thought

From 2 to 7 years of age the child progresses through the *preoperational thought* period. The preoperational thinker deals at a much higher level with symbols. The 2- to 7-year-old uses language and memory and has a growing understanding of past, present, and future. The word *preoperational,* however, indicates that the child is not capable of understanding the fundamental *relationships* between things or events.

Errors in Thinking

Preoperational thinking is irrational by adult standards and leaves the child with many misunderstandings and erroneous conclusions that may be quite surprising to older children and adults. The preoperational child cannot simultaneously coordinate several properties (e.g., size, color, shape, and number) of objects and events. For example, the preoperational thinker may correctly agree that object A is bigger than object B but at the same time deny that B is smaller than A. A child at this age, if given a marble and a penny, then a second marble and a second penny, and so forth one by one until there are an equal number of each, will report that there are more marbles than pennies because the marbles take up more space or perhaps that there are more pennies than marbles because the coins make a tall stack. This child cannot understand that if one takes two clay balls the same size and flattens one into a new shape, the two masses still contain equal amounts of clay. Piaget attributes these errors in understanding to the child's not having yet developed the concept of *reversibility,* or the ability to conceptualize that a completed process can also be performed in reverse order so that the materials involved are returned to their initial condition. Before age 7 or so a child does not grasp the basic relationship between objects or between events or understand the process of transition.

Preoperational thought is characterized by *egocentrism.* The preschooler is unable, and the early school-age child only poorly able, to take another person's point of view. Hence he is annoyed because another does not know what the child has dreamed, and he expects even a stranger to know a person or event that the child refers to in conversation. Preschoolers believe their experiences are universal and even that events revolve around them to the extent demonstrated by a preschool child who, when asked to explain the sun's daily movement across the sky, replied, "It follows me."

Another characteristic of preoperational thought is *centering,* which is the tendency to center attention on one feature of something and to be unable to see its other qualities. The child with the marbles and pennies attended only to the size of the collection and ignored its numerical features even though he was able to count the items. A child who is aware of the pain-producing potential of a hypodermic needle has great difficulty conceiving of its therapeutic properties.

7 to 11 Years: Concrete Operations

Between the ages of 7 and 11 cognitive development proceeds through the stage of *concrete operations.* The child gradually overcomes the earlier egocentrism and centering and masters the concepts of reversibility, mentioned above, and *conservation.* Conservation refers to the ability to understand that a thing is essentially the same even though its shape or arrangement is altered. The previously mentioned example of the clay masses is a problem in *conservation of mass.*

Conservation of number is demonstrated by Piaget's experiment in which a child watches as a fixed number of objects are clumped together or spread out over a surface; a preoperational child judges that the number of items is modified by their concentration in space, but a child in the stage of concrete operations does not make that mistake.

During the period of concrete operations the child becomes skilled at classifying objects by any of their several characteristics. After age 7 or so a child can say, for example, that dogs, people, and horses have in common the property of being alive; that apples, nuts, and meat are all edibles; that all spaniels are dogs but not all dogs are spaniels; and that parts are smaller than the whole they compose in combination. Obviously the child of 11 years has come a long way toward being able to observe, analyze, and understand.

The Final Stage of Intellectual Development: Formal Operations

The child does not attain a fully adult quality of thinking until the last stage of cognitive development, which Piaget called the *formal operations* period. According to Piaget's theory, there is a change between ages 11 and 15 years that enables the child to think introspectively about his own thoughts and to solve complicated, abstract problems such as those found in formal logic and calculus. The young person can now form and test hypotheses that require imaginative departures from reality but that are still within the range of the scientific method. This new capacity to imagine how things might be if they were not as they are has many consequences, including empathy and compassion ("How would I feel if it happened to me?") and idealism perhaps combined with intolerance ("There is obviously a better way."). The *content* of thought has become less important than the *form* of the abstract problem, and so the young person in the stage of formal operations becomes able to deal with the *structure* of thought sequences without being limited to "real-life" experiences. For example, a teenager will tolerate and answer a problem such as "If blue dogs have pink pups and Herman is a blue dog, what color will Herman's puppies be?"

whereas a younger child still in the concrete operations stage will regard the problem simply as nonsense and will be unable to process it.

Stimulus-Response Theory of Behavior

The basic premise of stimulus-response theory (also sometimes called learning theory, behaviorism, and behavior modification theory) is that behavior is *learned.* Behaviorists believe that the child initially behaves in random ways consistent with developmental capability and that the rewards and punishments that result from the action influence the child's subsequent behavior. Acts that bring pleasure are repeated in similar situations, while behavior that results in punishment, disappointment, pain, or frustration tends to be discontinued. Behavior thus is a consequence of experience, of *learning.*

Behaviorists believe activity results from a need which they call *drive.* Examples of drive are hunger and fear. A hungry or frightened animal or person goes into action in order to relieve hunger, get away from danger, or take some other goal-directed action aimed at reducing drive. Drive reduction is rewarding, and behavior that effectively reduces drive becomes learned and is repeated in future similar states of heightened drive.

Generalization is the phenomenon by which learning is transferred from the learning situation to other, similar situations. A young child who develops a fear of hospital personnel in white clothes may subsequently show the same fear response to barbers, grocers, or other people dressed in white. A child's response to the mother tends to generalize to a nursery school teacher, for example, in proportion to the extent to which the teacher resembles the mother in appearance, mannerisms, approach to the child, etc.

Learned behavior can usually be "unlearned" *(extinguished)* if the situation can be modified so that the reward previously associated with the behavior no longer results from the behavior. For example, children who

have learned that they can get what they want by having a tantrum theoretically will eventually give up tantrum behavior if it ceases to bring rewards.

Since people who espouse stimulus-response theory believe behavior is the product of experience with rewards and punishments, they believe behavior can be changed by a planned program of rewarding, punishing, or ignoring. Control over reward and punishment is the basis of behavior modification when the same principles and similar procedures are applied to human behavior. Praise or material reward consistently given when a child performs a socially desirable act generally has the effect of leading the child to repeat that act in order to gain additional reward. Ignoring or punishing an act tends to result in its discontinuation.

Typical Growth and Development Patterns
The Newborn (Birth to 1 Month)
Physical Development
Apgar Scoring

All newborn babies' well-being is evaluated at 1 and 5 minutes after birth with the Apgar assessment scale. This procedure provides a rapid and standardized method for identifying infants who are at risk and assessing the severity of their condition so that appropriate resuscitation can be started. The purpose of the 1-minute score is to evaluate the infant's response to birth and identify infants who need immediate assistance because their vital functions are depressed. The 5-minute score is a reevaluation and also shows how well depressed babies have responded to resuscitative measures.

The Apgar test consists of five observations made in the order in which they are listed in Table 2-1. The baby receives a score of 0, 1, or 2 for each of the five observations: heart rate, respiratory effort, reflex irritability (response to suction catheter stimulation of the nostril), muscle tone, and color. The Apgar score is the total of

TABLE 2-1 Apgar Scoring Chart

Observation	Score		
	0	1	2
Heart rate	Not seen, felt, or heard—external cardiac massage in progress	<100	>100 even if tachycardia or arrhythmias are present
Respiratory effort	Apneic (absence of respirations at 1 and 5 min)	Irregular, shallow, gasping, weak cry	Vigorous, sustained, regular, lusty-cry
Reflex irritability	No response	Frown, grimace	Facial grimaces, sneezing, coughing
Muscle tone	Completely flaccid	Some flexion of extremities; some resistance to extension of extremities	Good muscle tone, spontaneous flexion of extremities; resistance to extension of extremities
Color	Cyanotic or pale	Body pink, extremities blue (cyanotic)	Entire surface is pink

Source: V. Apgar, "A Proposal for a New Method of Evaluation of the Newborn Infant, *Current Researches in Anesthesia and Analgesia,* July–August 1953, pp. 260-267.

TABLE 2-2 Score Sheet for External Physical Characteristics of the Newborn, for Use in Estimating Gestational Age*

External Sign	Points					Score
	0	1	2	3	4	
Edema	Obvious edema of hands and feet; pitting over tibia	No obvious edema of hands and feet; pitting over tibia	No edema			_____
Skin texture	Very thin, gelatinous	Thin and smooth	Smooth; medium thickness; rash or superficial peeling	Slight thickening and peeling, especially of hands and feet	Thick and parchmentlike; superficial or deep cracking	_____
Skin color	Dark red	Uniformly pink	Pale pink; variable over body	Pale; pink only over ears, lips, palms, or soles		_____
Skin opacity (trunk)	Numerous veins and venules clearly seen, especially over abdomen	Veins and tributaries seen	A few large vessels clearly seen over abdomen	A few large vessels seen indistinctly over abdomen	No blood vessels seen	_____
Lanugo (over back)	No lanugo	Abundant; long and thick over whole back	Hair thinning, especially over lower back	Small amount of lanugo and bald areas	At least one-half of back devoid of lanugo	_____
Plantar creases	No skin creases	Faint red marks over anterior half of sole	Definite red marks over > anterior one-half; indentations over < one-third	Indentions over > anterior one-third	Definite deep indentions over > anterior one-third	_____
Nipple formation	Nipple barely visible, no areola	Nipple well defined; areola smooth, and flat, diameter < 0.75 cm	Areola stippled, edge not raised, diameter < 0.75 cm	Areola stippled, edge raised, diameter > 0.75 cm		_____
Breast size	No breast tissue palpable	Breast tissue on one or both sides, < 0.5 cm diameter	Breast tissue both sides; one or both 0.5-1.0 cm	Breast tissue both sides; one or both > 1 cm		_____
Ear form	Pinna flat and shapeless, little or no incurving of edge	Incurving of part of edge of pinna	Partial incurving whole of upper pinna	Well-defined incurving whole of upper pinna		_____
Ear firmness	Pinna soft, easily folded, no recoil	Pinna soft, easily folded, slow recoil	Cartilage to edge of pinna, but soft in places, ready recoil	Pinna firm, cartilage to edge; instant recoil		_____
Genitals Male	Neither testis in scrotum	At least one testis high in scrotum	At least one testis down			_____
Female (with hips one-half abducted)	Labia majora widely separated, labia minora protruding	Labia majora almost cover labia minora	Labia majora completely cover labia minora			
					External total	_____

*Score from this table is combined with score obtained from Table 2-3, and Table 2-4 is then consulted for gestational age determination.

Source: L.M.S. Dubowitz, V. Dubowitz, and C. Goldberg, "Clinical Assessment of Gestational Age in the Newborn Infant," *Journal of Pediatrics,* 77:1-10, 1970.

these five scores. A perfect score is 10, and the lowest possible is score 0. A baby whose score is 0, 1, or 2 is considered severely depressed and requires immediate resuscitation, including mechanical assistance with ventilation, and intensive care. A moderately depressed infant is one whose score is 3 to 6. This infant definitely needs close monitoring during the first 24 hours and may also have to be attached to a ventilator. Infants scoring 7 to 10 are in

TABLE 2-3 Instructions for Scoring the Neurological Assessment of the Newborn*

Posture
With the infant supine and quiet, score as follows:

Arms and legs extended	= 0
Slight or moderate flexion of hips and knees	= 1
Moderate to strong flexion of hips and knees	= 2
Legs flexed and abducted, arms slightly flexed	= 3
Full flexion of arms and legs	= 4

Square window
Flex the hand at the wrist. Exert pressure sufficient to get as much flexion as possible. The angle between the hypothenar eminence and the anterior aspect of the forearm is measured and scored according to Fig. 2-3. Do not rotate the wrist

Ankle dorsiflexion
Flex the foot at the ankle with sufficient pressure to get maximum change. The angle between the dorsum of the foot and the anterior aspect of the leg is measured and scored as in Fig. 2-3.

Arm recoil
With the infant supine, fully flex the forearms for 5 s, then fully extend by pulling the hands and release. Score the reaction according to:

Remain extended or make random movements	= 0
Incomplete or partial flexion	= 1
Brisk return to full flexion	= 2

Leg recoil
With the infant supine, fully flex the hips and knees for 5 s, then extend them by traction on the feet and release. Score the reaction according to:

No response or slight flexion	= 0
Partial flexion	= 1
Full flexion (less than 90° at knees and hips)	= 2

Popliteal angle
With the infant supine and the pelvis flat on the examining surface, flex the leg on the thigh and fully flex the thigh with the use of one hand. With the other hand extend the leg, then score the angle attained as in Fig. 2-3

Heel-to-ear maneuver
With the infant supine, hold the infant's foot with one hand and move it as near to the head as possible without forcing it. Keep the pelvis flat on the examining surface. Score as in Fig. 2-3

Scarf sign
With the infant supine, take the infant's hand and draw it across the neck as far across the opposite shoulder as possible. Assistance to the elbow is permissible by lifting it across the body. Score according to the location of the elbow:

Elbow reaches the opposite anterior axillary line	= 0
Elbow between opposite anterior axillary line and midline of thorax	= 1
Elbow at midline of thorax	= 2
Elbow does not reach midline of thorax	= 3

Head lag
With the infant supine, grasp each forearm just proximal to the wrist and pull gently so as to bring the infant to a sitting position. Score according to the relationship of the head to the trunk during the maneuver:

No evidence of head support	= 0
Some evidence of head support	= 1
Maintains head in the same anteroposterior plane as the body	= 2
Tends to hold the head forward	= 3

Ventral suspension
With the infant prone and the chest resting on the examiner's palm, lift the infant off the examining surface and score according to the posture shown in Fig. 2-3

*Score obtained by use of this table is added to the score from Table 2-2, and infant's estimated gestational age is found in Table 2-4. See also Fig. 2-3.

Source: L.M.S. Dubowitz, V. Dubowitz, and C. Goldberg, "Clinical Assessment of Gestational Age in the Newborn Infant, *Journal of Pediatrics,* 77:1-10, 1970.

good condition and generally require routine nursery observations and routine newborn care.

Estimation of Gestational Age

Full-term infants are those born between 38 and 42 weeks of gestation. Infants born before the thirty-eighth week are classified *preterm;* babies born later than 42 weeks of gestation are called *postterm.* These variations in maturity at birth are significant because both preterm and postterm infants have special physical vulnerabilities; consequently, they are classified as high-risk infants and are given special medical and nursing care. Special methods have been developed for assessing infants (ordinarily within the first 24 hours after birth) to identify their degree of maturity and hence to classify them as preterm, term, or postterm.

The Dubowitz method for estimating gestational age is presented in Tables 2-2 through 2-4 and Fig. 2-3. The Dubowitz procedure assesses the gestational age of healthy neonates and is considered accurate to within 2 weeks of actual gestational age. Certain aspects of the method are affected by illness in the newborn. Assessment of gestational age is discussed in more detail in Chap 17,

TABLE 2-4 Maturity Score Sheet for Estimating Newborn's Gestational Age*

Total Score	Gestational Age, Weeks
5	26
10	27
15	29
20	30
25	31
30	33
35	34
40	35
45	36
50	38
55	39
60	40
65	42
70	43
75	44

*For estimating gestational age after scores have been obtained for neurological characteristics (see Fig. 2-3 and Table 2-3) and external physical characteristics (see Table 2-2).

Source: L.M.S. Dubowitz, V. Dubowitz, and C. Goldberg, "Clinical Assessment of Gestational Age in the Newborn Infant," *Journal of Pediatrics,* 77:1-10, 1970.

Neurological sign	Points 0	1	2	3	4	5	Score
Posture							
Square window	90°	60°	45°	30°	0°		
Ankle dorsiflexion	90°	75°	45°	20°	0°		
Arm recoil	180°	90–180°	<90°				
Leg recoil	180°	90–180°	<90°				
Popliteal angle	180°	150°	130°	110°	90°	<90°	
Heel to ear							
Scarf sign							
Head lag							
Ventral suspension							

Neurological Total: _____

External Total: _____

TOTAL SCORE: _____

Gestation Age: _____
(in weeks)

FIGURE 2-3 Score sheet for the neurological characteristics of the neonate. Instructions for using this chart are presented in Table 2-3. The resulting score combined with the score obtained by the use of Table 2-2, and the gestational age is then found in Table 2-4. (*From L.M.S. Dubowitz et al., "Clinical Assessment of Gestational Age in the Newborn Infant," Journal of Pediatrics, 77:1-10, 1970.*)

TABLE 2-5 Body Size Measurements for Full-Term Infants at Birth

	Percentile		
	5th*	50th†	95th‡
Weight	2400 g (5 lb 4 oz)	3275 g (7 lb 3 oz)	4100 g (9 lb)
Length	44 cm (17.5 in)	48.5 cm (19.25 in)	53 cm (21 in)
Head circumference	32 cm (12.5 in)	34.5 cm (13.5 in)	37 cm (14.5 in)

*Only 5 percent of term infants are smaller than the figures in this column.
†This is the median (average) for both sexes. Boys are slightly bigger than girls on average by about 30 g (1 oz) and about 2/3 cm (1/4 in).
‡Only 5 percent of term infants are larger than the figures in this column.

"High Risk Neonates and Their Families," along with preterm and postterm newborns and their care.

Weight, Length, Head Circumference, and Vital Signs

Table 2-5 lists the normal range of weight, length, and head circumference for full-term babies at birth. The baby normally loses 5 to 10 percent of its weight within the first few days of life but returns to birth weight by 10 days of age. Thereafter weight increases by 150 to 180 g (5 to 6 oz) a week. Length increases about 4 cm (2 in) during the first month (Tudor, 1981, p. 296). By 1 month of age head circumference has increased by about 2.5 cm (1 in).

The baby's height, weight, and head measurement are recorded on a growth chart such as those included in Appendix B. A dot is placed at the intersection of the vertical line B (for *birth*) and the horizontal line corresponding to the baby's length, weight, or head circumference. The position of the dot reveals how the infant's size ranks in comparison to that of other infants of the same age. A baby at the 5th percentile is larger than only 5 percent of infants at that age, an infant at the 25th percentile is larger

TABLE 2-6 Normal Ranges of Vital Signs for Children and Adolescents

	Full-Term Newborn (Birth to 4 weeks)	Infant (1 to 12 Months)	Toddler	Preschool Child	School-Age Child	Adolescent
Temperature						
Axillary	36.0°C–37.0°C (96.8°F–98.6°F)*			35.5°C–36.5°C (96.0°F–97.8°F)†		⟶
Rectal	37.1°C–38.1°C (98.8°F–100.6°F)		⟵	36.8°C–38.1°C (98.2°F–100.5°F)†		
Oral	⟵ Not appropriate at this age ⟶			⟵ 36.5°C–37.5°C (97.7°F–99.5°F)†⟶		
Heart rate (increases with fever, stress, or activity; decreases in sleep)	120–160* (may be irregular)	120–160‡	80–140*	80–110‡	75–100‡	60–90‡
Respiratory rate (increases with fever, stress, or activity; decreases in sleep)	40–60* (may be irregular)	30–60‡	24–40‡	22–34‡	18–30‡	12–20‡
Blood pressure§						
Systolic	50–70 (12 h old) 60–90 (96 h old)	74–100	80–112	82–110	84–120	94–140
Diastolic	25–45 (12 h old) 20–60 (96 h old)	50–70	50–80	50–78	54–80	62–88

*M. Tudor, *Child Development*, McGraw-Hill, New York, 1981.
†L. Littlefield, "Antipyretic Therapy," in R.A. Hoekelman et al. (eds.), *Principles of Pediatrics: Health Care of the Young*, McGraw-Hill, New York, 1978.
‡From M.F. Hazinski, "The Cardiovascular System," in J. Howe et al. (eds.), *The Handbook of Nursing*, Wiley, New York, 1984.
§Ranges represent the 10th and 90th percentiles reported by National Heart, Lung, and Blood Institute's Task Force on Blood Pressure Control in Children, 1978; M. de Swiet et al., "Systolic Blood Pressure in a Population of Infants in the First Year of Life: The Bromptom Study," *Pediatrics*, 65:1028, 1980; and H. Versmold et al., "Aortic Blood Pressure during the First 12 Hours of Life in Infants with Birth Weight 610–4420 Grams," *Pediatrics*, 67:607, 1981.

than 25 percent, a baby at the 50th percentile is precisely average, and so on. Plotting length against weight gives an indication of the baby's body build in comparison to other infants.

Table 2-6 shows normal ranges of vital signs.

Motor Development
The full-term infant holds all four extremities in flexion and resists efforts by others to extend his arms, legs, and fingers. Placed in a prone position (on his abdomen), the baby flexes the knees under the abdomen and turns the head to one side.

The neck muscles are not strong enough to stabilize the head, but the extensors are stronger than the flexors. When the baby is held in a seated position, the head drops onto the chest but the infant attempts to lift the chin from the chest. If the baby is held in ventral suspension (balanced on his abdomen across the examiner's hand), the head is briefly held level in the same plane as the trunk. If a supine (back-lying) baby is pulled to a sitting position, neck control is completely absent and the head lags behind (follows) under the influence of gravity. However, the infant spontaneously rotates the head right and left when lying either prone or supine.

Reflexes The newborn's eyes open separately or together and shut in response to sudden bright light. Sucking and rooting reflexes are well established: If the cheek, lip, or corner of the mouth is stroked, the infant turns his head and moves the lips and tongue in attempt to grasp the stroking object in his mouth. The neonate resists removal of the nipple or other object from the mouth and moves the head in an effort to follow such an object if it is gradually withdrawn from the mouth. Some newborns can suck their thumbs, fingers, or fists. Additional neonatal reflexes are described in Chap. 20, "The Nervous System." Infant reflexes are very important indicators of the baby's neurological normality; hence they play a prominent role in assessment of the newborn.

Psychosocial Development
In the initial hour or so after birth the infant experiences a period of pronounced alertness. During this period the baby actively participates in developing a relationship with the mother if they are together and in close contact. Newborns are able to elicit care-giving responses from others (e.g., by behavior such as making eye contact and crying) and to respond to and thereby reward care-giving and comfort measures offered by others.

Parent-Infant Attachment
The process of forming a parent-child relationship is called *attachment* or *bonding*. Health care professionals have long realized that it is vitally important to promote parent-infant attachment, since faulty bonding places the child at risk for various developmental hazards ranging from life-threatening problems such as failure to thrive

and child abuse to difficulties in socialization and school achievement. In the interest of promoting bonding as well as for the humanitarian reason that it is inherently the right of new parents and the newborn to be together, it is now widely recognized that part of the nursing care of neonates and their families involves facilitating interaction between the baby and both parents *at birth and in the following hours and days.*

Infant Behavioral States

Infant behavior has been classified into six different behavioral states.

1. *Quiet sleep* The infant sleeps deeply without movements of the eyes, face, trunk, or extremities except for startles at rather regular intervals. Respirations are regular. The baby is not easily aroused by environmental stimuli.
2. *Active sleep (light sleep)* The eyes are closed, but rapid eye movements are noticeable. Respirations are irregular, often more rapid than in quiet sleep. There is some limb movement in addition to startles. Mouthing and sucking occur at times. The baby startles in response to environmental stimuli and may awaken.
3. *Drowsiness* The infant may open and close its eyes, but the eyes appear unfocused. The lids may flutter. The response to stimuli may be delayed. The infant moves from this dozing state into sleep or greater alertness. Mild activity (wiggling, writhing) occurs.
4. *Alert inactivity* The eyes are open and bright, and the baby seems to be concentrating on the environment. There is little movement.
5. *Alert activity* This state is characterized by a generally high level of motor activity, including bursts of arm waving and kicking. Respirations are irregular. The skin may be quite flushed. The baby's eyes are bright but not necessarily focused.
6. *Crying* The baby cries intensely. The face flushes, and the baby grimaces. Crying is accompanied by vigorous motor activity.

These six states of consciousness occur in all babies, but each infant has his own personal manner of combining and expressing them. Even in the first few days after birth each child demonstrates a unique behavioral style. There are wide normal variations among newborns in regard to the amount of time spent in each state, the rapidity of transition from one state to another, the ease with which the baby can be aroused or quieted, and the baby's usual number of changes from one state to another in a given time period. A newborn's characteristic manner of organizing and expressing his states of consciousness has been shown to influence his parents' feelings and behavior toward him.

The Brazelton Neonatal Behavioral Assessment Scale

The Brazelton Neonatal Behavioral Assessment Scale (BNBAS) (Brazelton, 1984) is a valuable tool for evaluating, among other things, a newborn's individual style of organizing behavioral states and a baby's characteristic way of interacting with the environment (including people in the environment). A limitation of the BNBAS in that the nurse or other professional must have special training at one of several centers (Brazelton, 1984) before using it. In clinical settings where a trained person is available to administer the BNBAS, the instrument is of great value in helping parents understand the new baby and also understand that a baby's behavior powerfully influences the ways in which his parents interact with him.

The BNBAS also helps parents become aware of the baby's own style of interacting with environmental stimuli and comforting himself when upset. It demonstrates the infant's way of showing excitement, level of irritability, and degree of cuddliness and consolability. New parents thus can be helped to "know" the baby's temperament and personality traits and to shape the environment and their interactions with the baby to maximize mutual satisfaction.

Perceptual-Cognitive Development

Newborns make numerous sensory discriminations and demonstrate certain preferences. They can discriminate between similar sounds, various tastes and odors, tactile sensations, and visual stimuli. Moving objects are distinguished from nonmoving objects, and newborns follow moving objects with their eyes, though only within their very nearsighted range of vision. Babies show a clear preference for looking at moving things and human faces. Human voices are a preferred sound, particularly higher-pitched voices.

Vision seems best about 8 in in front of the face and at the midline. During the first month the infant begins to stare intensely at the other person's face during interactions.

Development Through Adolescence

Developmental milestones from infancy through adolescence are depicted in Tables 2-7 through 2-16. Average ages for eruption of deciduous teeth are given in Fig. 2-4. In Fig. 2-5, average ages for loss of deciduous teeth and eruption of permanent teeth are displayed. Growth charts for infants and children are reproduced in Appendix B. Pubescent milestones for American girls and boys are noted in Figs. 2-7 and 2-8.

Text continued on p. 37.

TABLE 2-7 Developmental Milestones: 1 to 3 Months of Age

Physical	Psychosocial	Perceptual-Cognitive
Gains approximately 1 kg (2.2 lb) per month	Increasing periods of wakefulness with crying	Begins to recognize familiar faces, objects, and situations (such as feedings)
Length increases approximately 2.5 cm (1 in) per month	Cry becomes differentiated to express hunger, pain, fatigue, need for holding	Begins to show interest in environment (inspects)
Fixates visually on faces and objects	Growing awareness that cry brings parents	Begins to follow objects visually
Follows to midline		Begins to play with parts of body
Responds to sounds by quieting, turning head to look, or startling	Development of socially responsive smile	Begins to combine visual activities with grasping (hand to mouth)
Able to lift head when prone	Actively follows movements of familiar person and slowly moving objects	Begins to coordinate stimuli from various sense organs (e.g., looks in direction of sound)
Turns from stomach to back	Responds differently to different sounds	Begins to indicate awareness of strange or unfamiliar situations
	Visually searches to locate sounds of human voice	
	Beginning of prelanguage vocalizations: cooing, babbling	
	Vocalizes in response to voice of parent	
	Begins to laugh aloud	
	Maximal need for sucking pleasure	
	Responses initially governed by tension, grows toward more specific seeking of pleasure	
	Derives satisfaction from feeding, holding, rocking, tactile stimulation from both parents	
	Increasingly indicates desire to avoid unpleasant situations	
	Not yet able to act intentionally to elicit responses from others	

Source: Adapted from R.M. Benfield and D.M. Harris, "The Infant—1 to 12 Months," G.M. Scipien et al. (eds.), *Comprehensive Pediatric Nursing,* 2d ed., McGraw-Hill, New York, 1979.

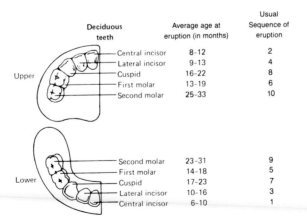

FIGURE 2-4   Average ages at which children acquire deciduous (primary, or "baby," teeth). These ages are taken from material distributed by the American Dental Association. *(From M. Barnard et al., Handbook of Comprehensive Pediatric Nursing, McGraw-Hill, New York, 1981.)*

TABLE 2-8 Developmental Milestones: 4 to 6 Months of Age

Physical	Psychosocial	Perceptual-Cognitive
Gains approximately 1 kg (2 lb) per month	Growing interest and enjoyment in image in mirror	Growing awareness of self as different from environment
Doubles birth weight by 5 months	Increasing vocalization which is self-reinforcing	Increasing interest and ability to respond to novel stimuli
Length increases approximately 2.5 cm (1 in) per month	Vocalizations vary according to mood	Actively interested in environment—activity becoming primary motive of experience
One tooth may erupt about 6 months	Growing enjoyment of play with people and objects	
Reaches for objects	Chuckles and laughs socially, especially when stimulated	
Rakes object with fingers	Demands and enjoys attention	
Passes objects from hand to hand	Infant is increasingly lovable and affectionate	
No head lag	Interest in mother generalized to include other members of the family	
Turns over completely	Attachment is more observable than before; infant prefers comfort from a familiar person, not a stranger	
Bears weight on legs	Shows anticipation and happy expectation as well as beginning ability to delay gratification	
Sits, initially with support and then alone	Beginning to explore mother's breast and body	
	Actively responds to highly stimulating play	

Source: Adapted from R.M. Benfield and D.M. Harris, "The Infant—1 to 12 Months," in G.M. Scipien et al. (eds.), *Comprehensive Pediatric Nursing,* 2d ed., McGraw-Hill, New York, 1979.

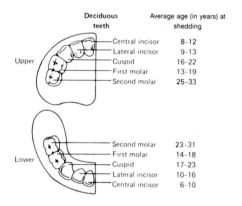

Deciduous teeth	Average age (in years) at shedding
Upper	
Central incisor	8–12
Lateral incisor	9–13
Cuspid	16–22
First molar	13–19
Second molar	25–33
Lower	
Second molar	23–31
First molar	14–18
Cuspid	17–23
Lateral incisor	10–16
Central incisor	6–10

Permanent teeth	Average age (in years) at eruption	Usual sequence of eruption
Upper		
Central incisor	7–8	4
Lateral incisor	8–9	6
Cuspid	11–12	12
First bicuspid	10–11	8
Second bicuspid	10–12	10
First molar	6–7	2
Second molar	12–13	14
Third molar	17–21	Variable; last
Lower		
Third molar	17–21	
Second molar	11–13	13
First molar	6–7	1
Second bicuspid	11–12	11
First bicuspid	10–12	9
Cuspid	9–10	7
Lateral incisor	7–8	5
Central incisor	6–7	3

FIGURE 2-5 Average ages at which children lose deciduous (primary) teeth and acquire permanent (secondary) teeth. These ages are taken from material distributed by the American Dental Association. *(From M. Barnard et al., Handbook of Comprehensive Pediatric Nursing, McGraw-Hill, New York, 1981.)*

TABLE 2-9 Developmental Milestones: 7 to 9 Months of Age

Physical	Psychosocial	Perceptual-Cognitive
Gains approximately ½ kg (1.1 lb) per month	Increasing babbling to produce vowels, consonants, and chained syllables	Beginning realization that objects exist even when out of sight (object permanence)
Length increases approximately 1.5 cm (½ in) per month	Begoins to say "da da," "ma ma," or equivalent	Beginning ability to play peek-a-boo
Although tooth eruption is extremely variable, one per month may erupt	Vocalizes to people differently than to things	Is able to reach an object by pulling a string
Thumb-finger grasp	Begins to respond to simple verbal requests	Begins to develop sense of space and depth
Transfers objects from hand to hand	Listens selectively to familiar words	Increasing interest in feeding self
Claps hands together	Enjoys music	Actively explores objects with multiple senses
Hitches (backward locomotion when seated)	Uses vocalizations to obtain desired object	Beginning ability to put objects in container
Crawls	Reaches out to be picked up	Begins to understand causality (a specific action becomes associated with its subsequent result)
	Growth toward participation in interactive games (peek-a-boo, patty cake, so-o big)	
	Increasingly aggressive orally—mouthing, biting—and determined about these activities	
	Strong attachment behavior emerges; threat of mother's loss elicits violent response	
	Shows growing desire to please mother	
	Stranger anxiety increases	
	Play becomes more pleasurable and purposeful to cope with stranger anxiety (such as attachment to pacifier, blanket, favorite teddy bear)	
	Begins to show fear of being left alone; bedtime becomes troublesome	
	Shows attachment to father as source of excitement and pleasure	

Source: Adapted from R.M. Benfield and D.M. Harris, "The Infant—1 to 12 Months," in G.M. Scipien et al. (eds.), *Comprehensive Pediatric Nursing,* 2d ed., McGraw-Hill, New York, 1979.

TABLE 2-10 Developmental Milestones: 10 to 12 Months of Age

Physical	Psychosocial	Perceptual-Cognitive
Gains approximately ½ kg (1.1 lb) per month	Responds to own name	Begins to imitate actions, vocalizations, etc.
Length increases approximately 1.5 cm (½ in) per month	Imitates definite speech sounds and facial expressions	Works to get toy that is out of reach
Although tooth eruption is extremely variable, one per month may erupt	Begins to communicate by pointing to desired object	Increasing curiosity and growing drive to actively explore the environment
Pincer grasp	Jabbers expressively, utilizing jargon speech	Begins to experiment to reach new goals
Pulls to stand	Uses "ma ma" and "da da" specifically for parents	Increasing interest in novelty
Stands alone momentarily	Begins to test parental responses, especially at bedtime and meals	Growing determination to eliminate barrier to desired activities or goals
Cruises (walks while holding on to furniture or hands of adult)		Growing concept of time, space, and causality

Source: Adapted from R.M. Benfield and D.M. Harris, "The Infant—1 to 12 Months," in G.M. Scipien et al. (eds.), *Comprehensive Pediatric Nursing,* 2d ed., McGraw-Hill, New York, 1979.

Continued.

TABLE 2-10 Developmental Milestones: 10 to 12 Months of Age—cont'd

Physical	Psychosocial	Perceptual-Cognitive
Beginning to have regular bowel and bladder patterns	Enjoys attention and repeats activities reinforced by others	Shows interest in picture books
Releases objects at will	Grows toward beginning use of a few simple words	
Puts objects in a container	Ceases behavior in response to "no, no" or own nname	
	Increasing drive toward independence, especially in feeding and locomotion	
	Reacts with frustration when limits are placed on curiosity and urge to explore	
	Need for parental approval fosters mastering of new situations (e.g., weaning)	
	Is able to show range of emotions: anger or frustration, affection, fear (especially of separation), anxiety (especially with strange situations or persons), and joy at mastering a new task	

TABLE 2-11 Developmental Milestones: 13 to 18 Months of Age

Physical	Psychosocial	Perceptual-Cognitive
Walks without holding on (awkwardly at first, with wide stance, irregular step length, arms abducted, and fingers spread)	Seeks adult companionship (searches, follows)	Obeys simple commands ("Look," "Roll me the ball")
Runs within a few weeks of walking (awkwardly in same ways as initial walking)	Fear of strangers is less than in late infancy	Points on request to pictures of familiar objects in books ("Show me the baby") by 18 months
Goes from sitting to standing without using hands (15 months)	Hugs and kisses familiar people and toys	Makes wishes known by pointing and jabbering (15 months); uses names of few things in addition to family members by 18 months (bottle, cookie, shoe)
Kneels without support	Imitates housework, "helps" clean house	
Climbs into adult chair and turns around to sit	Comforts self with "security blanket" or favorite toy	Spends all waking time actively exploring environment
Backs into child's chair to sit (18 months)	Uses "no" a great deal, even when compliant and cheerful	Remembers where things are kept and looks in those places for them
Pulls and pushes toy while walking; can bend at same time without losing balance	Tells self "no, no" in imitation of parent (beginnings of self-control)	Experiments by trial and error, repeating action many times and observing outcome
Climbs stairs on knees, descends by scooting on buttocks	Asserts independence, resists assistance and interference	Remembers: searches briefly for object that has been removed from view (believes object continues to exist even when out of sight)
Throws and drops toys for another to retrieve, especially around 15 months	Has little tolerance for frustration (tantrums occur) but is easily distracted from upsets	
Stacks 2 or 3 blocks on each other by 15 months, 3 or 4 by 18 months		Learns about own body and environment by touching, exploring (sensorimotor learning)
Scribbles, gets off paper		Knows and correctly uses names of parents (mama, dada, or the like)
Removes shoes and stockings		
Has 4 to 16 teeth		
Anterior fontanel closes by 18 months		

Source: Adapted from M. Barnard et al., *Handbook of Comprehensive Pediatric Nursing,* McGraw-Hill, New York, 1981.

TABLE 2-12 Developmental Milestones: 19 to 24 Months of Age

Physical	Psychosocial	Perceptual-Cognitive
Walks very well and without apparent concentration	Continues to be highly autonomous—wants to do things own way and without interferences or assistance	Varies experimentation, trying new methods of doing things
Still runs awkwardly but falls far less than earlier	Peak age for temper tantrums	Still repeats actions many times and observes outcomes
Throws overhand without losing balance	Becomes possessive about playthings	"Predicts" outcome of own actions on basis of earlier observation—knows what to expect
Can kick a small ball (tennis ball) placed on floor	Mimicry is well established—imitates others' gestures (an important precursor to the social learning to be required in the next months and years)	Searches longer for an object that has been moved from view (sense of object permanence increases)
Jumps in place (both feet)	Wish for approval begins to modify wish for self-assertion and gratification	Points on request to a few body parts ("Where is your nose?" "Show me your foot")
Turns book pages, several at a time	Plays beside rather than with other children	Combines two words in primitive sentences ("Daddy bye-bye")
Spoon and cup control are good; child eats without assistance except for cutting food and cleaning self afterward	Plays alone for extended period if adult is nearby	Names and points to familiar objects in pictures (dog, baby)
Undresses with little help except for buttons		Appropriately uses pronouns (you, me)
Crudely copies vertical lines from demonstration		Asserts ownership ("Mine!")
Has 16 teeth		Uses own name to refer to self
Height at 24 months is approximately ½ of adult height		Begins to show some understanding of time; responds to request to "wait just a minute"
		Is unable to attend to more than one characteristic of an object or situation at a time
		Begins to perceive and express discomfort over wet or soiled diaper
		Vision is approximately 20/60 by 24 months (Tichy, 1981)

Source: Adapted from M.U. Barnard et al., *Handbook of Comprehensive Pediatric Nursing,* McGraw-Hill, New York, 1981.

TABLE 2-13 Developmental Milestones: 2 Years of Age

Physical	Psychosocial	Perceptual-Cognitive
Walks up stairs, placing both feet on each step	Becomes ritualistic: is upset if a routine is not followed in detail	Knows own first and last name, age, and sex by 2½ to 3 years
Dresses self with help	Resists bedtime	Highly egocentric—thinks own opinion is the only one, cannot put self in another's place or see things from another's point of view
Piles 8 to 10 blocks atop each other	Awakens early and gets up alone	
Imitates horizontal pencil stroke	Separates easily from mother; tolerates her absence for several hours, as for nursery school	Language and symbolization increase; for example, knows meaning of tomorrow, yesterday, after your nap (sense of time); recognizes two-dimensional pictures of three-dimensional objects; and knows waving good-bye means the waver is about to leave
Can manipulate doorknobs, screw caps for bottles, and other simple fasteners	Generally cooperative about toilet training	
Pours from one container to another (spills)	Imitates abstract adult qualities, such as sex-role behavior	
Washes and dries hands (gets water on clothes and floor)		

Source: Adapted from M.U. Barnard et al., *Handbook of Comprehensive Pediatric Nursing,* McGraw-Hill, New York, 1981.   *Continued.*

TABLE 2-13 Developmental Milestones: 2 Years of Age—cont'd

Physical	Psychosocial	Perceptual-Cognitive
Climbing up and jumping off are favorite activities	Social conformity increases—is more agreeable, gets along better, and has fewer frustrations and temper displays	Identifies need for toileting, eating, drinking
Quadruples birth weight by 30 months	Parallel play progresses toward interactive play with other children, in which children participate in a shared play theme (house, cars, etc.); cooperation and sharing of toys is rare	Uses descriptive words: hot, cold, big, hungry
Jumps forward with both feet together (broad jump)		Animistic thought: believes inanimate objects (especially anything that moves) have life, consequently thinks elevators, cars, etc., have wishes and intentions
Pedals tricycle	Daytime bladder and bowel control are good—nighttime bed-wetting is diminishing	Magical thinking: believes that "wishing makes it so" and that own thoughts cause things to happen—feels omnipotent
Holds pencil with thumb and two fingers, like an adult		Reasons from the particular to the particular (transductively) rather than from the particular to the general (inductively) or from the general to the particular (deductively): thinks two things that have been observed to happen together will always happen together or are cuase and effect (for example, a nurse wearing a white uniform has caused the child pain; therefore, white and pain are believed to be associated, and the approach of someone in white causes the child to begin screaming)
Copies a circle after demostration		
Can walk several steps on tiptoe		
Stands briefly on one foot		
Walks up and down stairs, placing one foot on a step		
Has full set of 20 primary teeth		Symbolic thought enables child to pretend
		Vision is approximately 20/40 to 20/30 by 36 months (Tichy, 1981)

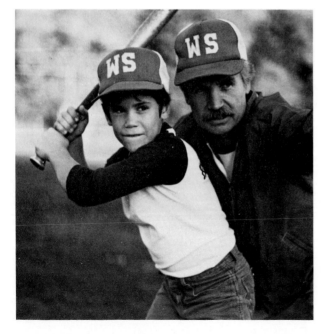

FIGURE 2-6 Adults other than parents are often admired by school-age children and sought out as role models and sources of personal values. *(Photo by Betsy Smith.)*

TABLE 2-14 Developmental Milestones: 3, 4, and 5 Years of Age

Physical	Psychosocial	Perceptual-Cognitive
3 Years Old		
Pedals tricycle	Develops concept of own identity and family	Has beginning understanding of past and future—"tomorrow" and "yesterday" still confusing
Walks backward	Imitates others	
Walks up and down stairs alone, alternating feet	Boy exhibits penis as if to affirm body intactness	Thinks anything that moves (e.g., car, moving parts of hospital equipment) is alive and has feelings and motives
Uses scissors with some success	Meets and accepts strangers	
Strings large beads	Demonstrates much sexual curiosity; "masturbates"; knows own sex	Does not distinguish fantasy from reality
Demonstrates good small muscle control by ability to copy circle and cross	Is jealous of sibling	Thinks own feelings (e.g., fear, hostility) are shared by everyone else; cannot take another's point of view
Tries to draw; may add an eye or leg when asked to draw a complete person	Is friendly, pleasing; alternates with periods of irritability, provocativeness	
Helps dry dishes	Partipates in simple games	
Unbuttons front and side of clothes	Cooperates in play with others; takes turns; plays spontaneously with a group	
Undresses and helps dress self	Enjoys reliving infancy through hearing stories	
Uses toilet; usually stays dry at night	Has many fears: animals, noises, darkness, strange shadows, TV villains, etc.	
Washes hands		
Feeds self		
May brush teeth		
4 Years Old		
Buttons front and side of clothes	Is very active and constantly on the move	Learning number concepts—counts to 3, repeats 4 numbers, counts 4 coins
Laces shoes, cannot tie	Uses language aggressively: lots of talking, questioning, teasing, silly language, mild profanities, name calling	Names one or more colors well
Brushes teeth	Stays with group activities longer	Has poor space perception
May bathe self with direction	Enjoys "dress-up," drawing, hammering	Thinks anything that moves is alive and has feelings and motives
Takes partial responsibility for toileting	Participates in much dramatic play	Poorly distinguishes fantasy from reality
May attempt to print letters	Likes to tell and hear stories	Thinks own feelings are shared by everyone else; cannot take another's point of view
Makes drawings with form and meaning but rarely detailed	Engages in cooperative play with peeers	Focuses on one aspect of a thing to the exclusion of its other traits
Represents person by head and eyes	Takes opportunities to do things for self	
Adds two parts to complete drawing of a person	"Helps" adults	
Throws ball overhand	Exhibitionistic, bids for attention; noisy; less pleasant in a group than 3-year-old	
Cuts out pictures	Fabricates, exaggerates, boasts, and tattles; dramatizes experiences	
Copies square	Has imaginary companion, often used to project blame for actions	
Builds 5-block gate from model	Is proud of accomplishments	
Can manipulate puzzle pieces	Volunteers to help group	
Moves with more graceful and rhythmic motion	Keen observer	
Jumps and climbs well	Persists in sexual curiosity	
Manages stairs unaided	Has good sense of "mine" and "yours"	
Hops on one foot	Can perform simple errands	
Can learn basic gymnastic skills	Interacts more with peers	

TABLE 2-14 Developmental Milestones: 3,4, and 5 Years of Age—cont'd

Physical	Psychosocial	Perceptual-Cognitive
	5 Years Old	
Dresses self except for tying shoes	Is cooperative and sympathetic; generous with toys	Copies a triangle
Washes self without wetting clothes	Evidences tension by nose picking, nail biting, whining, snuffling	Constructs a rectangle from 2 right triangles
Can learn to hit ball with bat	Is protective yet jealous of younger siblings and playmates	Does not fully understand time gradations
Runs with skill and plays at same time; runs on tiptoe	Is relatively independent	Knows weeks as units of time; names weekdays
Jumps rope	Is interested in kin relationships	Knows 4 or more colors
Skips well	Has dreams and nightmares	Knows age and residence
Skates on one roller skate	Is serious about self and abilities	Determines the heavier of 2 objects
Rides tricycle well	Is less rebellious than at 4	Beginning to understand kinship relations such as uncle, grandmother
Makes darwing of person including body, arms, legs, feet	Accepts responsibility for acts	Beginning to develop power of reasoning
Adds about 7 parts to complete drawing of person	Glories in achievements	Focuses on one aspect of a thing to the exclusion of its other traits
Puts 3 or more details in drawings	Desires a companion	Knows he is not serious when concocting tales
Drawings have more form; picture of person has more parts, clothes, and "personality"	Talks constantly	Understands simple letter and number games
Prints first name and maybe other words; forms letters well but sometimes backwards	Uses adult speech forms	
Handedness usually established	Finds speech more important than before in peer relationships	
May loose temporary teeth	Participates in conversation without monopolizing it	
	Asks for definitions	
	Asks fewer but more relevant questions	
	Laughs frequently during conversation	
	Generally tells the truth but may offer alibis to save face	

Source: Adapted from E. G. Nahigian, "The Preschooler—3 to 5 Years," in G. M. Scipien et al. (eds.), *Comprehensive Pediatric Nursing,* 3d ed., McGraw-Hill, New York, 1986.

TABLE 2-15 Developmental Milestones: 6 to 12 Years of Age

Physical	Psychosocial	Perceptual-Cognitive
Roller skating, ice skating	Becomes a member of the childhood peer society; forms strong friendships and loyalties among peers	Usually can tell clock time and understands its meaning at age 6; soon learns calendar time and days of week
Skateboarding	Influence of other children increases; influence of family members decreases somewhat	Develops concepts of cause and effect based on scientific principles but continue some supersitition and belief in magic or other illogical causes
Jumping rope		
Playing ball games of all types		
Swimming and diving	Adults other than parents are admired and become more influential than before; parents are compared to these new role models (Fig. 2-6)	Understands jokes, riddles, double meanings; abstractness and sophistication of humor increase with age
Horseback riding		
Bicycle riding		
Calisthenics	Relationships with parents become more adultlike and egalitarian	Becomes able to look at things from another's point of view and understand that varying opinions are possible
All self-care skills (independent care of teeth and hair, self-dressing, etc.)	Especially at 7 and 8, play groups and friendship pairs are of the same sex and show strong disparagement of the opposite sex ("Boys stink"; "Girls are so dumb"); same-sex friendships continue to predominate even after this phase of extreme criticism passes	Knows by 6 or 7 that some things that can move (e.g., machines, rolling stones) are nevertheless not alive
Fine motor games (marbles, jacks, etc.)		
Printing by 5 or 6, then cursory writing by 8		Learns to manipulate symbols according to established rules (e.g., arithmetic, spelling)
Jigsaw puzzles		
Playing musical instruments	Peer acceptance becomes of paramount importance, and child's self-concept fluctuates in accordance with ability to achieve peer status	After about age 7: Can classify objects into categories according to size, color, etc. Understands the concept of subcategories (e.g., all dogs are animals but not all animals are dogs) Understands that the amount of a substance does not change just because it is put into a new shape (e.g., a fixed quantity of water poured from a tall glass into a shallow pan does not become "more" or "less") Becomes able to consider simultaneously several qualities of a thing or situation (e.g., pros and cons, short-term and long-term effects)
Arts and crafts		
Electronic video games		
Using all the basic tools of society: telephone, hammer, pliers, scissors, needle and thread, knife, computer, etc.	Anxieties of school years are related to school performance, peer popularity, and physical strength or intactness in addition to family disruptions or other circumstantial happenings	
	Becomes more private about thoughts (fantasies, fears, jealousies, etc.), sharing more with friends than with adults	
	Anxiety over body injury may be greater than adults expect (adults may mistakenly think these children are "old enough to know better" than to fear "minor" procedures such as venipuncture and orthopedic cast removal)	
	Group activities (camping, ball teams, Girl and Boy Scout functions, etc.) are greatly enjoyed	
	Enjoys collecting (rocks, stamps, insects, etc.), especially at age 8	

Source: Adapted from M. U. Barnard et al., *Handbook of Comprehensive Pediatric Nursing,* McGraw-Hill, New York, 1981.

TABLE 2-16 Developmental Milestones: Adolescence

Physical	Psychosocial	Perceptual-Cognitive
Early Adolescence (11 or 12 to 14 Years)		
First sign of puberty is onset of rapid growth (adolescent growth spurt) in height and weight; extremities and neck lengthen before trunk does, causing gangly appearance	Often characterized by turmoil, uncertainty, wide mood swings, and outbursts of temper or emotion	Intellectual ability gradually matures so that by 14 or 15 years childhood cognitive processes are replaced by adult thinking (Piaget's stage of formal operations—See below)
Growth spurt begins as much as 4 or 5 years earlier in some children than in others of the same sex so that wide variation in size is common	Difficulty in adjusting to major physical changes and integrating new body into self-concept and body image	
Girls begin growth spurt about age 8½ to 11 years, about 2 years earlier than boys on average; onset of growth spurt is concurrent with the first pubescent changes (beginning breast development in females, increasing size of testicles and penis in boys)	Beginning interest in opposite sex: group dating may begin	
	Concerned about and dissatisfied with own body; exaggerates importance of real and imagined flaws	
Girls are often taller, heavier, and physically more mature than boys until about age 14, when boys become larger than girls	Ambivalent about own physical changes	
First menstruation usually between 10 and 16, with average 12 or 13	Very interested in social behavior and psychology as well as in physique and physical development of self and others	
First ejaculation usually between 12 and 16, with average 13 or 14		
Acne and oiliness of skin and hair common		
Middle Adolescence (14 to 17 or 18 Years)		
Trunk lengthens so that trunk and extremities assume more adultlike proportions	Strong need for contact with peers; discusses and tests ideas with friends before taking a position on anything	Piaget's stage of formal operations—see below
Growth in height is essentially complete by age 15 in girls and 17 in boys	Decreasing ties with family; family conflicts are at a maximum	
Sexual maturity (capacity for reproduction) follows menarche and first ejaculation by about 1 to 3 years	Establishes sexual identity and prepare for or adjusts to sexual relations; love feelings may be intense	
	Exploring self and temporarily imitating various others to establish sense of personal identity	
	Identifies mainly with persons outside the family	
	Preoccupation with own and peers' physical development subsides somewhat as adolescent becomes preoccupied with own personality and thought processes; this egocentrism leads to belief that other people are as interested in him as he is in himself	
	Idealistic; dissatisfied with status quo	
	Crushes on older person of opposite sex are common	
	Group dating is gradually replaced by double- or triple-dating and then by pairing off as a couple alone	

TABLE 2-16 Developmental Milestones: Adolescence—cont'd

Physical	Psychosocial	Perceptual-Cognitive
Late Adolescence (18 to 21 or 22 Years)		
Most girls experience few changes in height or weight; proportions are those of a mature young adult	Conflicts with siblings and parents decrease, and family relations become more like interactions between adults	Final stage of cognitive development (stage of formal operations) becomes established:
Boys continue to gain muscle mass and weight and to thicken and "fill out" for several years after full height is achieved	Has adopted adult social roles; is largely independent and able to provide for self without parental assistance and take responsibility for consequences of own behavior	Can think about hypothetical situations and imagine how things *could* be in a better world (Fig. 2-9)
Skin and hair oiliness and acne usually are greatly improved	Has begun career or is training for it	Can understand and apply the scientific method
Secondary sex characteristics become fully mature, but sex organs may not for a few more years, especially the uterus	Idealism becomes moderated somewhat as a result of experience; adolescent may become disillusioned and cynical	Can apply logical processes to hypothetical situations that are contrary to fact
	Identity becomes firmer than before, and so need for peer group decreases and is replaced by self-reliance and interdependence with one or a few close friends	Can understand metaphors
		Continues to accumulate experience that becomes useful in making judgments

Source: F. Anderson, M. Denyes, and A. Altshuler, "The Adolescent," in G. M. Scipien et al. (eds.), *Comprehensive Pediatric Nursing,* 3d ed., McGraw-Hill, New York, 1986; S. Nicholson, "Growth and Development," in J. Howe (ed.), *Nursing Care of Adolescents,* McGraw-Hill, New York, 1980.

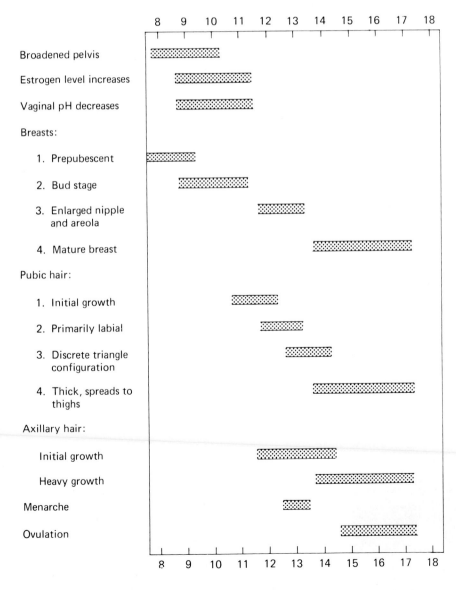

FIGURE 2-7 Average age at appearance of pubescent milestones in American girls. *(From G.H. Lowrey, Growth and Development of Children, Year Book, Chicago, 1973, pp. 299-302; J.M Tanner, Growth at Adolescence, Thomas, Springfield, Ill., 1962; Committee on Adolescence, Group for the Advancement of Psychiatry, Normal Adolescence, Scribner's, New York, 1968, pp. 105-110.)*

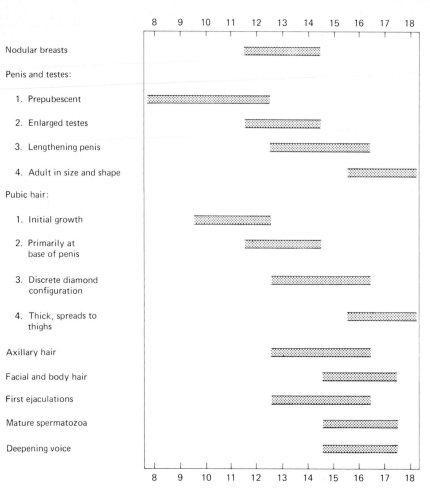

	8	9	10	11	12	13	14	15	16	17	18

Nodular breasts

Penis and testes:

  1. Prepubescent

  2. Enlarged testes

  3. Lengthening penis

  4. Adult in size and shape

Pubic hair:

  1. Initial growth

  2. Primarily at base of penis

  3. Discrete diamond configuration

  4. Thick, spreads to thighs

Axillary hair

Facial and body hair

First ejaculations

Mature spermatozoa

Deepening voice

FIGURE 2-8   Average age at appearance of pubescent milestones in American boys. *(From G.H. Lowrey, Growth and Development of Children, Year Book, Chicago, 1973, pp. 299-302; J.M. Tanner, Growth at Adolescence, Thomas, Springfield, Ill., 1962; Committee on Adolescence, Group for the Advancement of Psychiatry, Normal Adolescence, Scribner's, New York, 1968, pp. 105-110.)*

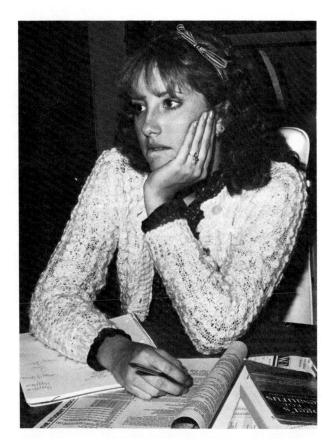

FIGURE 2-9   Daydreaming serves a real purpose in adolescence. *(Photo by Betsy Smith.)*

Learning Activities

1. Write a detailed description of a 2-minute observation of the behavior of a child or adolescent. Interpret the behavior in terms of Erikson's theory, Piaget's theory, or behavior modification theory.
2. Observe as your clinical instructor or another experienced professional estimates the gestational age of a neonate, using the Dubowitz method or another standardized method.
3. Over a period of several hours or a few days, keep a record of two young infants' behavioral states. Note the time of day at which each baby enters a new state, what patterns exist in the sequence and pace of changes of state, how long each state lasts, and what activities take place in the environment at those times. Talk with the parents about the baby's individual pattern and how it affects them and the ways they interact with the baby.
4. Interview the parents of an infant, toddler, preschooler, school-age child, and adolescent. Ask each parent to provide a capsule description of his or her child. How has the child changed in recent weeks or months? What are the parent's main concerns about or problems with the child at this stage of childhood? What actions has the parent taken to deal with the problems, and how effective were they? What are the pleasures of being the parent of a child this age? What developmental changes in the child is the parent looking forward to? When are the changes expected to occur? Are the expectations realistic in terms of developmental norms or the child's past patterns? What nursing actions are appropriate to promote the health and development of the child and parent?
5. Pretending you are an infant, toddler, preschooler, school-age child, or adolescent, look around your environment or other places you go for safety hazards. How can these places realistically be "child-proofed" to prevent accidents?
6. Look over the old records of your own or a friend's childhood (baby book, nursery or school periodic reports, family health records, etc.). Compare the child with the norms for height, weight, and behavior. If photographs are available, describe the child's appearance at various ages, paying special attention to body build, proportions, facial configuration, and other physical characteristics. What are your conclusions about the use of group norms for assessing an individual?
7. Take a listening walk with a preschooler or young school-age child. Have the child identify and explain the sounds in the environment. Encourage the child to fantasize about the sounds.
8. Conduct or attend a hospital orientation tour for a group of children.
9. Examine several children's books (check the local bookstore, supermarket, etc., or ask a librarian to recommend books). What general themes or main problems are dealt with (e.g., getting lost, making a moral decision, going to the hospital)? How does the author approach the theme or problem to help children cope?
10. Ask a hospitalized preschooler, school-age child, or adolescent to draw pictures of a hospital, a child in a hospital, and a nurse or doctor. Notice the comments the child makes while drawing. When the pictures are finished, ask the child to tell you about them.
11. Interview a school-age child or adolescent about any prominent current event (beginning of school year, holiday, news event). What are the child's opinions about why things are as they are, what would improve the situation, who worries about these things, and so on?

Study Questions

1. To help children reach their highest level of development, the nurse must:
   1. Understand how children change with time.
   2. Provide excellent physical care.
   3. Be familiar with hazards that threaten progress.
   4. Take the place of the child's parents when they are not making wise decisions.
      A. 1 and 2   C. 1, 2, and 3
      B. 2, 3, and 4   D. 1, 2, 3, and 4
2. It is usual for children of the same age to have similar:
   1. Physical skills.
   2. Measurements.
   3. Physiological characteristics.
   4. Behavioral qualities.
      A. 1 and 2   C. 1, 2, and 3
      B. 2 and 3   D. 1, 2, 3, and 4
3. Comparing an individual child with the norms for his age group:
   1. Is part of the pediatric nursing assessment.
   2. Identifies variations that indicate a problem.
   3. Is likely to demonstrate the child's individuality.
   4. Should be attempted only by highly trained specialists.
      A. 1 and 3   C. 3
      B. 2 and 4   D. 1, 2, and 3
4. Which of the following statements are compatible with Erik Erikson's theory of development?
   1. Infants should be trusted to make their needs known to their caretakers.
   2. Self-assertion is the major developmental issue for toddlers.
   3. Schoolchildren achieve their developmental tasks by using fantasy and pretending.

4. Adolescents normally behave quite differently from one time to another as they experiment with variosu roles and temporary identities.
   A. 1, 2, 3, and 4   C. 1, 2, and 3
   B. 2, 3, and 4   D. 2 and 4

5. Which of the following statements are compatible with Piaget's theory of development?
   1. Paralysis of the upper extremities in infancy would be expected to delay intellectual development.
   2. Playthings (toys, objects to handle, things to climb on, etc.) are nice for infants and toddlers but not really important to their intellectual development.
   3. By about age 7 or 8 years a child can learn to think logically, as adults do, if he is provided with good educational experiences and environmental stimulation.
   4. By about age 7 or 8 years a child is able to classify objects into categories and hence can manage a simple collection of rocks or autumn leaves.
      A. 1 and 2   C. 3 and 4
      B. 2 and 3   D. 1 and 4

6. Behaviorists believe that:
   1. Some children are born with more intelligence than others.
   2. Behavior depends on previous experience with rewards and punishments.
   3. Behavior that brings pleasure tends to be repeated.
   4. Adults can discourage undesirable behavior by simply ignoring it.
      A. 1, 2, and 4   C. 2, 3, and 4
      B. 1 and 3   D. 3 and 4

References

Brazelton, T.B.; *Neonatal Behavioral Assessment Scale,* 2d ed., Lippincott, Philadelphia, 1984.
Tichy, A.M.: "Sensory System," in M. Tudor (ed.), *Child Development,* McGraw-Hill, New York, 1981.
Tudor, M. (ed.): *Child Development,* McGraw-Hill, New York, 1981.

Bibliography

Harris, J.R., and R.M. Liebert: *The Child: Development from Birth through Adolescence,* Prentice-Hall, Englewood Cliffs, N.J., 1984.
Klaus, M.H., and J.H. Kennell: *Bonding: The Beginnings of Parent-Child Attachment,* Mosby, St. Louis, 1983.
Papalia, D.E., and S.W. Olds: *A Child's World,* 4th ed., McGraw-Hill, New York, 1987.
Segal, J., et al.: "The Infant—Ready and Able to Learn," *Children Today,* 14(2):19-23, 1985.
Tribe, C.: *Profile of Three Theories: Erikson, Maslow, Piaget,* Kendall-Hunt, Dubuque, Iowa, 1982.
Tudor, M. (ed.): *Child Development,* McGraw-Hill, New York, 1981.
Wadsworth, B.J.: *Piaget's Theory of Cognitive and Affective Development,* 3d ed., Longman, White Plains, N.Y., 1984.

3

Parenting and Functions of the Family

Objectives

After reading this chapter, the student will be able to:

1. State at least three reasons why it is important to direct nursing care toward the entire family rather than only toward the child.
2. Describe how family members can be included in each phase of the nursing process.
3. Define the term *heritage consistent health beliefs* and give at least one example for each of the following groups: far easterners (Chinese, Vietnamese, Cambodian, etc.), Hispanics (Mexican, Cuban, Haitian, etc.), Native Americans (Navajo, Cherokee, etc.), Indians, and Jews.

4. Define the following family types and state at least one benefit and one disadvantage of each: nuclear family, one-parent family, extended family, and blended family.
5. Use a systems theory perspective to list at least five effects a child's illness may have on the family.
6. Use a role theory perspective to list at least five effects a child's illness may have on the family.
7. Define *family developmental task* and give at least five examples.
8. List at least five ways parents can encourage the development of a child's self-esteem.
9. List at least three things a nurse must do to give good care to children and families from differing cultural backgrounds.

Chapter 2 focused on children and adolescents and on what they are like at each age. That information is an essential part of the background for pediatric nursing, but by itself it is incomplete. In addition to the developmental forces that shape children, there is another enormously powerful factor in every child's health and behavior: the family. Nursing care that fails to take account of this influence is likely to fail.

The Family Is the Client

The goal of nursing is to facilitate each child's attainment of his potential. This goal is not limited to the treatment of health problems but includes the promotion of good health. Nurses attempt to prevent illness and accidents and to lead the child to develop a life-style that supports robust mental and physical well-being. These ends can seldom if ever be attained without the inclusion of the family in the care plan, whether the client is a child, adolescent, or adult.

It is primarily in the family that children learn the health-related attitudes and behavior that affect their health throughout childhood and, more likely than not, the adult years as well. Attitudes and practices having to do with nutrition and weight control; safety; use of alcohol, tobacco, and other drugs; activity and rest patterns; coping with stress; mental health phenomena; and ways of using the health care system are initially developed at home.

Decisions about health care for children are made and implemented by family members far more often than by health care professionals. For example, a parent or other influential adult family member decides what is an appropriate diet, whether and when to consult a health care professional, and how closely to follow the professional's recommendations.

Nurses are increasingly recognizing that it is necessary to work with family units rather than individuals. Two points are becoming clearer.
1. The "patient," i.e., the one person who serves as the "reason" for seeking professional attention, is but a focal point for what is indeed a family health matter rather than an individual concern.
2. In the end it is the family members, not the professionals, who hold the power either to sabotage the care plan or to carry it out. The implication for practice is both clear and simple: *Clients (families) must be thoroughly involved in the development of the care plan.*

Part of the care in the *assessment* phase of the nursing process must be to find out what the family expects and wants to happen as a result of the child's involvement with the nurse. When client's expectations or priorities conflict with those of the nurse, negotiation must be undertaken in order to avoid either (1) the nurse's finding that the family does not cooperate with the plan or (2) the family's feeling that the plan is irrelevant, inappropriate, or an imposition.

The family must participate also in the *planning* stage of the nursing process. This is especially true when the interventions will be carried out by family members. It is obviously important not to make plans for the family members that they cannot or will not carry out.

The extent of family members' involvement in nursing *intervention* obviously varies greatly from family to family. The complexity of care and the child's capacity for self-care are important factors.

Family participation in the *evaluation* phase is necessary and appropriate. Clients very often have criteria different from those of professionals for measuring the success of treatment. Collaborative evaluation can avoid the too common situation of a dissatisfied client unsafely discontinuing what a professional considers an effective regimen.

In addition to these pragmatic reasons for involving clients in the nursing process, there are compelling ethical reasons as well. The patient rights issues that have emerged out of the consumer rights movement clearly point to the ethical necessity of informing people about assessment findings, treatment options, and expected outcomes. The health professions exist to provide service, and those who receive the services should of course play a major role in planning and evaluating the care provided.

Health and Illness

Since the family is the unit on which the nurse focuses, the child should be considered a subunit and must be regarded in the context of the family. Each family defines, interprets, and explains health and illness in terms of its experiences and expectations. The *heritage* of a given family, that is, the family's cultural, ethnic, and religious background, may determine these interpretations. The family learns from its *cultures,* its *ethos* (ethnicity), and its *religion* how to be healthy, how to prevent illness, and how to react to and treat illness. The *American Heritage Dictionary* (1975) defines these terms as follows:
1. *Culture:* "The totality of socially transmitted behavior patterns, arts, beliefs, institutions, and all other products of human work and thought characteristic of a community or population."
2. *Ethos:* "The disposition, character, or attitude peculiar to a specific people, culture, or group that distinguishes it from other peoples or groups; fundamental values or spirit."
3. *Religion:* "The expression of man's belief in and reverence for a superhuman power recognized as the creator and governor of the universe."

Culture

Culture deeply shapes a person's way of experiencing, perceiving, thinking, and speaking; it also teaches what to regard as important and unimportant. Many institutions, rituals, and practices contribute to the shaping of a culture, and the meanings are subtle and difficult to articulate. Culturally determined health beliefs stem from the "world view, symbols, values, and patterns of social conduct" that constitute group life, that is, from ethnic identity (Chrisman and Kleinman, 1980, p. 452).

Ethnicity

The phenomenon of ethnicity is complex, ambivalent, paradoxical, and elusive. The characteristics of an ethnic group include a common geographic origin, race, language or dialect, religious practice, traditions, values, symbols, food preferences, and internal sense of distinctiveness (Petersen, 1980).

There are at least 106 ethnic groups and more than 170 Native American groups in the United States that meet the above criteria. According to Chrisman and Kleinman (1980, p. 452), "the ethnic groups within this country quite often believe and practice within their original health care system and carry forth with their ancestral, or traditional, beliefs." People continue to immigrate to the United States. Today the main influx of immigrants is from the far east (Vietnam, Laos, and Cambodia) and from Cuba, Haiti, Mexico, and South America. "These immigrants . . . bring their unique health and illness beliefs and practices to this country' ' (Castillo, 1979).

Religion

Religion is a major reason for the development of ethnicity (Petersen, 1980). Numerous cults, sects, denominations, and churches exist in the United States. Ethnicity and religion are clearly related, and religion is quite often the determinant of ethnic membership.

Religion provides the family with a frame of reference and a perspective with which to organize information. Religious teachings about health and illness help construct a meaningful philosophy and system of health-related and religious practices. For example, many of the rituals practiced at birth, such as circumcision and baptism; numerous dietary practices, such as food restrictions and combinations; and rites of passage, such as confirmation, are tied to religious beliefs related to health.

Definitions of Health and Illness

The most widely held definition of *health* has historically been that stated in the constitution of the World Health Organization: "Health is a state of complete physical, mental, and social well-being and not merely the absence of disease" (World Health Organization, 1947). Currently there is disagreement regarding this definition, and other definitions are being developed. In describing *holistic health,* for example, the word *wellness* is widely used, as are the broad concepts of life-style, health-illness continuum, self-responsibility, adaptation, stress management, risk reduction, fitness, healthful environment, health promotion, and "internal balancing" of body, mind, and spirit (Salmon, 1984).

On the other hand, *illness,* "sickness of body or mind," has an obsolete connotation of "evil and wickedness" (*American Heritage Dictionary,* 1975). Illness can be described as abnormal functioning of body systems. Each person recognizes or defines illness by assessments of

what may be observed (objective assessment) and what may be believed (subjective assessment) to be wrong. The nurse may define illness in terms of cardinal signs and symptoms such as fever, pain, swelling, and so forth; the parent or child may see illness as the child's inability to do what he wants to do or to go to school.

Heritage Consistent Families

Health and illness are interpreted and explained in terms of the family members' personal experiences and expectations. From their heritage people learn (1) how to be healthy, (2) how to prevent illness, and (3) how to react to illness.

A family whose predominant life-style and behavior reflect major elements of its national, cultural, religious, and/or ethnic origins is described as *traditional* or *heritage consistent* (Estes and Zitzow, 1980). When the heritage consistent family interacts with nurses who (1) come from different national, cultural, religious, or ethnic orientations or (2) have become well socialized into the profession of nursing, there may often be differences of opinion, which may result in conflict, either overt or covert.

Among heritage consistent families there tend to be numerous "folk" beliefs that determine perceptions of health and illness. For instance, in the heritage consistent Chinese family, illness is believed to be a lack of harmony and an imbalance of yin and yang. Preventive measures are designed to maintain the balance between yin and yang. An illness believed to be caused by an imbalance of yin and yang may be treated by ingestion of a substance high in the missing factor; that is, a disease caused by too much yin would be treated with a yang food or medicine (Wallnöfer and von Rottauscher, 1972).

To the extent that any American black family has retained its African heritage consistent viewpoints, the family may define health as a state of personal harmony (between the body, mind, and spirit) that is in harmony with nature (Jacques, 1976). Illness may then be seen as disharmony. It may be attributed to the workings of demons, the devil, or evil spirits. Several methods may be utilized to prevent or treat these actions, among them the belief and practice of voodoo. Belief in both "white" and "black" magic exists to an unknown extent, and care is taken to avoid contact with magical elements (Jacques, 1976).

A Hispanic family with heritage consistent beliefs may describe health as the balance of the four humors "*blood*—hot and wet; *yellow bile*—hot and dry; *phlegm*—cold and wet; and *black bile*—cold and dry" (Currier, 1966, p. 251). Health may also be viewed as the result of good luck or as a reward from God for good behavior (Welch, Comer, and Steinman, 1973). Illness is an imbalance of the four humors, the result of bad luck, and/or a punishment from God for bad behavior. One factor is a "hot-cold imbalance," caused by improper diet. Foods are neither hot nor cold in the sense of temperature; rather, this terminology serves as a classification of given foods. Certain foods are known to be "cold" and others "hot." Examples of "cold" foods are chicken, honey, fruits, avocado, bananas, and lima beans. Examples of "hot" foods are chocolate, coffee, cornmeal, garlic, kidney beans, onions, and peas. Illness can occur if these foods are eaten in improper combinations or amounts. For example, *frialdad del estómago,* "cold stomach," is caused by eating too many foods classified as "cold." An infant who requires a formula that contains "hot" evaporated milk may be fed a "cold" food such as whole milk (Harwood, 1971).

Another agent believed to cause illness is the dislocation of body parts. An example of this is *caida de la mollera,* "fallen fontanel" (Saunders, 1958). This disorder is thought to be caused when a stranger touches a baby's fontanel. It is a complication of severe dehydration. A parent may avoid taking an infant for a well-baby checkup because of the fear that this illness will result (Lucero, 1975).

The heritage consistent Native American family may define illness as an indication of disharmony with self and nature. A family from the Hopi Nation may associate illness with evil spirits; consequently, care is taken to avoid or ward off these spirits (Boyd, 1974). One from the Navaho Nation may see illness as the reuslt of (1) displeasing the holy people, (2) annoying the elements, (3) disturbing animal and plant life, (4) neglecting the celestial bodies, (5) misuse of a sacred Indian ceremony, or (6) tampering with witches or witchcraft (Bilagody, 1969). A Cherokee family may describe illness as the imbalance of body, mind, and spirit that is brought on by excess in one domain and neglect of the other two areas. For example, a child who is a student and spends too much time in study—development of the mind—may neglect his body and spirit and therefore be vulnerable to disharmony, i.e., an illness of some sort (Spector, 1979b).

Prevention and Treatment of Illness

Prevention and treatment of illness depend on one's understanding of the cause of a given illness or set of symptoms. Among people who hold heritage consistent health and illness beliefs, ideas about the causation of illness differ vastly from the modern model of epidemiology.

In traditional epidemiology, illness is most often attributed to the *evil eye.* The evil eye belief is "primarily the belief that someone can project harm by looking at another's property or person" (Maloney, 1976, p. v). Belief in the evil eye "has existed in all times and in all countries" (Elworthy, 1958, p. 3). Belief in the evil eye is thought by some to be merely a superstition, but what is seen by one person as superstition may well be another person's religion.

The common characteristics of the evil eye belief include the following (Maloney, 1976, p. vii):

1. The power emanates from the eye or mouth and strikes the object or victim, frequently a newborn baby or young child.
2. The injury, whether illness or another misfortune, is sudden.
3. The person who casts the evil eye may not be aware of having this power.

4. The afflicted person may or may not know the source of the evil eye.
5. The injury caused by the evil eye may be prevented or cured with rituals or symbols.
6. The belief helps explain sickness and misfortune.

Prevention of illness may be undertaken with methods that ward off evil, by avoidance of people believed to cast the evil eye, or by maintenance of balance between body, mind, and spirit, yin and yang, or "hot or cold." Illness is treated with the use of traditional healers and traditional remedies (folk medicines). The following are examples of specific traditional methods used to prevent and treat illnesses.

Prevention

Amulets, objects such as charms or talismans, are worn on a string or chain around the neck, wrist, or waist to protect the wearer from the evil eye (Fig. 3-1).

1. *Azabache,* or *mano negro* ("black hand"): This small clenched fist is used by heritage consistent Puerto Rican parents to prevent the evil eye from harming a baby. It is placed on the baby throughout the first year of life, either on a chain around the neck or wrist or pinned to a diaper or shirt. If a *mano negro* is placed on the baby's shirt while the neonate is still in the hospital, the nurse must exercise great caution to make sure it is not lost.
2. *Corno,* or goat's horn: The *corno* is worn by people of Italian origin to prevent the evil eye. The charm in Fig. 3-1 is gold; others are larger and made from red plastic. Often a *gobbo* is inside. The *gobbo* is a hunchback with an umbrella, believed to block the evil eye. The *corno* is the most prevalent amulet against the evil eye.
3. Lucky 13: An amulet worn by Italian children to prevent the evil eye.
4. *Mano cornuta:* Another amulet worn by Italians to prevent the evil eye.
5. *Mano milagroso:* The "miraculous hand," worn by children of Mexican background to prevent the evil eye.
6. Hand of God: A charm worn by children of Semitic background, generally Jewish, to prevent the evil eye.
7. *Chai:* A Hebrew charm worn to signify and protect life.
8. Thunderbird: An amulet from the Hopi Nation worn to bring good luck and to protect the wearer from harm and evil.
9. *Milagros:* The arm and leg are Mexican amulets, worn to prevent harm and evil.
10. Talisman: The talisman, an object or amulet believed to possess extraordinary powers for the prevention of evil, is worn on a rope around the waist or carried in a pocket or purse. The one illustrated in Fig. 3-1 is worn or carried by believers in voodoo.
11. Bangles: These braclets, worn by both males and females, originated in Haiti and the West Indies. The silver bracelets are open to "let out evil" and closed to

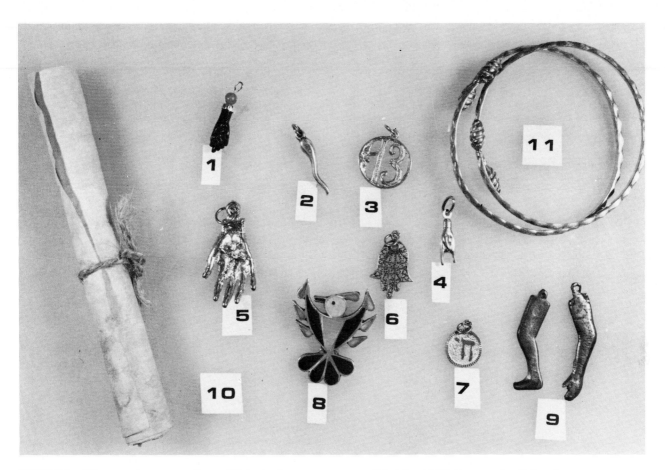

FIGURE 3-1   Objects used to prevent illness. (1) *Azabache,* or *mano negro*—"black hand." (2) *Corno,* or "goat's horn." (3) "Lucky 13." (4) *Mano cornuta.* (5) *Mano milagroso.* (6) "Hand of God." (7) *Chai.* (8) Thunderbird. (9) *Milagros.* (10) Talisman. (11) Bangles. *(From the private collection of Rachel E. Spector, R.N., Ph.D. Photo by Rob Schadt, Audiovisual Coordinator, Boston College, Chestnut Hill, Mass.)*

prevent evil from entering the body. These bracelets tend to tarnish and leave a black ring on the skin when person a is becoming ill. When this tarnish ring develops, the person knows he must rest, improve his diet, and take any other needed precautions. Many people believe that they are extremely vulnerable to evil and even to death whenever these bracelets are removed.

It is important for nurses to realize that if these bracelets or amulets are removed from a child, the parents and child experience a great deal of anxiety (Modestino, 1978).

In addition to amulets, certain substances are also used to ward off the evil eye and prevent illness. They are hung in the home, worn on the body, or ingested. Figure 3-2 illustrates some of these items.

1. Onion is often eaten raw to prevent illness.
2. Garlic may be hung in the home, worn on the body, or eaten raw. In the Azorean home, garlic may be hung over the front door, the back door, and a door in between to ward off the evil eye (Like, 1978).
3. Thousand year eggs. These eggs, used in the Chinese community, have been stored for a prolonged period

of time until the insides have gelled. They are eaten uncooked and are considered helpful in preventing illness and keeping the body healthy (Gaw, 1978).
4. *Corta maldad* is a powerful Indian oil worn to keep away evil.
5. *Baños del niño Fidencio* consists of herbs and leaves that can be carried or sprinkled around the home to protect the family from envy and to bring peace and good luck. The mixture comes from Nuevo León, Mexico, the home of a famous folk healer, Fidencio Constantino. Niño Fidencio practiced healing from the 1920s until 1938. He is the central figure of a widespread cult.
6. *Jabón de la mono milagroso* ("soap of the miraculous hand") is used to cleanse the body and protect it from evil.

Diet may also be used to prevent and treat illness. For example, in the Chinese home balance must be maintained between foods with yin and yang properties by eating them in certain specified proportions. In the Hispanic home "hot" and "cold" foods must be balanced. The kosher diet followed by traditional Jewish families and a similar Muslim diet mandate the avoidance of pig products

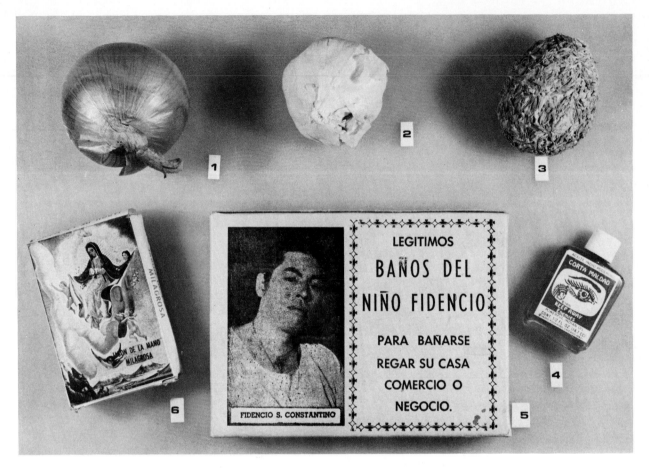

FIGURE 3-2   Substances used to prevent illness. (1) Onion. (2) Garlic. (3) Thousand year egg. (4) *Corta maldad.* (5) *Baños del niño Fidencio* (6) *Jabón de la mano milagroso. (From the private collection of Rachel E. Spector, R.N., Ph.D. Photo by Rob Schadt, Audiovisual Coordinator, Boston College, Chestnut Hill, Mass.)*

and shellfish. Furthermore, traditional Jews believe that milk and meat must not be eaten at the same meal.

Treatment

The admitted use of folk medicine is increasing, and the practice may be observed among families from all walks of life and backgrounds. The roots, herbs, and/or seeds that are used as medicines often transcend ethnic lines, and many of the same substances are used in multiple communities; other remedies are unique to a given community. Fig. 3-3 shows some folk remedies.

1. Essence of chicken with *tang wei:* This product from China is used to treat abdominal pain, headache, anemia after illness, postpartum weakness, dizziness, and poor appetite. It is interesting to note that chicken soup is used for these same purposes by a large number of families from many ethnic backgrounds.
2. Ginseng: The ginseng root, believed to be the best folk remedy of all, is used to allay fear, expel evil, brighten the eyes, open the heart, benefit understanding, and treat every kind of disease (e.g., persistent vomiting of pregnant women, chronic malaria, persistent fever, cough, and polyuria) (Chen, 1973). Ginseng ("sang") is

also found in the Smoky Mountains of North Carolina and Tennessee.

3. Linden tea: This tea is used to treat nervous disorders and facilitate weight reduction. Two cups must be drunk in the morning and one at night. A small amount calms a fussy baby.
4. Korean ginseng tea: This packaged preparation is dissolved in cold or hot water, mixed with sugar or honey, and used for the same purposes as the ginseng root.
5. Estafiate: This herb is brewed into a tea that is used to treat joint pains.
6. Anise: Anise is a tea used to treat flatulence or cough and to induce relaxation. It is often used to treat infant colic and is also rubbed on the gums of teething babies.
7. Herbal prescription: A combination of herbs is made into a tea and used to treat diarrhea.
8. Chinese tea: This tea is used to treat digestive problems.
9. Mandrake root: This root is used in combination with other herbs to treat liver and bowel problems, uterine disorders, and intermittent fever.

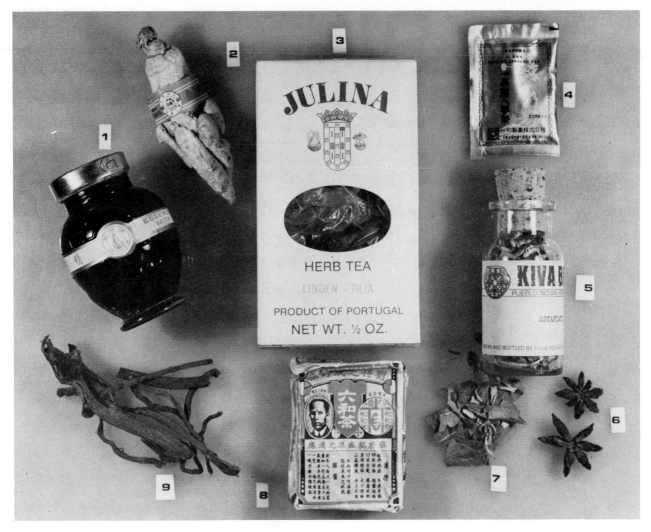

FIGURE 3-3 A sample of folk remedies. (1) Essence of chicken with *tang wei*. (2) Ginseng. (3) Linden tea. (4) Korean ginseng tea. (5) Estafiate. (6) Anise. (7) "Herbal prescription." (8) Chinese tea. (9) Mandrake root. *(From the private collection of Rachel E. Spector, R.N., Ph.D. Photo by Rob Schadt, Audiovisual Coordinator, Boston College, Chestnut Hill, Mass.)*

Healers

In the traditional context, healing is related to taking the source of illness away from the ill person. Within a given community there are specific people known to possess the power to heal. The healer, male or female, is most often a person who is thought to have received the gift of healing from a divine source.

A family in a heritage consistent community may consult a healer before or during the utilization of modern health care services because the relationship between family and healer is much closer than that between family and health professional. The healer understands the problem in the context of the family's traditional background, language, and social status (Spector, 1979a). The following are examples of healers:

1. Medicine man; the traditional healer of the Native Americans. The spiritual cause of the problem is sought using herbs and rituals.

2. *Señora:* a woman (Puerto Rican) especially knowledgeable in the causes and treatment of illness.
3. *Espiritista:* a folk practitioner (Puerto Rican) who is more knowledgeable in the causes and treatment of illness than the señora.
4. *Santero* (*santera* if female): a person (again Puerto Rican) consulted for psychiatric problems.
5. *Curandero* (*curandera* if female): a person (Mexican) with God-given abilities to heal; uses a religious and psychiatric approach to healing.
6. *Partera:* a midwife (Hispanic).
7. Yerbero: a herbalist (Hispanic).
8. Root worker: A person (black) who is able to determine the cause of an illness and the treatment.

There are numerous differences between physicians and nurses on the one hand and traditional healers on the other. Table 3-1 compares the two.

One must remember that traditional healers have been

TABLE 3-1 Differences between Modern Western and Traditional Healers

Modern Western	Traditional
1. Complaint-oriented	1. Illness-oriented
2. Organ-specific	2. Whole-specific
3. Bacterial and pathogen-caused	3. Imbalance—nature-caused
4. Technical diagnosis	4. Visionary diagnosis
5. "Hands-on" treatment	5. Theological treatment
6. Synthetic drugs	6. Natural drugs
7. Specialization by system	7. Specialization by function
(a) Internal medicine	(a) Herbalists
(b) Surgery	(b) Diagnosticians
(c) Orthopedics	(c) Lay persons
(d) And so forth	(d) And so forth
8. Learned by academic approach	8. Learned by practice approach
9. Communicated in narrative	9. Communicated in ritual

a part of human cultures for as long as humans have had communities. The methods they utilize to heal were developed over the years by trial and error. Today's traditional healers are knowledgeable and understand the deep-seated beliefs of heritage consistent families within their cultures.

Definitions of Family

A common definition of *family* is "people who are related by blood or marriage." Probably most people would accept the expanded definition that a family is people related by blood, marriage, or adoption. Some definitions specify two parents with their minor children.

Many people feel that their family includes others besides blood relatives and people legally adopted or married into the kin group. Children (and often adults as well) commonly include household pets in family drawings, plans for family outings, family lists, and the like. Members of a commune may consider all other members as family and may pool and distribute resources within the group as a whole. Some people have a neighbor or friend who is treated as family, perhaps being called uncle or aunt by children.

Murphree, an anthropologist, proposed that nurses define family broadly as "a socially organized group of two or more individuals of either or both sexes, including either adults or adults and children, functioning together to meet at least some portion of the basic human needs" (Murphree, 1979, p. 113). In the same spirit, Miller, a nurse, recommended that nurses define family broadly lest they overlook people who could be helpful in supporting the client and enabling the family to help itself. She proposed that in clinical nursing situations *family* be defined as "two or more persons who are joined by an agreement to share various aspects of life together" (Miller, 1984, pp. 79-80).

Types of Families

As in most aspects of human endeavor, people demonstrate wide variety in forms of family life. Some children live with both of their parents; some do not; some do, but not in the same place or at the same time. Some live with stepparents, with or without the stepparents' children from earlier marriages. In addition to (or instead of) their parents, some children live with other adults and perhaps also other children, some or all of whom may or may not be related to them. The membership of the households in which children grow up may take many forms. The point is not which is best or what is right but how to identify the strengths and risk factors of any child's family in order to exploit the strengths and compensate for the vulnerabilities. No one approach to family living is all "good" or all "bad." It is important to remember that personal values rather than objective facts are the basis of many of our own and everyone else's ideas about family life. Conflicts of values need not be a problem if one keeps in mind that the goal of the professional is to promote health, not to promote conformity to one set of beliefs.

Each family is unique and will not conform in every aspect to general descriptions. The types of families included in this discussion are as follows:

1. Nuclear family: a married couple living together with their own or adopted dependent child or children
2. One-parent family: one adult living alone with his or her own or adopted child or children
3. Extended family: either of the preceding types living with one or more members of the parents' family of origin, such as the parent's mother or father, sibling (with or without offspring and spouse), or grandparent
4. Blended family, also called reconstituted family and stepfamily: one or both members of a married couple who have brought children from their previous marriages to the present family
5. Other social configurations, including pairs or groups of adults with other relationships besides those listed above, and children.

Nuclear Family

Many people, especially of the white middle class, consider this the predominant and most legitimate family form. The traditional nuclear family, in which the husband is employed and the wife is not, is "a small minority of all families at any given time" and appears to be increasingly a thing of the past (Masnick and Bane, 1980, p. 95). Most Americans live in a nuclear family at some time during their childhood and/or as a parent, but it is by no means unusual for a person to spend a portion of the childhood years in some other type of family.

The nuclear family has a mixed reputation as a setting in which to live, love, and develop, whether as a child or as an adult. The benefits of the nuclear family include the following.

1. It receives social approval and is looked upon as the "normal" or desirable type of family.
2. The small family unit has great social mobility, being freer than some other family forms to change residence

if opportunities or changing interests lead them to move either down the block or across the country.

3. The role expectations of all members are generally well established, clear, and unambiguous. Everyone "knows" that in nuclear families the husband "should" be the sole or principle breadwinner; the wife "should" have primary responsibility for child care and home management, even if she is also employed outside the home; and the children "should" conform to parents' viewpoints and values, provide affection and a source of parental pride, and so forth.

4. Interpersonal ties within the nuclear family tend to be very close and strong.

5. Financial adequacy is sometimes considered a strength of nuclear families and is sometimes considered a weakness. Nuclear families fare rather well in comparison with one-parent families, who are limited to one adult's income and often have greater expenses for day care, housekeeping, home maintenance, or other services that two-parent families manage as do-it-yourself activities. On the other hand, nuclear families may have fewer resources and fewer personnel to absorb unexpected financial setbacks.

The nuclear family has been criticized for certain inherent disadvantages or weaknesses. Among the criticisms are the following.

1. Children have access to only two adults (the parents) as role models from whom to learn about family life and to learn how to behave when they become adults and parents. Furthermore, one or both of the parents are usually away from the child for most of the day and hence not available as role models. Children's opportunities to prepare for becoming parents are further lessened by the fact that nuclear families are often small and may not provide much experience in caring for brothers and sisters.

2. Child care (teaching, intellectual stimulation, affectional interactions, etc.) is hard for the small two-parent family to provide, especially when both parents work. Consequently, much of the care and rearing of even young children is delegated to baby-sitters or day care centers that may or may not be good at what they do.

3. The nuclear family is more vulnerable than larger groups to financial and emotional devastation if one adult becomes ill, dies, or leaves the family. Moreover, nuclear families appear to be somewhat cut off from backup resources that could be provided by extended families.

4. Because of the small number of people in the family and because intense relationships with people outside the family are often discouraged, family members become socially restricted and overly reliant on family members to meet all their needs. Possessiveness and selfish expectations easily limit others' freedom and engender resentment.

5. The rigid sex roles typical of nuclear families require both males and females to curtail development of their natural androgynous potential. This restriction not only limits personal potential but also discourages understanding of and empathy for members of the opposite sex.

One-Parent Family

There is a great diversity among one-parent families. Some function very well; others do not. The circumstances of one-parent families vary in many ways that influence their well-being. One important factor is the reason for the absence of the second parent—death, divorce, desertion, separation, nonmarriage, or single-person adoption. These different reasons have different effects on family functioning.

The one-parent family is usually considered a highly vulnerable family form. Little is said in its favor except for the following.

1. Many people think it is probably better than having the parents together if the parents have severe conflicts.

2. If the second parent was a liability for the other family members—abusive, a spender in excess of what he or she contributed to the family income, and so on—the family may fare better without that person.

3. Children from one-parent homes may develop considerable independence, responsibility, and social versatility if circumstances require that they take care of themselves and be responsible for helping the parent and siblings.

4. Since the tasks of managing the household, making a living, and caring for children are simply assigned to the available household personnel rather than according to traditional sex roles, some people consider that one-parent families have the advantage of discouraging sexual stereotyping.

But on the whole one-parent families appear to have more disadvantages than strengths. Some of the problems are as follows.

1. The one parent carries the load of trying to fulfill the parent roles and adult roles that are more or less a full-time job for two parents in a nuclear family. The resulting task overload causes fatigue and frustration, and some activities have to be skipped over in favor of more pressing priorities. If the parent works, the shortage of time is felt more acutely, and employment and child care sometimes compete harshly for the parent's attention. Before- and after-school hours, school vacations, and children's sick days create particular problems.

2. Money is in short supply for a great many one-parent families, particularly if the parent is a woman. The single source of income is often inadequate. Although men's earning potential generally exceeds women's, men who are single parents also frequently find finances a problem.

3. Because there are few people in the family and because they have experienced the loss of the other parent, the remaining parent and children are especially vulnerable to further loss. Particularly if there is only one child, parent-child relationships may become markedly possessive and dependent. The departure or death of a

family member can cause severe separation stress.

4. The children have exposure to only one parental model; thus they get a narrower experience in what adults believe, do, and are interested in than they would if they had both parents.

5. A solitary parent, in addition to being overtaxed by the demands of child care, employment, and household management, is likely to have unmet personal needs.

6. The parent often feels caught between the need to accept money, child care assistance, or other goods and services from his or her own parents and the wish to remain independent of them.

7. Children whose parents do not live together may feel stigmatized because of it. They may feel embarrassed and inadequate—"different"—when mothers and fathers are invited to school events, or when there is a class project to make Mother's Day or Father's Day gifts. Self-esteem often suffers an additional blow because children may believe that they are to blame for the other parent's absence or that they are "no good" as evidenced by the apparent fact that the parent rejected them and chose to leave them behind.

Extended Family

The nuclear or one-parent family living with relatives has the advantages of membership in a supportive social network if the adults are on good terms. The strengths of extended families include the following.

1. Rather than relying on only one or two parents, the extended family has a larger pool of personnel to provide the goods and services family members need. Housing costs, for instance, are lower for one large dwelling than for two or more smaller ones; clothing can be shared or passed along to younger children; and there is usually someone who can assist with the care and supervision of children.

2. The richer variety of role models helps the child develop a broader repertory of attitudes and behavior that may increase versatility and coping skills. Having a close relationship with several adults provides a broad base of love and does not place the child at risk to "lose everything" if one adult dies or goes away or if the child loses favor with one person.

3. With more people in the household, everyone's activities tend to become more visible to everyone else. Accordingly, children can acquire more experience in observing how people perform skills, express and resolve conflicts, evaluate outsiders in terms of their own value system, and so forth.

4. Family identity is generally prominent in extended families, since kinship is the underlying reason for group membership. Older children and adolescents reared with a strong sense of family identity may find it relatively easy to formulate their own sense of self (their personal identity) because they are part of the group.

5. Adults in extended families can be highly beneficial to one another. The companionship of other adults is a valuable source of stimulation and support.

Life in an extended family is not without its drawbacks, of course. Among the difficulties that can arise in this family form are the following.

1. There is a relative (and sometimes pronounced) lack of privacy.

2. Role clarification is commonly an issue, especially in three-generation households: Whose job (or privilege) is it to plan the menu, discipline the children, decide about major purchases, choose the activity for a family outing, and so on? When people have known each other for a long time (e.g., mother and adult daughter), the past relationship washes over into the present and old interaction patterns may continue.

3. Extended families are less mobile than smaller family units so that it is relatively difficult to move, for example, to a new town to take advantage of new employment opportunities.

Blended Family

The reconstituted, or blended, family (stepfamily) is a common phenomenon because so many widowed and divorced people with children remarry. The advantages of this family form include those of nuclear families and the avoidance of some of the problems of one-parent families. Economic security may be greatly enhanced by adding a second parent, but not necessarily. Loss of previous alimony income or other financial supplements for single parents and their children, combined with continuing outlay for alimony to previous marital partners, can create heavy expenses for the new family. New housing may have to be found in order to accommodate the larger family and the larger space can cost more.

Expectations for emotional security and satisfaction are often not fulfilled. While emphasizing that not all blended families experience serious interpersonal difficulties, Schulman (1972) very cogently identified numerous unrealistic expectations and other "myths" that place these families at risk for dissatisfaction, conflict, and emotional problems. Among them, as reported by Schulman, are the following.

1. Most or all family members have been traumatized in the earlier family. Both children and adults may feel strong needs for acceptance and love and may at the same time be overly sensitive to real or imagined slights or rejections. The adults may expect the children to show "instant love" for the new stepparent, whereas in reality this is an unrealistic expectation in any relationship. The children also make spoken or unspoken comparisons between the stepparent and the previous parent.

2. There is a cultural expectation that stepmothers will be "wicked" or cruel. Although most are neither, there can be a tendency for children and others to make unfavorable comparisons between the stepmother's behavior and the stereotyped selflessly nurturant role that women are often expected to enact.

3. The parents' motives for the marriage may predispose to conflict and disappointment. People with exaggerated hopes of being taken care of or those who enter

marriage primarily to secure a caretaker for their children may find that the tasks of family membership are greater than they can meet with equanimity.

4. The new stepparent may be seen by one or more children as an intruder into a previously well-established parent-child relationship. Adolescents are especially likely to feel that the newcomer is taking over some of their roles, particularly when the adolescent is of the same sex as the stepparent. Children are likely to underestimate how much the new spouse will fill the companionship needs of the natural parent, and feelings of being displaced can engender resentment. Adolescents can be quite unaccepting of the sexual aspects of the relationship.

5. Splinter groups may form when the parent blindly sides with the stepparent regardless of the justness of the child's dissenting point of view. There is a tendency for a parent to see his or her own children as better behaved, more deserving, and better adjusted than the spouse's children, which can lead to coalitions and scapegoating among children.

6. Children may feel that they are treated unfairly when parents allot chores and privileges unequally, when in fact the parents may be making their decisions according to the children's ages, sexes, or other individual traits. These feelings of persecution are especially common among stepsiblings and seem harder for parents and children in blended families to handle.

Other Groups

There are many other social configurations that function as families. Those who simply share a household— friends, boarders, unmarried lovers—may feel and act like a family, regardless of kinship, gender, and sexual involvement with one another. People who reside in the same neighborhood or housing development may relate as family members, sharing their resources, cooperating to solve their common problems, supporting one another in times of trouble, and engaging in recreation and other activities together. Groups of people who do not necessarily live very close to one another but who have some common value or background may also function as families. These groups include ethnic, national, and ideological subgroups, especially if the members feel isolated from or persecuted by mainstream society.

Finally, people who live in communes and/or have communal marriages generally operate as a family to a greater or lesser extent. Communes differ enormously in regard to purpose, size, stability, leadership, patterns, economic viability, sexual policies, ideologies, and health-related beliefs as well as in their child-rearing practices. Communal marriages, or group marriages (in which three or more adults have a long-term mate relationship, sharing a residence and economic resources and bringing up their children communally), also vary greatly. Overall the advantages include the following:

1. The ability to choose one's friends and to include them in one's family
2. The expanded pool of resources: personnel, services, emotional support, love, property, money, and so forth
3. The availability of multiple role models both for children and for adults
4. Companionship

The disadvantages commonly include the following:

1. Impermanence of individual members in the group
2. Lack of social and legal status, creating stigma and issues concerning legitimacy of children and inheritance rights
3. Lack of privacy and individual autonomy
4. Jealousy, especially if there are multiple sexual relationships
5. Many and conflicting demands placed on children, who may find it possible to avoid following through with any one set of behavioral expectations

Family Theories

While theories about individuals, such as the child development theories of Erikson and Piaget, have obvious merit, they also have limitations. Hence, it is important to realize that each client is continually influenced by family, friends, staff in the clinical setting, school or work groups, and various other small and large groups.

Systems Theory

Systems theory (Bertalanffy, 1968) is useful for nursing because it helps the nurse recognize and comprehend the complexity that inevitably characterizes human life. Systems theory undertakes to deal with *wholeness.*

A system is two or more elements (individual component parts) that interact with each other and together make up a whole. A body system, to use a familiar example, is a group of interrelated organs and tissues that together perform a particular set of functions. The cardiovascular system has as its components the heart and blood vessels, and they work together to circulate the blood. A social system is made up of people who interact to form a group that performs certain functions.

Families are systems. The elements of the family system are the individual family members: mother, child, father, grandmother, and so on. In addition to these individual elements of the system, there are also subsystems, subgroups of people who have a special relationship to one another. In families with more than one child, the children constitute a subsystem of which the siblings are the only members (Fig. 3-4). There may be further subdivisions within family systems. In a blended family, "his children" and "her children" are members of separate subsubsystems, and "their children" are yet another group, while all belong to the child subsystem of the family.

Systems theory states that there is constant and reciprocal interaction among the several members within a system; that is, all members continually influence and are influenced by all others. In the family system not only do the several parts of the system interact reciprocally with one another but any change brought to bear on one member of the system inevitably affects in some way all the other members of the system.

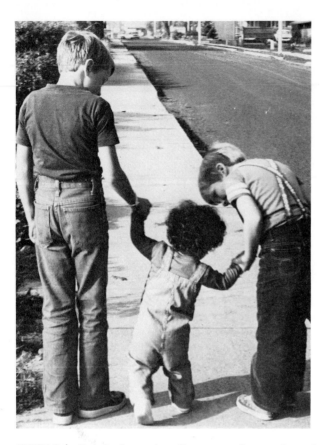

FIGURE 3-4 Each family member affects every other member and is affected in return. Siblings profoundly influence one another, and the sibling subsystem is a strong force in the larger family system. *(Photo by Betsy Smith.)*

A child who becomes ill or injured and requires hospitalization, for example, is by no means the only person in the family who is affected. The demands on parental concern, time, and finances require changes in resources available. Parents cannot be home while they are with a hospitalized child; substitute caretakers may be brought into the home; siblings may miss the absent child, worry, feel responsible for their sibling's misfortune, and resent the heightened attention he receives. Individuals and the family as a unit may be affected by changes in their interactions with *other* systems such as the health care institution, the parents' occupational systems, the children's school groups, and the extended family. The family system and its members undergo continual change as reestablishment of equilibrium is sought. No member of the family is unaffected, and none is only an actor or only a reactor.

Every system has certain functions to perform, and its activities are organized toward attaining its objectives. The family, for example, may include among its functions the economic support of its members, the education and socialization of its children, the provision of essential health care, and the giving and receiving of affection.

In striving to achieve its goals, a system consumes energy, information, services, and commodities from its environment and releases by-products into the environment.

Environment includes not only the natural and physical surroundings but also the economic and political situation, the cultural norms, and the other existing systems that impinge on the family: schools, health care agencies, public transportation facilities, mass media, public assistance programs, and so forth. In systems theory the materials and information taken in from the environment are called *input* while the things the system produces are called *output.* The system receives continual informative signals from within itself and also from the environment, called *feedback.* Feedback that causes the system to change its ways (i.e., indications that the system is not meeting its goals) is *negative feedback,* while information that results in a continuation of the status quo is *positive feedback.* The input-output-feedback mechanism gives the system the capacity for self-regulation.

A *closed system* is one that does not interact with its environment; in living things closed systems do not exist. *Open systems,* the alternative, are characterized by exchange of energy, information, personnel, services, commodities, and so on back and forth across the hypothetical *boundary* that separates the system from its environment. Family systems obviously interact with their environment, but some are more open than others; that is, some families more readily and more extensively relate to community agencies, natural resources, public events, other families, and so forth. It should be clear from this discussion that the family's ability to meet its goals depends on its ability to acquire what it needs (health care, employment, information, etc.) from its environment.

The essence of systems theory is that it views the system as being continually in flux. The individuals and subgroups within the family endlessly influencing one another and being influenced in return so that the system undergoes continuous internal change. Moreover, the system is set into an environment with which it also is in continuous mutual interaction; the family changes the environment and is reciprocally affected. No element within a system (e.g., no person within a family) can experience change without all other members of the system also feeling the impact in some way.

Role Theory

Role theory deals with the social expectations that accompany social position. *Position,* also called *status,* refers to a person's place in the social order—mother, wife, teacher, and so forth. One person generally occupies a good many positions at the same time. A particular child may be a son, grandson, Boy Scout, Japanese American, and Californian, for example, among other things.

Status can be acquired in a number of ways. Some positions are acquired at birth (son, Japanese American), some are awarded by other people (best friend, favorite child), and some are adopted (rescuer, invalid).

A *role* is a cluster of behaviors, attitudes, values, and beliefs that are expected to accompany a position. Members of the clergy, for example, are expected to conform to high moral standards, sacrifice their own comfort in service to those who need them, hold certain spiritual be-

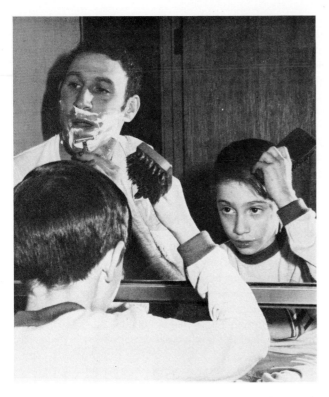

FIGURE 3-5 Role learning, from simple to complex, at home and elsewhere, is a major activity of childhood and adolescence. *(Photo by Betsy Smith.)*

liefs, and avoid unseemly activities; these beliefs, values, and behaviors compose the clergy *role*.

Roles are learned (Fig. 3-5). This learning results both from formal training such as that which takes place in the family, at school, and in church and from incidental experience such as occurs in the peer group, through watching television, and by making casual observations of other people.

For every role there is a complementary role played by someone else in the person's social setting. Thus, one cannot fulfill a nurse role unless someone will enact the client role; there cannot be a teaching role without someone to act as learner.

Family life includes many roles: caretaker, wage earner, disciplinarian, and many others, including sex roles, age roles, and sometimes sick roles, black sheep roles, scapegoat roles, and so forth. There are normative expectations that *go* with every role to define how people in those roles are "supposed" to behave.

A family or other social system functions smoothly as long as all the roles necessary to keep the system operating have been assigned to someone in the group and as long as those individuals are willing and able to enact them. Crisis may be expected when the family role structure has to be realigned because someone relinquishes his or her customary roles. If the wage earner dies or becomes incapacitated, for example, the family system undergoes a period of instability until provisions are made to reassign the role of wage earner to other family members. Role revision goes on continually in families because of

inevitable changes that occur with aging. Conspicuous role changes for both child and family members occur when a child begins school, begins adolescence, leaves home, gets married, and so forth.

Role conflict occurs when an individual feels forced to choose between two roles that are incompatible with each other. An adolescent, for example, may experience role conflict in a situation in which he desires to follow the behavioral standards that accompany his role as a member of his family and also wishes to gain the approval of his peers by carrying out some activity that is contrary to what his family would expect. A related concept is *role strain,* which refers to the feelings of inadequacy or guilt that are experienced when a person feels unable for some reason to fulfill one of his roles.

Family Development Theory

In this theory (Duvall and Miller, 1984) the family unit is viewed as moving through an orderly and predictable sequence of developmental stages as time passes, in the same way an individual progresses from one stage to another. At each of the family's developmental stages there are developmental tasks to be achieved (Fig. 3-6).

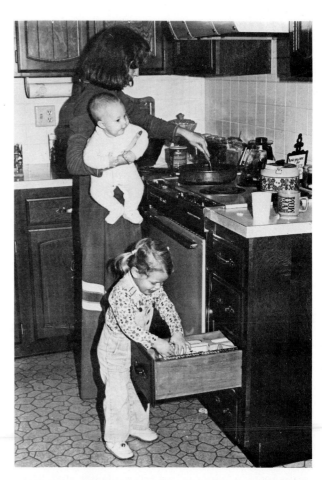

FIGURE 3-6 The family unit has a natural developmental progression ("family life cycle"). The major interests, problems, goals, and day-to-day activity patterns of the family change as the years pass. *(Photo by Betsy Smith.)*

In the first stage of family life the married couple have the developmental task of adjusting to living together and providing for their own needs as a couple. They must develop effective ways of dealing with their financial needs, housing, social relations, sexual relationship, recreational patterns, and the myriad other adjustments of being a married couple. They must also plan for their next developmental stage, that of childbearing.

The childbearing stage is considered to last from the birth of the first child until the child is 2½ years old. The family now focuses on the activities and challenges of nurturing an infant and toddler and revising the marital relationship to accommodate to the changes that result from adding a child or children to the family.

The third family stage is the span of time in which the oldest child grows from 2½ to 6 years of age, the child's preschool period. The family tasks at this stage are to provide a safe and stimulating environment that supports the maximal development of the preschool child and to make the further adjustments in their marital relationship that are required (because of lack of privacy as the child gets older, possible increasing need for living space and money, etc.).

The fourth stage spans the oldest child's school-age period. The developmental tasks for the family are to foster the child's adjustment to school, support the child's growing understanding of the world (use of money, moral development, social interactions with people outside the family, etc.), and maintain a supportive and gratifying marriage and home life.

The years between the first child's thirteenth birthday and the time when he leaves the parental home for marriage, work, or postsecondary education constitute the next phase in the family's development. The major tasks are to (1) facilitate the adolescent's development of independence and ability and to live responsibly as an adult, (2) promote the parents' readiness to release their adult child from the home, and (3) develop the parents' abilities to find productive and meaningful interests to engage them after the children are grown.

The "launching-center" phase of family development is the period between the oldest child's departure from the parental home and the last child's leaving. The tasks are to support the children as they move into career, marriage, or college and to revise the parents' home and life-style so that they have a satisfying day-to-day life as the children leave their household.

The seventh developmental stage is the period extending from the onset of the "empty nest" to retirement. The marital couple generally live alone together for the first time since they were newlyweds, perhaps 20 to 30 years earlier. The relationship requires readjustment, and each spouse needs new interests both for personal development and for sharing with the other. The husband and wife enter a new phase in their relationship with their own parents, whom they understand better after having reared children and whose advancing age requires new patterns of interaction as the older generation becomes more or less dependent upon their children. Grandchildren bring new gratifications as well as demands for revision of the new grandparents' self-concepts.

The final phase of the famiy developmental cycle is the period from retirement until the death of both spouses. Developmental tasks include adjusting to retirement, maintaining relationships with one's adult children and their families, and coping with widowhood and the prospect of one's own eventual death.

Developmental Tasks and Goals of Parents and Families

A *developmental task* has been defined by Havighurst (1979, p. 2) as "a task which arises at or about a certain period in the life of an individual, successful achievement of which leads to happiness and success with later tasks, while failure leads to unhappiness in the individual, disapproval by society, and difficulty with later tasks." *Individual developmental tasks* are categorized in a variety of ways but often include Erikson's eight stages of life as well as Piaget's stages of intellectual development, which were discussed in Chap. 2.

When two people join to become a family, they bring with them their own tasks to master and add to these the developmental tasks of a family. The tasks suggested by Hymovich and Chamberlin (1980) are:
Meeting the basic physical needs of the family
Assisting each family member to develop his individual potential
Providing emotional support and communicating effectively with all family members
Maintaining and adapting family organization and management to meet changing needs
Functioning in the community
Each of these tasks is appropriate to a family consisting of a childless couple or to a family with children. Obviously, the larger the family, the more complex the tasks to be mastered. It is also apparent that the opportunity exists for conflict as to whose needs will receive priority over the needs of others. In the United States, for example, there has been a long-standing cultural expectation that parents sacrifice their own needs for those of their children. This expectation has met with some resistance recently among adults who believe that they have the right to "find themselves" even though their children may be penalized. Unless parents recognize that their own unmet needs can continue to influence their child-rearing practices, they may unknowingly either try to meet these needs vicariously through their children's experiences or limit their children's opportunities in much the same way their own were curtailed.

As the family expands and the children grow, parents need new knowledge and skills to help each family member achieve optimum fulfillment. This purpose is facilitated when parents have clearly defined their long-range goals, but goals often remain diffuse or unspecified. For example, a mother who values imagination and creativity in her child and a father who values conformity will undoubtedly give their child mixed messages until they consciously clarify their goals.

The question parents need to answer is how they can rear a child who will become an adult valued by the parents themselves and by society. Schuster (1980) believes that successful adulthood is marked by (1) ability to cope flexibly and independently with the demands of the culture, (2) achievement of balance between personal rights and societal responsibility, and (3) respect for oneself and others. A fourth goal that is probably implicit in these three is to achieve high-level wellness. These accomplishments seem to be stated broadly enough that most people could agree to them as goals.

Parenting Styles

There is probably far less unanimity about child rearing now than there was before our society became so highly mobile. Parents tended to rear their children as they had been reared, and there was relatively little exposure to alternative methods. Child rearing has gradually moved away from these traditional approaches, and as a result, many adults lack confidence in their roles as parents. The search for answers has created a market for child-rearing "experts" to share their beliefs about competent parenthood. Bookstore shelves are amply supplied with "how to" books that claim to have the right answers to parents' problems.

It is easy to see why parents may have difficulty deciding how to rear their children. What guidelines can nurses use in helping parents develop effective parenting practices before crises occur?

First of all, there should be an attempt to match the natural inclinations of the parents with the particular child-rearing approach. It may be unrealistic and guilt-producing to expect some people to substitute active listening for immediate action or reaction. A temperamentally impatient parent would find it extremely difficult to tolerate impertinence while helping the child express negative feelings. Wise (1980) uses a model that could be useful in helping to decide the natural inclination of the parents. Rather than using single continuums ranging from permissive to strict or democratic to authoritarian, he suggests a three-dimensional model (Fig. 3-7) using three intersecting continuums: permissive-restrictive, loving-hostile, and anxious-calm. Thus several possible parenting styles emerge. Loving parents (right-hand side of Fig. 3-7) can range from highly permissive to very restrictive and may be emotionally involved or calm and detached. Parents who are basically hostile toward their children (left-hand side of Fig. 3-7) may express these feelings by indifference or dictatorial behavior and, again, may do so with anxiety or detachment.

Although the model was developed to explain the relationship between parental disciplinary practices and their effects on children, these same practices are usually consistent in other areas of child rearing. It can be seen from Table 3-2 that children who experience certain

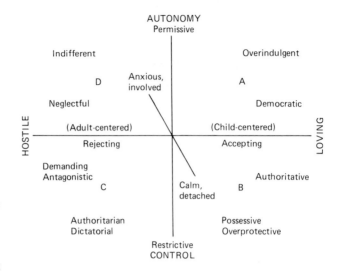

FIGURE 3-7 Three-dimensional hypothetical model of parental behaviors and attitudes toward the child ("anxious, involved" versus "calm, detached" is the arm of the third dimension). *(From C.S. Schuster and S.S. Ashburn, The Process of Human Development: A Holistic Life-Span Approach, 2d ed., Little, Brown, Boston, 1986, p. 368.)*

kinds of parental actions are more likely to display particular characteristics than are children exposed to other types of interactions (Wise, 1980). It is essential to remember that in Wise's studies, although relationships existed between parents' practices and children's responses, not *all* children responded in the predicted ways. There are always exceptions.

The values of the parents and the goals they hold for their children are also important considerations in selecting parenting approaches. People who value creativity and responsible freedom in their children can select child-rearing techniques which are relatively permissive, knowing that research findings tend to support the relationship between permissiveness and creativity (Wise, 1980). There is a possible danger in encouraging some parents to use the method with which they are the most comfortable. For example, Dobson (1982) advocates the use of physical pain in certain situations as an effective form of discipline. Parents who use spanking as the primary method of discipline may refer to Dobson's book to validate their practices without really understanding the safeguards he includes.

Doherty and Ryder (1980) proposed that parents who learn *techniques* for managing children may not appear genuine in their interactions and that children are quick to sense this. Parents may blame themselves for the "bad" approaches they use or think that new techniques can solve all the complex problems of family living. There is also a danger of marital conflict if one parent adopts a particular technique and then blames the spouse for using other approaches.

Since each child in a family may respond differently to parental management, it is advantageous for parents to

TABLE 3-2 Relationship of Disciplinary Practices to Personality Development

Type of Parental Discipline	Parent Behavior	Child Behavior
1. Permissive-accepting (a) Calm and detached	Allow freedom of choice consistent with age Establish rules cooperatively Use positive reinforcement and logical consequences Accept undesirable behavior in calm and detached manner Demonstrate love	Adopt adult roles Low hostility Extroverted Active Autonomous Creative Disrespectful toward adults Dominating and aggressive toward peers Periodic disobedience
(b) Anxious and involved	Overly indulgent	Behave on basis of feelings Seen as spoiled by outsiders Become sociable, achieving, highly motivated adults
2. Restrictive-accepting (a) Calm and detached	High expectations Exercise considerable control Serve as role models Demonstrate love Seek to earn right to exercise authority	Positive self-concept Highly motivated Self-directing Less creative More dependent More conforming More introverted
(b) Anxious and involved	Overly protective	Immature Dependent Introverted Resent control and solicitousness
3. Restrictive-rejecting (a) Calm and detached	Rigid control Arbitrary rules Frequent punishment Authoritarian	Repressed and internalized hostility Self-punishing Accident and suicide prone
(b) Anxious and involved	Demanding Antagonistic	Introverted Socially inept and unresponsive Shy and immature Less motivated Conforms onlyin presence of external controls
4. Permissive-rejecting	Indifferent Neglectful	Poor self-concept Hostile toward parents Impulsive and aggressive "Acting-out" delinquent behavior

Source: Wise,1980, pp. 407-410.

have a wide range of options and techniques at their disposal. For example, when a child's self-esteem is being damaged by a punitive teacher, some parents would attempt to change the teacher's behavior, some would move the child to a different teacher, and others might deal directly with helping the child cope constructively with the difficult situation. Each option is the right one in certain situations, but parents may need help to identify what options are available. In choosing disciplinary techniques, the parents need to take the child's developmental characteristics and temperament into consideration. A highly active 4-year-old who is seen hitting a friend may find it impossible to sit quietly for a 5-minute time-out but may understand why he can no longer play with that friend—a logical consequence of his misbehavior. A youngster who is very sensitive to parents' nonverbal messages may need no more than a stern look to quell misbehavior.

Certain child-rearing approaches have been recognized as unwise and ineffective (see Table 3-3). However, it should be apparent by now that there is no one way to rear children that will guarantee desired results. It is, rather, a case of deciding what each child needs to develop optimally and then deciding how to meet these needs. Wise (1980, p. 418) cited Garsee as the source for the five Ls of child rearing: Love, Limits, Learning, Liberty, and Liability. Children who turn out well as adults are believed to have done so because their parents provide them with these five Ls (see Fig. 3-7).

Love should never be conditional; each child should know with certainty that he is loved. Highly controlling parents can make it clear to a child that their restrictions and expectations are based on their love for the child, but no parent should withdraw love because a child misbehaves.

Limits can also be provided in a variety of ways. All

TABLE 3-3 Inappropriate Child-Rearing Techniques

Hazards to Effective Parenting (Ginott)	12 Roadblocks to Communication (Gordon)	Thou Shalt Not (Dodson)
Threats	Ordering, directing, demanding	Belittle
Bribes	Warning, threatening	Threaten
Promises	Moralizing, preaching	Bribe
Sarcasm	Advising, giving solutions	Extract promises of better conduct
Asking questions to which answers are already known	Lecturing, teaching, giving facts	Supervise overprotectively
Imposing responsibility	Judging, blaming, criticizing	Talk excessively
Encouraging denial, disowning, suppressing, or prettifying feelings	Praising, buttering up	Insist on blind and instant obedience
Insults	Name-calling, ridiculing	Pamper and overindulge
Name-calling	Interpreting, analyzing	Use inconsistent rules and limits
Prophesying	Reassuring, sympathizing	Use rules inappropriate to child's age
Bossing	Probing, interrogating, questioning	Use moralizing and guilt-inducing methods of discipine
	Withdrawing, diverting, distracting	Give any command you do not intend to enforce

Sources: Ginott, 1965, Chaps. 3 and 4; Gordon, 1976, p. 32; Dodson, 1970, pp. 213-217.

children need some limits for their own safety. Growing up without limits has been likened to driving across a high bridge without railings on either side. Permissive parents would provide low railings but would build the child's sense of confidence in managing his own life. Punitive parents would punish the child for getting too near the railing and not respecting their wishes. Controlling but nonpunitive parents might build high railings but allow the child freedom within those limits.

Learning includes the acquisition of knowledge about the child's world (the intellectual component) and the development of awareness of what behavior is acceptable in various circumstances and what the consequences are for misbehavior. Here, too, the content and rate of learning can vary according to the parents' approaches to child rearing. For example, the responsibility for completing homework in some permissive-accepting homes might be delegated to the child, but the parents would provide an appropriate setting and would take advantage of opportunities to give positive reinforcement. In permissive-accepting homes with overly involved parents, homework might be viewed as an infringement on the child's right to relax and have fun. In contrast, the anxious, involved parent in a restrictive-accepting atmosphere might stay with the child during homework and might supply some of the answers as a means of protecting the child from possible failure. Review Table 3-2.

Liberty and liability are closely intertwined, as are all the *L*s of child rearing. Children need liberty to make decisions consistent with their level of maturity and to experience the consequences of those decisions. Children have a right to try—and to fail—and to learn from these experiences. They also have a right to be protected from excessive failure.

Influences on Child-Rearing Practices

It has been well established through observation and research that parents tend to bring up their children as they

were brought up. If a child's two parents were reared in very different circumstances, difficulties in child rearing can result unless the couple's differences can be resolved. It is also true that education and experience can modify the effects of an individual's upbringing.

At the same time that expectant parents are making decisions and setting expectations about their future roles as parents, they are formulating expectations of the infant, including the characteristics they believe are desirable. Some may be glad for a baby of either sex as long as it is healthy. Others express a deep need for a boy to carry on the family name or to emulate the father's athletic or business prowess. Some mothers need a dainty, passive infant who responds to cuddling, while others enjoy an active, sturdy baby who appears ready to fight the world. When parents' expectations coincide with the qualities of the newborn, healthy parent-child relationships are apt to develop, but difficulties may arise when there is a conflict between expectations and reality.

In addition to expectations and goals, parents have certain attitudes, opinions, and beliefs about children and child rearing, which have been modified through exposure to public education about child rearing. These attitudes, opinions, and beliefs deal with such concerns as the role of the child in the home, how a youngster should behave in social situations, and the quality of school performance expected.

Parents begin child rearing with varying levels of knowledge about children's growth and development and about how to foster optimum well-being. If they have had experience in caring for young children, have observed the methods others use, and have read widely, they may have acquired a wide range of skills they can use flexibly as the situation demands. If knowledge is lacking, their choice of child-rearing practices may be limited. If they are fortunate enough to have children who respond well to these limited approaches, their expectations for the children can still be met. Parents who are more likely to have problems are those with insufficient knowledge or skill to cope with the particular problems presented by their children. For example, well-educated parents with high expectations for their children may not be able to adapt to a child who is temperamentally highly distractible and low in persistence.

The resources individuals bring to parenting include their ability to learn as well as their levels of confidence and feelings of self-worth. Parents who view themselves as competent tend to rear competent children. On the other hand, a parent who is timid about new experiences tends to restrict the child's experiences as well.

Resources for parenting of course include money and the goods and services for which money is used, including transportation, health insurance, housing, clothing, food, medical care, and such miscellaneous expenses as toys and baby-sitting. The financial cost of rearing a child is greater than parents may realize—$80,000 to $120,000 in a city or suburb, according to USDA figures, and more in outlying areas (Tuhy, 1983). Tuhy further stated that parents earning $50,000 in 1983 would spend $278,000 to bring up a son born that year to age 18 and an additional $17,000 to raise a daughter. The additional "cost" of lost wages if one parent did not work until the child started school could easily reach $116,000 ($20,000 yearly plus 5 percent inflation).

As parents begin the child-rearing process, another variable affects the way they rear their children: the influence the child and subsequent children have on the parents. As parents develop sensitivity to the changing needs of the infant, they learn to modify certain actions in order to comfort or bring pleasure to the baby. As the baby grows, they must be able to shift from providing complete care to nurturing the child's increasing independence.

Parenting and the Development of Children's Self-Esteem

The establishment of high self-esteem in early childhood is a foundation for successful attainment of developmental tasks throughout life. There are many definitions of self-esteem, some quite simple and others very complex and theoretical. In general it can be said that in order to have high self-esteem, people must believe that they are lovable and of value and that they are competent. The purpose of this section is to discuss ways parents can foster—or hinder—high self-esteem in their children.

There are a number of child-rearing principles (Felker, 1974) which are particularly important in facilitating high self-esteem. They are so important that they bear repeating.

1. Facilitate the child's mastery of each developmental task. An infant who learns that adults can be trusted to meet his needs is developing a sense of security and value. Knowledge of the developmental tasks which follow in the subsequent stages of development helps the parents tolerate the autonomy-seeking behavior of the toddler and accept the innovative ways in which the child later displays initiative or industry and searches for identity.

2. Provide verbal and physical expressions of love. Many parents assume that their children realize that they are loved, but children are often not able to make such inferences without help.

3. Help infants and young children develop behaviors which make it easy for them to elicit positive attention. Felker (1974) wrote that when his daughter was very young, both parents made it a point to elicit a smile from her before picking her up. The baby quickly learned to interrupt her crying to smile, and this smile continued to get attention from others in her environment.

4. Emphasize the many new things that have been learned and the possibility of additional learning. It must be discouraging at times for young children to be faced with so much they want to learn as well as what their parents want them to learn. Parents can point out the many accomplishments that have occurred and explain that the child will be able to learn other things with increasing growth. The amount of learning to be done is staggering, and a new element of competition is introduced along with systematic and pervasive evaluations by teachers, peers, and parents.

5. Provide a wide range of opportunities for learning and permit the child to risk failure and learn from failure. Each time a child copes successfully with a new experience, feelings of competence increase. Some risk is present for the child, and sometimes failure results. Wise parents can use the failure as a learning experience and provide the child with alternative actions for successful coping.

6. Provide the child with adult role models appropriate for the child's age. During the preschool years it is important that the child have a role model of the opposite sex; a few years later a same-sex role model is essential. It is important that children learn appropriate gender behaviors. Same-sex role models may be particularly important for school-age boys, since so many of their teachers are women. Children whose behavior is not appropriate for their sex may be subject to teasing or ridicule, which is damaging to their feelings of belonging to a peer group.

7. Help the child learn positive self-referent language. Children quickly absorb the words spoken to them and use the same words in talking to themselves or about themselves. The toddler who slaps his own hand and mutters "Bad boy" and the preschool child who sits passively waiting for an adult to help her while she repeats "Can't do it" are both on the way to a negative self-image. In order for them to talk to themselves in positive terms, they must hear positive words and must also know that it is acceptable to say positive things about themselves. As children learn to talk to themselves, they can be helped to praise others. (For parents who are uncomfortable with so much "praise," the word *encouragement* can be substituted.) Part of learning to praise oneself and others is realistic goal setting and evaluation. Parents whose

expectations are too high or who measure success only in terms of perfection set their children up for failure. Parents can help children set realistic goals for themselves within a time span that has meaning to the child. There are three important points here. The goal must be important to the child, it must be attainable, and it cannot require too much time.

8. Respect children's rights to their feelings. It is all too easy for adults to try to minimize feelings. "You don't really hate your teacher," "Things can't be all that bad," and similar admonitions are heard regularly by many children. Such comments say to the child that feelings are not important, and the next step in reasoning is that the child is not viewed as important, either. Children do need to learn how, to whom, and under what circumstances feelings can be expressed.

9. Avoid or minimize use of language or behavior which diminishes the child's feelings about his worth, competence, and belonging. Many of the child-rearing techniques listed as inappropriate in Table 3-3 are potentially damaging to self-esteem. Some of the actions imply that feelings are not important or that the child is not valued, while others can carry messages of rejection. The divorced mother who accuses her son of being just like his father is also sending a message that the boy does not belong.

10. Provide praise (encouragement, positive reinforcement, "strokes," etc.) for more than outcomes. Acceptable attitudes, feelings, ideas, decisions, methods, reactions (Felker, 1974), and even effort may all be worth acknowledging. Parents need to expand their vocabulary of adjectives which connote pleasure with a child. A pamphlet entitled *100 Ways to Say "Very Good"* (Sherzan and Todd, n.d.) gives many examples.

Child Rearing in Families with Special Circumstances

Many parents are faced with special child-rearing problems brought about by death, divorce, alcoholism or chronic illness in a parent or a developmental disability or illness in a child. These crises can force changes in life-style. Some parents elect a life-style different from that of the majority, such as communal living or a homosexual relationship. Although the basic needs of the children remain the same as in the average household, parents may have special difficulties in meeting these needs, the children themselves may be unable to benefit from their parents' usual approaches, or special circumstances may require additional attention.

Single-Parent Families

Providing children with sufficient *love* may be no problem if the parent and/or children have a good support system, if the other parent is still available, or if the one parent has an extraordinary capacity to give love. It is often difficult for a parent who has total responsibility for a household to continue to demonstrate love in ways that children can understand. There is a tendency in some homes to use one of the children as a parent's confidant and to expect more understanding and more mature behavior than the child's age warrants. A 5-year-old may take on heavy household responsibilities. Thus, *limits* consistent with children's ages are not established. Obviously, some responsibility is appropriate, but if a child's *liberty* or freedom to be a child is abridged, problems may develop later. Children from single-parent homes may experience more *liability* for their actions than they should have to handle. If they are given (or take on) responsibilities that are beyond their abilities, they are apt to encounter a number of failures. Single parents may also have difficulty facilitating their children's *learning*. A study (Morgan, 1980) of 18,000 children in 14 representative states found that children from single-parent homes were late to school more often, had a higher incidence of school absence and dropping out, and had lower academic achievement ratings. Such findings put an additional burden on single parents and point out the necessity for schools and society generally to provide more support for these families.

Divorce

Parents who are contemplating divorce are often very concerned about the effects it will have on the children. Some may seek professional help; others either are so absorbed in their own problems that they are oblivious to their children's problems or are so immobilized that they are unable to be of help. Other adults may be in a position to help the children directly or to provide sufficient assistance to the custodial parents to help them assist the children. Parents need to know that younger children tend to blame themselves for the divorce and that with increasing age one or the other parent is assigned blame and is the target of the child's anger.

Parents should also be aware of another common response: the fear of abandonment. One parent who loved him has abandoned the child, and the youngster has no reason to believe that the remaining parent might not do likewise.

Open lines of communication among family members are essential during the period of adjustment following a divorce. Children who can express their feelings and ask important questions are more likely to receive the love and reassurance they need. Parents should expect that questions and negative feelings may reappear periodically as children enter new phases of development.

Death of a Parent

When a family's single-parent status is brought about by death, the remaining parent's grief may make it exceedingly difficult to help the children understand what is happening. The tendency to protect children by sending them away at the time of a death or funeral is gradually being replaced by a sharing of the grief among family members. Although it may be painful for a child to see a parent cry, it can also help the child grieve appropriately. Children need someone who will explain what is going on in terms appropriate to their level of understanding. The presence of familiar friends and relatives, adherence to a routine familiar to the child, and repeated reassurance that the child is loved and will be taken care of will help early in the bereavement process. Parents need to be prepared for continued questions about death and for the new concerns that may arise. Grief can reappear when a father figure is needed to participate in Cub Scout activities or when a mother-daughter banquet is scheduled.

Teen-Age Parents

Approximately half a million babies are born each year to mothers under 20 years of age. Adolescents who become parents may have difficulty in carrying out appropriate child-rearing activities, in part because they still have a number of their own developmental tasks to meet. Activities with peers and the demands of school may provide stiff competition for the ever-present needs of infants.

When an adolescent and her infant continue to live in the young woman's family home, it is essential that lines of responsibility be clearly understood. The adolescent who wants to assume the mother role with her infant may have to compete with her own mother for the opportunity. She may also resent the demands her mother and her infant make on her. If the mothering is shared, the infant will benefit if both the mother and the grandmother have reached an agreement on child-rearing techniques, including limit setting.

The role of the adolescent father in parenting was underestimated in the past. However, in one study it was found that approximately a quarter of the young mothers and their infants were living with the fathers, and an additional 46 percent of the fathers were regularly involved with their babies (Zitner and Miller, 1980). Thus in many of these young families the father's beliefs about child rearing may be exerting a strong influence.

Adolescents typically have very little knowledge about normal growth and development, which makes it hard for them to know how to facilitate an infant's development. Other concerns are the bland or rejecting feelings some mothers display toward their infants and their tendencies to be overly casual about the babies' well-being (Grow, 1979). When limited knowledge and uncaring attitudes exist together, abuse or neglect may follow.

Stepparents

Not all single-parent households remain so throughout the children's growing years. Many new families consist of the mother and her biological children and a father who either has lost custody of his own children or has not had children, but other combinations are possible, each of them having a network of complicated legal, economic, sociological, and psychological issues which can be of concern to health workers. With whom does the school nurse confer if the child has a serious health problem? What is the protocol for giving emergency treatment while the child is visiting the noncustodial parent? What problems are faced by parents in stepfamilies in facilitating optimum growth and development in their children?

Assuming that each involved parent is eager to pro-

vide the children with the five Ls discussed earlier, what special considerations are involved? Too many stepparents try too hard to love their new children or try to force love from them. *Love* must grow; it cannot be forced, and it may not even be realistic to expect an adolescent ever to love a stepparent. At the same time, children of the biological parent may question whether they are still loved because of the attention given to the new spouse or the stepsiblings. Frequent verbal and physical manifestations of affection may help reassure the children that they are still loved and lovable.

Limits need to be established by the parents as to what behaviors are acceptable in the new family, who is to enforce those limits, and what the consequences are for exceeding them. It should be clear to everyone how each member is expected to share the various roles and responsibilities of a family. Parents must be sensitive to (and ready to limit) the ways noncustodial parents can use the children as intermediaries for securing information or carrying detrimental messages.

Children should have the freedom *(liberty)* to continue to love absent parents, grandparents, and significant others from their earlier lives. Depending on the ages of the children involved, they should have some choice in deciding how much time they want to spend with the noncustodial parents. As in other stressful family situations, some children may need protection against *liabilities* imposed by too many, or far different, expectations. It is still important for the children to experience liability for the decisions that are theirs to make.

Academic *learning* may be adversely affected while children are adjusting to a blended family. Teachers who are made aware of the new living arrangements and the stress involved can help the children cope with school. Stepchildren have a great deal to learn about building new relationships and maintaining old ones. They also need to learn that it is safe to express their feelings and reactions to being part of a stepfamily. It is quite possible for many stepchildren to learn that being a part of a stable stepfamily where the adults are committed to promoting optimum development is far better than being in their earlier milieu (Manosevitz, 1981).

Poverty

Parents who grew up in poverty may also rear children in poverty and perpetuate the cycle. Poverty implies a lack of material things, but there is frequently an accompanying impoverishment of psychological and cognitive development. This should become clear in the following discussion of the difficulties in providing the five Ls.

In order to truly *love* a child, parents need to have experienced (and must continue to experience) love themselves. Love has been likened to a savings account; one can continue to make withdrawals only as long as there is a reserve supply or new deposits. Thus some mothers, rather than giving love, expect to receive it from their infants and children. Sometimes when love is present the mother may get satisfaction from a cuddly infant, but as the child strives for independence she may need help to feel that the child still loves her. It should be pointed out that many deprived parents love their children dearly and sacrifice many of their own needs in order to provide for their children.

Limit setting in many homes is apt to be inconsistent and based on the amount of interference the behavior presents. As a result, children learn to listen for the tone of voice and the mood of the parent rather than focus on the message.

Liberty may be restricted in terms of providing the children with a variety of learning experiences which will help them cope with middle-class school systems and social institutions. On the other hand, parents may allow or expect greater responsibility from the children in terms of self-care or care of younger siblings. The kindergarten child who is expected to get himself ready for school may experience a great deal of *liability* for lack of cleanliness and inadequate clothing.

Because *learning* is such a broad topic, it is in this domain that parents have the most difficulty. Part of the problem stems from the way the parents themselves learned to use and transmit language skills.

Children learn language from their parents, but their attempts at language must be heard and reinforced. One mother thrust her 2-year-old on the examining table at the well-baby clinic with the words "She won't talk at all." Even in the strange clinic setting, Theresa used a great deal of jargon as well as several distinguishable words she repeated after the examiner. Educationally and economically deprived parents not only often fail to listen, they also characteristically do not direct much speech to the children. Their own limited education and low-socioeconomic-level life experiences are reflected in a smaller vocabulary which in turn limits the words the children hear. Many parents are apt to give instructions or reply to questions with a gesture or a very short response rather than with an explanation. The speech heard by these parents' children differs in quality and quantity from that heard by middle-class children. In addition, it is less likely that speech errors will be corrected or that appropriate responses will be rewarded. A child from such a home is unlikely to learn to listen to others. Often children and adults do not expect to be heard unless they yell; therefore, everyone yells. As a result, hearing discrimination may not be well developed. Also, poor children may not learn to come to adults for help or approval, which again limits their learning at home and, later, in school.

The poor may not be able to buy materials or take advantage of experiences advocated for furthering child development. More important, they do not always know how to utilize existing opportunities to teach their children. For instance, many items in an impoverished household have different textures or make various sounds from which an infant can learn. Plastic pants feel different from cloth diapers; a baby bottle used for pounding sounds different from a spoon. But for these early discrimination experiences to be meaningful, parents need to supply words and encourage curiosity, and they frequently do not do this. Parents and older siblings can help the toddler and preschooler begin to grasp concepts of numbers, color, and size. Does he want one or two pieces of candy? Can he count the people in the room? Daddy's shirt is bigger than his, but his shirt is bigger than the baby's. Socks can be matched for color, and the colors of items of clothing can be named when dressing the child. These suggestions may sound too simple, but for some low-income parents such actions do not come naturally.

Another area of potential difficulty is that of helping the children feel worthwhile. If the parents have been battered by society and feel powerless to change, these attitudes are transmitted to the children, leading them to expect failure before they even try. If they do reach school feeling good about themselves and they attend a middle-class school, it will not be long before they realize they are different. They will differ in appearance, in behavior, and possibly in ability to learn, not because they are intellectually inferior but because they do not have the same base of learning as the other children.

Dual-Career Families

The earlier controversy about *whether* both parents should work has largely been replaced with questions as to *when* women should return to work following the birth of an infant. Some child-rearing authorities are adamant that only dire necessity should force a mother to work during the first 3 years of each child's life. Studies to support these claims are almost nonexistent, although the evidence to date does suggest that high-quality and consistent mothering is important. Studies of school-age children point out differences in sex-role concepts among children of working and nonworking mothers but find no consistent evidence of differences in school performance.

The ways in which working parents provide the five *L*s should not differ substantially from those of families in which only one parent is employed, other than ensuring that the substitute caretakers provide care compatible with the beliefs of the parents. More emphasis on the quality of family interactions may be required.

Foster Parents

Foster parents are called upon to meet extraordinary needs of children in their care, often on an emergency basis. Such children may have been neglected or abused or may have suffered the loss of both parents, or this may be one more in a series of placements. It stands to reason that these children feel abandoned by their parents and may fear abandonment by the foster parents as well. If the children feel they have precipitated the abandonment by their own behavior, they may test the foster parents to the very limit—as if to rule out or verify their own worth.

It can be very difficult to provide an acting-out child with unconditional *love,* but many foster parents seem to have this capacity. Reminding themselves of all that the child has been through can help them develop more patience. There is a danger, of course, in letting sympathy interfere with *limit* setting. It is difficult to set limits on a child who may have been accustomed to very different limits in his own home or another foster home, but learning what is and is not acceptable is a necessary part of the child's adjusting to a family. Selecting a few essential limits might be a first step in order to provide the child a chance to experience success rather than overwhelming him with new expectations. A foster child needs the *liberty* to talk about his own family or earlier placements, and foster parents may need to remind themselves that the child may be idealizing these earlier experiences. Academic *learning* may have been disrupted by one or more placements, and special help may be needed as a result. Foster parents can help the child understand that someone will always be available to provide care and that the child was not responsible for the situation which precipitated placement. Activities to foster self-esteem are particularly relevant for foster children.

Adoptive Parents

Parents who adopt infants can expect to experience the same kinds of crises as do natural parents. One difference, however, is the need to respond differently to the child's curiosity about his origins. It is generally recommended that children be told early, even before they really understand, to minimize the trauma of accidental discovery. Parents may need to help children understand that they were in no way responsible for the placement decision. Unless this is done, children may believe their parents gave them up because they were not lovable. The child who grows up knowing that he was "chosen" may not experience any difficulties unless labeled as different by peers, relatives, or others. The most stressful time for parents may be during the adopted child's adolescence. When adolescents are struggling to develop their sense of identity, parents may become upset at their insistence on knowing about their families of origin. A calm acceptance of the need to know and assurance that in several states adoption records can be made available to the child at age 18 (not to the adoptive parents) may alleviate the problem.

Parents who adopt an older child may experience some of the same difficulties as foster parents. The child may feel shame or guilt for having created the need for placement and may fear abandonment by the adoptive parents, particularly if they tease or threaten to "send him back where he came from."

On the other hand, adoptive parents may have no more problems than other couples in providing their children with the five *L*s. Most children, whether born into a family or adopted, fantasize to some extent that they truly belong with someone else who is more famous, wealthier, or more ideal than their present parents. As in so many other situations, the parents' ability to meet the needs of their children is the crucial point.

Homosexual Parents

Homosexual couples who are rearing children have at least two problems to overcome in providing the children with the five *L*s. The first difficulty is in providing the children with opposite-sex and same-sex role models at the appropriate times in their development. This, of course, is important if the children are to learn expected gender-related behaviors. The second potential problem is that of ensuring peer group involvement, since there is a good possibility that the children will be taunted or ostracized because of their parent's different life-style. Without interactions and feedback from peers, learning can be curtailed. In some situations, children may be denied relationships with grandparents who are unable to accept the life-style of their grown child. There should be no particular difficulties in providing the other *L*s of child rearing except for protecting the child from feeling liable for the parent's behavior.

Parents with Special Problems

A variety of other impediments can be identified that have the potential to interfere with effective child rearing. These may arise when parents' goals and expectations for their children are markedly distorted, their value systems are divergent from the predominant ones in the community, there is a deficit in knowledge or skill, or the resources available to the parents are insufficient to meet the children's needs. Examples of situations where such impediments exist include parents' acute or chronic mental illness, chronic physical handicaps or diseases, addictions, and mental retardation or severe learning disorders. Some handicapped parents do a superb job of parenting in spite of various limitations of vision, hearing, mobility, energy, and so forth. Others with seemingly slight disabilities are unable to function effectively as parents. The extent to which a particular parent can provide the five *L*s must be carefully assessed.

Parents with Special Children

Some children's problems are such that ordinary child-rearing approaches are ineffective. In some instances the children's problems are so severe that even the best parents could not deal with them without assistance, and in other cases the problems may be less severe but beyond the resources of those particular parents. For example, all parents would need some professional guidance in managing a child with severe cerebral palsy, but relatively few parents would be totally unable to cope with an infant with a cleft lip. What are some of the barriers parents face in providing their special children with the five *L*s?

Before parents can *love* a developmentally disabled infant, they must have time to grieve for the loss of the perfect infant they had expected. If the infant's condition is such that the infant is unable to interact with the parents, love can be slow in developing. Thus the blind infant who cannot gaze back at the mother or the retarded infant who does not learn to smile *may* receive less love; the situation depends on the parents' ability to give unconditional love. Parents who depend heavily on their children's performance to receive gratification may have difficulty loving a child whose performance is below expected levels.

It can also be hard for parents to set *limits* for a disabled child. When they are unsure how much the child can comprehend, they may be reluctant to use any disciplinary measures, or they may feel the child deserves all the pleasure available, even at the expense of other family members. Lack of limits for the handicapped child can also lead to difficulties with siblings who must meet parental expectations. For many years parents were counseled to allow their children to behave in accordance with their mental ages rather than their chronological ages. It was considered acceptable for a severely retarded adult male to give his teacher a good-morning kiss, because his developmental level was that of a much younger child. As more retarded children are remaining in their home communities, more effort is being expended to teach them chronological-age-appropriate social behavior.

A natural tendency of parents with developmentally disabled children is to restrict learning opportunities and decision making. These youngsters have the same right as normal youngsters to try and to fail, although care must be taken to see that they experience a lot of success. The move to integrate children with handicaps into regular classrooms sometimes results in the retarded children's learning a great deal through imitating their normal peers.

Many communities offer home training programs for parents, and special services are usually available in schools. Learning how to behave when one has a disability can also be difficult. They need to learn that they are not to blame for having a handicap and that they are still lovable. Unfortunately, they are also expected to learn how to help normal people feel more comfortable in their presence (Goffman, 1963).

Although the majority of the needs of handicapped children are the same as the needs of their normal peers, parents frequently believe that they do not have the necessary skills to help these children learn. The nurse who points out the many ways that the child is like nonhandicapped children helps the parents apply their existing knowledge and skills in new ways.

Nursing Responsibilities

The nurse's role in fostering effective child rearing has been referred to occasionally throughout this chapter, but it is the purpose of this section to examine some of the ways nurses can assist parents in this developmental task. Obviously, the degree to which any nurse becomes involved depends on whether she is a neighbor, a casual friend, a community health or school nurse, or even a nurse in an intensive care unit.

Difficulties in child rearing are apt to occur when there are limitations in parental knowledge or skill, when resources are inadequate, or when incongruencies exist between the expectations, goals, and value systems of the family and those of the health professionals involved. Intervention, if it is to be successful, must be based on a careful appraisal of these limitations and incongruencies as well as on the strengths of the family.

Supporting Parents' Self-Esteem

An earlier discussion focused on how parents can help their children develop high self-esteem. A necessary pre-requisite for parents is that they feel good about themselves. When an adult's self-esteem is low or negative, the usual methods of increasing self-esteem may not work. People tend to incorporate only those words or actions which are consistent with their existing self-image. Thus, if the nurse compliments the mother, the mother may brush it off as of no consequence ("Anybody can do that") or believe that the nurse does not really mean what was said.

In spite of this tendency to negate positive statements about themselves, many people are hungry for evidence that others care about them. The nurse can demonstrate caring in a multitude of ways, and at some point the mother may begin to realize that she must be worth caring about. Helping such a mother view herself as competent may be facilitated by helping her select goals which are obtainable and carry meaning for her. For example, the low-income mother who has little concern for future events may not see immunizations as necessary for her infant. She might, however, attend well-child clinic if it gave her an opportunity to socialize with other mothers and receive positive feedback for being "a good mother who attends the well-child clinic." Recognition or praise is extremely important, but it must be appropriate and sincere. Praise should not be put off until a goal has been reached but, like praise for children, can focus on many aspects of daily living. Wearing a new shade of lipstick, calling for an appointment, or keeping the baby free from diaper rash would be examples worthy of praise.

A mother who feels incompetent tends to avoid situations she believes she cannot handle. Unfortunately, she also is likely to restrict the experiences her children have, which in turn limits their opportunities to experience success. The nurse may be able to find ways of helping such women cope with newness, such as accompanying them, telling them in detail what to expect, or finding someone else to accompany them. The mother might also be willing to practice making self-praising comments as a first step in preventing low self-esteem in her children. It is crucial that the self-perpetuating cycle of low self-esteem be broken.

Parent Teaching

How nurses share knowledge and skill is perhaps even more important than the actual information they share. Vocabulary must be appropriate to the individual's level of understanding, and the amount and complexity of the information must be based on what the individual wants to know. It is easy to assume that everyone is as interested as the nurse in knowing why children behave as they do when all the parent wants to know is what to do about it the next time it happens.

Learning is facilitated when new information is associated with facts already known. For example, the nurse might remind the mother of most people's nervousness about speaking to a group and liken this feeling to how a child who is slow to warm up feels before every new experience. It is also important to remember that relearning takes a great deal more energy than does learning something totally new, because the learner experiences more frustration and anxiety when having to rethink earlier learning.

Selecting the appropriate teaching methods is also crucial to learning. Some people prefer to read materials for themselves and only need suggestions as to sources. Others like to read materials and discuss them with someone. Still others want to have the facts given to them verbally. Some parents need to experience what they are learning about (e.g., through simulated exercises or role playing), while others profit from a variety of audiovisual media. Many parents would be interested in books written for children to help youngsters cope with special problems.

The status of the teacher is also important to some parents. Parents of a handicapped child often appreciate receiving help from parents who are in similar circumstances rather than from professionals.

Nurse and Family: Success in Spite of Differences

Professional health care workers frequently identify problems that are not similarly identified by the families themselves. This is usually a reflection of incongruence between the health worker and the family in respect to definitions or goals. Parents who define *health* as the absence of disease will not be interested in actions to achieve high-level wellness. The mother who defines *clean* in terms of a process she went through rather than the appearance of the cleaned product may react with indignation if the grayish but recently washed clothes are labeled as dirty. In families whose goal is to keep out of trouble with the law, child-rearing practices differ from those of families in which moral or religious values govern behavior. If these discrepancies are to be identified, the nursing assessment must include these less tangible aspects of child rearing. Goals can then be selected that are explicit, valued by the parent, and achievable in a reasonable time. The goals selected may not even resemble the ones originally held by the nurse.

The nurse who finds out what the parents plan to do in respect to a specific health practice and then helps them do it safely and efficiently will probably have great success in seeing the parents' goal met. Finding out what they know and how they plan to implement their knowledge enables the nurse to supplement their knowledge with ideas from her own reading and experience. Offering such suggestions tentatively enables the parents to accept or reject them without fear of penalty. Phrases such as "You might want to try . . ."; "Some people believe that . . ."; and "Other mothers have told me . . ." are usually more successful than a specific. "Why don't you try this?"

There are obviously times when a nurse cannot stand by and allow parents to harm their children by their actions or inaction. It is a nurse's responsibility to help a parent see that there is a problem which cannot be allowed to continue. The specific role is covered in Chap. 13, which deals with child abuse and neglect.

Whether nurses facilitate effective child rearing depends on the degree to which they establish helping relationships. A truly helping relationship

1. Is built on empathy for the parents and the problems they are facing, not on sympathy. Empathy leads to working through problems, whereas sympathy leads to reassurance which fosters denial.
2. Takes into consideration the nurse's attitudes, opinions, and beliefs as well as any biases or stereotypes which can unconsciously interfere with the relationship.
3. Views parents as self-directive and responsible and demonstrates this viewpoint by planning *with* parents and not by requiring parents to take specific actions to win the nurse's approval.
4. Requires that the nurse care about and respect the parents, as evidenced by reliance on descriptive words rather than evaluative ones.
5. Promotes personal growth and increased self-confidence in parents as well as increasing their ability to cope with future difficulties.

The nurse caring for children from various cultural and family backgrounds must:

1. Be aware of her own personal beliefs and practices regarding health and illness
2. Be conscious of how her earlier beliefs and practices may have changed with nursing knowledge
3. Recognize the various connotations of the words *health* and *illness* and the ensuing differences in practices among people
4. Understand the traditional beliefs regarding health and illness of heritage consistent families
5. Understand the sociocultural-historical milieu in which the family lives

---

Learning Activities

1. Tour the neighborhoods where families of cultures different from your own reside.
2. Meet with leaders of these communities and ask them to explain health practices and needs from the families' points of view.
3. Participate in community activities in these neighborhoods.
4. Read literature by authors from each ethnic group with which you are working.
5. Invite a small number of parents to be interviewed before your class or clinical seminar group. Include both mothers and fathers and both young and experienced parents if possible. Can they describe what characteristics they want their children to have as adults and the actions they will take to achieve these goals? Do they feel that the way they themselves were brought up has prepared them for child rearing? If there is more than one child in the family, how do they feel their child-rearing approaches vary in accordance with the characteristics of each child? What aspects of having a child have differed from their expectations?

6. List the roles you (or another person in your family) play in the family system (comedian, wage earner, errand runner, child care provider, health adviser, troublemaker, teacher, household maintenance person, director, producer, star, scapegoat, source of pride, source of conflict, scholar, invalid, etc.). How would the family be affected if you (or the other person you have described) became unwilling or unable to fulfill these roles?

Study Questions

1. Children acquire their attitudes toward health and illness and their health practices primarily from:
   A. Members of the family.
   B. Other children.
   C. Nurses and doctors.
   D. Schoolteachers.
2. Family beliefs and attitudes toward health-related matters are influenced mainly by:
   A. Sociocultural background.
   B. Health status.
   C. Economic status.
   D. Self-esteem.
3. Definitions of health and illness:
   1. Vary from family to family and from person to person.
   2. Are legally enforced by the World Health Organization.
   3. May not be the same in the nurse's mind as they are in the client's.
   4. Influence client cooperation (compliance) with recommendations made by health professionals.
   A. 1 and 4   C. 1, 3, and 4
   B. 2 and 3   D. 1, 2, 3, and 4
4. Heritage consistent folk beliefs may include the following ideas:
   1. Illness can be caused by external forces such as the bad will or evil wishes of other persons.
   2. Illness can be caused by unwise or disobedient behavior such as poor diet, envy, and breaking the rules of society.
   3. Illness can be prevented or treated by the use of special charms or jewelry items.
   4. Illness can be prevented or treated by special dietary combinations, herbs, or roots.
   A. 1 and 2   C. 3 and 4
   B. 2 and 3   D. 1, 2, 3, and 4
5. A nuclear family is:
   1. A man and woman who are married to each other living together with one or more of their own children.
   2. A man and a woman who are married to each other living together with their own children and children from their previous marriages.
   3. One or more children living with their grandparents.
   4. A man or woman living with one or more of his or her own children
   A. 1   C. 1, 2, and 4
   B. 2   D. 2 and 3
6. Systems theory includes which of the following ideas:
   1. Any change affecting one member of a family will inevitably cause all other members of the family to be affected in some way.
   2. Closed family systems last longer than open family systems.
   3. The family is affected by its environment, but the environment is not affected by changes in the family.
   4. All members of a family system are affected by all other members of the family system.
   A. 1, 2, and 4   C. 1 and 4
   B. 2, 3, and 4   D. 1 and 3
7. Role theory states that:
   1. Roles are pretenses that interfere with honesty in interpersonal interactions.
   2. For every role there are certain social expectations about how the person in that role ought to behave.
   3. Parents impose certain roles upon children, who then are caught in those roles until puberty.
   4. A person cannot carry out any particular role unless someone else is willing and able to adopt a role that complements it.
   A. 1, 2, 3, and 4   C. 1 and 3
   B. 2   D. 2 and 4
8. A *family developmental task:*
   A. Is a sign that a family is carrying out its necessary activities.
   B. Impedes progress by interfering with the happiness and adjustment of individuals.
   C. Changes from one time to another.
   D. Can be assigned by a health professional as a method of assessing the family.
9. A nurse can assist parents by:
   1. Selecting a good book on child rearing and advising all mothers and fathers to follow the book.
   2. Identifying successful parents that other mothers and fathers can learn to imitate.
   3. Helping mothers and fathers select realistic child care goals that seem worthwhile to them.
   4. Helping mothers and fathers reduce their fears and increase their self-esteem
   A. 1, 2, 3, and 4   C. 3 and 4
   B. 1 and 2   D. 1 and 4

References

American Heritage Dictionary of the English Language, Houghton Mifflin, Boston, 1975.
Bertalanffy, L: *General Systems Theory,* Braziller, New York, 1968.
Bilagody, H.: "An American Indian Looks at Health Care," in R. Feldman and D. Buch (eds.), *The Ninth Annual Training Institute of Psychiatrist-Teachers of Practicing Physicians,* Western Interstate Commission on Higher Education, Boulder, Colo., 1969.

Boyd, D.: *Rolling Thunder,* Random House, New York, 1974.

Castillo, L.J.: "Communicating with Mexican Americans—*Por Su Buena Salud,*" keynote address, Baylor University College of Medicine, Houston, 1979.

Chen, L.S.: *Chinese Medicinal Herbs,* trans. F.P. Smith and G.A. Stuart, Georgetown Press, San Francisco, 1973. (Originally published in China, 1578.)

Chrisman, N., and A. Kleinman: "Health Beliefs and Practices," in S. Thernstrom (ed.), *Harvard Encyclopedia of American Ethnic Groups,* Harvard University Press, Cambridge, 1980.

Currier, R.L.: "The Hot-Cold Syndrome and Symbolic Balance in Mexican and Spanish-American Folk Medicine," *Ethnology,* **5:**251-263, 1966.

Dobson, J.: *Dare to Discipline,* Bantam, New York, 1982.

Dodson, F.: *How to Parent,* Nash, Los Angeles, 1970.

————: *How to Discipline with Love,* New American Library, New York, 1978.

Doherty, W.J., and R.G. Ryder: "Parent Effectiveness Training (P.E.T.): Criticism and Caveats," *Journal of Marital and Family Therapy,* October 1980, 409-419.

Duvall, E.M., and B. Miller: *Marriage and Family Development,* Harper & Row, New York, 1984.

Elworthy, R.T.: *The Evil Eye—The Origins and Practices of Superstition,* Julian Press, New York, 1958. (Originally published by John Murray, London, 1895.)

Estes, G., and D. Zitzow: "Heritage Consistency as a Consideration in Counseling Native Americans," paper presented at National Indian Education Association Convention, Dallas, November 1980.

Felker, D.W.: *Building Positive Self-Concepts,* Burgess, Minneapolis, 1974.

Gaw, A.: "Health and Illness in the Chinese Community," lecture, Boston College School of Nursing, 1978.

Ginott, H.: *Between Parent and Child,* Macmillan, New York, 1965.

Goffman, E.: *Stigma,* Prentice-Hall, Englewood Cliffs, N.J., 1963.

Gordon, T.: *P.E.T. in Action,* Wyden, New York, 1976.

Grow, L.J.: *Early Childrearing by Young Mothers,* Child Welfare League of America, New York, 1979.

Harwood, A.: "The Hot-Cold Theory of Disease: Implications for Treatment of Puerto Rican Patients," *Journal of the American Medical Association,* **216:**1154-1155, 1971.

Havighurst, R.J.: *Developmental Tasks and Education,* 3d ed., McKay, New York, 1979.

Hymovich, D.P., and R.W. Chamberlin: *Child and Family Development: Implications for Primary Health Care,* McGraw-Hill, New York, 1980.

Jacques, G.: "Cultural Health Traditions: A Black Perspective," in M.F. Branch and P.P. Paxton (eds.), *Providing Safe Nursing Care for Ethnic People of Color,* Appleton-Century-Crofts, New York, 1976.

Like, R.: "Attitudes toward Mental Illness in a Rural Azorean Parish: A Preliminary Study," paper presented at First Congress of Azorean Communities, Angra Do Heroismo, Terciera, August 1978.

Lucero, G.: "Health and Illness in the Chicano Community," lecture, Boston College School of Nursing, March 1975.

Maloney, C. (ed.): *The Evil Eye,* Columbia University Press, New York, 1976.

Manosevitz, M.: *On Stepfamilies,* adapted from "The Human Condition" radio series, Hogg Foundation for Mental Health, Austin, Tex., 1981.

Masnick, G., and M.J. Bane: *The Nation's Families: 1960-1990,* Auburn House, Boston, 1980.

Miller, J.R.: "Family Assessment and Nursing Intervention," in J. Howe et al. (eds.), *The Handbook of Nursing,* Wiley, New York, 1984, pp. 79-80.

Modestino, G.: "Health and Illness in the Haitian Community," lecture, Boston College School of Nursing, March 1978.

Morgan, D.: "Children from Single-Parent Homes Have More School Problems: Study," *Des Moines Sunday Register,* Des Moines, Iowa, Sept. 14, 1980.

Murphree, Alice H.: "Cultural Influences on Development," in G.M. Scipien et al. (eds.), *Comprehensive Pediatric Nursing,* 2d ed., McGraw-Hill, New York, 1979.

Petersen, W.: "Concepts of Ethnicity," in S. Thernstrom (ed.), *Harvard Encyclopedia of American Ethnic Groups,* Harvard University Press, Cambridge, 1980.

Salmon, J.W.: "Defining Health and Reorganizing Medicine," in J.W. Salmon (ed.), *Alternative Medicines,* Tavistock, New York, 1984.

Saunders, L.: "Healing Ways in the Spanish Southwest," in E.G. Jaco (ed.), *Patients, Physicians, and Illness,* Free Press, Glencoe, Ill., 1958.

Schulman, G.I.: "Myths That Intrude on the Adaptation of the Stepfamily," *Social Casework,* **53:**131-139, 1972.

Schuster, C.S.: "The Holistic Approach," in C.S. Schuster and S.S. Ashburn (eds.), *The Process of Human Development: A Holistic Approach,* Little, Brown, Boston, 1980.

Sherzan, S., and J. Todd: *100 Ways to Say "Very Good,"* Iowa Council for Children, Parent Education Subcommitee, Des Moines, Iowa, n.d.

Spector, R.: *Cultural Diversity in Health and Illness,* Appleton-Century-Crofts, New York, 1979a.

————: *Hawk Littlejohn: Medicine Man of the Cherokee,* videotape interview, Boston State College, Boston, 1979b.

Tuhy, C.: "What Price Children?" *Money,* **12**(3):77-84, 1983.

Wallnöfer, H., and von Rottauscher, A.: *Chinese Folk, Medicine,* American Library, New York, 1972.

Welch, S., J. Comer, and M. Steinman: "Some Social and Attitudinal Correlates of Health Care among Mexican Americans," *Journal of Health and Social Behavior,* **14:**205-213, September 1973.

Wise, F.F.: "Concepts of Discipline," in C.S. Schuster and S.S. Ashburn (eds.), *The Process of Human Development: A Holistic Approach,* Little, Brown, Boston, 1980.

World Health Organization, "Constitution of the World Health Organization," *Chronicle of the World Health Organization,* **1:**29-43, January 1947.

Zitner, R., and S.H. Miller: *Our Youngest Parents,* Child Welfare League of America, New York, 1980.

Bibliography

Bagley, C., and G.K. Verma: *Multicultural Childhood,* Gower, Brookfield, Vt., 1983.

Bauwens, E.F.: *The Anthropology of Health,* Mosby, St. Louis, 1979.

Bernardo, S.: *The Ethnic Almanac,* Doubleday, Garden City, N.Y., 1981.

Bienenfeld, F.: *Helping Your Child Succeed after Divorce,* Borgo, San Bernardino, Calif., 1985.

Brandt, P.A.: "Stress-Buffering Effects of Social Support on Maternal Discipline," *Nursing Research,* **33:**229-234, 1984.

Clark, A.L.: *Culture and Child Rearing,* Davis, Philadelphia, 1981.

Dinkmeyer, D., and G.D. McKay: *The Parent's Handbook: Systematic Training for Effective Parenting (STEP),* Random House, New York, 1982.

Elling, R.H.: *Socio-Cultural Influences on Health and Health Care,* Springer, New York, 1981.

Goldzband, M.G.: *Quality Time: Easing Children through Divorce,* McGraw-Hill, New York, 1985.

Harwood, A. (ed.): *Ethnicity and Medical Care,* Harvard University Press, Cambridge, 1981.

Henderson, G., and Primeaux, M. (eds.): *Transcultural Health Care,* Addison-Wesley, Menlo Park, Calif., 1981.

Leininger, M.: *Transcultural Nursing: Concepts, Theories, and Practices,* Wiley, New York, 1978.

McGoldrick, M., J.K. Pearce, and J. Giordano: *Ethnicity and Family Therapy,* Guilford Press, New York, 1982.

Robbins, M., and T. Schacht: "Family Hierarchies," *American Journal of Nursing,* **82**(2):284-286, 1982.

Spector, R.E.: *Cultural Diversity in Health and Illness,* Appleton-Century-Crofts, Norwalk, Conn., 1st ed., 1979; 2d ed., 1985.

Thernstrom, S. (ed.): *Harvard Encyclopedia of American Ethnic Groups,* Harvard University Press, Cambridge, Mass., 1980.

4

Promoting the Health of Children

Objectives

After reading this chapter, the student will be able to:
1. Identify the recommended immunization schedule for normal infants and children and contraindications for giving immunizations.
2. Identify the recommended immunization schedule for children who were not immunized in the first year of life.
3. Be familiar with screening tests which are performed at various health promotion visits.
4. Apply the principles of physical, psychosocial, and perceptual-cognitive development at various stages to the promotion of development and health.

AAP Guidelines for Health Supervision

The focus of this chapter is on promoting children's health in community settings. The American Academy of Pediatrics Guidelines for Health Supervision are found in Table 4-3.

Immunizations

Several childhood diseases are preventable through immunization. Diphtheria and tetanus toxoid are combined with pertussis (whooping cough) vaccine and given intramuscularly as DTP. Three live-virus vaccines—parotitis (mumps), rubeola (measles), and rubella (German measles)—are combined as one vaccine (MMR) and given subcutaneously. Trivalent oral polio vaccine (OPV) is given by mouth. *Haemophilus* b polysaccharide vaccine (HBPV) is given subcutaneously. If the vaccine contains an adjuvant (aluminum compound), it is given intramuscularly (Committtee on Infectious Diseases, 1986).

The recommended schedule for immunizations is shown in Table 4-1. However, not all parents begin a child's immunizations in infancy. The recommended schedule for children under 7 years and over 7 years of age is given in Table 4-2.

If the primary series of immunizations is interrupted for any reason, it is not necessary to restart it. No immunizations are given to a child who is experiencing acute febrile illness; if a child already has a fever, febrile reactions from the immunization will be masked. The presence of gastroenteritis is a contraindication for administering OPV. The poliovirus must be colonized in the intestine to produce an immune response, and gastroenteritis may interfere with this activity. None of the live-virus vaccines are given to children who have leukemia, lymphoma, or immunologic disease or to those who are receiving radiation therapy, steroids, or antimetabolites. The immune system is depressed in such children, and serious reactions may result. MMR, particularly the rubella component, poses a threat to the developing fetus in the first trimester. Ideally, girls receive this vaccination prior to puberty. If a girl is of childbearing age and has not received MMR, it is imperative that she not become pregnant within 3 months of vaccination. If she is sexually active, a rubella titer should be done before MMR is given. A family history of allergies and determination of any allergies a child may have are important factors in selecting the viral vaccine preparation. Sensitivity to substances such as eggs and neomycin will result in reactions to substances in the vaccine. It is possible to receive passive immunity through blood transfusions. If a child has had a transfusion, 6 weeks must pass before MMR is given or the child will not form antibodies. Children who have a history of nervous system disorders have an increased probability of a serious reaction to pertussis vaccine.

Information forms for each immunization should be given to parents so that they know the possible side effects. This information is reinforced verbally. If parents agree to have the infant or child immunized, a consent form is signed.

TABLE 4-1 Recommended Schedule for Active Immunization of Normal Infants and Children

Recommended Age	Immunization(s)	Comments
2 mo	DTP,* OPV*	Can be initiated as early as 2 wk of age in areas of high endemicity or during epidemics
4 mo	DTP, OPV	2-mo interval desired for OPV to avoid interference from previous dose
6 mo	DTP (OPV)	OPV is optional (may be given in areas with increased risk of poliovirus exposure)
15 mo	MMR*	MMR preferred to individual vaccines; tuberculin testing may be done
18 mo	DTP,†‡ OPV‡	
24 mo	HBPV*	
4-6 yr§	DTP, OPV	At or before school entry
14-16 yr	Td*	Repeat every 10 yr throughout life

*DTP = diphtheria and tetanus toxoids with pertussis vaccine; OPV = oral poliovirus vaccine containing poliovirus types 1, 2, and 3; MMR = live measles, mumps, and rubella viruses in a combined vaccine; HBPV = *Haemophilus* b polysaccharide vaccine; Td = adult tetanus toxoid (full dose) and diphtheria toxoid (reduced dose) in combination.
†Should be given 6 to 12 months after the third dose.
‡May be given simultaneously with MMR at 15 months of age.
§Up to the seventh birthday.
Note: For all products used, consult manufacturer's package insert for instructions for storage, handling, and administration. Biologics prepared by different manufacturers may vary, and those of the same manufacturer may change from time to time. Therefore, the physician should be aware of the contents of the package insert.

Source: Committee on Infectious Diseases, American Academy of Pediatrics: *Report of the Committee on Infectious Diseases,* 20th ed., American Academy of Pediatrics, Elk Grove Village, Ill., 1986, p. 9.
Author's Note: A conjugate vaccine (diphtheria toxoid-conjugate) to prevent *Haemophilis* b infection recently licensed for use in children 18 months or older is now recommended for all children at 18 months of age. (Recommendations of the ACIP, 1988).

TABLE 4-2 Recommended Immunization Schedules for Children Not Immunized in First Year of Life

Recommended Time	Immunization(s)	Comments
Less than 7 Years Old		
First visit	DTP, OPV, MMR*	MMR if child ≥ 15 mo old; tuberculin testing may be done
Interval after first visit		
1 mo	HBPV*†	For children 24-60 mo
2 mo	DTP, OPV	
4 mo	DTP (OPV)	OPV is optional (may be given in areas with increased risk of poliovirus exposure)
10-16 mo	DTP, OPV	OPV is not given if third dose was given earlier
Age 4-6 yr (at or before school entry)	DTP, OPV	DTP is not necessary if the fourth dose was given after the fourth birthday; OPV is not necessary if recommended OPV dose at 10-16 mo following first visit was given after fourth birthday
Age 14-16 yr	Td*	Repeat every 10 yr throughout life
7 Years Old and Older		
First visit	Td, OPV, MMR	
Interval after first visit		
2 mo	Td, OPV	
8-14 mo	Td, OPV	
Age 14-16 yr	Td	Repeat every 10 yr throughout life

*DTP = diphtheria and tetanus toxoids with pertussis vaccine; OPV = oral poliovirus vaccine containing poliovirus types 1, 2, and 3; MMR = live measles, mumps, and rubella viruses in a combined vaccine; HBPV = *Haemophilus* b polysaccharide vaccine; Td = adult tetanus toxoid (full dose) and diphtheria toxoid (reduced dose) in combination.

†*Haemophilus* b polysaccharide vaccine can be given, if necessary, simultaneously with DTP (at separate sites). The initial three doses of DTP can be given at 1- to 2-month intervals; so, for the child in whom immunization is initiated at 24 months old or older, one visit could be eliminated by giving DTP, OPV, and MMR at the first visit; DTP and HBPV at the second visit (1 month later); and DTP and OPV at the third visit (2 months after the first visit). Subsequent DTP and OPV 10 to 16 months after the first visit are still indicated.

Source: Committee on Infectious Diseases, American Academy of Pediatrics: *Report of the Committee on Infectious Diseases,* 20th ed., Academy of Pediatrics, Elk Grove Village, Ill., 1986, p. 11.

With DTP, fever can occur within 24 to 48 hours. A localized reaction at the injection site is manifested by soreness, redness, and swelling. The infant may be fussy. Acetaminophen 10 to 15 mg/kg of body weight per dose is given for fever. A localized reaction is treated with the application of tepid or warm compresses to the site. Parents are advised to report unusual side effects, such as ur-

ticaria or loss of consciousness, immediately. MMR may produce fever. Symptoms of measles—anorexia, malaise, fever, and rash—may be manifested in 7 to 10 days, and a mild rubella rash may occur within a few days. In older children and adults particularly, joint swelling and pain may arise in approximately 2 weeks. Acetaminophen is given for fever and joint pain. All symptoms do disappear. The child is not contagious when these symptoms arise. Rarely, paralysis occurs within 2 months of receiving OPV, but the benefit of protection is believed to outweigh this risk. Haemophilus b vaccine is relatively free of side effects. However, within 24 hours of the injection, redness and swelling can occur and the child may develop a fever of 38.3°C (101°F) or greater. Side effects usually disappear quickly and are treated as described for DTP.

Promoting Development and Health

Physical, psychosocial, and perceptual-cognitive development at various ages is described in Chap. 2. In this chapter that information is applied to promoting development and health. Parents need to know what to expect at different stages in order to feel competent in caring for their children. Appropriate health education and anticipatory guidance cannot be provided without a data base. A pertinent history, physical examination, and appropriate screening tests provide the necessary knowledge. Exchange of information between family members and health care providers is imperative if the parents and/or the child are to be involved in decision making about the child's care. Some *general* nursing diagnoses for this area are as follows.

1. Injury, potential for
   (a) Related to parent/child lack of awareness of environmental hazards
   (b) Related to maturational age of the child (see Table 4-4 for a developmental approach to accident prevention)
2. Knowledge deficit, potential for
   (a) Related to development at various ages
   (b) Related to nutritional needs at various ages
   (c) Related to elimination patterns at various ages
   (d) Related to sleep patterns at various ages

The Neonate: Birth to 1 Month

A safe environment that will maintain extrauterine life and support growth and development is an obvious and overriding need of newborn infants. Neonates' neuromuscular immaturity leaves them highly vulnerable to environmental insults. They require conservation of body heat, maintenance of a clear airway, protection from injury and infection, and provision of nutrients.

For the well-being of both infant and parents, the parents need help in understanding the infant's care requirements and unique individual pattern of moving from one behavioral state to another. Parents (particularly the mother, who is recovering from pregnancy and delivery)

TABLE 4-3 AAP Guidelines for Health Supervision

Age[2]	* Infancy *						* Early Childhood *					* Late Childhood *					* Adolescence[1] *			
	By 1 mo.	2 mos.	4 mos.	6 mos.	9 mos.	12 mos.	15 mos.	18 mos.	24 mos.	3 yrs.	4 yrs.	5 yrs.	6 yrs.	8 yrs.	10 yrs.	12 yrs.	14 yrs.	16 yrs.	18 yrs.	20 + yrs.
History Initial/interval	●	●	●	●	●	●	●	●	●	●	●	●	●	●	●	●	●	●	●	●
Measurements																				
Height and Weight	●	●	●	●	●	●	●	●	●	●	●	●	●	●	●	●	●	●	●	●
Head Circumference	●	●	●	●	●	●														
Blood Pressure										●	●	●	●	●	●	●	●	●	●	●
Sensory Screening																				
Vision	S	S	S	S	S	S	S	S	S	S	o	o	o	o	S	o	o	S	o	o
Hearing	S	S	S	S	S	S	S	S	S	S	o	o	S³	S³	S³	o	S	S	o	S
Devel./Behav.[4] Assessment	●	●	●	●	●	●	●	●	●	●	●	●	●	●	●	●	●	●	●	●
Physical Examination[5]	●	●	●	●	●	●	●	●	●	●	●	●	●	●	●	●	●	●	●	●
Procedures[6]																				
Hered./metabolic[7] Screening	●																			
Immunization[8]		●	●	●			●	●	●			●					●			
Tuberculin Test[9]	←					●→	←			●	→						←		●	→
Hematocrit or Hemoglobin[10]	←				●	→	←			●	→			←		●	→	←	●	→
Urinalysis[11]	←			●		→	←			●	→			←		●	→	←	●	→
Anticipatory[12] Guidance	●	●	●	●	●	●	●	●	●	●	●	●	●	●	●	●	●	●	●	●
Initial Dental[13] Referral										●										

1. Adolescent related issues (e.g., psychosocial, emotional, substance usage, and reproductive health) may necessitate more frequent health supervision.
2. If a child comes under care for the first time at any point on the schedule, or if any items are not accomplished at the suggested age, the schedule should be brought up to date at the earliest possible time.
3. At these points, history may suffice: if problem suggested, a standard testing method should be employed.
4. By history and appropriate physical examination: if suspicious, by specific objective developmental testing.
5. At each visit, a complete physical examination is essential, with infant totally unclothed, older child undressed and suitably draped.
6. These may be modified, depending upon entry point into schedule and individual need.
7. Metabolic screening (e.g., thyroid, PKU, galactosemia) should be done according to state law.
8. Schedule(s) per Report of Committee on Infectious Disease, *1986 Red Book.*
9. For low risk groups, the Committee on Infectious Diseases recommends the following options: (1) no routine testing or (2) testing at three times—infancy, preschool, and adolescence. For high risk groups, annual TB skin testing is rcommended.
10. Present medical evidence suggests the need for reevaluation of the frequency and timing of hemoglobin or hematocrit tests. One determination is therefore suggested during each time period. Performance of additional tests is left to the individual practice experience.
11. Present medical evidence suggests the need for reevaluation of the frequency and time of urinalysis. One determination is therefore suggested during each time period. Performance of additional tests is left to the individual practice experience.
12. Appropriate discussion and counselling should be an integral part of each visit for care.
13. Subsequent examinations as prescribed by dentist.
N.B.: **Special chemical, immunologic, and endocrine testing** are usually carried out upon specific indications. Testing other than newborn (e.g., inborn errors of metabolism, sickle disease, lead) are discretionary with the physician.
Key: ● = to be performed: S = subjective, by history:
    o = objective, by a standard testing method.

Source: American Academy of Pediatrics Guidelines for Health Supervision II. American Academy of Pediatrics, Elk Grove Village, IL, 1988.

also need rest, health, and freedom from anxiety.

Parent-infant bonding, which is necessary for good parenting behavior and for the newborn's wellbeing and development, requires that the parents and baby be together and have assistance as necessary to make their interactions rewarding. The first weeks after delivery are taxing for most mothers, who feel fatigued, socially isolated, and burdened by the infant's constant care requirements (although most are reluctant to say so). Assistance is provided where possible, including contact with other empathic parents of young children. If relatives or others can help, it is recommended that they assist with household tasks rather than with the baby's care, which should be given by the mother or father for the most part in order to maximize bonding. Parental concerns include skin care and hygiene, nutrition, elimination, sleep, and crying. Health care providers must address these issues, along with stimulation, play, and safety.

Skin Care and Hygiene

Sponge baths are generally recommended until the umbilical cord is healed, after which tub baths can be given.

The hair and scalp, including the fontanels, should be shampooed once or twice a week. The use of oil on the hair and/or skin can cause a rash by clogging the pores of the skin; seborrhea, or "cradle cap," eventually results. Therefore, parents are encouraged to use nothing or a lotion rather than oil to moisturize the skin. The use of cotton applicators for cleaning the nose and ears is discouraged not only because they are unnecessary and unsafe (injury can result if the baby wiggles during the cleaning) but also because they pack wax against the typanic membrane. Washing the pinna and the opening to the external canal with a washcloth is adequate. A wick made of cotton can be used to stimulate the sneeze reflex in order to clear the nasal passages, and a soft rubber suction bulb can be used to aspirate mucus. Cleaning the nose before the baby eats or sleeps can ease breathing during feeding and resting.

Parents often are concerned that a newborn has a cold because he snorts and sneezes. Since the neonate's nasal passages are small, the normal amount of mucus produced blocks them. The neonate then sneezes (his method of "blowing his nose") to clear the nasal passages.

As a result of maternal hormones received transplacentally in utero, some female neonates have vaginal discharge and neonates of both sexes may have breast engorgement. These phenomena usually disappear by 6 weeks to 3 months of age. Daily removal of *smegma,* a white stick substance, from the clitoris and labia of female neonates can prevent adhesions of the labia and vagina.

Umbilicus

When the newborn is discharged from the hospital with his mother, the umbilical cord is still in place. Parents are taught to apply alcohol on a cotton ball to the cord stump and surrounding area with each diaper change to facilitate the drying process. As the cord separates, brown exudate is noted. Parents are instructed to cleanse the exudate from the umbilical area, using cotton and rubbing alcohol. The cord usually is separated completely in 7 to 10 days. Neonates are given sponge baths until the cord is off and dry. Parents are advised to report a large amount of drainage or any purulence, redness, swelling, or foul odor. The use of belly binders should be discouraged; they can hinder the healing process and are not recommended for the treatment of umbilical hernias.

Jaundice

Many newborns demonstrate physiological (normal) jaundice on or about the third day of life. The neonate will appear jaundiced because his immature liver is unable to handle the by-products of red blood cell destruction. Some babies also have bruising or a cephalhematoma, which may increase their bilirubin levels. Normally the jaundice begins to disappear by about the fifth to seventh day after birth. In some nurseries phototherapy is begun for all jaundiced newborns. Parents need reassurance that physiological jaundice is a normal phenomenon and that drawing the infant's blood to determine the bilirubin level is a common procedure. Jaundice appearing within the first 24 to 48 hours of life is not normal but is suggestive of a hematologic disorder (Chap. 17).

Circumcision

If a male newborn has been circumcised, it is important to instruct the parents to use petroleum jelly on the tip of the penis and around the foreskin until the skin has returned to a normal color (about 4 to 5 days). The foreskin of uncircumcised males should not be retracted forcibly since some *phimosis* (narrowing of the foreskin) is normal in the first 4 to 6 months. Gentle retraction should be demonstrated to the parents of a circumcised neonate after healing is complete (Chap. 29).

Nutrition

A foremost concern of parents is feeding the neonate. Ideally, both breast-feeding and bottle feeding are discussed in the prenatal period. Once the parents have decided on a method, the health care provider supports them in that decision. The supply of breast milk may not be established completely for 3 weeks. Breast milk contains all the nutrients the infants needs until 6 months of age. In the first 48 to 72 hours the breast produces *colostrum,* a yellowish fluid which contains antibodies against bacteria and viruses. The neonate breast-feeds every 2 to 3 hours in the first 1 to 2 weeks. The baby gradually lengthens the time between feedings to every 3 to 4 hours during the day and 5 to 7 hours during the night.

Bottle-fed babies begin by taking 2 to 3 oz every 3 to 4 hours during the first couple of weeks of life. They too gradually lengthen the time between feedings and by 1 month are consuming 24 to 26 oz per 24 hours. Full-term babies during the first 6 months of life need 110 to 120 cal/kg of body weight per day. Formula contains 20 cal per ounce; thus, the health care provider can easily compute the amount of formula an infant needs. Newborns generally adjust their intake to meet their individual requirements. Overfeeding is discouraged. Feeding of newborns is discussed in detail in Chap. 7.

Many neonates and infants hiccup, a normal phenomenon which requires no treatment, as hiccups are not harmful and will eventually go away. It does no harm and may be effective to offer the baby water during an attack.

Elimination

The number and consistency of bowel movements vary considerably among infants and are influenced by what the infants are fed and by their individual body rhythms. Breast-fed babies generally have looser and more frequent stools than do bottle-fed infants. Often an inexperienced parent considers this elimination pattern to be diarrhea. An infant can have between 1 and 12 stools per day or even miss 1 or 2 days and still be normal.

Constipation is another common concern of parents. Because the baby strains, grunts, turns red, draws up his legs, or even cries during a bowel movement, parents often believe that he is constipated. As long as the stools are soft, this behavior is normal. If the stool consists of hard balls, a diagnosis of constipation is correct. Constipation can be managed by adding 1 to 2 tsp of Karo syrup to 2 to 4 oz of water or formula each day until the stools become soft-formed. Treating an infant's constipation with laxatives or enemas is dangerous and should be very strongly discouraged because their use interferes with muscle tone and the later establishment of bowel habits. Parents are encouraged to call the health care provider if they think the baby is constipated.

Sleep

Prevention of behavioral problems begins at birth. Sleeping routines can be established early in life. Infants quickly associate bed with sleep if they are left to sleep once they have been changed, played with, and fed.

A newborn rarely sleeps for more than 3 to 5 hours without waking, usually wanting to be fed. Because the growth rate is so great in the first few weeks and the amount of milk consumed at any one feeding is relatively small, a neonate requires nourishment more frequently than does an older infant. The baby will sleep through the night as soon as he develops the capacity to maintain himself nutritionally for that length of time, usually by 4 or 5 months and in many cases by 1 to 3 months.

Crying

Babies cry more than parents expect. The crying of a baby can be very difficult for parents to tolerate; they may display many different reactions to prolonged crying. They may feel frustrated if they believe their caretaking is at fault. They may feel angry that the baby continues to cry despite their quieting attempts, and they may feel guilty about their anger.

Crying is the primary means for the newborn to communicate any of a number of problems. One of the most common reasons for crying is physical discomfort. The baby may be wet, cold, or hot; may have a rash; or may be demonstrating the symptoms of colic. The parent needs to decide the reason for the crying and then attempt to intervene appropriately (this is easier said than done).

There are specific quieting techniques which parents may employ to help stop the crying, such as picking up the baby, bathing him in warm water, taking him for a ride in the car, rocking him, or placing him in an infant swing. Sometimes a baby cries because he is overstimulated. Overstimulated babies require techniques such as being swaddled, being placed in a darkened room, or if all else fails, being left to cry alone for a period of 20 to 30 minutes. The occasional use of this last technique will not harm the infant. Indeed, some child psychologists favor this technique as a primary intervention. They explain that if parents pick the baby up every time he cries, he soon learns that when he wants to be held he must cry. Parents can prevent this expectation by touching, talking to, and playing with him while he is content. When he fusses, he is put to bed to sleep. Giving attention when he cries teaches him to cry longer and more frequently. Giving him attention when he is quiet can eliminate frequent crying.

Stimulation and Play

Visual, auditory, and tactile stimulation, including interaction with others, is important during waking states. Overstimulation to the point of restlessness or crying should be avoided. Play activities and equipment include face-to-face verbal and visual stimulation, singing, rocking, walking, stroking and patting, propping the baby upright in the infant seat at intervals, and crib mobiles.

Many researchers agree that both maternal care and infant well-being are enhanced when mother and newborn are not separated at birth but are allowed close bodily contact within the first hours after delivery. Mothers who have immediate close contact with their unclothed babies have been found to respond more positively to their infants than do mothers who have initial contact several hours later. There appears to be a brief period immediately after birth during which both mother and newborn are especially sensitive to and positively affected by direct contact with each other. Close contact appears to be a mutual need of mother and infant.

Safety

The first approach to accident prevention ideally occurs in the prenatal period. Prospective parents are asked whether they have considered buying a car seat. Car seats approved by the National Safety Council are recommended (Fig. 4-1), while the use of car beds and hook-type seats is discouraged. Holding a newborn or an infant in one's arms while riding in a car is not advocated. If the driver must apply the brakes suddenly, the infant can be propelled from the holder's arms and thrown against the dashboard or the windshield. Car seats are recommended from the time the neonate leaves the hospital until the child weighs 40 lb (between 3 and 5 years of age). Infant and child car seats have many advantages. They can prevent serious damage to infants and children in the event of a sudden stop or an accident.

The spacing of crib bars and mattress fit are also discussed with prospective parents. Crib bars farther apart than 2⅜ in are dangerous because the baby's body can slide through sideways. Since his head is too large to slide through, he can strangle. Bumper pads can prevent this accident. If the mattress does not fit the crib snugly, the baby can slide between the mattress and the bars onto the crib springs and impair his circulation or nerve function.

Parents need to be aware that newborns "scoot" (the crawl reflex). Thus, they are prone to falling from an elevated surface (e.g., bed) if precautions are not taken. Neonates also require protection against other environmental hazards, such as exposure to cold or excessive heat (e.g., a too warm bath, sun exposure), overly exuberant siblings or household pets, and pillows or other objects which can cause suffocation.

The Infant: 1 to 3 Months

Parenting is arduous and valuable work. It is important that the health care provider take time to explore parents'

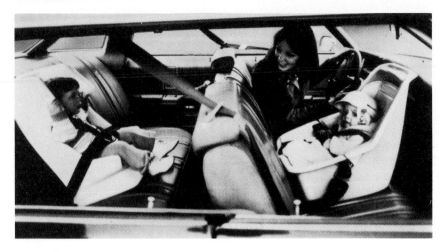

FIGURE 4-1   When riding in a car, infants and small children should be securely fastened to protect them in case of sudden stops or accidents. *(Photo courtesy of General Motors.)*

concerns and to point out where they seem to be doing well and commend them. The infant's developmental characteristics are discussed, and parents are taught what to expect and how to prepare for it.

The infant's social capacity increases noticeably during this period. Interaction with others, especially family members, is a necessary stimulant to psychosocial and cognitive development. Parents generally find the baby's social responsiveness (e.g., smiling, recognition, vocalizations, and laughter) very rewarding. They are usually quite aware of and pleased by the infant's changing physical size, strength, and motor abilities; this awareness makes most parents responsive to anticipatory guidance (teaching about what developmental changes will come next) in preparation for the continuing changes that can be expected in the coming days and weeks. Parental concerns include nutrition, sleep, and crying. In addition to discussing these topics, the nurse or other health care provider needs to include stimulation, play, and safety (Table 4-4). The first OPV and DTP are given at 6 weeks to 2 months of age. Side effects and appropriate interventions, as noted earlier in this chapter, are discussed with the parents.

Nutrition

The baby should be held for all feedings. Bottle propping invites aspiration and drastically reduces both the infant's opportunities for experience (social, cognitive, and sensory) and the parent's development of empathic and effective interactions with the infant. Nutrition is discussed in more detail in Chap. 7.

Sleep

Around 3 months of age most babies sleep through the night without a feeding. If they do not, parents are reassured that this event will soon occur. Most babies continue to take several long naps (2 to 3 hours) during the

day and early evening; however, some only engage in "catnaps" for 15 to 20 minutes several times a day.

Crying

Crying may continue to be of concern. The same techniques discussed in the section on newborns are explored to determine what may be effective with a particular baby.

Stimulation and Play

While awake, the infant should be placed where the activities of others can be seen and heard. Voices, music, and other environmental sounds provide auditory stimulation. An infant seat enables the baby to see much more than can be viewed from crib-lying positions. Crib mobiles are desirable for visual experience, learning, and motor practice for the upper extremities.

Play activities for this age include face-to-face conversation and facial gestures, stroking and patting, and carrying and rocking. Toys include things to listen to (rattle, bell, music maker, noisemakers), things to look at (mirror, picture books, toys that move such as mobiles and balls), and objects that provide tactile experience and comfort, such as stuffed animals.

Safety

Obtaining a developmental history at each visit is important for accident prevention. Some babies at 1 month continue to propel themselves involuntarily toward the top of the crib when lying on the abdomen (the crawl reflex). Parents need to be cautioned that infants must never be left on surfaces from which they can fall. By 2 months of age infants normally roll and thus cannot be left alone on an elevated surface.

As grasp and hand-to-mouth movements become more precise, parents need to be made aware of the necessity of keeping unsafe objects (e.g., sharp objects, hot drinks, and

TABLE 4-4 Promotion of Development: 1 to 3 Months of Age

Stimulation	Safety	Feeding*	Sleep
Touch: holding, cuddling, rocking, feeding, bathing, diapering, variation in positioning—prone, supine, upright; roughhousing (after 2 mo); toys to grasp *Sucking activity:* breast, bottle, hand, pacifier *Visual:* human face; colorful, moving objects *Auditory:* male and female voices; variety of sounds; singing; rattles *Olfactory:* breast, formula, father's and mother's bodies	Begin now to keep medicines, cleaning products, and other poisons out of reach Restrain infant while in an automobile in a recommended auto safety device (see Fig. 4-1) Avoid large crowds and exposure to infectious diseases Be certain that crib mattress is firm and there are no gaps between mattress and sides of crib Be certain that cribs and playpens have bars spaced 6 cm (2⅜ in) or less and that crib sides are secure Do not leave infant unsupervised on high surfaces (even in infant seats) Never prop bottle owing to risk of suffocation and/or aspiration	Breast-feeding (preferred) or prepared formula fortified with iron Formula intake at end of 2d month of approximately 29 oz in 24 h Formula intake at end of 3d month of approximately 33 oz in 24 h	4- to 10-h sleep intervals Frequent naps Increasing wakefulness with crying Behavioral clues given to indicate need for sleep Need for parents to accept individual sleep and wakefulness pattern of infant

*See also Chap. 7, "Nutritional Influences in Child Health."

Source: Adapted from R. M. Benfield and D. M. Harris, "The Infant—1 to 12 Months," in G. M. Scipien et al. (eds.), *Comprehensive Pediatric Nursing,* 2d ed., McGraw-Hill, New York, 1979.

lighted cigarettes) out of range of the infant's arm movements. A discussion of toy size and toys will small removable parts is imperative to prevent aspiration of foreign bodies. Nursing bottles must never be propped for feeding a baby who remains in a crib. Babies need to be held for all feedings so that they will not choke and will not be deprived of the interpersonal stimulation that occurs during feeding.

The Infant: 4 to 6 Months

Infants at this age are becoming more aware of themselves and the environment. They chuckle, laugh, and are quite vocal. They reach for and grasp objects, turn from abdomen to back and back to abdomen, and sit (first with support and then alone). The overriding parental concerns at 4 months are nutrition and drooling. Topics for discussion include these concerns plus stimulation, play, and safety (Table 4-5). The second and third sets of OPV and DTP are given at 4 months and 6 months of age. Information about side effects and interventions is reiterated.

Nutrition

Solid foods are begun during this age period if not earlier (Chap. 7). By 4 months the *extrusion reflex* (reflexive protrusion of the tongue to spit out involuntarily food that has been placed in the mouth) fades sufficiently so that the use of a spoon no longer triggers automatic spitting. Babies at this age may feed themselves crackers, and

at around 5 months they may drink from a cup if someone holds the cup. Infants hold their own bottles at about 6 months of age.

Feeding constitutes a large part of the child-parent interaction. Parents should be counseled to avoid coaxing, forcing, or overentertaining at meals; conflict started in infancy or childhood may distort eating behavior and the parent-child relationship for many years to come.

Drooling

At approximately 3 months of age the salivary glands are developed. The infant has not learned to swallow the saliva produced, and so he drools. Parents of infants between 3 to 4 months wonder if tooth eruption has begun. The nurse should explain that although teething can begin early, it usually starts at around 6 to 7 months of age or even later. She can then discuss the production of saliva at this age.

Stimulation and Play

Objects to hold and manipulate become an important part of the baby's experience at this age. Varied colors, textures, shapes, and sizes and things that make various noises (e.g., rattle, spoon with pan) help provide sensory stimulation *and* motor experience to support learning. Appropriate toys include rattles and other small objects such as blocks, which can be grasped, shaken, and banged together. Toys which "speak," imitate animal sounds, and present other auditory stimuli are enjoyed and probably

TABLE 4-5 Promotion of Development: 4 to 6 Months of Age

Stimulation	Safety	Feeding*	Sleep
Touch: opportunity to explore own body parts; holding, physical care; sitting with support; opportunity to explore mother's and father's bodies *Activity:* toys and objects to reach for and hold, space and incentive for turning over and creeping; play centered on infant's body (weight bearing, roughhousing, etc.); opportunity for some quiet time alone for self-directed play *Sucking activity:* breast, bottle, hand, objects to chew if teething *Visual:* mirror, changes in objects and environment (novelty), facial expression *Auditory:* rattles and other noisemaking toys, talking, singing, music	Be sure that all surfaces infant may mouth are free of lead-containing paint and other toxic substances Keep safety pins closed Destroy plastic garment bags because of risk of suffocation Do not put strings or chains around infant's neck Carefully label medications, formula, and any other feeding to avoid accidental ingestion of a toxic substance Have local poison control center number and syrup of ipecac on hand in case of accidental ingestion of toxic substance; use ipecac only under direction of health professional Inspect each toy to ensure that it is made of nontoxic substance, has no sharp edges, has no parts that could be swallowed, and will not break readily Never leave infant alone in the bath. To avoid tap water burns, household hot water temperatures need not exceed 49°C (120°F)	Breast-feeding (preferred) or prepared formula fortified with iron Formula intake of approximately 35-37 oz in 24 h Introduction of semisolid foods at 4 to 6 mo Beginning interest in self-feeding (messy)	Sleeps 8-12 h at night Takes 2-3 naps lasting 1-4 h Awakens at night occasionally (possible causes include noise, hunger, pain, wet, cold, illness) By 3 mo differentiates day from night

*See also Chap. 7, "Nutritional Influences in Child Health."

Source: Adapted from R. M. Benfield and D. M. Harris, "The Infant—1 to 12 Months," in G. M. Scipien et al. (eds.), *Comprehensive Pediatric Nursing,* 2d ed., McGraw-Hill, New York, 1979.

help the infant prepare for making the sound discriminations involved in receptive and expressive language. The infant actively responds to his image in a mirror.

An increasing ability to sit combines with maturing distance vision to enable the infant to see the surrounding environment. Parents and hospital nurses should take advantage of this expanding capacity for learning; visually stimulating surroundings should be presented, and the baby should be placed where he can watch other persons. Crib mobiles and cradle gyms which can be reached for and grasped help the baby develop eye-hand coordination, which will be essential for subsequent skills such as self-feeding and manipulation of objects.

Language stimulation is highly important, as the infant is beginning to discriminate meanings that will permit more mature behavior later (e.g., following instructions, using expressive language). Family members are encouraged to talk to the infant while he is feeding, bathing, crying, and so forth. Adults should address the baby by name, talk about what they are doing and what the baby is experiencing, and begin teaching the baby the names of things.

Safety

All attainable objects are mouthed, and so it is necessary to take precautions to prevent mouth injuries, poisoning, and aspiration. Falls and automobile accidents continue to be major hazards.

During the physical examination the health care provider can test the infant's hand-to-mouth coordination, ability to reach and grasp, ability to sit alone, and so forth. To prevent accidents, it is important to know which developmental tasks the infant has mastered. If he can sit alone, discussion of crawling and/or hitching is logical as a next phase. Accident prevention includes the covering of wall sockets. As the child becomes more mobile, his curiosity about his surroundings can be satisfied. Thus, he will stick his fingers into wall sockets, pull on cords, and "mouth" electrical cords. If his central incisors have erupted, he may even bite the cord. The home now must be "baby-proofed." Since his method of exploring is touch, taste, and smell, the parents should keep at least 1 oz of syrup of ipecac in the home (securely locked up) and place the number of the local poison control center on the wall by the phone.

TABLE 4-6 Promotion of Development: 7 to 9 Months of Age

Stimulation	Safety	Feeding*	Sleep
Touch: comforting, hugging, kissing, allowing body play (hands, feet, genitals, etc.) *Activity:* raisin or small pellet to improve grasp, opportunity for creeping, crawling, standing, exploring the environment, walking with assistance; some self-feeding Interactive games: peek-a-boo, patty cake, bye-bye, give and take Opportunities to respond to new and familiar adults and children Preparation for separation from mother, father (such as waving bye-bye) Container to hold smaller objects and to pour out Positive reinforcement for vocalizing and other tasks achieved	To avoid sunburn, expose infant gradually to sun for short periods Never leave child unsupervised in water Be careful that plants are out of reach and that poisonous plants are removed Clear floors of small objects, such as pins, matches, and other things that might be swallowed; have a plan for a choking emergency Choose nonflammable articles of clothing Remove untouchables and breakables from low tables Be cautious with tablecloths, electrical cord to coffeepot or iron, and other things an infant might grasp to pull objects onto self Use safety gates or blockades at stairs	Breast or prepared formula fortified with iron Variety of solids 3 times a day Ability to feed self biscuit	10- to 12-h sleep intervals 2-3 naps Bedtime accompanied by crying as infant fears loss of mother Occasional awakening at night for assurance of mother's presence

*See also Chap. 7, "Nutritional Influences in Child Health."

Source: Adapted from R. M. Benfield and D. M. Harris, "The Infant—1 to 12 Months," in G. M. Scipien et al. (eds.), *Comprehensive Pediatric Nursing*, 2d ed., McGraw-Hill, New York, 1979.

The Infant: 7 to 9 Months

Infants during this stage begin to realize that objects exist even when they are out of sight. Stranger anxiety, a normal phenomenon in most babies, may increase; this is sometimes puzzling to parents. Topics of concern to parents include nutrition, sleep, and stranger anxiety. Other issues for discussion are stimulation, play, and safety (Table 4-6).

Nutrition

To prevent dental caries (nursing bottle mouth) now that teeth are erupting, the use of sugar, fruit juices, milk, and carbonated beverages in the bottle is avoided, particularly at nap time and bedtime. Infant feeding is discussed in detail in Chap. 7.

Sleep

Parents may need to be counseled not to give in to the infant's protests about being put to bed. Adherence to a rational routine can prevent severe household disruptions due to sleep refusal in the months to come. If he awakens at night, the baby can be reassured with patting or talking. He need not be walked or taken to the parents' bed.

Stranger Anxiety

Babies who are afraid of strangers should not be confronted abruptly by or left with such persons, and parents and nurses need to ease the child into social situations. For example, the baby-sitter should come early so that the

baby can spend several minutes with the sitter *and* the mother and see that the mother "endorses" the sitter. When an item is to be given to the infant (e.g., medication, a gift, a developmental test item), it is wise to give it to the mother and let her hand it to him.

Stimulation and Play

The infant continues to need opportunities for physical and cognitive experience geared to his emerging capabilities. Verbal stimulation is highly important to the baby's social and cognitive progress. Health care providers should impress upon parents the importance of talking to the child. Peek-a-boo games and toys which disappear and reappear, such as a jack-in-the-box, and toys on strings that can be cast away and retrieved, are discussed. These activities help the infant learn that things continue to exist even when they are out of sight (the concept of object permanence) and help him master separation anxiety.

Safety

As the child becomes increasingly mobile, it is important to emphasize the provision of a safe place in which he can practice motor skills and exploration of objects. A playpen or expanding-perimeter "fence" allows sufficient space but prevents the baby from moving to unsafe areas. Increasing mobility and hand control call for rigorous precautions to prevent falls (e.g., gates at the head of stairways) and other injuries, poisonings, and aspiration of small objects. Parents are counseled to have syrup of ipecac on hand

TABLE 4-7 Promotion of Development: 10 to 12 Months of Age

Stimulation	Safety	Feeding*	Sleep
Touch: acceptance for expression of variety of emotions—assertiveness, frustration, affection, fear, anxiety, excitement—and for genital self-touch Games of pointing to body parts Experiences with different textures: clay, mud, sand, water *Activity:* increasing space and opportunity for locomotion and exploring (crawling)—use of soft flexible shoes or bare feet; objects to climb on; barriers to remove to reach goal Increasing opportunity for self-feeding Larger objects for play; ball, cups, spoons Positive reinforcement for accomplishments: verbalizations, attempts to sing, expressions of independence and autonomy Increasing interaction in games; allow for self-directed play *Sucking activity:* table foods with increasing texture; weaning from pacifier to teething objects *Visual:* baby books, pointing to pictures in books *Auditory:* increasing use of simple requests and directions *Olfactory:* variety of objects to smell	Use a locking-lid garbage can for hazardous refuse Empty all wastepaper baskets frequently Keep all extension cords unplugged while infant has access to them Shield heaters and fans from infant's reach As the infant crawls, be sure medications, household cleaning agents, and other caustics are out of reach Have syrup of ipecac on hand in case of accidental ingestion of toxic substance Have number of local poison control center near telephone Be sure sharp instruments, such as knives, are out of reach Set the crib mattress at the lowest adjustment when the infant can pull to standing Discontinue use of the crib once height of siderail is less than ¾ of height of infant Do not leave items in crib which could be climbed upon to get out of crib	Breast or prepared formula fortified with iron Increasing self-feeding: pincer grasp of food (bite-size pieces), finger foods Introduction of food with eruption of teeth for chewing Decreasing appetite at this age	10- to 14-h sleep interval at night 1-2 naps (1-4 h in duration) Possible refusal to take morning nap Difficulty with bedtime and naptime as infant does not wish to cease activities Short crying periods; release of tension

*See also Chap. 7, "Nutritional Influences in Child Health."

Source: Adapted from R. M. Benfield and D. M. Harris, "The Infant—1 to 12 Months," in G. M. Scipien et al. (eds.), *Comprehensive Pediatric Nursing,* 2d ed., McGraw-Hill, New York, 1979.

and keep the telephone numbers of the physician and poison control center by the telephone. Once children pull themselves up to stand, tablecloths, electrical cords, and sharp-edged coffee tables must be eliminated from the environment.

The Infant: 10 to 12 Months

Infants at this age begin to imitate and strive toward independence. Fine motor skills become more apparent. The baby does not tolerate extended separation from the mother well, and so separations exceeding a few hours should be avoided if possible. Discipline becomes a prime concern of parents. Other topics of interest are nutri-

tion, elimination, sleep, stimulation, play, and safety (Table 4-7).

Discipline

Punishment and other forms of discipline for tantrums are totally beyond the infant's developmental level. Distraction and nonreinforcement (ignoring) are effective, appropriate, and supportive to further development.

Nutrition

Weaning to the cup is well under way by 12 months, but the infant may take a bedtime bottle for several more months. To prevent caries, sugar-containing liquids, including milk, in the bedtime bottle are avoided. Self-feeding is messy but highly important for developing a sense of self and for entry into the next developmental period, toddlerhood, which has been called the stage of autonomy. The child is given a spoon and allowed to help with feeding. Finger foods are served, and the child is permitted the use of the hands for self-feeding of foods (e.g., mashed potatoes) which adults eat only with utensils.

Elimination

Bowel movements decrease to one or two daily, but attempts to toilet train are best deferred until at least 24 months, when the child's maturation and understanding will facilitate faster progress with less frustration for parent and child.

Stimulation and Play

As motor, social, and perceptual-cognitive development expands, the infant needs and seeks gradually broadened experience. The restrictions imposed by playpen, crib, and other constrained environments must not be overdone. Play activities involving disappearance and return (peek-a-boo, jack-in-the-box) are still developmentally appropriate. Putting one thing into another and taking it out again is a favorite play activity; nesting toys, small (but too large to aspirate) objects such as baby blocks, and containers such as coffee cans are provided. The child uses toys that can be pushed or followed (cars, balls) and containers whose lids can be removed and replaced. Old magazines to look at, ruffle, and crumple are good toys.

Safety

As at earlier (and later) ages, the child needs protection from environmental hazards and parents should have anticipatory guidance to ensure safety as successive developmental changes take place. Crawling and walking expose the child to new hazards, while most of the old dangers of earlier infancy (e.g., falls, burns, drowning, poisoning, auto accidents) continue.

The Toddler: 13 to 18 Months

Dealing with toddlers is quite different from dealing with infants. Toddlers have different needs and give different rewards, and parents vary in the ease and enthusiasm with which they make the transition from caring for a relatively dependent, controllable infant to parenting an assertive, mobile toddler. The nurse should be sensitive to parental concerns and frustrations and provide information and guidance where needed.

Stranger anxiety has diminished, and the child is intent upon exploring the environment, walking, running, and climbing onto furniture. *No* is a favorite word. Parents may have questions about the child's decreased appetite. The greatest parental concern is negativistic behavior; it is addressed when discussing the child's activity and mobility with the parent. Other topics included at this time are stimulation, play, and safety. The MMR vaccine is given at 15 months of age, and the booster OPV and

DTP are due at 18 months. *Haemophilus* b conjugate vaccine is also recommended at 18 months of age. Side effects and appropriate interventions are discussed with parents.

Nutrition

A mixed diet of cut adult foods should be well established during this period. Milk intake generally should be limited to 2 or 4 cups daily in order to avoid overweight and leave room for sufficient amounts of the necessary nutrients provided by other foods. The child becomes insistent upon self-feeding, refusing food offered by others. The growth rate slows in comparison to infancy; parents may worry about decreased appetite and may need help determining appropriate amounts of food. Additional information about nutrition is covered in Chap. 7.

Activity and Mobility

Walking and being on the go are an obsession for toddlers, especially when walking is a new accomplishment. Meals, treatments, and other interferences with mobility will be met with protest. Within reason, the child's developmental urgency to keep moving is accommodated: Parts of meals can be supplied as finger foods "to go," treatments requiring restraint should be administered as quickly as possible, and physical restrictions should not be used unnecesarily.

Negative Behavior

Parents may need help to understand and tolerate the child's apparent stubbornness and negativeness. They should be reassured that this behavior is natural, that it is necessary as a part of the developmental progress toward more mature behavior, and that it will pass. Engaging in struggles of will is discouraged. The child is allowed freedom from restriction when it is safe and reasonable to do so. Controls are imposed firmly and kindly as needed. The establishment of rituals can help. For example, going to bed, which is commonly a focus of parent-child conflict, can be preceded by predictable routines, such as bath, bedtime story, and hugs for family members, which terminate in being put irrefutably to bed.

The child's "short fuse" is dealt with directly. Parents are advised not to deceive the child in order to avoid confrontation. For example, parents are cautioned against "sneaking out" when leaving the child with a baby-sitter. The best procedure is to tell the child that they are leaving, say good-bye and tell him that they will return later, and go without returning to check on things. Repeated experience with honest, reliable adults who do as they say builds confidence and security.

Temper Tantrums

Temper tantrums are not uncommon as the developing child reaches the stage of autonomy. They are best ignored. Giving the child attention, whether positive or negative, teaches him that temper tantrums are a means of gaining the parents' attention.

Stimulation and Play

Receptive vocabulary is considerable at this age, and the child understands a great deal even though his expressive use of language is very limited. Parents are encouraged to talk to the child about his surroundings and experiences and are told that the child's understanding is a payoff for their verbal stimulation in the past.

The transition object (favorite toy, blanket, or other security object) serves an important psychological function in helping the child establish the ability to separate from the primary caregiver, as is necessary for continuing development. Parents' inclination to take the object away from the child is discouraged even though it is worn out or embarrassing to them.

Play activities include objects which involve mobility: pull toys, sit-upon toys with wheels, and things to push. Stories and story books with large pictures of familiar objects, people, and animals are very important for intellectual and linguistic development (Table 4-8). It is important for parents and nurses to understand that during the sensorimotor stage (infancy and toddlerhood) children cannot learn except by direct firsthand experience.

Safety

Ingestion of harmful substances remains a major problem. Syrup of ipecac is discussed again with parents. The need for supervision, especially in regard to streets, traffic, wading pools, and swimming pools, is stressed.

The Toddler: 19 to 23 Months

The toddler becomes increasingly mobile, and parents may need help in understanding such an active child. Toilet training is of utmost concern to many parents. These topics, along with stimulation and play, are discussed.

Activity and Mobility

Mobility continues to be a major means of learning and coping. Accordingly, mobility should not be restricted unnecessarily. The child is intensely eager to perform newly acquired developmental skills and seems driven to repeat new activities unendingly in spite of parental wishes. Parents may need an explanation that this preoccupation with whatever is new (e.g., washing hands, opening doors) is a natural phenomenon that is necessary to ensure developmental progress. Arranging the home environment to minimize safety risks, breakage, and frustration on the part of all parties involved is discussed with the parents. Anticipatory guidance at all ages includes assisting parents in accepting and accommodating within reason to the child's preoccupation with his new abilities. However, the toddler period may be especially taxing because the child is so much more mobile than in infancy and because the child's reasoning and judgment are so much less mature than at later ages.

Since negative behavior can still present problems, choices are limited (a few crayons, not dozens) to reduce confusion, frustration, and out-of-bounds behavior. Choices are not offered when in fact none exist. For example, the child is asked, "Do you want milk or water with your medicine?" rather than, "Are you ready to take your medicine?"

Elimination

Many parents believe that their children are now mature enough to begin toilet training. Parents are helped to evaluate the child's readiness for toilet training and are counseled against too early or too rigorous attempts, which can put parents and child at cross-purposes.

In order to be "toilet trained," a child must show signs of readiness. Neither children nor adults can urinate or

TABLE 4-8 Play Activities for Toddlers

13-18 Months	19-24 Months	25-36 Months
Toys that are pushed or pulled while child walks or runs	Sand with buckets, shovels, spoons, sieve, cupcake pans, etc.	Same as at 19-24 mo
Blocks: child can stack 2 or 3 by 15 months, 3 or 4 by 18 months	Water with buckets, measuring cups, sponges, dolls to bathe, etc.	Simple songs, especially with accompanying hand gestures or other body movements
Containers of all kinds and things to put in them and take from them	Activities that involve pouring of liquids or dry materials	Rhymes
Imitation of housekeeping activities—"helps"	Large motor activities: running, jumping, climbing, crawling	Blunt scissors with paper of various colors and textures, paste
Favorite toy or other comfort object ("security blanket")	Play-Dough and cookie cutter	Pegboard with hammer
Social games with theme of departure and return: peek-a-boo, peeking around corner, throwing toy for adult to fetch and return to be thrown again	Dolls (for children of both sexes)	Crayons and paper
	Large jigsaw puzzles (approximately 3 pieces)	Tricycles
Sit-upon toys with wheels	Large beads for stringing	Swings
Stories and story books	Play telephone	Simple dress-up clothes (hats, shoes, purses, etc.)
Nesting toys (boxes, cylinders, etc., that fit into one another)	Picture books, stories	
Low structures for climbing	Blocks	
	Balls	
	Toy cars	
	Safe climbing equipment	

Source: Adapted from M. U. Barnard et al., *Handbook of Comprehensive Pediatric Nursing,* McGraw-Hill, New York, 1981.

defecate on command. The child must have a sufficient bladder capacity to hold his urine for several hours. He must be able to tell the parent either verbally ("wet," "dry," "potty") or nonverbally (pointing, going to potty chair) that he needs to urinate or defecate. In order to be independent, he must know how to raise and lower his pants.

Parents can help their children with this task by teaching them to grasp the waistband of the pants in the middle, front and back, in order to lower and raise them. If the child is taught to grasp on either side, he will have difficulty trying to bring his pants over his protruberant buttocks. The period between the time he feels the urge to urinate or defecate and the time he *must* do so is short. The child is taught this method of raising and lowering the pants during regular dressing and undressing sessions. Trying to learn this task at "potty" time can be frustrating to the child and the parent, since a child may have an "accident" before lowering the pants. Before toilet training begins, the child must be able to follow simple directions. If a potty chair is not used, the child may need a stool to climb onto the toilet and to rest his feet on once he is sitting on the toilet.

There are numerous methods of toilet training. Most people agree on the fundamentals necessary to attempt this training: (1) one or two significant people who are willing and able to devote time and effort to establishing patterns of toileting, (2) a mutual communication system between the child and the significant person, (3) reinforcement for success, and (4) no harsh punishment for failure.

Some difficulties related to toilet training seem to be associated with the child's desire to accomplish the task. It is not that the toddler does not want to please the significant person or demonstrate an ability to control his own excretory function, but other interests tend to keep the child from reaching the toileting facilities until it is too late. More severe problems exist when the toddler manipulates the parent through overcontrolling his body functions, either retaining over prolonged periods or expelling in forbidden places.

As the toddler progresses toward the second birthday, bowel movements become more regular and are preceded by specific, recognizable behavior. An alert mother can predict when her child is about to have a bowel movement and begin the learning sequence by placing the child on a potty chair or a piece of similar furniture at those times. She becomes trained to pick up the child's cues. Only then can awareness on the child's part follow and develop into the ability to inform the mother of the need to eliminate.

Stimulation and Play

Play activities can often be designed to permit the child to practice new skills and interests in a safe way that does not lead to conflict with the parents. Water play in the backyard, for example, may be substituted for water play in the bathroom or kitchen. Favorite and developmentally appropriate play materials are listed in Table 4-8.

The Toddler: 24 to 35 Months

Both fine and gross motor control increase, and accident prevention becomes a major concern. Safety, nutrition, elimination, sleep, self-stimulation, self-comfort, stimulation, play, activity, and mobility are discussed.

Safety

Because of the toddler's increasing motor skills, acute curiosity, and expanding environment, accident prevention takes on new dimensions. Parents' awareness of safety hazards needs continual updating. As comprehension increases with age, the child can and should be increasingly instructed in safety regulations and precautions ("Do not pet the dog until she has finished eating," and so forth). Two-year-olds, however, cannot be relied upon to remember and obey warnings, and so a safe environment and excellent supervision are necessary. The early morning hours, when toddlers may awaken and get out of bed before family members are awake, present hazards that do not exist for younger children, who remain in their cribs.

Accidents are the leading cause of mortality and morbidity in toddlers. Ingestion of harmful substances is still a major problem in spite of safety caps for bottles and educational campaigns urging parents to keep unsafe materials out of children's reach. Young children taste and swallow countless substances. Acetaminophen is involved in more childhood poisonings than is aspirin. Other drugs, plants, cleaning liquids and powders, and petroleum products (e.g., kerosene, gasoline, charcoal starter, and oil-base polishes) frequently are ingested. Medications kept in women's handbags are a hazard to curious children, as are toxic plants kept about the lawn and house.

Many poisonings follow seasonal and geographic patterns. In spring the toddler is likely to find fertilizers, cleaning agents, and paints. Summer brings gardening chemicals and plants, many varieties of which are poisonous. In the fall and winter heating oils and antifreeze present ingestion hazards for the toddler. In cooler climates ingestion of heating oil and road salt is common, while in warmer climates poisonings from lawn and household plants are more common. Inner-city dwellings and old, low-income rural residences may still have paint containing lead, which is a serious hazard for young children who chew windowsills, crib rails, plaster flakes from walls, and the like.

Prevention of ingestion accidents, of course, consists of keeping toxic products out of the reach of children who are too young to be taught that these substances are unsafe (Fig. 4-2). All hazardous substances should be placed in locked cabinets, and poisonous plants should be given away or destroyed during the child's toddler years. Placing drugs in a high cabinet or in drawers is an insufficient precaution because the toddler is learning to climb and explore. Medicine should never be referred to as candy, and inedible substances should never be stored in soft drink bottles or other containers that may make them look like food products. Nurses and parents need to know how to contact the nearest poison control center for

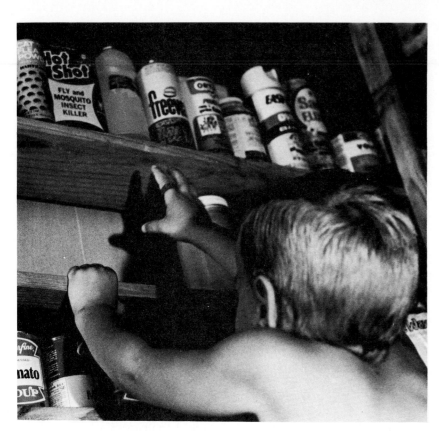

FIGURE 4-2   Poisons and caustics must be placed where young children cannot reach them. *(Photo by George Lazar.)*

prompt advice and treatment in case preventive efforts fail. Syrup of ipecac should be on hand, and parents need to be reminded of the poison control number.

Another common preventable accident of the toddler years is the aspiration, ingestion, or insertion of objects into body orifices. Toddlers (and preschoolers) aspirate or swallow coins and aspirate peanuts; stuff peas, beans, gravel, or small candies into their noses, ears, and navels; and aspirate or swallow buttons or eyes chewed off toys.

In anticipation of these potential accidents, the nurse should counsel parents about prevention. Playthings that have breakable or removable parts small enough to aspirate or put into body openings should be strictly avoided. Stuffed animals must be examined to ascertain whether the eyes and buttons are securely attached; if they are not, they can be taken off and replaced with paint or embroidery. Coins call for special precautions. Children learn early that money is a valuable acquisition. Knowledge that coins can secure many desired objects enhances the desire to get and keep money. Almost all toddlers occasionally handle coins. Introduction to money as a valuable item helps the young child become oriented to a value necessary in society and in itself is not to be discouraged; however, the child can be taught to hold and examine a coin for a short supervised period and then to place it in a bank, purse, or box to be kept out of reach until retrieved by an adult for further use.

Children like to climb inside boxes and other enclosures. The environment should be such that they cannot enclose themselves or lock themselves in. For example, if there is an old refrigerator nearby, its doors must be removed.

Accidents resulting in injury, mutilation, or death are a major health problem for children of all ages. Toddlers, however, are particularly at risk for traumatic injuries because they cannot envision the outcomes of their behavior and because they put few voluntary restrictions on themselves. A few of the more common accidents are those caused by falling, running in front of cars, running while carrying pointed objects, being burned by fire or hot objects, and being injured as a passenger in an automobile.

Adequate supervision of play can prevent most accidents to toddlers. Supervision can be by direct observation or by confining the child to a safe play area and eliminating harmful toys. Since constant observation is impossible, the nurse's objective should be to have parents become aware of the potential danger of the objects with which toddlers can come in contact. The stick left over from a sucker or Popsicle can injure the eyes, mouth, or throat; children's swings, occupied or empty, can severely injure a toddler who does not get out of their way; stairways are fascinating places but are not safe; and the open street, which is very attractive to toddlers, presents the hazards of vehicles, dogs, and other children who play too vigorously for the toddler's safety.

Most families have cars, and transporation of children begins early in infancy. The young infant is placed in a safety seat and restrained while the parent is occupied with driving the car. Because the toddler rebels against all restraints, parents tend to abandon the use of safety seats in the interest of a peaceful ride. However, the development needs of the toddler lead to manipulation of the window handles, door handles, door latches, cigarette lighter, and even the ignition key that dangles so irresistibly.

Despite the availability of child-size safety seats and belts (Fig. 4-1), injuries to toddlers who fall from moving vehicles continue to be a major problem. Furthermore, accidents occur because drivers are distracted by toddlers moving about or behaving dangerously inside the car. A nurse working with the parents of toddlers should emphasize the need for proper safety restraints for children riding in a car. Children behave better when restraints are used. They are unable to stand up, find it difficult to hang the upper body out a car window, and cannot climb over the driver. Being elevated in a car seat, the child can see out the window. Parents can point out interesting sights, holding the child's attention and perhaps increasing his vocabulary. The nurse also needs to stress to parents that safety seats are required by law in some states. As with all safety equipment, proper and consistent use can prevent injuries and, in the case of toddlers, can even prevent automobile accidents.

Nutrition

Nutritional assessment and parental guidance continue to be an important aspect of preventive health care for 2-year-olds. The toddler's loss of baby chubbiness may combine with pickiness and appetite jags to raise parental concerns about undereating (Chap. 7).

Elimination

Neuromuscular maturation must be reached before successful toilet training is accomplished. Daytime bowel and bladder control usually can be attained by age 30 months. Nighttime control is harder to master and can be a problem through the preschool years. Suggestions for reducing bed-wetting include reducing fluid intake after the last meal of the day, extending the quiet period before bedtime, and awakening the child for toileting during the night.

Sleep

Sleep requirements gradually decrease from infancy on. By 2 years of age the child needs 10 to 14 hours of sleep daily. Some children no longer need a mid-morning nap, but most continue to sleep for part of the afternoon. It is not unusual for 2-year-olds to resist going to bed, particularly at night. Parents complain that toddlers fight sleep, scream to stay up, and climb out of bed repeatedly.

To help develop workable sleeping patterns for a toddler, the nurse must first find out what sleep and activity schedules are currently being used. Perhaps the awakening hour is unrealistically early or late, and perhaps household activity interferes with the child's bedtime. The entire activity schedule should be evaluated before any plans are made to work on the child's sleeping patterns. Overall suggestions for encouraging sleep include reduc-ing stimulation prior to the desired nap time, providing quiet toys for bedtime use, and above all not using bed as a punishment. The toddler's age-typical love of ritual can be utilized to everyone's advantage through the establishment of a bedtime routine which helps the child become accustomed to a predictable chain of events ending in going to bed. After-dinner bathing, selecting and dressing oneself in pajamas, saying good night to family members, choosing a bed toy, hearing a prespecified number of stories in bed, turning on his own night-light, and being left to play with a chosen toy is a bedtime ritual than can be adapted to the needs and preferences of any family. Firm adherence to such an established procedure can do much to ensure that the toddler gets the rest that is needed without the insecurity he feels when allowed to exasperate his parents.

Self-Stimulation and Self-Comfort

Self-stimulation is an outgrowth of the child's interest in learning about his own body. In touching and manipulating parts of the body the toddler experiences feelings of pleasure and thus returns to the pleasure-giving body areas for repeated effect. Probably the most common form of self-stimulation or self-consolation is thumb or finger sucking, which is especially frequent when the toddler is distressed or tired and ready for sleep.

Another form of stimulation observed in this period is masturbation. Tight diapers and inadvertent touching of the penis lead the young boy to discover his penis and the pleasure that accompanies manipulation of it. This behavior is not exclusively male, as little girls also discover similar pleasure in clitoral stimulation, but sexual arousal is more obvious in boys because of visible erections. The only harm in genital self-stimulation is that it upsets parents and others and hence subjects the child to punishment or ridicule that the toddler poorly understands and that may subsequently interfere with his self-concept.

Stimulation and Play

The rapid growth of language and concept learning calls for exposure to a stimulating interpersonal environment. Toddlers need to be talked to and in that way helped to expand their vocabulary and begin to understand basic concepts such as colors, numbers, and relative size. Play with other children, including age-mates, gives a great boost to learning about social expectations and the natural outcomes of various kinds of behavior. Play activities include coloring, large jigsaw puzzles, building blocks, sand and water play, large motor activities such as running and jumping, riding a tricycle, climbing, participatory group activities such as singing simple songs with accompanying gestures, picture books and stories, rhymes, and dramatic play (dolls, dishes, dress-up clothes, and other simple props). Other recommendations are given in Table 4-8.

Activity and Mobility

Mobility is a major means of coping, especially while language skills are limited. Unnecessary confinement, especially during hospitalization or other periods of increased stress, is avoided.

The Preschool Child

Preschool children seem to have an insatiable curiosity which is reflected in their activities, questions, and boasting as they explore reality. Important topics of discussion with parents include stimulation and play, curiosity and imagination, discipline, safety, sex education, and death. Parents may also have questions related to nutrition and sleep. The fifth OPV and DTP are given some time between 4 and 6 years of age.

Stimulation and Play

Peer experience, particularly with children close in age, is very important for social and cognitive development. Children who do not have neighborhood or kinship play groups should be enrolled in nursery school or day care programs.

Interaction with parents and other adults teaches young children language, social rules and regulations, conscience, sex roles, effective manipulation of things in the environment, affectional relationships, and numerous other necessary lessons about becoming socialized members of human society. Stimulation should include stories and readings, guided experience with new activities and new settings (zoo, farm, bus rides), and simple demonstrations of how things work.

Play activities should include games designed to support perceptual and intellectual development. Games that involve concepts and sensory discrimination include matching things according to size, texture, shape, and color; counting; recognition of simple likes and opposites ("Baby is little, Daddy is _____"; "Ice cream is cold, cocoa is _____"); and sensory discrimination games such as identifying unseen objects (behind a screen or in a paper bag) by the sounds they produce or the way they feel. Other toys and play activities appropriate for this age group are crayons and coloring books, blunt-tipped scissors and paper, materials to pour (e.g., sand, water), toy tool chests, dress-up clothes, dolls, household equipment for imaginary play, musical records and cassettes, and (especially for 5-year-olds) simple games based on following rules, such as musical chairs, "May I?" and "red light, green light."

Curiosity and Imagination

The 4-year-old's incessant questions can be taxing to adults, and parents may need help understanding that tolerant listening is more important than providing precise explanations. Similarly, the 4-year-old's boasting and exaggerations can be upsetting to adults who perceive him as lying. Responses which neither accuse the child of telling untruths nor encourage belief in outlandish ideas may be helpful as a middle ground for parents. For example, a parent might say, "Wouldn't it be wonderful if people could really do that?" or "I used to think that when I was a child."

Sexual curiosity is best viewed in the context of the young child's general curiosity about the world and the differences and occurrences observed. Explorations of the child's own and others' bodies are a developmentally typical part of all children's interest in what they and others are like.

Discipline

Discipline is essential during the preschool years to protect the child from endangering his health and safety, to help him avoid social condemnation, and to prevent the psychological insecurity children experience if they are permitted to feel that they are "bad" and out of control. Good discipline promotes respect for, not fear of, safety regulations, societal standards, and adults. In time the well-disciplined child develops *self*-control that further ensures his physical, psychological, and social well-being. The following guidelines are helpful to parents and others in relating to preschoolers.

1. Discipline should be motivated by love and should have as its objective the child's long-range best interest.
2. Discipline should be consistent. Limits imposed on the child's behavior must be consistent across time and among his disciplinarians. Discipline should also be consistent with the child's developmental level so that disciplinary methods and expectations for this behavior are suited to his abilities and change as he matures. Without unnecessarily departing from the goal of consistency, it is appropriate to consider mitigating circumstances, such as unusual fatigue and periods of special stress.

The best discipline is that which is also consistent with the nature of the child's infraction. A child who abuses others' property may be forbidden to use it for a time, for example, or one who takes intolerable risks with a particular piece of playground equipment in spite of instruction may be restricted from using it.

Since the objective of discipline is to teach the child safe and socially acceptable ways of operating within his environment, discipline also should be consistent with the standards expected by his family and the larger sociocultural setting in which he must operate successfully.

3. The child should know why he is being disciplined and should be helped to identify acceptable alternatives to his misbehavior. Unexplained or misperceived discipline misses its target and may engender hostility and retaliation.
4. Ineffective measures should be corrected. Repeating discipline which has been unsuccessful only frustrates both child and adult and can damage the self-concept of both as well as their appraisals of one another's competence.
5. The parent or other disciplinarian should understand his motivations in the disciplinary situation and try not to punish while angry.
6. Discipline should be limited to hazardous activities affecting the physical, emotional, or social well-being of the child.

Good behavior deserves at least as much attention as misbehavior and should be acknowledged and rewarded. Preschoolers enjoy pleasing others, but their rigid self-expectations often cause them to distrust anyone who insists on praising their lesser attempts. It can also frustrate the preschooler to be told repeatedly that he is "good" when he knows he has entertained "evil" wishes. As with discipline, praise is necessary to the growing child but ought to be offered thoughtfully and purposefully.

Safety

Accident prevention is a big part of preventive health for preschool children. Four-year-olds are particularly at risk for accidental injury and death because they are so exuberant and vigorous and have such exaggerated notions about their capabilities. Preschool children's accidents include both pedestrian and passenger mishaps involving motor vehicles, poisoning, drowning, burns, falls, lacerations, ingestion and aspiration of foreign substances, strangling by accidental hanging, and suffocation (for example, in discarded refrigerators). Supervision is essential to prevent accidents; so is safety instruction, particularly as children get older. The example set by parents and others is highly influential.

Sex Education

Preschoolers are highly curious about life, from the tiniest insect upward. Most of all, as their self-awareness grows, they become curious about themselves and their origin.

As part of the child's quest to understand the mystery of life he conducts personal research through physical exploration of self and playmates, usually to the distress of adults, who have forgotten or find little consolation in remembering their own curious childhood experiments. This type of learning can be used positively as a stepping-off point for explaining sex differences and socializing the child to cultural and family standards of privacy.

It is important to remember that the preschooler is not yet either moral or immoral. Morality develops later, after the child has identified himself and established social values. Parents are advised to approach sex education on a rather neutral and forthright plane from the earliest days, perfecting their explanations as opportunities and the child's needs present themselves.

Terminology for body parts offers an objective avenue to instruction related to the body and its functions. A parent would never call an arm, eye, or tongue by a "more neutral" term; the practice of devising an "acceptable" term for the genitals is unwise and tends to encourage attitudes of unacceptability toward genital and excretory matters.

Hesitancy about the body, and about sex in particular, is easily communicated to a child even on a nonverbal level. Consequently, whether or not he has been given an accurate explanation of life and birth, he may deny and repress portions of his lesson and construct his own explanation to complete the gaps. Nevertheless, the inevitable question usually surfaces, "How did I get made?" Finding out the child's reason for asking is the best initial action

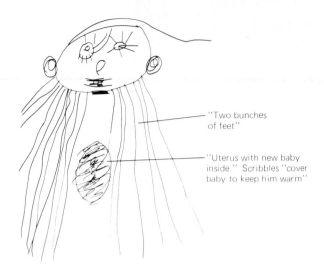

"Two bunches of feet"

"Uterus with new baby inside." Scribbles "cover baby to keep him warm"

FIGURE 4-3   A picture of "Mommy" drawn by a preschooler.

for the parent. From there, the parent should proceed with the realization that the child cannot retain many details in one hearing and will require repetition and expansion from time to time.

A mother's pregnancy prompts a preschooler's fantasy and questions. A simple initial statement that a baby has started to grow in a special place inside Mommy is acceptable to the preschooler, who will then signal his parents when he wants additional information. One preschooler experimented with what this would be like a few days after his mother's initial statement. He curled up next to his mother, covered himself totally with a sheet, and announced, "I'm inside your uterus." He explored further by making use of art, drawing a rather apt representation of his mother (Fig. 4-3).

The preschooler needs realistic preparation for the baby's arrival. He needs to know that the baby is coming and what babies are like. He also needs to know where and by whom he will be cared for at the time of the birth. It is helpful to him to participate in age-appropriate ways in making the household arrangements preparatory to the baby's joining the family.

The natural sequel to these fantasy explorations is the reality of the baby's arrival. The preschooler's responses to the infant may include great curiosity, demonstrated by questioning, looking, and touching; displeasure about the baby's noises and demands on the parents' time; affection; regression or regressive imitation of the baby; and jealous or rivalrous behavior. The child needs to be assured of his parent's continuing love for him, and he needs acceptance of and assistance with his natural feelings of jealously (Fig. 4-4).

Understanding Death

Another undeniable part of the human condition is mortality. Rather than attempting to explain death to preschoolers, parents may prefer to hide it. It is unnecessary and unfair to deny the child the experience of learning about death and the ways people react to it. Death is not simple to explain; it is in fact a difficult concept for young children to understand and frequently is fraught with emotion. Full human sharing requires the sharing of loss, and family life seems the appropriate setting in which to learn this lesson.

As with the beginnings of life, opportunities to help a child understand and deal with death present themselves subtly and often. Perhaps a crushed insect will initiate his questioning.

Commonly the first test arises when a pet dies. The parents' first inclination may be to substitute a similar animal before the child realizes his loss. This practice deceptively intimates that life never ends and denies the child the opportunity for practice with the natural and inevitable experience of loss. Equally unwise is the immediate promise of and acquisition of a new pet to forestall the child's reaction. When this method is used, the child is again denied a normal human need to express a sense of loss. Later, when he has been helped to be reconciled to his loss, it is more appropriate to let the child participate in selecting a new pet.

Parents, siblings, grandparents, and friends die. When these realities occur, they cannot and should not be concealed. Occasionally, in an attempt to comfort a child, an adult may suggest that a new parent, sibling, grandparent, or friend can be acquired to make up for the loss. This

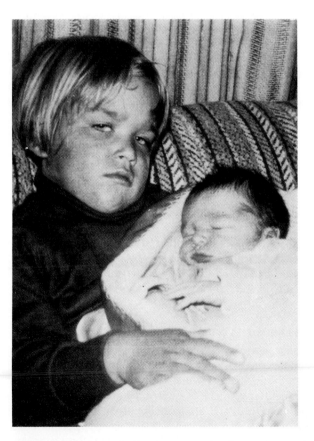

FIGURE 4-4 The preschooler meets a new brother or sister with mixed feelings.

suggestion is obviously unwise. In addition to being unrealistic and disrespectful of both the child and the deceased, it may lead the child to infer that he too could be replaced readily in the affections of family and friends if he were to die.

Most families subscribe to a belief which conceives of life as continuing beyond its finite limits. For such families this belief provides a basis for helping the child deal with death, especially when it promises eternal reward and offers the hope of eventual reunion.

When a parent dies, the explanation may be particularly difficult, but it must be given if only to preclude the child's fantasies about what might have happened. A preschool child may otherwise imagine that his own wishes or actions have caused the death or that the parent has abandoned him voluntarily.

Nutrition

Nutritional assessment and parental guidance as needed to prevent obesity and other forms of inadequate nutrition are important health maintenance measures. The child requires about 1250 cal/d at 3 years of age, about 1400 at 4, and about 1600 at 5. Complete guidance about diet can be found in Chap. 7.

Sleep

Preschool children require about 12 hours of sleep daily. Most 3-year-olds take an afternoon nap. A well-established bedtime routine is advisable to minimize reluctance to go to bed and encourage uninterrupted sleep. The bedtime routine can be adapted for each household, but for most children it should include (1) an established bedtime that is the same every night, (2) a physically tired child, (3) avoidance of excitement for a half hour before bedtime, (4) a satisfying evening meal but no snacks immediately before sleep, (5) a predictable series of events such as songs, stories, prayers, turning on the night-light, and getting into bed, and (6) an expectation that the child will comply. Factors tending to disturb sleep may include bad dreams, fears, and bed-wetting.

The School-Age Child

School-age children engage in a great deal of physical activity. Peer group and same-sex friendships are important. Children may be anxious about school performance, physical abilities, and family situations. Parents are concerned about sex education, discipline, helping the child develop a sense of responsibility, and adjustment to school. Accident prevention continues to be of prime importance. Since the child spends so many hours in school, the school nurse may be providing the health education and anticipatory guidance to the child and including the parents as problems arise. Mental health problems may occur in this age group.

Safety

Accidents are the leading cause of death in school-age children of both sexes. Health professionals must give safety education a prominent place in their interactions with children, parents, and appropriate others (e.g., school personnel, city council members, sports and recreation program personnel).

Automobile and Traffic Safety

Children need to be taught to cross streets at corners and understand traffic signals. Children out after dark should wear reflective patches on their jackets or coats.

The use of seat belts is essential and should be encouraged for all family members at each health maintenance visit. Any child over 22.5 kg (50 lb) should use adult seat belts, but shoulder straps should be avoided until the child is at least 140 cm (55 in) tall (a shorter child could strangle on the shoulder strap). Children should never be allowed to ride in the open back of a pickup truck.

Bicycle Safety

If a child is old enough to ride a bicycle, he is old enough to know and follow the rules of the road, which are the same for bikes as for cars. Reflective tape is readily available and should be placed in several sports on the bicycle. In addition, cyclists should be taught not to carry passengers, hitch rides by holding on to moving vehicles, and dart from behind parked cars. Children need to be informed that automobile drivers have blind spots, particularly the right rear and the side of the car.

Burns

Common causes of severe burns among the school-age population include improper use of matches and acci-

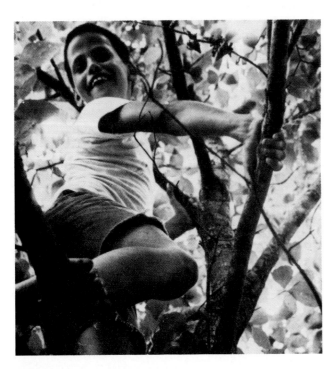

FIGURE 4-5 Safe climbing in trees includes avoiding slippery shoes and weak or dead limbs as well as keeping a secure handhold. *(Photo by George Lazar.)*

dents involving carelessness with campfires, barbecue grills, and fireplaces. Additionally, numerous children are injured each year by igniting firecrackers despite the fact that they are prohibited by law in many states.

Children need to be taught respect for fire as well as the appropriate ways of dealing with campfires, matches, and so forth. Children should always be supervised by an adult when they are using matches or are near fires.

Falls

School-age children enjoy climbing. Despite parental warnings, many children fall from trees, roofs, and playground equipment. As a result, many suffer from fractures during the middle years. Children should be cautioned about the risks, but it is not realistic to demand that they not climb trees or swing from branches (Fig. 4-5). Excessive restrictions can make children fearful and hesitant to try new things or can make them deceitful.

Swimming and Water Safety

All children should be given the opportunity to learn to swim. Parents should be encouraged to seek information regarding community resources for swimming lessons when they are not provided by the school system. Regardless of their ability to swim, children should be warned against swimming alone and should know that they must heed warning signs in areas where swimming is prohibited. They should be restricted to swimming only in areas where a lifeguard is present. From a very young age, children should be taught by parental example to follow safe boating rules; regardless of their ability to swim, they should wear a safety jacket whenever boating.

Calling for help as a joke and other kinds of horseplay are to be discouraged stringently. One must never dive into water of an undetermined depth; diving where the water is shallower than expected or where there are underwater objects such as boulders or fallen trees is a common cause of neck fractures.

Firearms

School-age children should be informed about gun safety rules. At a minimum, all children should know never to assume that a gun is unloaded and never to point a gun at anyone. Safety instruction about gun handling is necessary for all children who handle guns for hunting or target shooting. Children should never use firearms without adult supervision. Safe storage of guns and ammunition when they are not in use is an important part of safety instruction.

Adjustment to School

School adjustment is a major developmental task of the school-age years. School adjustment includes the development of productive work habits and essential academic skills and enjoyment of one's own ability to solve problems and produce things. Supportive interventions as needed with parents, children, and school personnel are important aspects of mental health promotion.

School Readiness

A crisis can be described as a major change in one's life-style or a period of disequilibrium. Entrance into school can indeed be called a crisis. The health care provider can assist the parents of children entering school by providing anticipatory guidance at the preschool health mainte-nance visit.

For many children, the most fearful aspect of starting school is the actual separation from their mothers. Parents can lessen this separation anxiety by exposing a child gradually to the "outside world." Children enjoy visits to the zoo and to museums and libraries, and in doing so they become familiar with people and places outside the home and family.

Children should have the experience of being away from their parents for several hours at a time before start-ing school. Overnight visits to friends as well as play ses-sions at a friend's house help a child learn that he can sur-vive without his parents. He develops confidence in him-self and learns to relate to other adults. Today many moth-ers seek employment outside the home, and from a very early age children are sent to day care or preschool. Cop-ing with separation occurs earlier for these children. Be-fore beginning school, the child should know his name, address, and phone number; he also needs to know how to cross streets and, specifically, how to get to school. These things give the child a sense of security and control of the new situation.

A child who has an established routine at home has lit-tle trouble adjusting to the routines at school. Schoolwork requires concentration and diligence. A child who has had projects and tasks to accomplish at home finds it easy to do the same at school.

In general, a child who has been given the opportunity to make friends and spend some time away from home finds school an exciting new adventure. Parental attitudes about education greatly influence the child's readiness and also influence his attitude about the teacher and the school.

School Progress

Asking the child what he likes best and least about school should provide the health care provider with important information about academic achievements as well as the child's perception of himself. A child who feels he does poorly in school and has no best subject is likely to have a low self-concept. Many times such a child has learning problems or problems with adjustment. The school nurse can be a valuable resource in such instances and can facil-itate evaluation of the child's problems within the school setting.

Parents can unwittingly contribute to a child's poor self-concept when their expectations are unrealistic. Par-ents who focus on high academic achievement sometimes need to be reminded that not all children are capable of receiving all A's. A child who sincerely struggles to learn and earns C's should be rewarded for his efforts. Parents need to work closely with teachers to identify the child's

strengths as well as weaknesses. Parents need to provide encouragement for the child's area of talent instead of fo-cusing only on areas in which he is weak.

Stimulation and Play

While the child's need for stimulation is perhaps not as obvious in the school years as it was earlier, it is still im-portant to realize that high-quality social, physical, and in-tellectual input are essential for high-quality development during this large and important segment of life. School-age children naturally engage in a great deal of stimulating in-teraction with one another and with the objects and ideas they encounter in the environments of home, school, and the ever-widening social and physical world. They require adult guidance to select their activities and interpret their experiences.

Television

The effect of television on children's behavior and atti-tudes remains a matter for debate. Television is a strong influence with the potential both to enhance and to im-pair the kinds of people children become. The extent and quality of the influence of TV and other media undoubt-edly depend on how events are portrayed.

Violence on TV has been singled out as an important issue. Other influences on children's development pre-sumably include the ways the media portray sex roles, health and illness, affectional relationships, power, status, authority, drug use, attitudes toward wealth and material possessions, and so on.

All children watch TV or are otherwise influenced by the media. Social scientists have calculated that a great many youngsters actually spend more time in front of the television than in classrooms and that they witness thou-sands upon thousands of criminal assaults and murders as well as violent acts of retribution carried out against of-fenders by supposedly justified "good guys" such as pri-vate detectives, police officers, and the military. What is less well understood is the ability of parents and others to soften or reverse the values and behavior portrayed in the media.

It would be unjust to conclude that television viewing has no positive influence on children. Television can in-deed expand children's experience outside the home and family. Some believe that the viewing of TV violence en-ables children to discharge rather than act out aggressive feelings. It has also been postulated that TV viewing en-hances a child's language development.

It is ultimately the responsibility of parents to guide and evaluate children's television viewing. When TV is used as a baby-sitter, it interferes with creativity and ini-tiative. Time spent watching TV is time away from physi-cal activities, reading, conversation, and other valuable pursuits.

Special programs designed to enlighten, educate, and, of course, entertain children can serve as an excellent ad-junct to development. Parents need to be selective about TV viewing and take the time to watch programs with their children. In this manner parents can discuss the child's perceptions and clarify misconceptions so that TV can be a positive experience.

Play

Play activities include individual and group sports and games of all sorts (volleyball, horseback riding, gymnastics, hopscotch, tennis, rope jumping), cognitive activities (dominoes, cards, other table games, science kits, collections), activities which involve producing things (crafts, cooking, gardening, art, photography, kite making), and imaginative activities (children's theater, reading, movies, puppetry, magic sets). Play continues to be an excellent and natural modality for developing needed skills (cognitive-perceptual, motor, and social) and for working through experiential and emotional problems.

It has been said that play is a child's work. The functions of play are many. By "trying on" various roles, the child is assisted in establishing sex-role identity. Through competitive sports, the child learns to cope with failure as well as success. A sense of comradeship is developed through team activities and clubs. Hobbies and special interests expand the child's knowledge of his universe.

Sex-typed play originates during the preschool years, but it becomes more evident during the middle years. Boys more than girls seem to avoid playing with objects traditionally associated with the opposite sex. Today, however, children seem to be more interested than children were a few years ago in the type of play generally associated with the opposite sex. Girls nowadays are frequently involved in team sports such as baseball and soccer; boys are less hesitant to learn about cooking and baking.

The kind of play a child engages in changes with his developmental needs. Generally the school-age child becomes physically more active in play. Running, tumbling, and climbing help the child develop coordination as well as gross motor skills. As skills improve, the child's confidence is increased and advanced forms of play such as roller skating and skipping rope become favorite pastimes.

The child in this age group engages in more cooperative forms of play than do preschoolers. The young school-age child of 6 or 8 generally designs his play activities around the familiar aspects of home and family. Playing house is among his favorite activities. The child tries on roles such as doctor, nurse, fire fighter, and police officer. As the child's imagination flourishes, he becomes a cowhand or astronaut. The 6- to 8-year-old generally imitates people of the same sex. As the child matures, he needs less parental involvement and can amuse himself for long periods of time with activities such as drawing, reading, and puzzles.

The child of 8 becomes a collector. While younger school-age children also enjoy collecting things, the 8-year-old pays more attention to quality than to quantity. He classifies and organizes his collection, which may include anything from insects and rocks to fantasy characters and pictures of sports heroes. Table games and loosely organized clubs gain interest, but the 8-year-old hates to lose and often changes the rules or cheats in order to win.

By 9 years the child has developed some basic reading skills and enjoy reading and music lessons. Television and movies are favorite passive activities, but participation in organized events takes up a good part of the child's free time. A great sense of satisfaction can be achieved by becoming part of a team. Competition and its relationship to the child's sense of self-esteem depend largely on the quality of supervision. There is a great deal of controversy about the value of adult-organized activities. When adults assist children in playing fair and following rules, the activities provide the children with an opportunity to experience success as well as failure and maintain a sense of self-esteem. When parents place too much emphasis on winning, the activities are no longer fun and the child becomes anxious and in many instances loses self-confidence and enthusiasm (Fig. 4-6).

By 9 to 11 years companionship becomes more important than play. Around this time the child has identified a "best friend"; gangs develop, and peer group acceptance becomes extremely important.

The 12-year-old is characterized by enthusiasm and impulsive behavior. The child acts without considering consequences and finds himself in situations never before experienced. At the same time the 12-year-old is able to accept limited responsibility and enjoys taking on jobs such as baby-sitting and delivering newspapers. Chores and realistic responsibilities give the preadolescent the opportunity to become self-sufficient and confident as he approaches adolescence and adulthood.

Sex Education

Sex education can be defined as learning about oneself as a sexual being. Children need to know that both sexes have similar feelings and potential and that sex is more than a physical experience. A great deal of controversy exists as to who should provide sex education (parents, teachers, health professionals, or others) and what should be taught. It is to be hoped that the old question of *whether* children should receive this kind of education has now been answered. The fact is that all children form attitudes and beliefs about sexuality. If they do not have access to reliable and accurate information from adults, they depend instead on other children, on what they may read or observe, and on fantasy and conjecture. The outcome in this case is unpredictable and probably inadequate. Parents, educational institutions, and professionals all have roles to play in sex education, just as they have in all other aspects of providing safe and sufficient resources to meet the needs of children.

Intentionally or not, parents are the child's first and possibly most influential teachers with regard to sexuality. Parents who are demonstrative and openly show affection to each other teach children that such behaviors are healthy and good. Conversely, parents who do not display affection for each other or show embarrassment when "caught" being affectionate teach children to view sexuality with embarrassment and negative connotations.

In what they do and say, adults willingly or unintentionally teach about sex roles—what is expected and acceptable behavior for males and for females. Sex-role stereotypes seem to be diminishing, and new and different sex-role options are available for both boys and girls. The caring, gentle, and sensitive male is no longer widely viewed as weak or inadequate. Girls compete in athletic activities, and academic excellence is reinforced for them as well as for their male counterparts. New freedoms exist for all, and this encourages children to pursue their interests and attain success in the areas best suited to them.

School-age children have questions and concerns about their bodies as well as about their sexuality. It would seem that their education should be shared by the parents, the schools, and the health professional so that it will be as complete and accurate as possible. Since parents may lack knowledge or feel uncomfortable discussing these issues with their children, the nurse can be a major resource person in this area.

Children need to know that a healthy sexual experience should take into consideration the partner's feelings, values, and beliefs as well as their own. Sexuality is surely more than sexual intercourse, and whichever institution or combination of institutions is chosen to educate the child, he needs to learn more than anatomy, physiology, and biology.

Values clarification may be an effective way of enabling children to establish at least a baseline personal code of sexuality; they can then use this baseline to assess new information and new experience. While it is inevitable and appropriate that a child's attitudes will change as he or she matures and acquires more experience of sexuality, the original baseline is helpful as at least a point of reference to reduce confusion and assist with coping. In addition to helping children establish values, sex education for school-age children must include basic factual information about healthy sexuality and reproduction, ways to deal with sexual advances by adults, and preparation for pubescent changes. Information on sexual abuse is covered in Chap. 13, "Abused or Neglected Children."

Understanding Death

Before 5 years of age children view death as temporary. Although the idea of death disturbs the young child, he views it mainly as a separation from those he loves. The child from 5 to 9 years of age realizes the finality of death and associates it with monsters, creatures, and other frightening characters. However, the child believes he has power over death and can avoid it or, conversely, can cause it to happen. Children in this developmental stage need to be reassured that bad thoughts or angry feelings toward another person cannot cause death. This issue needs to be addressed especially when a child experiences the death of a close family member or friend. Children need to know that anger and jealousy are normal feelings and are not the cause of sickness, injury, or death.

After the age of 9 the child's understanding of death is more adultlike. The child knows that death is inevitable and associates it with leaves falling and flowers dying. At this age children are curious about death. Depending on their religious upbringing, they may relate it to an afterlife, a permanent sleep, or coffins and cemeteries.

Most children experience the death of a significant person or pet. Depending on the child's age and developmental level, various behaviors are seen as the child experiences grief. Depression is as normal for a child as it is for an adult, and the child needs special support at such a time, but denying him the right to participate and grieve openly only deprives him of the opportunity to recognize that feelings of sadness and depression are healthy and normal.

Smoking and Drugs

Most school-age children are exposed in various ways to drugs and tobacco. Children model the behaviors of adults, and as they mature and try to "grow up," they take on adult behaviors and habits. It is difficult to warn children about the hazards of drugs and tobacco when parents smoke and depend on liquor and drugs to get them through a day or a bad situation.

It is unrealistic to expect that most children will not experiment with drugs and tobacco at least once. The health care provider needs to communicate in an open, honest fashion when discussing these issues with the child. Factual information about the effects of drugs (including alcoholic beverages and tobacco) should be shared with the child. The child needs to know that the

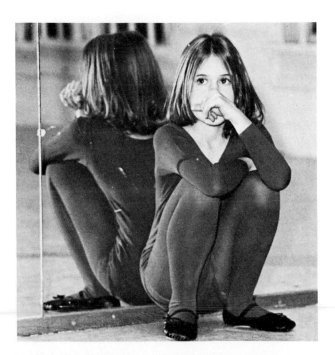

FIGURE 4-6   Self-esteem is a critical issue in the school-age years. Feelings of inferiority readily arise when the child does not feel successful. *(Photo by Betsy Smith.)*

discussion is confidential and that the health care provider is nonjudgmental but truly concerned about the child's well-being. Children need to be warned about the dangers of materials distributed by strangers or older students in the school yard.

Open communication with parents is essential for the school-age child since peer pressure and acceptance are so important at this time. Parents need to establish a good communication system early so that the child will feel free to discuss such matters. Parents also have to be aware of the signs of trouble so that help can be obtained as early as possible. It is during these years that the school-age child must have both gentle guidance and trust from his parents as well as constant support and positive reinforcement in order to avoid the pitfalls of drug experimentation. The child also needs good adult role models.

Discipline

Parents must establish clear guidelines for a child's behavior in language that the child can understand. For example, "Behave yourself" is ambiguous and unclear to a child. Instead, the parents must define clearly what is expected of the child: "I expect that you will make your bed before coming to breakfast"; "I want you to take your bath before nine o'clock."

Children need positive reinforcement for good behavior. Praise and encouragement are much better learning tools than are spankings and punishment. For example, the parent might say, "I really appreciate it when you make your bed like you did today." The child who receives attention only by being "bad" quickly learns that "bad" behavior wins attention. Such reinforcement establishes a vicious cycle between the parent's scolding and the child's acting out.

All children test parents to be certain of established limits. When the child breaks a rule or behaves in an unacceptable manner, the punishment should be swift, should be delivered with matter-of-fact attitude, and should be appropriate for the deed as well as the child's age. Sending a school-age child to his room for 20 minutes or taking away a privilege has infinitely more impact on the child than does spanking or screaming. It is also important to communicate that the child's behavior, not the child himself, is unacceptable or disappointing. The courteous, thoughtful parent who praises and supports a child's good behaviors will reap the many rewards and satisfactions that come from a well-behaved, confident, and likable child.

Responsibility

The school-age child is attempting to master the developmental task of *industry*. Previously the child worked at accomplishing certain tasks exclusively through play. Now he has a desire to do important, meaningful work—the work of the real, adult world.

To become a responsible adult the child needs to have chores, or tasks, assigned to him. Parents need to communicate their expectations clearly and provide the knowledge and guidance necessary for the child to complete the task successfully. The child takes pride in a job well done but needs praise and encouragement in order to satisfy his desire for recognition. When faced with unrealistic expectations and tasks that are too complex, he feels he has failed. He perceives himself as inferior and may give up trying, never realizing his goal.

Chores appropriate for school-age children range from making beds and hanging up clothes to dish washing and lawn mowing. Parents vary in their systems of rewards; some simply praise the child for the completed tasks, while others reward the child with special favors or money. Regardless of the method chosen, it is important for parents to remember that children need and deserve positive feedback.

Health Education

Now that they are less often under the supervision of the family, children need to be taught to provide increasingly for their own health and safety. Health education should stress participation in their own preventive care, with an explanation of how responsibility for health and safety can be expected to be rewarded with good physique, function, and appearance. All these traits are highly desired by school-age children, whose peer status system is based to a large extent on physical function and appearance, and so these kinds of expected payoffs can be used as motivators for good health practices. Health instruction should include anatomy and physiology, hygiene (including dental self-care), accident prevention, nutrition, sexuality, fire escape plans, the Heimlich maneuver, and values clarification about tobacco and drugs (including alcohol). Most school-age children are quite interested in anatomy and physiology and are responsive participants in health education programs geared to their development level.

Nutrition

The average school-age child requires about 80 kcal/kg/d, or 1600 to 2200 kcal/d. The child's diet should consist of the following:
Two or more servings of meat and eggs
Three cups of milk
Four servings of fruits and vegetables (including one dark green or deep yellow)
Four servings of bread and cereals
More information is provided in Chap. 7.

Sleep

Children need about $10\frac{1}{2}$ hours of sleep at age 6; the requirement gradually decreases to about $8\frac{1}{2}$ hours by age 12. Guidance and limit setting may be necessary to ensure sufficient sleep.

Mental Health

Mental health problems are not uncommon among school-age children; health professionals need to know how to recognize socioemotional difficulties. The children who should attract particular concern are those whose behavior deviates from the norms for their cultural and chronological peer group; those who are in trouble with the law, school, or other authorities; those who do not have friends; and those who are subjected to situational stress such as parental death, chronic illness, or child abuse. Mental health is discussed in Chap. 14, "Emotional Disorders of Childhood and Adolescence."

Adolescent

Adolescents undergo many physical and psychological changes. Self-concept is revised from questions about being normal to self-identity to values and beliefs. Behavior can be erratic, and peers are of prime importance. As with the school-age child, the school nurse has a primary role in providing health education and anticipatory guidance to the adolecent. The Td (adult tetanus toxoid and diphtheria toxoid) vaccine is given between 14 and 16 years of age (10 years after the last DTP).

Mental Health

Mental health upsets are common, especially while the adolescent's self-esteem and self-confidence waver and social and academic pressures seem unmanageable. Adolescents vigorously attempt to achieve peer acceptance and conformity to peer values. Real or imagined differences from the peer group standards, for example, late sexual development, may cause great emotional distress.

Early developers and especially late developers need honest information about the range of normality, the influence of familial patterns on the age of puberty, and the fact that final body size as established by individual genetic potential is not altered by early or late puberty.

Fears and anxieties about being in some way abnormal are pronounced in early adolescence and continue to some extent thereafter. Teenagers need factual information about the wide range of normality in body configuration, social uncertainty, sexual curiosity, emotional variability, and so forth. They also need a nondirective, nonjudgmental adult with whom to explore questions and examine alternatives.

Nurses of adolescents must inform themselves about recognizing and intervening in presuicidal behavior. Suicide is the third leading cause of death in adolescence. Mental health assessment and necessary interventions are major parts of health promotion in adolescents. Young people who particularly should attract concern are those whose behavior deviates from the norms for their peer group; those who are in trouble with the law, school, or other authorities; those who are subjected to situational stress such as family problems, school failure (real or imagined), or social failure (real or imagined); those who have a chronic illness or physical deviation from peer standards; and those who have no friends. Mental health is discussed in Chap. 14, "Emotional Disorders of Childhood and Adolescence."

Sex Education

In light of current statistics on premarital intercourse, sexually transmitted diseases, and pregnancy, sex education should be an important component of health care. Some people believe sexual information and attitudes should be taught by parents in the privacy of the home. In a national survey of adolescents, 70 percent responded that their parents did not discuss sex freely in the home; two-thirds said their parents have never discussed topics such as contraceptive methods, masturbation, and venereal disease. Others believe adolescents are adequately informed about sex through their peers. Myths and inadequate information are widespread. More than 25 percent of adolescents 16 years and over expressed the belief that if a girl does not want a baby, she will not become pregnant even without contraceptives! (Conger, 1979.) These findings continue to be relevant today. Many adolescents believe that the odds are against pregnancy, since they "only did it a few times," and so contraceptives are not seen as necessary.

Nurses can be important sources of information about sex and sexuality. They can work with parents in providing information and support since parents are often uninformed or embarrassed. Nurses can support and guide parents in their attempts to discuss sexual issues with adolescents, perhaps acting as an adjunct information source. Nurses can also offer sex education in health care and school settings.

Sex education includes values clarification about attitudes and motivation, the role of sexuality in interpersonal relations, and predictable consequences of alternative courses of action. (Adolescents are not future-oriented.) The kinds of information appropriate for adolescents include such topics as the anatomy and physiology of reproduction, normal sexual feelings and behavioral responses, normality and benefits of masturbation, pros and cons of various contraceptive means, available community resources, description of venereal disease, and implications of adolescent pregnancy and abortion. Education about sexuality involves teaching adolescents how to think rather than what to think. Since adolescents are cognitively capable of sophisticated problem solving, they should be encouraged to use those skills rather than given pat answers. The nurse's attitude toward sexuality and adolescent sexual behavior is important. The modeling effects, positive or negative, can far surpass the informational effects. It is important to encourage adolescents to discuss their sexual feelings and to give them a supportive environment in which to make decisions about sexual behavior.

Alcohol, Tobacco, and Other Drug Use

Increased use and abuse of drugs, including alcohol and tobacco, has been observed in recent years. This trend is not specific to adolescents but rather extends to all of society. Research has shown that adolescents whose parents significantly use such drugs as alcohol, tranquilizers, tobacco, and sedatives are more likely than are other adolescents to use marijuana, alcohol, and other drugs. While the majority of adolescents are not serious drug users, the use of marijuana, alcohol, and tobacco is widespread. The majority of adolescents reported some alcohol use in the month prior to one survey, while only a small percentage reported daily use (Bachman, Johnston, and O'Malley, 1981.) About 5 percent of high school adolescents are considered problem drinkers on the basis of the criterion of getting drunk once a week or more. Marijuana users account for the greatest percentage of adolescents who have experimented with illicit drugs. It is estimated that more than half of all American adolescents have at least experimented with marijuana.

More than one-fourth of the seniors in a study by Bachman, Johnston, and O'Malley (1981) reported using an illicit drug other than marijuana during the previous year. Illicit drugs are used in combination with alcohol, which produces an increased capacity for altered mood states and lethality.

Several reasons for adolescent drug use have been identified. Bachman, Johnston, and O'Malley (1981) found the life plans and life-styles were related to drug use. High school seniors who anticipated completing college reported lower use than did seniors with no college plans. Grades were negatively correlated with smoking and drug use. Truancy and school absenteeism were positively correlated to substance use. The frequency of evenings out with friends also correlated positively with the use of drugs, especially marijuana and alcohol. These authors noted that drug use is highest among adolescents least influenced by adult-operated institutions: school, home, and church. Experimentation with drugs may take place out of curiosity and a sense of daring. Peer group influences, boredom, recreational use of drugs, rebellion against parents, escape from life pressures, alienation, and emotional disturbance facilitate substance use. Differences are apparent between regular drug users or abusers, who use drugs to escape life, and drug experimenters, who seek new aesthetic or sensual experiences. The adolescents most likely to become addicted or dependent on drugs are those with personal, emotional, social, and family problems (Rice, 1981).

Nurses can contribute to the prevention of adolescent drug and alcohol abuse. First, nursing assessment should include how adolescents feel about drugs and alcohol and why they choose to use them. This information determines whether they are becoming responsible users or problem users. Second, nurses can help adolescents with responsible decision making about drug and alcohol use. If adolescents choose to use these substances, they must decide what, how much, under what circumstances, and with whom to drink or use other drugs. Third, providing information about the physiological, psychological, and legal effects of drug and alcohol use can assist adolescents in making informed choices. Fourth, compassion and responsiveness to individual adolescent needs can prevent substance users from becoming substance abusers.

Safety

Serious accidents increase during adolescence, often as a result of identity-seeking experimentation ("How fast can I drive?"; "How much can I drink?") and risky activities undertaken to get or keep peer esteem. As in the earlier age groups except infancy, accidents are the leading cause of death. Since adolescents are so often unsupervised and in charge of their own decisions and behavior, accident prevention in this age group depends largely on voluntary adoption of safety practices. The example set by adults, particularly adults the teenager finds attractive and identifies with, is important. Safety instruction, like other kinds of health education, must emphasize the short-term benefits to be gained by observing safety precautions and must employ a rationale that the adolescent can respect. Areas of safety instruction should include skateboards, motorcycles, automobiles, swimming and diving, firearms, and safety practices related to the use of alcohol and other mind-altering drugs. Drivers' education courses should be encouraged.

Understanding Death

It is during adolescence that the individual first develops an adultlike concept of death. School-age children come to understand that death is permanent and inevitable for everyone, but they commonly fantasize the existence of a personified, supernatural skeleton or bogeyman who collects souls or otherwise causes death (Gronseth et al., 1980). Adolescents may still have mistaken ideas about the causes and physiology of death, but they are clear about the fundamental understanding that dying is a natural and universal outcome for all living things and that they themselves will someday life (Gronseth et al., 1980). The emotional consequences of this understanding and responses to the fatal illness or death of someone the adolescent knows vary from horror and denial to philosophical acceptance, just as in adulthood. Nursing issues associated with death and dying are discussed in Chap. 16.

Play and Recreation

Play takes on a different dimension during adolescence. More sex-specific interests are developed; moreover, younger adolescents have interests different from those of older adolescents. During early adolescence both boys and girls are interested in watching television. This activity allows diversion from uncomfortable thoughts and feelings and may facilitate fantasies of adventure, romance, and heroism. Listening to a loud radio tuned to a popular music station is a frequent practice among adolescents. Movies, particularly with sexual themes, and stories about adolescent conflicts or teen idols are also very popular activities. Some adolescents are interested in hobbies such as reading, mechanical or electrical devices, and homemaking arts such as cooking and sewing.

By middle adolescence young people seek the companionship of persons of the opposite sex. They become interested in dating, dancing, and parties.

School sports activities are of interest to early and late adolescents. As noted by Nicholson (1980), until recently girls were primarily involved as spectators and cheerleaders. Federal requirements for increased spending for female athletic programs and court decisions allowing girls to play on baseball teams have encouraged girls' participation in sports. Boys are usually interested in training, competing, and excelling in sports activities such as football, basketball, baseball, swimming, gymnastics, and soccer.

Much of an adolescent's time is spent with friends, either on the telephone or in activities. What may appear to be endless telephone conversations permit the teenager to enhance social skills, develop a support system with peers, practice different ways of behaving, and exchange ideas, thoughts, and feelings.

Play and recreational activities popular with teenagers include group and individual sports and games emphasizing physical skill and/or strategy (Ping-Pong, chess, other ball games and board games), arts (painting, drawing, sculpture), crafts (weaving, pottery, carving), collections (stamps, autographs), other hobbies (model construction, car repair, ham radio, photography), hunting, and fishing. Interests become as diverse and abilities as well developed as in adults.

Health Education

Health education needs to be geared toward self-care. Information and values clarification are necessary with regard to general health maintenance (e.g., diet, exercise, hygiene, rest, dental care), sexuality, mental health, anatomy and physiology, and the use of drugs (including alcohol and tobacco). Alcohol abuse is *not* rare among young people of high school and college-age, and undoubtedly it is much more common than are problems with so-called stronger or more dangerous substances.

Problems such as nearsightedness, astigmatism, and caries are common and can arise quickly. Thus, visual and dental checkups are recommended at least yearly.

Caloric requirements in adolescence vary with the stage (rate) of growth the young person is experiencing. The Recommended Dietary Allowance, a figure designed as an average for groups of adolescents and obviosly not suitable for every individual, specifies 2100 to 2200 cal daily for female adolescents and 2700 to 2800 for males. Dietary practices have to be adjusted to meet the new needs of the adolescent period of rapid growth. Special circumstances such as athletics, pregnancy, obesity, and chronic illness further modify nutritional requirements. Both undernutrition and obesity are relatively frequent in adolescence. Unbalanced weight-loss diets, which are likely to appeal to adolescent girls, are particularly hazardous because they do not provide the nutrients needed either for the young woman's growth or for the preparation of her body for a successful pregnancy in the forthcoming several years. The emphasis of nutrition education in adolescence must be upon self-care (Chap. 7).

Adolescents are highly present-oriented, and so health education and health care should be designed to produce short-term, prompt rewards whenever possible. For example, a teenager may discontinue smoking because it interferes with athletic performance or lessens his appeal to the opposite sex, not because it causes respiratory disease in later years.

Adolescents are quick to perceive and reject the biases of adults, especially in the realm of thou-shalt-nots, for example, safety precautions, sexual behavior, marijuana, and alcohol. Teaching and demonstration can be effective in supporting good health attitudes and practices, but preaching is unlikely to succeed with young people, whose developmental progress requires making up their own minds.

Once a girl reaches Tanner stage 2 for breast development (about 12 years), breast self-examination is taught. Testicular examination is taught to boys at 14 years of age. Both self-examinations are reviewed at subsequent health visits.

Health education should include preparation for the role of health care consumer. Igoe (1980a, 1980b) described health education curricula that incorporate this goal. She also identified teaching approaches that succeed with adolescents and encouraged the involvement of teenagers as volunteer workers in school health screening and teaching programs.

Summary

The focus of this chapter is the promotion of the development and health of children and adolescents during wellness visits. It is important for nurses to realize that the topics discussed can be raised with parents and children in settings other than the physician's office or the well-child clinic. For example, if a child is hospitalized and his immunizations are not up to date, the nurse can talk with the parents about the importance of protecting children against childhood diseases. The school nurse can discuss accident prevention, sexuality, and common health problems with school-age children and adolescents; can perform vision and hearing screening; and can make referrals as appropriate. Preparing parents and children for various diagnostic tests and for surgery is also part of health promotion. (These topics are covered in Part 3.) Thus, promoting children's health involves not only keeping the child well but also preventing further problems when a child is ill.

Learning Activities

1. Prepare an outline for discussing accident prevention with the parents of infants, toddlers, and preschoolers. Ask several parents who have children in one of these age groups to join you for a group discussion.
2. Arrange to visit a school nurse. Ask her to share with you the way in which she promotes children's health in her school district.
3. Arrange to spend time with a pediatric nurse practitioner. Determine the types of health education she provides to parents and/or children.

Study Questions

1. The recommended age at which to begin the diphtheria, tetanus, and pertussis (DTP) and polio (OPV) vaccines is:
   A. 1 month.   C. 3 months.
   B. 2 months.   D. 4 months.

2. A 15-month-old infant has received DTP and OPV at 2 months and 4 months of age. The parents ask what immunizations are due now. The nurse answers that:
   A. The series must begin again since more than 10 months has passed since the last immunizations.
   B. The child is up to date for DTP and OPV but needs the MMR shot.
   C. The child needs the third OPV, third DTP, and MMR.
   D. The child is not due for any immunizations at this age.

3. The first scoliosis screening examination is done at age:
   A. 7 years.   C. 9 years.
   B. 8 years.   D. 10 years.

4. The mother of a 2-week-old boy tells the nurse that her baby sneezes. She wonders if the baby has a cold. The nurse explains that:
   A. Sneezing is his way of blowing his nose.
   B. If he has a fever, he does have a cold.
   C. She needs to contact the physician immediately.
   D. He needs to see an allergist.

5. A father asks the nurse how long car seats should be used. The nurse explains that car seats are recommended:
   A. From 1 month to 12 months.
   B. From the time the newborn leaves the hospital until the child weighs 40 lb.
   C. Only in states in which car seats are required by law.
   D. For the first 2 years of life.

6. The parents of a 6-week-old infant ask the nurse at what age babies usually begin to sleep through the night. The nurse answers:
   A. At 1 month.   C. At 2 months.
   B. At 6 weeks.   D. At 3 months.

7. Language stimulation is important in 4- to 6-month-old infants because:
   A. The baby now can smile in response to a voice.
   B. Hearing is now well developed.
   C. The infant is beginning to discriminate meanings.
   D. The infant now knows that objects exist even when they are out of sight.

8. During the toilet-training process, the best time to teach children how to raise and lower their pants is:
   A. At "potty" time.
   B. During regular dressing and undressing sessions.
   C. After nap time.
   D. Just before bedtime.

9. Four-year-old children are particularly at risk for accidental injury and death because:
   A. They are exuberant, are vigorous, and have exaggerated notions about their capabilities.
   B. They engage in so much horseplay.
   C. They are seeking peer esteem and are engaged in identity-seeking experimentation.
   D. They have not developed prehension.

10. The parents of a 5½-year-old boy are discussing school readiness. They explain that the child has had various experiences of being away from them for several hours at a time; knows his name, address, and telephone number; knows how to cross streets and get to school; and has had many opportunities to make friends. They wonder what else might be helpful. The nurse explains that:
    A. From what they have said, the child should not experience separation anxiety.
    B. There is nothing more to be done to help in his future adjustment to school.
    C. They need to help him establish a sense of security prior to school.
    D. Experience with established routines and projects and tasks to accomplish at home is helpful in later adjustments to school.

11. Adolescent myths regarding pregnancy following sexual intercourse are related to lack of information and:
    A. Their orientation to the present.
    B. Their lack of values.
    C. Their use of drugs.
    D. Their many physical changes.

References

American Academy of Pediatrics: *Guidelines for Health Supervision,* American Academy of Pediatrics, Elk Grove Village, Ill., 1981.

————: *Guidelines for Health Supervision,* American Academy of Pediatrics, Elk Grove Village, Ill., 1985.

American Academy of Pediatrics: *Guidelines for Health Supervision II,* American Academy of Pediatrics, Elk Grove Village, Il., 1988.

Bachman, J.G., L.D. Johnston, and P.M. O'Malley: "Smoking, Drinking, and Drug Use among American High School Students: Correlates and Trends, 1975-1979," *American Journal of Public Health,* **71:**59-69, 1981.

Barnard, M.U., M.A. Chard, J. Howe, P.J. Phillips, and G.M. Scipien: *Handbook of Comprehensive Pediatric Nursing,* McGraw-Hill, New York, 1981.

Charney, E.: "Well Child Care as an Axiom," in E. Charney (ed.), *Well Child Care,* Ross Laboratories, Columbus, Ohio, 1986.

Committee on Infectious Diseases, American Academy of Pediatrics: *Report of the Committee on Infectios Diseases,* 20th ed., American Academy of Pediatrics, Elk Grove Village, Ill., 1986.

Conger, J.: *Adolescence: Generation Under Pressure,* New York, Harper & Row, New York, 1979.

Gronseth, E.C., D.P. Geis, M.A. Anglim, and I.P. Martinson: "Dying and Death," in J. Howe (ed.), *Nursing Care of Adolescents,* McGraw-Hill, New York, 1980.

Igoe, J.B.: "Health Counseling and Teaching," in J. Howe (ed.), *Nursing Care of Adolescents,* McGraw-Hill, New York, 1980a.

————: "School Health Programs," in J. Howe (ed.), *Nursing Care of Adolescents,* McGraw-Hill, New York, 1980b.

Nicholson, S.W.: "Growth and Development, in J. Howe (ed.), *Nursing Care of Adolescents,* McGraw-Hill, New York, 1980.

"Recommendations of the Immunization Practices Advisory Committee (ACIP) Update: Prevention of *Haemophilus influenzae* type b," *American Journal of Diseases of Children,* 142 (4):419–420, 1988.

Rice, F.P.: *The Adolescent: Development, Relationships, and Culture,* 3d ed., Allyn and Bacon, Boston, 1981.

The Nursing Process: A Systematic Approach to Pediatric Health Care

Objectives

After reading this chapter, the student will be able to:
1. Outline the five steps of the nursing process.
2. Differentiate between subjective and objective assessment data.
3. Identify the components of a nursing history.
4. Formulate nursing diagnoses.
5. Describe a method for setting priorities.
6. Write client goals in terms of measurable client behaviors.
7. Discuss involvement of the client and family in planning and implementing the nursing care plan.
8. Explain different methods of documentation.
9. Describe the purpose of evaluation and revision in a nursing care plan.

The nursing process is an organized, systematic approach to nursing practice. It is a deliberate intellectual activity that enables the nurse to diagnose and treat the actual or potential health problems of pediatric clients in any health care setting. Using the five components of the nursing process—assessment, diagnosis, planning, implementation, and evaluation—the nurse can provide effective nursing care.

Assessment

Nursing assessment entails the collection of data, the organization of data, and the analysis of data. A thorough and accurate data base is obtained through interviewing, observation, and laboratory and diagnostic studies. Clustering data within an organizational framework facilitates the process of analysis. Relevant findings are extrapolated from the organizational framework to identify the child and family's strengths and problems requiring intervention.

Collection of Data

The subjective portion of the data base is the nursing history. The nursing history consists of information obtained from the child or caregiver regarding the physical and emotional state of the child and family. The quality of the history is a function of the trust that the historian has in the interviewer. The nurse's ability to establish rapport affects the client's ability to relate a thorough and accurate history. Other factors that affect the history include limitations of memory, comprehension, and language; emotional stress due to anxiety; and fear or guilt regarding the child's illness (Korsch and Aley, 1973, p. 6).

The objective portions of the data base are the observations made by the nurse of client behaviors, child-family interactions, physical assessment, and laboratory and diagnostic findings. Observation is the means by which one takes notice of something through the five senses of sight, hearing, taste, smell, and touch. Through sight, the nurse may view tearing in the child's eyes, increased respirations, or the caregiver rocking the child in an upright position. Through touch and hearing, the nurse may percuss dull lung sounds and auscultate decreased breath sounds. Laboratory and diagnostic chest findings may reveal decreased oxygen levels and consolidation in the left lower lobe. Observation, then, is the process of noting objective facts about the client.

Interviewing

The nursing history is obtained through interviewing the child and his caregivers. Such an interview can be defined as a goal-directed communication between the client and the nurse in which the child and family share information about themselves. In an effective interview this sharing takes place in an accepting and understanding atmosphere created by the nurse. Guidelines for an effective interview are listed in Table 5-1.

Observation

Observation is an ongoing process that begins during the first encounter with the child and family. The process of observation occurs any time the nurse is with the client: in the context of a formal interview or casual conversation, during a physical examination, at the time of a treatment or procedure, or in silence at the client's bedside. Observation can and does occur in the absence of verbal exchange and certainly should occur simultaneously with verbal interaction. During conversation the nurse observes nonverbal behavior because the client responds at both verbal and nonverbal levels. Both assist the nurse in guiding the interview and understanding the needs of the client. In addition, the nurse observes parent-child inter-

---

TABLE 5-1 Guidelines for Client Interviews

Environment

1. Provide privacy: Seek a remote corner of the room or draw the curtains
2. Minimize environmental distractions: Reduce the noise level of the radio or television; control interruptions and ask visitors to wait outside
3. Introduce yourself: Give your name and role
4. Greet the child by name with a smile and direct eye contact: Get down at the child's level
5. Greet the parent or guardian: Explain the purpose of and time frame for the interview
6. Maintain an unhurried image: Listen attentively; spend a few minutes in play
7. Provide age-appropriate toys to occupy the child during the interview

Interviewing techniques

1. Increase the child's level of comfort: Demonstrate interest, affection, respect, and acceptance
2. Use self-disclosure by relating a personal experience or telling the child some information about yourself
3. Use open or closed questions depending on the information required: Open question—"What do you think is wrong with your child?" Closed question—"Has your child ever been to the hospital before?"
4. Use direct or indirect questions: Direct question—"Do you have any allergies?" Indirect question—"I am wondering how you feel about having to stay in the hospital longer."
5. Avoid leading questions which interject the interviewer's values: "You do not spank your children, do you?"
6. Avoid double questions which preclude alternative answer: "Do you employ a baby-sitter while you work or do you use day care services?"
7. Use language that is clearly understood
8. Allow sufficient time for the child and family to respond
9. At the conclusion, ask the client if there is anything else which has not been discussed or if there are any further questions

Interviewing the parent

1. Explore the caregiver's main concern: "What is it that worries you the most about your child's condition?"
2. Establish the caregiver's expectations of the health provider: "What is it that you expect to have done for your child at the clinic or hospital?"

Interviewing the child

1. Assess the child's cognitive development
2. Ask why the child thinks he is in the clinic or hospital and what he has been told about the visit
3. Determine whether the child should be interviewed with or without his caregivers: Toddlers tend to be more comfortable in close proximity to their parents, whereas adolescents divulge more information when interviewed separately and then together

---

actions in order to gather data about the parent's feelings toward the child and vice versa. Through observation of their interaction during play or in the examining room, the nurse can see who controls the parent-child relationship and note the child's usual behavior and the ways in which the parent copes with it. Guidelines for making observations are listed in Table 5-2.

TABLE 5-2 Guidelines for Making Observations

1. Be aware of bias, attitudes, and values which contribute to stereotyped beliefs about clients
2. Guard against the tendency to generalize
3. Make descriptive observations; report specific, observable, and nonjudgmental factors or behaviors
4. Validate observations with the child, family, and/or health team members
5. Look for themes or patterns in the observations
6. Note verbal and nonverbal data when making the observations
7. Note the environment or situation within which the behavior occurs

Organization of Data

The interview and observational data must be organized in a meaningful way. Many pediatric interview guides and assessment tools are available to the nurse; these formats will direct the nurse to areas of importance which need to be covered. Familiarization with these areas can help the nurse prepare for an interview. However, rigid adherence to an assessment tool may make the interview stilted and artificial.

Content of the History

The history includes identifying data, the chief complaint, a history of the present illness or complaint, the past health history, the family history, and functional health patterns. The nurse may be responsible for obtaining a complete history or only components, depending on the particular setting and situation. A comprehensive history should be obtained on the child's first visit to the health provider as well as during hospitalization. The guideline below is appropriate for a child's history.

1. Identifying Data The child's name, age, birth date, sex, and address are obtained.

2. Date of Admission

3. Admitting Diagnosis

4. Chief Complaint This is the child's or caregiver's statement of the reasons for seeking health care. It is recorded in the client's own words.

5. History of Present Illness This is the client's description:

Symptoms
  Onset
  Duration
  Intensity
Treatment instituted
Factors that aggravate or relieve symptoms
Caretaker's specific concerns.

The historian should be allowed to describe the chief complaint and the history of the illness without interruption. It is likely that many of the nurse's questions will be answered as the client tells the story, obviating the need to bombard the child with questions.

6. Past Health History The past medical history includes the areas shown below.

Childhood medical and psychiatric illnesses
Developmental milestones
  Motor
    Rolling over, sitting, crawling, standing, walking, sports
  Social and cognitive
    Smiling, first words, sentences, playing, school
Immunizations
  DTP, polio, measles, mumps, rubella
Allergies
  Drugs, foods, contactants, inhalants
Accidents and injuries
Hospitalizations

For infants and young children, information about prenatal and perinatal events is particularly important. Information about the pregnancy helps establish the adequacy of the child's intrauterine environment, particularly with regard to fetal nutrients and blood supply. Exposure to potential teratogens is also assessed (history of medication, alcohol, illness, and radiation exposure). A description of labor and delivery is helpful in determining the possibility of neurological insults due to prolonged fetal distress or neonatal hypoxia.

7. Family History The family history includes the age and health status of the child's family. Data are collected about parents, grandparents, and siblings.

Questions regarding health status focus on the family's history of inheritable diseases and conditions with familial tendencies. Examples are diabetes, cancer, sickle cell anemia, heart disease, allergies, and cystic fibrosis. It is helpful to be aware of the family's significant illnesses and their effect on the family's functioning. Health status or cause of death of the grandparents is recorded.

8. Functional Health Patterns One method of eliciting the child's and family's level of function or dysfunction is to obtain a history of life-style patterns. The nurse assesses the child and family with reference to each of the 11 functional health patterns. Gordon's (1987a) Functional Health Pattern Assessment Tool for Infant and Early Childhood is presented in Table 5-3.

Analysis of Data

The nurse reviews the information collected, drawing from the body of nursing knowledge and personal experiences, to identify client responses that are healthy and those which are not. The data may be sorted to reflect the strengths and weaknesses of the pediatric client and family. The conclusions derived from the nurse's assessment of the client's strengths and weaknesses are referred to as nursing diagnoses.

Nursing Diagnosis

The transition from the data base to a list of diagnostic statements is a critical step in the utilization of information for planning and implementing client care. A nursing

TABLE 5-3 Functional Health Pattern Assessment: Infancy and Early Childhood

Use a parent report until the child can answer the items. The following includes some screening items related to parent assessment, or use adult assessment.

I. Health-perception–health-management pattern
  A. Parents' report:
    1. Pregnancy/labor/delivery history (this baby, child)?
    2. Health status since birth?
    3. Adherence to routine health checks? Immunizations?
    4. Infections? Frequency? Absences from school?
    5. If applicable: Medical problem, treatment, and prognosis?
    6. If applicable: Actions taken when signs/symptoms perceived?
    7. If appropriate: Been easy to follow things doctors or nurses suggest?
    8. Preventive health practices (diaper change, utensils, clothes, etc.)?
    9. Parents smoke? Around baby?
    10. Accidents? Frequency?
    11. Crib toys (safety)? Carrying safety? Car safety?
    12. Safety practices (household products, medicines, etc.)
  B. Parent (self): Parents'/family's general health status?
    1. General appearance of infant/child
    2. General appearance of parent(s)
II. Nutritional-metabolic pattern
  A. Parents' report of
    1. Breast-feeding/Bottle? Estimate of intake? Sucking strength?
    2. Appetite? Feeding discomfort?
    3. 24-hour intake of nutrients?
    4. Supplements?
    5. Eating behavior?
    6. Food preferences? Conflicts over food?
    7. Birth weight? Current weight?
    8. Skin problems: Rashes, lesions, etc.?
  B. Observation
    1. Height?
    2. Weight?
    3. Skin color, hydration, rashes, lesions
III. Elimination pattern
  A. Parents' report of
    1. Bowel elimination pattern (describe). Frequency? Character? Discomfort?
    2. Diaper change routine?
    3. Urinary elimination pattern (describe). Frequency of diaper change?
    4. Estimate of amount? Stream (strong, dribble)?
    5. Excess perspiration? Odor?
IV. Activity-exercise pattern
  A. Parents' report of
    1. Bathing routine? (When, how, where, type of soap?)
    2. Dressing routine? (Clothing, inside/outside home)
    3. Crib or other? Describe
    4. Typical day's activity (hours spent in crib, carrying, play, type of toys)
    5. Active? Activity tolerance?
    6. Perception of baby's/child's strength ("strong/fragile")?
    7. Child: Self-care ability (bathing, feeding, toileting, dressing, grooming)?
    8. Parent (self) child care, home maintenance activity pattern
  B. Observation
    1. Reflexes (appropriate to age)
    2. Breathing pattern; rate, rhythm
    3. Heart shounds; rate, rhythm
    4. Blood pressure
V. Sleep-rest pattern
  A. Parents' report of
    1. Sleep pattern: Estimated hours?

    2. Restlessness? Nightmares?
    3. Infant: Sleep position? Body movements?
  B. Parent (self): Sleep pattern?
VI. Cognitive-perceptual pattern
  A. Parents' report of
    1. General responsiveness?
    2. Response to talking? Noise? Objects? Touch?
    3. Following objects with eyes? Response to crib toys?
    4. Learning (changes noted)? What teaching baby?
    5. Noises/vocalizations?
    6. Speech pattern? Words? Sentences?
    7. Use of stimulation: Talking, games, etc.?
    8. Vision, hearing, touch, kinesthesia?
    9. Child: Name, tell time, address, telephone number?
    10. Pain? Discomfort? (Describe?
VII. Self-perception–self-concept pattern
  A. Parent's report of
    1. Mood state?
    2. Child's sense of worth, identity, competency?
  B. Child's report of
    1. Mood state?
    2. Many/few friends? Liked by others?
    3. Self-perception ("Good" most of time? Hard to be "good"?)
    4. Ever lonely?
    5. Fears (transient/frequent)?
  C. Observation
    1. Child: Eye contact, speech pattern, posturing
  D. Parent (self)
    1. General sense of worth, identity, competency?
VIII. Role/relationship pattern
  A. Parent's report of
    1. Family/household structure?
    2. Family problems/stressors?
    3. Family members/infant (or child) interaction?
    4. Infant/child response to separation?
    5. Child: Dependency?
    6. Child: Play pattern?
    7. Child: Temper tantrums? Discipline problems?
    8. Child: School adjustment?
  B. Observation
    1. Smiling response (infant)?
    2. Social interaction (child)? Aggressive/withdrawn?
    3. Response to vocalizations? Requests?
  C. Parent (self)
    1. Role engagements? Satisfaction?
    2. Work? Social? Family? Relationships?
IX. Sexuality-reproductive pattern
  A. Parents' report of
    1. Child's feeling of maleness/femaleness?
    2. Questions regarding sexuality? How respond?
  B. Parent (self)
    1. If applicable: Reproductive history?
    2. Sexual satisfaction/problems?
X. Coping-stress tolerance pattern
  A. Parents' report of
    1. Child's pattern of handling problems, frustrations, anger, etc.? Stressors? Tolerance?
  B. Parent (self)
    1. Strategies for handling problems?
    2. Use of support systems?
    3. Life stressors? Family stress?
XI. Value-belief pattern
  A. Parent (self)
    1. Things important in life? Desires for the future?
    2. If appropriate: Perceived impact of disease on goals?

Source: M. Gordon, *Nursing Diagnosis: Process and Application,* 2d ed., McGraw-Hill, New York, 1987, p. 443-445. Used with permission.

diagnosis is a statement of an actual or potential health problem "which nurses, by virtue of their education and experience, are capable and licensed to treat" (Gordon, 1976, p. 1299). The most discriminating criterion for a nursing diagnosis is whether the nurse can intervene, or treat the problem, independently.

Diagnostic labels should be clear, concise, well-defined statements directing the major elements of the care plan. The diagnoses should guide the nurse in selecting nursing interventions, preventing potential problems, making decisions about referrals, and initiating discharge planning.

Formulation of Diagnostic Statements

There are three generally accepted components of nursing diagnosis: (1) the client's actual or potential diagnostic statement, (2) the related or risk factors (i.e., the cause), and (3) the defining characteristics.

The Nursing Diagnosis

The diagnosis describes an actual or potential problem of the child and family. An *actual* diagnosis refers to a situation that exists in the present. For example, an adolescent with facial lacerations from a motor vehicle accident may have an actual problem of body image disturbance. A *potential* diagnosis "refers to a situation which may cause difficulty in the future" (Atkinson and Murray, 1983, p. 21). Early recognition may prevent the problem or lessen its consequences. A child on bed rest with skeletal traction is at risk for boredom related to immobility and long-term hospitalization. Anticipating the effects of bed rest, the nurse may identify a problem of potential diversional activity deficit.

The Related or Risk Factors

The related or risk factor describes probable factors causing or maintaining the client's health problem. The specific factor must be identified, as several probable factors may relate to the same nursing diagnosis. For example, an actual fluid volume deficit in a child may be related to fever, diuresis, decreased fluid intake, hemorrhage, or diarrhea. Knowledge of the specific cause is critical to the selection of appropriate nursing interventions or referral for medical treatment.

The term *related factor* is used to identify causes of *actual* nursing diagnoses. The term *risk factor* is used to identify possible causes of *potential* nursing diagnoses.

The related or risk factor is connected to the diagnostic statement by the phrase *related to*. Thus:

Potential for injury *related to* disorientation

The Defining Characteristics

The third component consists of the defining characteristics. Noting the defining characteristics relative to each diagnostic statement assures the nurse that the diagnosis is valid and is based on assessment data. The diagnosis may be validated by verifying the information and conclusions with the child and family. Peers may also validate a diagnosis by processing the data and arriving at the same conclusions. When the nurse cannot specify the defining characteristics, potential diagnoses may be written to assure the continuance of further client assessment.

The North American Nursing Diagnosis Association (NANDA) has generated several diagnostic statements. The list of nursing diagnoses approved at the eighth national conference in 1988 is given in Table 5-4. As the classification system is still evolving, "it is expected that

---

TABLE 5-4 North American Nursing Diagnosis Association Approved Nursing Diagnoses, 1988

Activity intolerance	Knowledge deficit (specify)
Activity interolance, potential	Mobility, impaired physical
Adjustment, impaired	
Airway clearance, ineffective	Noncompliance (specify)
Anxiety	Nutrition, altered: less than body requirements
Aspiration, potential for	Nutrition, altered: more than body requirements
	Nutrition, altered: potential for more than body requirements
Body image disturbance	
Body temperature, altered, potential	Oral mucous membrane, altered
Bowel incontinence	
Breastfeeding, ineffective	Pain
Breathing pattern, ineffective	Pain, chronic
	Parental role conflict
Cardiac output, decreased	Parenting, altered
Communication, impaired verbal	Parenting, altered, potential
Constipation	Personal identity disturbance
Constipation, colonic	Poisoning, potential for
Constipation, perceived	Post-trauma response
Coping, defensive	Powerlessness
Coping, family: potential for growth	
Coping, ineffective family: compromised	Rape-trauma syndrome
Coping, ineffective family: disabling	Rape-trauma syndrome: compound reaction
Coping, ineffective individual	Rape-trauma syndrome: silent reaction
	Role performance, altered

From North American Nursing Diagnosis Association, 1988.

Continued.

TABLE 5-4 North American Nursing Diagnosis Association Approved Nursing Diagnoses, 1988—cont'd

Decisional conflict (specify)	Self-care deficit, bathing/hygiene
Denial ineffective	Self-care deficit, dressing/grooming
Diarrhea	Self-care deficit, feeding
Disuse syndrome, potential for	Self-care deficit, toileting
Diversional activity deficit	Self-esteem disturbance
Dysreflexia	Self-esteem, chronic low
	Self-esteem, situational low
Family processes, altered	Sensory/perceptual alterations (specify) (visual, auditory, kines-
Fatigue	thetic, gustatory, tactile, olfactory)
Fear	Sexual dysfunction
Fluid volume deficit (1)	Sexuality patterns, altered
Fluid volume deficit (2)	Skin integrity, impaired
Fluid volume deficit, potential	Skin integrity, impaired, potential
Fluid volume excess	Sleep pattern disturbance
	Social interaction, impaired
Gas exchange, impaired	Social isolation
Grieving, anticipatory	Spiritual distress (distress of the human spirit)
Grieving, dysfunctional	Suffocation, potential for
Growth and development, altered	Swallowing, impaired
Health maintenance, altered	Thermoregulation, ineffective
Health-seeking behaviors (specify)	Thought processes, altered
Home maintenance management, impaired	Tissue integrity, impaired
Hopelessness	Tissue perfusion, altered (specify type) (renal, cerebral, cardio-
Hyperthermia	pulmonary, gastrointestinal, peripheral)
Hypothermia	Trauma, potential for
Incontinence, functional	Unilateral neglect
Incontinence, reflex	Urinary elimination, altered patterns
Incontinence, stress	Urinary retention
Incontinence, total	
Incontinence, urge	Violence, potential for: self-directed or directed at others
Infection, potential for	
Injury, potential for	

nurses will modify, delete, and add to the currently accepted listing" (Gordon, 1987b, p. 4).

Priority Setting

Once nursing diagnoses have been identified, priorities are established. The nurse rank-orders the diagnoses from the highest priority to the lowest priority. Maslow's hierarchy of needs is useful in priority setting. Physiological and safety needs take precedence over belongingness, esteem, and self-actualization needs. Life-threatening problems such as airway obstruction, circulatory collapse and shock, and hemorrhage will obviously be first priorities. However, physiological needs may not always have the highest priority. For example, a young child may refuse to eat and may become withdrawn when separated from his family. If the family meets the child's needs for security and affection, the physiological nutrition need will probably resolve.

Priorities are assigned in collaboration with the child and family. If the child or family members do not view the problem as a priority, little may be accomplished in trying to solve the problem. Differences between nurse and client priorities can be resolved through open communication; however, life-threatening and safety needs take precedence over client preferences.

Other factors also affect priority setting. Values held by the child and family, policies of the institution, finances, time and personnel requirements, and other resources necessary to achieve the client goals all have to be considered.

Planning

The planning phase of the nursing process is dependent on an adequate nursing assessment and valid nursing diagnoses. With these necessary steps completed, the nurse is ready to begin developing the nursing care plan. There are several actions which must take place during the planning phase.

1. Problems which can be resolved or lessened by nursing intervention are differentiated from those which must be referred to others, must include others for resolution, or can be managed by the child and family.
2. Short- and long-term goals for the child and family are developed collaboratively.
3. Alternative nursing interventions are considered, and specific ones are selected.
4. The care plan is written to include the nursing diagnoses, client goals, and nursing interventions.

Goal Setting

Client *goals,* are developed for each identified nursing diagnosis. The goal statement consists of the desired or realistically expected correction of the client's problem within a specified time period. The outcome will indicate specific criteria, in the form of client behaviors or clinical manifestations, that indicate that the problem is resolved or lessened or has been prevented.

Short-term and long-term goals need to be considered in the process of identifying client outcomes. Short-term goals (STGs) are the steps that lead to the attainment of long-term goals (LTGs); they are the immediate needs of the client. Long-term goals are the ultimate desired client behaviors and are usually stated in more general terms.

Formulation of Goal Statements

The goal statement contains the subject, verb, criteria of performance, and condition under which the client performs the outcome; in other words, the who, what, how, and when and the condition necessary for goal achievement. In reading the goal statement, it should be clear who the subject is. The *subject* may be the child or any part of the child, the parent, or another caregiver. It is not appropriate to designate the nurse in client outcome statements.

The *verb* specifies what behavior the client will perform. It should be written in positive, measurable terms. For example, verbs may include *walking, verbalizing, demonstrating, explaining,* and *reporting.* The nurse should avoid vague words like *knowing* or *understanding* and negative words like *not exceeding.*

In addition, the goal statement must indicate how the nurse will know when the performance has been satisfactorily accomplished. The how and when components of the statement are the *criteria* used for measurement of outcome. The how criterion can be compared with baseline data or with the results of ongoing monitoring. The criterion may specify how much, how far, how well, or how long. When—the time frame for attainment of the outcome—is essential in the evaluation of client progress. The statement may indicate when the goal is to be met by including such phrases as *within 1 week, upon completion of this module,* and *prior to discharge.*

One more item must be considered before the outcome statement is complete. The nurse must identify any special *conditions* affecting the performance of client behaviors. Examples of conditions may include the use of assistive devices (cane, eye-glasses, commode), specific dietary regimes (1200-cal diet, nutrition supplements), procedural techniques, family assistance, and personnel assistance and/or supervision.

Examples of goal statements follow.

The parent (subject) will demonstrate (verb) the preparation of insulin injections using aseptic technique by tomorrow afternoon (criteria).

Using the necessary equipment, the adolescent will

change the ostomy appliance according to the procedure taught prior to discharge.

Jim will walk the length of the unit corridor unassisted six times a day by the end of the week.

As nurses learn to assess, plan, and write orders to achieve specific goals, there is a danger of presuming to control the client's life. Regimens imposed on children and their families with the best intentions but without their participation in the planning are destined to a high rate of failure. Goals must be realistic, mutually planned, and valued by the child and family.

Implementation

When the expected outcomes (client goals) have been determined, the nurse is ready to develop the strategies or nursing interventions which will assist the child and family in achieving those outcomes. The nurse will draw upon her knowledge and experience to delineate alternative actions and select the strategies which will best solve the identified problem and effect the desired outcome. In addition, consideration will be given to the safety and comfort of the child, available staff and resources, time constraints, institutional policy, and client preference when safety permits.

Nursing interventions are written only for problems which can be solved with nursing care or problems which require the involvement of nursing and other disciplines. The interventions provide clear direction for the nursing staff in implementing care for the child and family.

Formulation of Nursing Intervention Statements

Nurses all too often use generalities on nursing care plans. Such phrases as *force fluids, turn and position,* and *ambulate client* are inadequate. Nursing intervention becomes haphazard when caregivers interpret the phrases differently. The nurse writing the intervention must clearly specify the action in writing.

Nursing interventions are statements containing a verb, recipient, objective, condition under which the nurse performs the action, and frequency and time indicators. The nursing intervention begins with an action *verb* identifying the behavior to be performed. Examples include *assess, encourage, discuss, record, assist,* and *supervise.* The *recipient* of the action is specified in the nursing intervention unless it is clearly understood to be the child. Family members or significant others may be recipients of nursing interventions. The *objective* describes what is to be assessed, encouraged, discussed, and so on. Skin integrity, fruit juice, and dressing procedures are examples of objective measures. The intervention should indicate the *conditions* (how) under which the action is to be performed, for example, "using a flashlight" or "according to injection site rotation chart." The *frequency* and specific *time* at which the action is to be carried out should be stated in the intervention statement. Phrases such as "daily" and "every shift" are inadequate. Times should be stated as clock hours, in relation to other activities ("prior to meals" or "during bath"), or with phrases such as *on even hours.*

The following are examples of complete nursing intervention statements:

Using a flashlight (condition), assess (verb) skin integrity beneath cast (objective) bid (frequency), at 8 A.M. and 8 P.M. (time).

This evening, discuss with parents sterile dressing procedures according to procedure manual for home care of central venous catheter.

The Care Plan

The nursing care plan is intended as a communication tool for other members of the health care team. The care plan facilitates the decisions the nurse has made with the client and practitioners of other disciplines. Written care plans avoid duplication and omission of client problems and nursing actions. They also document the nursing care provided for clients and their families.

The major components of the care plan are the identified problems or nursing diagnoses, the client goals or expected outcomes with deadlines, and the nursing interventions. The content of the care plan should be individualized to meet the specific needs of the child and family and should be consistent with the total plan of care. The amount of information that is required for each care plan will depend on the complexity of the client's problems.

The format of the care plan may vary but should be easily accessible and organized to be used effectively by those providing nursing care in a given agency or institution. The care plan should be as clear and concise as possible but should have space for needed information. One nurse must assume responsibility for writing the care plan, including all necessary updates and/or revisions. In some institutions nursing care plans are written in ink, signed by the accountable nurse, and accepted as part of the client's legal medical record.

Standard Care Plans

As nurses care for children and their families, the individual approach is vital to excellence in nursing practice. However, care can be standardized for selected types of clients or for given common problems and teaching needs. The standard care plan has its greatest value when used for children and families for whom no unusual problems are anticipated. For example, nursing care of a school-age child who undergoes a routine appendectomy may be planned and implemented using a standard care plan. The postoperative monitoring is routine, diet and ambulation progress is expected, and discharge planning requires only a follow-up check by the physician. The standard care plan should contain an area for individual client preferences in order to personalize the care. Standard care plans can facilitate planning, conserve time, and ensure quality nursing care.

Implementing the Plan

The *implementation* step of the nursing process begins once the nursing care plan has been developed. The planning phase is the responsibility of the nurse in collaboration with the client and family. Implementation of the plan may involve the nurse, the child, the family, and significant others. The giving of nursing care, continuing data collection, and documenting the care plan are the three components of implementation.

Giving Nursing Care

The nurse will utilize her intellectual, technical, and interpersonal skills, along with creativity ingenuity, to implement the nursing care plan. In the pediatric setting, adapting a given action to the age and cognitive level of the individual child is particularly important. A sound knowledge of growth and development is vital to the implementation of safe, effective care with an approach that makes the experience as positive as possible for the child and family. Specific strategies which work well for an individual child should be documented and become part of the nursing care plan. For example, a young child's intake of fluids may be facilitated if lines are drawn on a cup or if the child has another concrete way of assessing his own progress. Ingenuity and creativity, while necessary for all clients, are essential components of implementing nursing care in a pediatric setting.

Note: Nursing care plan 5-1 is not all-inclusive. With an ongoing assessment of Lisa's status, her responses to the interventions implemented, and her family's reactions, the care plan will need to be evaluated, revised, and expanded. Additional diagnoses, goals, nursing intervention, and evaluations will be necessary for postoperative and home-care planning.

Continuing Data Collection

During the implementation phase the nurse uses her skills of observation and listening to continue collecting data about the child and family. The expression of feelings and responses to nursing interventions provide information for determining progress, identifying new problems, reordering priorities, and altering the care plan if necessary.

Documenting the Care Plan

Documentation of nursing interventions and of the child's and family's responses is necessary from a legal standpoint, from a communication standpoint, and for the evaluation of nursing care as it relates to the attainment of client goals. Client responses and nursing actions must be recorded in a meaningful manner.

Flow Sheets

Many routine and repeated nursing actions can be easily documented on a flow sheet or treatment sheet. Actions such as baths, vital signs, dressing changes, mouth care, and urine tests performed on a regular basis can be quickly documented in this manner. Time is conserved,

NURSING CARE PLAN 5-1

Identifying data: Lisa, B., 21 mo (11/8/85), white, female

Date of admission: 8/3/87

Admitting Diagnosis: Left congenital hip dysplasia

Chief complaint: Mother reports Lisa is coming into the hospital for traction therapy and an operation on her hip.

History of present illness: At 15 mo of age, Lisa was noted by neighbors to be limping and occasionally falling, and they questioned the possibility that one leg was shorter than the other. The parents took Lisa to their local pediatrician, who referred them to an orthopedist. X-rays were taken, and the family was referred to the medical center for treatment.

Past health history: Developmental milestones have been met at normal times, with walking occurring at 13 mo. Bilateral myringotomy tubes were placed in her ears at 10 mo of age because of recurrent serous otitis media. There have been no subsequent problems. There are probable allergies to penicillin, ampicillin, and disposable diapers; rash and itching have been noted after their use. Immunizations are up-to-date.

Family history: The paternal grandfather has a history of diabetes mellitus and kidney stones, the father had amblyopia, and a paternal second cousin had "some kind of hip problem." History is negative for other problems.

Functional health patterns

Health perception–health management: The mother's pregnancy, labor, and delivery were uneventful. Lisa was born 3 weeks prematurely, weighing 2.7 kg. There were no prenatal problems.

Nutrition-metabolic: Current weight is 11.0 kg, her appetite is usually good, breakfast is her best meal, and most foods are accepted well. Lisa uses a cup without assistance and uses a spoon but prefers finger feeding.

Elimination: Toilet training has not started. Diapers are changed approximately 6 to 8 times per day, of which 1 to 2 have soft-formed stool.

Activity-exercise: Walking very well, runs awkwardly with occasional falls, likes to turn pages in book, "dance" to music, throw ball, play with blocks, and assist with dressing.

Sleep-rest: Lisa sleeps about 10 hours at night (8:30 P.M. to 6:30 A.M.), takes an afternoon nap of 1 to 2 hours, and sometimes takes a morning nap. Bedtime routines consist of a story while being held and tucked in with her doll and teddy bear.

Cognitive-perceptual: Says several words and uses 2- to 3-word phrases. Points to body parts and familiar objects in picture books.

Self-perception–self-concept: "Lisa insists on doing things herself." Does not like to share toys with her friends.

Role relationship: Lisa lives with her father (age 29), her mother (age 27), and her sister (age 4) in a small town 75 miles from the medical center. The mother reports that Lisa plays well with her sister and has been an easy child to care for. She has not been separated from her parents except for short periods with a baby-sitter while parents went out in the evening. The mother plans to room-in with Lisa, the father will visit weekly, and the grandparents will care for Lisa's older sister.

Sexuality-reproductive: Lisa frequently imitates mother's behavior at home (e.g., clean house, cook). Parents have observed occasional periods of genital self-stimulation, which they ignore or divert attention to another activity.

Coping–stress tolerance: Continues to use the word "no" frequently, has temper tantrums (screams, hits, kicks) when she does not get her own way. Mother usually removes her from the situation and tries to ignore Lisa until behavior has subsided.

Value-belief: Baptized Catholic, attends church regularly with parents and sister.

Physical assessment: The exam was within normal limits except for (1) bilateral myringotomy tubes, (2) left leg 0.6 cm shorter than right, and (3) limited abduction of left hip.

Parents' understanding of the treatment plan: Parents state they know Lisa is to be in traction for several days and that she is to have hip surgery followed by a long time in a cast. They voice concerns about how she will adapt to all of this.

1. Split Russell's traction, probably 2 to 3 weeks
2. Arthrogram after approximately 14 days in traction
3. Surgical correction of dislocated hip
4. Hip spica cast for 6 months or longer
5. Eye and ENT consultations to rule out amblyopia and check ears

---

and the progress note will indicate any change or deviation related to an identified problem. The nurse must decide which problems are appropriate for flow sheet records, which data to include, and the frequency of monitoring. For example, many of the nursing care actions and findings in monitoring physiological stability can be easily documented on flow sheets (Table 5-5). In most institutions vital signs are recorded on a standard form. In the pediatric setting an intake and output form should also be used to record hourly measurements of intravenous therapy, nasogastric feedings, and the like.

Progress Notes

The information necessary for documenting progress or lack of progress toward outcome achievement is recorded in a narrative progress note. The use of a problem-oriented system facilitates the writing of meaningful nursing documentation. The progress notes may be part of an

DEVELOPMENT OF NURSING DIAGNOSES

Client's Strengths	Client's Problems:	Nursing Analysis	Nursing Diagnosis

Immunizations up-to-date
 	
Adequate nutrition
	Possible allergies
	  Penicillin
	  Ampicillin
	  Disposable diapers
		With multiple allergies, the potential for the appearance of additional allergies increases. The nurse infers that there is a potential problem of an allergic response, but the statement lacks an etiology; therefore, it is not a nursing diagnosis.	

Active Adequate rest Mother rooming-in	History of ear infections, bilateral tubes in ears Paternal history of amblyopia	With a previous history of serous otitis media and a paternal history of amblyopia, there may be a potential problem of these two sensory deficits. However, gross vision and hearing tests are normal, language is appropriate for age; therefore, the nurse awaits the results of the eye and ENT consults before considering either to be a problem.	
	Exerts independence with "no" and temper tantrums	Although Lisa's mother is planning to room-in, the mother fears that events will prevent her from holding and cuddling her child, especially at this age (21 mo), and may interfere with the normal parent-child relationship. Lisa will be in traction 14 to 21 days, then will have a hip spica cast applied following surgery. Mother fears that Lisa's responses to immobility may alter their usual pleasant relationship.	Parental role conflict related to separation from child due to illness
	Parental concerns about hospital procedures and child's adaptation to traction and cast	During the admission interview, the nurse realizes that Lisa's parents lack in-depth knowledge about the diagnostic and surgical procedures to be performed. They are unable to project the problems they may encounter in caring for Lisa during and after hospitalization.	Knowledge deficit, related to parents' lack of information about hip dysplasia and its treatment

Note: The initially identified priorities relate to to helping the toddler and mother cope with the hospitalization and imposed immobility. The first two diagnoses are interrelated. The interventions for them are aimed at attaining the ultimate outcome of minimizing the effects of hospitalization: immobility, surgery, casting, which affects the parentations is identified as the next level of priority, and the expected outcome is that there will be no complications.

Client's Strengths	Client's Problems:	Nursing Analysis	Nursing Diagnosis
	Left left 0.6 cm shorter than right leg, limited abduction of left hip	The physician's treatment plan calls for the use of Russell's traction followed by surgical repair and application of a hip spica cast. All these treatments interfere with Lisa's mobility. The nurse recognizes the multiple physiological effects of immobility and the potential complications that can result. In this case, a broad diagnosis is phrased with several subheadings.	Potential impaired skin integrity related to immobility Potential constipation related to immobility Potential altered tissue perfusion related to immobility Potential loss of motor function secondary to pressure on nerves in legs related to immobility

Nursing Diagnosis	Client Goals	Nursing Orders	Evaluation
1. Parental role conflict related to separation from child due to illness	LTG: The parent and child will maintain a positive attachment and trust relationship throughout the period of hospitalization. STG: Lisa will exhibit behaviors expected of a toddler during the protest phase of separation (crying, tantrums, negativism). STG: Parents will verbalize feelings and concerns about the effects of hospitalization and treatment on Lisa. STG: Parents will participate in Lisa's care. STG: Parents will verbalize feelings of satisfaction about their role in care and Lisa's ongoing response to them.	1. Foster a positive rooming-in experience for mother throughout period of hospitalization 2. Encourage weekly visition by father and sibling and grandparent visits once or twice during hospitalization 3. Encourage family photographs, drawings, audiotape recordings, and favorite objects from home (toys, blankets, clothes). 4. Provide simple, truthful explanations to Lisa. 5. Provide parents with time and privacy to verbalize their feelings and concerns on a weekly basis, every Saturday. 6. Include parents in bathing, feeding, and playing with Lisa every day. 7. Discuss Lisa's response to immobility and treatment as behaviors are anticipated or occur. 8. Provide positive feedback for parent involvement in and success with Lisa's care.	8/4—Mother oriented to unit. 8/4—Father unable to visit this week. 8/10—Mother stated that Lisa has done better than she expected and that she was pleased with Lisa's response to her care. 8/8—Lisa continues to protest separation from parents for treatments or procedures and clings to mother afterward.

Nursing Diagnosis	Client Goals	Nursing Orders	Evaluation
2. Knowledge deficit related to parents' lack of information about congenital hip dysplasia and its treatment	LTG: Parents will correctly describe Lisa's condition and treatment regimen. STG: Parents will verbalize an understanding of congenital hip dysplasia and of diagnostic and surgical procedures within 2 weeks. STG: Parents will verbalize an understanding of post-operative and home care for a child in a spica cast prior to discharge.	1. Assess parents' current understanding of diagnosis and treatment within next 2 days. 2. Correct any misinformation and misunderstandings on an ongoing basis. 3. Provide explanations and literature about Lisa's condition and treatment by 8/7/87. 4. Answer questions and refer to physician as appropriate. 5. Content will include (a) Routine hospitalization and traction care. (b) Diagnostic procedures (laboratory and radiology studies) (c) Perioperative procedures, postoperative care, and pain management (d) Spica cast and Bradford frame hospital and home care	8/5—Mother able to repeat information concerning Lisa's condition and diagnostic procedures. States she shares this information with husband over the telephone. 8/5—Mother assisting with bathing and feeding of Lisa. 8/7—Mother performing skin care to lower extremities when Lisa is out of traction.
Potential impaired skin integrity related to immobility Potential constipation related to immobility Potential altered tissue perfusion related to immobility Potential loss of motor function secondary to pressure on nerves in legs related to immobility	LTG: Lisa will be physiologically stable throughout the period of immobility in traction. STG: Vital signs will be within the normal ranges for Lisa as measured every 8 h. STG: Toes will be pink and warm with brisk capillary filling when tested every 4 h. STG: Skin will be pink, warm, and intact upon daily observation during bath. STG: Lisa will maintain a fluid intake of 1000 ml daily. STG: Lisa will have soft-formed stool daily.	1. Measure vital signs at 0900, 1500, and 2100 hours. 2. Perform neurovascular check of lower extremities every 4 h at 0100, 0500, 0900, 1300, 1700, and 2100 hours. 3. Check all skin areas during bath. 4. Keep sheepskin under child when in traction. 5. Remove traction tid (1 h for bath and 30 min at two other times as determined in planning with mother); while out of traction, give skin care and massage lower extremities. 6. Give daily fluids to an intake of at least 1000 ml. Record intake and output. Measure specific gravity every shift. 7. Check with mother and record daily stools at 0900.	8/6—Vital signs table. 8/4—Toes pink, warm, brisk capillary filling, able to move all and respond to touch. 8/7—Skin is warm, pink, and intact. 8/7—Intake adequate, specific gravity 1.014. 8/7—Lisa's having difficulty with bowel movements. Prune juice and high-fiber foods added to diet. Daily stool softener prescribed.

TABLE 5-5 Treatment Flow Sheet

Treatment	Problem #	8/4/87	8/5/87	8/6/87
1. Neurovascular check q 4 h at 0100, 0500, 0900, 1300, 1700, 2100	3	JS JS PT 01 05 09 PT 13		
Toes pink and warm		+ + + +		
Capillary filling		+ + + +		
Movement		+ + + +		
2. Skin check (intactness) daily during bath	3	JS 09 +		
3. Traction off for skin car tid 0900-1000, 1230-1300, 1930-2000	3	JS 09-10		
4. Check for daily BM (normal consistency)	3	JS 09		

overall formal problem-oriented medical record system or part of the nursing documentation system. In either system documentation relates to the identified nursing diagnoses and client goals. The progress note is written documentation of the child's and family's responses to nursing intervention and provides current information in a continuous, ongoing form. Each progress note should relate to a specific problem (by number and title) and should contain client and family responses, additional data obtained, assessment of status, and ongoing plans for intervention. Thus, progress notes usually contain four specific parts: (1) subjective data, (2) objective data, (3) assessment statement, and (4) plan. The four parts are designated by the acronym SOAP.

Subjective data (S) should include data reported by the child and family in relation to feelings, thoughts about care or problems, requests for action, or observations they have made. Verbal reports may be written as quotes where applicable or as interpretations of reports from the child and family. Examples are "I want my Mommy," and "I like apple juice."

Objective data (O) should include data which the nurse observes or measures in a quantitative way. Examples are weight, vital signs, physical examination findings, frequency of pain medications, laboratory results, and size of a decubitus ulcer.

The *assessment statement* (A) is a summary of the nurse's thoughts about the specific problem. It is the cognitive analysis of current data to determine client progress and effectiveness of intervention, providing the basis for ongoing evaluation. It should not be confused with the nursing process assessment component of data collection. Examples include "Client correctly demonstrated three-point crutch-walking gait" and "Increased parental anxiety regarding finances, receptive to social service visit."

The *plan* (P) section should indicate continuation of the present plan if it is deemed effective, identify the need for additional data collection to delineate the problem or management, state additional plans for nursing intervention, or indicate a change in the plan. Examples include "Assess parental motivation and readiness to care for child on peritoneal dialysis," "Teach child to test own urine for sugar and acetone," "Check results of blood drug levels,"

TABLE 5-6 SOAP Note

8-17-87	#4	Obesity
1000	S:	"I'm not as hungry anymore. I can eat a lot of things I like but not as much."
	O:	Weight 79.4 kg down from 82.3 kg on admission. No longer seeks food between meals.
	A:	Losing weight on 1200-cal diet and exercise program.
	P:	Continue present plan. Acknowledge weight loss with verbal praise.

and "Continue present plan." The signature and title of the person writing the note completes the progress note. An example of a narrative SOAP note is given in Table 5-6. Examples of Progress Notes for Lisa are:

8-8-87 #1 Potential alteration of parent-child relationship
1400
S: "I feel more comfortable taking care of her in the traction." "She sure likes to be held when she's out of traction."
O: Mother bathing, changing, and feeding Lisa. Lisa cuddles, smiles, talks, and plays with mother when held. Cries and clings to mother when nurse or physician comes close to her.
A: Parent-child interaction positive. Lisa's response to caregivers normal for age.
P: Continue plan as outlined

M. Brown, R.N.

Discharge Summary

In any setting, the child and family must have a nursing evaluation and statement of status at discharge. The summary should identify continuing problems, indicate the level of understanding about home care management, state to whom referrals are being made, say whether return appointments are necessary and when, and identify other special arrangements such as telephone follow-up.

Evaluation

The evaluative process involves comparing a measurement with a standard or norm and making a decision about the relationship (Mager, 1973, p. 8). Client goals serve as standards for evaluating the child's and family's responses to the plan of care. The nurse determines the extent to which client goals have been achieved.

Formulation of Evaluative Statements

An evaluative statement consists of two components: (1) the extent to which the client has achieved the goal and (2) the expected outcome which supports this achievement. The nurse determines the level of client achievement. At the time specified in the goal statement, the nurse will state whether the goal has been met, partially met, or not met and include the child's and family's responses to validate this assessment.

Examples of evaluative statements (based on the previous examples of goal statements) follow.

Goal partially met, mother demonstrated the preparation of insulin injections using aseptic technique, father was unable to attend practice session.

Goal met, adolescent changed ostomy appliance using correct procedure and equipment.

Goal unmet, Jim refuses to walk unit corridor.

Formative Evaluation

Formative evaluation is an ongoing process. As the nurse implements the care plan, the client's responses to the plan are evaluated. If the goal has been met and the problem has been resolved, the nurse indicates this in writing on the care plan and discontinues related nursing actions. However, if the nursing diagnosis has not been resolved even though the goals have been met or if the goals have been partially met or are unmet, reassessment of the care plan must always be done. Using problem solving, the nurse determines why the nursing diagnosis has not been resolved. All five of the nursing process steps are examined to decide if they are appropriate. Questions the nurse should explore during this reassessment phase are listed in Table 5-7. After this, the care plan will be revised, reimplemented, and reevaluated, enhancing the continuous nature of the nursing process.

Summative Evaluation

The summative, or final, evaluation of client outcomes is reflected in the discharge summary. Goals to be attained before the time of discharge are determined by the client and nurse. The status of the client in relation to goal achievement must be considered at the time of discharge if appropriate follow-up care is to be determined. The

evaluation will indicate problem resolution and/or identify new and continuing nursing diagnoses. This information can then be communicated to the community health nurse or other health care provider or agency as a basis for ongoing postdischarge intervention.

Learning Activities

1. Select two or three charts of hospitalized children. Read the admission histories and critique them for clarity and comprehensiveness.
2. Develop several questions to be used in a functional health pattern assessment tool for adolescents.
3. Compare and contrast three different pediatric nursing assessment tools.
4. For your assigned clients, identify their strengths and weaknesses, determine appropriate nursing diagnostic statements, and prioritize.
5. Evaluate the nursing care plan and progress notes of one client. Choose one nursing diagnosis and search for evidence of
   a) Client and family involvement in planning
   b) Determination of achievable outcomes
   c) Criteria which will reflect goal attainment
   d) Progress notes which reflect ongoing assessment of client progress
   e) Solution or referral of the problem
6. Interview a community health nurse to determine what information is expected from the referral source and whether it is usually sent with the referral of children and their families.

Study Questions

1. Which component of the nursing process is represented when the nurse measures a client's vital signs upon admission?
   A. Assessment. C. Intervention.
   B. Planning. D. Evaluation.
2. The results of a client's vital signs represent which kind of data?
   A. Subjective. C. Ancillary.
   B. Objective. D. Personal.
3. Nursing diagnosis is a statement that describes a client's:
   A. Pathological condition.
   B. Potential strengths.
   C. Health problem.
   D. Desired outcome.
4. Client situations which may cause difficulty in the future are referred to as:
   A. Potential health problems.
   B. Actual health problems.
   C. Probable health problems.
   D. Valid health problems.

TABLE 5-7 Reassessment Questions for Revisions

Was the initial assessment incomplete or inaccurate?
Did the nurse correctly identify the client's health care needs?
Were there incorrect or omitted nursing diagnoses?
Were the goals inappropriate or unrealistic for the client?
Were the nursing interventions ineffective or inappropriate?
Was the evaluation of the client's responses accurate?

5. Which of the following is an example of a correctly written nursing diagnosis?
   A. Inability to purposefully move within the physical environment.
   B. Impaired physical mobility related to traction
   C. Traction related to a motor vehicle accident.
   D. Peripheral vascular assessment for uncompensated musculoskeletal impairment.

6. The components of a goal statement include the client, a verb, a condition, and:
   A. An action.   C. A characteristic.
   B. An etiology.   D. A criterion.

7. The written nursing care plan should be completed *prior* to which step of the nursing process?
   A. Assessment.   C. Implementation.
   B. Planning.   D. Evaluation.

8. The purpose of evaluation is to:
   A. Ensure that the diagnosis is related to the health problem.
   B. Decide whether the goal has been attained.
   C. Determine whether nursing actions were performed correctly.
   D. Document the nursing care being given.

References

Atkinson, L.D., and M.E. Murray: *Understanding the Nursing Process,* Macmillan, New York, 1983.

Gordon, M: "Nursing Diagnosis and the Diagnostic Process," *American Journal of Nursing,* 76(8):1298-1300, 1976.

————: *Nursing Diagnosis: Process and Application,* 2d ed., McGraw-Hill, New York, 1987a.

————: *Manual of Nursing Diagnosis 1986-1987,* McGraw-Hill, New York, 1987b.

Griffith-Kenney, J., and P.J. Christensen: *Nursing Process: Application of Theories, Frameworks, and Models,* 2d ed., Mosby, St. Louis, 1986.

Korsch, B.M., and E.F. Aley: "Pediatric Interviewing Techniques," *Current Problems in Pediatrics,* 3(7):3-42, 1973.

Mager, R.F.: *Measuring Instructional Intent,* Fearon, Belmont, Calif., 1973.

Mayers, M.G.: *A Systematic Approach to the Nursing Care Plan,* 3d ed., Appleton-Century-Crofts, East Norwalk, Conn., 1983.

McLane, A., K. McFarland, and M. Kim: *Classification of Nursing Diagnosis: Proceedings of the Seventh National Conference,* Mosby, St. Louis, 1987.

Bibliography

Alfaro, R.: *Application of Nursing Process: A Step-by-Step Guide,* Lippincott, Philadelphia, 1986.

American Nurses' Association: *Standards of Nursing Practice,* American Nurses' Association, Kansas City, Mont., 1973.

Dossey, B., and C.E. Guzzetta: "Nursing Diagnosis," *Nursing 81,* 11(6):34-38, 1981.

Fortin, J., and J. Rainbow: "Legal Implications to Nursing Diagnosis," *Nursing Clinics of North America,* 14(3):553-561, 1979.

Mager, R.F.: *Preparing Instructional Objectives,* 2d ed., David S. Lake, Calif., 1984.

Marriner, A.: *The Nursing Process: A Scientific Approach to Nursing Care,* 3d ed., Mosby, St. Louis, 1983.

6

Physical Assessment

Objectives

After reading this chapter, the student will be able to:
1. Discuss the developmental approach for performing physical assessments in the pediatric population.
2. Discuss the importance of length and weight measurements in relation to head circumference measurements.
3. List the historical questions that pertain to each body system.
4. Describe and list the normal findings for each system of the body.
5. Demonstrate the use of distraction in performing physical assessments of children at different ages.

The physical assessment of a child is one of many sources that provide the health team with data about the child and his present health status. If done properly, it will be the objective documentation of the subjective information obtained through the interview of the child and his family. However, if not done properly, it most likely will lead to a frustrating experience for the child, the family, and the nurse performing the physical assessment, thus creating a negative experience for the child and family and lessening the likelihood of obtaining accurate information. Reliable information from the interview and physical assessment is essential to the identification of an accurate problem list and nursing diagnosis that will allow the health care providers to implement appropriate plans and interventions. Without these steps, the accuracy of the evaluation and any subsequent interventions can be questioned. In this section physical assessment of children at the various development stages are described as a means of making the assessment experience a positive one for the child, his family, and the nurse.

The Art of Physical Assessment of the Child

Physical assessment of the child is accomplished through the use of play, observation, auscultation, palpation, and percussion. A physical assessment that is performed in conjunction with appropriate age-related play most likely will lead to a positive interaction with a cooperative child and his parents. If a child is frightened or is constantly moving, it may be difficult to distinguish between normal and abnormal findings. Observations should be started from the time the child enters the health care environment.

Unlike observation, the interview may or may not start at the point of entrance of the child and family into the health care environment. In the majority of instances the interview will begin in the examining room and will be extended during the physical assessment as a means of obtaining information and a way to develop rapport with the child and family. Observation and interview are difficult to separate since observation is one of the means by which the nurse documents information regarding the child's and parent's responses to certain questions and statements. It is also used to collect data about the interaction between the child and family. Finally, observation is used to determine the ways in which the child reacts to the specific techniques used during his physical examination.

General Considerations and Rules in the Physical Examination

Physical examination of the child is a very involved, unique skill. Much of it can be carried out while the nurse interviews the parent, in the child's presence—just by observing the child and his actions and reactions to the environment and the individuals in the environment. At the start of the actual examination, the age of the child and his previous experience with examinations must be taken into consideration in order to determine what part of the body to inspect first and to decide whether the child is to be held on his mother's lap (Table 6-1). If developmental milestones are taken into consideration, one should be able to eliminate the anxiety that many children go through when the privacy of their bodies is intruded upon. The nurse should not assume that the child will not be embarrassed or frightened by having a physical examination performed.

The significant difference between the examination of an adult and that of a child is that the basis of the entire physical examination of the child is growth and development. The nurse should know the changes a child goes through at different stages of development and their significance in identifying normal and abnormal characteristics during the examination. At no time should the child be considered a small adult.

Realizing that any approach toward the child may precipitate a crying spell, the examiner must keep in mind that the time to elicit as much information as possible is while the child is feeling calm and not threatened. For example, while the child is sitting in the security of his parent's lap, the examiner may want to count respirations, watch for color changes, and observe developmental tasks. Conversely, the examination of the newborn may start with auscultation of the chest and heart so that an accurate examination can be done before the neonate is awakened and starts crying. The examination of a young child begins with the least threatening part of his body, for example, the extremities, and proceeds to the most threatening. The examination of an older school-age child or adolescent can be performed in a systematic manner very similar to that used with an adult. In all interactions with the pediatric client, the examiner should bear in mind that the age of the child and/or the developmental level determines the approach to be taken.

Before making any attempt to perform the examination, there are certain rules to be followed.

1. The examination room should be decorated with bright colors and pictures that are familiar to children.
2. Age-appropriate toys should be used before an interview and exam are begun as well as throughout the interview and history.
3. A toy, such as a hand puppet, can be used with infants, toddlers, and preschoolers as a means of gaining cooperation during the use of certain instruments (Fig. 6-1).
4. Rattles or keys can be used as a means of gaining an infant's cooperation.
5. It is helpful to encourage mothers to have a child bring his favorite stuffed animal or doll so that certain examination techniques can be demonstrated on it.
6. A calm, unhurried manner during the interview and examination is reassuring to the child and his parents.
7. Abrupt and quick, jerky movements should be avoided.
8. The nurse should interact with the patient throughout the examination. Children of all ages enjoy such interaction, and it is a good distractor.
9. During the examination, the examiner's smiling face can help allay fears.
10. It is important to maintain eye contact with children while talking to them, although avoidance of eye contact with an older infant may be necessary in order to stop his crying.
11. The parent is allowed to undress and dress an infant or young toddler so that the nurtse can observe their interactions.
12. The examination is performed in accordance with developmental levels, starting with the least distressing

TABLE 6-1 An Approach to the Routine Physical Examination

Physical Examination*	Approach

0-4 Months

Physical Examination*	Approach
1. Observe general appearance, body proportions, and development	Approach while infant is asleep or quiet
2. Observe color and respirations	
3. Count respirations, auscultate heart, count apical pulse, auscultate chest	
4. Palpate anterior and posterior fontanels	Place infant in parent's arms
5. Measure head circumference	
6. Palpate abdomen and femoral pulses	Give infant bottle; have infant supine on table or in parent's lap
7. Examine genitalia and rectum	
8. Examine eyes, ears, nose, mouth, and throat	Place infant in parent's arms or supine on table
9. Examine extremities	Observe and examine infant on table
10. Test CNS development; test primary reflexes	

4-12 Months

Physical Examination*	Approach
1. Observe general appearance, body proportions, and development	Place infant in parent's lap; distract infant with bottle, rattle, or toy
2. Observe color and respirations	
3. Auscultate heart and chest	Place infant first in upright position in parent's lap and then lying down
4. Palpate anterior and posterior fontanels and measure head circumference	
5. Examine abdomen, genitalia, and rectum	Examine in parent's lap
6. Examine eyes, ears, nose, mouth, and throat	
7. Test CNS development	

1-3 Years

Physical Examination*	Approach
1. Observe for general appearance, body proportions, and development	Allow child to play with familiar tools, e.g., tongue blade, flashlight, stethoscope, or toy
2. Examine extremities and nervous system	
3. Examine neck	Have child in parent's lap or walking in examining room; allow child to have a security object and to be in parent's lap or on examining table
4. Examine chest and heart	
5. Examine abdomen	
6. Examine genitalia and rectum	Use parent's and examiner's laps before using the examining table for examination of the abdomen and genitalia and, in some cases, eyes, ears, nose, throat, and mouth.
7. Examine head, eyes, ears, nose, throat, and mouth	

3-6 Years

Physical Examination*	Approach
1. Evaluate nervous system development	Talk to the child
2. Examine head, neck, chest, heart, abdomen, extremities	Use flattery
3. Examine genitalia, urinary meatus, and rectum	Allow child to sit in parent's lap if so desired
	Use familiar instruments, e.g., stethoscope
	Allow child to play with instruments

6-9 Years

Physical Examination*	Approach
Perform physical examination in orderly fashion with genitourinary and rectal last	Let patient choose whether parents should remain in room
	Use flattery
	Ask child questions
	Familiarize patient with instruments
	Encourage cooperation

9 Years-Adolescence

Physical Examination*	Approach
Perform physical examination in orderly fashion with genitourinary and rectal last	Let patient choose whether parents should remain in room
	Ask patient questions
	Educate patient regarding body, instruments, and findings
	Encourage patient to ask questions or talk about himself and his activities

*Developmental assessment is done throughout entire history and physical examination and should be used first on physical examination for building rapport. Patient and/or parents are educated regarding body, instruments, examination, and findings throughout physical.

Source: M. U. Barnard et al., *Handbook of Comprehensive Pediatric Nursing,* McGraw-Hill, New York, 1981, p. 25.

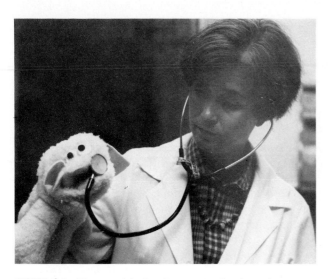

FIGURE 6-1   The use of the hand puppet in the physical examination. *(Courtesy of Molly U. McKinley.)*

activities and ending with the most distressing or embarrassing tasks (Table 6-1).

13. Older toddlers, preschoolers, and early school-age children should be allowed to undress and dress themselves so that the nurse can observe important developmental tasks.

14. The examination room should have furniture that allows the examiner to interact with the child patient at eye level. At times it helps if the examiner interacts with the child while being at a lower level than the child (Fig. 6-2).

15. A second opinion is always sought for any positive findings on physical examination as well as for any questionable findings.

16. Education and age-appropriate anticipatory guidance are provided throughout the physical examination. The examiner describes what she is doing and what will follow. It is also helpful to help the parents anticipate the type of physical assessment to expect at the next visit and the type of response to expect from the child. For example, when examining a cooperative 6-month-old infant, it may be helpful to tell the parent, "Because infants become frightened of strangers at around eight months, you might expect Tommy to cry and be more frightened of these procedures and of me at his nine-month well-baby check."

17. Cold hands are warmed before the examination begins.

Young Infant: 2 Weeks to 6 Months

Much of the objective information that is needed from a young infant can be obtained while he is in his parent's arms, whether asleep, awake, or feeding. In this position the infant is warm, secure, and most likely comfortable. At the same time the parent may feel he or she has some control of the bodily intrusion being experienced by the baby.

Observation of the baby during this time produces information about parent-infant interactive qualities and about the presence of pain and/or tenderness which may be experienced by the infant during invasive procedures. Vital signs, such as the respiratory rate, can be taken while the newborn is at rest; the nurse should also observe any color change, retractions, nasal flaring, or restlessness. Range of motion of the extremities is also noted at this time.

Auscultation of a young infant's chest can be accomplished while he is in the security of his parent's arms. A receiving blanket can be wrapped around an exposed chest so that the infant is kept warm, and the chest can be exposed without much intrusion. *Auscultation* is the technique of listening with either the naked ear or a stethoscope. Obviously, if the child is comfortable and not crying, the examiner will hear better. Any audible wheezing, congestion, hyperperistalsis, etc., can be detected by sitting on a low stool (Fig. 6-2) next to the parent's chair so that the examiner is at the level of the lap in which the baby is sitting. At this same time, retractions can be detected and the respiratory rate can be counted.

Palpation, the technique of applying the hands to parts of the patient's body to determine underlying deviations from the normal, can be done very successfully while the infant is feeding, resting, or sleeping in his parent's arms. In general, palpation follows observation. An exception is examination of the abdomen, in which case it follows observation and auscultation. The young infant's abdomen can be observed, auscultated, and lightly palpated while he is quiet in his parent's lap. A much deeper palpation can be performed after the infant is placed on the examination table. Another approach to examining the abdomen of a young infant is simply to place him on the examining table with the parent standing next to the examiner. The parent then interacts with the infant while the examination is carried out. This also is an excellent time for the examiner to role-model interactive skills with

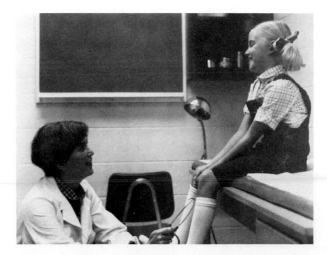

FIGURE 6-2   Use of a stool by the examiner to be at a lower level than the child. *(Courtesy of Molly U. McKinley.)*

the infant as well as provide education and anticipatory guidance for the parent.

Older Infant: 6 to 12 Months

The smiling, cooperative, cooing infant of the first 6 months of life may now turn into a crying, anxious, frightened client. The sequence of the examination is from the least frightening to the most frightening (Table 6-1). Most of the examination is performed while the infant is in the lap of a parent or familiar adult. Much time should be spent interacting with infants of this age through play so that rapport can be established. At this time the examiner should be on eye level with the infant and should constantly chatter in a low-pitched voice. Color, respiratory rate, and type of respiration can be observed simply by having the parent lift the undershirt of the infant or pull back a blanket or shirt that is wrapped around the upper torso. It is usually much better to have the parent take off the T-shirt at the beginning of the interview (history) than at the time of the examination. The infant does not seem to be as aware or frightened of the intrusion if it is done this way.

Any auscultation should be carried out in a slow manner, with constant chattering from the examiner. Distraction techniques can be used by either the examiner or the parent to lessen the fright associated with the stethoscope. The examiner should place the stethoscope on distal portions of the body first to demonstrate to the infant that the stethoscope does not hurt. The foot is a good site to place the head of the stethoscope first, followed by placing it up the leg at several points, such as mid-lower leg, knee, and midthigh. Usually the infant will then allow the examiner to listen to the front part of the chest. As the posterior part of the chest is examined, the infant may again question the objective of the examiner. The infant can be placed over the parent's shoulder with the parent or an assistant distracting him during the examination

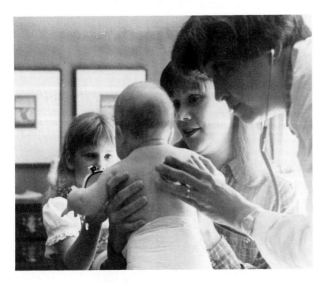

FIGURE 6-3 Distracting the infant when he is placed over the parent's shoulder. *(Courtesy of Molly U. McKinley.)*

(Fig. 6-3), or he can be placed sideways so that at all times he can watch the movements of the examiner. In some instances the examiner may have the parent place the stethoscope at certain points on the chest while the examiner makes the infant aware of the examiner's hands.

The examination of the abdomen follows and is performed in the same way as for the younger infant. However, if the infant will not allow the examiner to auscultate or palpate the abdomen, the examiner can again obtain the assistance of the parent, asking the parent to remain always in the sight of the infant. The parent can be asked to place the stethoscope lightly on the four quadrants of the abdomen, thus enabling the examiner to auscultate. If there is concern about tenderness, the parent can repeat the sequence with the stethoscope, pressing to see if any pain or tenderness is elicited. Following this maneuver, the nurse can perform a much deeper examination. In most instances the infant will have become accustomed to having his chest and abdomen touched. If crying occurs, deep abdominal palpation can be obtained with each inspiration. It is of the utmost importance that the parent remain within the infant's field of vision so that at no time will the infant think his parent has left him.

Toddler

As with the older infant, the least distressing procedures are carried out after some time is spent playing and talking with the toddler. Again, the use of the parent's lap may be necessary for the young toddler, but the older toddler may agree to be examined on the table. The key is to make sure the parent is at least physically near the toddler while the examination is being carried out. Being at eye level and explaining what will be done is of great importance, since the toddler's receptive language is more advanced than his expressive language.

As the physical examination progresses, the toddler should be allowed choices between things that are going to be done. For example, the nurse may ask, "Do you want me to look at your eyes or mouth first?" Having a choice allows the toddler to feel he has control over the situation. Nurses must guard against giving him a choice that cannot be fulfilled or asking him a question to which he may answer no.

Nudity may or may not be an issue; if it is, the toddler is allowed to remove or help remove the clothing that covers the part being examined. In this case the removal of the shoes and socks for examination of the feet should be the starting point, since this is obviously the least distressing point. The examination is then carried out as described in Table 6-1.

Preschooler

Because of the specific developmental tasks the preschooler is experiencing, the examiner should address the physical examination slowly and with much explanation along the way. The exam can usually take place on the examination table unless the preschooler is extremely frightened. If such a situation should arise, part of the examination can take place in the parent's lap.

When the child comes into the environment in which the examination will occur, it is important to decrease his fantasies, for example, by allowing him to play with the instruments that are being used, having him participate in the examination itself, and asking him to hold the stethoscope head or squeeze the bulb during the pneumoscopic examination of the ear. The examiner may also allow the preschooler to examine her, for example, look into her mouth, or to use the patellar reflex hammer on her. Each part of the examination should be explained very carefully so that at no time does the preschooler believe his body is being mutilated or that he is being punished for a wrongdoing.

If the preschooler is ill, an explanation is very important so that he does not think the illness is the result of wrongdoing. The use of the body outlines, along with simple explanations, is helpful in decreasing the chances that fantasy will take over the preschooler's thoughts about the examination.

The approach to the body parts varies from the approach used with infants and toddlers in that the examination can be done in a more orderly fashion, leaving the genitourinary and rectal exam for last. Certainly some preschoolers will react more like toddlers in the examination of their bodies; for them the approach taken with toddlers may have to be adopted.

Whether the preschooler will be modest depends on the individual. Some consider the examination a major intrusion, while others cooperate fully. Appropriate gowning and draping of the preschooler should be carried out on an individual basis.

Some examination techniques may be bothersome to preschoolers. During percussion of the thorax and abdomen they sometimes feel they are being hit. Demonstrating the technique on a desk or table may help alleviate this misconception. Palpation of the abdomen may be difficult in a ticklish patient. For ticklish children, much distracting conversation should be used while having the patient place both hands (with the fingers spread apart) on the abdomen. Palpation can take place between the fingers; this approach tends to lessen the ticklish response.

School-Age Child

The approach to the school-age child should take the privacy, modesty, and anxiety of the patient into account. Every opportunity should be taken to explain to the child what is being done, since most school-age children have little knowledge about their bodies but are eager to learn. The school-age child comprehends the components of the examination best with the use of body outlines, pictures, and the opportunity to familiarize himself with the instruments used as well as actually perform part of the physical assessment on the examiner, e.g., use the otoscope to look in the examiner's ears.

The examination proceeds from least embarrassing to most embarrassing; it can be performed in the presence of

the parents or without the parents, depending on the choice of the child. The examiner should not expect the school-age child to react to the examination as an adult would. This misconception is one of the most common mistakes made with children of this age.

Adolescent

Regard for an adolescent's independence and rapidly changing identity should be kept in mind as the examination is planned. Adolescents like to be considered old enough to be examined without the presence of a parent. However, the nurse should always give the adolescent the choice of whether he wants his parents present, since on occasion, especially in illness, he may want a familiar adult present during the exam.

Because of the adolescent's rapidly changing body image, the physical examination can serve as a time for education and reassurance that certain changes (or lack of change) are normal. Again, the use of visual aids is an excellent method of enhancing the adolescent's knowledge about his body. Since he is very interested in his physical and emotional changes, the time spent examining him provides an excellent opportunity for teaching him about health and wellness.

Summary

The approach to physical examination should be based on the age, development, level of wellness, and past experiences of the child with the health system. These considerations, along with the rules of the physical examination enumerated earlier in this chapter, should lead to a very informative and satisfying experience for all involved.

Performing the Physical Assessment
Linear Measurements: Height, Weight, and Head Circumference

Length/stature and weight should be measured and plotted on a standardized anthropometric chart (Figs. 2-5, 2-6, 2-8, and 2-9 in Chapter 2) at each physical assessment. These linear measurements are obtained at least five times during the first year of life and then yearly through adolescence. As a baseline, an initial assessment for length and weight should be performed on the newborn. The average length for a newborn infant is 46 to 51 cm (18 to 20 in); the male infant is on the average longer than the female. The average weight of the newborn infant ranges from 3175 to 3400 g (7 to 7½ lb). The male infant is usually heavier than the female. Weight is evaluated in relation to length. At no time can a 6-lb newborn be regarded as small for his age or an 8-lb newborn be considered heavy. Consideration must be given to the ratio of weight to length; only then can the full-term newborn be regarded as normal, heavy, thin, or malnourished. This ratio can be calculated according to Rohrer's ponderal index:

$$\frac{100 \times \text{weight in grams}}{(\text{Length in centimeters})^3}$$

The ponderal index describes how heavy the baby is for his length and age; larger numbers indicate a heavy baby for his length, and smaller numbers describe an infant who is thin for his length (Table 6-2).

Standardized charts demonstrate the growth profile of a patient over time and indicate whether the child maintains his own growth pattern on the growth grid. Any child who is plotted on the chart and is found to be in the 5th percentile or lower or in the 95th percentile or higher requires a careful evaluation. Length, weight, and head circumference must be evaluated in relation to one another. A careful assessment based on subjective and objective data should be made for growth tendency or for familial (parents and grandparents) tendency; nourishment; and heart, psychosocial, endocrine, renal, and metabolic problems. Normal growth covers a wide range and individual children tend to have growth spurts at different times. A child who has been in the 5th percentile all his life may be found to be perfectly normal, but a child who has been in the 50th percentile and suddenly drops below the 10th percentile has to be considered for thorough evaluation. The most common causes of a child's growth deviations from the norm on a standard chart are related to nourishment and the genetic influences of both parents and grandparents.

In addition, the crown-to-rump length should be calculated to determine whether the individual has child or adult body proportions (Fig. 6-4). This appraisal is calculated by placing the child in a sitting position and measuring from the vertex of the head to the point at which the child's buttocks touch the table. Crown-to-rump length

makes up 70 percent of the total length at birth, decreases to 60 percent at 2 years of age, and finally becomes about 52 percent at 10 years of age. The child is thought to have infantile stature if the sitting height is greater than one-half the standing height. However, if the sitting height is one-half of or slightly less than the standing height, the child is said to have adult stature. If the child has adult stature before 10 years of age, problems such as dwarfism and sexual precocity should be suspected. Conversely, if the child is late in developing adult stature, hypothyroidism or other serious pathological problems should be suspected and thoroughly evaluated.

Children who are found to be very high on the growth grids are rare but should be evaluated thoroughly for nutritional status. Obesity may be due to psychological factors. Conversely, the most common cause of failure to gain weight is malnourishment. Pathological problems must be kept in mind as possible causes for any of these deviations.

The next measurement that should routinely be taken and plotted on the standardized chart is the head circumference. This appraisal, in comparison with the chest circumference, weight, and length, should help the nurse determine whether head growth is progressing normally or indicates the presence of a pathological condition. At birth, the average head circumference is 37 cm (14½ in) and the average size of the chest is 35 cm (13¾ in). During the first 3 months of life, 2 cm (just over ¾ in) of growth in head circumference per month can be anticipated. At 4 to 6 months, 1 cm per month of increase in head circumference should be expected; from 6 to 12 months, 0.5 cm per month should be expected. The measuring tape is placed around the greatest circumference of the head (over the occiput and over the supraorbital ridges). The chest circumference is measured midway between inspiration and expiration; the tape should be placed across the nipple line. Measurements should be taken immediately after birth, then 3 to 4 days later to de-

TABLE 6-2 Rohrer's Ponderal Index Range

3.00 = heavy for length
2.54 = average
2.21 = light for length

FIGURE 6-4 Average crown-to-rump length for a newborn, a 2-year-old, and a 10-year-old.

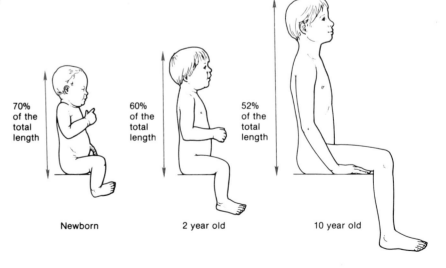

70% of the total length — Newborn

60% of the total length — 2 year old

52% of the total length — 10 year old

termine the head circumference after the edema and molding processes have resolved, and then on subsequent clinic visits. Head circumferences should be taken routinely on patients up to 2 years of age and plotted along with the length/stature and weight.

Vital Signs

Temperature

The normal temperature for a child is 37.6° C (99.6° F) rectal, 37° C (98.6° F) oral, and 36.3° C (97.4° F) axillary. These temperatures can vary greatly in a child with the least disturbance of the metabolic rate. The temperature should be taken rectally in children up to 5 years of age and then orally unless for some reason the child may harm himself. Axillary temperature can also be used if the need arises. The temperature should be taken before the newborn or child has been disturbed. The length of time of taking a temperature depends on the method and can range from a few seconds with an electronic thermometer to 3 minutes, which should be allowed for the rectal temperature.

After the birth, the newborn's temperature drops and varies with the temperature of his environment. Usually the temperature does not stabilize before the first week of life. Hypothermia in the newborn may indicate infection, just as hyperthermia does in older infants and children.

If fever exists, the nurse should make every attempt to identify the cause. Low-grade or high-grade fevers are of great significance and should be followed with careful evaluation by a qualified nurse or physician. It may be important for the nurse to have the parent keep a record of the child's temperature for several days; these notations may give important diagnostic information. It should be kept in mind that some children tend to have convulsions with febrile episodes. To prevent convulsions, every attempt should be made to identify the cause of the fever and determine whether there is a history of febrile convulsions.

Heart and Respiration Rates

The pulse rate is also of significance. It is usually obtained in children either apically or radially. Taking the temporal, carotid, pedal, popliteal, and femoral pulses is also impor-

TABLE 6-4 Descriptive Terms in Assessing Skin

Term	Description
Turgor	Skin normally smooth and firm when 1 to 2 in of skin and subcutaneous tissue over the abdominal wall is grasped between thumb and forefinger, squeezed, and allowed to fall back in place; with poor turgor, it remains suspended and creased for a few seconds
Edema	Abnormal amount of extracellular fluid; pitting edema noted when, following finger pressure, impressions remain in skin for several seconds
Skin lesions	
Primary	
Macules	Circumscribed, flat discolorations 1 cm or less in size
Patches	Like macule, but greater than 1 cm in size
Papules	Circumscribed, elevated, solid but superficial discolorations 1 cm or less in size
Wheals	Edematous, transitory papules, or plaques; usually erythematous
Plaques	Like papules but greater than 1 cm in size
Nodules	1 cm or less in size and solid with depth; above, level with, or beneath surface
Tumors	Like nodules but greater than 1 cm
Vesicles	Circumscribed elevations filled with serous fluid 1 cm or less in size
Bullae	Like vesicles but greater than 1 cm
Pustules	Circumscribed elevations of various sizes filled with purulent fluid
Petechiae	Circumscribed elevations containing blood or blood pigments, 1 cm or less in size
Purpura	Like petechiae but greater than 1 cm
Secondary	
Scales	Shedding, dead epidermal cells, either dry or greasy
Crusts	Variously colored deposits of skin exudates
Excoriations	Superficial and traumatic abrasions
Fissures	Linear, sharply defined breaks with abrupt walls
Ulcers	Excavations into the column; irregular size and shape
Scars	Connective tissue formations which replace tissue lost through disease or injury
Keloids	Hypertrophied scars

Source: M. Chard and G. S. Dudding, "Common Skin Problems in the Newborn and Infant," *Issues in Comprehensive Pediatric Nursing,* 1:29, 1975.

tant in evaluating circulatory status. In a young child the pulse should be counted for a full minute, since there are some normal irregularities. If an older child is being evaluated for cardiac status, his pulse should be taken for 1 minute. In addition to rate and rhythm, the location of the pulse (apical, radial, or specified other) should be noted (Table 6-3).

Respirations are the next measurement. Rate, rhythm, and any retractions should be noted at this time. Again, it is preferable to count for a full minute, especially in an infant or ill child. Like the pulse, these measurements

TABLE 6-3 Normal Pulse and Respiratory Rates for Specific Ages*

Age	Pulse per min	Respirations
Newborn	100-160	30-40
2 years	100-140	28-32
4 years	90-96	24-28
6 years	80-90	24-26
8 years	80-84	22-24
10 years	80-84	22-24
12 years	78-80	18-20

*These ranges are averages only and vary with the sex of the child.

should be compared with the norms for the age of a particular child (Table 6-4).

Blood Pressure

The blood pressure should be taken after all other vital signs have been measured and before the child has a chance to become excited (Fig. 6-5). Blood pressure can be measured by auscultation, or palpation. The size of the blood pressure cuff is important in all these methods, and its width should never be less than one-half or more than two-thirds the length of the part of the extremity used. A narrow blood pressure cuff will give an abnormally high reading, and a wide cuff will give an abnormally low reading. Usually the arms are used for measuring the blood pressure; however, with a cardiac or suspected cardiac patient the blood pressure should be taken in all four extremities for purposes of comparison and to identify a patient who has coarctation of the aorta.

General Appearance

The general appearance of the child should be included next in the physical examination. It can be evaluated by simply looking at the child during the history taking, while the child is playing, and while the physical examination is being performed. The nurse should observe the child for acute distress, cleanliness, alertness, spontaneity, mood, color, size, proportions, and interactions with the parent or health care provider.

Skin

Newborn The examination can be conducted when the baby is nude and under the warmer.

Infant The examination can be conducted when the baby is dressed (initially, and then removing one piece of clothing at a time) and in the parent's arm. The parent changes the position of the baby as required. Older infants are observed for indications of restlessness or other signs of itching.

Toddler and Preschooler The examination can be conducted with the child in panties and examining gown. If there is a rash, involved parts are exposed with the help of the parent to determine the distribution of rash. The child is observed for itching—restlessness and scratching.

School-Age Child The child is dressed in an examining gown, and skin is examined as various parts are exposed during the examination sequence. The child is asked to point out areas of skin problems and describe stages by pointing to lesions that are at different stages. This is done with the help of a parent in the case of an early school-age child.

The first or last evaluation performed is that of the skin, although most of it is done throughout the entire examination. The skin gives very important clues to the presence or absence of disease. All areas should be examined carefully for color, abrasions, cuts, infections, burns, and bruises at different stages of healing. A thorough in-

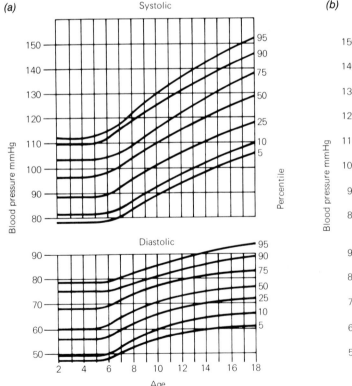

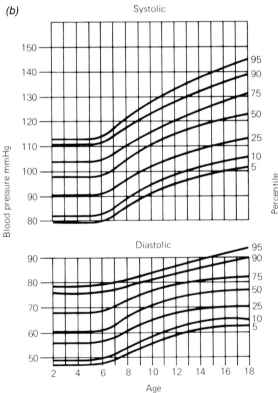

FIGURE 6-5   Percentiles of blood pressure measurements in *(a)* boys and *(b)* girls. *(From "Report of the Task Force on Blood Pressure Control in Children," Pediatrics, 59, (suppl.): 803, 1977.)*

spection may alert the examiner to possible neurological problems, cardiac problems, and the possibility of child abuse.

The head, forehead, ears, and skin creases of the newborn and infant should be examined for the presence of seborrheic dermatitis (cradle cap). In addition, the newborn's skin should be examined for milia, lanugo, vernix caseosa, petechiae, moles, café au lait spots, and any birthmarks. Newborns may have erythema toxicum neonatorum, but this rash can be considered normal. Moles and birthmarks are evaluated by identifying the location and measuring the size.

Color is carefully appraised next. Any cyanosis, pallor, and flushing should be noted, and their relation to the child's activity should be considered (see Chap. 24). The presence of jaundice is determined. It is most easily identified if pressure is applied to the skin using the flat surface of a glass slide. Pressure empties the capillary bed of the skin and helps the nurse observe for jaundice. This examination is best carried out in direct sunlight (Gundy, 1981). If jaundice is present in the newborn, the examiner should note how many days after birth it began. A bilirubin determination can be made by means of laboratory tests.

Skin texture should be carefully evaluated for dehydration, malnourishment, edema, dryness, and scaliness. Turgor can best be evaluated over the sternal area and the medial malleolus. Edema found in dependent areas and around the eyes should have further medical evaluation.

Skin rashes are common in infants and children and may indicate allergic reactions, infectious disease, or heat rashes. These lesions should be differentiated from petechiae, which may be indicative of a blood dyscrasia or meningococcal meningitis. Lesions should be identified and described according to their location and characteristics (Chap. 19) (Table 6-4). The history should elicit information about any new allergens or individuals with communicable disease to whom the patient has been exposed.

Diaper rashes should be examined carefully to determine the presence of a monilial infection. Usually these infections are found in the crease folds of the buttocks as well as the general diaper area. If there is any question of an infection such as staphylococcal infection, a culture should be done.

Pustulovesicular lesions, which are commonly found on the upper lip but also on other areas of the body, may be impetigo. If the cause of the lesions is questionable, a skin culture is done. Herpes simplex is commonly found around the mouth and at times on the genitals. A referral is made for follow-up medical care. The skin should also be carefully examined for tinea, which is commonly found in the scalp and on the feet.

Pityriasis is another disease commonly found in children. The pruritic papulosquamous eruption found in skin creases may last 2 to 8 weeks. Any dermatologic disorder should have medical follow-up.

The adolescent is examined for acne. History may elicit information that shows what aggravates this condition.

The hair and nails are also included in the examination of the integumentary system. Hair over the entire body should be examined for amount, distribution, and texture. Any sign of alopecia or dry or oily hair may be indicative of other systemic disorders. A child who exhibits early pubertal hair (before $9\frac{1}{2}$ years of age) needs further evaluation to ascertain the presence of other signs of precocious puberty (see Chap. 29).

Finally, the nails should be examined for nail biting, color, concavity, pitting, fissures, leukonychia, consistency, and inflammation. Ingrowing of the toenails is found in newborns and is frequently a point of infection. Ingrown toenails may also be seen in older children who have not trimmed them properly.

Head

Newborn The examination should take place while the newborn is in a semisitting position and is quiet. It can be done most easily while the neonate is in the arms of a parent.

Infant The position is the same as that for the newborn; the examiner may want to measure the head just prior to examination of the ears, nose, and mouth. Peek-a-boo and similar games should be used with the older infant to gain cooperation. A parent may have to place the tape around the patient's head the first time to decrease stranger anxiety in the older infant.

Toddler The examination is probably most successfully done in a parent's lap. An explanation and demonstration should be carried out before the toddler's head is measured (Fig. 6-6). For example, the examiner may measure her own head, a doll, or stuffed animal's head.

Preschooler If head circumference is still measured at this age, the guidelines for explanation and demonstration used for the toddler are applicable.

School-Age Child and Adolescent Head circumference is not routinely done. If it is appropriate, it is done first in the examination sequence. The examiner explains what is being done.

Measurement of the head has been discussed above. Head control should be noted at the beginning of the examination. The amount of control depends on the age of the infant during the first 4 months of life. The newborn has little or no head control. Head lag is obvious: When the infant is pulled to a sitting position, the head remains hyperextended or hyperflexed. If placed on his abdomen, the newborn can raise the chin off the mattress and turn the head; if placed in the supine position, he will lie with the head to one side and will be capable of slightly elevating the head occasionally from the mattress. Not until the infant is 3 months of age will the examiner begin to see some head control, and by the end of the third month good midline head control should be evident. If there is a failure to gain head control by the end of the third month and there is persistence of the tonic neck reflex past 4

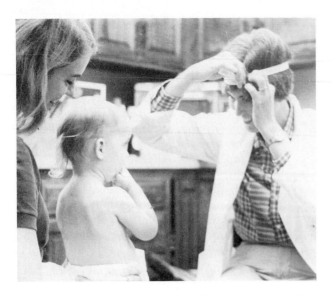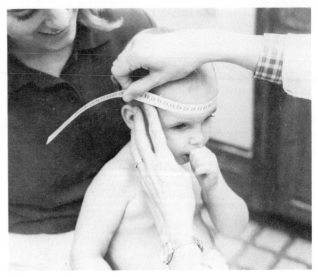

FIGURE 6-6   Measuring the head circumference. *(Courtesy of Molly U. McKinley.)*

months, the possibility of a pathological condition must be considered. These manifestations can be the earliest symptoms of cerebral palsy. In addition, the fontanels should be measured. The examination and measurement of the head should be done while the infant is calm and in an upright position.

The anterior fontanel is the first to be measured. This diamond-shaped opening can increase in size during the first 6 months of life and then start to diminish. Measurements vary among children, averaging about 1.5 to 2 cm. This fontanel can be as large as 4 or 5 cm and still be normal, but if it is this big, the infant may be referred to a physician for an evaluation. The anterior fontanel usually closes between 12 and 18 months, but it can close as early as 9 months. The posterior fontanel, a triangular-shaped opening, can be found in the midline of the occiput and usually is about the size of the end of an average-sized adult's index finger. It can be expected to close by 2 to 3 months of age (Fig. 6-7).

Bulging, tense, full, or sunken fontanels should be identified. A bulging fontanel can denote serious problems such as hydrocephalus, hemorrhage, or other causes of increased intracranial pressure. Conversely, a sunken fontanel may indicate dehydration or malnourishment. If the sizes of the head and chest are disproportionate, increased intracranial pressure and microcephaly should be considered, depending on whether the head is large or small in comparison with the chest. Fontanels must be checked when the child is not crying. If a fontanel is bulging when the child is crying, the examiner must be sure that it returns to normal tensity when the crying has stopped. During the examination of the anterior fontanel, a slight pulsation may be seen or felt and can be considered normal unless it is bounding.

In addition to examination of the fontanels, the suture lines must also be closely palpated and observed. Suture lines may overlap shortly after birth. However, this over-

lap disappears in a few days, and the sutures can be palpated as small ridges until about 6 months of age. Abnormal sutures that are extremely wide should make the examiner suspect hydrocephalus or other causes of increased intracranial pressure. Premature closure of the sutures (craniosynostosis) can be detected through palpation and measurement and by noting the shape of the infant's head. The examiner will see an increase in the longitudinal plane with premature closure of the sagittal suture and an increase in the lateral plane with early closure of the coronal sutures. Obviously, for detection of these shapes, the examination of the head must be done from all angles and the shape of the face must be carefully scrutinized.

The head is also inspected and palpated for any abnormal ridges, caput succedaneum, cephalhematoma, craniotabes, asymmetry, growths, bruises, scratches, alopecia, or flattening. These findings may indicate other types of pathological conditions. For example, flattening of the occiput may be due to (1) lying in one position, (2) the intrauterine position, (3) premature suture closure, (4) torticollis, or (5) abnormal intracranial growth.

Percussion of the head can determine the possibility of a subdural hematoma. This technique is done in the same manner in which other body parts are percussed and should take place over the sagittal suture. Dullness is a positive sign for diagnosing subdural hematoma.

The skull can also be auscultated with the bell of the stethoscope for bruits. Continuous or systolic bruits can be heard over the orbital and temporal areas in children up to 4 years of age and still be normal. However, any time a bruit is heard, it should be evaluated by a physician even though bruits are usually not pathological until after age 4.

Additionally, the need for transillumination of the skull may arise any time there is a question about head circumference or shape or fontanel size. To transilluminate,

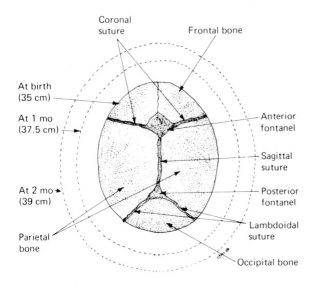

FIGURE 6-7 Head circumference and anatomic points.

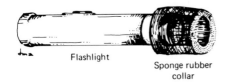

FIGURE 6-8 Flashlight for transillumination of the head.

sponge rubber is fitted around the head of a flashlight so that there is a tight fit when the flashlight is placed against the skull (Fig. 6-8). The procedure is carried out in a dark room with the child in the parent's lap. The flashlight is then turned on and placed snugly at different points on the head. Increased luminosity may be indicative of a subdural hematoma, hydrocephalus, or other causes of increased intracranial pressure.

The scalp should be checked for cradle cap, nits, ticks, scabies, and tinea capitis. Hair should also be inspected and palpated for dryness, oiliness, and distribution.

Face

Newborn Same as for examination of the head; in addition, facial movements while resting, feeding, and crying are observed.

Infant Same as for the newborn. Eye contact is limited with the older infant since it may stimulate an anxiety reaction.

Toddler and Preschooler Position is the same as for examination of the head; facial movements can be examined during conversation elicited from the toddler or preschooler and at the time crying or laughing occurs.

School-Age Child and Adolescent Examination follows that of the head. Observations are made throughout the entire exam, during conversation, smiling, or crying.

The face is first observed for shape, symmetry, proportions, and evidence of paralysis. The facial shape and di-

mension change during the first 10 years of life. Any unusual shape may be indicative of certain syndromes or congenital defects. For example, when the newborn cries, the nurse should observe for failure of one eye to close, which may indicate Bell's palsy. The older child should be able to smile and wrinkle his forehead so that the examiner can determine whether paralysis is present. Any twitching or tics should also be observed at this time. The examiner then attempts to elicit Chvostek's sign.

Color is evaluated next. Any cyanosis, jaundice, or pallor should be identified. Dark circles under the patient's eyes may signify allergies or fatigue. These dark circles should be differentiated from bruising.

Local edema around the eyes and over the parotid area should be looked for and palpated. During the examination of the parotid area, the child is sitting upright and looking at the ceiling while the examiner runs a finger downward from the zygomatic arch to palpate for swelling. The child is then asked to lie down. If swelling is present, the parotid gland falls back and moves the pinna of the ear forward. The sublingual glands and submaxillary glands should also be palpated for enlargement. Any identified enlargement should be seen by the physician; since these glands are usually not enlarged, enlargement may indicate local infection, cystic fibrosis, or one of many other pathological conditions.

Eyes

Newborn The examination can best be carried out while the newborn is feeding or quiet in a bassinet or in a parent's lap. The newborn's response to the examiner's or parent's face and to colored and black and white objects is observed. A sleeping newborn can be held in an upright position; this usually stimulates the newborn to open his eyes.

Infant The infant is examined in the parent's lap or while quiet or feeding and lying in a crib or on an examination table. The older infant is best examined while in the security of his parent's lap. A flashlight with a rubber figure over the head (Fig. 6-9) is good for assessing the in-

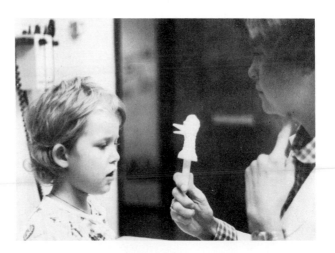

FIGURE 6-9 Flashlight with animal head for use in checking the eyes of a young child. *(Courtesy of Molly U. McKinley.)*

fant's tracking of brightly colored objects and moving objects. Bright objects, such as the yarn ball from the Denver Developmental Screening Test, can also be used to test the baby's focusing on and following of brightly colored objects. A hand puppet or stuffed animal is also excellent for checking the infant's ability to follow objects and ability to accommodate. If darkness is required for an eye examination, a dimly lit room is preferred by the older infant.

Toddler and Preschooler The examination of ocular movements and accommodation can be done while the toddler is playing or talking with the examiner. A more thorough examination of the eye, such as for corneal light reflex or pupillary reflex, can be carried out while the toddler is in the security of the parent's arms. This appraisal should be preceded by a demonstration on a doll, stuffed animal, or parent. Some toddlers will allow this to be done while sitting at eye level on the examination table. Appropriate restraint should be used for safety if the toddler is uncooperative.

School-Age Child and Adolescent The examination should be preceded by an explanation of what the patient can expect and why the examination is being done. During and after the examination careful explanation of the findings should be provided. Appropriate visual aids should be used.

The external examination of the eye should include observation of the eyelids, the eyelashes, and the orbital area around the eye, along with the tear ducts, tear glands, conjunctiva, sclera, iris, and pupil. Any tics or abnormalities are noted. The ophthalmoscope is used to determine lens opacity and examine the fundus. The examination is not complete until vision screening is included. In addition, the examiner should palpate the eyes for turgor. A flashlight should be used to check the reactions of the pupils to light and the equality of the pupils.

The eyes should be examined for edema. Questions should be aimed at identifying specific times of the day when the edema appears. If edema is present, the patient should be referred for medical evaluation, especially in relation to renal problems. Other causes of swelling include injury, drugs, allergies, and cellulitis. The eyelid can be palpated to identify poor tensity, tenderness, or pain. The eyelashes should be checked for position and to determine whether the child has been losing them or pulling them out. Observation for styes, lid nodules, ptosis, foreign objects, infection, and scabies should also be included. Suborbital dark circles may indicate allergy or inadequate rest.

The nurse should note the lacrimal ducts for presence, position, patency, and infection. Excessive tearing or drainage should be identified. In the drainage is green or purulent, a culture should be done. The cause of tearing, such as the presence of a foreign body, should be identified. Education about the function of the lacrimal ducts should be offered.

The conjunctivae should be examined for color and any type of abnormal growth. The sclerae should be checked for hemorrhage, discoloration, moles, or jaundice. The newborn's sclerae may have a blue tint and still be normal. However, deep blue sclerae may indicate a much more serious problem, such as osteogenesis imperfecta. Sclerae may also have an occasional conjunctival hemorrhage during the first 2 to 3 weeks of life. Injected sclerae may be indicative of an allergy, conjunctivitis, beginning glaucoma, eyestrain, or a foreign body.

The child is screened for extraocular muscle balance, central nervous system problems, and blindness by checking the movements of the eyes and the pupillary light reflex. The young infant is held at arm's length and then rotated slowly in one direction. The infant will look in the same direction in which he has been turned. When the rotation is stopped, the infant's eyes look in the opposite direction after a few quick nystagmoid movements. If the nystagmus is sustained during this maneuver or when the infant is at rest, blindness or central nervous system problems must be suspected (Gundy, 1981). In older children the movements of the eyes are evaluated by examining extraocular movements. The patient is asked to follow the examiner's finger through the six cardinal fields. When the eyes are in the upper and lateral positions, any evidence of nystagmus should be noted. Nystagmus in this part of the examination may be normal, but it should also alert the examiner to other signs and symptoms of a pathological state.

The final examination of a movement of the eyes is for convergence. The examiner performs the cover test by sitting directly in front of the patient and holding a light 0.66 to 1 m (2 to 3 ft) in front of the patient's eyes. The patient is asked to focus on the light. The examiner then covers one of the patient's eyes, making sure that the child continues to watch the light steadily for a short period of time. The examiner should quickly remove the cover from the covered eye without moving the flashlight. If the eye just uncovered moves to look at the flashlight, a deviation such as strabismus, esotropia, exotropia, hypertropia, or hypotropia is suggested (Fig. 6-10). Absence of movement of the uncovered eye means that there are no abnormal deviations. The test is repeated with the other eye. The pupillary light reflex is obtained by shining a light from approximately ½ m (1½ ft) in front of the face into both eyes at the same time. If the child is looking directly at the light, the reflection of the light should be at the same point on both pupils. A deviation may suggest strabismus, exotropia, esotropia, hypertropia, hypotropia, or a tumor of the eye. Any deviation should always be referred to a pediatrician or ophthalmologist for evaluation (Fig. 6-11).

The examiner then proceeds to rule out exophthalmos and endophthalmos. If either is found, the child should be referred to a physician. Endophthalmos should not be mistaken for ptosis, which may be an important neurological symptom. Exophthalmos is indicated when the eyeball appears to protrude; endophthalmos, when the eyeball appears to be sunken. These conditions can also be identified by noting what part of the eyes the lids cover. A disorder such as a tumor of the eye or thyroid

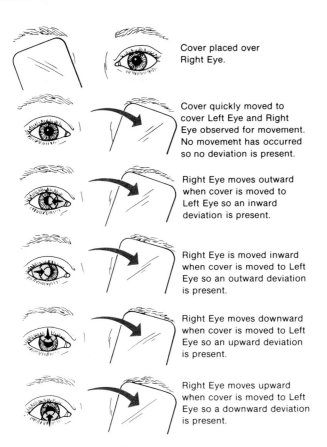

Cover placed over Right Eye.

Cover quickly moved to cover Left Eye and Right Eye observed for movement. No movement has occurred so no deviation is present.

Right Eye moves outward when cover is moved to Left Eye so an inward deviation is present.

Right Eye is moved inward when cover is moved to Left Eye so an outward deviation is present.

Right Eye moves downward when cover is moved to Left Eye so an upward deviation is present.

Right Eye moves upward when cover is moved to Left Eye so a downward deviation is present.

FIGURE 6-10   Cover test diagram.

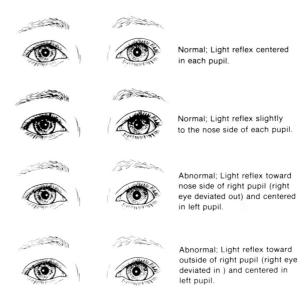

Normal; Light reflex centered in each pupil.

Normal; Light reflex slightly to the nose side of each pupil.

Abnormal; Light reflex toward nose side of right pupil (right eye deviated out) and centered in left pupil.

Abnormal; Light reflex toward outside of right pupil (right eye deviated in) and centered in left pupil.

FIGURE 6-11   Pupillary light reflex diagram.

disease may be identified by noting the presence of exophthalmos. The position of the eyes also should be noted. If the eyes appear to be below the lower lid, the child may have the setting-sun phenomenon. This finding can be normal in a preterm infant and in some normal full-term newborns, but it may also be a sign of hydrocephalus.

Finally, examination of the fundus should take place. Many children must be sent to the ophthalmologist for this test so that their eyes can be dilated for accurate and thorough examination of the retina.

The child is placed directly in front of the examiner; a very young or frightened child should be placed in his parent's lap. The child is asked to look directly across the room. The examiner proceeds with the evaluation by sitting in front of the child and using the right eye to examine the patient's right eye and the left eye to examine the patient's left eye. The examiner should first select a +8 to a +2 lens for examination of the cornea, iris, and lens. The child is reassured that he will see a bright light but that it will not be painful. The examiner begins by shining the light on the pupil and moving close to the child. The examiner should immediately see the red reflex unless the lens is not clear. With a non-Caucasian child, the examiner will note that the red reflex is paler. If this red reflex is absent, cataracts or another pathological condition should be suspected. As the examiner moves close, she will change the lens to a 0 to −2, making the landmarks of the retina much clearer (Fig. 6-12). Abnormalities of the

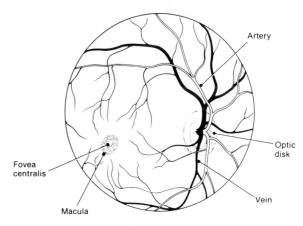

FIGURE 6-12   Normal eye ground.

retina are then observed for, such as a pale retina, blurred disk edges, papilledema, or a spot of blood that may indicate a retinal hemorrhage. The size of the veins and the arteries should be noted. They may be about equal size, or the veins may be slightly larger. The vessels should then be noted for abnormal dilation or abnormal pulsation. Next it should be noted whether they cup or dip down into the disk. These situations may indicate a pathological condition, and the child should be referred to a physician.

In the fundus examination of the newborn, the red reflex is usually all that is noted under normal conditions.

Absence of the red reflex is a good indicator of congenital cataracts.

Finally, vision screening is carried out. Vision screening can begin very early in life and should be continued with routine examinations. The vision of the very young child can be tested by watching him track moving objects such as bright lights and bright colors. The child's pupils should also be observed to note accommodation. Peripheral vision is well developed in newborns. Central vision begins to develop in the first month of life. Infants are hyperopic, and 20/20 vision is not reached until approximately 4 to 6 years. Any developmental retardation or lack of interest in the environment should induce the examiner to carry out a very thorough screening. Vision in the older child may be screened by the Snellen test or the Titmus test. Any questions about the adequacy of the child's vision should be followed by referrals.

Ears

Newborn Examination of the ears is most easily done if the newborn is on his back and his head is restrained by an assistant.

Infant Safety is of the utmost concern in the examination of the ear. If the examination can be conducted in the parent's lap, the infant will feel secure, especially if he has developed stranger anxiety. However, many times an assistant is needed to hold the head securely for removal of cerumen and examination of the tympanic membrane. When the assistant is restraining the head, the parent can hold the infant's or child's legs by placing his or her hands above the patient's knees (Fig. 6-13).

Toddler Same as for infant; much explanation should be included, along with constant chattering when looking into the toddler's ear. The toddler, like the preschooler, should be allowed to touch the otoscope to lessen his fears of the instrument. It is also helpful to demonstrate the procedure on his parent, a doll, or a stuffed animal before the examination.

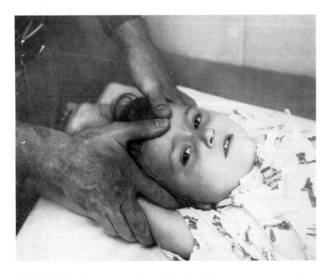

FIGURE 6-13 Restraining the child's head for an ear examination. *(Courtesy of Molly U. McKinley.)*

Preschooler Same as for toddler. In addition, an ear model can be used to demonstrate what is inside the ear. Older preschoolers may not need to be restrained. All preschoolers need feedback about what is being done and what is being seen. A cooperative preschool child can also be taught how to squeeze the bulb during a pneumoscopic examination for tympanic membrane mobility.

School-Age Child Usually children of this age need no restraining, but the examiner may have to place a single finger on the side of the head to remind the child not to move. If restraint is required, an assistant and parent can participate in the procedure in the same way as for the younger child. A thorough explanation using appropriate visual aids should be offered.

Adolescent The examination follows the same sequence as that for adults. Appropriate explanation with visual aids should be used to explain procedures and findings.

The examination of the ear includes its position, the area immediately surrounding the ear, the outer auricle, the external canal, and the tympanic membrane. The presence of tenderness or pain should be noted.

To begin, the examiner should always observe the position of the ears. Low-set ears in newborns should lead the examiner to suspect the possibility of internal renal anomalies or trisomy. The top of the auricle should be even with the level of eyes; that is, an imaginary line can be drawn from the top of the auricle to the outer angle of the eye. In addition, the nurse should note whether the auricle stands out, which may indicate an outer ear infection, mumps, cellulitis, mastoiditis, or the possibility of congenital anomalies.

The area around the ears should then be inspected and palpated for preauricular cysts and any type of fistula. If these are present, the child should be referred for surgical removal of these abnormalities so that future infections can be avoided. The examiner notes important landmarks for abnormalities in shape.

The observer then will look for any evidence of dried drainage in the outer auricle. If drainage is found, the examiner should suspect otitis media or otitis externa. It is important while taking the history to learn how long the drainage has been present and to rule out the chance that the "drainage" consists of dried tears, dried milk, or melted cerumen.

At this point the otoscopic examination should be initiated. The first and most important requirement is an excellent light source. The ear can be manipulated by the examiner; while doing so, she should note whether there is any pain. The nurse should use the largest speculum that will still allow visualization of the tympanic membrane. This size selection will avoid puncturing the membrane with the speculum. The otoscope is held firmly in one hand, and the same hand rests on the child's head to prevent the speculum from going through the membrane if the child moves suddenly (Fig. 6-14). The child's head is tilted slightly away from the examiner. In a child under

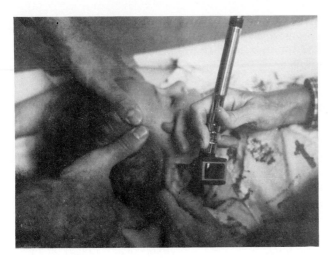

FIGURE 6-14   Position of the hand in examination of the ear. *(Courtesy of Molly U. McKinley.)*

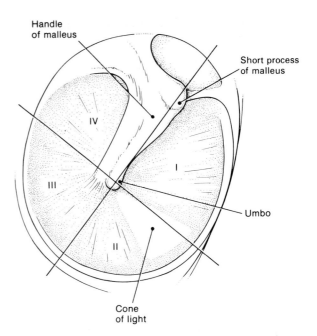

FIGURE 6-15   Normal tympanic membrane.

3 years of age, the auricle is *pulled down and back* in order for the examiner to view the eardrum. In the older child the auricle is *pulled up and back* for better visualization of the membrane. These manipulations are done because of the different ways the canal is positioned in children at different ages. The speculum is then placed very gently in the outer portion of the external canal to enable the examiner to visualize the outer canal. Pain during manipulation or while the speculum is being put into position may indicate the presence of a furuncle or otitis externa. At this time the examiner observes for erythema of the canal, which may indicate the presence of an infection or disease. If the membrane cannot be visualized because cerumen is present, a larger speculum may increase the field of vision sufficiently to view the eardrum and its landmarks. If this does not work, the experienced examiner should use a wire loop to remove the cerumen or irrigate the ear with tepid water or saline. An irrigation should never be done if there is any question that the eardrum may be perforated or if a foreign body is present. Dizziness and vomiting may follow the irrigation.

The examination should be continued so that the tympanic membrane is viewed. The landmarks of the eardrum should be identified: the light reflex, umbo, handle of malleus, and short process of the malleus (Fig. 6-15). The eardrum itself is a pearl-colored membrane that is translucent or opalescent. The membrane may be injected because of infection, crying, manipulation, or force. The light reflex starts at the umbo and proceeds anteroinferiorly at the same angle as the jaw on the side of the head on which the ear is being examined. In an infected ear the light reflex will be dulled, distorted, or absent. In addition, the translucency of the drum will be dull or absent. The drum may be bulging (from fluid), or there may be some injection of the membrane, and the handle of the malleus will not be clearly outlined. Conversely, the membrane may be retracted, as indicated by prominence of the bony landmarks. All these signs require referral for treatment.

Mobility of the eardrum can be tested, usually by the physician or a specially trained nurse. A tight-fitting speculum is needed. Air insufflation is conducted by means of a rubber tube which is connected to the outside of the otoscope, and air is gently blown or squeezed into the canal. The examiner observes the mobility of the drum. Absence or decrease of motion indicates disease, such as serous or suppurative otitis media.

The pre- and postauricular nodes are palpated. The tip of the mastoid is tapped, and the child is observed for indications of pain. Pain or tenderness may indicate mastoiditis.

Hearing tests are performed as the final part of the examination. The examination can be done by determining whether the child can hear a watch ticking. Making statements to the child when he is not watching the examiner or when his back is turned may also help identify hearing loss. A tuning fork can be used to identify either bone or air conduction losses. The vibrating fork is placed against the child's mastoid process until he can no longer hear the vibrations. Next the examiner places the vibrating tuning fork about 1 in from the ear. The child should hear the air-conducted vibrations longer and louder than the bone-conducted ones. Finally, the vibrating fork is placed in the middle of the child's forehead. Normally the sound of the vibrations in both ears should be equal. However, if it is heard better in one ear than in the other, this discrepancy again indicates a neurosensory loss or a conductive loss. In unilateral conduction hearing loss the hearing is better in the good ear. If neurosensory deafness is present, the hearing is better in the affected ear.

Finally, the vestibular function test may be performed to rule out any brainstem or vestibular disorder. This test is done by injecting cold water [18.33°C (65°F)] in the ear, after which nystagmus should occur. An alternative test is to turn the child around several times, after which nystagmus should occur. The absence of nystagmus in either test can be a definite sign of disease. Any positive findings on hearing or vestibular function tests require a referral of the child to an audiologist or physician for further evaluation.

Nose

Newborn The newborn is examined while sleeping, feeding, or lying on his back in a bassinet or his parent's arms.

Infant This examination should be carried out while the infant is in the parent's arms.

Toddler This examination should be carried out while the toddler is in the parent's lap. Some toddlers may allow it to be done while sitting on the examination table. An age-appropriate explanation should be included.

Preschooler Most preschoolers will allow this assessment to take place while seated on the examination table. If the preschooler is frightened, he is allowed to sit in the security of his mother's lap.

School-Age Child and Adolescent This appraisal is done during the normal examination sequence. Appropriate explanations and demonstrations should be given.

A much-neglected area of the physical examination is the nose, which should be checked with the same care as any other part of the body. To begin, observation should determine whether the patient is breathing through his nose or his mouth. A newborn should have a stethoscope placed on the sides of both nares to determine their patency. This appraisal is done by blocking one side while listening to the other side. Any newborn with blockage of one or both sides of the nose must be considered to be at risk for respiratory distress. A child who constantly breathes through his mouth may prove to have enlarged adenoids, allergies, polyps, or a deviated septum.

The shape of the nose is then examined. A nose with a flat or saddle-shaped bridge may indicate trisomy, congenital syphilis, cleft palate, or other conditions.

The alae nasi should be observed for flaring. Flaring may indicate respiratory distress. The patient should also be observed for the "allergic salute," in which he keeps rubbing the tip of the nose because of itching, rhinorrhea, or rhinitis.

The mucosa is observed either with a speculum or by gently pushing the tip of the nose upward. The mucosa should be pink. Paleness or extremely red or gray mucosa indicates a pathological condition. Children with allergies have pale mucosa, whereas red mucosa may indicate an infection. Gray mucosa may be a manifestation of chronic rhinitis.

The characteristics of the secretions should be observed. Whether they are thin, watery, purulent, or bloody should be noted. Cultures are done if purulent discharge is present. Epistaxis should be noted. The point of bleeding is usually found in the lower anterior tip of the septum. The cause may be trauma, allergy, dryness, or a blood dyscrasia.

Finally, palpation and percussion should be performed over maxillary and ethmoid sinuses. Tenderness may indicate sinusitis and require medical follow-up. Transillumination is usually unsatisfactory in young children; e.g., the frontal sinuses cannot be visualized prior to 7 years of age.

Mouth and Throat

Newborn and Infant This is one of the few times when crying can facilitate the examination. While the baby is crying, the examiner quickly visualizes as much of the mouth and throat as possible. The child is examined in his bassinet, on the examining table, or in the parent's arms.

Toddler The examiner asks the toddler to open his mouth so that visualization can take place without the use of a tongue blade. The appraisal is demonstrated on a parent or favorite doll or stuffed animal before any attempt is made to look at the child's throat.

Preschooler Same as for toddler. In addition, the preschooler is allowed to examine the mouth of the examiner so that he can see what it looks like and learn how the examination is done.

School-Age Child and Adolescent The child is allowed to look at the mouth of the examiner. An explanation of what is being done and what the findings are is given with the use of age-appropriate language and visual aids.

A careful examination of the mouth is frequently overlooked. The child should be in a sitting position, facing the examiner. The young child should preferably be in his parent's lap with the parent restraining the head by placing a hand on the child's forehead (Fig. 6-16). If the child is uncooperative, the hands and feet should be restrained.

The examiner should ask the child to open his mouth.

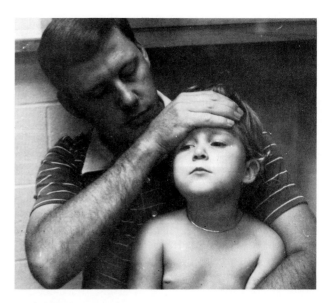

FIGURE 6-16 Restraint of a child while in the lap of a parent for examination of the mouth and throat. *(Courtesy of Molly U. McKinley.)*

Sometimes gentle stroking of the submandibular region helps the child relax and follow directions. As the examination proceeds, the lips and the area around the mouth should be examined for pallor, cyanosis, dryness, fissures, edema, and sores. The lips are thoroughly examined for any asymmetry.

Proceeding to the mouth, the examiner should ask the child to lift, move, depress, and stick out the tongue as much as possible without the assistance of the tongue blade. If a tongue blade is used, it should be placed at a 45° angle across the tongue to minimize the chance of gagging. It is important for the examiner to give the child a tongue blade to play with and examine first.

Any peculiar odors of the child's breath should be noted, as they may indicate the presence of caries, diabetes, mouth breathing, or poor oral hygiene. The buccal mucosa is now inspected for moisture, distended veins, lesions, trauma, thrush, Koplik's spots, sores, cysts, or tumors. The gums are inspected for tenderness, inflammation, bleeding, edema, and hypertrophy. Raised or receding areas of the gums should be noted. In addition, a black line at the margin of the gums may indicate some type of metal poisoning, such as lead poisoning.

The teeth are inspected for number, caries, fractures, abnormal formation, color, position, and hygiene. Teeth with flattened edges may be found in children who grind their teeth. The gums should be looked at to see whether they are inflamed or receding at the base of the tooth.

Salivation is inspected next. The consistency, amount, color, and odor of the saliva should be noted. Excessive drooling or the absence of salivation is a significant symptom at certain ages. Drooling, however, is evident around 3 to 4 months of age and at the time of teething. Absence of saliva may be considered normal before 3 months of age.

The tongue should be inspected carefully. The dorsal, inferior, and lateral aspects are inspected for unusual color, sores, birthmarks, moisture, atrophy, and tumors. The size and position in the mouth is carefully noted. The patient should be asked to protrude the tongue so that the nurse can note any deviation or tremors; an older child should be asked to protrude the tongue and move it laterally against a tongue blade to test the tongue's strength. The frenulum should be examined to make sure it is of appropriate length. The tongue is examined for abnormal dryness, deep furrows, or scars.

Finally, the hard and soft palates are inspected for clefts, Epstein's pearls, abnormal areas of hypertrophy, and an abnormally high arch. All clefts, regardless of size, must be referred to a physician. A highly arched palate and hypertrophy of the palate may indicate potential for speech impediments.

The throat is then examined. Rotating the tongue blade from a 45° angle back over the posterior aspect of the tongue, the examiner will most likely elicit the gag response. It may be necessary for the child to say "ah" with a short *a* sound. At this time a quick but thorough inspection should take place. The epiglottis is observed during the gag for edema and erythema. If they are present, med-

ical follow-up is indicated. The posterior aspect of the pharynx should be observed for drainage, erythema, edema, and abnormal growths or vesicles. The tonsils are assessed for edema, erythema, and the presence of exudate or a pseudomembrane. Red tonsils with an exudate may indicate a streptococcal infection, and redness without an exudate is most likely a viral infection. A culture follows most examinations where erythema is present.

The uvula is then inspected for mobility and length. When the patient says "ah" (with a hard *a*), both the uvula and the soft palate should move. Lack of motion may be an early neurological sign.

Finally, the examination is conducted when the patient is asked to speak. Abnormal hoarseness merits follow-up. For the older child who has difficulty pronouncing certain letters, a speech evaluation should be considered.

Neck

Newborn The examination can be done while the newborn is in the parent's lap or reclining on his back.

Infant and Toddler The examination should be done while the infant is secure in his parent's lap. This exam follows examination of the chest. Some toddlers will allow this to be done while sitting on the examination table.

Preschooler This examination is performed while the preschooler sits on the examination table or in his parent's lap. Simple age-appropriate explanations should be offered.

School-Age Child and Adolescent This appraisal is done in a normal examination sequence and is accompanied by age-appropriate explanations and demonstrations.

After examination of the salivary glands, the nurse can proceed to the examination of the lymph nodes of the neck. Inspection of the neck may help the nurse identify enlarged nodes prior to the palpation of the neck. In order to inspect for the nodes, the examiner can have the patient move his neck in a full range of motion. Then, with the neck flexed toward the side being examined, palpation for the various nodes can begin. Using the index and third fingers, the examiner can move the skin over the underlying tissue rather than moving the fingers over the skin. Beginning with the occipital or preauricular nodes, the examiner can proceed through the various chains.

Children normally have palpable lymph nodes up to about 12 years of age. The nodes may become enlarged with any infection of the throat or scalp. Enlarged nodes should be measured and palpated for tenderness, and their location should be noted. Nodes that are tender and enlarged should be checked by a physician.

The neck should be inspected carefully for abnormalities of size and shape which may be indicative of syndromes, (e.g. Turner's syndrome) underlying muscular problems, or other disorders. Any tilting, stiffness, rigidity, or painful motion require further medical examination. Both sternocleidomastoid muscles should be observed and palpated for atrophy or signs of a mass. Stiffness and nuchal rigidity always indicate the need for a medical examination.

The trachea is palpated and inspected to note any deviation. The examiner's thumbs are placed on each side of the trachea above the suprasternal notches, and the sides of the trachea are carefully palpated in an upward direction. A deviation can indicate pneumothorax.

The thyroid is also inspected and palpated. The examiner should first stand behind the patient with the patient's neck hyperextended. Placing the fingers over the thyroid's lateral borders, the examiner asks the patient to swallow. Any enlargement or nodules can be felt. Following this, the examiner can stand facing the patient, inspecting for any fullness in the neck. Palpation of the gland should follow after location of the thyroid isthmus below the cricoid cartilage.

Chest

Newborn This part of the examination is done while the newborn is asleep or feeding. It can be accomplished while he is in his parent's arms or in a bassinet. Obviously, the number of retractions is determined before auscultation is started. The anterior chest wall is examined first, followed by placing the newborn over the parent's shoulder so that the posterior chest wall can be auscultated.

Infant For the young infant the examination is the same as for the newborn. The older infant is examined in the same manner, but if he is anxious, he should be placed sideways so that he can constantly watch what is being done to him. Rattles or teething rings can be given to the older infant so that he is distracted from the examination (Fig. 6-17).

Toddler Most toddlers feel secure if the examination takes place in a parent's lap. Auscultation should be preceded by the nurse's listening to the chest of a favorite stuffed toy or a parent. Giving the toddler a choice of whether the examiner will listen to his front or back first gives him some control over the situation and usually re-

sults in his cooperation. Sometimes the exam can be carried out while the toddler is seated on the examination table. Constant feedback is necessary. Most auscultation is done while the child is at rest. Usually a child of this age is too young to understand taking a deep breath and blowing out.

Preschooler The preschooler can usually be examined on the examination table. Because he usually holds his breath when asked to take a deep breath, the examiner must instruct him to blow out on a tissue after taking the deep breath. "See how high it will go" will usually keep the deep inspiration and expiration going so that the entire examination can be done. The preschooler may consider percussion an attack on his body; one stated, "He hit me." Percussion is first demonstrated on his favorite stuffed toy; then his foot, knee, and hand; and finally his chest.

School-Age Child The chest is examined in a normal examination sequence. Taking a deep breath and blowing it out should first be demonstrated by the examiner, and then the child is allowed to practice before the examination is started. Age-appropriate education and visual aids will enhance the examination.

Adolescent This appraisal is performed in a normal examination sequence. Education and the use of visual aids should be included during and at the end of the examination so that techniques as well as findings are understood by the adolescent client.

The examination of the chest begins with observation of the anterior and posterior aspects of the thorax. First the shape of the chest is noted. A funnel chest, pectus excavatum, pigeon chest, barrel chest, or any other abnormalities merit careful consideration.

Any retractions are identified as to type and degree, along with asymmetrical respiratory movements (Fig. 6-18). At the same time, any signs of respiratory distress should be identified. Any tachypnea (see Table 6-3), grunting, rales, rhonchi, or wheezing should be noted.

Next, the chest should be palpated to rule out cysts, tumors, or other abnormal growths. Intrathoracic lesions are ruled out by inspecting and palpating for tracheal deviation (in the young infant the trachea may deviate slightly to the right and still be normal) and observing for unequal respiratory movements. Areas of percussion that are dull or flat and abnormal fremitus may be indicative of a lesion. The clavicles should be palpated as intact. Axillary and clavicular areas are examined to determine node enlargement.

Next the hands are placed at subsequent times over the lower chest, both anterior and posterior, with the thumbs adjacent to each other. The patient is asked to inhale, and the examiner notes any asymmetry of the onset and depth of the inspiratory movement. This procedure should also be carried out over the lateral aspects of the chest and over the shoulders below the clavicles as the patient is approached from behind.

The final technique of palpation should be to note the quality of vocal and tactile fremitus. This appraisal is done

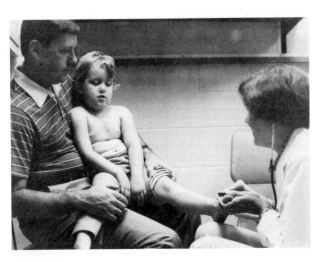

FIGURE 6-17 Placement of child in parent's lap for examination of chest and heart. *(Courtesy of Molly U. McKinley.)*

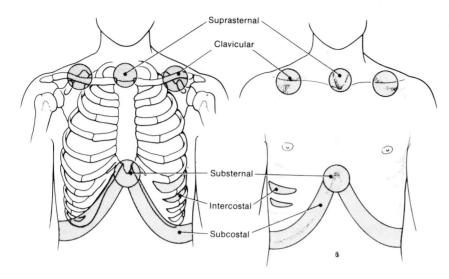

FIGURE 6-18   Areas of respiratory retractions.

using the ulnar surface of the palm or the flat surface of the hand. Symmetrical palpation, using the lateral aspects of the hands, follows when the examiner asks the patient to repeat the words *one, two, three,* and *ninety-nine.* The vibrations from the larynx should be transmitted to the thorax. The frequency of the voice should match the frequency felt in the thorax; this phenomenon is known as tactile fremitus. The frequency of the voice should also match the frequency heard in the thorax, which is the vocal fremitus. The match is poor in adolescent females, but there are good matches in male children. Any modification or absence of vocal or tactile fremitus indicates that either obstruction or consolidation of the respiratory tract may be present and should be considered a significant pathological sign.

Percussion can identify any abnormalities of the percussion note. Abnormalities indicate the possibility of some disorder such as pneumonia, pleural effusion, enlargement of the heart, atelectasis, neoplasms, and birth defects.

Auscultation is the final part of the chest examination and is most likely the most threatening. It, too, is done symmetrically over the anterior, posterior, and lateral aspects of the thorax. The auscultation of the thorax may be preceded by listening with the bell of the stethoscope in front of the nose or mouth; thus, evaluation of breath sounds can begin to take place before the sleeping infant or child is disturbed.

The chest is then auscultated to note breath sounds. The child is asked to breathe through his mouth deeply. A younger child may be asked to blow on an object such as a tissue to accomplish deep breathing. Children's breath sounds are almost always bronchovesicular or even bronchial. Decreased breath sounds may indicate pneumothorax, atelectasis, pneumonia, pleural effusion, or empyema. Increased breath sounds may be a sign of pneumonia. Breath sounds heard over the sternum or vertebral column may signify the presence of a foreign body, a mass, or some type of consolidation.

Abnormal sounds, such as rales, rhonchi, pleural rub, wheezing, and grunting, should be identified as either inspiratory or expiratory. Rales that disappear after coughing are not significant.

Rhonchi, originating in the larynx or trachea, should be distinguished from rales. Any sounds that are equal in intensity over the entire chest and resemble those from the nose most likely originate from the larynx or trachea.

Heart

Newborn Examination of the heart should take place when the baby is quiet, i.e., sleeping, feeding, or comfortable in his parent's arms. The stethoscope should be warm. Reassurance for the mother during auscultation is important since examination of the heart may take some time. An example of verbal reassurance is "Your little one sure has a good ticker."

Infant The appraisal is best done prior to examination of the chest and possibly as the first part of the physical examination. It is essential that it be done while the infant is quiet. Reassurance as well as education should be given to the parent during the examination.

Preschooler A slow, informative approach is best, with the preschooler in the presence of a parent. Allowing him to listen to the examiner's heart and then his own prior to the examination of his heart usually lessens any fantasy he might have about what is being heard through the stethoscope (Fig. 6-19). The blood pressure is an important part of the examination and can be tested by allowing the preschooler to inflate the cuff so that he feels he has some control over the situation.

School-Age Child This appraisal is included in the normal examination sequence. The child should have education regarding the examination and the accompanying findings. The school-age child is allowed to listen to his heart. During measurement of the blood pressure he is allowed to listen to what is being heard either on his arm or on the examiner's arm. Age-appropriate feedback should be included throughout the examination, especially about diet, exercise, and smoking and their effects on the heart.

Adolescent The teenager is allowed to listen to his

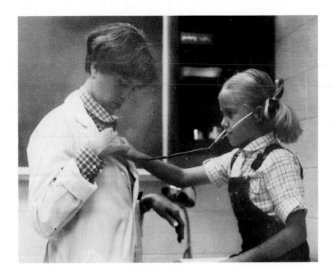

FIGURE 6-19   Child listening to examiner's heart. *(Courtesy of Molly U. McKinley.)*

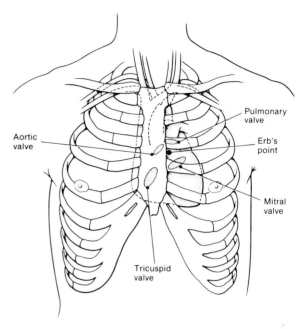

FIGURE 6-20   Areas of heart sounds.

TABLE 6-5 Grades of Murmur

Grade I	Barely audible murmur on auscultation
Grade II	Slight murmur heard in all positions; heard after exercise
Grade III	Moderate murmur; not accompanied by thrill
Grade IV	Loud murmur, accompanied by thrill
Grade V	Very loud murmur heard with stethoscope barely on chest; accompanied by thrill
Grade VI	Audible murmur heard with stethoscope a distance from chest wall and without stethoscope; accompanied by thrill

Sources: M. Green and J. B. Richmond, *Pediatric Diagnosis,* Saunders, Philadelphia, 1962, p. 98; L. A. Barness, *Manual of Pediatric Diagnosis,* Year Book, Chicago, 1972, pp. 119-120.

heart. Smoking, drinking, obesity, exercise, and their effects on the heart are discussed with him.

Examination of the heart usually follows auscultation of the chest; however, in the quiet newborn or infant it may precede it. The pulse is counted (apical in infants). A blood pressure reading is included in the appraisal at 3 years of age and thereafter.

The patient should be examined in the upright, supine, and left-lateral positions. Examination should also take place when the patient is leaning forward. The environment needs to be extremely quiet during the auscultation process. For the newborn and the infant, auscultation of the heart is done during sleep if at all possible.

The rate (see Table 6-3), rhythm, intensity, and any abnormality of heart sounds are noted over the aortic, pulmonary, tricuspid, and mitral regions and at Erb's point. A slight speeding of rhythm during inspiration and a decrease during expiration is known as a normal sinus arrhythmia. Any other tachycardia or bradycardia suggests a pathological condition.

Next the location of heart sounds must be determined to rule out any heart displacement (Fig. 6-20). The first heart sound is systolic; the second is diastolic. A third heart sound is heard in many children. If three heart sounds are heard, they must be distinguished from gallop rhythm, which is indicative of congestive heart failure and can be felt over the apex of the heart. This differentiation may be made by palpating the chest. The gallop rhythm can be palpated, but the third heart sound cannot. Also, the gallop rhythm would be present only if other signs of heart disease were present.

Sometimes there is turbulence of the flow of blood in the heart which is identified as a murmur. If a vibration is felt, it is known as a *thrill.* Since it is difficult to determine whether a murmur is organic or functional, murmurs should always be evaluated by a physician.

The nurse needs to locate the murmur, which heart sound it follows, point of maximum intensity, pitch, transmission, duration, quality (blowing, rapsy, rumbling, soft, harsh, whistling, etc.), and regularity. She should also note whether it disappears or increases after the child cries, exercises, or sits up. In addition to the aforementioned characteristics, murmurs are graded on a scale of I to VI (Table 6-5). By no means does the intensity of the murmur correlate with its seriousness. Any loud, continuous diastolic murmur requires medical follow-up; however, it can be an innocent murmur.

Innocent, or functional, murmurs can usually be described as transient, systolic, soft, or blowing. They are found along the left sternal border in the pulmonary area. They may disappear or decrease in intensity after exercise, crying, and eating, or they may change during the respiratory cycle, although the opposite may occur.

After auscultation, the nurse should determine

whether there is excess precordial activity. Then the point of maximal impulse (PMI), where the apex of the heart hits the chest wall, should be identified. The PMI is usually found inside the nipple line at the fourth to fifth intercostal space. In younger infants it may be found outside the nipple line. If the PMI cannot be felt, fluid or air may be present between the heart and the chest wall. Thrills may also be found during this palpation procedure.

A thrill can be described as similar to the feel of a cat purring. Thrills should be identified as to time of occurrence during the cardiac cycle. Thrills are usually associated with grade IV to VI murmurs. Systolic thrills radiating from the aortic area to the right side of the neck may be the result of aortic stenosis, and systolic thrills radiating to the left side of the neck may be the result of pulmonary stenosis. Continuing thrills also felt in this area may be indicative of patent ductus arteriosus. A diastolic thrill felt at the apex of the heart is very likely caused by mitral stenosis.

Percussion outline, the cardiac margins. This may give the examiner some idea of the size of the heart, but it has limited value. Dullness heard over the precordium during percussion may be suggestive of pericarditis.

Examination of carotid, radial, femoral, popliteal, and pedal pulses should identify presence, regularity, and intensity. Absence of any of these pulses suggests a pathological condition. For example, the femoral pulse is often absent in children who have coarctation of the aorta. In addition, cold, cyanotic, or pale extremities suggest the possibility of cardiac disease. In the older child, clubbing of the fingers should be identified.

The child should also be observed during or after exercise and feeding for color changes, excessive sweating, and exceptional fatigue. Growth grids are important in assessment of the heart because growth failure may accompany organic heart disease.

Breast

Newborn through School-Age Child This examination takes place at the same time as the examination of the chest.

Adolescent In the late school-age period and in adolescence examination of the breasts of girls is an occasion where modesty is of major concern. The examination is conducted, and the patient is taught how to perform self-examination. This instruction should be followed with a return demonstration.

Breasts are examined in both male and female children. Engorgement is commonly found in newborns of both sexes. "Witch's milk," the equivalent of colostrum, can be expressed from some newborns' nipples.

Regardless of the age or sex of the patient, the breasts should be examined for infection, abnormal growths, abnormal size, and tissue amount. Any child whose breasts develop before the usual time should be observed for other signs of precocious puberty.

With the patient in sitting and lying positions the breasts are observed for symmetry, dimpling, masses, color, discharge, and skin problems. These observations are repeated with the patient's hands raised above the head, with the hands pressed over the lateral aspects of the waist, and with the patient leaning forward. Palpation should take place while the patient is upright as well as reclining. When reclining, the patient should have a folded towel placed under the shoulder on the side on which the breast examination is being performed. The breasts are divided into several pie-shaped areas. In each area examination takes place from the distal portion of the breast to the nipple and should include axillary, pectoral, supraclavicular, infraclavicular, and subscapular nodes. The epitrochlear nodes should also be palpated over the medial epicondyle of the humerus. The areola is inspected and palpated for abnormalities. Finally, the nipple is compressed between the index finger and thumb around the entire circumference; there should be no discharge.

The male should also be examined for similar abnormalities and to note any increased size of the breasts, which may indicate an endocrine disorder. An increase in the size of the male's breasts at the time of puberty may be a normal deviation.

Abdomen

Newborn The newborn should be examined while he is sucking, sleeping, or quietly lying in his parent's lap. The examiner should have warm hands.

Infant The infant, like the newborn, is examined best while quiet and sucking. The infant is placed either on the laps of the parent and the examiner or on the examination table, and his thighs are held in a flexed position so that deep palpation is possible (Fig. 6-21).

Toddler Usually by this age the patient has begun to be ticklish and may be frightened or uncomfortable. Examination can be successfully carried out by placing the child on the table, flexing his knees, and talking to him as the abdomen is auscultated with a warm stethoscope. After auscultation the examiner can use the hand which is already holding the stethoscope and begin light and then

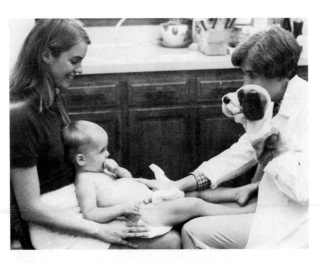

FIGURE 6-21 Using the mother's and examiner's laps for examination of the abdomen. *(Courtesy of Molly U. McKinley.)*

deeper palpation. Conversation should continue throughout the examination.

Preschooler The approach used for the toddler can be taken with the preschooler. Additionally, if the child is moving or is ticklish, the examiner can place the child's hand between hers and the abdominal wall and proceed with the palpation. Tenderness can be elicited using this method. A very ticklish child can also be examined by placing his hands on his own abdomen and spreading his fingers. Palpation is then conducted between the fingers.

School-Age Child and Adolescent The same techniques are used with the school-age child, but much conversation centered on subjects other than what is being done should be carried out. Deep palpation may be more successful if it is performed when the child takes a deep breath. At the conclusion of the examination, information regarding the findings can be shared with the patient.

The presence of a concave abdomen suggests a diaphragmatic hernia, and a convex abdomen suggests some type of obstruction. The neonate's umbilical cord should be observed for one vein and two arteries and for signs of bleeding, infection, or granuloma. The older child's abdomen is examined for size, contour, and skin abnormalities. The contour should be examined while the child is standing and then in a reclining position. Children under 4 years of age usually have a "potbelly" appearance. Masses, feces, air, or fluid must be suspected if the distention is generalized. It is not uncommon to see protrusion of the infant's umbilicus. Normally the protrusion disappears after the first 2 years of life or by the time the child begins to walk. It may be present up to the first 7 years of life in black children. The examiner should inspect the child's abdomen for diastasis of the rectus muscles. Such a defect in the wall should be measured periodically. It is considered a normal variant if the defect is no more than 5 cm (2 in) wide.

Auscultation is carried out after inspection if at all possible so that palpation or percussion will not disturb the bowel sounds. Auscultation is done to determine the presence or absence of peristalsis. Hypoactive peristalsis suggests peritoneal irritation. Bowel sounds may increase with the conditions of peritonitis, obstruction, gastroenteritis, and anxiety. Absence indicates some obstruction, such as paralytic ileus; bowel sounds are also absent immediately after abdominal surgery.

The entire abdomen is percussed in an orderly fashion. Possible points of tenderness are percussed last. A tympanic sound is usually found. A dull percussive sound over the liver helps outline its borders; dullness over the other parts of the abdomen suggests abnormal growths or fecal masses. Percussion in a child with appendicitis may result in rebound tenderness.

Infants are observed for visible peristaltic waves, which may indicate an obstruction, such as pyloric stenosis, or congestive heart failure. These waves may be considered normal finding in preterm or small newborns.

Palpation begins with the lower chest or the inguinal area. The beginning point should be the point least likely to cause difficulty. First, palpation should focus on superficial masses. All four quadrants of the abdomen are palpated lightly. The examiner should note tenderness (as exhibited by guarding), softness, or hardness. At this time it is important to note whether the spleen can be felt. The spleen can be further palpated lightly after the child has been placed on the right side. Usually the spleen should not be felt. If it is palpable, a pathological condition is suggested. Conversely, the liver is easily felt 1 to 2 cm below the costal margin up to 1 year of age in thin children. This finding can usually be considered normal but should be interpreted in association with other signs and symptoms.

A hungry infant should be given a pacifier or bottle when his abdomen is palpated for a pyloric tumor. The tumor can be found below the right costal margin just to the right of the midline of the abdomen. The entire abdomen is then palpated for other superficial masses. Deep palpation follows over the entire abdomen in the same orderly fashion as for superficial palpation.

Kidneys and deep abdominal masses are best felt on deep palpation when the child is inhaling or exhaling thoroughly. Bimanual palpation by ballottement is useful for feeling retroperitoneal masses. One hand is placed above the area being examined and one below the area. The ballotting hand should quickly be thrust into the area being examined. Rebound tenderness may be elicited, and masses may be felt.

Finally, inguinal areas are examined for lymph node enlargement and other masses. A mass in the inguinal area is always abnormal. Masses may be tumors, hernias, or undescended testicles, and the child should always be referred to a physician.

Genitalia

Newborn and Infant The appraisal is performed at the same time as the abdominal examination. The examiner should be sure that her hands are warm.

Toddler If there is a possibility of undescended testicles in a male toddler, he is placed in a squatting position on the floor. The scrotum and inguinal canal are then palpated for the presence of the testicle. The warm, soapy hands of the examiner help guide the testicle into the sac. The female toddler should be placed in a semirecumbent position on her mother's lap. The mother is facing the examiner, and their knees are in contact. The child's feet are placed against the examiner's knees. The mother is then asked to spread the labia majora apart so that the genitalia can be assessed by the examiner. The toddler may be less apprehensive if all clothes but her underpants have been put back on. Appraisal of the genitalia should be the last part of the examination.

Preschooler The examination position for the preschool girl is the same as for the female toddler, but instead of having the mother spread the labia majora, the nurse can instruct the preschooler to place both index fingers on the labia. Then the examiner places her index fingers on top of the child's and guides the child's fingers to spread the labia major. At this point the preschooler is asked to cough, thus making the genitalia more visible. A preschool male can be asked to squat or can be placed on the examining table with his legs crossed, thus eliminating the cremasteric reflex.

School-Age Child The examination of the genitalia in the school-age child should be one of the last parts of the exam. Young girls like having their mothers present during this exam, and boys usually prefer having it done without a parent present. Boys should be given anticipatory guidance that an erection during an examination is a normal response. If testicles are to be examined, the examiner's warm, soapy hands will facilitate manipulating the testicle down into the scrotal sac. If the cremasteric reflex is strong, the examiner can ask the boy to sit cross-legged on the table or on a towel on the floor. Not only does this position lessen embarrassment for the patient, it also eliminates the cremasteric reflex (Hoekelman, 1980, p. 352).

Adolescent The examination usually is done while the parents are not present. It should be performed with gloved hands. Testicles may ascend into the inguinal canals, and an erection may occur as a result of their being examined. Appropriate education should be provided regarding this reflex. In addition, instruction about self-examination of the testicles should be provided during this part of the examination and followed by a return demonstration. The pelvic examination of the adolescent girl is discussed in Chap. 29. It is not done routinely in the pediatric setting but should be done routinely in a setting providing health care for adolescents. The genital examination gives the examiner the opportunity to educate the patient about the normal pubertal changes taking place. Teenagers, being unfamiliar with their body parts and changes, often fear that normal changes are pathological.

The genitalia of both males and females are carefully inspected with gloved hands for abnormalities. Female patients are examined for synechia vulvae, enlarged clitoris, masses in the labia majora, and imperforate hymen. The presence and distribution pattern of pubic hair should be noted not only at the time of pubertal changes but also prior to puberty so that endocrine disorders can be detected. A vaginal or urethral discharge may indicate the presence of foreign bodies or some type of infection. Discharge in the newborn girl is almost always normal, even if it is tinged with blood.

Male patients should be examined for the size of the penis. The position of the urethral meatus is observed to rule out epispadias and hypospadias. A urethral discharge should also be looked for in the examination. If uncircumcised, the penis should be inspected for phimosis and infection. The circumcised male's penis is checked for adhesions of the remaining foreskin and infection.

The scrotum should be examined for the presence and size of each testis. See Chap. 29 for more details on the examination and a review of the Tanner stages of sexual maturation. The examiner should note any pain upon palpation. If the scrotal sac is enlarged, transillumination should be used to determine whether the enlargement is a hydrocele, a hernia, or a mass. An irreducible, transilluminated mass is usually a hydrocele. A mass that cannot be transilluminated may be a hernia. However, bowel filled with air in the scrotum can be transilluminated. Any acute swelling of the scrotum should be seen by a physician since it may be due to torsion of the spermatic cord or another more serious disorder.

Finally, the cremasteric reflex is tested by stroking the inner aspect of each thigh. If the testis does not rise within the scrotum, one must consider it a positive neurological sign.

Perineum and Rectum

Newborn The newborn is placed on his back with the hips flexed, and the anus is gently exposed and lubricated. The little finger, covered by a well-lubricated finger cot, is used for this examination. The examiner explains to the parents that crying may occur and that the examination may stimulate the passage of stool. The parents may be told that use of the little finger is comparable to the insertion of a rectal thermometer.

Infant This examination is uncomfortable for the infant. It is performed in much the same way as in the newborn. Some infants, especially older ones, are more cooperative if placed prone on a parent's lap with the legs dangling. The infant can be distracted with talking and toys while the examination is performed. This appraisal should be the last part of the examination.

Toddler Most toddlers do not like having this examination done. The lap position described for the infant can be used for the young toddler. Sims's position is also very convenient and seems less threatening. If the rectal examination is being used to rule out appendicitis, the toddler should be placed on his back with the legs and hips flexed. The mother should be near the child's head to comfort him during the examination. The examination can be compared to having a rectal temperature taken.

Preschooler The preschooler needs to have the rectal examination explained to him by equating it to having his temperature taken. The little finger is generally still used; however, some examiners prefer the index finger in larger preschool children. Sims's position is the most comfortable position as long as the child can see his parent during the exam. If appendicitis is being ruled out, the child is examined while on his back. The lubricant used for the examination should be shown to him before it is applied to the anal area. He is allowed to touch it as well as put a finger cot on his finger. The examiner begins by first applying the lubricant to the anal area and then very gently inserting the lubricated finger into the rectum while at the same time asking the child to take a deep breath. The examiner tells the child that he may feel like he is having a bowel movement. Supportive and encouraging conversation throughout the examination will result in a cooperative, relaxed child unless pain is elicited.

School-Age Child Some younger school-age children prefer having a parent with them during the examination, while older ones prefer having the parents out of the room. The approach to the actual examination is the same as that for the preschooler, with the exception that the index finger is used in place of the fifth finger. Age-appropriate education should be done before, during, and after the examination. Engaging the child in topics of conversation which are interesting to him may help him relax during the exam, especially if he is anxious.

Adolescent The adolescent usually finds the rectal examination the most uncomfortable part of the physical examination. The male adolescent can be asked to assume either the knee-chest position or Sims's position, or he may wish to bend his upper body over the examination table while he stands. The latter two are usually preferred. The female usually prefers Sims's position, but at times it is necessary to include the rectal examination during the pelvic examination. As with the school-age child, it is necessary to explain to the adolescent in detail what to expect from the examiner and what it will feel like. The lubricant and the type of glove to be used should be shown to the patient. The teenager is asked to take a deep breath during the time of finger insertion. Once this has been done, the teen is encouraged to talk by being asked questions so that his attention is diverted. Appropriate education regarding the findings should follow the examination.

The perineal area in both sexes should be examined for abnormal growths and signs of scratching. Scratching may indicate the presence of pinworms.

The anal region should be observed for abnormal masses, rectal prolapse, and mucosal tabs. A well-lubricated finger is then used to perform the rectal examination. Any tear found in the mucosa indicates an anal fissure. If any fissures are present, bleeding may follow the examination. The tone of the anal sphincter should be noted. A tight sphincter may be indicative of anal stenosis and may result in constipation and pain upon defecation.

A shelflike mass several centimeters above the anus may indicate aganglionic megacolon. It is also possible to palpate a retrorectal mass and the uterus during the rectal examination. The presence or absence, amount, and consistency of feces in the rectum should be assessed by palpation. Absence of feces in an ill child may indicate obstruction. Large amounts of feces may indicate anal stenosis, psychological problems, or constipation. By means of a bimanual rectal examination (using the index finger in the rectum and the other hand on the abdomen), points of abdominal tenderness may be identified. For example, a rectal examination is used in ruling out appendicitis. The inserted finger is not initially pointed toward the area of suspected tenderness, since pain can cause the child to quickly lift his buttocks off the table. At the conclusion of the examination, however, the examining finger is directed toward the area of suspected tenderness.

Neuromuscular System, Extremities, and Spine

The approach described will encompass the examination of both the central nervous system and the musculoskeletal system, since both involve testing the same parts of the body and watching the child at play. Developmental considerations are as follows.

Newborn and Infant The child is examined during both waking and sleeping periods for the assessment of these systems. The appraisal may be conducted on the examination table, in the bassinet, or in the parent's arms.

Toddler and Preschooler The toddler should be evaluated as he walks into and in the health care environment. He is given toys to play with during both the interview and the physical examination. When evaluated, these observations will give the nurse valuable information regarding the use of his extremities and spine and the status of his central nervous system.

School-Age Child The school-age child should be observed when he is being weighed and measured and as he walks in the health care environment. During the interview, body posture, response to questions, and emotional status give valuable information pertaining to these systems. Following the interview, a systematic evaluation of the neuromuscular system is integrated throughout the physical exam. Age-appropriate explanations of the examination and the examiner's findings should be given to the patient during and at the completion of the exam.

Adolescent Same as for the school-age child.

Extremities and Spine

The examination of the musculoskeletal system takes place from the time the history and physical examination begin. Initially, the child's ability to move is observed in relation to his developmental stage. The absence of movement as a result of a musculoskeletal deformity, injury, or disease is noted.

Throughout the history and examination the examiner should listen for complaints of pain. Types of pain are good indicators of the types of disorders present. For example, pain that occurs with the movement of a part and is relieved with rest is usually the result of injury to that part. Beall (1977, p. 2) noted that a "loose fragment of bone in a joint will give sudden, severe pain of short duration. In the event of infection in a part, the pain is severe and is not relieved by rest." In addition, tumors of the bone can "cause a similar constant pain which frequently will awaken the patient at night."

The initial inspection of the musculoskeletal system should focus on limited motion, deformities, asymmetry (due to swelling, atrophy, or shortening), and inflammation. The child is observed while walking, both during play and as the result of a command, from all points of view, with an emphasis on the lateral view. During this time the two phases of the walking gait—stance and swing—are inspected for any deviation, with particular attention paid to the phase involved in the deviation. The stance "includes heel strike, midstance with the entire foot on the floor, and toe-off." The swing phase involves "foot acceleration, swing-through and deceleration" (Beall, 1977, p. 2). The child's lower extremities are examined for varus or valgus deviations, torsion of the legs, or clubbing of the feet. These conditions are discussed more thoroughly in Chap. 22. The cause of toeing-in and toeing-out with ambulation should be determined.

The neck, torso, and extremities are put through first

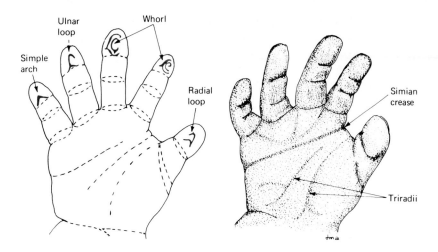

FIGURE 6-22 Geographic creases of the palms.

active and then passive range of motion. The neutral zero method is the one most commonly used to measure joint motion. That is, "the anatomic position is the position of full extension and is considered to be the zero point. All movements are measured in increasing degrees of arc from this point" (Beall, 1977, p. 2). When the joints are being put through range of motion, the joint is palpated to determine whether there is crepitus or catching. Swelling, heat, inflammation, or atrophy of these parts is noted. Length of extremities should be measured. True limb length is measured by selecting two bony prominences as constants; e.g., "to measure the length of legs one should measure from the anteriorsuperior iliac spine to the level of the medial malleolus" (Beall, 1977, p. 6). Circumferential muscle mass is measured at the same points on both arms and at the same points on both legs.

Next, the extremities should be observed for abnormal masses, sores, deviation, or extra digits. The temperature of the skin is noted, and all the pulses (cited earlier in this chapter) are palpated. The hands and soles of the feet should be checked for normal geographic creases or the presence of simian creases. A simian crease may be normal or abnormal. Signs of generalized edema should be noted (Fig. 6-22).

In an infant, the hips should be abducted passively to 180° to rule out hip dislocation. Each hip can be rotated only to a 45° angle if dislocation is present. To be complete, an Ortolani test should be done. The index finger is placed just below the inguinal ligament over the greater trochanter. The examiner then abducts and lifts the lower extremity being examined. A "click" is felt as the hip is reduced and is considered a positive finding. Allis's sign can be elicited by placing the patient supine with the feet flat on the examining table and the hips and knees flexed. The examiner, standing at the foot of the table, determines whether the knees are at different levels. If this observation is positive, a dislocated hip is suspected. Allis's sign can be checked not only in infants but also in older children with suspected hip problems (Beall, 1977).

After the extremities have been assessed, the neck and spine are examined for limitations in motion and for de-

formities. When examining the spine, the examiner asks the child to sit, stand, and bend over. In this way a curvature can be detected. During the time the patient is standing for observation of the spine, the presence or absence of Trendelenburg's sign is noted.

The sacrococcygeal area is the last part to be examined. Any type of postanal dimple should be checked thoroughly to rule out neurological and cord defects. Any mass, open areas, drainage, or signs of inflammation should be examined by a physician.

Central Nervous System

A thorough developmental and emotional history is taken of the parents and/or the child. A history of behavioral problems, gait deviations, dizziness, febrile convulsions, ataxia, muscle weakness, loss of muscle control, twitching, loss of any special sense, or meningeal irritation is reason for a more thorough neurological examination.

The basis for the neurological examination of the newborn through the preschool child is development. A very thorough developmental history and evaluation should be performed, including the areas of gross motor, fine motor, language, and social development. If at any time there are abnormal deviations in any area of development, a more thorough neurological examination should be performed. It is of the utmost importance that examination of the eye grounds be included in the neurological examination. During the developmental/neurological history and examination of the older child, emotions, behavior, level of consciousness, reading ability, speech patterns, and intellectual responses should be elicited and evaluated.

The newborn should be examined for the presence of the primary reflexes. The reflexes should start to diminish at around 3 months of age and be completely gone at 4 to 6 months. Any residual primary reflexes should be considered as positive neurological signs. More detail about this examination is given in Chap. 20.

The primary reflexes present are walking, stepping, rooting, crawl, Bauer's, suck, grasp, Moro, tonic neck, sole plantar, and spinal curvature. The normal newborn should be in a flexed position, have good muscle tone, and show no signs of muscle paralysis. Parts of this examination can be carried out while watching a newborn in his parent's arms. The reflexes should be tested systematically.

Along with evaluation of the primary reflexes, the newborn's deep tendon reflexes and state of consciousness are of equal importance. The state of consciousness is evaluated in the awake and asleep states.

The older child's neurological examination includes developmental history and evaluation of cerebral functioning, cranial nerves, cerebellum, special senses, and motor development. Ankle clonus should be noted and considered within normal limits in the very young infant and abnormal in the older infant (over 7 months) and child. If strong deep tendon reflexes are found in the infant and child, the nurse should have a neurologist follow up with a more thorough examination to rule out a pathological condition.

Meningeal irritation should be suspected if an older child complains of a stiff neck and resists flexing it or if a newborn or infant suddenly cries when the legs are lifted for a diaper change. This resistance to bending the neck may not always be present in children with meningeal irritation. The examiner should also attempt to elicit Kernig's sign and Brudzinski's sign. If either is elicited, the examiner should suspect meningitis.

Testing

To supplement the history and physical assessment, certain standard tests should be performed. Some are routine for any age group, while others are used when the child attains a certain age. Obviously, the standard tests are either supplemented or replaced by others if certain findings result from the history and physical examination. Testing in this context involves the use of standardized procedures for measuring the biochemical, physical, psychological, and developmental status of an individual. The order in which various tests are done is not always the same. Some which are considered routine can be done before, during, or after the history and physical examination. The purpose of these tests is to identify children at risk for developmental deficits or other problems. Testing provides a method of determining the developmental level at which the child is functioning.

Test Selection

Most developmental tests (screening and diagnostic) are based on samples of social behavior, gross and fine motor skills, and communications skills. It is extremely important that the nurse select tests that (1) are standardized for a large population, (2) have a high reliability (measure what they claim to measure), and (3) are valid (perform well related to outside nontest criteria). Nurses should be familiar with sources which report information about standardization of the tests they select and discuss the level of competency necessary to administer and evaluate the tests. Examples of such sources are Buro's *Mental Measurements Yearbook* and Anastasi's *Psychological Testing.*

Assessment by testing may be done routinely (e.g., developmental testing on all well babies, toddlers, and preschoolers) or selectively, when a deviation is suspected (e.g., language development testing, emotional development testing). To exercise judgment regarding the selection of tests, the nurse must be aware of the various purposes tests serve. For example, tests may perform the following functions:

1. Provide baseline data for future comparisons.
2. Provide baseline data for ongoing nursing and health care team action
3. Obtain data not otherwise readily available by observation, examination, or history
4. Distinguish between the individual's present and potential functioning
5. Determine the area and level of dysfunction
6. Assist in determining intervention by nurses or other members of the health care team
7. Provide information on the basis of which the nurse may wish to make a referral

Another consideration in test selection is whether indirect or direct evaluation of the child is more advantageous. In an indirect approach, for example, the examiner asks specific questions of the parent (or responsible person) about the child's behavior. Typical questions are (1) Is your child able to (or at what age did your child) climb? skip? jump? unwrap covers? fasten shoes? (2) Is your child able to (or at what age did your child) help with the simple tasks? play competitively? singe harmoniously? (3) Does your child (or at what age did your child) imitate or echo your sounds and words? talk in phrases? describe and share events? (4) Does your child (or at what age did your child) mind? get a drink? toilet self? The Prescreening Developmental Questionnaire and the Preschool Attainment Record (PAR) are examples of this approach to assessment and are used extensively by developmental specialists when direct observation of the child may not be expedient because of illness of the child, absence at the time of interview, or other reasons. Data from this approach are not obtained by observing the child directly.

The major approach to developmental testing is for the examiner to observe the child's behavior directly when he is asked or induced to perform specific and predetermined acts. Examples include the following: (1) placing the infant on his abdomen and observing whether he lifts his head and chest (age 2 to 4 months), (2) telling the child to walk backward and observing whether he can take two or more steps while retaining balance (age 12 to 22 months), (3) asking the child to hop on one foot and observing whether he can do so two or more times (age 3 to 5 years), (4) placing a block in each of the child's hands and encouraging the child to bang the blocks together (age 7 to 12 months), (5) asking the child to show his eyes, ears, and nose to the examiner (age 13 to 21 months), (6) placing colored blocks on the table and asking the child to identify the red block, the blue block, and so on (age 2½ to 4½ years), (7) giving the child a toy and gently pulling it away, observing whether the child resists having the toy taken away (age 4 to 10 months).

The direct observation approach enables the examiner to note the child's behavior pattern in relation to parents and examiner, thus providing additional clinical information. The Denver Developmental Screening Test (DDST) is an example of this approach. Both the direct and indirect approaches to developmental assessment are well-accepted procedures, and the choice depends on time available for testing, cost, convenience, and examiner preference.

Test Considerations

Testing may be done in the eco-setting (home or school), clinic, or inpatient hospital unit. The nurse should be aware of several considerations before proceeding with testing, including the following four major considerations:
1. Age of child
   (a) Short testing periods are needed for infants and toddlers as they tire easily.
   (b) A frequent change of activity for preschool children is useful because of their short attention span.
2. Eating and sleeping patterns
   (a) Infants may regurgitate if tested in the area of mobility after eating.
   (b) Preschool and school-age children should be tested 1 to 2 hours after eating in order to elicit maximum effort at the time of high energy levels.
   (c) School-age children need to be tested early in the school day. Fatigue and the need for creative play are high after school hours.
3. Facilities
   (a) The environment should be regulated for light, temperature, and noise. Distractions may alter test results at all age levels.
   (b) Adequate space should be available before testing developmental levels requiring movement or the placement of objects at specified distances.
4. Health of child
   (a) Physical well-being is necessary to maximize the child's ability to perform the requested tasks. Testing is deferred when the child is ill.
   (b) Stress in the testing situation is a normal response, but testing should be deferred if the child has suffered shock or physical or emotional trauma in the week preceding the examination.

Attending to these considerations increases both the validity and the reliability of the test results and provides the most satisfactory milieu for the nurse to focus on the child and his parents.

Laboratory Tests

Laboratory screening tests are also used to supplement information gathered through the history, developmental testing, linear measurements, and physical examination. Blood tests, such as hematocrit and hemoglobin, and urine analysis and cultures can be either routine or sup-

plemental to certain preliminary findings. Other blood tests and cultures may be ordered, depending on the findings and the plan of action. These tests are all considered standardized and have specific normal values for the national population as well as for the institution in which the tests are being performed.

Graphic Testing

Graphic testing is also done to supplement the information derived from the tests described above. Such tests as the electrocardiogram and electroencephalogram are selected to accompany a nurse's referral to a specific physician or nurse or preparatory to a nurse-physician consultation.

Radiological Testing

Radiological studies may be ordered by a nurse in consultation with a medical colleague in order to obtain additional information about specific problems.

General Comments

The purposes of any of these tests can be summarized as follows:
1. To augment information gathered during the history and physical examination
2. To obtain additional data when referring a patient for medical, nursing, or other professional consultation
3. To provide data for making a nursing diagnosis
4. To provide additional data for planning a nursing intervention
5. To provide additional data to evaluate outcome

In making efforts to gather additional information through tests that are not considered routine, much discretion and consultation should be used.

Study Questions

1. The major difference between examination of an adult and examination of a child is:
   A. The examination is more lengthy with a child.
   B. The child's parents assist with the examination.
   C. The size of the child.
   D. The examination is based on growth and development.
2. The least threatening place for an examination of an infant, toddler, or preschooler is:
   A. A brightly colored examination room.
   B. A toy-filled examination room.
   C. On a parent's lap.
   D. His own home environment.
3. Height and weight measurement should be:
   A. Obtained at least five times during the first year of life.
   B. Plotted each time it is obtained.
   C. Done at each physical examination.
   D. All of the above.

4. When evaluating height and weight, one must:
    A. Evaluate them in relation to each other.
    B. Evaluate them in relation to head circumference.
    C. Plot them on standardized charts.
    D. All of the above.
5. Blood pressure measurements are accurate if:
    A. The BP cuff is not less than half the width of the upper arm.
    B. The BP cuff is not greater than two-thirds of the width of the upper arm.
    C. The bladder of the cuff encompasses the arm.
    D. All of the above.
6. A pulse rate in a young child should be counted for:
    A. 10 seconds.   C. 30 seconds.
    B. 15 seconds.   D. 60 seconds.
7. The anterior fontanel can be expected to close at:
    A. 2 to 3 weeks.   C. 12 to 18 months.
    B. 3 to 4 months.   D. 24 to 36 months.
8. Transillumination of the skull should be conducted:
    1. Routinely.
    2. If there is a question about the size of a fontanel.
    3. If the head circumference is abnormal.
    4. If the shape of the head is normal.
        A. 1, 3, and 4
        B. 2, 3, and 4
        C. 1, 2, 3, and 4
        D. None of the above
9. The cover test is a test for:
    A. Strabismus.
    B. Convergence.
    C. Pupillary light reflex.
    D. Color blindness.
10. In a child less than 3 years of age the otoscopic exam is conducted by:
    A. Allowing the auricle to maintain its natural position.
    B. Pulling the auricle down.
    C. Pulling the auricle up.
    D. Pulling the auricle down and back.
11. The purpose of air insufflation during the ear examination is to:
    A. Determine the patency of the ear canal.
    B. Observe the mobility of the drum.
    C. Determine hearing levels.
    D. Rule out the presence of a tumor.
12. When a tuning fork is used for hearing tests, it is placed against the mastoid process and subsequently 1 in from the ear. The child should hear the:
    A. Air-conducted vibrations longer than the bone-conducted ones.
    B. Bone-conducted vibrations longer than the air-conducted ones.
    C. Bone-conducted vibrations louder than the air-conducted ones.
    D. Bone-conducted vibrations and air-conducted vibrations equal lengths of time.

13. A newborn with blockage of one side of the nose must be examined:
    A. For a cleft palate.
    B. For a possible sinus tumor.
    C. For respiratory distress.
    D. None of the above.
14. For examination of the mouth, the young child should be:
    A. Placed in a reclining position.
    B. Restrained with his hands under his back.
    C. Restrained on the lap of a parent.
    D. Placed in a mummy restraint.
15. Children normally have palpable nodes up to about 12 years of age.
    A. True
    B. False
16. Rales are considered abnormal chest sounds:
    A. Whenever they are heard with the naked ear.
    B. Unless they disappear after coughing.
    C. Unless they remain after coughing.
    D. When they are found only in one lobe.
17. A thrill is defined as a:
    A. Turbulence of the flow of blood heard during the heart examination.
    B. Turbulence of the flow of blood heard by the patient when he is resting.
    C. Turbulence of the flow of blood heard over a shunt.
    D. Turbulence of the flow of blood felt as a vibration over the heart.
18. A grade VI murmur is:
    A. Audible without a stethoscope.
    B. Audible only after exercise.
    C. A moderate murmur accompanied by a thrill.
    D. A murmur not accompanied by a thrill.
19. Regardless of the age or sex of patients, the breasts should be examined.
    A. True
    B. False
20. If a concave abdomen is detected during the physical examination of a newborn, one should consider:
    A. An intestinal obstruction.
    B. A hiatal hernia.
    C. A diaphragmatic hernia.
    D. It normal.
21. If a 1-year-old child's liver is felt 1 cm below the costal margin, this is:
    A. Indicative of an obstruction of the biliary tract.
    B. Indicative of congestive heart failure.
    C. Considered normal for this age.
    D. Considered normal for any age.
22. The examination of the genitalia of an adolescent, whether male or female, should be performed with gloved hands.
    A. True
    B. False

23. A rectal examination can be used for:
    A. Ruling out appendicitis.
    B. Examination of the anus.
    C. Ruling out obstruction.
    D. All of the above.
24. During an examination of the hips of a newborn the examiner should be able to abduct them passively to:
    A. 45°.   C. 180°.
    B 90°.   D. 200°.
25. The primary reflexes of a newborn should disappear by:
    A. 1 month.   C. 6 months.
    B. 3 months.   D. 8 months.

References

Beall, M.S.: "Evaluation of the Musculoskeletal System in the Pediatric Patient," *Issues in Comprehensive Pediatric Nursing,* 2(4):1-13, 1977.
Hoekelman, R.A.: "The Pediatric Physical Examination," in B. Bates (ed.), *A Guide to Physical Examination,* 2d ed., Lippincott, Philadelphia, 1980.

Bibliography

Baer, E., M. McGowan, and D. McGivern: "How to Take a Health History," *American Journal of Nursing,* 77(7):1090-1133, 1977.
Benjamin, A.: *The Helping Interview,* Houghton, Mifflin, Boston, 1974.
Bernstein, L., R. Bernstein, and R. Dana: *Interviewing: A Guide for Health Professionals,* 2d ed., Appleton-Century-Crofts, New York, 1974.
Brammer, L.: *The Helping Relationship: Process and Skills,* Prentice-Hall, Englewood Cliffs, N.J., 1973.
Brown, J.: *Telephone Medicine,* Mosby, St. Louis, 1980.
Dunn, L.J.: "Legal Aspects of Communication with and about the Pediatric Patient," *Issues in Comprehensive Pediatric Nursing,* 4(5-6):13-18, September-December 1980.
Erikson, E.: *Childhood and Society,* 2d ed., Norton, New York, 1963.
Gundy, J.H.: *Assessment of the Child in Primary Health Care,* McGraw-Hill, New York, 1981.
Piaget, J.: *The Origins of Intelligence in Children,* International Universities Press, New York, 1952.
Smith, J., and M. Felice: "Interviewing Adolescent Patients: Some Guidelines for the Clinician" *Pediatric Annals,* 9(6):38-44, 1980.

7

Nutritional Influences on Child Health

Objectives

After reading this chapter, the student will be able to:
1. Describe two critical growth periods.
2. Discuss the different caloric needs of infants, children, and adolescents.
3. Identify the variables which influence a child's nutritional status.
4. Describe the special nutritional needs of preterm and low-birth-weight neonates.
5. Discuss the pros and cons of breast-feeding and formula feeding.
6. Identify the components of a pediatric nutritional assessment.

Nutrition in the healthy child includes consideration of nutritional needs for growth as well as psychosocial and developmental influences on dietary habits. For ill children, the impact of disease on nutritional status is also an important factor. The role of early dietary practices in the prevention of obesity, hypertension, cancer, and atherosclerosis has not been defined (Committee on Nutrition, 1986b). However, the impact of nutritional status on growth, susceptibility to infection (Puri and Chandra, 1985), and recovery from trauma has been established. Nutritional intervention in the pediatric setting involves both nutritional support during illness and nutritional education for the promotion of health. The purpose of this chapter is to review nutrition in fostering children's health.

Role of Nutrition in Growth

Nutrition and Physical Growth

Increases in physical size are the most visible signs of growth in infants, children, and adolescents. Growth in physical size, body organs, and tissues occurs as a result of sequential increases in the number or size of cells. Growth is influenced by genetic, behavioral, environmental, hormonal, and nutritional factors (Vaughan, 1983).

Critical Periods of Growth

Growth in children has classically been measured in terms of weight and height. Growth from infancy to adolescence involves incremental increases in weight, height, and head circumference which vary with age. Accelerated weight gain and linear growth peak during two critical periods including infancy (Vaughan, 1983) and adolescence. Head circumference has been used as a measure of brain growth in children during the first years of life. The critical period of cellular growth in which malnutrition may alter brain development occurs between mid-pregnancy and the second year of life (Dobbing, 1974).

Catchup growth is a phenomenon used to describe accelerated weight gain or linear growth in a child with a history of growth failure (Ashworth and Millard, 1986). A chronic history of inadequate calories and protein may adversely affect a child's growth potential in both weight and height. To achieve "normalization" of growth, nutrients must be provided in excess of normal needs to allow for the increased requirements for accelerated weight gain and linear growth. Severely malnourished children may grow at rates 20 times the normal weight gain for healthy children of the same age (Ashworth and Millard, 1986).

Serial measurements of weight and height are used to monitor the adequacy of growth in a child from birth to adolescence. Reference standards for physical growth are used to compare growth in an individual with sex and age-adjusted percentiles. The reference standards (Hamill, 1979) established by the National Center for Health Statistics (NCHS) include growth charts for: (1) weight, length, and weight for length in the birth to 36-month age group, and (2) weight, height, and weight for height in the 2- to 18-year age group. The growth charts are presented in Appendix B.

Body Composition

Weight provides a gross measure of nutritional status but does not differentiate between the contributions of adipose tissue and lean body mass (muscle mass) to total body weight. There are sex- and age-related differences in body composition which occur between infancy and adolescence (Fomon, Haschkes, Ziegler, and Nelson, 1982). For example, the adipose content of the body is highest between 4 and 6 months of age (Fomon, Ziegler, and O'Donnell, 1974) and the onset of puberty (Forbes, 1978). Sexual differences in lean body mass (muscle mass) and adipose tissue are most evident in adolescence.

During puberty, growth of lean body mass is greater in males while accumulation of adipose tissue is greater in females (Forbes, 1978).

Nutrient Intake and Utilization

The nutritional needs of children are determined by requirements for maintenance of normal body function, growth, and physical activity. Nutritional status has been defined as "the condition of the body resulting from utilization of the essential nutrients available to the body" (Boerma, 1975). The nutritional status of a child is affected by three factors: (1) intake of essential nutrients, (2) requirements for nutrients, and (3) the body's utilization of the consumed nutrients.

The Recommended Dietary Allowances (RDAs) are guidelines for the average nutrient needs of a healthy population. THE RDAs are not intended for use in determining individual needs and do not account for altered requirements in acute or chronic disease. The nutrient requirements established by the RDAs provide a margin of safety above minimal needs.

Energy Needs

The body utilizes the energy provided by foods in the form of carbohydrates, protein, and fats. The caloric content of each of these sources of energy is as follows:

1 g fat = 9 cal
1 g protein = 4 cal
1 g carbohydrate = 4 cal

A kilocalorie, or "calorie," is the amount of energy necessary to raise one kilogram of water one degree Celsius.

The caloric needs of infants, children, and adolescents are based primarily on requirements for maintenance, growth, and physical activity. Maintenance of normal body function or basal metabolism contributes to approximately 50 percent of total caloric needs. Energy allowances for growth vary with age. Physical activity is a significant factor to consider in computing the caloric needs of children. In the 2- to 10-year-old age group, physical activity accounts for almost one-third of energy needs compared with less than 5 percent of energy requirements in adults.

In Table 7-1 the caloric needs of infants, children, and adolescents are summarized. Energy requirements are highest in the first 6 months of life, remain constant from 4 to 10 years of age, and vary in adolescence depending on an individual's stage of physical maturity. Caloric requirements in adolescents are most appropriately based on height rather than chronological age to reflect physiological needs during different stages of the growth spurt (Mahan and Rosebrough, 1984).

Guidelines for an Adequate Diet

The essentials of an adequate diet include selection and consumption of foods which provide adequate amounts of nutrients and energy for the maintenance of normal body function and growth. The use of a variety of foods in opti-

TABLE 7-1 Caloric Needs of Infants, Children, and Adolescents

Age Group	Caloric Needs
Infants	
Birth-6 mo	115 kcal/kg
6-12 mo	105 kcal/kg
Children	
1-3 yr	100 kcal/kg
4-6 yr	85 kcal/kg
7-10 yr	86 kcal/kg
Adolescents	
Males	
11-14 yr	17 kcal/cm height
15-18 yr	16 kcal/cm height
Females	
11-14 yr	14 kcal/cm height
15-18 yr	13 kcal/cm height

Source: Adapted from Food and Nutrition Board (1980).

mal amounts is the best assurance of an adequate diet.

Table 7-2 includes the major nutrient sources and physiological functions of 10 key nutrients which if consumed in appropriate amounts provide the other 40 essential nutrients required by the body. In addition to selecting a wide variety of foods, it is important to distinguish between foods of high versus low nutrient density. Foods of high nutrient density, or "protective" foods, provide major nutrient contributions, while foods of low nutrient density provide mainly calories. For example, high-nutrient-density foods include milk, meat, fortified and enriched whole grains, dark green or yellow vegetables, and citrus fruits, whereas low-nutrient-density foods include soft drinks, candy, cookies, and chips. The recommended number of servings from each food group for children and teenagers is enumerated in Table 7-3.

Carbohydrates

Carbohydrates in the diets of children include polysaccharides (starches), disaccharides (lactose, sucrose), and

---

TABLE 7-2 Nutrients for Health

Nutrient	Important Sources of Nutrient	Provide Energy	Build and Maintain Body Cells	Regulate Body Processes
			Some Major Physiological Functions	
Protein	Meat, poultry, fish Dried beans and peas Eggs Cheese Milk	Supplies 4 cal/g	Constitutes part of the structure of every cell, such as muscle, blood, and bone; supports growth and maintains healthy body cells	Constitutes part of enzymes, some hormones and body fluids, and antibodies that increase resistance to infection
Carbohydrate	Cereal Potatoes Dried beans Corn Bread Sugar	Supplies 4 cal/g Major source of energy for central nervous system	Supplies energy so protein can be used for growth and maintenance of body cells	Unrefined products supply fiber—complex carbohydrates in fruits, vegetables, and whole grains—for regular elimination; assists in fat utilization
Fat	Shortening, oil Butter, margarine Salad dressing Sausages	Supplies 9 cal/g	Constitutes part of the structure of every cell; supplies essential fatty acids	Provides and carries fat-soluble vitamins (A, D, E, and K)
Vitamin A (retinol)	Liver Carrots Sweet potatoes Greens Butter, margarine		Assists formation and maintenance of skin and mucous membranes that line body cavities and tracts, such as nasal passages and intestinal tract, thus increasing resistance to infection	Functions in visual processes and forms visual purple, thus promoting healthy eye tissues and eye adaptation in dim light
Vitamin C (ascorbic acid)	Broccoli Oranges Grapefruit Papaya Mango Strawberries		Forms cementing substances, such as collagen, that hold body cells together, thus strengthening blood vessels, hastening healing of wounds and bones, and increasing resistance to infection	Aids in utilization of iron

Source: National Dairy Council, *Guide to Good Eating,* 4th ed., Rosemont, Ill., 1985.

TABLE 7-2 Nutrients for Health—cont'd

| Nutrient | Important Sources of Nutrient | Some Major Physiological Functions | | |
		Provide Energy	Build and Maintain Body Cells	Regulate Body Processes
Thiamin (B$_1$)	Lean pork Nuts Fortified cereal products	Aids in utilization of energy		Functions as part of a co-enzyme to promote the utilization of carbohydrates; promotes normal appetite; contributes to normal functioning of nervous system
Riboflavin (B$_2$)	Liver Milk Yogurt Cottage cheese	Aids in utilization of energy		Functions as part of a co-enzyme in the production of energy within body cells; promotes healthy skin, eyes, and clear vision
Niacin	Liver Meat, poultry, fish Peanuts Fortified cereal products	Aids in utilization of energy		Functions as part of a co-enzyme in fat synthesis, tissue respiration, and utilization of carbohydrate; promotes healthy skin, nerves, and digestive tract; aids digestion and fosters normal appetite
Calcium	Milk, yogurt Cheese Sardines and salmon with bones Collard, kale, mustard, and turnip greens		Combines with other minerals within a protein framework to give structure and strength to bones and teeth	Assists in blood clotting; functions in normal muscle contraction and relaxation and normal nerve transmission
Iron	Enriched farina Prune juice Liver Dried beans and peas Red meat	Aids in utilization of energy	Combines with protein to form hemoglobin, the red substance in blood that carries oxygen to and carbon dioxide from the cells; prevents nutritional anemia and its accompanying fatigue; increases resistance to infection	Functions as part of enzymes involved in tissue respiration

monosaccharides (fructose, glucose). Carbohydrates provide the most readily available source of energy, and they should be supplied on a regular basis to prevent the depletion of body stores and the onset of ketosis. *Ketosis,* or the mobilization of fat stores for energy, occurs in children when carbohydrate sources provide less than 10 percent of the total caloric intake (Committee on Nutrition, 1985).

The selecton of carbohydrate sources is important in terms of nutrient density and the contribution of sucrose to caries. Complex carbohydrate sources, including enriched and fortified grains, contain B vitamins and iron, while fruits and vegetables are important sources of ascorbic acid, vitamin A, folic acid, and minerals. In contrast, simple carbohydrate sources (soft drinks, candy, sugar, cookies) contain large amounts of sucrose which provide

only calories and contribute significantly to the development of dental caries (Committee on Nutrition, 1985).

The use of diets containing increased amounts of dietary fiber has not been accepted widely in the pediatric setting. (Committee on Nutrition, 1985, 1981), although epidemiological studies have shown a decreased incidence of diverticular disease, colon cancer, and coronary heart disease in adults on high-fiber diets. Certain aspects of dietary fiber including (1) relatively low caloric density, (2) increased bulk or volume, and (3) adverse effects on mineral absorption contribute to concern about the use of high-fiber diets in children (Committee on Nutrition, 1985). The American Academy of Pediatrics (AAP), Committee on Nutrition, currently recommends a moderate intake of whole grains, fruits, and vegetables for normal laxation in children over 1 year of age. The use of

TABLE 7-3 Recommended Number of Servings from Each Food Group for Children and Teenagers

Food Group	Child	Teenager
Milk	3	4
1 cup milk, yogurt, *or*		
Calcium equivalent:		
1½ slices (1½ oz) cheddar cheese*		
1 cup pudding		
1¾ cups ice cream		
2 cups cottage cheese*		
Meat	2	2
2 oz cooked, lean meat, fish, poultry, *or*		
Protein equivalent:		
2 eggs		
2 slices (2 oz) cheddar cheese*		
½ cup cottage cheese*		
1 cup dried beans, peas		
4 tbsp peanut butter		
Fruit-vegetable	4	4
½ cup cooked, or juice		
1 cup raw		
Portion commonly served such as a medium-size apple or banana		
Grain, whole grain, fortified, enriched	4	4
1 slice bread		
1 cup ready-to-eat cereal		
½ cup cooked cereal, pasta, grits		

*Count cheese as serving of milk *or* meat, not both simultaneously.

Source: National Dairy Council, *Guide to Good Eating,* 4th ed., Rosemont, Ill., 1985.

high-fiber diets which exclude sources from major food groups is not advised (Committee on Nutrition, 1985).

Protein

The protein requirements of children vary with age and parallel needs for growth. Requirements are highest in infancy and in adolescent males (Food and Nutrition Board, 1980). Protein needs are altered by diseases in which specific amino acids may need to be restricted or increased. Examples include inborn errors of metabolism (restricted) and children with protein depletion (increased).

The RDAs for protein in children allow for the increased requirements associated with growth. Providing adequate calories is essential to "spare" amino acids for synthesis of tissue and other metabolic functions. Protein is utilized as an energy source when caloric needs are not met. Protein requirements in adolescents are most appropriately based on height rather than chronological age to reflect physiological needs during different stages of the growth spurt (Mahan and Rosebrough, 1984).

The amino acids are classified as essential and nonessential, categories that do not indicate their indispensability to growth and repair of body tissue but only the body's ability to synthesize them. *Essential amino acids* are

those which the body cannot synthesize and which therefore must be obtained in the diet. Protein sources that contain optimal quantities of all eight essential amino acids are known as *complete proteins*. Protein sources that do not contain all the essential amino acids are *incomplete proteins*. Protein sources such as eggs, meat, dairy products (milk, cheese, yogurt), fish, and poultry are complete proteins while grains, legumes, and vegetables contain incomplete proteins. A mixed diet has complete and incomplete protein sources in which different foods "complement" one another to provide all the essential amino acids.

Vegetarianism

Vegetarianism in the pediatric setting is influenced by parental philosophy and religious, health, or economic factors. Vegetarian diets range from diets excluding only red meats to severely restrictive diets in which protein is restricted to foods of plant origin. A classification of vegetarian diets is given in Table 7-4.

The use of a strict "vegan" diet is of particular concern in pediatrics since children require proportionately increased amounts of calories, protein, and micronutrients per kilogram of body weight. While lactovegetarian and lacto-ovo-vegetarian diets may be nutritionally adequate for use in children, strict vegan diets may be deficient in calories, protein, calcium, iron, zinc, riboflavin, and vitamin B_{12} (Truesdall and Acosta, 1985). Nutritional deficiencies among children on vegetarian diets are due to (1) decreased nutrient intake, (2) high bulk and low caloric density of foods in the diet, and (3) decreased absorption of minerals (calcium, zinc, iron).

Nutritional counseling for individuals on a vegetarian diet should focus on methods of maximizing the nutrient density of the foods consumed. Guidelines for increasing the content of nutrients which are commonly deficient in vegetarian diets are given in Table 7-5.

Fats

Fats are important in the diets of infants, children, and adolescents to provide a concentrated source of calories

TABLE 7-4 Classification of Vegetarian Diets

Diet	Recommendation
Total vegetarian ("vegan")	Restrict all animal sources of protein; protein from plant foods only
Lactovegetarian	Restrict meat, poultry, fish, and eggs; protein from milk, milk products, and plant foods
Lacto-ovo-vegetarian	Restricts meat, poultry, and fish
Semivegetarian	Restrict some groups of animal foods (i.e., red meats); protein from dairy products, eggs, and plant foods
New vegetarian	Restrict some groups of animal foods with emphasis on "organic" and unprocessed foods

Source: American Dietetic Association (1980).

TABLE 7-5 Nutrient Guidelines for a Vegan Diet

Nutrient	Food Sources
Calories	Legumes, legume spreads, nuts, nut butters, dried fruit, avocados
Riboflavin	Fortified soy formula, almonds, brewer's yeast,† wheat germ, leafy green vegetables
Calcium	Fortified soy formula, legumes, green leafy vegetables
Zinc	Legumes, nuts, tofu, miso
Vitamin B_{12}	Fortified soy formula, meat analogs, miso, brewer's yeast,† B_{12} supplement
Iron*	Fortified soy formula, green leafy vegetables, enriched and fortified grains
Vitamin D	Exposure to sunlight

*Ascorbic acid enhances absorption.
†Brewer's yeast not appropriate for infants.
Source: Adapted from Truesdall and Acosta (1985).

and essential fatty acids and to function as carriers for fat-soluble vitamins. They should contribute a minimum of 30 percent of total calories in infants (Committee on Nutrition, 1976b) and approximately 30 to 40 percent of energy intake in children and adolescents (Committee on Nutrition, 1986b). Excessive intakes of fats are inadvisable for infants, children, and adolescents because they may depress the appetite for other foods, lead to ketosis, and may contribute to obesity.

The essential fatty acids (EFA) are necessary for growth, development of cell membranes, synthesis of prostaglandins, and metabolism of cholesterol (Friedman, 1980). The EFA are not synthesized by the body and are provided by vegetable oils (soybean, safflower, corn) in the diet. The AAP Committee on Nutrition (1976b) has recommended that 3 percent of the calories in infant formulas be contributed by linoleic acid. The risk of EFA deficiency is increased in children receiving fat-free parenteral nutrition regimes and in instances of fat malabsorption (i.e., cystic fibrosis).

The effects of early restriction of cholesterol and saturated fats on children have not yet been defined (Committee on Nutrition, 1986b). Diet is only one component contributing to cardiovascular risk. Among children, obesity and aerobic fitness are more important determinants of coronary heart disease (Fripp et al., 1985) than is the dietary intake of cholesterol and saturated fat (Weidman et al., 1978). The restriction of cholesterol and saturated fat as recommended for adults is not applicable to children because the effects on growth are unknown and the beneficial impact on CHD has not been proved (Committee on Nutrition, 1986b). The issue of modifying dietary fat intake in children also involves the nutritional implications of restricting dairy products and meat. Each of these major food groups provides key nutrients, including protein; calcium and iron are obtained from dairy products and red meats, respectively. The AAP Committee on Nutrition (1986b) does not recommend restriction of cholesterol and saturated fat in children less than 2 years of age.

Noncaloric Nutrient Needs
Vitamins and Minerals
Unlike the nutrients discussed above, vitamins and minerals do not produce energy. No one food contains all the vitamins and minerals needed by the body; therefore, a varied diet is essential to provide an adequate intake of each of these substances.

Vitamins function as cofactors in a wide range of metabolic reactions, including the synthesis of RNA and DNA. They are grouped according to their solubility in either water or lipid mediums.

Fat-soluble vitamins (A, D, E, and K) can be stored by the liver and adipose tissue and therefore do not have to be consumed on a daily basis. However, since these vitamins are stored by the body, large doses may be toxic (Mahoney, 1980; Committee on Nutritional Misinformation, 1974). Fat-soluble vitamins follow the same route of digestion and absorption as do dietary fats. Conditions that interfere with the absorption and utilization of fats may increase dietary needs and necessitate supplementation of fat-soluble vitamins.

Water-soluble vitamins (vitamin C, thiamine, riboflavin, niacin, vitamin B_6, folate, and vitamin B_{12}) are not stored by the body to any appreciable degree and must therefore be consumed on a daily basis. Although excessive amounts of water-soluble vitamins do not usually cause toxicity, adverse reactions have been reported from the ingestion of large amounts of vitamin C and vitaimin B_6 (Schaumburg et al., 1983; Rudman and Williams, 1983).

Minerals play a vital role in water and acid-base balance, nerve impulse transmission, and muscle contraction and act as catalysts for enzymatic reactions. The essential minerals can be divided into two subgroups. Macro, or major, minerals include calcium, phosphorus, magnesium, sodium, potassium, and chlorine. The micronutrients, or trace minerals, are iron, copper, zinc, iodine, and fluoride. Most minerals are not stored in the body and must be supplied in the daily diet.

Deficiencies of vitamins and minerals can be either primary or secondary. A primary deficiency results from inadequate intake of a nutrient. In a secondary or indirect deficiency, the intake is adequate but the absorption, excretion, or function of a nutrient may be altered (Table 7-6). Infants and children who are ill or receive certain medications may require supplementation of specific vitamins and minerals.

Iron
A constituent of hemoglobin and myoglobin, iron is necessary in the transport, storage, and utilization of oxygen (Bothwell, 1962). The accumulation of iron in the body is regulated by the intestinal mucosa. When stores of iron are abundant, it is taken up by the muscosal cells, retained, and later returned to the intestinal lumen by desquamation. In the event of iron deficiency, iron crosses the intestinal mucosa into the circulation and little is desquamated by the musocal cell (Finch, 1977).

The absorption of iron is a complex process that is in-

TABLE 7-6 Noncaloric Nutrient Needs

Nutrient	Functions	Sources	Pediatric Concerns
Fat-Soluble Vitamins			

Vitamin A (precursor, carotene)	1. Component of photosensitive pigment of the eye
	  (a) Rods—rhodopsin (visual purple)
	  (b) Cones—iodopsin
	 2. Maintains integrity of epithelial membranes
	 3. Essential to bone and tooth development
		Liver, fish oils, whole milk, egg yolk, fortified margarine, butter
		 Carotenes from dark green and yellow vegetables and fruits
			Attention should be given vitamin A status in gluten enteropathy, obstructive jaundice, cystic fibrosis, biliary atresia, and cirrhosis
			 Can be toxic when taken in excessive amounts; supplementation should not be necessary with the use of whole milk, formula, or breast milk; after infancy and often during adolescence, intake may be marginal, but unnecessary supplementation should be avoided

Vitamin D	Maintenance of calcium homeostasis and skeletal integrity: aids in absorption and utilization of calcium and phosphorus; regulates level of serum alkaline phosphatase	Fish oils, yeast-fortified or irradiated milk, fortified oleomargarine; some cereals and diet foods may be fortified; vitamin D content of the diet should be basis for supplementation Exposure of skin to sun	Hypervitaminosis may develop with intakes of 1000-3000 IU; excessive intake associated with idiopathic hypercalcemia of infancy Absorption is hindered in cystic fibrosis, gluten enteropathy, short-bowel syndrome, colitis
Vitamin E (alpha tocopherol)	Antioxidant: stabilizes lipid portion of cell membrane, preventing oxidative deterioration and cellular damage; protects vitamin A, which is easily oxidized	Vegetable oils are a major source Proprietary infant formulas Baby foods highest in content are peaches, apricots, squash, sweet potato, spinach	Negligible placental transfer of this vitamin results in low reserves in the newborn Supplementation is indicated with preterm, low-birth-weight infants, and with malabsorption
Vitamin K	Catalyzes synthesis of prothrombin in the liver (anticoagulants interfere with utilization)	Synthesized by intestinal bacteria Widespread in food, green leafy vegetables, pork, liver	Due to sterile intestinal tract of the newborn, vitamin K is lacking for prothrombin formation; deficiency is associated with hemorrhagic disease of the newborn Supplementation is indicated with malabsorption and prolonged diarrhea Prolonged use of antibiotics interferes with intestinal synthesis
Water-Soluble Vitamins			
Ascorbic acid (vitamin C)	1. Provides intercellular cementing substance necessary to formation and maintenance of bone matrix, cartilage, dentine, collagen, and connective tissue 2. Related to metabolism of phenylalanine, tyrosine, and trytophan 3. Makes iron available for hemoglobin and maturation of red blood cells 4. Facilitates action of folic acid 5. Apparent role in resistance to bacterial infections and body's ability to cope with stress	Citrus fruit, tomato, cabbage, potato, strawberries, melon	Breast milk has sufficient ascorbic acid if mother's intake is adequate; supplementation is necessary with unfortified formula preparations Citrus is a common allergen; delayed introduction advisable (after 6 mo); when 2 oz of undiluted juice is tolerated, supplementation may be discontinued

Source: Adapted from Tables 4-4 and 4-5 in G. M. Scipien et al., *Comprehensive Pediatric Nursing,* 3d ed., McGraw-Hill, New York, 1986. p. 58-61 and 64-65.

TABLE 7-6 Noncaloric Nutrient Needs—cont'd

Nutrient	Functions	Sources	Pediatric Concerns
Minerals			
Minerals Calcium	1. Bone and teeth formation 2. Participates in blood coagulation 3. Initiates muscle contraction; vital to contraction and relaxation of cardiac muscle 4. Necessary to normal nerve transmission	Milk, cheese, dairy products Secondary sources are green leafy vegetables, legumes, nuts, and whole grains	Hypocalcemic tetany may accompany the following: Newborn given too large an initial feeding Vitamin D deficiency Celiac disease Late stages of renal insufficiency Acute pancreatitis Prolonged immobilization leads to calcium resorption and increased serum calcium levels
Iron	1. Constituent of hemoglobin and myoglobin; involved in O_2 and CO_2 transport 2. Component of cellular oxidative systems which release energy from the metabolic breakdown products of food	Liver, meat, green vegetables, whole or enriched grains, legumes, nuts Excellent baby food sources are dry infant cereals, quick-cooking Cream of Wheat, strained liver, strained beef with beef heart Drinking water Plant and animal foods vary according to soil and water	Iron-deficiency anemia is the most common hematologic disease of infancy and childhood; chronic iron-deficiency anemia may result from lesions of the GI tract, Meckel's diverticulum, polyps, or hemangioma; absorption is hindered by steatorrhea Supplements should not be used where water supplies over 0.7 ppm; fluoride content in excess of 2.0-2.5 ppm produces a mottling of enamel

fluenced by many variables. A major factor is the nature of iron in the ingested food (Layrisse, 1968). There are two types of iron in food, heme and nonheme iron. *Heme iron* is contained in hemoglobin and muscle myoglobulin and is therefore obtained exclusively from meats. Heme iron is absorbed relatively well. *Nonheme iron,* which is found in both animal and vegetable food, is less well absorbed. Its absorption is strongly influenced by the presence of other foods ingested at the same meal (Cooke, 1972). Ascorbic acid and an unknown component in meat are the most potent enhancers of the absorption of nonheme iron.

Certain dietary and medicinal substances are known to decrease the absorption of iron. Specific items include antacids, tannic acid (in tea), calcium and phosphate salts, edetic acid (EDTA), phytates (in cereal grains), oxylates (in spinach), and phosvitin (in egg yolk) (Monsen, 1978). When the iron status of a child is compromised, inordinate consumption of these substances should be avoided since they may substantially decrease iron absorption.

In the full-term infant, iron deficiency usually is not seen before the age of 4 to 6 months because of adequate iron stores at birth. Low-birth-weight infants exhaust their iron stores at an earlier age (2 to 3 months) because of lower stores and a more rapid rate of postnatal growth.

Therefore, the requirements for iron are greater in low-birth-weight infants than in term infants.

According to the AAP Committee on Nutrition (1985), iron supplementation should begin in full-term infants between 4 and 6 months of age and in preterm infants no later than 2 months of age. Sources of iron supplementation include iron-fortified commercial infant formula and/or servings of iron-fortified infant cereal. In preterm infants who are formula fed, iron-fortified formulas usually provide an adequate source of iron. However, breast-fed preterm infants should receive iron in the form of ferrous sulfate drops at a dose of 2 to 3 mg/kg/d (of elemental iron) to a maximum of 15 mg/d (Committee on Nutrition, 1985).

The iron content of human milk is similar to that of cow's milk; however, more of the iron from human milk is absorbed (Saarinen, Siimes, and Dallman, 1977a). Breast-feeding provides partial protection against the development of iron deficiency anemia in full-term infants (Saarinen and Siimes, 1977b). As a substitute for human milk during the first 9 to 12 months, the AAP Committee on Nutrition (1985) recommends commercial infant formula over fresh cow's milk.

In preschool and preadolescent children iron intake generally increases as a result of the greater opportunity

TABLE 7-7 Foods High in Iron

Good Sources	Excellent Sources
Egg	Liver
Prunes	Pork, beef, veal
Strawberries	Navy beans, lima beans, soybeans,
V-8 juice	lentils, split peas
Broccoli	Prune juice
Collards	Tomato juice
Green peas	Oatmeal
Sweet potato	Bran flakes with raisins
Sweet potato	Cream of Wheat
	Spinach
	Molasses
	Corn syrup
	Wheat germ

Source: Committee on Nutrition, American Academy of Pediatrics, G. B. Forbes and C. W. Woodruff (eds.), *Pediatric Nutrition Handbook,* American Academy of Pediatrics, Elk Grove Village, Ill., 1985.

TABLE 7-8 Good Sources of Ascorbic Acid

Food	
Orange juice, frozen concentrate, diluted as directed	Liver, calf, cooked
Strawberries, fresh	Asparagus, cooked
Broccoli, fresh, cooked	Potato, white, baked
Broccoli, frozen, cooked	Cranberry juice cocktail
Orange	Tomato juice, canned
Grapefruit juice, canned	Spinach, frozen, cooked
Cantaloupe	Winter squash, mashed
Grapefruit	Sweet potato, baked
	Liver, beef, cooked

Source: P. A. Kreutler, *Nutrition in Perspective,* Prentice-Hall, Englewood Cliffs, N.J., 1980.

to obtain more iron from a mixed diet. Although milk is an excellent source of many nutrients, it is a poor source of iron. Drinking large amounts of milk displaces other, more iron-rich foods from the diet, and it also decreases the availability of iron for absorption.

One point which must be made in parent education is the need for iron-rich foods and reasonable (nonexcessive) use of milk (Table 7-7). The addition of a source of ascorbic acid to every meal and/or consumption of meat, poultry, or fish enhances the availability of iron in the diet significantly (Table 7-8).

Fluoride

Fluoride is important in dental health because it acts both systemically and topically on teeth. Systemically, fluoride is incorporated into the enamel of the tooth prior to eruption. Fluoride acts topically (i.e., directly on erupted teeth) by limiting demineralization and encouraging remineralization of enamel (Holloway and Levine, 1981), thereby reducing the opportunity for tooth decay (Aasenden, 1974; Adair and Wei, 1978).

Recommendations for dosage regimens are determined by the fluoride content of the local water supply and the age of the child. The goal of supplementation is to provide adequate fluoride for prevention of caries (between 0.05 and 0.07 mg/kg/d) (Forrester and Schulta, 1974) while avoiding an excess (greater than 0.1 mg/kg/d) (Forsman, 1977) that may cause dental mottling. In locations where fluoridation is inadequate (less than 0.7 ppm), the Committee on Nutrition (1986a) recommends that fluoride supplements be given to all children beginning at about 2 weeks of age.

Fluoridated toothpastes are an important source of topical fluoride. However, parents need to know the danger of excessive fluoride intake and to teach children to avoid swallowing toothpaste.

Water

Although not considered a food, water is a vital nutrient which plays many roles in the proper function of the human body. Water functions as an essential component of cell structure and as a solvent for cellular changes. It acts as a medium for ions, transports nutrients and waste products, and assists in the regulation of body temperature.

The principal pediatric consideration is the infant's large body water content (70 to 75 percent of body weight) compared with the adult's (60 to 65 percent) (Behrman and Vaughan, 1983). This difference makes infants vulnerable to dehydration and subsequent electrolyte imbalances. As a result, a baby must consume large amounts of fluid per unit of body weight to maintain water balance. In addition, water turnover is closely related to metabolic rate. The metabolic rate per kilogram of body weight in the infant is greater than that of the adult. Therefore, the increased products of metabolism require more water for excretion.

Water balance becomes a primary concern in infant feeding when any of the following situations exist: (1) relatively low fluid intake (less than 100 ml/kg/d), (2) lowered renal concentrating ability, (3) excessive losses (fever, diarrhea, vomiting, polyuria, hot climate, diuretic use, and increased respiratory and metabolic rates), (4) comatose patients or those unable to communicate thirst, and (5) a diet with a high renal solute load. Solutes that must be excreted by the kidney are referred to collectively as the renal solute load. Electrolytes and nitrogen are the principal solutes to be excreted, and protein is therefore the primary dietary contributor to renal solute load. A diet with a high renal solute load obligates more water for the excretion of nitrogenous end products.

The requirement for water is deermined by the amount lost in the stool and urine and from the skin and lungs. In addition, a small amount of water is needed for growth.

Fluids in liquids and foods are the primary sources of water. Foods typically consumed in infancy and childhood have high fluid contents. Water is also obtained from the oxidation or metabolism of protein, carbohydrate, and fat.

Under normal environmental conditions, formula

which is prepared properly and breast milk supply an adequate quantity of water for infants; thus supplemental water is not necessary. During very hot weather, however, the infant may require additional water.

Nutrition and the Preterm and Low-Birth-Weight Infant

The nutritional goal for feeding low-birth-weight infants is not definitely known. According to the Committee on Nutrition (1977), "achieving a postnatal growth that approximates the in utero growth of the normal fetus at the same postconceptual age appears to be the most logical approach at present." A major consideration in feeding a preterm or low-birth-weight infant is that the nutritional reserves of the infant have been interrupted at the point in gestation at which delivery occurred.

Nutrients can be provided parenterally, enterally, or by a combination of routes. Parenteral glucose, lipid, and amino acids are essential in the nutritional management of low-birth-weight infants when enteral feedings are not feasible because of medical conditions or when feedings must be advanced so slowly that the daily nutrient needs cannot be met enterally. The mode of enteral feedings must be individualized for each infant and based on the gestational age, birth weight, and clinical state.

The caloric needs of low-birth-weight infants vary. They are based on requirements for maintenance and growth.

The protein requirement for low-birth-weight infants is between 2.2-4.0 gm/kg/day. There has been controversy about whether breast milk provides sufficient protein to accommodate the rapid growth of a low-birth-weight infant. The type of protein, whey versus casein, also is a consideration in providing adequate protein to low-birth-weight infants. Whey-predominant formulas have been shown to be better tolerated (Committee on Nutrition, 1977).

The ability of low-birth-weight infants to digest and absorb fats, particularly saturated fats, is relatively poor (Davidson and Bauer, 1960). This limitation is associated with liver immaturity and decreased synthesis of bile salt (Watkins et al., 1975). The inclusion of medium-chain triglyceride as part of the fat in formulas has been shown to improve fat absorption in low-birth-weight infants and to increase weight gain, calcium absorption, and nitrogen retention.

The low-birth-weight infant's utilization of carbohydrate differs slightly from that of the full-term infant. The intestinal disaccharidases maltase and sucrase develop early in fetal life, while lactase reaches mature levels at term. Therefore, the low-birth-weight infant may digest lactose incompletely during the first few days of life (Boellner, Beard, and Panos, 1965). Formulas which are designed specifically for preterm infants also contain glucose polymers which have the advantage of adding less osmotic activity to the feeding than do lactose and monosaccharides.

Formulas and human milk which provide 20 kcal/oz

are recommended for full-term infants. However, more concentrated formulas (25 kcal/oz) are often used to facilitate increased caloric intake in low-birth-weight infants who may have a limited gastric capacity. Several studies have shown that feeding low-birth-weight infants formula with a higher caloric density results in faster growth (Committee on Nutrition, 1977). If low volumes (less than 120 kcal/kg/d) are given, insufficient water may be provided for renal excretion.

Recently, there has been renewed interest in the use of human milk for preterm infants. Some investigators believe that it may help prevent necrotizing enterocolitis and contributes to the immunologic and physiological benefits of colostrum and human milk.

Infant Nutrition

Feeding the vigorous term newborn normally is relatively simple. Breast milk is considered the preferred feeding, since its unique composition meets the nutritional requirements of full-term infants for the first several months of life. When breast-feeding is unsuccessful, inappropriate, or terminated early, the best alternative for meeting nutritional needs during infancy is commercially prepared infant formula.

Breast-Feeding

Breast-feeding has become more common. Not only is there an increase in the number of mothers choosing to breast-feed, more mothers are continuing to nurse for a longer period of time. The increased incidence of breast-feeding is not limited to better-educated, higher-income women; it is also seen among lower-income families, women with elementary and high school educations, and mothers in the Women, Infants, and Children (WIC) program (Martinez and Nalezienski, 1982).

Factors that influence the chemical composition of human milk at any given time include the stage of lactation, the mother's diet, the time of day, and the time of sampling during a given feeding. For instance, colostrum is different from mature milk, and fat content is higher at the end of the feeding than at the beginning.

Colostrum, a thick, yellowish fluid with a mean energy value of 67 kcal/100 ml, is readily available at delivery if the mother is multiparous. It is higher in protein, fat-soluble vitamins, minerals, sodium, potassium, and chloride than mature milk and has a high ash content. Fatty acids are synthesized quickly by the breasts. Colostrum, which is extremely rich in vitamins A and E and carotenoids, has an abundance of antibodies. It also facilitates passage of meconium and growth of normal flora in the intestine.

The next stage of lactation is the transitional period that terminates in the production of mature milk. This transition occurs gradually, beginning about 7 to 10 days postpartum, and lasts until the fourteenth day postpartum. During this stage the total protein and immunoglobulins decrease, as do fat-soluble vitamins. Water-soluble vitamins increase, as do fat content, lactose, and total caloric content. Following this transition, mature milk is produced.

Thirty to 55 percent of the kilocalories in human milk are fats in the form of globules or droplets. Milk lipids include triglycerides, diglycerides, monoglycerides, free fatty acids, phospholipids, glycolipids, sterols, and sterol esters. Oleic, linoleic, linolenic, and palmitic acids are the major fatty acids present in human milk. The diet of the mother does not affect the total amount of fat but does influence the composition of the fat content.

Forty percent of human milk protein is casein. Casein commonly is called curds. Sixty percent of the protein is lactalbumin, or whey. The major constituents of whey proteins are alpha-lactalbumin and lactoferrin. Alpha-lactalbumin is a part of lactose synthetase. Human milk has high levels of alpha-lactalbumin. Lactoferrin is iron-binding; it also inhibits iron-dependent bacteria in the intestine.

Lactose, the major carbohydrate in breast milk, is sometimes called milk sugar. Galactose and glucose make up this disaccharide, which is synthesized by the breast.

Vitamins found in human milk are sufficient for the infant, except for vitamin D. It is recommended that breast-feeding be supplemented with vitamin D (Committee on Nutrition, 1976b). Since iron is available in human milk, the administration of a supplement is debatable. Fluoride supplementation may be provided from birth.

It is well known that human milk affords protection from disease. Mortality and morbidity rates in breast-fed infants are lower than those in formula-fed babies (Cunningham, 1977). Several anti-infectious factors in human milk are known to decrease infection, inhibit colonization of the bowel, and destroy the cell walls of bacteria. Breast-feeding has been associated with a lower incidence of food allergies than has artificial feeding (Atherton, 1978).

Since breast milk is species-specific, it is generally non-allergenic for the human infant and macromolecules from breast milk are not usually absorbed. However, it has been shown that allergens from the mother's diet may enter her breast milk and cause an allergic reaction in a sensitive infant (Frieds, 1981). Although heredity plays a part in the development of allergy, the prophylaxis of breast-feeding combined with diet or hypoallergenic foods in infants with a strong history of allergy may be beneficial.

Formula Feeding

Infant formulas are manufactured from nonfat cow's milk which has been modified to reduce the solute load and heat treated to produce an easily digested protein. In addition, combinations of vegetable oils and carbohydrates are added to increase the caloric concentration to approximate that of human milk (20 kcal/oz). Complete information on the nutrient content of human milk and commercially prepared infant formulas is provided in Table 7-9.

Protein

Protein is a source of essential and nonessential amino acids. It is recommended (Fomon, Ziegler, and O'Connell, 1974) that a growing infant receive between 6 and 16 percent of total calories as high-quality protein. Milk-based formulas provide protein within this range.

Fat

Infant formulas contain 48 to 50 percent of their calories as fat by replacing the butterfat with a blend of vegetable oils, which improves the absorption of fat. Formulas also furnish an adequate amount of the essential fatty acid linoleic acid, necessary for the development of cell membranes and as a precursor for prostaglandins (Elliott, 1979). Intake of at least 3 percent of total calories as linoleic acid is sufficient to prevent essential fatty acid deficiency (Woodruff, 1978).

Carbohydrate

Carbohydrate is the second largest source of energy in milk-based formulas and human milk. Lactose is the main carbohydrate in milks. Formulas provide 41 to 43 percent of the total calories as carbohydrate.

Vitamins and Minerals

Commercial formulas are fortified with vitamins and minerals to meet the requirements of the Infant Formula Act of 1980. Concentrations of nutrients in formulas are often higher than mean values for breast milk to compensate for the superior bioavailability of human milk.

Other Types of Milk

In addition to the standard infant formulas (Similac, Enfamil, and SMA), there are a variety of specialized formulas available for medical conditions such as malabsorption and formula intolerance. Table 7-10 suggests formulas for problems frequently seen in infancy and gives the rationale for their use. Formulas made from recipes which have not been evaluated for nutritional adequacy are not recommended for infant feeding. Imitation and filled milks are not intended for use as infant feedings since kwashiorkor has been reported in infants fed a nondairy creamer as a substitute for milk (Sinatra, 1981). Raw milk may be contaminated with pathogenic bacteria and is therefore not advised for infants.

Goat's milk does not contain adequate amounts of iron, vitamin D, and vitamin C and also is not recommended for routine infant feeding during the first year of life. In addition, infants fed exclusively with goat's milk are at risk for megaloblastic anemia because of the inadequate folate levels in goat's milk.

Whole cow's milk which is unmodified is not suitable for the human newborn. It is deficient in iron, fluoride, and vitamins A, C, and D. The appropriate age at which cow's milk can be introduced safely into the infant's diet is unknown and remains an area of controversy. Excessive amounts of cow's milk have been associated with (1) iron deficiency anemia, (2) occult bleeding from the gastrointestinal tract, (3) protein intolerance, and (4) high renal solute load. Although human milk and infant formulas are recommended for infant feeding, the Committee

TABLE 7-9 Content of Human Milk and Commercially Prepared Formulas

Type	kcal/oz	Protein, g/100 ml	Carbohydrate, g/100 ml	Fat, g/100 ml	Na, meq/ liter	K, meq/ liter	Ca, meq/ liter	P, meq/ liter	Fe, meq/ liter
Breast milk	20	1.1-1.2	6.8-7.0	3.8-4.5	7	13-14	17 (340 mg/ liter)	8 (162 mg/ liter)	5.0 (1.5 mg/ liter)
Vitamin-mineral considerations: Vitamin D and ascorbic acid may need to be supplemented when the maternal intake is low; before 3-6 mo the need for additional iron is determined by adequacy of birth stores									
Cow's milk, whole†	20	3.3-3.5	4.8-4.9	3.7	22-25	35	58.5 (1240 mg/ liter)	35 (950 mg/ liter)	0.5 (1 mg/liter)
Vitamin-mineral considerations: Cow's milk does not supply iron, ascorbic acid, or fluoride and must be fortified with vitamin D									
Cow's milk, skim†	10	3.5-3.6	4.8-5.1	0.1-0.2	23-26	34-37	60 (1240 mg/ liter)	61 (1010 mg/ liter)	Trace
Vitamin-mineral considerations: Skim milk does not supply iron, ascorbic acid or fluoride; during processing, vitamins A and D are destroyed; therefore, skim milk is enriched with vitamin A and fortified with vitamin D									
Proprietary formulas Similac 20 (Ross)	20	1.5	7.2	3.6	10-10.9	18-19.2	25.5 (510 mg/ liter)	25 (390 mg/ liter)	Trace (with iron, 12)
Vitamin-mineral considerations: Proprietary formulas are completely vitamin-enriched, but they may not provide iron. Read labels carefully.									
SMA (Wyeth)	20	1.5	7.2	3.6	6.5-7	14-14.4	22 (420 mg/ liter)	21 (312 mg/ liter)	12
Enfamil (Mead Johnson)	20	1.5	7.0	3.7	12	18	27.5	20.6	1.5 (with iron, 12)
Special formula preparations						*Vitamin-mineral considerations:* Same as for proprietary formulas.			
Prosobee (Mead Johnson)	20	2.5	6.8	3.4	18-18.3	19	40 (788 mg/ liter)	34 (525 mg/ liter)	12.7 (13 mg/ liter)
Neomulsoy (Syntex)	20	1.8-1.86	6.5-6.6	3.6	16.1-17	23.1-25	42 (800 mg/ liter)	40 (600 mg/ liter)	10 (10 mg/ liger)
Cho-Free (Syntex) (with added carbohydrate)	20	1.8	6.4	3.5	15-15.8	22-22.6	44 (850 mg/ liter)	44 (640 mg/ liter)	8.3 (10 mg/ liter)
Lofenalac (Mead Johnson)	20	2.2-2.32	8.8	2.7	13.9	17-19.4	32 (630 mg/ liter)	30.3 (473 mg/ liter)	12.7 (13 mg/ liter)
Meat Base (Gerber)	20	2.9	6.1	3.2	7.9	9.9	50	43	16
Nutramigen (Mead Johnson)	20	2.2	8.8	2.6	14	17.4	32 (630 mg/ liter)	30 (473 mg/ liter)	12.7 (13 mg/ liter)
Portagen (Mead Johnson)	20	2.4	7.8	3.2	13.9	24	32	30	12.7
Pregestimil (Mead Johnson)	20	2.2-2.36	7.74-8.8	2.8-3.2	14	19.4-21	32 (630 mg/ liter)	30 (473 mg/ liter)	12.7 (13 mg/ liter)

*Fluoride supplementation must be considered. The appropriate age of supplementation is under evaluation.
†Included in the table for purposes of composition comparison, but they are not suitable for infant feeding.
‡When used for infant formula, 13 oz of evaporated milk is diluted with 18 oz of water, and 30 g of carbohydrate is added.

Sources: S. J. Fomon, *Infant Nutrition,* Saunders, Philadelphia, 1974. *Infant Formulas,* Mead Johnson & Company, Evansville, Ind., 1977. *Product Handbook,* Ross Laboratories, Columbus, Ohio, 1977. Syntex Laboratories, Palo Alto, Calif., 1977. *Nutrient Values, Gerber Baby Foods,* Gerber Products Company, Fremont, Mich., 1977. *Harriet Lane Handbook,* 8th ed., Johns Hopkins Hospital, Medical Publishers, Inc., Chicago, 1978. Adapted from table prepared by E. Getchell and R. Howard for G. M. Scipien et al. (eds.), *Comprehensive Pediatric Nursing,* 2d ed., McGraw-Hill, New York, 1979.

TABLE 7-10 Indications for Use of Infant Formulas

Problem in Infancy	Suggested Formula	Rationale
Allergy to cow's milk protein or soy protein	Protein hydrolysate (Nutramigen or Pregestimil)	Protein sensitivity
Biliary atresia	Portagen	Impaired intraluminal digestion and absorption of long-chain fats
Cardiac disease	SMA, Enfamil	Low electrolyte content
Celiac disease	Pregestimil, followed by soy-based formula, followed by cow's milk formula	Advance to more complete formula as intestinal epithelium returns to normal
Constipation	Routine formula, increase sugar	Mild laxative effect
Cystic fibrosis	Portagen	Impaired intraluminal digestion and absorption of long-chain fats
	Pregestimil	Whey protein and disaccharide digestion and absorption impaired
Diarrhea:		
Chronic nonspecific	Routine formula	Appropriate distribution of calories
Intractable	Pregestimil	Impaired digestion of intact protein, long-chain fats, and disaccharides
Failure to thrive (when intestinal damage is suspected)	Pregestimil	Advance to more complete formula as intestinal epithelium returns to normal
Gastroesophageal reflux	Routine formula	Thicken with 1 tbsp cereal/oz; small, frequent feeds
GI bleeding	Consider soy-(?) or cow's milk-free formula	Milk toxicity in infants
Hepatitis:		
Without failure	Routine formula	Impaired intraluminal digestion and absorption of long-chain fats
With failure	Portagen	
Lactose intolerance	Soy-based formula (e.g., Isomil, Prosobee)	Impaired digestion or utilization of lactose
Necrotizing enterocolitis (after resection)	Pregestimil (when feeding is resumed)	Impaired digestion
Renal insufficiency	PM 60/40	Low phosphate content, low renal solution load

Source: W. A. Walker and K. M. Hendricks, *Manual of Pediatric Nutrition,* Saunders, Philadelphia, 1985, p. 73.

TABLE 7-11 Satiety Behaviors in Infants

Age, weeks	Behavior
4-12	Draws head away from nipple
	Falls asleep
	When nipple is reinserted, closes lips tightly
	Bites nipple, purses lips or smiles, and lets go
16-24	Releases nipple and withdraws head
	Fusses or cries
	Obstructs mouth with hands
	Increases attention to surroundings
	Bites nipple
28-36	Changes posture
	Keeps mouth tightly closed
	Shakes head as if to say no
	Plays with utensils
	Increases hand activity
	Throws utensils
40-52	Typically includes 28 to 36 week behaviors
	Sputters with tongue and lips
	Hands bottle or cup to mother

Source: P. L. Pipes, "Health Care Professionals," in G. Garwood and R. Fewell (eds.), *Educating Handicapped Infants,* Aspen Systems, Rockville, Md., 1982. With permission of Aspen Systems Corp.; modified from A. Gessell and F. L. Ilg, *Feeding Behavior of Infants,* Lippincott, Philadelphia, 1937.

on Nutrition (1983) has approved the use of whole cow's milk after infants reach 6 months of age provided that they are consuming one-third of their calories as supplemental foods. Reduced-fat cow's milk (2 percent or skim milk) is not recommended during infancy.

Feeding Technique

Formulas may be given to infants at room temperature or even directly from the refrigerator without any harmful effects. If warmed the temperature of formulas should always be tested before feeding.

Health professionals caring for children must be aware of the dangers of using microwave heating, since liquids may become dangerously hot while the container remains cool to the touch. Incorrect heating may causes burns and lacerations secondary to exploding containers (Puczynski, Radmaker, and Gatson, 1983).

Ideally, the infant should be allowed to regulate his own schedule. Feeding an infant when he signals hunger is called demand feeding. With this method of feeding, the infant's physiological needs can be met promptly and feeding will not be associated with prolonged hunger and crying. It will help avoid feeding problems such as gulping the milk because of extreme hunger or an inadequate in-

TABLE 7-12 Feeding Guidelines for Infants During the First 6 Months*

	0-2 Weeks	2 weeks-2 mo	2 mo	3 mo	4-5 mo	5-6 mo
Formula						
Per feeding	2-3 oz	3-5 oz	5 oz	6-6½ oz	7-8 oz	7-8 oz
Average total	22 oz	28 oz	30 oz	32-34 oz	32 oz	28 oz
Number of feedings	6-8	5-6	5-6	5	4-5	4-5
Food texture	Liquids	Liquids	Liquids	Liquids	Baby soft	Baby soft
Food additions						
Apple juice†						3-4 oz
Baby cereal, enriched					2-2½ tbsp, B & S	3 tbsp, B & S†
Strained fruits					1½-3 tbsp, B, L, & S	2-3 tbsp, B, L, & S
Strained vegetables					1-2 tbsp, L	2-3 tbsp, L
Strained meats						1-2 tbsp, L
Egg yolk or baby egg yolk						½ med or 1 tbsp
Teething biscuit						½-1
Total calories	440	560	600	660-680	729-788	791-870
Recommended cal/kg	410	410-608	608	667	725-784	784-878
Oral and neuromuscular development related to food intake	Rooting, sucking, swallowing	Rooting, sucking, swallowing	Rooting, sucking, swallowing	Extrusion reflex diminishes; sucking becomes voluntary	Learning to put hands to mouth; develops grasp	Chewing begins; can approximate lips to rim of cup

*Calculations based on male growing at the 50th percentile for height and weight.
†Offer from the cup.
‡B = breakfast, L = lunch, S = supper

Source: Table prepared by E. Getchell and R. Howard for G. M. Scipien et al. (eds.,), *Comprehensive Pediatric Nursing,* 2d ed., McGraw-Hill, New York, 1979.

take due to exhaustion from crying. Successful infant feeding requires a correct interpretation of the infant's hunger and the realization that babies cry for reasons other than hunger. Infants do not need to be fed every time they cry.

Since it takes approximately 1 to 4 hours for an infant's stomach to empty, an infant will become hungry at different times of the day. In general, infants must be fed every 3 to 5 hours throughout the first year of life. Weak or small infants may require more frequent feeding, at 2- to 3-hour intervals. By the end of the first month most infants will have established a regular feeding schedule.

The amount of milk consumed at each feeding varies. It is recommended when bottle feeding that each bottle contain more than the average amount taken at a feeding. This allows the infant to regulate his own intake. Infants should not be urged to drink more than they desire just to empty the bottle. Parents need to recognize satiety behaviors in their infants in order to avoid overfeeding (Table 7-11). The length of time a feeding takes depends on the age and degree of hunger. Feedings generally require 10 to 25 minutes. Tables 7-12 and 7-13 give feeding guidelines for infants during the first 12 months of life.

Adding Solid Food

Recommendations for the addition of solid foods to the infant's diet have changed over the years. Supplemental foods were seldom fed to infants less than 1 year of age in the 1920s. By the 1950s, however, solid foods were added to the diet as early as 1 to 2 weeks of age, and by 3 months many children were on a full range of baby foods. At the present time the recommended age for adding baby foods is about 4 to 6 months.

There is no nutritional advantage to the early introduction of solid foods. A major reason parents add food to the diet of their infants is the hope that they will sleep through the night, a commonly held belief that has proved to be false.

Current recommendations for the addition of solid foods to the diet are based on the infant's developmental readiness to progress to foods with texture. The development of feeding skills and the feeding behavior that the child should be accomplishing from birth up to 3 years of age are given in Table 7-14.

Defining developmental readiness is important in establishing realistic feeding goals for children. The development of feeding skills proceeds in a predictable sequence which depends on the maturation of the child's

TABLE 7-13 Feeding Guidelines for Infants 6 to 12 Months Old*

	6-7 mo	7-8 mo	8-9 mo	9-10 mo	10-11 mo	11-12 mo
Whole milk						
Per feeding	8 oz†	8 oz	8 oz	8 oz	8 oz	8 oz
Average total	28 oz	28 oz	24 oz	24 oz	24 oz	24 oz
Number of feedings	3-4	3-4	3	3	3	3
Food texture	Gradual increase ⟶		Mashed table ⟶			Cut fine
Food items						
Orange juice	4 oz	4 oz	4 oz	4 oz	4 oz	4 oz
Fortified cereal	⅓ cup, B‡	⅓ cup, B	½ cup, B	½ cup, B	½ cup, B	½ cup, B
Fruit, canned or fresh	4 tsp, B, L, & S	4 tsp, B, L, & S	2 tbsp, L & S	2 tbsp, L & S	3 tbsp, L & S	3 tbsp, L & S
Vegetables	1½ tbsp, L & S	2 tbsp, L & S	2 tbsp, L & S	2 tbsp, L & S	3 tbsp, L & S	3 tbsp, L & S
Meat, fish, poultry	1 tbsp, L & S	2 tbsp, L & S	2 tbsp, L & S	2 tbsp, L & S	2½ tbsp, L & S	2½ tbsp, L & S
Egg yolk or baby egg yolk	1 med yolk, or 2 tbsp	1 med yolk, or 2 tbsp	1 med yolk, or 2 tbsp	1 whole egg	1 whole egg	1 whole egg
Teething biscuit or bread	1 biscuit	1 biscuit	½ slice bread	½ slice bread	½ slice bread	½ slice bread
Starch: potato, rice, macaroni				2 tbsp, S	2 tbsp, S	2 tbsp, S
Desert: custard, pudding						2 tbsp, S
Butter			1 tsp	1 tsp	1 tsp	1 tsp
Total calories	859	876	937	974	1037	1069
Recommended calories (108 kcal/kg)	810-864	864-918	918-972	972-1015	1015-1048	1048-1083
Oral and neuromuscular development related to food intake	Begins using cup ⟶	Sits erect with support ⟶ Feeds self biscuit ⟶		Without support ⟶ Holds bottle	Picks up small food items and releases	Will hold and lick spoon after it is dipped into food; self-feeding

*Calculations based on male growing at the 50th percentile for height and weight.
†Offer small amounts (2-4 oz) when milk is presented from the cup.
‡B = breakfast, L = lunch, S = supper.

Source: Table prepared by E. Getchell and R. Howard for G. M. Scipien et al. (eds.), *Comprehensive Pediatric Nursing,* 2d ed., McGraw-Hill, New York, 1979.

central nervous system. Fine, gross, and oral motor skills influence the infant's ability to eat solid food. The developmental readiness to begin consuming food occurs at around 5 to 6 months of age, when the tongue thrust disappears and the ability to swallow semisolid foods is more coordinated. It is essential for infants to be able to communicate a desire for food by moving toward it and opening the mouth and to indicate satiety by leaning back and turning away. Head control and the ability to sit with support are necessary for feeding.

Once a solid food has been introduced to an infant, no other should be given for 4 to 7 days to determine whether there is an allergic response to that particular food. A single-grain cereal such as rich is an excellent choice for the first solid supplemental food since it is well tolerated and provides additional iron and calories. Adding new foods each day can result in a variety of allergic reactions (rash, diarrhea, respiratory problems). When a number of different foods are introduced simultaneously and an allergic response is evident, the cause of the appar-

ent allergy is difficult to determine. Introducing a single new solid and giving it to an infant for several days can prevent a significant problem. Potentially allergenic foods should be offered in small quantities. The order of introduction of other solid foods such as vegetables, fruits, and meats is not critical. Good protein sources such as meats should be introduced earlier in breast-fed infants than in formula-fed infants because of the lower protein content of human milk.

A variety of foods should be introduced gradually to produce a nutritionally balanced diet. There is no reason to force a child to eat a particular food that is disliked.

Either commercially prepared foods for infant feeding or homemade foods may be used. Home-prepared infant foods typically contain more calories than do commercial foods. Spinach, beets, carrots, turnips, and collard greens should not be used for making homemade infant foods since they may contain sufficient nitrate to cause methemoglobinemia (Committee on Nutrition, 1980). Commercially prepared infant foods no longer contain added salt.

TABLE 7-14 Development of Feeding Skills

Age	Oral and Neuromuscular Development	Feeding Behavior
Birth	Rooting reflex Sucking reflex	Turns mouth toward nipple or any object brushing cheek
	Swallowing reflex	Initial swallowing involves the posterior of the tongue, by 9-12 weeks anterior portion is increasingly involved, which facilitates ingestion of semisolid food
	Extrusion reflex	Pushes food out when placed on tongue; strong the first 9 weeks By 6-10 weeks recognizes the position in which he is fed and begins mouthing and sucking when placed in this position
3-6 mo	Beginning coordination between eyes and body movements	Explores world with eyes, fingers, hands, and mouth; starts reaching for objects at 4 mo but overshoots; hands get in the way during feeding
	Learning to reach mouth with hands at 4 mo	Finger sucking; by 6 mo all objects go into mouth
	Extrusion reflex present until 4 mo	May continue to push out food placed on tongue
	Able to grasp objects voluntarily at 5 mo	Grasps objects in mittenlike fashion
	Sucking reflex becomes voluntary, and lateral motions of the jaw begin	Can approximate lips to rim of cup by 5 mo; chewing action begins; by 6 mo begins drinking from cup
6-12 mo	Eyes and hands working together	Brings hand to mouth; at 7 mo able to feed self biscuit
	Sits erect with support at 6 mo	Bangs cup and objects on table at 7 mo
	Sits erect without support at 9 mo	
	Development of grasp (finger to thumb opposition)	Holds own bottle at 9-12 mo Pincer approach to food Pokes at food with index finger at 10 mo
	Relates to objects at 10 mo	Reaches for food and utensils including those beyond reach; pushes plate around with spoon Insists on holding spoon not to put in mouth but to return to plate or cup
1-3 yr	Development of manual dexterity	Increased desire to feed self: *15 mo:* begins to use spoon but turns it before reaching mouth; may hold cup; likely to tilt cup rather than head, causing spilling *18 mo:* eats with spoon, spills frequently, turns spoon in mouth; holds glass with both hands *2 yr:* inserts spoon correctly, occasionally with one hand; holds glass; plays with food; distinguishes between food and inedible materials *2-3 yr:* self-feeding complete with occasional spilling; uses fork; pours from pitcher; obtains drink of water from faucet

Source: Table prepared by E. Getchell and R. Howard for G. M. Scipien et al. (eds.), *Comprehensive Pediatric Nursing,* 2d ed., McGraw-Hill, New York, 1979.

The addition of salt or sugar to foods for home use and the use of canned foods which contain large quantities of salt and sugar are not recommended.

Combination foods should be fed to older infants only after tolerance for the individual ingredients has been determined. These foods are generally more expensive than single-item foods and may contain fewer nutrients.

During the latter part of the first year the child gradually changes to the family's diet. Mashed or chopped foods of suitable texture should be introduced to the infant generally by the age of 6 or 7 months. The textures of the foods given are diverse and progress toward the time when the child will consume meals with the family. Finger foods are given at 6 or 7 months of age and help improve hand-to-mouth coordination. Hard toast and teething biscuits help reinforce positive finger-feeding experiences. As the skills increase, the infant should be encouraged toward independent feeding and given foods for self-feeding such as small pieces of cooked vegetables, fruits, meats, and cheese sticks.

Foods offered to infants and children should require a minimum amount of chewing to avoid choking and aspiration. A number of deaths have occurred in infants and toddlers who were eating such foods as hot dogs, nuts, grapes, carrots, and round hard candies (Food and Drug Administration, 1985).

As mashed or chopped foods are introduced in the diet, weaning from the bottle or breast to the cup should be considered. Although there is no special time for weaning that is best for every infant, most infants show signs of developmental readiness after 6 months of age. By the time the infant is 1 year of age, he usually can hold and drink from a cup with assistance. Weaning should be done gradually by replacing one bottle or breast-feeding at a time. The last feeding to be discontinued is usually the nighttime one.

Prolonged bottle feeding can lead to a severe form of dental decay known as nursing bottle caries. This condition can be avoided if milk and juices are not used as pacifiers at nap time or bedtime. Delaying the introduction of fruit juices until the infant is able to drink from a cup has been suggested as a means of preventing tooth decay. The marketing of juices in ready-to-feed bottles may prolong the infant's attachment to the bottle and contribute to caries.

Feeding time for infants should be pleasurable for both the infant and the parent, taking place in a calm, comfortable environment free from distractions. Infants should be held while feeding with the bottle positioned so that air does not flow through the nipple. Bottle propping is *not* an acceptable method of feeding because of the risk of aspiration.

When solids are introduced, the infant's position is very important. Initially the infant is held in an upright position. Once the infant has coordinated the intake of solid food with swallowing, an infant seat may be used. As the infant gains body and head control a high chair is used; however, parents need to be reminded to take proper precautions. It is important to restrain the infant in order to avoid very serious safety problems.

Feeding problems frequently encountered during the first year of life include spitting up and vomiting, diarrhea, constipation, and food allergies. For a summary of practical approaches to infant feeding problems, see Table 7-15.

Food allergies are most common during childhood due to the physiologic immaturity of the gastrointestinal tract and to the high exposure to many new food antigens. All foods are potentially allergenic, but wheat, milk, eggs, and corn are the chief offenders. Others include chocolate, oranges, soy, legumes, rice, fish, beef, pork, and chicken. Allergic responses to food vary and may include vomiting, diarrhea, eczema, irritability, and hyperactivity.

The most common nutritional allergy in infants is allergy to cow's milk. Milk protein allergy is manifested by vomiting, diarrhea, and colic. The diagnosis of milk allergy is based on the clearing of symptoms after milk products have been removed from the diet. The diagnosis should be confirmed after milk is reintroducd in the diet to ascertain whether the symptoms reappear. Once the diagnosis of milk protein sensitivity is established, a diet free of milk and milk products is indicated. Infants who are not fed human milk and are sensitive to cow's milk should be given a soy-based or protein hydrolysate infant formula (Table 7-10).

Nutrition for Toddlers and Preschool Children

The toddler and preschool periods are marked by "plateauing" of the growth rate. Parents need to be reminded that since growth is slower, the appetite will not be as robust as it was during infancy. The toddler years can be a troubled period as weaning occurs and the toddler moves from a predominantly milk diet to progressively more solid foods. Parents need reassurance and instruction from nurses and other health care professionals regarding adequacy of intake and achievement of desirable meal patterns.

The toddler and preschool years are important years for the development of food habits. Researchers who have studied large numbers of children believe that what happens during the first few years of life is of paramount importance in eating behavior later in life. Desirable food habits include the following:

1. Willingness to accept a sufficient quantity of foods and a variety of foods.
2. Development of independent feeding skill
3. Willingness to try new foods in small portions
4. Having structured mealtimes rather than eating all day long

A factor that is extremely important in the development of good food habits is a proper environment. Mealtimes should be pleasurable and supportive rather than times for family arguments and discipline. For some children, socializing during mealtime may be too distracting; therefore, feeding the child before the rest of the family eats may be appropriate. The child must be given sufficient time to eat at his own pace. Children also may become restless and fidgety when required to sit during long meals. It is important to allow a child ample time to settle down from play before a meal begins. An additional problem is fatigue. Children who are overly tired may find it difficult to eat.

Parental and sibling behavior has a tremendous impact at this time of increased imitation and sex-role identification. Attitudes about food and interactions among family members are observed and imitated accurately. A parent who refuses to eat vegetables cannot expect the child to be enthusiastic about vegetables.

Most toddlers are picky, fussy easters with strong taste preferences. Food jags are common. Children may have a voracios appetite one day and eat almost nothing the next. They often are influenced by factors other than the taste of food. Consequently, the manner in which food is served is important.

1. New textures and flavors should be introduced gradually.
2. Servings should be small and should be placed on child-sized dishes.
3. Children should always sit securely on a sturdy, well-balanced chair with their feet well supported on the floor.
4. Utensils that are the appropriate size for the small hands of the 2- to 5-year-old child should be used.
5. Menus should be simple, and foods should not be too difficult to chew.
6. Color should be a consideration in the food that is served, since most children have a natural interest in color.

It is important to realize that in teaching young children good food habits, it is usually easier to change the food than it is to change the child. For instance, young children who may have trouble swallowing a dry food, such as mashed potatoes, will find it acceptable if extra milk is added to it.

Nutrition for School-Age Children

School-age children are not without nutritional problems. As children spend the day in school they adjust to a more

TABLE 7-15 Practical Approaches to Infant Feeding Problems

Problem	Signs and Symptoms	Management
Intake of formula too large	Regurgitation Vomiting Diarrhea or frequent large stools Normal or excessive weight gain History of excessive intake for age	Reduce formula intake at feedings Explain problem in detail to parents and give reassurance
Intake of formula too small	Irritable Underweight Hungry Constipated History of inadequate intake for age	Increase amount and frequency of formula and possibly calorie content of feedings
Improper technique of feeding	Any of the above signs and symptoms Following errors frequently encountered: 1. Hole in rubber nipple too small (providing too-long feeding period) or too large (causing excessive swallowing of air, discomfort, and regurgitation)	A puncture with a needle will not increase size of aperture; discard and use a new one
	2. Formula too hot	Moderately cold or room-temperature formulas are well tolerated
	3. Improper placement of nipple in mouth	Place nipple far enough back in mouth
	4. Failure to bubble the infant	After feeding, hold infant erect against shoulder to expel swallowed air
	5. Improper position of infant during feeding, such as horizontal or with propped pillow	Position should be inclined to at least a 45° angle
	6. Nursing from an empty bottle	Formula should fill the nipple throughout feeding, and ½-1 oz should be left in the bottle at termination of feeding
	7. Improper sterilization technique	Check sterilization technique; for terminal sterilization: 1. Scrub bottles, nipples, equipment 2. Measure and mix formula 3. Pour mixture into bottles 4. Place bottle on rack in sterilizer and boil gently for 25 min 5. Store capped bottles in refrigerator
Improper composition of formula	Carbohydrate: Excessive amounts may produce diarrhea	Added carbohydrate in the form of corn syrup to evaporated milk formula need rarely exceed 1 oz, or 2 tbsp, per 24-h volume
	Protein: Allergy to protein in cow's milk; allergic infants may have vomiting, irritability, diarrhea, with or without blood in stool; onset 2-4 weeks after initiating formula; history in other family members is significant	A few days' trial with a cow's milk substitute such as soybean milk, Nutramigen, or Cho-Free, with subsequent alleviation of symptoms, indicates milk allergy
	Fat: Improper fat digestion causes large, bulky stools; digestion of cow's milk butterfat may be less complete than that of fat in breast milk	Substitute a formula free of butterfat, such as Similac or Enfamil
Emotional problems in the family	Irritability Colic Spitting up Vomiting Failure to gain weight	Explanation, education, patience, and understanding are needed along with constant reassurance and considerable tact

Source: Adapted from W. T. Hughes and F. Falkner, "Infant Feeding Problems: A Practical Approach," *Clinical Pediatrics,* 3:65, 1964. Table prepared by E. Getchell and R. Howard for G. M. Scipien et al. (eds.), *Comprehensive Pediatric Nursing,* 2d ed., McGraw-Hill, New York, 1979.

orderly routine, gain mastery in motor skills, and expend energy in various sports programs. Currently, most children also learn about food and nutrition in school. Feeding guidelines for school-age children are given in Table 7-16.

Nutritional Requirements of Adolescents

Increased nutritional requirements in adolescence parallel the adolescent's need for accelerated skeletal growth and deposition of lean body mass and adipose tissue. The growth spurt spans 18 to 24 months during which nutri-

TABLE 7-16 The Basic Four Food Groups Throughout the Growing Years

Food Group	Servings per Day	Average-Size Servings for Age			
		Toddler	Preschool	School-Age	Adolescent
Milk or equivalent	4	½-¾ cup	¾ cup	¾-1 cup	1 cup
½ cup milk equals					
2 tbsp powdered milk					
1 oz cheese					
¼ evaporated milk					
½ cup cottage cheese					
1 serving custard (4 servings from 1 pt milk)					
½ cup milk pudding					
½ cup yogurt					
Meat, fish, poultry, or equivalent	2 or more	3 tbsp	4 tbsp	3-4 oz (6-8 tbsp)	4 oz or more
1 oz meat equals					
1 egg, 1 frankfurter					
1 oz cheese,* 1 cold cut					
2 tbsp peanut butter, cut meat					
¼ cup tuna fish or cottage cheese*					
½ cup dried peas or beans					
Vegetables and fruits to include	4 or more				
Citrus fruit or equivalent	1 or more	4 oz	4 oz	4-6 oz	4-6 oz
1 citrus fruit serving equals					
½ cup orange or grapefruit juice					
½ grapefruit or cantaloupe					
¾ cup strawberries					
1 med orange					
½ citrus fruit serving equals					
½ cup tomato juice or tomatoes, broccoli, chard, collards, greens, spinach, raw cabbage, brussels sprouts, 1 med tomato, 1 wedge honeydew					
Yellow or green vegetable or equivalent	1 or more	4 tbsp	4 tbsp	⅓ cup	½ cup
1 serving equals					
½ cup broccoli, greens, spinach, carrots, squash, pumpkin					
5 apricot halves					
½ med cantaloupe					
Other fruits and vegetables	2 or more				
Other vegetables including potatoes		2-3 tbsp	4 tbsp	⅓-½ cup	¾ cup
Other fruit including apples, banana, pears, peaches		½ med apple	½-1 med apple	1 med apple	1 med apple
Breads and cereals or whole grain or enriched equivalent	4 or more				
1 slice bread equals		½ slice	1 slice	1-2 slices	2 slices
¾ cup dry cereal		½ cup	¾ cup	1 oz	1 oz
½ cup cooked cereal, rice, spaghetti, or macaroni		2 tbsp	¼-½ cup	½-1 cup	1 cup or more
1 roll, muffin, or biscuit					

*If cottage or cheddar cheese is used as a milk equivalent, it should not also be counted as a meat equivalent.

Sources: Infant Feeding Guide, for use by professional staffs, Washington State Department of Social and Health Services, Health Services Division, Local Health Services, Nutrition Unit, 1972. Table prepared by E. Getchell and R. Howard For G. M. Scipien et al. (eds.), *Comprehensive Pediatric Nursing,* 2d ed., McGraw-Hill, New York, 1979.

tional requirements may be doubled compared with other periods of adolescence (Mahan and Rosebrough, 1984). The peak in growth coincides with sexual maturity and occurs in Tanner stage 3 and stage 4 among females and males, respectively. Since wide variations of growth occur during this period, the requirements for energy and pro-

tein are based on height and reflect physiological needs (Table 7-1).

Nutrients which are of particular concern in adolescence include calcium, iron, zinc, vitamin A, ascorbic acid, folic acid, and vitamin B_6. Accelerated growth increases the adolescent's requirements for calcium, iron, and zinc. Calcium needs are increased 50 percent above prepubertal and adult requirements to provide amounts sufficient for skeletal growth and deposition of lean body mass. Diets may contain inadequate amounts of calcium for teenagers who consume soft drinks as a substitute for milk and females who restrict dairy products for weight-reduction purposes. Requirements for iron are increased in response to increase in blood volume, muscle mass, and menstruation in females. Iron supplementation may be indicated in adolescent females who are at risk for iron deficiency on the basis of increased requirements, marginal dietary intake, and increased losses with menstruation. Zinc requirements are increased because of the role of zinc in growth and sexual maturation.

A paucity of information exists regarding vitamin requirements during adolescence. Vitamins which are frequently low in the diet of adolescents include vitamin A, ascorbic acid, and folic acid (Truswell and Darnton-Hill, 1981).

Dietary Habits

The dietary habits of teenagers typically are characterized by irregular meal consumption, snacking and frequent intake of fast-food meals. The eating behavior of adolescents is influenced by (1) family dietary practices, (2) peers, and (3) the media. Dietary habits during this period also reflect psychosocial development in which increased autonomy is manifested in irregular meal consumption and eating meals away from home. These patterns increase from early to late adolescence (Story, 1984).

Snacking frequently is used as a substitute for meals among adolescents. Between-meals snacking can make significant contributions to nutrient requirements depending on the quantity and quality of food consumed. Between-meals snacking may contribute approximately 25 percent of total caloric intake in addition to significant amounts of protein, riboflavin, thiamine, and ascorbic acid (Thomas and Call, 1973). The nutrients most limited in snacks include vitain A, calcium, and iron. Frequent eating of fast-food meals by adolescents contributes to a high intake of saturated fat, cholesterol, and sodium (Story, 1984). Fast-food meals contain limited amounts of calcium when the menu selection includes soft drinks in place of milk or a milkshake. Since snacking and consumption of fast-food meals are integral aspects of adolescent eating behavior, nutritional intervention should focus on the selection of food sources with high nutrient density according to individual food preferences. Basic food requirements for the adolescent are identified in Table 7-16.

The maintenance of adequate hydration during exercise is critical in optimizing athletic performance and minimizing the risk of heat stroke. Dehydration with fluid deficits of 4 to 5 percent can reduce muscle work capacity by 20 to 30 percent (Bergstrom and Hullman, 1972). Severe fluid deficits of 7 to 10 percent can precipitate circulatory collapse and heat stroke (Committee on Nutritional Misinformation, 1974). Electrolytes lost during exercise and competitive events can be replaced through a normal diet; therefore, the primary concern is to maintain adequate hydration (American Dietetic Association, 1980a). The use of diuretics, fluid, and/or caloric restriction to promote rapid weight loss increases the risk for dehydration and electrolyte imbalances and compromises athletic performance (Smith, 1976). Substances often used to increase the ability to work have not been shown to enhance athletic performance (American Dietetic Association, 1980a) (e.g. wheat germ, vitamin E, lecithin, gelatin, honey, bee pollen, and brewer's yeast). Guidelines for a preperformance meal should include (1) consumption of foods and fluid 3 to 4 hours before competition, (2) use of protein and complex carbohydrate sources, and (3) restriction of high-fat sources which contribute to delayed gastric emptying (American Dietetic Association, 1980a).

Nutritional Assessment

Factors That Influence Nutritional Status

Many factors increase or decrease certain nutritional needs. When ignored, they can influence a person's nutritional status adversely. They include periods of rapid growth, stress, disease states, metabolic errors, some medications, and socioeconomic factors such as poor housing, inadequate income, and lack of food. These factors particularly affect children who are in periods of very rapid growth and are especially vulnerable to nutritional deficits. It is important to consider theses variables in the assessment of a child's nutritional status.

Assessment of Nutritional Status

Nutritional assessment in children involves four components: anthropometric, biochemical, clinical, and dietary indexes. The components of nutritional assessment are presented in Table 7-17.

Anthropometric Assessment

Serial measurements of weight and length/stature are used as parameters of physical growth. Comparing those data with reference standards (Appendix B: National Center for Health Statistics growth percentiles) allows a nurse to identify abnormalities in growth. Progressive deviations from a given percentile (Owen, 1973) should alert the nurse to a potential growth abnormality.

TABLE 7-17 Components of Nutritional Assessment

A:	Anthropometric: weight, length/stature, head circumference, triceps skinfold, midarm muscle circumference
B:	Biochemical: serum albumin, hemoglobin, hematocrit, mean corpuscular volume, specific vitamin and minerals levels as indicated
C:	Clinical: physical signs of nutrient deficiencies
D:	Dietary: diet history, recent weight loss, N/V/D, fever, surgery or illness, oral/motor feeding problems, multivitamin and mineral supplements, drug-nutrient interactions

Source: Table prepared by S. Malone for G. M. Scipien et al. (eds.), *Comprehensive Pediatric Nursing,* 3d ed., McGraw-Hill, New York, 1986.

Weight and Weight for Length/Stature

Weight for length/stature is used as an indicator of a child's short-term nutritional status. In comparing a child's actual weight with the ideal weight (50th percentile weight for height), the data provide information about the adequacy of that weight. Weight measurements between the 10th and 90th percentiles on the NCHS growth charts are considered normal, while those below the 10th percentile or above the 90th percentile may indicate inadequate or excessive weight, respectively. Infants and children less than 36 months old are always weighed without clothes. Children over 36 months are weighed with minimal clothing (i.e., underwear) on a balance beam scale. It is important to balance the scale before use.

Length/Stature

Serial measurements of length/stature are used as indicators of growth and long-term nutritional status. For example, children with chronic malnutrition demonstrate varying degrees of growth retardation. Errors in length or stature measurements frequently occur as a result of using inappropriate measuring techniques (scale measurement stick, in bed with measuring tape). In obtaining a recumbent length, it is essential to use a measuring board and sliding foot piece in children less than 2 years of age.

Head Circumference

Serial measurements of head circumference are used to measure brain growth. Measurements below the 5th percentile may be indicative of chronic undernutrition. It is extremely important to identify landmarks on the skull to ensure that all nurses are measuring the same circumference. Errors occur when different angles are used in acquiring this measurement.

Body Composition

Serial measurements of the upper arm's triceps skinfold and midarm muscle circumference are used to assess subcutaneous fat stores and muscle mass respectively. Measuring these sites is useful when (1) weight is falsely elevated (fluid retention, solid tumors), (2) weight is unobtainable (e.g., multiple trauma patient in traction), and (3) definitions of relative fat and muscle mass contributions to total weight are indicated. Body composition measurements above the sex- and age-adjusted 15th percentile are considered normal; values below the 15th percentile indicate depletion (Gray and Gray, 1980).

Biochemical Assessment

A variety of biochemical laboratory tests are used to provide objective measurements of a child's nutritional status and to monitor a child's metabolic responses to nutrition support (tube feeding, total parenteral nutrition). Biochemical indicators of nutritional status may confirm deficiencies which are suggested by anthropometric, clinical, and/or dietary assessments.

A serum albumin level traditionally has been used as an indicator of visceral protein status. While serum albumin is the most specific indicator of protein depletion, it is insensitive to acute changes. The relatively long half-life of 21 days and large body pool contribute to its lack of sensitivity. Serum albumin levels may be decreased by nonnutritional factors including over-hydration, liver disease, inflammatory bowel disease, nephrotic syndrome, and burns. Serum albumin levels less than 3.6 g/dl are indicative of visceral protein depletion (Jensen et al., 1983).

Immune function is compromised in the malnourished child with protein depletion. A synergistic relationship exists between malnutrition, decreased immunocompetence, and susceptibility to infection (Puri and Chandra, 1985).

In addition to laboratory indexes of visceral protein status and immune function, levels of specific nutrients may be measured in children with suspected deficiencies on the basis of inadequate intake or absorption or increased requirements.

Clinical Assessment

Clinical assessment of nutritional status refers to physical manifestations of nutritional deficiencies. In general, the clinical signs of these deficiencies occur in the later stages of depletion. These clinical signs may range from overt wasting of subcutaneous fat and skeletal muscle in the extremities to dry, flaky skin. Clinical signs of nutritional deficiency are frequently nonspecific and require a trained observer for accurate assessment.

Dietary Assessment

Dietary assessment includes an evaluation of the feeding history and a child's "typical" intake. The feeding history is used to evaluate the introduction of solids in infants, use of breast-feeding or formula feeding, food intolerances, behavioral or oral/motor feeding problems, and food preferences. The diet history provides an estimation of present intake and may be compared with the RDA as a "guideline" for nutritional adequacy. The diet history and other methods of collecting food consumption data including 3-day food records, 7-day food records, and 24-hour recalls are subject to multiple limitations. Children may be placed on "calorie counts," which require the documentation of every spoonful of food ingested and fluids taken. The next day, a nutritionist computes the child's caloric intake for the previous day. The reliability of the informant, commitment to maintain food records, and description of "typical" intake all contribute to the validity of dietary assessment. Methods for collecting dietary data are presented in Table 7-18.

In summary, nutritional assessment serves multiple functions in both the hospital and outpatient settings. Basic screening indexes including weight for length/stature, hemoglobin, and a diet history suggestive of nutritional risk factors (e.g., recent weight loss, anorexia, nausea, vomiting, diarrhea) aid in identifying children who are need of nutritional intervention. In addition, an ongoing nutritional assessment in children who require nutritional intervention is critical in monitoring changes in nutritional status and determining the effectiveness of the nutritional support plan.

TABLE 7-18 Dietary Assessment Guidelines: Methods

Methods of Assessment

1. Daily recall: The interviewer makes a detailed listing of foods consumed during the previous 24 h, obtaining estimates of the quantity of each food consumed during this period
2. Food records: A record is kept of everything consumed for a given period (3-7 days)
3. Dietary questionnaire: The following information is considered pertinent in determining actual food intake:
   (a) Social situation: family size, family economics, family feeding problems, family weight problems, ethnic background
   (b) Developmental stage: feeding age, texture of food, ability to chew, suck and swallow
   (c) Growth: birth weight, height, weight gain, weight loss
   (d) Feeding behavior: food appetite, fluid consumption, favorite food, food dislikes, mealtime behavior problems, meals per day at home, meals out, school lunch, school hours, snacks per day, hungriest time of day
   (e) Food frequency per day: meat, fish, poultry (including cold cuts, hot dogs, tuna fish) _____, milk _____, eggs _____, potato, macaroni, rice, noodles _____, crackers _____, fruit and fruit juices _____, vegetables _____, puddings, ice cream, custard _____, cookies, _____, cake, pies _____, doughnuts, pastry , candy _____, potato chips, pretzels _____, tonic, Kool-Aid _____, vitamin supplementation

Analysis

1. Intake may be compared to food guide, such as basic four food groups
2. Nutrient content may be calculated using tables of food composition
3. Nutrient analysis made from a report of food actually consumed

Evaluation

Nutrient intake is compared to some standard; in the United States the standard most frequently used is the Recommended Dietary Allowances of the National Research Council

Limitation

1. Reliability of informant
2. RDA standard cannot be applied to individuals. Child's intake applies only to groups of children

Source: Table prepared by E. Getchall and R. Howard for G. M. Scipien et al. (eds.), *Comprehensive Pediatric Nursing,* 2d ed., McGraw-Hill, New York, 1979.

Learning Activities

1. Visit a day care center during mealtime. Observe the menu being served and the portion sizes of various foods. If possible, select two children of different ages, obtain height and weight, and record their food intake. Plot the height and weight on growth charts. Calculate the caloric and protein content of the meal. What comments could you make about feeding skills, dietary intake, and growth?
2. Visit a supermarket and select foods for a 6-month-old infant. Calculate the cost for feeding an infant for a day.
3. Visit either an elementary school lunch or high school lunch period. Record your observations about the students' acceptance of the lunch. How many students appeared of normal weight, underweight, obese? What recommendations could you make about the menu or environment?

Study Questions

1. The most rapid growth periods in order are:
   A. (1) 0-12 months, (2) 12 months-24 months.
   B. (1) 6 years-8 years; (2) 13-16 years (females) and 16-18 years (male).
   C. (1) 0-12 months, (2) 9-13 years (females) and 12-16 years (males).
   D. (1) 9-13 years (females) and 12-16 years (males), (2) 0-3 months.
2. The best indicator of growth is:
   A. Weight.   C. Weight-to-height ratio.
   B. Height.   D. Skinfold thickness.
3. The critical period(s) for attaining one's potential height occur(s) during:
   A. Fetal life.   C. Adolescence.
   B. Infancy.   D. All of the above.
4. Catch-up growth is considered to be:
   A. The growth the child has after growth hormone therapy.
   B. Growth toward the natural curve following interference with growth.
   C. The weight a preterm infant gains after he or she is dismissed from the hospital.
   D. The weight that an obese child regains after being on a weight-loss program.
5. _____ provide 40 to 50 percent of the energy consumed by individuals in the United States.
   A. Fats.   C. Carbohydrates.
   B. Proteins.   D. Fats and carbohydrates.
6. Protein needs are the greatest during:
   A. Fetal development.
   B. The first year of life.
   C. The prepubescent period.
   D. The adolescent period.

7. A diet which contains fat is:
    A. Discouraged because of the coronary risk.
    B. A carrier of vitamins A, D, E, and K.
    C. A source of glycogen.
    D. A very high source of bile salts.

8. During infancy at least _____ percent of the calories must be provided from fat.
    A. 0.   B. 20.   C. 33.   D. 50.

9. Iron-defiency anemia is quite common:
    A. Before 4 months of age.
    B. From 9 to 24 months of age.
    C. From 8 to 9 years of age.
    D. In adolescence.

10. Fluoride may produce adverse effects, which include:
    A. Skin rashes.
    B. Mottling of tooth enamel.
    C. Diarrhea.
    D. Central nervous system depression.

11. Newborns with a family history of allergies should be:
    A. Placed on a soybean formula.
    B. Placed on an evaporated milk formula.
    C. Breast-fed.
    D. Encouraged to nurse in any way the mother desires.

References

Aasenden, R., and T.C. Peebles: "Effects of Fluoride Supplementation from Birth on Human Deciduous and Permanent Teeth," *Archives of Oral Biology,* **19**:321-326, 1974.

American Dietetic Association: "Nutrition and Physical Fitness," *Journal of the American Dietetic Association,* **76**:437-443, 1980.

————: "Position Paper on the Vegetarian Approach to Eating," *Journal of the American Dietetic Association,* **77**:61-69, 1980b.

Ashworth, A., and D.J. Millard: "Catchup Growth in Children," *Nutrition Reviews,* **44**:157-163, 1986.

Atherton, D.J.: "A Double-Blind Controlled Crossover Trial of Antigen-Avoidance Diet in Atopic Eczema," *Lancet,* **1**:401, 1978.

Behrman, R.E., and C. Vaughan (eds.): *Nelson Textbook of Pediatrics,* 12th ed., Saunders, Philadelphia, 1983.

Boellner, S.E., A.G. Beard, and T.C. Panos: "Impairment of Intestinal Hydrolysis of Lactose in Newborn Infants," *Pediatrics,* **36**:542, 1965.

Boerma, A.H.: "The 30 Years War against World Hunger," *Proceedings of Nutrition Society,* **34**:145, 1975.

Bothwell, T.H., and C.A. Finch: *Iron Metabolism,* Little, Brown, Boston, 1962.

Committee on Nutrition, American Academy of Pediatrics: "Iron Supplementation for Infants," *Pediatrics,* **58**:765, 1976a.

————: "Commentary on Breast-Feeding and Infant Formulas, Including Proposed Standard for Formulas," *Pediatrics,* **57**:279, 1976b.

————: "Nutritional Needs of Low Birth Weight Infants," *Pediatrics,* **60**:519, 1977.

————: "The Use of Whole Cow's Milk in Infancy," *Pediatrics,* **72**:253, 1983.

————: *Pediatric Nutrition Handbook,* 2d ed., American Academy of Pediatrics, Elk Grove Village, Ill., 1985.

————: "Fluoride Supplementation," *Pediatrics,* **77**:758-761, 1986a.

————: "Prudent Life-Style for Children: Dietary Fat and Cholesterol," *Pediatrics,* **78**:521-525, 1986b.

Committee on Nutritional Misinformation, Food and Nutrition Board: "Water Deprivation and Performance in Athletes," *Nutrition Reviews,* **32**:314-316, 1974.

————: "Hazards of Overuse of Vitamin D," *American Journal of Clinical Nutrition,* **28**:412, 1975.

Cooke, J.D., M. Layrisse, C. Martinez-Torrez, R. Walker, E. Monsen, and C.A. Finch: "Food Iron Absorption Measured by an Extrinsic Tag," *Journal of Clinical Investigation,* **51**:805-815, 1972.

Cunningham, A.S.: "Morbidity in Breast-Fed and Artificially Fed Infants,'" *Journal of Pediatrics,* **90**:726, 1977.

Davidson, M., and C.H. Bauer: "Patterns of Fat Excretion in Feces of Premature Infants Fed Various Preparations of Milk," *Pediatrics,* **25**:375, '1960.

Dobbing, J.: "Infant Nutrition in Later Achivement," *American Journal of Clinical Nutrition,* **41**:477-484, 1985.

Dobbing, J.A.: "The Later Development of the Brain and Its Vulnerability," in J.B. Davis, and J. Dobbing (eds.) *Scientific Foundations of Pediatrics,* 2d ed., Heinemann, London, pp. 744-759, 1974.

Elliott, R.B.: "Fats and Fatty Acids," in *PEdiatric Nutrition Handbook,* American Academy of Pediatrics, Committee on Nutrition, Evanston, Ill., 1979, pp. 1-472.

Finch, C.A.: "Iron Nutrition," in N.H. Moss and J. Mayer (eds.), *Food and Nutrition in Health and Disease, Annals of the New York Academy of Science,* **300**:221, 1977.

Fomon, S.J., F. Haschkes, E.E. Ziegler, and S.E. Nelson: "Body Composition of Reference Children from Birth to Age 10 Years," *American Journal of Clinical Nutrition,* **35**:1169-1175, 1982.

Food and Drug Administration: A Report to, held in Elkridge, Md., August 4-5, 1983. Foods and Choking in Children," in G.B. Forbes and C.W. Woodruff (eds.), *Pediatric Nutrition Handbook,* American Academy of Pediatrics, Committee on Nutrition, Elk Grove Village, Ill., 1985.

Food and Nutrition Board, National Research Council: *Recommended Dietary Allowances,* 9th ed., National Academy Press, Washington, D.C., 1980.

Forrester, D.J., and E.M. Schulta (eds.): International Workshop on Fluorides and Dental Caries Reductions. Baltimore, University of Maryland, 1974, in Committee on Nutrition, American Academy of Pediatrics: "Fluoride Supplementation," *Pediatrics,* **77**:758-761, 1986.

Forsman, B.: "Early Supply of Floride and Enamel: Fluorosis," *Scandinavian Journal of Dental Research,* **85**:22-30, 1977.

Friedman, Z.; "Essential Fatty Acids Revisited," *American Journal of Diseases of Children,* **134**:397-408, 1980.

Fripp, R.R., J.L. Hodgson, P.O. Kwiterovich, J.C. Werner, H.G. Schuler, and V. Whitman: "Aerobic Capacity, Obesity, and Atherosclerotic Risk Factors in Male Adolescents," *Pediatrics,* **75**:813-818, 1985.

Getchell, E.L.: "Special Concerns; The Low-Birth-Weight Infant," in R.B. Howard and D.H. Herbold (eds.) *Nutrition in Clinical Care,* McGraw-Hill, New York, 1978.

Gray, G.E., and L.K. Gray: "Anthropometric Measurements and Their Interpretations: Principles, Practices and Problems," *Journal of the American Dietetic Association,* **77**:534-538, 1980.

Hamill, P.V., T.A. Drized, C.L. Johnson, R.D. Reed, A.F. Roche, and W.M. Moore: "Physical Growth: National Center for Health Statistics Percentiles," *American Journal of Clinical Nutrition,* **32**:607-629, 1979.

Holloway, P.J., and R.S. Levine: "The Values of Self-Applied Fluorides at Home," *International Dental Journal,* **31**:232-239, 1981.

Jensen, T.G., D.M. Englert, and S.J. Dudrick (eds.): *Nutritional Assessment,* Appleton-Century-Crofts, Norwalk, Conn., 1983.

Layrisse, M.C., and C. Martinez-Torres: In E.B. Brown and C.V. Moore (eds.), *Progress in Hematology,* Grune & Stratton, New York, 1968, vol. 7, pp. 137-160.

Mahan, L.K., and R.H. Rosebrough: "Nutritional Requirements and Nutritional Status Assessment in Adolescence," in L.K Mahan and J.M. Rees (eds.), *Nutrition and Adolescence,* Times/Mirror/Mosby, St. Louis, 1984, pp. 40-76.

Mahoney, C.P., M.T. Margolis, T.A. Knauss, and R.F. Labbe: "Chronic Vitamin A Intoxication in Infants Fed Chicken Liver," *Pediatrics* **65**:893, 1980.

Martinez, G.A., and J.P. Nalezienski: "The Recent Trend in Milk Feeding among WIC Infants," *American Journal of Public Health,* **71**:68, 1982.

Monsen, E.R., L. Hallberg, M. Layrisse, D.M. Hegsted, J.D. Cook, W. Mertz, and C.A. Finch: "Estimation of Available Dietary Iron," *American Journal of Clinical Nutrition,* **31**:134-141, 1978.

Puczynski, M., D. Rademaker, and R.L. Gatson: "Burn Injury Related to Improper Use of Microwave Oven," 'Pediatrics, **71**:714, 1983.

Puri, S., and R.K. Chandra: "Nutritional Regulation of Host Resistance and Predictive Value of Immunologic Tests in Assessment of Outcome," *Pediatric Clinics of North America,* **32**:499-515, 1985.

Rudman, D., and A.J. Williams: "Megadose Vitamins: Use and Misuse," *New England Journal of Medicine,* **309:**488, 1983.

————, and M.A. Siimes: "Iron Absorption from Infant Formula and the Optimal Level of Iron Supplementation," *ACTA, Paed Scand,* **66:**719, 1977.

————: M.A. Siimes, and P.R. Dallman: "Iron Absorption in Infants: High Bioavailability of Breast Milk Iron as Indicated by the Extrinsic Tag Method of Iron Absorption and by the Concentration of Serum Ferritin," *Journal of Pediatrics,* **91:**36, 1977.

Schaumburg, H., J. L. Kaplan, A. Windebank, N. Vick, S. Rasmus, D. Pleasure, and M. J. Brown: "Sensory Neuropathy from Pyridoxine Abuse: A New Megavitamin Syndrome," *New England Journal of Medicine,* **309:**445, 1983.

Sinatra, F.R., and R.J. Merritt: "Iatrogenic Kwashiorkor in Infants," *American Journal of Diseases of Children,* **135:**21, 1981.

Smith, N.: "Gaining and Losing Weight in Athletics," *Journal of American Medical Association,* **236:**149-151, 1976.

Stoch, M.B., and P.M. Smythe: "The Effect of Undernutrition during Infancy on Subsequent Brain Growth and Intellectual Development," *South Africa Medical Journal* **41:**1027, 1967.

Story, M.: "Adolescent Life-Style and Eating Behavior," in L.K. Mahan and J. Rees (eds.), *Nutrition of Adolescence,* Times/Mirror/Mosby, St. Louis, 1984, pp. 77-103.

Thomas, J., and D. Call: "Eating between Meals: A Nutrition Problem among Teenagers," *Nutrition Reviews,* **31:**137-139, 1973.

Truesdall, D.D., and P.B. Acosta: "Feeding the Vegan Infant and Child," *Journal of The American Dietetic Association,* **85:**837-840, 1985.

Truswell, A.S., and I. Darnton-Hill: "Food Habits in Adolescents," *Nutrition Reviews,* **39:**73-86, 1981.

Vaughn, V.: "Growth and Development," in R. Behrman and V. Vaughn (eds.), *Nelson Textbook of Pediatrics,* 12th ed., Saunders, Philadelphia, 1983, p. 16.

Watkins, J.B., P. Szczepanik, J.B. Gould, et al.: "Bile Salt Metabolism in the Human Premature Infant," *Gastroenterology,* **69:**706, 1975.

Weidman, W.H., L.R. Elveback, R.A. Nelson, P.A. Hodgson, and R.D. Ellefson: "Nutrient Intake and Serum Cholesterol Level in Normal Children 6 to 16 Years of Age," *Pediatrics,* **61:**354-359, 1978.

Woodruff, C.W.: "The Science of Infant Nutrition and the Art of Infant Feeding," *JAMA* **240:**657-661, 1978.

Woodruff, C.W., and J.L. Clark: "The Role of Fresh Cow's Milk in Iron Deficiency: I. Albumin Turnover in Infants with Iron Deficiency Anemia," *Am. J. Dis. Children,* **124:**18, 1972.

8

Legal and Ethical Issues

Objectives

After reading this chapter, the student will be able to:
1. Define the term *emancipated minor.*
2. Define *partial emancipation.*
3. Describe informed consent.
4. Describe the conditions under which parents have the right to refuse to consent to medical care for their minor children.
5. Describe the legal issue in privacy for the children receiving treatment.
6. Describe the legal issue surrounding confidentiality for children receiving treatment.
7. Describe the nurse's role as an advocate.

The legal and ethical literature dealing with pediatrics is extensive, and so it is important for the reader to understand that the content of this chapter is not all-inclusive. Instead, the more common situations which involve a pediatric nurse are explored. They include the diverse legal classifications of adolescence, the treatment of minors, the utilization of minors as research subjects, and children's access to health care, along with other topics which pertain *only* to children. Any of these subjects can stimulate a lengthy discussion or take up a semester of study.

Clinical practice has changed appreciably in the last 20 years. Influenced by technological progress and the capability to sustain life beyond former expectations, nurses confront a variety of ethical dilemmas daily, and these quandries have no easy answers. Also, there are nursing standards which need to be met and a nursing code which governs the activities of members of the profession. It is critical for nurses to know the parameters of clinical practice as they meet their day-to-day responsibilities.

Nurses who care for infants, children, and adolescents are facing issues among the most complex dealt with in any speciality area. Legal and ethical issues in pediatric nursing deal with the broad issues of the limits of personal and family autonomy in our diverse society. Pediatric nurses confront the conflict between the legitimate protection of the best interests of the child and the sometimes seemingly meddling interests of the state of health care system. These questions merit thoughtful analysis by pediatric nurses from both a legal and an ethical perspective.

Children, Health, and the Law

Pediatric nurses care for children as they move from an infant's dependency and legal incapacity through the process of physical, intellectual, and legal maturation in childhood and finally to adolescence, when they progress from parental control to adult self-determination. As a democratic society, we place a high value on self-determination. The rights movement (prominent in health care) has focused on careful determination of the elements of informed consent for adults and for minors as they move toward adulthood. In caring for children and in functioning as advocates for children in the health care system, it is important for nurses to develop a historical perspective on the position of minors under the law.

Historical Perspective

The legal tradition of the United States has its roots in the English system of common law. The right of self-determination under English common law has long suffered the distortions of paternalism. Historically, in the English patriarchal society and under English common law, children and adolescents were considered chattels, an expression derived from and connoting ownership similar to owning cattle. Children were in every sense of the word the possessions of their parents. The wife's rights were subordinate to and merged with the rights of the husband, who as head of the household had complete legal control of the family. The Latin expression *parens potestas* meant that parents had full power over their minor children, as they did over their cattle. This concept gradually gave way to the notion of *parens patriae,* which in common law in England and later in the United States meant that in legal issues relative to children there were actually three parties: the parents, the child, and the state. Despite the fact that it was recognized early in our legal tradition that the state has an interest in minors, they were traditionally unable to receive health care without the consent of their parents.

Consent to Treatment of Minors

The general rule of law, having its roots in the tradition of English common law, is that a minor may not be treated without parental consent. Treating a minor without parental consent may give rise to a civil action for assault and battery brought by the parents against the nurse or her employer even if the treatment was not negligent, was in the minor's best interest, and yielded a positive outcome (*Zaman* v. *Schultz,* 1933). The general rule of the requirement of parental consent to treatment has some clear exceptions. As the family structure has changed in the twentieth century, women have been granted more equality under the law and the individual rights of children have become more and more a focus of statutory law and judicial decree. Today's law represents an intricate balance between the rights and responsibilities of the parents, the child, and the state. It is significant that the age of majority has been reduced to 18 years during the past two decades in all U.S. jurisdictions.

When May a Child Be Treated without Parental Consent?

Emergency Exception

The most notable exception to the general rule requiring parental consent for the treatment of minors is the emergency care exception. This exception holds that a minor may always be treated without parental consent if delay in treatment would cause a risk of serious harm or further injury. In emergency situations it has always been accepted practice to treat first and ask questions later. Most jurisdictions have adopted clear provisions which support this emergency exception. For example, in Massachusetts a minor may be treated without parental consent "when delay in treatment will endanger the life, limb, or mental well-being of the patient" (Mass. Gen. Laws ch 112, §12E). Courts have held that parents may not recover damages for proper treatment without consent in any emergency (*Lecha* v. *Lawrie,* 1912). In nonemergency situations, if there is no parental consent, no treatment is possible. In nonemergencies such figures as grandparents and siblings who have reached majority may not be consenting parties for the treatment of minors.

Emancipated Minors

The most clearly defined class of children who have the capacity to consent to their own care are adolescents defined as emancipated minors. A minor who is emancipated is free from the care, custody, and services of his parents. Many jurisdictions have adopted statutory provisions regarding emancipated minors (*Hospital Law Manual,* 1981). It is generally recognized that a minor of either sex may give consent to his medical and dental care if

1. He is married, widowed, or divorced.
2. He is the parent of a child, in which case he may also consent to the child's care.
3. He is a member of the armed forces.

4. He is living separate and apart from his parents or legal guardian and is self-supporting and managing his own financial affairs.

Such jurisdictions have broadened their concept to include minors who are self-supporting even though they may be living at home. As noted above, a married minor is generally held capable to consent to his own treatment and the treatment of any minor child of his marriage. If the marriage is dissolved, the capacity to consent remains unless the dissolution is the result of an annulment based on the incapacity of the parties to consent to the marriage (Holder, 1977).

Mature Minors

The mature minor rule permits a minor to obtain health services without parental consent if he is capable of giving informed consent (that is, if he is capable of understanding the nature of treatment, including the concurrent risks, benefits, and alternatives) and if the health services are for the minor's benefit. At least four states have enacted the mature minor rule by statutory provision, and many more by judicial decree. The Mississippi statute states that "any unemancipated minor of sufficient intelligence to understand and appreciate the consequences of the proposed surgical or medical treatment or procedure may consent to such treatment" (Miss. Code Annotated 541-41-3H).

In jurisdictions where the mature minor rule has been established by case law, the criterion for inclusion of individual minors has been vague. At best, it involves the careful assessment of the minor by one or more health professionals using, when appropriate, an institutional protocol in order to determine the "maturity" of the minor.

Some criteria which have been suggested (Wadlinton, 1973) for health care providers to take into consideration when making this assessment are as follows.
1. How close to majority is the minor?
2. Is the treatment undertaken for the minor's own benefit rather than that of a third party?
3. Does the minor have sufficient mental capacity to understand the nature and importance of the proposed treatment?
4. Is the medical procedure major (e.g., invasive)?
5. Is the minor fully or partially self-supporting?
6. Is the minor living apart from parents?
7. Have the parents failed to meet their legal responsibility?

The mature minor rule appears to be supported by the American Law Institute's *Restatement of the Law of Torts,* which says, "If a child . . . is capable of appreciating the nature, extent and consequences of the invasion (of his body) his assent prevents the invasion from creating liability, though the assent of the parent, guardian, or other person is not obtained or is expressly refused" (*Restatement,* 1971).

It is worth noting that there have been no reported cases in which hospitals or other providers have been held liable for the performance of accepted therapeutic procedures on minors over the age of 15 years without parental consent; this fact is probably an indication of the general movement of the law toward an expanding concept of the *mature minor rule* (Pilpel, 1972). Parents have been unsuccessful in the cases which have been litigated with regard to this issue (*Younts* v. *St. Francis Hospital and School of Nursing,* 1970). It is likely that case law in this area in the next few years will become increasingly complex as courts grapple with the issue of informed consent and a minor child's competency to make reasoned decisions at different ages. There is little consensus on what children at different ages can reasonably understand. There is substantial need for policy-oriented research teams representing the medical, nursing, and legal professions to work in conjunction with child development experts in order to better define, as a basis for legislation, children's capacities for understanding at various age levels.

Partial Emancipation

The doctrine of partial emancipation allows minors to have a partial capacity for consent. Statutes vary significantly in this area from state to state, but essentially the doctrine recognizes that children may still be subject to parental control for some purposes and emancipated for others.

Partial emancipation is a statutory construction, and typically statutes in this area list specific diseases or conditions that a minor can consent to have treated. Such conditions often include pregnancy, need for contraception, alcoholism, drug abuse, and venereal disease. These statutes have generally been adopted by state legislatures in an effort to reduce barriers of access to treatment for minors when a "state interest" has existed in assuring their care. For example, in Massachusetts a minor who is or believes himself or herself to be suffering from or to have come in contact with any disease defined as dangerous to the public health may consent to care related to the diagnosis or treatment of the disease (Mass. Gen. Laws ch. 112, §12E). Many minor treatment statutes have been enacted as a result of the advocacy of concerned health professionals. A case in point occurred in 1967 when the American Medical Association (AMA) became concerned that adolescents were not receiving adequate treatment, especially for venereal disease. The AMA leadership took a stance which can only be described as radical and encouraged civil disobedience among it members. Neither radicalism nor civil disobedience is a characteristic which nurses often associate with the AMA. The association, through its journal, encouraged physicians to treat venereal disease without consent of the parents. The association newsletter published the following in April 1967:

> The inability to obtain parental consent to treat a minor for venereal disease should not cause a physician to withhold treatment if in his professional judgment treatment is immediately required. This applies even though action might appear to make a physician liable for a technical charge of assault and battery (*AMA News,* 1967).

At the time the AMA took its stand, only eight states had dispensed with the requirement of parental consent for venereal disease treatment. Ten years later all 50 states had abolished the requirement of parental consent, to the credit of the AMA and other interested groups. In a few states there is a requirement or a privilege of notifying parents, but in most jurisdictions there is neither.

Informed Consent

The doctrine of informed consent requires that health professionals fully describe to patients the risks, benefits, and possible alternatives to the treatment to which they are being asked to consent.

In part, the requirement of parental consent for treatment of minors is based on the presumed incapacity of a child to understand that there are risks and benefits of treatment. Courts have held recovery for patient plaintiffs who have suffered untoward results following treatment when the possible result had not been described in the process of obtaining informed consent, even when the treatment was not negligent. For example, in a 1972 case, *Canterbury* v. *Spence,* the court held recovery for a 19-year-old who was paralyzed after a laminectomy. The court rejected the defendant surgeon's claim that it was not common practice in the community to disclose the risks of paralysis and held that it was the physician's duty to disclose all material risks, all serious inherent and potential hazards, alternative methods of treatment, and the likely results of going without treatment.

Disclosure of risks is particularly important in treating minors without parental consent. In some cases courts have held that less than full disclosure to adult patients may sometimes be appropriate when knowing more might upset the patient sufficiently to have an adverse effect on recovery. This concept of therapeutic privilege should not be applied to minors treated without parental consent. If the minor's full knowledge of the risks and benefits of treatment may have a negative effect on the course of treatment, the minor's parents should be notified whenever possible.

Parental Refusal to Consent

Parents have a legal obligation to provide necessary medical care for their minor children. Courts have held failure to do so a criminal abuse under child abuse statutes and have ordered necessary care in the absence of parental consent. The legal issues hinge on the notion of "necessary care." All jurisdictions have ordered blood transfusions for children whose parents, often Jehovah's Witnesses, have refused consent of such transfusions even though the blood was intended to save the child's life (*Hoerner* v. *Bertinato,* 1961).

Some courts have ordered treatment of minors despite the parents' refusal to give consent when the medical treatment has been "highly desirable" although not "necessary" to save the child's life. For example, in the Chad Green case (*In re Custody of a Minor*) in 1978 the court ruled that where there is a substantial chance for a cure and a normal life for a child suffering from leukemia if he undergoes chemotherapy, limited custody of the child may be given to the Department of Public Welfare for the purpose of ensuring treatment, where parents objected to such treatment. While the court recognized that there exists under the Constitution a private realm of family life which the state should not enter, family autonomy is not absolute and may be limited when it appears that parental decisions will jeopardize child's life.

Courts have in some cases ordered surgery to correct deformities on the theory that refusal to consent to the surgical procedure constituted neglect because the child was being unreasonably deprived of the opportunity for a normal educational and social life (*In re Sampson,* 1972). In other instances courts have refused to order surgery when the condition was not life-threatening. The courts have held that weighing the risks of radical or dangerous surgery against the possible benefits is fully within the scope of parental authority and responsibility.

In the case of mature minors the court will consider the minor's wishes in cases in which parents refuse to consent to treatment. In *In re Seifertn,* 1955, the court considered the wishes of a 15-year-old boy whose parents refused on religious grounds to consent to surgical repair of his cleft lip and palate. The boy also refused to have the surgery. When the welfare department filed a petition for neglect, the court honored the wishes of the boy and his parents. However, the judge noted in his opinion that if the boy had wished to have the surgery, he would have overridden the parental veto on his behalf.

Courts have uniformly looked at the "best interests" of the child in making determinations of parental neglect. In cases where parental religious conviction has prevented treatment of a child, courts have uniformly preempted the parents' First Amendment rights in favor of the minor's best interests. Justice Holmes wrote in *Prince* v. *Massachusetts* in 1944 that although religious beliefs may make a martyr of a parent, "he is not free to make a martyr of his child." In all circumstances, courts have ordered treatment for minor children whose condition was life-threatening and whose prognosis was for a normal or nearly normal life-style if such treatment was instituted.

The case of Baby Jane Doe has brought to national attention the question of parents' rights to refuse life-prolonging medical treatment for their children. The original case and two other lawsuits, one filed by the federal government, the other by right-to-life attorney Lawrence Washburn, have focused the courts and public debate on procedural concerns regarding the treatment of gravely impaired newborns (*Weber* v. *Stony Brook Hospital*). The case posed the dilemma of how to best protect the interests of handicapped children while respecting the parents' right of privacy, interpreted both as a right to be left alone and as a right to decide on the treatment they deem best for the child. The case involved an infant suffering from spina bifida and hydrocephaly whose parents, following consultation with neurological experts, nurses, religious counselors, and a social worker, declined to consent to proposed surgery and chose to use antibiotics to protect against infection of the spinal column. The parents' decision was opposed and, following lower court action, was presented to the United States Supreme Court. The Court declined to hear the case, letting stand the decision of the New York Court of Appeals that the parents of the infant had the right to withhold life-prolonging surgery. The case acted as a catalyst for national debate on the procedural aspects of federal policy regarding the legal rights of seriously impaired newborns. The decision itself reiterates prior court opinions regarding parental consent: "that judicial proceedings touching the family relationship should not be casually initiated" (Steinbock, 1984, p. 19).

Parental Inability or Unavailability to Consent

When the parents of a minor child are unable to consent to care as a result of absence, abandonment, or incompetency, permission of the court must be sought to treat the child unless there is a medical emergency. The court may appoint a guardian ad litem to make a recommendation on behalf of a child in a given instance, or a permanent guardianship may need to be established. Consent to treatment must be obtained from the appropriate state authority for children who are wards of the state and for whom the state holds legal custody even though physical custody may be with the parents or a foster family.

Where parental consent is necessary and the parents are legally separated or divorced, the parent with legal or actual custody has a clear right to consent to medical treatment without the approval of the other parent. In informal separations, the parent who has personal possession of the child may consent to the child's care whether or not custody has been formally awarded to the parent. In cases where one parent is absent (for example, traveling or working away from home), the custodial parent has the right to consent to the child's treatment.

College Students

A college student living away from home, even though he may be financially dependent on his parents, is generally considered emancipated for the purposes of consent to treatment (Holder, 1977). Many campuses participate in blood drives; it should be noted that since blood donations are not for the benefit of the donor, in the absence of statutory authority minors cannot consent to donate blood prior to the age of majority.

Runaways

A runaway adolescent is away from home without parental consent. Therefore, no sanction by the parents of independent decision making can be inferred. If the runaway adolescent refuses to identify his parents or allow notification of them, it can be inferred that the runaway has the capacity to consent to necessary medical care. Health professionals finding themselves in this circumstance are well advised to document carefully in the medical record that the adolescent refused to allow notification and to include a statement to that effect signed by the runaway minor.

The Right to Refuse Treatment

The corollary of an adolescent's capacity to consent to his own care is his capacity to refuse treatment. An emancipated or mature minor's consent must be obtained for treatment. No case law currently exists in which a malpractice action has been brought by a minor against a health care provider for unwanted treatment. However, it is easy to imagine such an action in the future. Courts have held that mature minors cannot be forced to submit to care requested by their parents. For example, in a 1973 Connecticut case, *Melville* v. *Sabbatino,* the court ordered that a 16-year-old boy who had been admitted by his parents to a psychiatric facility as a "voluntary" admission had the right to leave the hospital when he wished to. The court's decision was based on a statute which allowed minors age 16 and older to seek psychiatric care on the basis of their own consent. The court reasoned that if the minor was capable of consenting to his own care, he was also capable of refusing such care.

Another example of the principle that a minor capable of consenting is also capable of refusing can be found in a 1972 case from Maryland, *Matter* v. *Smith.* In this case, a mother wanted to force her 16-year-old unmarried pregnant daughter to have an abortion over the minor's objections. The state had a statute giving emancipated minor status to minors seeking prenatal care. The court ruled that treatment concerning pregnancy included abortion and said that

> The minor, having the same capacity to consent as an adult, is emancipated from control of the parents with respect to medical treatment within the contemplation of the statute. We think it follows that if a minor may consent to medical treatment or advice concerning pregnancy, the minor, and particularly a minor over 16 years of age, may not be forced more than an adult to accept treatment or advice concerning pregnancy . . . the one consenting has the right to forbid.

The Contraception and Abortion Controversy

The legal and ethical issues involved in adolescents' right of access to contraception and abortion have been hotly debated in the United States for the past two decades. The debate over the access of minors to these services is a mirror of the debate over the access of adult women to these same services. Adolescent reproductive health care has become one of several political footballs in the raging war between "pro-choice" and "pro-life" forces. Decisions which are most appropriately made between the adolescent and her family and/or health care provider have been thrown into the political arena and into the courts.

Until 1965 it was by no means clear that even adults had the right to consent to contraceptive care. In 1965 in a Connecticut case, *Griswold* v. *Connecticut,* a statute forbidding the distribution of contraception devices within Connecticut state borders was overturned. The United States Supreme Court upheld the decision and held for the first time that a constitutional right of privacy existed. This right was held to be based on other specific guarantees in the Bill of Rights and further held to apply to sexual relations between spouses. Members of Planned Parenthood Association and the American Civil Liberties Union united to seek test cases to expand the notion of privacy, and in 1972 in a Massachusetts case, *Eisenstadt* v. *Baird,* the United States Supreme Court held the right to privacy is not just a right to marital privacy but a right to privacy in all matters relating to marriage, family, and sex. In the Massachusetts case the recipient of the birth control device was admittedly unmarried but not a minor. The question of a minor's legal right of access to contraception has never been the subject of a decision by the Supreme Court. Most authorities have supported the position that both the interest of a state and the interest of sexually active adolescents are served by adequate access of adolescents to contraceptives. Professional organizations have consistently held that the individual practitioner should have the right to make contraceptives available to minors. The AMA has stated

> Consistent with responsible preventive medicine and in the interest of reducing the incidence of teenage pregnancy . . . the teenage girl whose sexual behavior exposes her to possible conception should have access to medical consultation and the most effective contraceptive advice and methods consistent with her physical and emotional needs (AMA House of Delegates, 1971; see Jordan, 1974).
>
> The opposite perspective in this controversy argues that adolescent access to contraception increases sexual activity among teenagers and destroys parental control of the family. When a statute was passed by the California legislature specifically granting teenagers the right of access to medically prescribed contraceptives, it was vetoed by then Governor Ronald Reagan, who said the bill "represented the unwarranted intrusion into the prerogatives of parents . . . and would endanger the traditional vital role of the family structure in our society . . ." (Bodine, 1973).

On January 22, 1973, in *Roe* v. *Wade,* the United States Supreme Court decided that first-trimester abortion was part of the right to privacy. The Court held that during the first 3 months of pregnancy whether to abort was the decision of the woman and her physician and that the only restriction the state could impose was that the abortion be done by a physician. This right applied to adults, and in a footnote to the decision the Court specifically declined to comment on whether parental or spousal consent would be required.

Part of the issue has been resolved by the United States Supreme Court and lower courts, which have consistently ruled that a minor has the same rights to privacy as an adult and consequently the same right to abortion. Courts have held parental consent requirements unconstitutional, but the issue of whether something less than parental consent will be held constitutional, e.g., a court order in the absence of parental consent, has still not been heard by the Supreme Court (*Planned Parenthood Association* v. *Danforth,* 1975).

In a conservative posture that may be a bellwether for other jurisdictions, the Massachusetts legislature in the 1980 legislative session passed a law known as the Informed Consent Act, which has major implications for minors seeking abortion services. The implementation of the statute is still on appeal by the Planned Parenthood League of Massachusetts. The Massachusetts statute is the most restrictive to date with regard to consent to abor-

tions for minors. The law requires that unmarried women under 18 years of age obtain superior court approval for abortions unless (1) both parents have consented, (2) one parent has died or is unavailable within a reasonable time and in a reasonable manner and the other parent has consented, (3) both parents have died or are unavailable within a reasonable time or in a reasonable manner and the girl's guardian has consented, or (4) the girl's parents have divorced and the parent with custody has consented. Minors may elect to seek judicial approval if they do not want to ask for parental consent.

In a related matter also involving minors' rights to contraception, the United States Supreme Court in July 1977 held unconstitutional a New York statute which made it a crime to display or advertise contraceptives either inside or outside a drugstore and which further provided that contraceptives could be sold only in drugstores and only to persons over 16 (*Population Services International* v. *Wilson,* 1975).

Minors as Research Subjects

In examining legal concepts related to minors as research subjects, it is important to draw a distinction between therapeutic and nontherapeutic research. Therapeutic research is defined as activities undertaken for the systematic collection of data, in accordance with a designated protocol, that are intended to improve the health of the subject by diagnostic or treatment methods that depart from standard practice. Nontherapeutic research, in contrast, is undertaken for the systematic collection of data in accordance with a designated protocol but *not* for the direct benefit of the child.

A parent may consent to therapeutic research on a child in the same manner as he or she may consent to any other treatment. The burden lies on the caregiver to fully inform the parent that the treatment is experimental and to ensure that the parent understands completely its risks, benefits, and alternatives. Courts have awarded damages to parents without proof of negligence in cases in which children have been harmed in experimental procedures and the parents were not fully informed of the research aspect of the care (*Fiorentino* v. *Wenger,* 1966). Parents' capacity to consent to dangerous research, despite a therapeutic intent, is less clear. Parents and caregivers could probably be held in violation of the child abuse laws where effective and safer treatment is known to exist. For example, experiments at the Willowbrook State School, where institutionalized mentally retarded children were used as research subjects to test the effectiveness of an experimental vaccine for hepatitis, came under heavy fire as representing a gross departure from both legal and ethical standards regarding research with children (Golby, 1971).

With regard to nontherapeutic research, authorities have generally agreed that a parent cannot give a valid consent for any medical procedure on a child which is not for the direct benefit of the child and may carry some risk of harm. Authorities are divided on the issue of parental authority to consent to procedures which are of no direct benefit to the child and which carry no risk of harm. Ramsey (1974) argued that nontherapeutic research, while it may not be harmful, reduces the child to the status of "an object" and is therefore unethical. Those supporting nontherapeutic research in which there is no discernible risk of harm cite the need for such research and its general benefit to society. Curran and Beecher (1969) advocated that children under 14 years of age may be involved in nontherapeutic research with parental consent if (1) there is a strong reason in professional judgment for using children (as opposed to adults) in the research and the research has firm medical support and justification and promises important new knowledge of benefit to science and (2) there is no discernible risk to the child subject. Curran and Beecher also supported more hazardous research on minors over age 14 who are capable of understanding the nature and purposes of the experiment and its risks, as long as both minor and parent consent.

Responsibility for Paying for Minors' Health Care

As a general rule the party consenting to treatment is responsible for paying for the care. Parents are held responsible under the law for the necessary expenses of their children, which include routine and emergency health care. Traditionally, fathers have been the family wage earners and have been held responsible for their children's medical expenses. This rule is still held generally true even in the absence of a court order for child support. As a practical matter, if care is consented to by the custodial parent of the child in the absence of the other parent, the custodial parent may be held responsible for the cost of the care by the care provider. The custodial parent may have a right of recovery against the absent parent for the cost of the care. As a general rule, when both parents are available, it is necessary to have both parents consent to the care; therefore, the parents could hold joint financial responsibility for the cost of the care.

When care is consented to by a minor who is deemed capable of consent by virtue of either emancipation or partial emancipation or under the mature minor rule, the cost of the care is the financial responsibility of the minor, not of the parents.

Mental Health and Mental Retardation

The issue of a requirement of parental consent or, conversely, of the adolescent patient's right to refuse treatment has been a particularly thorny issue in mental health and mental retardation services. Most states have statutory requirements which allow for partial emancipation for purposes of minors' consent to psychiatric care and treatment of drug abuse problems. Minors who have the right to consent to care as voluntary patients also have the right to refuse such care. Historically, the more problematic issues have involved cases where parents have demanded commitment of their children to state institutions. The days of wholesale commitment of children and adolescents to large state psychiatric and mental retardation facilities are over. The United States Supreme Court examined procedural protections in the commitment of children in a 1979 case, *Parham* v. *J.R.* Lawyers representing the minor children in *Parham* argued that the interests of the parents and their children are not the same in regard to hospitalization. Therefore, they argued, minors should be afforded representation independent of their parents and the opportunity for a due process hearing to contest the judgments of their parents and mental professionals who view hospitalization as appropriate. The Court held in its majority opinion that without evidence of clear-cut abuse and neglect by parents or evidence that the psychiatrists who had admitted the children had acted in bad faith, there was no constitutional necessity for requiring complex procedures to review the admission of children. Review of the parents' request for admission by a neutral and independent physician is, however, constitutionally required. The Court drew no distinction between children who lived with their parents and children who were juvenile wards of the state, a distinction which had been supported in an amicus brief by the American Psychiatric Association and in the Court's minority opinion.

Legal Issues in Privacy and Confidentiality in the Treatment of Children

Confidentiality, or as otherwise stated, the right to information, is a complex issue in the care of children and adolescents. The rights of minors and their parents to access to information regarding care roughly parallels the right to consent to care implies a therapeutic contract between the health care provider and the patient or parents giving consent. This therapeutic contract further implies a fiduciary relationship between the care provider and the recipient which by definition is confidential. Owing to the heritage of paternalism in medical care, it has often been difficult for adult patients and the parents of minors to obtain direct access to medical records. Massachusetts is the only jurisdiction in which patients have absolute freedom of information. By statute in some jurisdictions, patients (or in the case of minors, their parents, if they are the consenting parties) have an absolute right to access to their medical records, including copies of these records (Mass. Gen. Laws ch 111, §70E). In general, in other jurisdictions patients have a right to such information as is necessary to provide informed consent, and it follows that anyone who can legally consent to his own care has a right to a confidential relationship with his health care provider. In a jurisdiction in which an older minor can consent to his own care, once he has done so, the parents would not need the information for consent purposes. In such a situation the physician, nurse, or other provider should not without consent of the minor disclose confidential information to the parents, including even the most basic data, such as whether the patient is enrolled for treatment. If the parents have consented to treatment of the minor and confidentiality between the provider and

Accountability in Pediatric Nursing Practice

the patient is desirable to encourage the patient to disclose all relevant information without worrying that embarrassing information will be disseminated, the burden falls upon the provider to negotiate the degree of access to information between the minor and the parents. If the provider intends to inform the parents about any aspect of the minor's care, the provider should at the outset of treatment make it clear to the adolescent that the parents will have access to information regarding the care. An adolescent who can consent for himself has a right to refuse to speak to a provider or to submit to examination or treatment, in the absence of an emergency, until the provider agrees not to tell his parents about his care. These agreements must be handled on an individual basis and should be clearly documented in the medical record.

The Committee on Youth of the American Academy of Pediatrics has drafted model legislation ("Model Act," 1973) regarding the consent of minors to health services. The model act suggests that if a minor is to be treated without parental consent and the procedure involves "major surgery, general anesthesia, or a life-threatening procedure," consultation with another physician is advisable to provide another opinion on the ability of the patient to understand the potential risks. The model act appears not to hold confidentiality in high value. Section 3 (4) addresses the treatment of minors without parental consent and recognizes the value of a minor's self-determination in situations in which "by informing them (the parents) the minor will fail to seek initial or future help. . . ." Unfortunately, the section further provides that

> After the professional establishes his rapport with the minor, then he may inform the patient's parents or legal guardian unless such action will jeopardize the life of the patient or the favorable result of the treatment.

Disclosure of confidential information to unauthorized persons about any patient, whether adult or child, without his consent may give rise to a successful action for damages (*Hammer* v. *Polsky,* 1962). Even if consent has been obtained, if the information communicated to a third party is untrue, the health care provider may be liable for defamation of character (*Vigil* v. *Rice,* 1964). Defamation of character is a communication by one person (for example, a health care provider) about a second person (a patient) conveying information which is untrue and diminishes unjustifiably the reputation of the person discussed. Defamation may be oral, as in slander, or written, as in libel.

Public health records should be awarded the same degree of privacy as private health records. Unfortunately, very few jurisdictions have statutes which protect the confidentiality of public health records. One problem that exists with health departments (and less frequently in private practice) is disclosure of personal information in the course of dissemination of statistical data about groups of patients for research or other studies. A health care provider in a public institution or teaching hospital has no greater right to publish articles about a patient without the patient's knowledge and consent than he or she would in a private practice (*Massachusetts* v. *Wiseman,* 1969).

Two recent trends in nursing practice have focused on increasing nurses' accountability for nursing practice: primary nursing and nursing diagnosis. Primary nursing is a decentralization of decision making for clinical practice to the staff nurse level at the bedside. Primary nursing requires nurses to take responsibility for their decisions and to acknowledge the risks inherent in decision making. A primary nurse needs and receives responsibility, both legal and ethical, for nursing care given a patient 24 hours a day, 7 days a week (Kozier and Erb, 1987).

In a legal sense, and for better or worse, pediatric nursing *is* quite simply what pediatric nurses do. The standard of care to which pediatric nurses are held is the standard of their peers. The legal yardstick by which a nurse's actions are measured is the so-called reasonable nurse standard of what a similarly educated and experienced pediatric nurse would have done in a similar clinical situation. Maternal-child health is measured as a clinical specialty not only by what maternal-child health nurses do but also by what they *should* do, specifically by what they have established as their standards of care.

Standards of care are a mixed blessing for a profession. Clearly defined standards of care are among the most powerful tools available for increasing the quality of services rendered to children and adolescents. The corollary is, of course, that to raise the standard of care is to raise the level of accountability to which nurses are legally held. Written standards of care are fully and commonly admissible as evidence in courts of law to prove malpractice. Both primary nursing and nursing diagnosis are standards of care. Primary nursing supports the nursing process and clarifies the responsibility of the individual nurse for clinical judgment and decision making.

Nursing diagnosis has become an accepted and now often expected part of nursing practice. As such, it raises some specific legal issues. These issues center on the use and definition of the generic term *diagnosis* in nursing practice and the implications of an evolving taxonomy of nursing diagnosis. As nurses develop a taxonomy for nursing diagnosis in pediatric nursing, they are raising the standard of care and defining more clearly than ever before what it is that they do and how they do it.

The term *diagnosis* originated from and is commonly associated with the medical profession. Centuries ago medicine was the first profession to use the term to refer to the judgment derived from the assessment of patients' illnesses. The lay public, lawyers, and judges have not understood the meaning of the term in the context of the nursing profession. Therefore, an assumption has developed that when nurses make a nursing diagnosis, they are mimicking medicine. The term as used in nursing was never meant to be borrowed from medicine but was the term most descriptive of a vital step in the nursing process. There is a difference in *focus* in the use of the term by the medical and nursing professions. Medicine uses it to describe specific diseases; nursing focuses on human responses to actual or potential health problems.

Leaders in the development of the concept of nursing diagnosis have suggested a number of definitions of the term. According to Marjory Gordon (Gordon, 1987), nursing diagnosis is both a product and a process. She views nursing diagnosis as "a concise term representing a cluster of signs and symptoms and describing an actual or potential health problem or state-of-the-patient which nurses, by virtue of their education and experience, are licensed and able to treat." For purpose of discussing the legal implications in nursing practice of nursing diagnosis, Gordon's definition is the most useful. It is operational and attempts implicitly to clarify the distinction between nursing diagnosis and medical diagnosis.

The legal issues in nursing diagnosis are further confused by the fact that there are times when it is both appropriate and necessary for nurses to make a medical diagnosis. Nurses who practice in an expanded role, for example, pediatric nurse practitioners, may make medical diagnoses and initiate treatment on the basis of protocols developed collaboratively with physicians. The accountability, legally and ethically, is shared between physician and nurse when the nurse makes a medical diagnosis and initiates treatment based on protocols. The nurse alone is accountable for nursing diagnosis and intervention. Nurses in medical emergencies, for example, cardiac arrest and shock, have always been required to make rapid assessments which are in fact medical diagnoses and to begin appropriate intervention, such as cardiopulmonary resuscitation. In the absence of training and experience in an expanded role or emergency situations, medical diagnosis is not an appropriate nursing function. Nurses who make a medical diagnosis in other than the aforementioned circumstances may be liable in a criminal action for practicing medicine without a license.

The legal regulation of nursing and other health care professions has traditionally fallen to the individual states, which have held responsibility for the health and welfare of their citizens, under the "police power" granted to them by the United States Constitution. In efforts to maintain high-quality health care, and specifically nursing care, beginning in the late nineteenth and early twentieth centuries, states enacted statutes regulating the licensure and training of professional nurses. These statutes came about as a result of organization and lobbying by early nursing leaders who were concerned about maintaining the standards of nursing care received by the public. Early statutes followed a medical model and defined practice largely in relation to medicine (Bullough, 1980). As nursing practice has expanded and become more precisely defined, nurse practice acts have been redrafted to reflect more clearly the current standards and definitions of nursing.

Changes in the law follow changes in practice. The new frontier today appears to be those jurisdictions which have by regulation or statute adopted some form of prescription-writing authority for nurses. The issue of prescriptive privileges for nurses is a classic example of professional and public confusion over the distinctions between medical practice and nursing practice. Some jurisdictions, notably Washington and Oregon, have been successful in achieving medically independent prescriptive authority for some nurses, who have been certified by the state's Board of Registration in Nursing as having authority to prescribe on the basis of a preestablished formulary. In other jurisdictions the function is medically dependent to varying degrees and seen as a delegated medical function.

Nurses are not licensed in any jurisdiction to treat medical problems independently but are licensed to practice nursing. Some state nurse practice acts, New York's, for example, specifically refer to nursing diagnosis in the language of the statute; in other states the function can be and will be inferred. A taxonomy for nursing diagnosis can provide significant assistance in evolving legal definitions of nursing practice.

Nurses are not immune to criminal or civil liability for their practice. Criminal liability as it relates to nursing practice and nursing diagnosis has at times focused on the implications of the generic term *diagnosis* and specifically on the differences between medical diagnosis and nursing diagnosis.

Civil liability for nursing practice falls into the area of tort law. A *tort* is an action brought by an individual on the basis of harm done to him or her by another, a civil wrong. Torts may be intentional, as in defamation, or unintentional, as in negligence. It is the unintentional tort of negligence which presents the greatest concern for nurses. Negligence, a common law category of tort, includes negligent malpractice. Negligence may be an act or the omission of an act which causes harm to another. Nursing malpractice is an act or failure to act by a nurse which causes harm to a patient.

To prove malpractice, a patient plaintiff must be able to show each of the following elements:
1. The defendant nurse owed the patient a duty of care.
2. The defendant nurse breached the duty of care.
3. The breach was the direct or proximate cause of harm to the patient.
4. The patient was really harmed or damaged.

For a patient plaintiff to prove a breach of the duty of care, the appropriate standard of care must first be established. The standard of care has traditionally been the so-called reasonable nurse standard: The defendant nurse's conduct is measured by the standard of what a nurse with the same training and experience would have done in a comparable situation.

The plaintiff's counsel has traditionally introduced evidence to prove the standard of care by having nurses testify as expert witnesses and by introducing documents such as the American Nurses' Association's *Standards of Practice*. Expert nurse witnesses are called to provide testimony regarding the generally expected standard of practice. The expert witness's testimony is expected to include the components of an adequate nursing assessment, the nursing diagnosis, and the appropriate nursing interventions and expected outcomes. Failure to assess adequately, formulate a judgment, and intervene appropriately has long been established as evidence of breach of a duty of care.

Many other issues must be considered in establishing a standard of practice and the breach of that standard. For example, the individual patient's or institution's reliance may be on the nurse to perform specific nursing functions. The reliance reflects the predictability of harm to the patient plaintiff if the defendant nurse acts or fails to act in a particular manner. The law is interested in outcomes, not processes. The absence of an adequate nursing assessment, the failure to make an appropriate nursing diagnosis, and the failure to treat a problem do not in themselves generate nursing malpractice liability. The failure must have led to documented harm to the patient plaintiff. Poor practice in the absence of a damaged patient does not constitute negligence in a legal sense.

Pediatric nurses are familiar with the case of *Norton* v. *Argonaut Insurance Co.* (1962), in which a Louisiana appellate court held a nurse liable for administering a fatal dose of digitalis to an infant by injection. The dose would not have been fatal if it had been administered orally. The physician did not specify the route and was also held liable in the wrongful death action. In regard to the nurse, the court said

> As laudable as her intentions are conceded to have been on the occasion in question, her unfamiliarity with the drug was a contributing factor in the child's death. In this regard, we are of the opinion that she was negligent in attempting to administer a drug with which she was not familiar. . . . Not only was Mrs. Evans unfamiliar with the medicine in question, but she also violated what has been shown to be a rule generally practiced by the members of the nursing profession in the community and which rule, we might add, strikes us as being most reasonable and prudent, namely, the practice of calling the prescribing physician when in doubt about an order for medication.

Negligence may be found in an action or in a failure to act. A successful malpractice action may be brought against a nurse for failure to assume professional responsibility. That responsibility may be a nursing responsibility or may be a delegated medical function. For example, in *Collins* v. *Westlake Community Hospital,* a 1974 Illinois case, a pediatric nurse was held liable for failure to follow the express written orders of a physician. In *Collins* a 6-year-old child had suffered serious injuries in a bicycle accident and had been admitted to a community hospital. An orthopedic surgeon treated the child's fractured leg with traction and left written instructions in the chart to "watch condition of the patient's toes." For the next 2 days the nurses' notes reflected careful attention to the child's circulation and the color of his toes. Then, on the evening of the second day, the nurse apparently failed to check the circulation. No entries were made in the patient's chart between 11 P.M. and 6 A.M. By morning a serious impairment of circulation was noted, and emergency surgery was done. A blood clot was removed, but not in time to prevent ischemic necrosis, and it was necessary to amputate the child's leg.

The appeals court, reversing a decision of the trial court, held that the night nurse's failure to follow the express written orders of the physician represented a clear-cut breach of the requisite standard of care and ordered a new trial on the issue of negligence. Since it is a routine practice for nurses to check the circulation of any patient with an orthopedic injury, failure to do so in this case would probably have constituted negligence even without an express written order. Nevertheless, the legal issue in this case was the nurse's responsibility to execute the physician's specific written order.

The general rule requiring a nurse to execute all lawful orders of a physician is tempered by the commonsense exception that the nurse must not execute an order if there is reasonable certainty that it will result in harm to the patient (*Toth* v. *Community Hospital at Glen Cove,* 1968).

A nurse must always exercise judgment in practice and must provide "reasonable care" to patients. When execution of an otherwise proper order appears contraindicated by the patient's observed condition, the standard of safe care may require that a nurse stop a prescribed course of therapy and contact the physician promptly to obtain modification or reconfirmation of the written orders. If the physician refuses to revise the order and if the nurse believes there is a possibility of harm to the patient, the nurse should firmly decline to carry out the order and immediately bring the matter to the attention of the immediate nursing supervisor or other appropriate hospital authority. Thorough documentation of the nurse's assessments and the communications in such a circumstance is critical in avoiding liability and protecting patients from harm.

Under the common law doctrine of *respondeat superior,* literally translated "the master shall be held responsible for the crimes of the servant," the nurse's employer is liable in any civil action for malpractice occurring during the course of the nurse's employment. The nurse is also liable, legally and ethically, for personal malpractice. In some circumstances the nurse's immediate supervisor may also be held liable, either indirectly for the injury to the patient or more directly for negligent supervision. When the nursing malpractice is related to a physician-delegated responsibility, for example, if a nurse has given a harmful dose of a medication which was prescribed in error by a physician, both the nurse and the physician may be held jointly liable. In practice settings where nursing students are involved in clinical responsibilities, both the students' nursing instructor and the nurse clinically in charge of the unit on which the students are providing care may be held liable for any student malpractice.

Pediatric Nurses as Expert Witnesses

Expert opinions are increasingly being sought after in the litigation of nursing malpractice cases. The plaintiff patient must begin by establishing the first two elements of negligence: first that there was a duty of care and second that there was a breach of the duty. In order to prove these elements, the standard of care which was applicable in the particular patient's care must be established. For example, if the claim is that the nurse negligently administered an injection, the plaintiff must introduce evidence to show the proper technique for the procedure and demonstrate that this technique was not followed. Historically, few cases have used or required nurses to serve as expert witnesses, in part because courts have not readily recognized that nursing is a profession with an independent body of knowledge and hence have often allowed physicians to give expert testimony on the appropriate standard of nursing care (Northrop and Mech, 1981). Some recent cases have supported not only the need for expert opinion in nursing malpractice cases but also the requirement that the testifying witness be a nurse. In *Vassey* v. *Burch* (1980), the plaintiff patient alleged that emergency room nurses were negligent for failing to recognize that he was suffering from appendicitis and for failing to report that fact to the physician. To show the applicable standard of care, the plaintiff introduced the statement of a physician, outlining the tests which would be done when a patient presents with the plaintiff's symptoms. In rejecting this evidence, the court stated

> Although the [physician's] affidavit . . . may be sufficient to establish the accepted standard of Medical care for a doctor in his office, it does not establish the standard of care for a nurse in a hospital.

In addition to acting as witnesses regarding standards of care in nursing malpractice cases, expert nurse witnesses may testify to the value of nursing services, the safety of nursing procedures, the quality and quantity of nursing services, and the standards of nursing education and administration. Nurse experts may be requested to provide in-court testimony or act as consultants to attorneys.

The following principles are suggested for consideration when an expert witness is preparing to give testimony (Kraft, 1977):

1. The expert must be completely objective and truly impartial rather than serving as a surrogate advocate.
2. The expert should simply answer questions clearly and firmly and should not volunteer any extraneous matter.
3. The expert should avoid arguing with the opposing attorney.
4. The expert should be prepared for the possibility that the opposing attorney will try to make the nurse angry to undermine the nurse's credibility.
5. The expert should avoid public comment to the press, radio, television, or other media.
6. The expert should avoid trying to answer all questions with certainty. There will always be some questions the expert cannot answer, and the expert should say so.

Ethical Issues

Ethical as well as legal dimensions are present in all nursing practice settings. Ethical and legal standards differ in their goals, duties, establishment, and sanctions.

In their goals, legal standards ensure a minimum level of competence for safe practice whereas ethical standards seek to promote practice that is both moral and of high quality. In relation to duties, legal standards relate to acceptable practices; ethical standards, to what ought to be. Legal standards are established by legislative, executive, or judicial actions; ethical standards are established by the professional association. Legal standards are enforced by a unit of state government; ethical standards are enforced by professional associations.

Sanctions for violation of either legal or ethical standards range from censure to suspension or expulsion, but they relate to licensure for legal standards and to membership in the professional association for ethical standards. Sanctions for nonmembers are limited to censure. Penalties may be imposed in civil cases for violations of both the legal standards and the ethical standards of practice.

One of the many obligations of the nursing profession is to provide its members with guidelines for professional activity, including ethical decision making. According to Barber (1979), professional behavior may be defined in terms of three essential and independent variables:

1. A high degree of generalized and systematic knowledge.
2. Primary orientation to the community rather than to individual self-interest.
3. A high degree of self-control or autonomy effected through a code of ethics internalized in the process of work socialization, through the use of informal peer controls, and through voluntary associations organized and operated by the work specialists themselves.

Barber further noted that the autonomy of a profession is never absolute but is regulated by the public and its political representatives to some degree, which ensures the public service behavior of the profession.

Professions develop codes or standards of conduct and relationships that govern professional activities as part of the self-disciplinary process. In nursing, the American Nurses' Association first adopted the Code for Professional Nurses in 1950 for all members of the profession. This code was revised and the present Code for Nurses adopted in 1985 (Table 8-1). The present code continues to represent the philosophy that the recipient of care is the primary consideration in any conflict of interest. The Code for Nurses was among the first national standards developed and adopted by the American Nurses' Association.

Many situations that arise in the course of pediatric nursing practice and research require not only legal but also ethical decisions. Practice settings are filled with ethical dilemmas: Who should decide what to do with children with serious birth defects? Should nurses ever lie to their patients? When should children be used as experimental subjects? Nurses often find themselves in the position either to make decisions or to influence the decision making. Ethical issues in the area of nursing practice and research are at present largely unsettled and sometimes even unexplored. Although there is hardly a topic on which a moral consensus exists, the demands of practical decision making often generate a force that presses the nurse for immediate solutions. Nursing ethics at this time

---

TABLE 8-1 Code for Nurses

Preamble

The Code for Nurses is based on belief about the nature of individuals, nursing, health, and society. Recipients and providers of nursing services are viewed as individuals and groups who possess basic rights and responsibilities, and whose value and circumstances command respect at all times. Nursing encompasses the promotion and restoration of health, the prevention of illness, and the alleviation of suffering. The statements of the code and their interpretation provide guidance for conduct and relationships in carrying out nursing responsibilities consistent with the ethical obligations of the profession and quality in nursing care.

1. The nurse provides services with respect for human dignity and the uniqueness of the client unrestricted by considerations of social or economic status, personal attributes, or the nature of health problems.
2. The nurse safeguards the client's right to privacy by judiciously protecting information of a confidential nature.
3. The nurse acts to safeguard the client and the public when health care and safety are affected by the incompetent, unethical, or illegal practice of any person.
4. The nurse assumes responsibility and accountability for individual nursing judgments and actions.
5. The nurse maintains competence in nursing.
6. The nurse exercises informed judgment and uses individual competence and qualifications as criteria in seeking consultation, accepting responsibilities, and delegating nursing activities to others.
7. The nurse participates in activities that contribute to the ongoing development of the profession's body of knowledge.
8. The nurse participates in the profession's efforts to implement and improve standards of nursing.
9. The nurse participates in the profession's efforts to establish and maintain conditions of employment conducive to high quality nursing care.
10. The nurse participates in the profession's efforts to protect the public from misinformation and misrepresentation and to maintain the integrity of nursing.
11. The nurse collaborates with members of the health professions and other citizens in promoting community and national efforts to meet the health needs of the public.

Source: American Nurses' Association, "Code for Nurses with Interpretive Statements," American Nurses' Association, Kansas City, Mo., 1985.

---

is an area in which there are more legitimate questions than satisfactory answers.

One of the most common areas in which nurses confront ethical dilemmas is the area of infants born with severe physical defects and deformities. The birth of such a child confronts the parents with difficult decisions at the time when they are least prepared to reason clearly. No one involved in the care of these infants can escape the agony. Parents often turn to nursing staff members for support and information when trying to make difficult decisions, for example, whether their baby should continue on life-support machines. Davis (1981a, p. 1035) suggested that the ethical and legal obligations in the decision making belong to the parents but further reasoned that "it is the ethical obligation of the staff caring for the baby to ensure that the parents receive all the necessary information and emotional support they need in order to come to grips with this profound dilemma and to make an informed decision." The further nursing responsibility is to provide the type and amount of care that evolves from whatever decision the parents make. Davis pointed out that parents need nonjudgmental support in this decision-making process. The information needed from staff is not what should or should not be done but the best professional opinion as to what the infant's life might be like with life support and what his death might be like without it. If there is reason to believe that the parents are either unwilling or unable to act in a responsible manner, it becomes the responsibility of the courts to guarantee that the interests of the infant are served. In practice this situation has usually meant ordering that the life of the infant be saved.

Another area in which pediatric nurses often confront ethical dilemmas is the are of the patient's or parents' ac-

cess to information. Not uncommonly parents or patients, particularly adolescent patients, request information about their illness or care which the physician has decided to withhold. This circumstance causes the nurse to be caught squarely between the conflicting demands of the patient or parents and the wishes of the physician. It raises the issue of how extensive the nurse's responsibility is to be consistent with the medical plan to withhold information. The nurse has a clear obligation to inform the physician of the patient's or family's concerns. If the decision of the physician remains to withhold information, the nurse has to weigh the ethics of going along with this decision against the ethics of having the patient informed. If a nurse goes along with the decision, then that nurse will have reasoned that the ethical principle of doing no harm is more important than the patient's or parents' right to autonomy (Davis, 1981b). Alternatively, there are numerous strategies the nurse may use to ensure that information is not withheld, ranging from involving others and generating peer pressure to directly informing the patient or parents.

Sometimes nurses may need to deal with conflicting expectations and intents of parents with regard to the child's care. Parents may disagree as to the proper course of action in treatment. For example, one parent may wish to proceed with a course of treatment. Davis (1980) noted that the parent may feel it would be in the child's best interest to withhold the treatment. Davis (1980) noted that the manner in which staff members handle these situations is critical to a satisfactory outcome. She suggested that staff members need to have meetings among themselves and with the parents to effectively identify the issues and agree on a course of action. She further encouraged conservative initial treatment in such situations to "buy time" to analyze the dilemma and evaluate alternatives.

Advocacy

Legal and ethical dilemmas in nursing practice raise issues about the nurse's role as advocate. Advocacy is the act of pleading the cause of another. The term *advocate* has historically been synonymous with lawyer. Lay advocates and advocates from professions other than the law, such as nursing, emerged in the late 1950s and early 1960s as part of a general trend toward the protection of individual constitutional rights. While the term is most often associated with the law, advocacy is essentially an ethical perspective.

Nurses who see their role as involving patient advocacy value patients' rights, specifically a patient's right to self-determination. Nurses holding this value perceive themselves as assisting patients in achieving their goals and meeting their needs, even if the needs and goals of the patient may not be the same as those of the patient's physician or of the health care institution (Murphy and Hunter, 1982). There is often enormous potential for conflict between the interests of health care institutions and those of patients. Nurses are generally caught squarely in the middle.

The question raised by nurses working as hospital employees is whether they can ever function as true patient advocates if employed by someone other than the person for whom they are advocating. In the purest sense the answer is no. If nurses are employed by institutions, they cannot advocate effectively for patients, particularly when such advocacy may place them in opposition to those institutions. Advocacy implies at least the potential of an adversarial position.

Nurses are intimately familiar with the ethical bind inherent in attempting to act as an advocate for an individual patient while employed by an institution. The ethical dilemma is clear: The institutional value is the value of the "greatest good for the greatest number," the so-called utilitarian value. In institutional settings, where most nurses are employed, this value stands in direct opposition to an advocacy or rights model of "the greatest good for an individual patient."

Mitchell (1981) conceptualized this dilemma as an assault on the integrity of the nurse. She argued that this moral dilemma of being caught in the middle is a substantial contributor to the burnout syndrome and to nurses leaving nursing. The problem of integrity arises out of a basic conflict inherent in the health care system. On one hand, the system is organized from the top down to carry out the medical mission of curing, healing, and saving patients' lives. On the other hand, the health care system is conceived of as structured from the base up to meet the multiple needs of patients, a patient advocacy model. Patients' needs include sympathetic care, comfort, teaching, and encouragement in addition to medical treatment. From the top down, it is the nurse who carries out the treatments which are crucial to the success of the medical mission. From the base up, it is the nurse who is most constantly involved in patients' daily care and who discovers and relays vital information about patients' needs to the health care team. Called upon to maximize first one and then the other conception of health care, she is prevented from acting with integrity under either system.

In pediatric nursing practice the problem is even more complicated. Not only does the medical mission influence care, other parties do as well—the parents and the state. Advocacy becomes an increasingly complex issue when the nurse is confronted not only with institutional demand but also with the sometimes conflicting desires of the patient and the parents. The state also has a significant interest in the welfare of children and in some instances becomes a primary actor in decision making regarding the care of children. As noted earlier in this chapter, the state's interest in the welfare of children goes back to common law England, where the king or queen had legal authority to act as a general guardian of orphans and was required to protect the welfare of the wards. The power, called *parens patriae,* is the legal cornerstone of today's child welfare system, including child abuse laws.

Practicing nurses who wish to work in an advocacy model must seriously confront the ethical considerations which arise from the numerous persons and institutions involved in making decisions that affect the children for whom they care. Gadow (1980) described advocacy in the decision-making process as helping the patient or parents noncoercively reach a decision through discussion aimed at helping clarify their values.

Nurses have the right legally as promulgated by nurse practice acts and the responsibility ethically as determined by appropriate standards of practice to act as patient advocates. To do so effectively, they must reach their own solution to the integrity dilemma. The nurse who acts as a patient advocate in clinical practice will be protected by the nurse practice act and professional standards to the extent that the advocacy is within the bounds of the nurse's legal authority.

Study Questions

1. A minor may be treated without parental consent:
   A. If delay in treatment would cause a risk for serious harm or further injury.
   B. Under no circumstances.
   C. Only if death is possible.
   D. If delay of treatment is greater than 2 hours.
2. In nonemergency occurrences and where no parental consent can be obtained for treatment by a minor:
   A. No treatment is possible.
   B. Grandparents may consent to treatment.
   C. Siblings over 16 years may consent to treatment.
   D. The minor may consent if over 7 years of age.

3. An emancipated minor is a minor who:
   A. Is married.
   B. Is not living with both parents.
   C. Is free from care, custody, and services of his or her parents.
   D. Has graduated from high school and has his or her own job.
4. Partial emancipation refers to the:
   A. Minors of divorced parents.
   B. Minor's right to have a partial capacity for consent.
   C. Minor's right to consent to medical treatment in emergency situations only.
   D. Minor's right for treatment of venereal disease only.
5. Informed consent refers to the requirement that:
   A. Minors sign for any treatment they will receive in a hospital setting.
   B. Parents sign for all minors' treatment.
   C. Health professionals fully describe the treatment to which patients are being asked to consent.
   D. Parents of minors sign consents for release of information.
6. Courts have ruled that a minor:
   A. Must accept treatment recommended by a physician.
   B. Has the right to refuse treatment.
   C. Does not have right to refuse treatment unless parents consent.
   D. May refuse treatment only if there is question of an abortion.
7. Generally, the party consenting to treatment is:
   A. Responsible for paying for the care unless the party is the minor.
   B. Responsible for paying for the care unless it is a stepparent.
   C. Responsible for paying for the care.
   D. None of the above.
8. Parents of an older minor who has consented to his own care have:
   A. A right to the confidential information related to their child's care.
   B. A right to sue the physician for allowing the minor to consent to his own care.
   C. No need for information for consent purposes.
   D. A right to request another physician if they have not consented for the care offered by the first physician.
9. Disclosure of confidential information to unauthorized persons about any child patient without his consent may result in:
   A. Legal action for damages.
   B. Legal action only if the information is untrue.
   C. No legal action since it involves information about a minor.
   D. None of the above.
10. When a pediatric nurse practitioner makes a medical diagnosis and initiates treatment based on protocols:
    A. The physician she collaborates with is always legally responsible.
    B. The nurse is involved in malpractice.
    C. The accountability is shared between a physician and nurse.
    D. The nurse alone is held accountable.
11. Nurses are ———.
    A. Sometimes licensed to treat medical problems independently.
    B. Usually licensed to treat medical problems independently.
    C. Never licensed to treat medical problems independently.
    D. None of the above.
12. It is an ——— which presents the greatest concern for nurses.
    A. Intentional tort of negligence.
    B. Intentional commission.
    C. Unintentional commission.
    D. Unintentional tort of negligence.
13. If a nurse believes that carrying out a physician's order could possibly harm a patient the following action should take place:
    A. Contact the physician.
    B. The nurse should firmly decline to carry out the order.
    C. Bring the matter immediately to the attention of her supervisor.
    D. All of the above.
14. A physician is considered to be an expert witness:
    A. Only in cases where standards of care are being determined for a physician's practice.
    B. When establishing the standard of care for a hospital nurse.
    C. When establishing a standard of care for a nurse in an expanded role.
    D. Only in those cases where standards of care are being determined for a nurse working in an office practice.

References

AMA News, April 17, 1967, p. 4.

Barber, B.: "Control and Responsibility in the Powerful Professions," *Political Science Quarterly,* 93(4):601-603, winter 1978-1979.

Bodine, N.: "Minors and Contraceptives: A Constitutional Issue," *Ecology Law Quarterly,* 3:859, 1973.

Bullough, B.: *The Law and the Expanding Nurse Role,* 2d ed., Appleton-Century-Crofts, New York, 1980.

Curran, W.J., and H.K. Beecher: "Experimentation in Children," *Journal of the American Medical Association,* 210(1):77, Oct. 6, 1969.

Davis, A.J.: "When Parents Disagree on Treatment," *American Journal of Nursing,* 80(11):2082, 1980.

———: "A Newborn's Right to Life vs. Death," *American Journal of Nursing,* 81(5):1035, 1981a.

———: "To Tell or Not," *American Journal of Nursing,* 81(1):156-158, 1981b.

"Disclosure of Confidential Information," *Journal of the American Medical Association,* 216(2):385, Apr. 12, 1971.

Gadow, S.: "Nursing Perspectives on Decision-Making Procedures," paper presented at conference on Dilemmas of Dying: Policies and Procedures for Decisions Not to Treat, Medicine in the Public Interest, Apr. 27-28, 1980, Boston.

Golby, S.: "Experiments in the Willowbrook State School," *Lancet,* i:749, 1971.

Gordon, M.: *Nursing Diagnosis Process and Application,* 2d ed., McGraw-Hill, New York, 1987.

Holder, A.R.: *Legal Issues in Pediatric and Adolescent Medicine,* Wiley, New York, 1977, p. 139.

Hospital Law Manual, Health Law Center, Aspen Systems Corporation, 1981. See for full tables of all minor treatment statutes as of the dates of publication.

"Independence of Nursing Function Affirmed by New York State Legislature," *American Journal of Nursing,* 71(6):1901-1902, 1971.

Jordan, E.: "A Minor's Right to Contraceptives," *University of California at Davis Law Review,* 7:270, 1974. (See for Proceedings of the AMA House of Delegates, June 20–24, 1971, pp. 55-56.)

Kozier, B., and G. Erb: *Fundamentals of Nursing,* 3d ed., Addison-Wesley, Menlo Park, Calif., 1987.

Kraft, M.: "Using Expert Witnesses in Civil Cases," Practicing Law Institute, New York, 1977, pp. 32-34.

Mitchell, C.: "New Directions in Nursing Ethics," *Massachusetts Nurse,* 50:7-10, July 1981.

"Model Act," *Pediatrics,* 51(2):293, February 1973.

Murphy, C., and H. Hunter: "Models of the Nurse-Patient Relationship," in C. Murphy and H. Hunter (eds.), *Ethical Problems in the Nurse-Patient Relationship,* Allyn and Bacon, Newton, Mass., 1982.

Northrop, C., and A. Mech: "The Nurse as Expert Witness," *Nursing Law and Ethics,* 2(3):1-6, March 1981.

Pilpel, H.S.: "Minors' Right to Medical Care," *Albany Law Review,* 36:466, 1972.

Ramsey, P.: *The Patient as a Person,* Yale University Press, New Haven, Conn., 1974.

Restatement of the Law of Torts, American Law Institute, sec. 59a, 1971.

Steinbock, B.: "Baby Jane Doe in Court," *The Hastings Report,* 40(1):13-19, February 1984.

Wadlington, W.: "Minors and Health Care: The Age of Consent," *Osgood Hall Law Journal,* 115(1), 1973.

Statutory References

Massachusetts General Laws, ch. 111, § 70E.
Massachusetts General Laws ch. 112, § 12E
Massachusetts General Laws ch. 112, § 12S.
Mississippi Code Annotated 541-41-3H.

Bibliography

American Nurses' Association: *Ethics in Nursing: References and Resources,* American Nurses' Association, Kansas City, 1982.

———: *Nursing—A Social Policy Statement,* American Nurses' Association, Kansas City, December 1980.

———: *Standards of Maternal and Child Health Nursing Practice,* American Nurses' Association, Kansas City, December 1983.

Annas, George J.: "Parents, Children and the Supreme Court," *Hastings Center Report,* 9(5):21-23, October 1979.

Creighton, Helen: "Action for Wrongful Life—Law for the Nurse Supervisor," *Supervisor Nurse,* 8(4):12-15, April 1977.

Curran, W.J.: "Law-Medicine Notes—Research and Children," *New England Journal of Medicine,* 299(18):1001-1002, November 1978.

Eldrige, Theresa: "Adolescent Health Care: The Legal and Ethical Implications," *Pediatric Nursing,* 5(2):51-52, March-April, 1979.

Haller, J.S., Jr.: "Newborns with Major Congenital Malformations—Can the Anguish of Decision Regarding Management Be Shared," *AORN Journal,* 27(6):1070-1075, May 1978.

Hoffman, Adele D.: "Legal and Social Implications of Adolescent Social Behavior," *Journal of Adolescence,* 1:25-33, 1978.

Jellinek, B.: "Adolescents' Knowledge of Consent Laws in a Massachusetts Community," *Pediatric Nursing,* 6(2):21-23, March-April 1980.

Jonsen, A.R.: "Research Involving Children: Recommendations of the National Commission for the Protection of Human Subjects of Biomedical and Behavioral Research," *Pediatrics,* 62(2):131-136, August 1978.

Karpel, M.A.: "Family Secrets: 1. Conceptual and Ethical Issues in the Relational Context. 2. Ethical and Practical Considerations in Therapeutic Management," *Family Process,* 19(3):295-306, September 1980.

Kohnke, Mary F.: "The Nurse as Advocate," *American Journal of Nursing,* 80(11):2038-2040, November 1980.

Mancini, Margaret: "Nursing Minors and the Law," *American Journal of Nursing,* 78(1):124-126, January 1978.

Murphy, Catherine P.: "The Moral Situation in Nursing," in E.L. Bandman and B. Bandman (eds.), *Bioethics and Human Rights,* Little, Brown, Boston, 1978, pp. 313-320.

"Parental Consent Requirements and Privacy Rights of Minors: The Contraception Controversy," *Harvard Law Review,* 88(5):1001-1020, March 1975.

Shartel, B., and M. Plant: "The Law of Medical Practice," Thomas, Springfield, Ill., 1959, p. 26.

Tiano, L.V.: "*Parham v. J.R.*—Voluntary Commitment of Minors to Mental Institutions," American Journal of Law and Medicine, 6(1):125-149, Spring 1980.

Torres, A., J.D. Forrest, and S. Eisman: "Telling Parents: Clinic Policies and Adolescents' Use of Family Planning and Abortion Services," *Family Planning Perspectives,* 12(6):284-292, November-December 1980.

Trandel-Korenchuk, D., and K. Trandel-Korenchuk: "Minor Consent, Part 1," *Nurse Practitioner,* 5(2):50-51, March-April 1980.

———: "Minor Consent, Part 2," *Nurse Practitioner,* 5(3):48, 50, 54, May-June 1980.

Special Problems in Caring for Children

The Hospitalization of a Child

Objectives

After reading this chapter, the student will be able to:
1. Discuss the process involved in admitting a child to a pediatric unit.
2. Describe the effects of pain, sensory deprivation, and sensory overstimulation in the course of an infant's hospitalization.
3. Identify and elaborate on five factors which influence a toddler's response to hospitalization.
4. List four types of play activities which can be used in working with hospitalized preschoolers.
5. Identify four variables which affect the hospitalization of adolescents.
6. List and discuss all the components of discharge planning.

In the hospital a nurse spends more time with a sick child and his family than does any other health care worker. In this role the nurse can help create a positive adaptation to hospitalization by the child and family. Awareness and consideration of the family's experience with illness, hospitalization, and discharge can increase a nurse's effectiveness and result in a much more positive outcome for the child and family.

Hospitalization is an interruption of a child's active cycle of growth and development and of his and his family's life-styles. The child is removed from the daily routines of home life, and contact with siblings, relatives, and peers may be limited. The child may experience strange and painful events and may have to communicate with strangers.

Preparation for such dramatic change is essential for both the child and his parents. The first contact with the hospital can set the tone for the rest of the hospital stay, and so the admission procedure should be planned and implemented carefully. The hospital environment should be designed to provide comfort for the ill child and his family as well as to meet their emotional and developmental needs.

Unplanned or emergency admissions are common, however, and effective communication between the nurse and the family can prevent the development of a crisis situation. Diagnostic and therapeutic procedures may occur so quickly that parents have little time to understand the process. The nurse can help family members understand the sequence of events and encourage their participation as much as possible.

Preparing for Hospitalization

Preparation prior to hospitalization can make the transition from home to hospital as nondisruptive as possible. Every family should be told what to expect when a child is admitted to the hospital. The child's developmental level and relationship with his parents determine when preparation should begin and in how much detail it should be carried out.

A physician is the primary source of facts concerning the purpose, therapeutic plan, and expected outcome of hospitalization. The information the physician offers should include a description of the physiological and/or psychological aspects of treatment which will be carried out as well as an estimation of the length of stay in the hospital.

Parents who know the strengths and weaknesses of the child and can communicate with him can help prepare the child for admission and interpret for him the events that will take place in the hospital. Parents rightfully may express and feel inadequacy in accompanying the child upon admission. However, with support from the nurse, a parent may be able to accompany the child. Whatever the circumstances, the child needs a familiar and understanding person to prepare him for and support him during admission to the hospital.

Preadmission

Preadmission preparation is most effective when the admission is planned and there is enough time for the nurse to provide necessary information to the child and the parents and make sure they understand it. The parent should be the main interpreter and supplier of information for the child. Through direct participation in learning about what hospitalization will be like, the parent may find his or her own anxiety alleviated somewhat. As the parent communicates with the child, he or she gains information which may answer many of his or her own questions, allowing the parent to support the child more constructively.

Many hospitals provide a booklet which describes the routines of the pediatric unit. The family should receive such materials before admission to help them plan for hospitalization. The information in preadmission booklets should be written for the parents and the child. Through simply written, factual information that can be easily read by people with elementary reading skills and through pictures of the pediatric unit, a story can be communicated. Families need to know what to bring with them to the hospital and what the physical accommodations will be. They also need to know who will be taking care of the child. The booklet may be written with simple words in large print and have pictures to color or a puzzle related to the hospital.

Printed materials, movies, slides, and a variety of playthings can help prepare the child for hospitalization. The nurse can provide or recommend any of several books about going to the hospital which are written especially for children. Some suggestions can be found in Books For Families at the end of this chapter. The nurse also may instruct the parents in simple play techniques that will help the child understand what will happen in the hospital. For example, if a child is to have a tonsillectomy, the nurse can demonstrate for the mother what will happen before and after the operation, using dolls that represent the child (patient), nurse, doctor, and others involved in the hospital care. Then the child's mother can enact this drama with the child at home to teach what to expect.

Children should be told openly that they are going to the hospital. Preparation depends on when and how the child's parents usually prepare him for a new experience. The child's ability to conceptualize time may be used as a guide for determining when to tell him about going to the hospital. In general, children over 7 years of age may be told as much as 2 weeks in advance of admission, as they are able to comprehend how far in the future "2 weeks" will be. The younger the child is under the age of 7, the shorter should be the interval between the time when he is told he is going to the hospital and the day he is admitted.

The child needs to participate as much as possible in planning his hospital visit. Depending on his age, he may want to choose which toys he will take with him, explain to his friends why he will be gone from school for a few days, or pick out new pajamas to wear. He may also participate by packing his own bag.

Admission Procedure

Admission to the pediatric unit and helping the family learn about their new surroundings are nursing responsibilities. The nurse is the best person for answering the family's questions about all aspects of hospital life and can, during the admission procedure, detect possible problem areas in the family and assess ways of dealing with them.

Two objectives should be carried out during admission: (1) acquainting the family with the physical facilities and services of the hospital and (2) exchanging information with the family about the child's care.

In order to accomplish the first objective, specific activities must be carried out at admission to ensure that the family is oriented to all aspects of the new environment. The nursing staff members on each unit should plan an admission procedure which is specific to their own unit facilities and to the needs of the families it serves. A list of all activities which should be carried out at admission is a helpful tool. This list might include items such as "orient to facilities in room, explain visiting and rooming-in policies, introduce family to staff, and show child the playroom."

Orientation to the Pediatric Unit

When the family arrives at the pediatric unit the parents should be shown the room where the child will stay and the toilet facilities he will use. If the bathroom is "down the hall," a landmark pointed out may be helpful in remembering which way to go. It is important to demonstrate exactly how the faucets turn on and off and how the toilet is flushed, as they may work differently from the ones the family uses at home.

The approximate times when meals are served to children should be provided for the family. This information may be particularly important for parents who plan their visiting time to coincide with the time when the child eats. For the child, knowing when meals will be served provides the beginnings of a routine for the day, and mealtime can become a way for him to judge the passage of time. Children need to know that "snack food" is available, and they can be shown the kitchen and snack supply on the unit.

It is important to discuss special dietary preferences, such as religious restrictions and the availability of vegetarian meals, with families on admission. If meals cannot be made available to them in the child's room, parents need to know where they can eat their meals. They should have directions about how to get to the cafeteria or coffee shop and the hours these facilities are open. It may also be important to give an estimate of food cost to some families.

Showing the child the playroom soon after he comes to the pediatric unit will let him know that there is a place in his new environment which may seem somewhat familiar. Children want to explore the playroom immediately and will relax noticeably amid toy trucks, dolls, books, and blocks. It is comforting for parents to know that there is a play facility to help them entertain the child.

Soon after admission it is important to explain to parents and children where and how they can call a nurse if they need help. The nurses' desk or charting station should be identified as a place where parents can get help. The call button or intercommunication system in their own room should be demonstrated, and it is a good idea to have the family participate in using this equipment as it is explained. If there is no phone in their room, the family should be shown the closest phone that may be used. Having a phone available is particularly important for family members who must be separated during hospitalization.

Providing for Parents

In many hospitals parents are encouraged to stay with their children 24 hours a day. There may be facilities which allow them to "live in" with the child, or they may spend varying amounts of time with the child. If a living-in arrangement is not available for the parents, the nurse should explore with them how much time they will spend with the child and how they will manage this time away from the rest of the family. They may need to know about available housing close to the hospital and about convenient transportation. If the family members (parents) must drive in and out of a large city, they may want to know the easiest route to and from the hospital. A small map of the hospital that shows how to get to the child's room may also be helpful.

When living-in is possible, parents need to know how their daily living needs will be met. They should have a clear understanding of the particular facilities available to them, such as those for eating, sleeping, and bathing. Knowing which parts of the pediatric unit and hospital are "out of bounds" as well as those which they may utilize makes the family feel more comfortable and secure.

Facilities where parents can relax or socialize with other parents should be pointed out. It is important that parents who spend a lot of time with a sick child have an opportunity to engage in some type of recreation or diversion. A list of churches and synagogues in the immediate area may be given to families, and they should be shown the hospital chapel.

One of the first questions parents ask upon arrival at the unit is, When are visiting hours? The family needs time schedules as well as suggestions regarding who may visit and how often. It is also a good moment to explain anticipated reactions of the child to having them leave and return for visits.

The Nursing Interview

The second objective of admission—exchanging information—is accomplished by conducting a nursing interview with the parents and the child. At this time the nurse can learn why the child has come to the hospital and the concerns and expectations he and his parents have about this experience. During this interview the nurse can communicate to the parents what they can expect of her and what she will expect of them.

Guidelines for the Nursing Interview
Identification
    Hospital identification stamp
    Child's nickname
    Chronological age and birth date
Health and physical development
    Length, symptoms, and nature of illness
    Past illnesses and health care
    Allergies to medications, food, or other substances
    Immunizations
    Names of medications child has taken
    Form in which medication was given and how child accepted it
    Gross motor development, i.e., sitting, walking, jumping

Fine motor development, i.e., eye movements, grasping, writing

Sensory development, i.e., vision, hearing, smell, taste, touch

Hospitalization

When and where previous hospitalizations occurred

Helpful or harmful incidents during previous hospitalizations

Treatments and procedures performed

Preparation for present admission

Expectations for hospitalization

Experiences with hospitalization and illness of family members

Social-cultural

Geographic and neighborhood setting

Type of dwelling

Ethnic background

Religious preferences

Parental and family relations

Who makes decisions about child

People important to parents and child

Recent changes in environment and family relations

Present level of personal-social development

Educational level of child and parents

Economic status

Hospitalization financing

Nutrition

Twenty-four-hour recall

Types of food, fluid, and formula

Current food and fluid likes and dislikes

Special diets

Mealtime patterns

Ability to feed self

Elimination

Frequency of bowel movement and urination

Constipation problems and remedies

Level of bowel and bladder control

Sleep

Sleeping arrangements, i.e., type of bed and with whom child sleeps

Hours for daytime and nighttime sleeping

Wakeful or sound sleeper

Communication

Level of language development

Special words, i.e., words for bowel movement, urination, hunger

Behavior

Habits or rituals

Reaction to stress and comforting measures

Parental reaction to stress

Methods of discipline and reaction to discipline

Behaviors for which punished

Types of punishment

Interaction with others

Play

Playmates and pets

Special games and hobbies

Favorite playthings

Playthings brought to the hospital from home

Giving information is just as important as acquiring information in the nursing interview. As information is obtained in each area of the history, the nurse should explain to the family how that information will be used to meet their individual needs during hospitalization.

Reinforcing Information

Although a great deal of information is exchanged between nurse and family during the orientation and the interview, the nurse cannot assume that all this information will be retained by the family. It is therefore important to provide reinforcement of information, particularly throughout the first days of hospitalization. Whenever appropriate, all members of the nursing staff can reinforce information which they know is a part of the admission procedure.

Developmental Impact of Illness and Hospitalization

Hospitalization and the possibility of living in the hospital environment are stressful situations for most families. Illness, separation, decreased mobility, enforced dependence, unfamiliar routines, fears, and misunderstandings can cause varying degrees of anxiety. The nurse can help a hospitalized child and his family maintain normality by sustaining an environment which will meet their physical and emotional needs and contribute to their growth and development.

Neonates
Parent Participation

The newborn's immediate surroundings are usually limited to his crib and his parents' arms. The sensations he receives are mainly visual, tactile, auditory, and oral, and through these modes he learns in the first few months of life to identify his mother. Therefore, it is important for the basic development of trust that the neonate's needs for food, warmth, and love be met by his mother or a constant mother figure throughout infancy.

Maintaining the parent-infant relationship is particularly important not only for the baby but also for his parents when the neonate must be hospitalized. For some parents, demands at home rightfully may take precedence over staying at the hospital with the baby. In this situation nursing management should be planned to allow the same person to care for the newborn each day so that his needs are met with a consistent approach.

A rooming-in or living-in arrangement which allows at least one parent to stay with the baby 24 hours a day is the best way to continue the close relationship necessary during this period of development. There are also other advantages in this type of arrangement. Parents are available to participate in the care, making them feel that they are providing a real contribution to helping the neonate get well. Having parents present also gives the nursing staff an opportunity to assess more closely family strengths and weaknesses and to teach parents to give care that will be necessary after discharge.

Living-in also allows for more informal contact with the nursing staff and contributes to a freer exchange of information. Families can give each other support as daily contacts bring them closer together. A lounge or small corner with table, comfortable chairs, and coffeepot can help stimulate informal interaction among parents, families, and staff.

Interruptions of Parent-Child Attachment

Illness and hospitalization create threats to parent-infant bonding. In order to form the mutual ties necessary for establishing a relationship in which parents give love and babies thrive, both parents and newborns need to be together and to be healthy enough to participate in these parent-child interactions. Ill or malformed babies and especially small preterm neonates often require hospitalization, frequently in a neonatal intensive care unit (Fig. 9-1). There they can receive lifesaving medical and nursing care, but contact with parents tends to be curtailed severely.

It has been known for years that separating mother from newborn can create great difficulties for the development of the mother's love, concern, and compassion for the baby. Klaus and Kennell (1970) observed that although maternal feelings of attachment begin before birth (for example, with confirming that one is pregnant, feeling the fetal movements, and giving birth), in some women such feelings are readily disrupted in the first day or days after the delivery. Disturbances in mothering long have been noticed in mother-child couples separated in the first postpartum days or weeks, including alterations in handling and holding the infant, inability to provide nurturing, neglect, failure to thrive, and even child abuse (Klaus and Kennell, 1983).

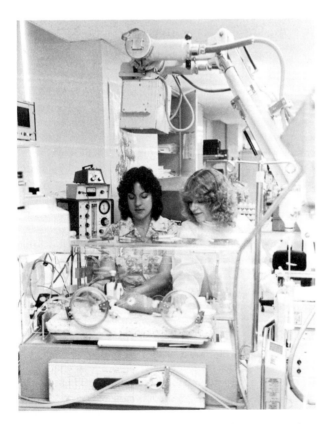

FIGURE 9-1 Parents may be overwhelmed by the vast array of equipment and personnel required to care for their infant.

Pain, Sensory Deprivation and Sensory Overstimulation

Illness and hospitalization may alter the neonate's sensory experiences greatly. The newborn's ability to perceive pain is not known with certainty. Babies cry less in response to pain in the first days and weeks of life than they do later, and crying newborns are easily distracted and comforted. However, most health professionals have abandoned the old belief that procedures, injections, circumcision, and the like are painless or nearly so. In many neonatal intensive care units babies are given medication for postoperative pain. Newborns react to a pinprick by moving their arms and legs, crying and grimacing. Pain research about infants and children is obviously difficult and sparse because of the inherent ethical problems, including involvement of minors in research and the issue of informed consent for minors (see Chap. 8, "Ethical and Legal Issues in Child Health"). It may be that the newborn's *perceptual* system permits babies to *feel* pain but that *motor* system immaturity prevents them from making clear, observable *responses* to show that they are experiencing pain.

The kinds and amounts of sensory stimulation neonates need for normal development may be absent during illness or hospitalization. Oral deprivation occurs if babies are unable to take oral feedings. Normal patterns of sucking and swallowing may be difficult to establish later, when feedings can begin. Sensory experiences normally acquired by being held against the parent's body, carried, rocked, talked or sung to, and held up to the parent's direct eye-to-eye gaze (the *en face* position) are prevented to some degree in ill and hospitalized babies (Fig. 9-2). These activities have been shown to be important for infant growth, early childhood IQ, language, motor coordination, and social development as well as for parenting (Klaus and Kennell, 1983). Bilateral eye patches, which are necessary for babies being treated with ultraviolet light for jaundice, eliminate visual intake, including the parent's face.

Hospitalized neonates, especially those in intensive care units, are very likely to receive continuous high-intensity sensory stimulation that may constitute overstimulation. Monitors, respirators, humidifiers, and other kinds of equipment produce round-the-clock noises that do not vary. The lights are bright at all times of night and day. Any handling by a staff member is motivated toward accomplishing a task rather than providing comfort, as by stroking and patting which parents usually provide.

Interventions for Hospitalized Neonates

The principal way to minimize the developmental hazards created by illness and hospitalization is to normalize parent-infant interaction and the neonate's stimulation as far as possible. Parents of an ill or preterm newborn must be taught (and *shown* by the nurse's example) how they may safely touch, embrace, and provide at least part of the care for the baby and how to speak and sing to the child without embarrassment. The incidence of infection in the nursery is not increased by parents' or other family mem-

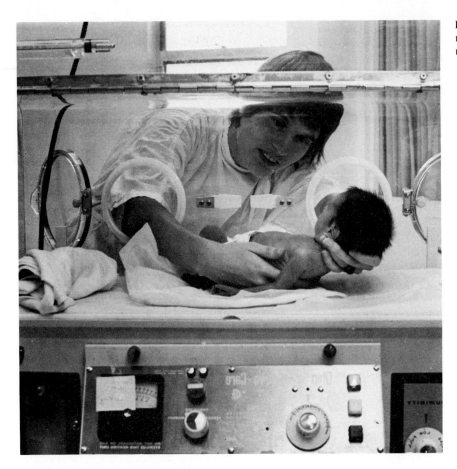

FIGURE 9-2   If her baby is in an incubator, the mother must overcome physical barriers to achieve the *en face* position.

bers' visiting as long as they practice careful hand washing and gowning and avoid visits when they have transmissible infections. Mothers and fathers need to be made welcome in hospitals, including intensive care units, and should be encouraged and assisted in assuming their rightful and central place as parents. The neonate's level of sensory stimulation should be regulated. Under- and overstimulation should be avoided, and painful, monotonous stimuli should be minimized.

Infants

Illness must not be allowed to interfere unnecessarily with the infant's growth and developmental progress. A sick baby, like a healthy one, needs empathic care, stimulation, and consistent interactions with parents. To the greatest extent possible nurses should make provisions so that the parents or other customary caregivers can continue their usual relationship with the infant. This participation involves providing for extensive (preferably unlimited) visiting when the baby is in the hospital and enabling parents (as far as possible) to give feedings, baths, and all other appropriate aspects of care. Parents need instructions about how to comfort and tend to the baby if the infant is receiving oxygen or IV fluids, how to interact with an infant in a mist tent, and so forth.

When infants must be hospitalized, it is difficult to understand fully how they may be reacting because they cannot describe their feelings. Infants 6 months or older show more pronounced signs of disturbance when hospi-

talized or receiving treatment than do younger infants. *Stranger anxiety* may be severe, especially around 8 months of age. If the parents do not stay with the baby, *separation anxiety* leads to frightened and angry crying. Babies separated from their parents may be difficult to console for the first few hours and may then become withdrawn, depressed, and indifferent toward their caregivers and surroundings. When the parents return after several hours or longer, the infant may burst into hard crying as soon as they come into view. This apparent increase in the baby's distress when the parents come back must not be misinterpreted to mean that the baby would be better off if the parents stayed away.

Sick infants, particularly small ones, may need to use all their energy to cope with the illness. In almost all instances where development has been proceeding normally, it can be expected that during the acute phase of an illness this development will appear to slow or stop completely. If the illness is relatively short, if the infant continues to be cared for (to the extent possible) by the mother or another familiar person, and if a stimulating environment is provided, there is no reason to believe that the illness will slow the attainment of developmental tasks significantly.

The sick infant may be unable to take his usual part in reciprocal interactions with his caregivers. The parents and other caregivers need to work together to observe small cues from the infant that he is comfortable or uncomfortable. Caregivers must recognize that they will have to work harder to provide the stimulation necessary to maintain the developing (1) locomotion abilities, (2) ability to take solid foods, (3) nonverbal and verbal communication, and (4) emotional relationships with family members and others. The illness may make it difficult or impossible for the infant to be as responsive and appealing as he normally would be, and thus the incentive for the adults to keep providing stimulation is reduced.

Interventions for Hospitalized Infants

The primary way to support the coping mechanisms of an infant is to support the parent. The infant cannot comprehend explanations of how and why certain things are done to him. There is every reason to believe, however, that the presence of a familiar, caring person decreases fear, relieves tension, and promotes the infant's sense of trust in people.

Although the infant cannot comprehend an explanation of a procedure, it is most desirable for the nurse to tell an infant that she is about to do something before she does it, just as the nurse would tell any other patient. The explanation provides verbal stimulation to the infant, the tone of voice can indicate caring, and of course the infant gradually will understand more and more of what is being said to him. If the parents are present, they will see that nurses talk to infants and will feel less ridiculous doing it themselves. The explanation to the infant reinforces what has been told to the parent. For example, an infant can be told he is going to receive an injection to help him get better. Although he is being hurt, his mother is there to comfort him.

Every attempt should be made to limit the number of people primarily responsible for the infant's care, especially if the parent is not staying with the infant in the hospital. Singing or other rhythmic music, holding, rocking, and providing a pacifier are effective comfort measures after a frightening or painful procedure.

Sometimes parents believe that if they are present during an unpleasant procedure, the infant will associate them with pain. The role of the parent as someone who supports the infant through good and bad times can be discussed. Also, the parent can be helped to realize that the infant associates the parents with many more comforting and pleasing experiences than unpleasant ones. If parents do not wish to be present during certain procedures, their wishes should be respected and they should be told that the infant will be cared for and comforted by the hospital staff until the parents return.

Toddlers

Toddlers are active, autonomous little children who under normal circumstances are occupied full time with exploring and interacting with the objects and people around them. Independence becomes the main theme of their behavior. Being ill, injured, or disabled can interfere with these activities. If hospitalization is necessary, the risks are even greater. Nurses and parents need to be well informed about the toddler's developmental characteristics and individual factors in order to promote his well-

being in spite of the stresses imposed by hospitalization. Many variables contribute to each toddler's reaction to health problems, including the following:

1. *His family:* past experiences, current relationships, reaction to illness, and ability to support him during his illness
2. *His unique developmental level:* sense of autonomy and independence, language skills and deficits, bowel and bladder control, neuromuscular coordination, and cognitive ability
3. *His personality:* adaptability, temperament, and coping skills
4. *His past and current life experiences:* family stresses including birth of a new sibling, divorce, a move, death of a significant person or pet; separation experiences with baby-sitters, nursery schools, extended family, or foster placement
5. *His previous illness, hospital, and health care experiences:* relationship with primary care provider, emergency room contacts, number and length of past hospital admissions, and type of preparation given for all health care experiences
6. *His current illness and related experiences:* type of illness, amount and types of diagnostic tests and treatments, amount and type of preparation for hospitalization and treatments, and required length of hospital stay

The nursing history should include this information, the strengths and weaknesses of the family, and the child-parent relationship so that the nurse can plan appropriate interventions. Some of the items which should be included in a toddler's care plan are separation anxiety, rituals and routines, independence and autonomy, communication, fears about body integrity, mobility, regression, and play.

Interventions for Hospitalized Toddlers
Separation Anxiety

The most obvious source of stress for a hospitalized toddler is separation. His relationship with his mother has become very intense and meaningful, and he feels secure in her presence (Fig. 9-3). He longs for constant attention from her and is fearful when she is gone. He develops a close relationship with his father; his siblings become important.

The reactions seen in the toddler experiencing separation anxiety include protest, despair, and detachment (Robertson and Robertson, 1972). During the protest phase the toddler cries, screams, and uses other overt behavior to let everyone know that he does not want his parents to leave. When they are gone, he lets the nursing staff know that he wants his parents back immediately. This protesting behavior can easily be misunderstood by the nursing staff and by the parents as well. Not understanding what he is trying to communicate, they may insist that he should be a good little boy. This request tells him that he should not be expressing these deep and significant emotions. Some toddlers have even been punished for continued crying.

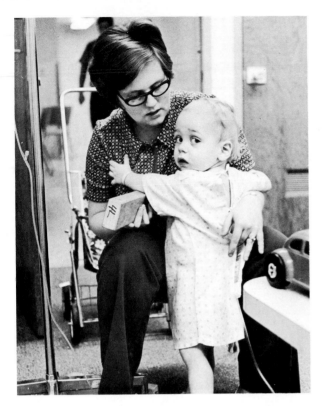

FIGURE 9-3 A hospitalized toddler experiences separation anxiety when his parent leaves.

Sometimes parents are afraid to visit their children because they feel that their visits are upsetting to them. Parents need help in understanding the normality of the toddler's protestations. They also need to know how they can best help the child cope with the separation. Leaving a familiar item which belongs to his mother or father with the child, returning as often as possible and staying as much as possible, and telling the child truthfully that they are leaving and that they will return are ways of helping the grieving child cope with the loss.

Nursing intervention with parents and toddler should take place at the time of the parents' departure. Such attempted consolations as "I'll be your mommy for a while" should never be used. They add to the child's fear that he has lost his mother.

If the parents cannot return frequently or cannot stay long because they have other pressures at home or must travel a long distance from the hospital, the toddler will need special help from the nursing staff. He may seek out a certain nurse and follow her around for the entire shift, protesting when she leaves. Ideally the toddler is assigned to one or two nurses who see him consistently and establish a trusting relationship with him. He will also need love, attention, cuddling, and diversional activity such as play. Some hospitals have established a Foster Grandparent program in which retired persons are available to provide continuity in a caring relationship with the child. The nurse may need to help the assigned foster grandparent know how to handle the protesting and grieving toddler. The separated toddler also needs constant reassurance

that his mother and father love him, will return to see him, and will take him home eventually so that he does not feel abandoned.

When the parent does not visit the child frequently and consistently and when he does not receive attention and consistency from the nursing staff, the child may exhibit the second and third stages of separation anxiety: despair and detachment. Despair is characterized by withdrawn, depressed behavior. The child may refuse to eat, leave his room, or relate to anyone. When his mother arrives, he may cry intensely or react with anger and distrust. Some children may reach for the nurse in preference to the mother. Detachment is evident when the child appears not to care when his mother and father return. He may ignore them, reach for another adult instead, or remain quietly in his crib. Nursing staff members often erroneously interpret this phase as positive adjustment to the hospital, since the child cries less and relates more to the staff. Because he forms superficial relationships with many staff members, he may become the ward favorite. He really needs the opportunity to form a trusting relationship with one individual to foster his psychosocial development.

Increasing use of rooming-in facilities, lengthening of visiting hours, and shortening of hospital stays for toddlers have minimized the problems which stem from separation anxiety. However, it is important to remind nurses that the toddler still experiences stress from separation—separation from the rest of his family and from the familiar surroundings of his home. All these losses create feelings of insecurity and grief. In the midst of separation from familiar family members and familiar surroundings, the toddler is faced with unfamiliar frightening surroundings and daily interactions with many strangers. The importance of consistency of personnel cannot be overemphasized.

Grandparents or friends should be allowed to visit and also stay overnight so that they can relieve the parents from their bedside vigil. If the hospitalization is a long one and if the child's condition becomes stabilized, he should be allowed to visit siblings or talk with them on the telephone. It also helps if photographs of siblings, grandparents, parents, pets, and his home are hung on his walls. Other familiar objects from home, such as favorite toys, blankets, and clothes, are also helpful.

Rituals and Routines

Another source of stress for the toddler during an illness and hospitalization is the major change in his daily routines and rituals which occurs in the hospital environment—an environment which imposes a new set of routines and rituals on him. The routines of his daily life are important to the toddler's sense of security; he knows what to expect and when to expect it. Even a vacation can be very upsetting to him. Because of the loss of familiar routines, he may exhibit many different behavioral changes, such as night fears or regression to bedwetting.

In addition to routines, toddlers tend to set up precise and involved rituals around the important activities of eating, sleeping, and bathing. A ritual is a rigid pattern of procedures which the toddler expects his parents or baby-sitters to follow. These rituals assure him that he can know what to expect and allow him to exert some control over the situation.

When planning nursing care for a toddler, it is important to learn about his special rituals and usual routines so that plans can be made to attempt to follow some of them during his hospitalization. Bedtime for toddlers often includes such rituals. Even when rituals are carried out the hospitalized toddler may have difficulty sleeping during naptime and at night.

Another area in which loss of rituals and familiar surroundings becomes important is that of eating. Eating patterns in a toddler are easily affected by changes in himself, the person who feeds him, and the environment. Since the toddler's appetite is erratic anyway, the effects of change may lead to refusal of food. Certainly hospitalization creates a change in the environment, feeding person, time, and food received. In addition, the toddler's illness or the drugs he is taking may cause some anorexia or nausea. Thus, a decrease in appetite can be expected until some adjustments are made by the child and his physical condition improves. It is not uncommon for him to eat only one good meal a day, and so it helps to know what he has eaten at previous meals. Attempting to force a toddler to eat will be unsuccessful, as eating is one activity he can control. It will help if the nurse attempts to follow the ritual used at home, have a familiar person help with the meals, and let the toddler feed himself as much as possible.

Closely related to the problems created by the changes in routines and rituals is the toddler's poor time sense. Nurses and parents need to realize that telling a toddler something will happen at a certain time means nothing to him. However, if he is told that something will happen after his nap, he will have a clearer idea of the time. Time schedules for a toddler revolve around his activities, not around a clock.

Independence and Autonomy

One of the outstanding features of this period is the toddler's egocentric view of life. He feels that the world should revolve around his desires and wishes. His egocentrism is closely related to his developing sense of independence and autonomy. He is the focus of his world. When events do not go exactly as he expects and wants them to go, the toddler is prone to react through the familiar mode of temper tantrums. He is trying to express his desire to be respected as an individual and his desire to control the world.

This type of negativistic behavior is quite evident in a hospitalized toddler. Hospitalization and illness, as already discussed, impose many restrictions on his behavior, his activities, and ultimately his independence. Painful and frightening things are done to him without his having any control over the situation. In many hospital settings he is consulted about nothing and given no choice in what hap-

pens, not even an explanation. The result is a negativistic, hostile toddler.

The toddler needs help in finding appropriate outlets which allow him to maintain some sense of independence and autonomy, thereby decreasing his negativistic outbursts. He needs to be allowed the privilege of making choices whenever and wherever possible, helping to preserve his sense of independence and autonomy.

Physical settings for toddlers ideally should encourage their independence by making it easy for them to eat, dress, and use the bathroom by themselves. A potty chair near the bed, feeding tables, and an accessible area for clothes and belongings help. Another way of helping toddlers increase their sense of autonomy is to let them explore their environment within the limits needed for their safety. The will feel more independent when they know that they can leave the room, go to the playroom themselves, and find the nurse when they want her.

Despite the nurse's efforts to allow some control, there are still many aspects of hospitalization which lead to temper tantrums and negativism. Toddlers may express this behavior mainly with their parents, who are "safer." They may express negativism at meals, an activity with which they feel a sense of control. Handling of the negativistic toddler is a highly individual problem, depending on the child and the situation. Some toddlers respond to being ignored at this time; some need to be held firmly until they gain control. Diversion through play or another activity such as showing the child an interesting toy, directing him to look out the window, or getting him to help another person with something may also be successful.

Communication   The toddler's parents are the nurse's most important resource in attempting to establish communication. It is important to find out from the parents the important words in the child's vocabulary and his unique way of communicating his needs and concerns both verbally and nonverbally. For the toilet-trained toddler it is vital that the words used to communicate toileting needs are understood. He becomes frustrated when the nurse does not respond to his need and then chastises him for wetting the bed.

Nonverbal behavior is a very important avenue of communicating with the toddler. His facial expressions, body movements, and body restrictions can be clues that help the nurse understand how he feels about a situation. Nonverbal communication is a two-way exchange; nurses must remember that their feelings and frustrations are communicated to the toddler by facial expression, tone of voice, body movement, and gentleness or roughness of handling.

In communicating with toddlers, it is important to do the following:

1. Give one direction at a time, using simple words that have meaning for them.
2. Be gentle in manner and tone.
3. Approach them on their level—*verbally and physically.*

4. Be positive by suggesting what to do rather than what not to do.

Fears about Body Integrity The toddler rapidly is becoming more aware of his external body. He has started to name body parts and is becoming aware of and interested in the bodies of others. Because of his new awareness about his body, injury or loss of a body part tends to create concern about his body integrity (wholeness). Thus, the toddler is concerned about the slightest injury. He shows his injured part to everyone he sees and may demand that it be covered up with a bandage to restore his sense of body wholeness.

Explanations given to him are understood in a very egocentric, limited manner. It is hard to assess just what he is thinking about the situation; he may attach all sorts of fantasies to the experiences and explanations or may feel that he has done something wrong. He may also blame the illness experience on his parents, who until now have been his protectors.

Nursing and parental support of the toddler are very important in helping him overcome his fears and fantasies. The toddler feels supported if he knows that his parents and nurses understand some of his fears. For the older toddler, simple, basic explanations about his illness and about diagnostic and treatment measures should be given by his parents or his nurse. Even if he does not understand exactly what is said, he will be comforted by knowing that the significant adults in his world do understand what is happening. Staying with the toddler when procedures are being done is also a very important means of support. He needs to have someone he trusts hold his hand and allow him to express his fear and anxiety through crying, holding on tight, or talking. Since explanations are ineffective in comforting the child after a painful procedure, physical and psychological comfort can be provided instead by holding him for a short period.

Mobility If an illness or hospital experience imposes a restraint on this very important activity, one can expect great frustration. Bed rest, casts, traction, and other types of restraints which limit walking and mobility are a source of stress for the young child. He may react by fighting against the experience: climbing over siderails, tearing off a restraint, or trying to walk with the cast. Some toddlers react verbally by screaming and crying for hours on end. A few toddlers may react by withdrawal and depression.

An important rule for the nurse to remember regarding immobilization is to replace the lost activity with another form of motion. Walking can be replaced by other means of motion such as a stroller, wheelchair or by moving the bed. In some hospitals there are special carts for young children who need to move around despite the presence of casts or an order for bed rest. Keeping a toddler on bed rest is almost impossible (Fig. 9-4). He is much quieter and happier if held or put on a moving cart and taken to the playroom, where he can be a passive observer of others' activities.

If an arm or leg restraint is necessary because of intravenous therapy, surgery, or equipment, the restraint

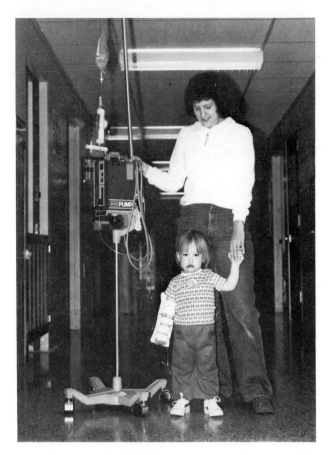

FIGURE 9-4 Mobility may be accomplished in various ways.

should be removed several times a day under close supervision so that the child can exercise the limb (unless movement is contraindicated) and the nurse can examine and care for the skin. Restraints on a toddler are often overused when simple explanations or other means of protection are less traumatic and more successful.

Immobility may decrease the child's opportunity to learn about himself, other people, and his environment through tactile, kinesthetic, and visual means. He needs the opportunity to develop through these sensory modalities. Water play, mirrors, body games, and back rubs are helpful replacements. Lack of mobility also decreases the toddler's opportunity to use his abundant energy and express his aggressive feelings. Activities such as tearing paper, pounding, and throwing balloons should be offered.

Regression Since the toddler so recently has acquired new abilities and more mature behavior, the stresses of illness and hospitalization can cause a regression in behavior. Regression can be expected in the areas of toileting, self-feeding, verbal communication, thumb sucking, and an increased need for security objects. Regression may be increased by undue anxiety, type of illness, or poor communication between child and staff members. Nursing staff members may also encourage regression by not accurately assessing the individual toddler's level of development. Toddlers are often automatically placed in diapers, fed by the nurse, or given a bottle.

The toddler's parents or nurse may expect him to maintain prior behavior at a time when this is very difficult or impossible. They may scold him, thus increasing his feelings of insecurity and inadequacy. Assessing the toddler's individual developmental levels and planning care accordingly may prevent regression. When regression occurs, the best approaches to helping the child are accepting his behavior, assuring him that he is understood, and helping him overcome the regression when he is ready.

Play The need for play does not cease in the hospital but becomes even more important. Play is helpful in making the hospital a more familiar place—toys are a universal sign of friendliness. Play can help in the establishment of a trusting relationship with a toddler, and it can serve as a means of communication with him. Through play he may express many nonverbal feelings. Play can serve as a diversion from the pain and fears he is experiencing. Play can become a replacement for mobility and can be helpful as an outlet for anger and frustration. It can also help the toddler feel more independent by giving him control over something and providing a sense of accomplishment. Thus, the toddler needs to have an opportunity for play in the hospital environment: play in a supervised playroom, play in his bed, play with his parents, and play with his nurses.

Play activities for the toddler must be chosen with regard to safety needs, limitations caused by illness, developmental level, and individual personality. Specific goals such as muscle strengthening, increasing coordination or dexterity skills, and learning about hospital routine and procedures may also be considered in selecting play activity.

Preschoolers

Preschoolers are very interested in the appearance and functions of the body. They become curious and upset about persons with visible handicaps or abnormalities. Even minor injuries or blemishes are likely to arouse anxiety. Preschool children are fearful about personal injury. They typically display their fear with crying and obvious upset whenever they get hurt, especially if there is bleeding

It is difficult for a preschooler to believe that injections, measurement of blood pressure or rectal temperature, and other health care procedures are not injurious and are motivated by good intentions. Young children's personal experiences and the common fantasies of their developmental stage lead them to believe that they may be annihilated (like television cartoon characters and balloons?) if punctured or broken (like toys and dolls?) if squeezed hard, as by a blood pressure cuff. They also believe that a person who deliberately performs acts that inflict pain or fear is motivated by hostility and a wish to punish.

Preschoolers have heard the warnings "Don't eat that or you'll get sick" and "Don't do that or you'll get hurt." When they are hurt or sick, they suppose they are to blame for having brought it on themselves. Therefore, preschoolers imagine that illness and injury are punishments for "bad" behavior, that the punishment is deserved, and that the unpleasant aspects of treatment constitute additional deserved punishment. The child also may perceive the hospital as a kind of jail where parents abandon disobedient children to be mistreated. A child may also have other troublesome ideas about hospitals. For example, he may think that, like someone else he has heard about, he will die in the hospital or will be given a baby to take home.

Under the stress and anxiety of these kinds of misperceptions, preschool children commonly display regression, denial, or other defense mechanisms. Less frequently a child will become aggressive in an attempt to "defend" himself against supposedly hostile nurses, physicians, and collaborating parents. Such children may shout abusively, call names, and even bite or kick.

Interventions for Hospitalized Preschoolers

It is difficult for any child to be sick and hospitalized, but many preschoolers continue positive growth and development throughout their confinement. This progress is to be encouraged so long as it does not exert additional stress on the child. When he can be permitted fairly normal motility and when his intrusive questioning and behavior are respected, the preschooler can learn a tremendous amount about himself, the hospital environment, and new relationships, even at his relatively immature level of comprehension. His ability to tolerate separation can be extended, and his coping devices can be enhanced.

Play

Ill or hospitalized preschool children need to play in order to improve their coping abilities and their understanding of what is happening to them. Play activities that are appropriate and helpful include but are not limited to the following:

Group activities with one other child or a small group

Telling stories, including stories about the child's own infancy

Singing songs, especially with accompanying body movements

Dressing up as adults or fantasy characters

Playing house

Coloring, cutting, and pasting

Throwing, hitting, or kicking balloons, beanbags, or other noninjurious soft toys

Riding toys: tricycle, wagon, scooter, fire truck

Pounding: hammer and peg toy, modeling clay

Pouring: fluids, sand, pebbles

Working with clay or Play Doh

Drawing pictures, finger painting, easel painting

Playing with toy cars and trucks, toy animals, dolls

Playing with small pets, watching goldfish

Playing outdoors

"Helping" adults

While all kinds of self-directed play are helpful, certain

play activities are specially designated as *therapeutic play.* In therapeutic play the nurse or other play therapist gives a child an opportunity to use toys and equipment with little or no instruction or interference while the therapist observes. The child's behavior during play expresses his fantasies, fears, and concerns, bringing them forward so that (1) the child can benefit directly by expressing anxieties and hostilities that might otherwise have remained "hidden" and (2) the therapist can take note of the attitudes and perceptions that the child reveals. A nursing care plan can then be designed to deal with issues revealed in the play setting, such as separation anxiety, guilt, and fear of mutilation.

It is common for children to move hesitantly and gradually into using the toys. They may glance at the nurse periodically for reassurance that it is permissible to "give shots" to the dolls and in other ways symbolically act out anger or curiosity (as by undressing the adults). In examining and manipulating syringes and other equipment and controlling the behavior of dolls, the child works toward achieving understanding and mastery of his experiences. In taking the role of other persons, the child is able to exert temporary control. These effects of play can help reduce anxiety and stress. In addition, play is indirectly ben-

eficial because the nurse can use the themes of the child's play as part of a nursing care plan. Misconceptions can then be corrected by means of age-appropriate teaching. Apprehensions can be reduced by means of truthful reassurances or changes in the way people interact with the child. It is important to note that the nurse does not interrupt the child's play to teach or otherwise intervene; interventions are made at a later time.

Drawings

Projective techniques are methods by which persons are able to reveal fantasies, anxieties, and attitudes through the use of symbols. A familiar example of a projective technique is the Rorschach test, in which a person makes up stories in response to pictures which resemble symmetrical inkblots. The stories are interpreted by a psychotherapist with special training in Rorschach testing. Simpler projective techniques can be used in the nursing care of children. The play kit described above is one such technique.

Drawings are another projective method that many small children can use, especially at ages 4 and 5 (and older). The self-portraits of a 5-year-old girl are shown in Fig. 9-5. Changes in her self-concept are evident from the

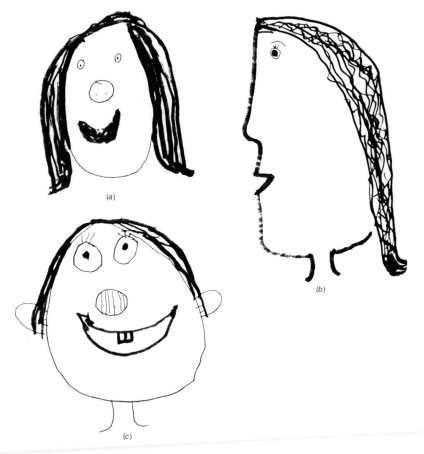

(a)

(b)

(c)

FIGURE 9-5   A 5-year-old was asked 7 days after neurosurgery for astrocytoma to draw three pictures of herself. Note how each picture differs from "year" to "year." (*a*) Herself "last year." Note her smile and long hair. (*b*) Herself "today." The profile may suggest her inability to look directly at herself or to have others see her. (*c*) After first drawing an imaginary X across the page, the child then drew this rather clownlike representation of herself and stated, "I'm sick of long hair." (Her hair had been cut preoperatively.)

drawings and the remarks she made as she drew. The nurse, aware of the child's loss of self-esteem, can arrange activities which bolster self-worth. Nurses also can offer attractive head coverings while reassuring the child that the hair will grow back.

Storytelling

Fictitious stories can be created to help preschoolers work through their experiences of sickness, injury, and hospitalization. It is important to end such stories happily with health and homecoming if that is consonant with the child's prognosis. A more difficult situation would invoke a chronically ill child. The stories told to such children should have realistic endings such as community programs or other social group activities which are available to them.

The nursery rhyme "Humpty Dumpty" may aggravate fears for an injured child who thinks that the doctor may be unable to "put him back together again." Cognitive immaturity requires that the preschooler have the story placed in perspective. A suggested concluding comment is the following: "But little boys and girls are different from eggs. When their bones break, they can be fixed. Besides, mommies and daddies could never find someone to replace their boy or girl. Mommies and daddies tell the doctor to do a good job, and then they take their children home when they're better."

School-Age Children

School-age children, especially those 6 through 9 years old, respond to illness or injury with many of the fantasies and misperceptions that are typical of preschoolers. It is a mistake to suppose that just because children have the intelligence and maturity for school they also automatically have an accurate understanding of their bodies and of illness and treatment. However they tend to conceal their ignorance and fears as they try to appear confident and grown-up.

Like younger children, school-age children believe that illness or injury is brought on by disobedience or other "bad" behavior and that the unpleasant treatments are punishments which they deserve because of their behavior. The health problem may have a fairly obvious self-induced component, as in the case of an accidental injury which occurred when the child was doing something he had been told not to do. In other cases the "cause-and-effect" link is illogical and known only to the child; for example, a child may imagine that he has gotten sick as a punishment for stealing or for hateful feelings toward a family member. In any case, guilt adds unnecessarily to the child's burden and interferes with coping. It is important to explain in understandable terms the cause of the problem and the reasons why the different treatments are being used. Parents and others also may believe that illness and accident are somebody's fault or punishments from God for someone's guilt. Since children commonly adopt their parents' beliefs, nurses need to be sensitive about finding out the parents' views as well as the child's.

School-age children frequently regress under the stress of illness or hospitalization. Unlike younger children, however, they usually find their own regressed behavior (and even the desire to regress) threatening and unacceptable to themselves. They place great value on acting grown-up and independent. They are likely to find "acting like a baby" and "being treated like a baby" very embarrassing. Being assisted with bathing or being bathed in bed, wearing pajamas all day instead of getting dressed, having urine or feces collected and inspected (or even mentioned), having the perineum exposed or examined, and sleeping in a bed with railings are among the experiences the school-age child equates with being treated like a baby or "little kid." Parts of his own behavior that he may find immature and therefore threatening and embarrassing include feeling afraid rather than brave, wanting to be held and comforted, and experiencing any loss of control over bodily functions such as bedwetting, fecal soiling, or vomiting on clothing or bedding. Privacy and modesty are important and must be respected.

Privacy and modesty are also major issues among older school-age children and those who are approaching puberty. However, their concern is more likely to relate to sexuality than to being regressed or babyish.

The loss of contact with friends is a serious threat to the school-age child, whose self-esteem is heavily dependent on continuous feedback from his peer group. When the health problem affects the child's appearance or physical function, the threat of losing status and even of being rejected or ridiculed compounds the child's anxiety and sorrow. Children also may fear that they will lose their place in the friendship group or even in the family if they are out of contact or incapacitated for very long.

Fears of disability and death are common even in children with minor illnesses and an excellent prognosis for complete recovery. Fantasies and misunderstandings abound. It is important to tell the child what is expected, if anything, in the way of residual defect or impairment after treatment and how long it is expected to last.

The hospital setting may seem bizarre and frightening even to children in the upper school-age years. This is especially true whenever perceptual accuracy is diminished, e.g., in semidarkness at night, when a child's vision or hearing is impaired, or when anxiety is high. Hospitals have many kinds of unfamiliar devices that look and sound scary. The sights (body casts, amputation, traction, gauze wraps "like a mummy") and sounds (respirators, suctioning, floor polishers, elevators, intercom systems) are also sometimes frightening and easily misconstrued. The nurse must be aware of the setting from the child's point of view and must give explanations even if the child has not asked. The nurse should emphasize the therapeutic purpose of the equipment or procedure to forestall misconceptions about punishment or torture and the fact that treatment is specific to each patient's needs so that the child will not mistakenly suppose that he too will have to undergo the same procedure or use a similar machine. For example, a nurse explaining leg traction might say that the ropes and weights are being used to hold a broken bone in place temporarily so that the bone can heal straight and that traction equipment is used only for people with broken bones.

Support of Hospitalized School-Age Children

Children of school age have many misconceptions and unrealistic fears related to their illnesses and injuries. The nurse should anticipate that fears are present even if the child masks them and should provide factual information (explanations, demonstrations, simulations, etc.) to reduce fantasy and anxiety.

Projective Techniques

Although school-age children's cognitive skills and language are more mature than those of younger children in terms of expressing what they think and what they fear, school-age children also are far more self-conscious and eager to save face by appearing to be well informed and unafraid. As a consequence, after age 5 years or so many youngsters keep their uncertainties and worries to themselves. Such children often can be led into conversation about their questions and fears if the nurse makes it clear that they are not the only ones who find the situation perplexing. Lead-in statements such as "Most children who come here wonder . . ." or "Lots of children worry about . . . because they have heard . . ." followed by facts to correct misinformation may be well accepted by school-age children. When they find the nurse accepting and sympathetic, they may take advantage of an invitation to ask their own questions if prompted by a statement such as "Maybe there is something else you would like to know about what we do here."

When simple conversation fails, the well-prepared nurse takes alternative routes to elicit the child's concerns and facilitate coping. If one is alert to the environment, projective devices "appear"; for example, television, books, and games frequently afford an opportunity to encourage verbalization of thought.

Therapeutic play as described for preschoolers can be used effectively with some school-age children, but in offering a play kit to a school-age child, the nurse must be prepared for the child's refusal to play. Playing with toys and dolls, especially while being observed, is too much like "kid stuff" for most school-age children, who are intent upon appearing more grown-up and try to avoid activities they consider childish. However, children of every age usually take advantage of opportunities to examine patient care equipment or models, including dolls that have been given sutures, chest tubes, and casts, provided that the materials are realistic and are presented as an educational experience rather than as play (Fig. 9-6). Romero (1986) described a technique using autobiographical scrapbooks and art to enable children to reveal and cope with their feelings about hospitalization.

A technique devised by Gellert (1962) has been employed to elicit data regarding the school-age child's un-

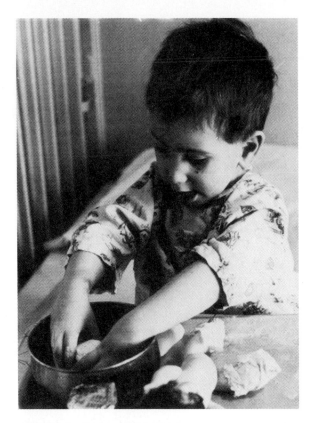

FIGURE 9-6   Child casting a doll as preoperative preparation. (*Courtesy of James Whitcomb Riley Hospital for Children, Indianapolis; Photo by G. Dreyer.*)

derstanding of his body and his illness. The child is asked to name the parts of his body under his skin, then to state the function of those body parts, and finally to suggest what would happen if each of the parts was missing (Figs. 9-7 and 9-8).

Children of this age enjoy creating puppet shows. Sometimes a little initial direction removes any potential threat; the nurse might suggest, for example, that a child devise a skit to orient him to the good and bad parts of being hospitalized.

Familiarizing Children with the Hospital

Familiarity with the hospital beyond the incidental tour of the department conducted on admission is helpful to the school-age child. Tours of the cardiac catheterization laboratory have been used in some hospitals to acclimate children who remain awake for the procedure. The tour can serve as a means to elicit questions and comments from children and parents regarding the procedure. When the tour is accomplished the day before catheterization, the school-age child has time to allay personal anxiety and prepare for the unavoidable test. Such a tour should be conducted only if the nurse later follows it up with supportive personal attention. An explanatory picture book about hospital areas serves a similar purpose for those reluctant to participate in a tour.

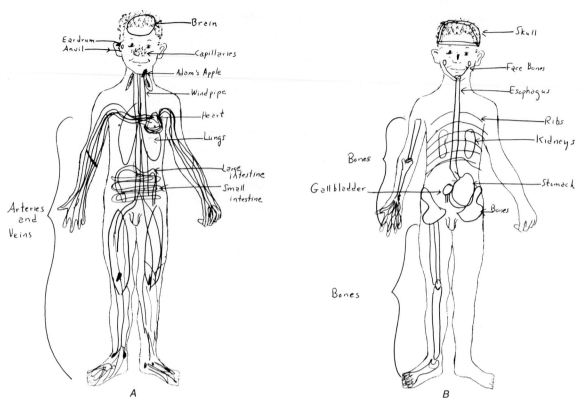

FIGURE 9-7   Richie's physiological drawing. (*a*)Rather precise completion of the outline. (*b*) Without a stomach or intestines, "you'd die."

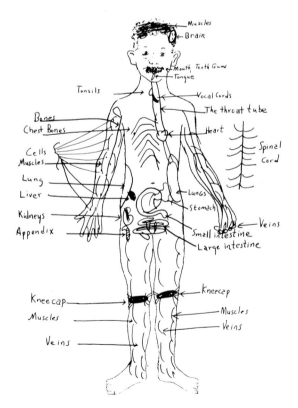

FIGURE 9-8   Eddie's physiological drawing. Muscles are important because "If you couldn't move you'd probably have a heart attack."

Providing Acceptable Outlets for Energy

Legitimate opportunities for self-expression of a rowdy nature are required. Ideally these opportunities take the form of playroom activities of punching, throwing, pounding, and general noise-making. However, any nurse caring for school-age children should anticipate being subjected to ridicule, disobeyed, and mimicked and should assume that her policies will sometimes be ignored. The probability of such behavior does not mean that letting children take over is desirable or that limits are not to be set and maintained; it merely calls for common sense and mature judgment based on awareness of the reasons behind the child's antagonistic behavior. A nurse with a firm self-concept can maintain equanimity and avoid involvement in petty quarrels with the children by applying developmental theory and remaining aware of the effect of hospitalization on behavior. The normal industriousness of the school-age child can be redirected cleverly to constructive activities which actually will satisfy the child more than misbehavior. Perhaps a child can be enlisted to make decorations for an unhappy child. Children of this age may also respond to an opportunity to calculate their own intake and output or determine caloric intake.

Organized Activities   Anxieties associated with illness, hospitalization, and their accompaniments are eased somewhat when the child is not left to flounder aimlessly in his strange environment. Organized activity, whether related to recreation or to schooling (preferably both), structures an otherwise seemingly random world of strange events. A recreation director, a school program, a library cart, planned events such as weekly movies or visits from celebrities, and a selected time in the playroom just for school-age children are some of the many successful methods of facilitating adjustment.

Members of social and benevolent organizations usually want to entertain sick children on special holidays or provide them with gifts. Since too much of this kind of activity in a short span of time proves too stimulating and disorganizing for the children, it would seem wiser to encourage interested persons to space their generosity throughout the year so that more children would benefit.

Adolescents

Interventions for Hospitalized Adolescents

The nursing care of adolescents needs to be designed in accordance with each patient's developmental traits and personal characteristics and background. Major developmental themes of the adolescent years that greatly influence the ways adolescents react to illness, disability, and health care are identity (self-concept, sex role, vocation, peer status, development of a personal value system, etc.), independence from parents, and establishment of interdependence in a love relationship. Individualistic factors such as the adolescent's family situation, past experiences, and adequacy of social supports for coping as well as the nature of the health problem also determine how each teenager responds to illness and hospitalization.

For ill adolescents, as for healthy ones, the basic question remains, Who am I? Despite the threat to their well-being posed by illness, they will continue to strive to adapt to the physical changes occurring in their bodies, clarify their sexual identities, realign their roles within the family and community, identify and refine meaningful personal value systems, select goals and prepare for future careers, and use their expanded intellectual skills more fully.

Knowledge about adolescent development and understanding of the goals toward which these young people are striving enable the nurse to view as strengths many behaviors that might otherwise be perceived as limitations. Nurses can provide knowledgeable care by focusing on the developmental strengths adolescents possess for dealing with illness and treatment.

The major physical changes that occur during adolescence have a great impact on the course of adolescents' physical illness states and on their psychosocial adaptation to them. Nurses must recognize and support the developing awareness and concern about bodily changes expressed by hospitalized adolescents.

Behavioral Responses

Often nurses become disturbed by the behavior they observe and move in impulsively to counter the actions of adolescents. In so doing, nurses fail to recognize that if they are patient enough to wait even a few minutes, adolescents are likely to alter their behavior to a tolerable, more balanced, mature level without assistance.

Adolescent behavior is one characterized by an exuberant and undaunted approach to life situations often resulting in overextension of self-sufficiency to provoke anxiety and fear. Suddenly the assertive, enthusiastic youngsters may retreat in fear and regress while reassessing what is happening to them. Once they recognize that they have regressed, they may feel a sense of guilt because they acted like babies and gave up the drive for independence. That recognition of what has happened spurs them on to strike out again toward adulthood. When both dependent and independent drives are expressed and accepted, adolescents have energy to assert themselves again and restart the cycle of behavior.

Understanding this pattern of behavior makes it possible for the nurse to recognize it, bear it, and respond in helpful ways. If adolescents are being assertive, the nurse can support this behavior by encouraging the self-assertion but protecting them from overextending to a degree where they are totally unable to manage themselves. In the face of regression, time must be allowed for the self-reassessment and problem solving that can take place if adolescents are protected from feelings of loss of self-esteem and guilt related to regression. The supported self-reassessment and problem solving strengthen adolescents' inner resources, helping them deal more effectively with new situations. Eventually the adolescents gain energy to reassert themselves and thus to learn and grow more effectively.

Maintaining Independence

The realignment of roles within the family and community that normally occurs during adolescence is an important consideration in caring for ill teenagers. In the presence of chronic illness in particular, the move from dependence on parents toward interdependence is sometimes slow and difficult. Strengths in adolescents that reflect striving toward independence can be identified and used to help hospitalized teenagers grow, as can strengths in their parents.

Throughout this discussion, it has been implied that adolescents possess an ability to solve problems. Too often intellectual skills are not identified on the list of strengths that this age group has available for dealing with illness and hospitalization. Adolescents, having developed to the highest cognitive level, can use thought processes to manipulate pieces of information and achieve solutions to problems. Once they find solutions to problems, they can consider the consequences without actually having to act them out. Frequently adolescents lack the pieces of information that they need for problem solving and the extensive experience that would assist them in deciding whether their solutions will achieve their goals.

Illness and hospitalization may interfere with intellectual growth by restricting the usual learning opportunities available to adolescents. Nurses can offset this problem by providing care that assists adolescents in identifying their problem-solving abilities, using these abilities, and gaining confidence in the use of their intellectual skills. Adolescent intellectual capacities can be stimulated by the multiple and varied problems encountered in the hospital environment.

Adolescents are often best equipped to know which actions will fit most comfortably into their own life-styles. They know their home routines and school days better than anyone else, and they need to help determine what actions are reasonable and workable for them in their own lives and settings.

It is obvious that adolescents need to be included in plans for their treatment, accepted as vital members of the health care team, and given the kind of information they desire and need to enable them to participate in their own care. They can be helped to decide what kinds and amount of information and supports are most appropriate in helping them prepare for and deal with potentially traumatic experiences. As they learn to recognize the actions that have been most helpful to them, they can begin to think them up by themselves and thus to expand their repertoire of methods to help themselves. By recognizing adolescents' ability to work with ideas and to solve problems skillfully and by encouraging them to practice these skills, the nurse enables them to resolve perplexing problems independently. In so doing, they are also helped to heighten their self-esteem, reduce their dependence upon others, become increasingly explicit in problem solving, and thus grow toward maturity.

Enhancing the Hospital Experience

The character of the environment in which the adolescent must come to terms with illness and treatment is another major factor in determining how effectively he will cope with problems. The concern of the persons around the adolescent and the support they are able to provide are important influences on the formation of adaptive responses to both long- and short-term experiences with illness. Groups of peers who support the ill adolescent provide assistance in maintaining a sense of self-esteem and a meaningful place in the world. A family that understands and cares provides the adolescent with strength and stability to cope with illness. Knowledgeable and concerned school, clinic, and hospital staff members can help the young person gain new skills to deal with change and crisis.

When treatment necessitates hospitalization, great strain may also be put on the teenager's ability to cope with the demands of a concurrent natural developmental crisis. Such stress is a further reason why it is so necessary that the hospital setting be designed to provide a growth-enhancing environment for adolescents. When groups of adolescents are cared for in one location, staff members can be recruited who are knowledgeable about their care and who find working with this age group an exciting, enjoyable, and challenging experience. A staff with both male and female members can give adolescents an opportunity to have experiences with those persons they can relate to most comfortably. A staff composed of persons with a variety of interests and talents can also help to develop each other's skills in such areas as purposeful listening, teaching, and use of humor (not teasing or ridicule, however). They can also share those methods of guidance which they have found most helpful in working with an adolescent population.

Through hospital school programs adolescents can be challenged to keep up with their classmates and make progress in achieving their educational goals. Such programs also help provide a semblance of normality in an adolescent's disrupted life-style. Recreational programs also are of help in overcoming boredom, releasing tension through activity, obtaining pleasure from sharing with others, and producing something of special value to adolescents. Nurses can play an important role in collecting data to substantiate a need for such programs or to point out the benefits to both lay and professional people.

When possible, an area of the hospital should be set aside where teenagers can enjoy the kinds of music, games, and socializing that are especially meaningful to them. For example, a lounge equipped with a Ping-Pong or pool table, record player, television, books and magazines, and pinball machines is very helpful to teenagers. If an outdoor area is available, a basketball and a place to shoot baskets will be used widely, even by adolescents confined to wheelchairs.

When units for adolescents do not exist, deliberate efforts will need to be made to provide individualized school and recreational programs which interest and stimulate teenagers' involvement. It is helpful for a nursing staff to compile a list of resource people who can be brought in to provide such services to adolescents in general hospital units. Such a list might include high school teachers or tutors, nurse specialists, recreation workers, and volunteers who have expertise in working with teenagers.

The adolescent may want to participate in making the decision whether to be admitted to a pediatric or an adult unit when no adolescent unit exists. Many teenagers find real satisfaction in being able to share their experiences as a means of helping to prepare other patients for special procedures, tests, or experiences in the hospital or clinic. They may enjoy and benefit from recognition of any contributions they can make in the hospital setting. They may want to help feed or entertain an elderly or a young patient. They may want to deliver the mail or help with some of the clerical work at the nurses' station. One student in an art school proudly donated several of his paintings to decorate the unit on which he had been hospitalized.

Flexibility of institutional rules, made with respect for the growing sense of independence and responsibility on the part of adolescents, also can be of help. Hospitalized adolescents enjoy sending out for a pizza together, watching a late television program, and having their need to "sleep in" the next morning respected. Through these activities the worth of teenagers is respected, a sense of caring about them as individuals is conveyed, and the staff's ability to bend institutional tradition to provide for the satisfaction of personal needs is demonstrated.

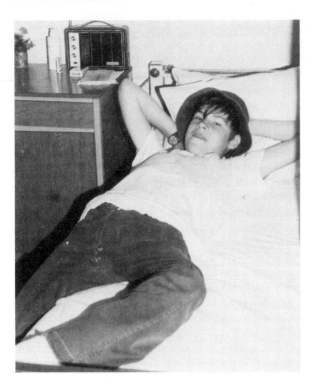

FIGURE 9-9   Whenever possible, adolescents should wear their own clothes during hospitalization.

Adolescents have to maintain their sense of identity in the face of a changed body, an unfamiliar setting, new expectations, and difficult problems. Making it possible for them to wear their own clothes and to decorate their beds and rooms to express themselves and to make them uniquely theirs also manifests respect for their personal likes and dislikes (Fig. 9-9). Bulletin boards at each bedside can allow for hanging favorite posters or cards. When possible, provision of a space for privacy where adolescents can be alone if they feel the need is also of importance. A quiet conference room for private conversations and provision for privacy while bathing, dressing, and being examined and treated are essential to meet the needs of teenagers. Access to mirrors in rooms and bathrooms also is needed and especially valued by both sexes.

Most teenagers are dependent on their peer group for support. When they are ill and hospitalized, access to friends is important. Whenever teenagers' conditions permit, their friends should be welcomed in the hospital and space should be provided where they can meet without disturbing others. Adolescents usually are quick to make new friends in the hospital and frequently derive much support from peers who are coping with similar problems. This characteristic can be supported by appropriate selection of roommates, provision for regular meetings of teenagers in the hospital, and the setting up of group meeting hours in clinics for adolescents with similar health problems (Fig. 9-10). School nurses can play a vital role in helping adolescents meet and support each other with health-related issues. Bedside telephones are invaluable to hospitalized teenagers, allowing them to maintain contact

with their friends at home and continue to receive their support. Telephones also serve to preserve interest in an activity which was probably an important part of their life-style at home.

Discharge Planning

In the effort to provide comprehensive nursing care for the hospitalized pediatric patient and his family, nursing intervention involves several interrelated functions. The nurse is concerned with providing (1) direct physical care, (2) psychological support for the child and his family, and (3) appropriate activities to promote the continued growth and development of the child and utilize his capabilities fully. These activities are necessary whether the child is acutely or chronically ill.

The long-range goals in the care of a child hospitalized with an acute illness are (1) returning the child to the highest possible level of physical and emotional health and (2) maintaining the family integrity. With a chronically ill child, the long-range goal is the maintenance of the highest possible level of physical and emotional health for both child and family. If the child and family are faced with a terminal illness, the long-range goal is keeping the child at home for as long as possible while providing support for both the child and family in order to maximize coping abilities and family function. With any hospitalization, one of the goals is also to minimize the psychological trauma to the child.

When these long-range goals are part of the care plan during hospitalization, the integration of the components

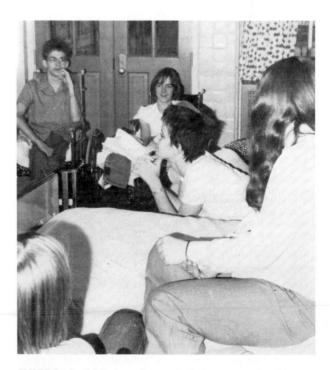

FIGURE 9-10   Adolescents frequently derive support from discussions with peers who are coping with similar problems.

of the nursing process includes planning for discharge. The pediatric nurse needs to be concerned with what happens to the child and family upon discharge and return home. The nurse assumes a leadership role in assessing the need for ongoing care after discharge and is also instrumental in the planning, implementation, and evaluation of discharge and postdischarge care. Increasingly, institutions are utilizing community health specialists to meet the complex needs of patients and families in this area.

Factors that Influence Discharge Planning

Discharge planning involves (1) connecting families with community resources to promote continuity between the hospital and the home and (2) adapting institutional therapies to the home setting. Often the nurse on the unit is responsible for family teaching while the continuing care nurse works with outside agencies to develop a home plan for services and support for the family's transition to the home.

Planning for discharge begins with the admission of the child. During the admission interview the nurse obtains information that will be useful in this planning.

Throughout the child's hospital stay additional information is gathered which will help the nurse identify learning needs and determine the capabilities of the child and family. Several variables will influence the specifics of the discharge planning as it evolves. Consideration must be given to physical needs related to the illness, to growth, and to developmental, emotional, social, and environmental needs. The delineation of the priority of needs will be influenced further by (1) the age of the patient, (2) the severity of the health problem, (3) the patient and family response to medical and nursing intervention, (4) the strengths and resources of the family in providing for the child's continuing care needs, and (5) the involvement of the child and family in the planning for discharge.

Components of Discharge Planning
Assessment

Identification of learning needs and assessment of the family's ability to provide care and cope with the illness ramifications supply the core of the discharge plan. How does the nurse identify the learning needs of the child and family? Some needs will be identified easily. If the child is a newly diagnosed cardiac or diabetic patient, the need to understand medication and diet management is obvious. The ability of the child and/or family to understand the disease process, deal with acceptance of the illness or injury, and provide long-term care at home is less easily determined. Observations of the child and family and involvement of them in care during the hospitalization are necessary if needs are to be adequately identified.

Other learning needs will be established as the child or family members ask direct questions of the nurse. Will Johnny's activity be limited when he gets home? How am I going to keep a 4-year-old quiet for a month? Where can I buy the special formula my baby needs? What should I do if the tube comes out?

Learning needs related to direct physical care are determined more easily by both the nurse and the family. However, the nurse must remember that many families are hesitant to ask questions. Careful listening to the parents as they talk to the nurse and to the parent and child as they interact will help the nurse further identify needs to be met in preparation for discharge.

Observation of the behavior of the child and family may provide the nurse with additional information. Comprehensive nursing care involves assessment of the parent-child relationship. Parents may need teaching and anticipatory guidance so that they can provide discipline, achieve realistic expectations for the child's behavior, manage his fears and anxieties, and cope with his normal developmental tasks.

Assessment of the family's ability to provide care and cope with the ramifications of illness will need to include consideration of additional factors such as the family constellation and whether a support system is present or there are stresses which may be increased because of the child's illness and hospitalization. In discharge planning, family relationships and means of assisting the parents and child must be considered.

What are the job responsibilities and the financial status of the family? If the mother has to work, is a competent caregiver available? If the father is a single parent, who cares for the child while he works? Does the substitute caregiver need instruction? Are funds available to the family to pay for necessary continuing services, special equipment, or dietary supplements? Planning must be realistic.

What care is required? Can it be carried out by the family members? If not, what resources are available to the family in the local community? Needs must be anticipated early in the hospitalization if realistic goals for discharge and follow-up care are to be determined and intervention is to be planned accordingly.

Planning and Goal Setting

The family and the child, if old enough, must be involved actively in the goal setting and planning for discharge. They are the source of much of the information mentioned above. They also need to know what is to be accomplished before discharge and what will be needed after discharge if they are to make realistic plans and family arrangements. Teaching the mother a particular procedure is not enough if the grandmother cares for the child much of the day. Plans must include obtaining special equipment, food, medications, and the like.

In most instances at least two disciplines—medicine and nursing—are involved in the care of a child. In many cases several disciplines are involved. Communication between the physician, nurse, and other health team members is vital to the preparation for discharge. Cooperative identification of needs and determination of goals will allow for the contribution of each discipline. Coordination of discharge planning is a responsibility of the nurse and can be accomplished most easily when one nurse plans the child's care throughout the hospitalization. The primary nurse has the greatest opportunity to implement teaching and to reinforce it with the child and family. The nurse is also best able to assess readiness for discharge and must assume responsibility for communicating this assessment to other members of the team.

In addition to effective verbal communication and cooperative planning, a written plan for discharge is essential. It should include the goals for the individual child and family and specific instructions necessary to carry out the plan. Movement toward the goals and completion of specific parts of the plan also are indicated in writing. This written plan allows for consistency between disciplines and between the shifts of nursing personnel providing care to the child and family.

Intervention

Teaching the Child and Family

Since teaching is a primary tool utilized by the nurse in preparing the child and family for discharge, a brief review of some of the basic principles of teaching as discussed by Redman (1980) is appropriate.

Learning goals can be classified into three domains. The cognitive domain focuses on understanding; the affective domain, on attitudes; and the psychomotor domain, on motor skills. Teaching in preparation for discharge most commonly involves all three domains. The nurse is concerned with the child's and family's understanding of the illness process or injury, the acceptance of the illness or injury by the child and family, and the development of the motor skills needed for management. Specific learning goals will vary with the individual child's or family's abilities and situation. Goals for the child and the teaching methods used must take into consideration his intellectual level, motor skill ability, and psychosocial development.

Motivation is required if the individual is to learn. Telling the child or family about the illness process or treatment method does not ensure learning. Learning is most effective when the individual is ready to learn. Motivation and learning readiness must be assessed continually by the nurse in planning for and implementing the teaching for discharge.

In the hospital situation, several factors can interfere with or delay the readiness of the child or family to learn. The process of adaptation will vary with the severity of illness and its implications for the child and family. Early in the adaptation process, denial or disbelief is often present. Even though the nurse must begin planning for discharge upon admission, it may take several days of support and reinterpretation of information before acceptance begins to occur and the child and family are ready to begin learning. Helping the child and family to reach this point is a part of the preparation for discharge. The child or family faced with birth defects, diabetes, leukemia, or serious trauma such as burns, head injuries, or multiple system injuries may have a prolonged adaptation period.

The nurse will also need to consider the hierarchy of human needs when assessing readiness to learn. Maslow lists physiological needs as most basic, followed by safety, love and belonging, self-esteem, and self-actualization. A child who is in pain or who is frightened of all that is happening to him will not be receptive to teaching. A family that is extremely insecure and anxious cannot be attentive to teaching. A mild level of anxiety is helpful in learning, but increasing levels are detrimental.

Closely intertwined with the emotional readiness to learn is experiential readiness. Learning moves most easily from the known to the unknown. Does the child or family possess the knowledge needed as a basis for learning a new skill? Are attitudes present that will interfere with learning? Assessment of prerequisite knowledge and behaviors is necessary if the nurse is to carry out teaching in a manner that is meaningful to the learner.

The material to be learned must be presented in a form that can be understood by the child and family. A variety of teaching methods are available to the nurse. One-to-one or group discussion can be used and supplemented with audiovisual materials such as booklets and filmstrips. Often the nurse will have to use ingenuity in adapting materials to fit the situation. When the requirement is the learning of physical skills, demonstration, return demonstration, and practice are the most effective. The materials the family will be using at home should be utilized. As a part of discharge preparation, the nurse will plan with the family to allow time for practice. The child and family must be able to "get into the act" if changes in behavior, development of understanding, and competency in motor skills are to occur. Perhaps the best way to accomplish this mutuality is to have the parent(s) room with the child and assume responsibility for care while the nurse is available for support and assistance.

It is also important for the nurse to remember that materials to be learned should be presented in small parts and in sequential order. It is easy for the family to be overwhelmed by having "so much to learn." An overview of what needs to be accomplished before discharge is helpful, but this information must be coupled with the assurance that the objectives will be accomplished "one step at a time." The learner needs to receive feedback as to his accomplishments and progress toward the goals. Positive feedback and successes will provide motivation to continue the learning process.

Communication at Discharge

Telephone communication with resources in the child's community can be utilized during the planning for discharge and at the time of discharge. A complete written referral form or discharge summary which includes family data, goals for the child and family, known or anticipated assistance needed, teaching carried out in the hospital, and current status of the child and family should be immediately available to those providing follow-up care. It is also important that the family and person or agency providing care know whom to contact at the hospital if they have questions. Many questions related to the day-to-day care of the child at home can be answered best by the nurse who has cared for the child during hospitalization. Parents need to know that they may call and seek assistance at any time. The family needs clearly written in-

Discharge Planning for a Toddler

Katie, 2 years old, was admitted for treatment of pneumonia. She lived with parents and a 4-year-old brother, and she was cared for by her grandmother while her mother worked. She was followed by a pediatrician for routine child care. Management of the acute illness and support during the crisis episode were the focus of most of the nursing interventions. Katie would not be discharged until the chest x-ray and other clinical data indicated that the pneumonia had been treated adequately. Her mother was rooming-in so that separation anxiety was minimized. Discharge planning, however, had to include consideration of the following factors: (1) iron-deficiency anemia discovered on admission, (2) follow-up for the pneumonia, (3) learning needs of the grandmother in caring for Katie, and (4) anticipatory guidance relative to behavior changes in Katie and her brother which might occur because of disruption of the family during the hospitalization. Setting of appropriate goals with the family and determination of behaviors indicating attainment of goals were necessary.

Need: Knowledge about iron-deficiency anemia
Goals: Prior to discharge parents and grandmother will be able to
1. Describe the causes of iron-deficiency anemia
2. Name specific foods important in Katie's diet

3. Demonstrate accurate measurement of the iron supplement
4. State time and method of administration and side effects

Need: Anticipatory guidance relative to behavior changes in Katie and her brother upon family reintegration
Goals: Prior to discharge parents and grandmother will be able to
1. Describe specific behaviors which might occur, such as regression in developmental behavior, clinging and anxiety upon separation from parents, fear of strangers, and night fears
2. Discuss reasons for the behavior
3. Describe their method of management

Need: Follow-up of the acute illness episode
Goals: Prior to discharge the parents will be able to
1. Describe the signs and symptoms which might indicate a recurrence of the illness
2. State when Katie is to return to her doctor for follow-up care

It was decided that a referral to the community health nurse was not indicated. A copy of the hospital course summary and the discharge summary were sent to the physician.

---

structions and information regarding medications, dressing changes, exercises, activity, and any other procedure they are expected to carry out.

Evaluation

Teaching requires that some method of evaluation be used to determine its effectiveness. The nurse may want to use a variety of methods such as oral questions and answers, written quizzes, and return demonstrations, during the hospitalization to determine one's teaching effectiveness. Evaluation is continued after discharge to determine the persistence of the change in behavior and evaluate the ability of the child and family to continue care in the home setting. Feedback from the community health nurse, evaluation at later visits to the clinic or physician's office, or other communication with agencies providing care is necessary if improvement is to occur in discharge preparation. Thorough planning for discharge is exemplified in the cases described above and on p. 199.

Learning Activities

1. Assume the role of a hospitalized adolescent who is overweight. Ask another student to play the role of a nurse who is discussing goals and outcomes with the teenager. Have the remaining students critique the amount of patient involvement in the planning and attaining of the goals which were developed.
2. Interview the parents of a toddler who is hospitalized in order to identify the emotions they are experiencing.
3. Review several hospital books for children and lead a group discussion to evaluate them. Determine the accuracy of content, appropriateness, and appeal to children.
4. Identify potential safety hazards in the pediatric clinical setting and determine how they can be alleviated or how children can be protected from them.

School-Age Child with Accidental Injury

Paul, a 7-year-old, was admitted following an accident. He had been hit by a car while riding his bicycle. His presenting problems were a fracture of the left femur, multiple abrasions, and a mild cerebral concussion.

Past Medical History Paul had had measles, chickenpox, and the usual colds and gastrointestinal upsets but no illnesses requiring hospitalization. Immunizations were up to date.

Social History Paul lives with his mother, father, and a sister age 4. All family members were in good health. His father was employed as a maintenance man for the local telephone company, and his mother was a homemaker. They had insurance which would cover most of the hospital costs.

Treatment Paul's condition was relatively stable on admission. Physical and developmental assessment revealed no abnormal findings other than the fracture, abrasion, and concussion. He was responsive but frightened unless his mother was close by. The abrasions were cleansed, and the left leg was placed in Russell's traction to maintain immobilization and alignment. The physician explained to the parents that Paul would be in traction for 2 to 3 weeks and then would be placed in a spica cast for several weeks. He would probably be discharged a day or two after the cast was applied.

With the overall goals of returning the child to the highest possible level of physical and emotional health and maintaining the family integrity, much of the care in the hospital was carried out with preparation for discharge in mind.

Need Paul's parents were both anxious and guilty. They verbalized, "We shouldn't have let him ride his bike in the street."

In-hospital intervention and application to postdischarge care Listened, empathized with normal concerns for Paul's safety. Reinterpreted normal activity levels of 7-year-old, need for independence, and impossibility of their watching him constantly. Reassured them that the accident was not their fault. Allowed parents to verbalize feelings about the accident. Prevented overprotection and limitation of activity and independence after recovery.

Need Paul was worried about missing schoolwork and not being able to ride his bike again.

In-hospital intervention and application to postdischarge care Assured Paul that he would be able to ride his bike again. Explained in simple terms the need for the leg to rest and get better. Used appropriate pictures of bones and casts. Arranged for Paul's family to bring in his books and assignments from school so that the hospital schoolteacher, family and nursing staff could continue his lessons. (If hospital teacher is not available, contact local school system for tutoring.) Allowed for clarification of the temporary nature of the immobility and helped Paul understand the reason for the traction and cast. Maintained intellectual stimulation and developmental level, making return to school easier.

Need Paul's mother felt she needed to bathe him and help him with every meal.

In-hospital intervention and application to postdischarge care Care by the mother was permitted early in the hospitalization, with discussion of the need for Paul to help himself as much as possible. Fostered independence and self-care as much as possible during hospitalization and after discharge.

Need Immobility interfered with need for activity and industry, occasionally leading to anger and frustration.

In-hospital intervention and application to postdischarge care Provided activities for release of aggressive or angry feelings—punching bag suspended from traction bar. Provided activities to foster creativity within the confines of the traction—construction projects, painting, drawing, scrapbook. Met needs for activity and industry in the hospital and showed mother ways of meeting these needs at home.

Need Paul's immobility and hospitalization interfered with his sibling and peer contact.

In-hospital intervention and application to postdischarge care Used telephone and parents to maintain home and sibling contact. Encouraged mother to have classmates and friends send cards and letters. Fostered reintegration of the family and peer group relations after discharge and recovery. Maintained contact with the outside world.

Need Home assessment was needed in preparation for discharge.

In-hospital intervention and application to postdischarge care Explored the living situation at home. Paul's bedroom was upstairs. A daybed was available downstairs, and Paul's father felt he could carry him up and down. A bed board was to be obtained by the family. The family car was a station wagon, and so transportation to and from the hospital and inclusion of Paul in some family outings would not be a problem. A bedpan and urinal were also obtained by the family. Because discharge needs were anticipated, the family was prepared to leave the hospital ahead of schedule.

Need The family needed to feel comfortable and competent in caring for Paul in his cast.

In-hospital intervention and application to postdischarge care The mother was involved with his care after the hip spica was applied. Teaching included the care of the cast, observation of toes for circulation, observations of the cast which might indicate an infection underneath, inspection of skin for irritation from cast edges, checking for small objects which might become lodged underneath the edges of the cast, and the proper method of turning and positioning. Instructions titled "Going Home in a Cast" were also given to the family.

Since Paul's mother could not move him by herself, a referral was made to the visiting-nurse association to provide a daily home health aide and weekly community nurse visits to assess Paul's progress and support the family. The family members were given the unit number to call if problems arose.

Preparation for the discharge of Paul focused primarily on assisting the mother in meeting the physical and psychosocial needs of a 7-year-old who was to be immobilized for several weeks.

Study Questions

1. Prior to a scheduled hospitalization:
   1. The child should know he is going to the hospital.
   2. The child should be told at least 2 weeks before the date of admission.
   3. The child's age should determine when he is told about the hospitalization.
   4. The child needs to participate in planning the hospital visit as much as possible.
      - A. 1 and 2
      - B. 1 and 3
      - C. 1, 3, and 4
      - D. 2 and 4

2. The objectives of an admission procedure are to:
   1. Acquaint the family with the physical facilities and services of the hospital.
   2. Detect possible problems
   3. Exchange information.
   4. Support the family.
      - A. 1, 2, and 3
      - B. 1 and 4
      - C. 1 and 3
      - D. 1, 2, 3, and 4

3. An infant's needs can best be met by:
   - A. A rooming-in arrangement which allows a parent to stay 24 hours a day.
   - B. Open visiting hours which allow parents to come and go freely.
   - C. A hospital which provides primary nursing.
   - D. Nurses who maintain close relationships with parents.

4. Prior to doing a procedure on an infant the nurse should:
   - A. Hold the baby for a few minutes.
   - B. Proceed quickly so that the infant can be comforted.
   - C. Advise the parents away from the infant about what is to be done.
   - D. Tell the baby what is to be done even though he cannot comprehend.

5. In helping a toddler cope with a painful procedure the nurse should:
   1. Calmly explain why the procedure was done.
   2. Comfort the child physically.
   3. Remain with the toddler afterward.
   4. Encourage the parents to stay even though they do not wish to be there.
      - A. 1, 2, 3, and 4
      - B. 2 and 3
      - C. 2, 3, and 4
      - D. 1, 2, and 3

6. A hospitalized preschooler's development can be nurtured during hospitalization through:
   1. Normal play.
   2. Orientation to the hospital environment.
   3. Therapeutic play.
   4. Detailed explanations.
      - A. 1, 2, and 3
      - B. 1 and 2
      - C. 2 and 3
      - D. 1, 2, 3, and 4

7. The role which illness may play in the life of an adolescent depends on:
   - A. The developmental strengths of the adolescent.
   - B. The nature of the illness and the treatment plan.
   - C. The quality of support systems available.
   - D. All of the above.

8. In working with the hospitalized adolescents, it is important for a nurse to remember that they need:
   1. Privacy.
   2. Space for personal belongings.
   3. An area where they can gather for meals and activities.
   4. An atmosphere with structure so that they know boundaries.
      - A. 1 and 2
      - B. 1, 2, and 3
      - C. 2 and 3
      - D. 1, 2, 3, and 4

9. Planning for the discharge of a school-age child begins:
   - A. Several days before he goes home.
   - B. When the family is available.
   - C. On the day of admission.
   - D. The morning of the discharge date.

10. The effectiveness of teaching done by a nurse can be evaluated by:
    - A. Oral questioning.
    - B. Written quizzes.
    - C. Return demonstrations.
    - D. All of the above.

References

Erickson, F.: "Play Interviews for Four-Year-Old Hospitalized Children," *Monographs of the Society for Research in Child Development,* 23(3):69, 1958.

Gellert, E.: "Children's Conception of the Content and Function of the Human Body," *Genetic Psychology Monographs,* 64:293-405, 1962.

Harris, C.J.: "The Neonate," in G. Scipien et al. (eds.), *Comprehensive Pediatric Nursing,* 3d ed., McGraw-Hill, New York, 1986, pp. 339-364.

Klaus, M.H., and J.H. Kennell: "Mothers Separated from Their Newborn Infants," *Pediatric Clinics of North America,* 17(4):1015-1037, 1970.

————: *Bonding: The Beginnings of Parent-Child Attachment,* Mosby, St. Louis, 1983.

Redman, B.K.: *The Process of Patient Teaching in Nursing,* Mosby, St. Louis, 1988.

Robertson, J., and J. Robertson: "Young Children in Brief Separations—A Fresh Look," in *Psychoanalytic Study of the Child,* Quadrangle, New York, 1972.

Romero, R.: "Autobiographical Scrapbooks: A Coping Tool for Hospitalized School Children," *Issues in Comprehensive Pediatric Nursing,* 9(4):247-258, 1986.

Bibliography

Ack, M.: "Psychological Effects of Illness and Hospitalization and Surgery," *Association for the Care of Children in Hospitals Journal,* 11(4):132-136, 1983.

D'Antonio, I.: "Therapeutic Use of Play," *Nursing Clinics of North America,* 19:351-359, 1984.

Garot, P.A.: "Therapeutic Play: Work of Both Child and Nurse," Journal of Pediatric Nursing, 1(2):111-116, 1986.

May, B., and M. Sparks: "School-Age Children: Are Their Needs Recognized and Met in Hospital Settings?" *Association for the Care of Children in Hospitals Journal,* 12(3):118-121, 1984.

Nadler, H.: "Art Experience and Hospitalized Children," *Association for the Care of Children in Hospitals Journal,* 11(4):160-164, 1983.

Poster, E.: "Stress Immunization: Techniques to Help Children Cope with Hospitalization," *Journal of Maternal-Child Nursing,* 12(2):119-134, 1983.

Thompson, R.H.: *Psychosocial Research on Pediatric Hospitalization and Health Care: A Review of the Literature,* Thomas, Springfield, Ill., 1985.

Yaros, P.S., and J. Howe: "Responses to Illness and Disability," in J. Howe (ed.): *Nursing Care of Adolescents,* McGraw-Hill, New York, 1980.

Zurlinden, J.K.: "Minimizing the Impact of Hospitalization for Children and Their Families," *American Journal of Maternal-Child Nursing,* 10(3):178-182, 1985.

Zweig, C.D.: "Reducing Stress When a Child Is Admitted to the Hospital," *American Journal of Maternal-Child Nursing,* 11(1):24-26, 1986.

Books for Families

Bach, A.: *Waiting for Johnny Miracle,* Harper & Row, New York, 1980.

Elliot, I.G.: *Hospital Roadmap: A Book to Explain the Hospital Experience to Young Children,* Resources for Children in Hospitals, Belmont, Mass., 1984.

Masoli, L.A.: *Things to Know Before You Go to the Hospital,* Silver Berdett, Morristown, N.J., 1984.

Reit, S.: *Jenny's in the Hospital,* Golden Books, New York, 1984.

————: *Some Busy Hospital,* Golden Books, New York, 1984.

Stein, S.: *A Hospital Story: An Open Family Book for Parents and Children Together,* Walker, New York, 1984.

10

Common Pediatric Nursing Procedures

Although some people consider children to be miniature adults, pediatric nurses know that anatomic, physiological, psychosocial, and cognitive differences typify this client population and are responsible for the challenges of this clinical specialty. No changes in a human being's existence are as dramatic as those which occur from birth through adolescence. Even though body size is an obvious variable, the age and developmental stage of a child determine a nurse's actions, interventions, and strategies. The specific growth and developmental aspects of the six stages of childhood are described fully in Part I.

Nurses must be creative in dealing with children. For example, as a result of variations in body size, pediatric equipment is not standardized as it is for adults, and so nurses must be resourceful in adapting equipment to meet the highly individualized needs of an infant or child.

Safety is a major concern too; children may not under-stand the nature of certain pieces of equipment, and so it may be necessary to protect them from the equipment or protect the equipment from them. Children often do not behave the way an adult would, and a nurse needs to anticipate childhood responses to certain occurrences. For example, a toddler usually resists intravenous therapy, and although the needle is securely placed, restraints frequently are needed to ensure continued patency.

Children's differences in body size are conspicuous, and this variation complicates accurate computation of intravenous fluids and medications. Fluid requirements are calculated on the basis of weight, surface area, or caloric needs. In the past a variety of formulas were used to compute drug doses, but they were completely inadequate for neonates. Also, dosages based on age alone were inaccurate because of tremendous variations in the body size of children within the same age group.

Fluid and electrolyte needs and medication dosages can be determined more accurately if they are based on body surface area (BSA), especially in smaller children, who have a greater BSA in relation to volume than do larger children. Height and weight are plotted on a nomogram, and the line which intersects with the surface area column identifies the child's BSA. The value is expressed in meters squared (m^2). An appropriate pharmaceutical dose is calculated by multiplying a patient's BSA by the dosage of the drug per square meter (Shirkey, 1973).

Teaching is critical to the restoration, maintenance, and promotion of health. In pediatrics, the cognitive level of the learner identifies the focus of the nurse's efforts. With a client who is less than 2 years old and in Piaget's sensorimotor stage (Chap. 2), the emphasis is on teaching parents or other adult caretakers. However, age-appropriate teaching strategies are gradually transferred to and involve other toddlers, preschoolers, and school-age children as their ability to comprehend develops. Adolescents, who are in the formal operations period, are cognitively mature and should be treated accordingly.

Pediatric nurses also deal with clients whose body systems are at various maturational stages; this accounts for differences in laboratory values, nutritional requirements, and vital signs at various stages of childhood. Certainly all these variables contribute to the challenges of pediatric nursing. In essence, children are different.

Administration of Medications

Drugs travel to all parts of the body by means of absorption, distribution, metabolism, and excretion. Many medications are given to infants and children by mouth and are absorbed in the small intestine. Any changes in intestinal motility, gastric pH, or intestinal enzymes can affect drug uptake by the blood. Neonates have decreased intestinal motility and gastric pH as well as delayed development of intestinal enzymes. Therefore, for this age group a drug's effectiveness, toxicity, and dosage requirements may be affected.

Once a medication has reached the bloodstream, it is delivered to the body tissues. During infancy and childhood the continual change in relative tissue mass which results from normal physical growth influences the uptake of a drug.

The liver is extremely important in metabolizing drugs. In the first 2 or 3 weeks of life immature hepatic enzymes affect a newborn's ability to metabolize some drugs. The liver of a neonate constitutes 4 percent of total body weight, whereas the adult liver constitutes only 2 percent of total body weight. Relative liver size is important in regard to the rate at which metabolized drugs are eliminated. Thus infants and children metabolize drugs more rapidly than adults do.

The kidneys are very important in excreting drugs. In the first 3 to 4 weeks of life the glomerular filtration and tubular secretion and reabsorption capabilities are impaired. Mature renal function occurs sometime around the fifth to seventh month of age. Therefore, drug toxicity is a very real danger during the neonatal period.

Computing Correct Dosages

The same general precautions one would use with adults (e.g., checking the correctness of the drug, dosage, time, and route) are used with children. Since there are no unit dosages for children of various ages and weights, nurses must calculate dosages from standard doses. For example, an infant is to receive erythromycin 120 mg as a liquid preparation that contains erythromycin 200 mg in 5 ml of liquid. The nurse can use the "desired over at hand" method to determine how many milliliters will contain the desired 120 mg:

$$\frac{\text{Desired amount}}{\text{Amount at hand}} = \frac{120 \text{ mg}}{200 \text{ mg}}$$

This fraction is reduced to ⅗, and ⅗ of the original 5 ml is 3 ml. An alternative method of performing this calculation is to set up the known and unknown quantities as a ratio: 120 mg is to χ ml as 200 mg is to 5 ml; $200\chi = 600$; $\chi = 3$ ml.

The most accurate methods of calculating pediatric dosages are based on either BSA or kilograms of body weight (e.g., 10 mg/kg/dose, or 40 mg/kg/d) (Fig. 10-1). Nurses can estimate the accuracy of children's dosages in several ways. The three most frequently used estimation methods are

$$\frac{\text{Weight of Child in pounds}}{150} \times \frac{\text{average adult dose}}{} = \text{estimated childs dose}$$

$$\frac{\text{BSA of Child}}{\text{BSA of adult}} \times \text{adult dose} = \text{estimated child's dose}$$

BSA of child in m^2 × dose per m^2 = estimated child's dose

Methods of Administering Medications

Administering medications to children may be fraught with danger. Nurses *must* know the drugs they are giving and how to calculate the correct dose, prepare fractional doses, identify toxic symptoms, and recognize untoward reactions. Nurses need to know that the immaturity of organs affects the rates of absorption and excretion. They must rely on observations to evaluate the effectiveness of the drug or identify its toxic signs, since some children cannot describe symptoms due to their age or condition.

The routes of administering medication to children are oral, ophthalmic, otic, nasal, intramuscular, subcutaneous, and intravenous. The approach a nurse selects depends on the physician's order, the child's stage of development, and the successful methods parents have used. In Table 10-1 specific growth and developmental principles, modes of administration, and effective nursing approaches according to stages are identified.

Intravenous Medications

Children who need intravenous medications must have an intravenous infusion in place. The site selected varies with

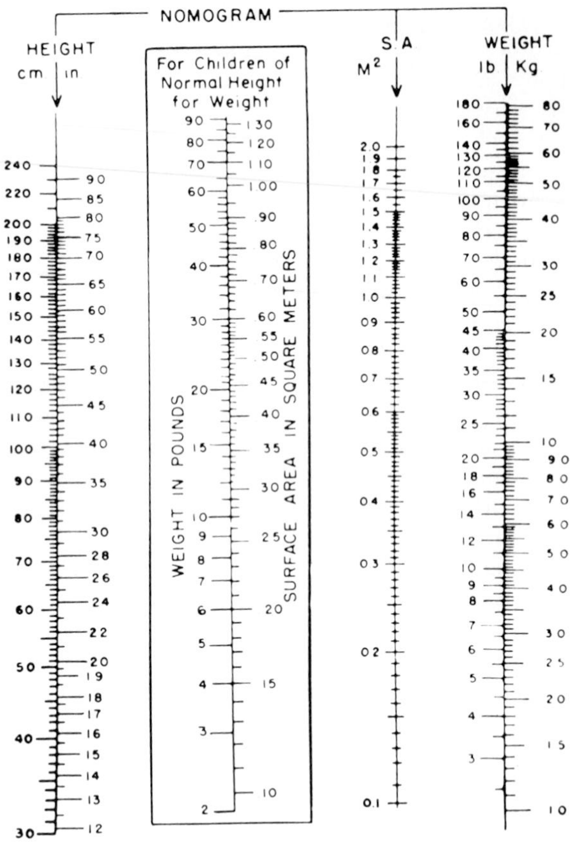

FIGURE 10-1 West nomogram for estimation of surface areas. The surface area is indicated where a straight line connecting the height and weight intersects the surface area (SA) column or, if the patient is roughly of normal proportion, is estimated from the weight alone (enclosed area). [*Nomogram modified from data of E. Boyd by C.D. West, from H.C. Shirkey in V.C. Vaughan and R.J. McKay (eds.) Nelson Textbook of Pediatrics, 10th ed., Saunders, Philadelphia, 1975, p. 1713. Used with permission.*]

TABLE 10-1 Administration of Medications

Growth and Development	Mode of Administration	Nursing Approach
	Infant	
Development of trust		Determine successful parental methods; talk to and touch infant; hold to comfort (parent or nurse) if infant cries following administration
Presence of swallow reflex	Oral route Elixirs and syrups	Use plastic syringe without needle; place syringe in mouth to one side; apply gentle pressure to expel small amount of contents; allow infant to swallow; repeat until all medication is given
	Tablets	Crush between two spoons; mix with syrup, honey, or fruit; give by spoon
	Capsules	Dissolve contents in small amount of water or mix with syrup, jelly, or fruit; give by spoon
		If gentle restraint is necessary, guard against aspiration; always give oral medications with infant in semireclining position
Elicitation of blink reflex when attempting to separate lids	Eye drops	Rest hand holding dropper on infant's forehead; release drops on inner canthus; the blink reflex will allow drops to come in contact with conjunctivas (see Fig. 10-2)
Straight external auditory canal	Ear drops	Turn infant's head to unaffected side; rest hand holding dropper on infant's head; pull pinna gently downward and backward with other hand; instill drops; keep infant in position for several minutes to allow medication to come in contact with surfaces of canal (see Fig. 10-3)
Nasal breather	Nose drops	Place infant in supine position; slightly extend neck (hyperextension causes strangling sensation); instill drops; maintain position for 1 min; instill 5 to 10 min before feeding so that infant can breathe through nose when sucking (see Fig. 10-4)
Less total muscle mass, particularly gluteus maximus Less predictable sciatic nerve placement	Intramuscular injection	Inject in vastus lateralis or rectus femoris muscle (see Figs. 10-9 and 10-10); may also use deltoid, but muscle mass is limited (see Fig. 10-11); rotate sites

TABLE 10-1 Administration of Medications—cont'd

Growth and Development	Mode of Administration	Nursing Approach
		Toddler
Development of autonomy Limited language skills and nonverbal communication Need for acceptable substitute behavior to express anger		Determine successful parental methods; approach child positively and firmly; give him simple instructions; gently restrain if necessary (he may kick or flail arms); tell him it is all right to cry; provide therapeutic play so that he may express anger
Same as infant Cup rather than bottle	Oral route	Same as infant
Blink reflex as drops instilled	Eye drops	Rest hand holding dropper on child's forehead; separate lids with other hand, forming "cup" with lower lid; instill drops onto lower palpebral conjunctiva; release lids
Same as infant	Ear drops	Same as infant (see Fig. 10-3)
Nose and mouth breather	Nose drops	Same as infant except drops do not necessarily have to be instilled 5 to 10 min before feeding
Same as infant	Intramuscular injection	Same as infant; ventrogluteal area also provides good muscle density (see Fig. 10-12)
		Preschooler
Wish for body integrity Fear of being attacked or mutilated Fantasy activity		Determine successful parental methods; provide choices; allow child to cry; gentle restrain if necessary; provide therapeutic play to act out fears of bodily harm
Ability to swallow and chew	Oral route	Same as toddler (although some children can swallow and chew tablets at an early age, resistance to medications may result in aspiration; thus, tablets are not recommended whole until 5 years of age); do not tell the toddler that medicine is candy or that it is tasty when in fact it is not; the child may choose who will hold the medicine cup or push the plunger, himself or the nurse; he may also decide substance in which medication will be mixed
Same as toddler	Eye drops	Same as toddler
Curved external auditory canal	Ear drops	Turn child's head to unaffected side; rest hand holding dropper on child's head; pull pinna upward and backward with other hand; instill drops; keep child in position for several minutes
Same as toddler	Nose drops	Same as toddler
Same as toddler	Intramuscular injection	Same sites as toddler; allow the preschooler to have choices; if it is the first in a series of injections, allow child to decide which thigh will be used (sites must be rotated therafter) or allow child to decide who will wipe injection site and who will compress muscle mass, child or nurse; place decorated bandage strip over injection site; do not tell child that injections will not sting or will stop hurting momentarily; allow him to squeeze adult's hand; distract him by having him count or wiggle toes
		School-Age Child
Concrete thought		Explain to child what medicationis and how it is expected to work
Ability to swallow easily and chew pills independently	Oral route	Offer pills and tablets whole; give elixirs and suspensions by medicine cup; allow choices, e.g., who will hold the medicine cup; children may need to be taught methods for swallowing pills, e.g., place toward back of tongue and take drink of water
Same as preschooler	Eye, ear, nose drops	Same as preschooler; allow him to instill his own drops if he wishes
Development of muscle mass	Intramuscular injection	Add posterior gluteal muscle mass as a site (see Fig. 10-13); allow choices as with preschooler; suggest that he may want to say "ouch," count, or wiggle toes

Continued

TABLE 10-1 Administration of Medications—cont'd

Growth and Development	Mode of Administration	Nursing Approach
		Adolescent
Difficulty in accepting authority; ability to solve problems (formal operational thought)		Explain what the medication is and how it is expected to work; describe how often it must be taken and at what intervals; ask adolescent to decide with nurse methods of achieving goal of taking medications
Same as school-age child	Oral route; eye, ear, and nose drops	May decide he wishes to give his own
Same as school-age child	Intramuscular injection	Same sites as school-age child; may decide he wishes to give his own or assist nurse, e.g., swab injection site, compress muscle mass, push down plunger, or remove needle from muscle once medication is injected

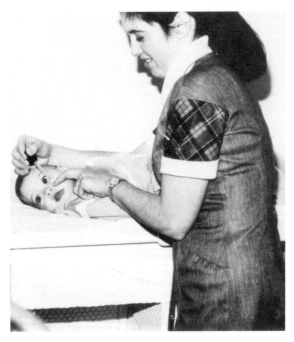

FIGURE 10-2 Instillation of eye drops. *(Photo courtesy of David Stewart, M.D.)*

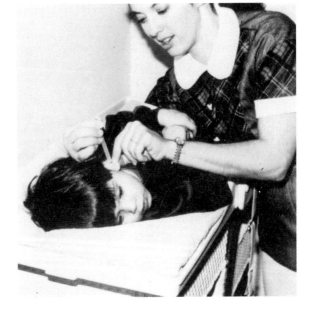

FIGURE 10-3 Instillation of ear drops. *(Photo courtesy of David Steward, M.D.)*

age. A scalp vein or superficial vein of the wrist, hand, arm, or foot is the preferred site for infants, while in older children any available vein may be chosen. Scalp veins are often used in infants: these veins have no valves, and so they can be infused in either direction (Fig. 10-5). In addition, the head can be moved freely by the infant without the danger of dislodging the needle.

A microdropper (60 drops per milliliter) and a calibrated volume control chamber are used to prevent volume overload. Once the desired amount of fluid is in the control chamber, tubing from the bottle to the burette is closed securely so that no more fluid will enter the control chamber. The chamber must be monitored frequently for flow rate and refilling.

Several devices are used in pediatric infusion therapy. An infusion pump is shown in Fig. 10-6. A syringe pump is used when a small amount of fluid is needed over a specific period of time (Fig. 10-7). Regardless of the apparatus used, the infusion site must be monitored frequently for infiltration and phlebitis. These observations may be difficult because the gauze and tape placed over the site to prevent dislodging of the needle make it difficult to examine the adjacent tissue. The amount infused is recorded hourly.

Immobilization of a body part may have to be implemented, especially for a very young infant, toddler, or otherwise uncooperative child who is receiving intravenous therapy. *Padded* arm or leg boards and padded tongue

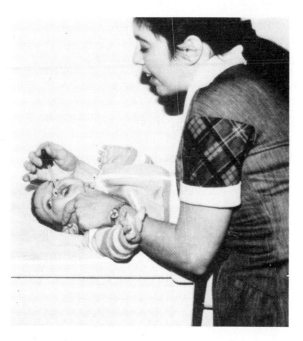

FIGURE 10-4   Instillation of nose drops. *(Photo courtesy of David Stewart, M.D.)*

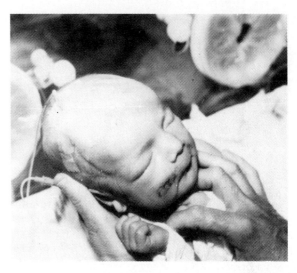

FIGURE 10-5   Infant with a scalp vein infusion. *(Photo courtesy of David Stewart, M.D.)*

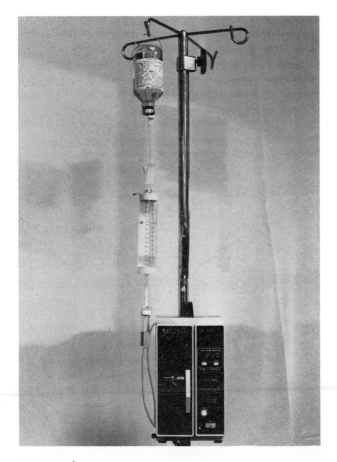

FIGURE 10-6   An IV motor pump. *(Photo courtesy of Bob Thiefels.)*

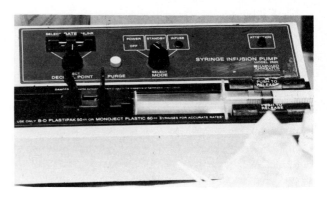

FIGURE 10-7   A syringe infusion pump. *(Photo courtesy of Bob Thiefels.)*

blades for small infants as well as covered sandbags are all effective in decreasing the activity of a body part. If additional restraints are necessary, they should be released every 2 to 3 hours, *one extremity at a time,* for exercise.

Intravenous medications may be added to the bag, bottle or burette, or they may have to be administered through a secondary setup. In all instances sterile technique is used. A nurse *must* check the specific dilution, the amount of the drug to be given, the diluent to be used, the compatibility of the drug with other drugs being given intravenously, the time period necessary for administration, and the rate of flow *before* giving the medication.

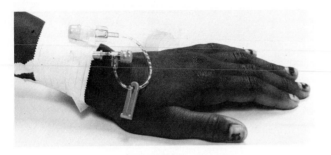

FIGURE 10-8   A heparin lock in place. *(Photo courtesy of Bob Thiefels.)*

It is important to assess the patency of the infusing line at all times, but especially before adding a drug. The nurse must ensure that the correct solution is being infused, check the site for infiltration and phlebitis, accurately record the rate and volume received (at least hourly), and label each bottle or bag which is hung with the date and time. All the tubing is changed every 24 to 48 hours and labeled with the date, time, and the initials of the nurse who is doing these tasks. All tubing connections should be checked routinely. At some medical centers each connection is taped to decrease the risk of separation.

The burette should never contain more than a 2-hour supply of fluid, especially in small infants, in whom fluid overload is a constant concern. There are times when a volume control chamber cannot be used because the patient is to receive more fluid in an hour than the chamber can hold, e.g., for an older child with asthma or one in sickle cell crisis. The time at which the bag or bottle is hung is an important notation.

Heparin Lock

When a cooperative child is to receive a lengthy course of antibiotics, the team may decide to convert continuous intravenous therapy to intermittent therapy by inserting a *heparin lock* (Fig. 10-8). The most obvious advantage for a child is increased mobility.

After the dressing is removed and the site is exposed, the intravenous tubing is detached from the hub of the needle and the heparin lock infusion set is inserted. Heparin, 10 units per milliliter, which then is injected into the setup, prevents the blood from clotting between the doses of antibiotics. Heparin must be instilled whenever the site is used. The area is wrapped securely for protection.

When an antibiotic is to be given, the heparin lock must be flushed with normal saline before antibiotic administration. The dilute heparin is instilled after the drug is given. The needle needs to be inserted in the center of the heparin lock diaphragm to decrease the likelihood of damage. Whenever a child has a heparin lock in place, the sterility of the intravenous system used to administer drugs *must* be maintained. The rubber diaphragm of the

heparin lock must be cleaned thoroughly with an antiseptic swab before use. The tubing also must be changed every 24 to 48 hours. If the child is receiving more than one antibiotic, separate systems are used for each drug. The site has to be assessed for infiltration or phlebitis, the tubing must be checked for patency, and the drug should be diluted adequately and administered within the prescribed time period, usually an hour or less.

Intramuscular, Intradermal, and Subcutaneous Injections

The technique for administering intramuscular, intradermal, and subcutaneous injections in children is the same as that used for adults (Figs. 10-9 and 10-14). Since they have less muscle mass, infants and small children have fewer available intramuscular sites. The posterolateral aspect of the gluteal area (Fig. 10-13) is another site which may be used with older children. As in adults, sites are rotated to prevent muscle fibrosis and subsequent contracture. A child may have to be restrained before the injection is given. A Band-Aid decorated with a happy face placed over the puncture mark can be comforting to the child. Children may wish to squeeze an adult's hand during the procedure. They may be distracted by having them count or wiggle their toes.

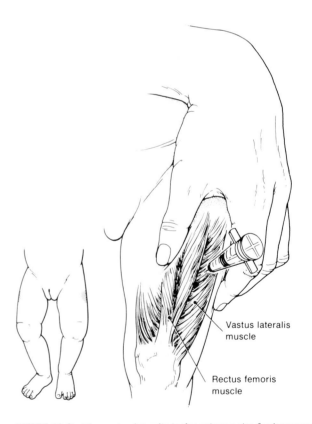

FIGURE 10-9   The vastus lateralis is the primary site for intramuscular injections in the thigh. The needle penetrates the midlateral anterior thigh on a front-to-back course. The thigh is grasped as shown to stabilize the extremity and concentrate muscle mass.

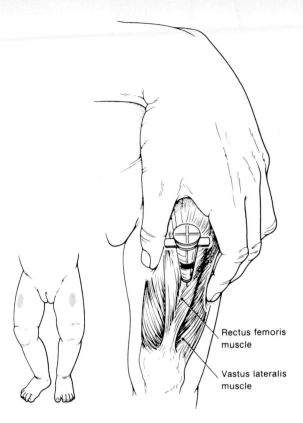

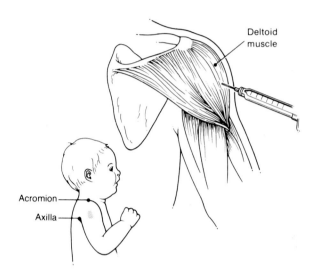

FIGURE 10-10 An alternative site for intramuscular injections in the thigh is the anterolateral surface. The needle is directed distally into the rectus femoris muscle. The thigh should be compressed as suggested in Fig. 10-9.

FIGURE 10-11 The injection site is determined by the acromion and the axilla, as shown. Because muscle mass is limited in the mid-deltoid area, repeated injections and large quantities of medicine are not recommended. Muscle mass should be compressed before insertion of the needle.

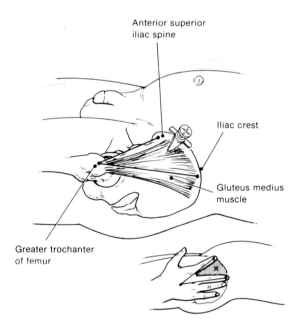

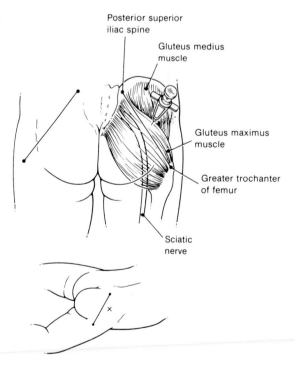

FIGURE 10-12 The ventrogluteal area provides good muscle density and is free from major nerves and vessels. If the injection is to be given on the child's left side, the right hand is used to determine landmarks, and vice versa. The palm is placed on the greater trochanter, the index finger on the anterior iliac spine, and the middle finger on the posterior edge of the iliac crest. The intramuscular injection is given in the center of the V, or triangle, formed by the hand, with the needle directed upward toward the iliac crest.

FIGURE 10-13 The posterolateral aspect of the gluteal area is located by palpating the posterior superior iliac spine and the head of the greater trochanter. An imaginary line is drawn, and the needle is inserted on a straight back-to-front course as shown.

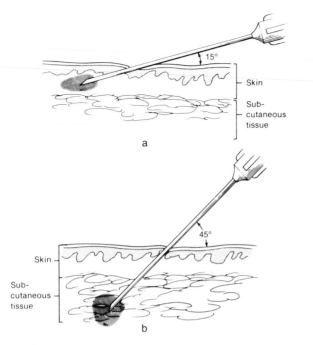

FIGURE 10-14 *(a)* Intradermal injection. Note the angle and placement of the needle. *(b)* Subcutaneous injection. Note the angle and placement of the needle.

Nasogastric Intubations

Inserting a Nasogastric Tube

A nasogastric (NG) tube may be needed to instill medication or feedings, remove gastric contents, obtain gastric secretions for diagnostic tests, remove amniotic fluid in the neonate, and decompress the stomach pre- and postoperatively. A polyethylene French catheter of the smallest diameter which will function for the purpose is preferred; however, a straight rubber French catheter may be used. For example, a No. 5 feeding tube is used for preterm infants, a No. 5 to No. 8 for infants, and a No. 10 to No. 16 for older children. Measurement for insertion orally is the length from the tip of the child's nose to the earlobe and down to the xiphoid process. This length can be marked on the tube with tape or an indelible marking pen. The tip is lubricated with lubricating jelly before insertion. Oily substances should not be used because of the danger of oil aspiration. Insertion is smoother if the tube is rolled into a tight circle, which allows the plastic material to follow the natural contour of the oropharynx into the stomach. As the tube is gently but steadily threaded, there should be no resistance; however, the child will experience gagging. Swallowing water may help an older child pass the tube more easily. Difficult passage, resistance, choking, coughing, and color change are indications for withdrawing the tube for reinsertion.

Escape of air via the tube as it reaches the stomach is not heard with the small-lumen tubes used for infants. The placement of the tube can be tested by aspirating the stomach contents (which are replaced) or by instilling 1 to 3 ml of air into the tube with a syringe as the nurse listens with a stethoscope for the air rushing into the stomach.

If the tube is to remain in place, it is usually inserted in the nose and should be taped *flat* as it leaves the naris. In no circumstances should the tube be pulled up and against the tip of the nares or against nasal mucosa, where it will cause irritation and tissue breakdown. Narrow adhesive tape fits around the tube and across the cheeks in one strip, preventing the tube from slipping out of place. It should be changed every 2 to 5 days.

Gavage Tube Feedings

Gavage feeding is an important procedure in supplying adequate nutrition to infants too small, and to any child too ill, to tolerate oral feedings. Infants with respiratory distress, cardiac anomalies or nasopharyngeal anomalies may need tube feedings. On occasion, the fluid given for nutrition (such as an elemental diet fluid) is objectionable in taste to a child or must be given in a constant flow via drip or a feeding pump (as for severe malnutrition or burns). Oral insertion of the tube for feeding causes less irritation, less chance of aspiration, and a less adverse gag reflex. Preparation should always include a recheck of tube position, aspiration and replacement of stomach contents, and aspiration of air from the tubing. For preterm babies, the amount of aspirate retained in the stomach from the previous feeding, the *residual,* is often subtracted from the amount to be given to avoid distention of the stomach. The feeding should be given slowly. It is best to hold the baby and allow him to suck on a pacifier, thereby simulating a normal feeding, so that he does not lose the satisfaction of bottle feedings. If the baby cannot be held, he should be positioned on his side or abdomen with the head slightly elevated. He needs to be burped during and after the feeding.

Once it has been determined that the NG tube is in the stomach and the aspirated stomach contents have been replaced, a syringe without a plunger is attached to the tubing. The feeding is allowed to flow into the stomach by gravity, about 1 ml/min in preterm and young infants and 10 ml/min in older infants and children. If the feeding does not start to flow by gravity, a *gentle* push with a plunger is helpful. The rate of flow depends on the size of the NG tube.

When the specified amount has been given, the tube is flushed with a small amount of water, which clears the tube, keeps it cleaner and patent, and renders it a poorer medium for bacterial growth. The tube is pinched off, and the syringe is removed. While it is preferable to remove the tube, the tube may remain in place after it is capped or clamped. If the NG tube is to be removed, it is pinched off and removed *quickly.* The amounts of residual and feeding are recorded. Oral and nasal hygiene are important nursing interventions which decrease the likelihood of upper respiratory and ear infections.

Gastric Lavage and Postoperative Decompression

Gastric lavage is done to remove certain harmful substances from the stomach as rapidly as possible. The size of the NG tube depends on the size of the child; however, the lumen cannot be so small as to prevent fragments of the ingested substance from being removed from the stomach. The child is placed on the left side, with the head down to decrease the possibility of vomiting and aspiration. The NG tube is passed, and correct placement is verified. Then saline solution is injected into the tube with a large syringe (30 or 50 ml). The amount instilled depends on the size of the child. The fluid is aspirated and placed in a large basin. This procedure is carried out repeatedly until the returns are clear.

Insertion of a nasogastric tube *before surgery* prevents vomiting and decompresses the intestine, making it easier to handle during surgery. Immediately after surgery, there is no peristalsis and bowel function is static. Therefore, *postoperative decompression* is necessary to prevent abdominal distention caused by swallowed air and gastric and intestinal secretions. Abdominal distention elevates the diaphragm, placing tension on abdominal and intestinal wounds and creating unnecessary complications. If the tube is blocked, the child may vomit and aspirate. Maintaining tube patency is a nursing responsibility; the tube is irrigated with a specified amount of saline solution every 2 hours. The nurse must check for position, flow, and contents returned and note unusual fluctuations in the amounts for each measured period of time (for example, between irrigations).

Drainage may be accomplished by attaching the tube to intermittent machine suction, gravity drainage, or in-the-bed level drainage. Continuous suction damages, stomach mucosa, and it is never used. The tube should not be clamped unless it is ordered by the physician for specific periods to test the child's tolerance. These NG tubes are removed when bowel function returns. Some indicators are passage of stool, flatus, and bowel sounds, and diminished amounts of fluid drained.

Gastrostomy Tube Feedings

To prevent esophageal reflux and avoid the hazards of prolonged nasogastric intubation, gastrostomy feedings may be used. It may be the feeding method of choice after gastrointestinal surgery and is used after surgery for esophageal atresia and tracheoesophageal fistula. Insertion requires general anesthesia; therefore, the procedure is done in the operating room.

The tube is placed halfway down the greater curvature of the stomach and is secured by a purse-string suture. The stomach itself is sutured to the anterior peritoneum, creating a gastrostomy. A mushroom catheter, size 16 to 18, with the tip cut off is preferred to a Foley catheter; the large balloon of the Foley catheter causes crowding within the stomachs of small children. The tube must be fixed firmly to the skin by the use of a cut nipple and silk suture. If the mushroom catheter comes out, it is replaced by a short Foley catheter. Infection may occur postoperatively at any time, and steps to prevent skin breakdown are based on keeping the area dry and clean (Fig. 10-15). While dressings may be used, one of the most effective

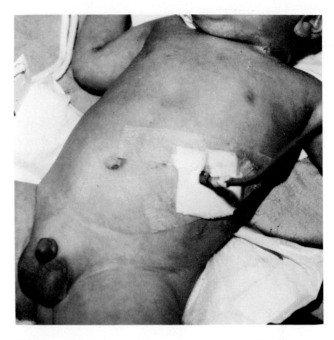

FIGURE 10-15 An infant with a gastrostomy tube in situ. *(Photo courtesy of David Stewart, M.D.)*

measures available is a covering of karaya powder and glycerine, which is mixed to a hot fudge consistency and placed around the gastrostomy site. This covering can be reinforced as needed; however, it is completely replaced only once daily.

Immediately after the surgical procedure, the gastrostomy is placed on gravity drainage for about 24 hours, with the child in a 45° semiupright position. The tube may be irrigated with saline solution, depending on the physician's orders. The fluid drained is collected into a floor bottle, a bag, or a test tube, depending on the amount and the gravity pull desired. Machine suction may pull the opposite stomach wall; therefore, it is not a desirable method.

Feedings begin after the tube has been attached to a syringe and elevated to the top of the incubator or a short distance above the child in a bed (Fig. 10-16). Progression takes place from initially lowering the gastrostomy to straight drainage between feedings, next to continuously elevating the tube, and eventually to clamping the tube between feedings. Glucose water is the first fluid given, followed by dilute formula. A slow, regular rate of instillation of the feeding is achieved by varying the height of the tube. When elevated, the height of the fluid column is the maximum pressure that can be exerted upon the stomach. Mechanical or manual force should never be used. A Y tube is sometimes used for simultaneous decompression during feeding. For optimum feeding, an infant should be held and given a pacifier. In many situations when oral feedings are begun, they are given concurrently with the gastrostomy feedings, which are gradually decreased as oral feedings are increased in amount. Within 7 to 10 days

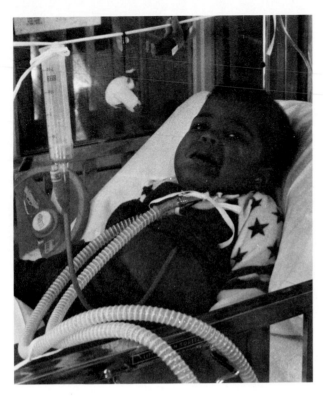

FIGURE 10-16   A toddler receiving a gastrostomy feeding.

after a gastrostomy tube is removed, the opening will close by contracture.

Chest Physical Therapy and Postural Drainage

Viscid secretions do not drain easily by gravity, and different procedures need to be performed on infants and children who are having difficulty removing them from the tracheobrochial tree. With these techniques, secretions can be moved toward the trachea so they may be coughed up or suctioned out. The maneuvers used to enhance the mobilization of these secretions, thereby facilitating their removal, include deep breathing, thoracic "squeezing," "clapping," vibrating, and reinforced coughing. During expiration, a nurse supplies brief, firm pressure with the hands compressing the sides of the thorax (*thoracic "squeezing"*). In *reinforced coughing,* after the child has taken a deep breath and coughed a couple of times as hard as possible, a nurse compresses the lower half of the child's chest and asks the child to cough again.

While postural drainage (PD) and chest physical therapy (CPT) may be preceded by the administration of medications in nebulizers approximately half an hour beforehand, a nurse needs to organize these activities to maximize their benefits for the infant or child. They should *not* be done immediately before meals, since the child may not want to eat because of a loss of appetite. They should not be done immediately after meals because the child may experience nausea and vomit. Timing is important.

Clapping or percussion is done in the positions demonstrated in Fig. 10-17 for 1½ to 2 minutes, while vibrating is done two or three times in all those positions. Sometimes the hand of a nurse is too large to percuss; in those instances a padded disposable nipple or small anesthesia mask (with the hole taped closed) may be used. A padded electric toothbrush may be used to give CPT to neonates. Although these maneuvers are usually done every 3 to 4 hours, the particular health problem of the infant or child determines the order of positions, the frequency, and the duration. If a reddened area is observed over the percussion site, the treatment must be discontinued immediately because an inadequate amount of air is being trapped within the cupped hand or the patient is being slapped instead of tapped. In either case the treatment is ineffective.

In patients with chronic conditions such as cystic fibrosis, PD should be done early each morning to remove secretions accumulated during the night. It should be performed just before bedtime to ensure more restful sleep.

Older children assume the same basic positions taken by adults. It is important to remember that the area to be drained is elevated with the brochus vertical to assist in removal. These youngsters are usually encouraged to cough and breathe deeply after each positional change.

Proper positioning is critical, and so pillows are used extensively for older children; infants may be placed on an adult's lap and legs. Infants cannot cooperate by taking deep breaths. Since an infant usually cries when placed in position, coughing can then be stimulated and the reinforcement technique can be applied. Since children are not able to cough effectively until they are about 4 years old, it may be necessary to suction infants and toddlers in order to remove their secretions.

While a patient is being percussed, air is trapped between the cupped hand and the chest, producing a hollow sound. A nurse should place one layer of a bath blanket, shirt, towel, or baby blanket between the cupped hand and the chest.

CPT can be especially stressful for a preterm infant or neonate, who may have an increased respiratory rate and changes in color for some time after the procedure. When children are unable to tolerate CPT, it may be more advantageous simply to hold them in various PD positions for a brief period of time.

It is critical for a nurse to do a respiratory assessment to determine the effectiveness of the procedure. The pulmonary fields should be auscultated *before* and *after,* and respiratory and apical rates should also be monitored prior to and immediately following the percussion. The child's color and overall activity level should be noted.

At many medical centers a physical therapist is consulted about the positions to be used in the therapy. All steps are demonstrated to the nursing staff members before they assume this responsibility. Generally the therapist also teaches parents the method they should use after the child is discharged. Frequently all positions are taught, regardless of the extent of involvement. This method is especially valid in the case of a child with cystic fibrosis,

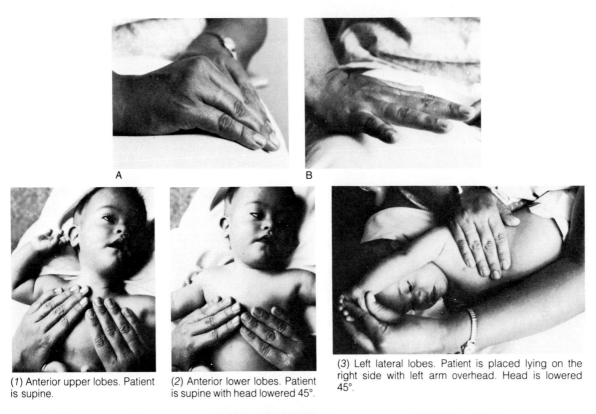

A   B

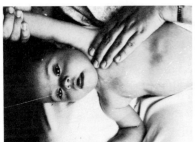

(*1*) Anterior upper lobes. Patient is supine.

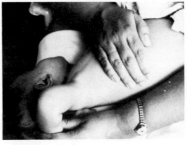

(*2*) Anterior lower lobes. Patient is supine with head lowered 45°.

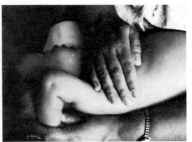

(*3*) Left lateral lobes. Patient is placed lying on the right side with left arm overhead. Head is lowered 45°.

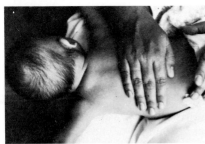

(*4*) Left lingual lobe. Patient is placed with half side lying on right with left arm over head. Head is lowered 45°.

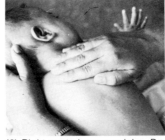

(*5*) Right lateral lobe. Patient is placed lying on right side with left arm over head. Head is lowered 45°.

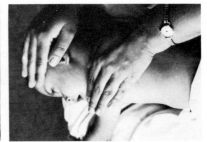

(*6*) Right middle lobe. Patient is placed with half side lying on left with right arm over head. Head is lowered 15°.

(*7*) Posterior lower lobes. Patient in prone position with head down 45°.

(*8*) Right posterior upper lobe. Patient prone with left shoulder elevated 30°.

(*9*) Left posterior upper lobe. Patient prone with left shoulder elevated 45°.

FIGURE 10-17   Positions for postural drainage and percussion. (*a*) Cupped hand position for percussion, which is done in all positions for 1½ to 2 minutes. (*b*) Hand position for vibration, which is done two to three times in all positions. (*From M. Smith et al., Child and Family: Concepts of Nursing Practice, McGraw-Hill, New York, 1982, p. 383. Used with permission.*)

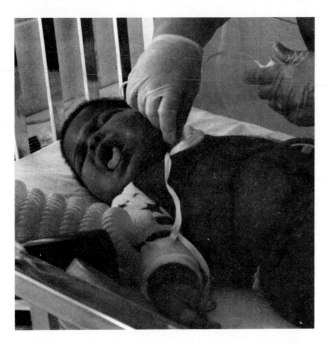

FIGURE 10-18 The gag reflex is demonstrated before suctioning is started. The nurse's thumb controls the suction pressure, which is not applied during insertion of the catheter. *(Courtesy of the Pediatric Nursing Department, Boston City Hospital, Boston, Mass.)*

in whom PD is an integral part of long-range care. The parents must do these procedures often and should be comfortable and knowledgeable about all their aspects.

Suction

Excessive amounts of mucus in the upper airway interfere with oxygenation. Suction is an effective method of eliminating or decreasing the respiratory distress an infant or child is experiencing.

A rubber bulb syringe can be used to remove mucus from the mouth or nares of a newborn or young infant. The bulb is depressed with the thumb and then inserted into the mouth or a nostril. The thumb is released gradually, providing the pressure for suctioning. It is not a sterile procedure.

When more vigorous suctioning is required, a disposal suction kit is used. Small suction catheters are used in neonates or infants to avoid traumatizing anatomic structures in the passage of the tube. For example, it is necessary to use a No. 5 or No. 6 French tip catheter when suctioning a preterm newborn and a No. 8 or No. 10 catheter in a full-term neonate. Vigorous and prolonged suctioning can result in hypoxemia and bradycardia.

A sterile catheter and a sterile glove are used. The catheter, lubricated in a water-soluble substance, is passed through the nose *without suction* until coughing is stimulated. At that point, *suction is applied* and the catheter is rotated gently and then gradually withdrawn (Fig. 10-18). Suction is applied for 10 seconds or less. It is important for a nurse to monitor the infant's appearance and

heart rate during the suctioning. Another nurse may help monitor the infant's apical rate.

Because of the possible unfavorable outcomes of suctioning, oxygen is frequently administered by mask before and after the procedure. When suctioning has been completed, the secretions are examined by a nurse, who records the color, consistency, and amount.

Restraints

Restraints are used as a safety measure for young children. They may be necessary after head or neck surgery, during intravenous therapy, to facilitate an examination or treatment, and in collecting a 24-hour urine specimen from an infant.

Restraints are used only when necessary. All restraints must be applied properly. Since the purpose of using them is to restrict movement, care must be taken to protect the skin and prevent impaired circulation. They must be checked frequently to ensure that they are in the correct place, that there is no circulatory impairment, and that the skin is free of irritation. Restraints are tied to the bed only, never to siderails. Slipknots are used for quick, easy release. They should be removed every 2 to 3 hours so that the restrained extremities can be exercised.

Since parents are frequently in attendance, they should be taught how to apply the child's restraints properly, when to remove them, and how to help the child perform exercises before reapplication. It is important for parents to understand why restraints are necessary. Instructing them to release one extremity at a time decreases the likelihood that a toddler will pull out an NG or intravenous needle. Parents can be especially helpful if they have the basic knowledge to manage the restraints.

Elbow Restraints

While this type of restraint prevents flexion of both elbows, it allows an infant or toddler to move the upper extremities freely (Fig. 10-19). It is used after the repair of a cleft lip or during a scalp vein infusion. Clean tongue blades are inserted into parallel pockets of a wraparound restraint made of soft material such as flannel, muslin, or cotton. The nurse pulls the patient's shirtsleeve or pajama top down the length of the arm, places the elbow in the center of the restraint, wraps the restraint around the child's arm, and secures it with the attached ties. Pulling the padding (shirtsleeve or pajama top) over the edge of the restraint and pinning it to the restraint prevents the device from slipping off the arm.

When elbow restraints are used, it is necessary to check both the axilla and the wrist frequently. Excessive rubbing can result in skin irritation.

Mummy Restraints

When a jugular puncture is to be done or an NG tube must be inserted, this type of restraint can facilitate immobilization of the trunk and upper as well as lower extrem-

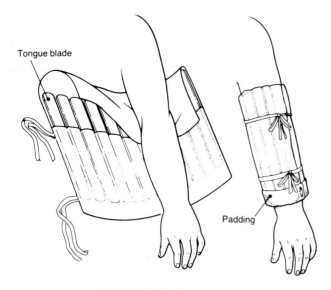

FIGURE 10-19   Elbow restraints.

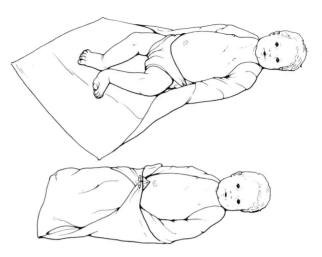

FIGURE 10-21   Alternative method of applying a mummy restraint, which exposes the infant's chest.

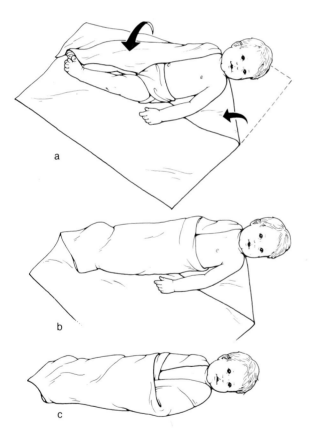

FIGURE 10-20   Mummy restraint. *(a)* and *(b)* Material is first folded over the right arm, and then the corner is tucked under left side. *(c)* The opposite corner is then folded over the infant's left arm and tucked under the right side to secure.

ities (Fig. 10-20). A small blanket is placed on the crib, and one corner is folded down toward the center. The infant is placed on his back on the blanket so that the shoulders are at the level of the fold and the arms are at the sides. The blanket is wrapped over the right arm and

tucked under the left side. The opposite blanket corner is then placed over the left arm and placed securely underneath the right side of the infant's body.

An alternative method of applying a mummy restraint can be used when it is necessary to expose an infant's chest (Fig. 10-21). First a blanket corner is placed around the right arm and tucked underneath, and then the left arm, is enveloped in the opposing blanket corner and secured. The remaining corner of the blanket, below the infant's feet, is brought up to the abdomen and pinned, leaving the chest exposed and accessible.

Clove Hitch Restraints

This type of four-point restraining measure (Fig. 10-22) is used on the extremities of toddlers and some older children. A clove hitch is not a slipknot. The wrists or ankles are always padded with shirt or pajama sleeves, pants legs, or gauze squares before application. Roller gauze or strips of muslin can be used.

A figure eight is made with the material selected. The clove hitch is slipped carefully over the padded wrist or ankle and then gently tightened at both ends. A slipknot is used to tie the ends to a stationary part of the crib or bed. These restraints should never be attached to siderails. If the clove hitch is applied properly, a finger can fit into the space between the padding and the clove hitch knot. It is extremely important to check frequently for any constriction which may impair circulation or cause unnecessary pressure.

Abdominal and Ankle Restraints

This type of restraint is commonly used to immobilize an infant. It is a large piece of muslin with abdominal binder flaps and long ties (Fig. 10-23). The infant is placed on his back in the middle of the restraint. Each half of the abdominal binder is wrapped around the infant's torso and pinned securely at the midline. It is stabilized by using

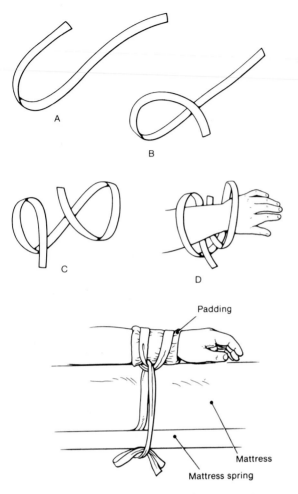

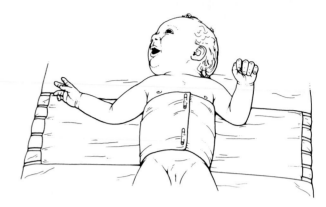

FIGURE 10-23 Abdominal restraint. The middle section is pinned around the infant's torso. The restraint is stabilized by securing the ends over the mattress to the crib springs or frame on both sides.

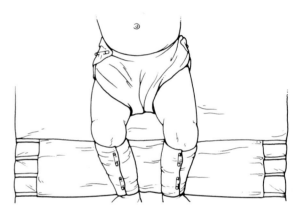

FIGURE 10-22 The clove hitch restraint. A figure eight is formed with gauze and then placed over padding on an extremity and tied by a slipknot to a stationary part of the crib.

FIGURE 10-24 Ankle and lower leg restraint. (Application technique is the same as for the abdominal restraint shown in Fig. 10-23.)

slipknots to tie it to the crib springs or frame.

The ankle restraint is used when it is necessary to immobilize the lower extremities (Fig. 10-24). Its application is the same as that of the abdominal restraint described above.

Restraining for Procedures

There are situations which necessitate physically restraining an infant or toddler to ensure safety and a successful venipuncture or spinal tap. Proper positioning is critical. The procedure must be explained to the child at an age-appropriate level or to the parents if the patient is not capable of understanding.

Jugular Venipuncture

This method of obtaining a blood specimen is used with infants and toddlers (Fig. 10-25). The angle achieved is the most conducive to entering the jugular vein when other attempts have been futile; however, it is essential that the head be held absolutely immobile. When the needle has been removed, pressure must be applied to the site for several minutes to prevent the formation of a hematoma.

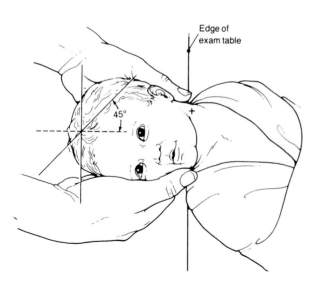

FIGURE 10-25 Correct position for jugular venipuncture procedure. The puncture site is indicated by x. The mummy restraint shown in Fig. 10-20 is used.

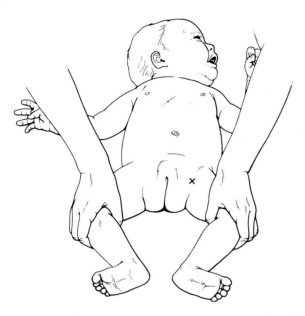

FIGURE 10-26   Position for femoral venipuncture procedure. The X indicates the puncture site.

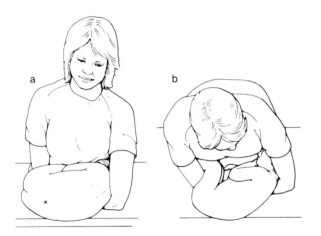

FIGURE 10-27   (*a*) Correct position for lumbar puncture procedure with the infant at or over the table edge. The X indicates the puncture site. (*b*) View of lumbar puncture restraint from above.

Femoral Venipuncture

It may be necessary to use the femoral vein to obtain a blood sample. The infant should be placed on his back with the legs in a froglike position (Fig. 10-26). Gentle pressure is applied to the knees for stabilization. When the baby is held in this manner, the nurse's upper arms also tend to restrict the activity of his upper extremities. The genital area is covered to prevent urinary contamination of the puncture site. When the procedure has been completed, pressure is applied to the site.

Lumbar Puncture

An infant or toddler needs to be held securely whenever a lumbar puncture is performed (Fig. 10-27). The child is

positioned at the edge of an examining table, on his side, facing the nurse. It is necessary to place the neck and knees in a flexed position to enhance the spinal flexion curvature and facilitate entry. Since the neck is flexed, it is important to observe the infant for respiratory distress, which can result from tracheal occlusion during neck flexion. If the patient is an active toddler, it is wise to wrap the lower extremities in a blanket beforehand. At the conclusion of a lumbar puncture, pressure is applied and a sterile bandage strip is placed over the site.

Methods of Dealing with Increased Body Temperature

The temperature control center is in the anterior hypothalamus. Heat-sensitive neurons in the hypothalamus and skin temperature receptors transmit messages to this control center to either lower or raise body temperature in accordance with ambient (environmental) temperature. If there is a rise in ambient temperature, skin blood flow increases to allow body heat to be released. During cold weather, skin blood flow is governed by the musculature of arteriovenous anastomoses. Constriction lessens venous plexus blood flow, and relaxation increases it.

Body heat is lost through radiation, conduction, convection, and evaporation. Methods of dealing with increased temperature are based on these mechanisms.

If core and skin temperature are higher than ambient temperature, more heat is radiated from than to the body in the form of infrared rays (radiation). If core and skin temperature are lower than ambient temperature, more heat is radiated to the body.

As cold air or a cold object is brought into contact with the skin, heat is lost from the skin surface to the air or to the cold object (conduction) by the transfer of thermal energy. The body surface gains heat by contact with a substance which is warmer than the skin.

A continuous supply of cool air is provided through convection. Since warm air is less dense than cool air, it rises and is replaced by cool air. Thus, heat is conducted to the air and then lost through the movement of air. This process is enhanced by wind or a fan.

If the ambient temperature is higher than the skin temperature, core temperature increases through radiation and conduction. Sweat is then deposited on the skin surface to provide cooling by evaporation. The heat required to change sweat from liquid to gas is absorbed from the body's surface, thereby cooling it. The flow of air current promotes evaporation. Increased humidity decreases air flow, and thus the speed of loss of body heat through evaporation is decreased.

Fever is produced by substances known as pyrogens. These proteins are secreted by bacteria or by injured tissue and are released in the blood. They act directly on the hypothalamus to increase heat production until the thermostat is reset at a higher point. Antipyretics (e.g., acetaminophen) lower body temperature during febrile states.

Newborns may be afebrile but septic. Young infants (up to 3 months) may or may not be febrile when infection is present. Thereafter and up to 3 years of age, even mild infections may produce a high fever. In some infants and young children a precipitous rise in temperature is accompanied by convulsions. The reason for this reaction is unknown.

General Measures for Reducing Fever

Once a fever is produced, several measures may be instituted to reduce it. If the fever is low-grade [38 to 38.3°C (100 to 101°F) rectally], lightweight loose clothing and removal of blankets and other covers may suffice. This type of clothing allows adequate movement of air and thus promotes reduction of core temperature not only through convection but also by evaporation if perspiration is present. If the fever is moderate [38.9 to 39.4°C (102 to 103°F rectally], minimal clothing (underpants or diaper) and no blankets or other covers are advised. Lowering of environmental temperature through minimal covering promotes reduction of core temperature through radiation and evaporation. If the fever is high [40°C (104°F) and above rectally] or if a fever of 39.4° (103°F) does not respond to temperature-regulating measures within an hour, a tepid-water sponge bath is advised to increase heat loss through evaporation. Ten minutes is generally sufficient for a tepid bath in the first year of life, and 20 to 30 minutes is enough for older children. Too rapid a decrease in temperature can result in chilling and/or peripheral collapse and subsequent shock.

Methods of fever reduction by conduction include the application of cool towels or cloths and the use of a thermal blanket. As noted above, convection can be enhanced by the use of a small fan. Care should be taken to avoid chilling, which can precipitate shivering. Shivering is a mechanism which produces more body heat, thus defeating the purpose of the treatment.

Excessive sweating can decrease plasma volume and alter electrolyte balance. Thus additional fluid intake during febrile states is needed to replace that which is lost through perspiration. Clear liquids are given every 30 minutes.

Antipyretics

The use of antipyretics varies with physicians. Some begin acetaminophen for a child with a fever as low as 38.3°C (101°F) rectally. Others do not advise its use until the temperature has reached 38.9°C (102°F) rectally. Still others wait until it is 39.4°C (103°F) rectally. The temperature is taken 20 to 30 minutes after the administration of an antipyretic. General fever reduction measures are used with antipyretics (Table 10-2).

Acetaminophen is contraindicated in infants and children who have G6PD deficiencies, since hemolysis may

TABLE 10-2 Methods of Dealing with Increased Temperature

Mechanism	Methodology	Nursing Responsibilities
Radiation: emission of heat from body as infrared rays get to areas or objects of lower temperature Conduction: loss of heat from warm skin surface to cool air or object Convection: replacement of warm air by cool air	Decreased environmental temperature Minimal clothing, no covers Thermal blanket Application of cool towels or cloths Lightweight loose clothing, no covers for low-grade fever Minimal clothing, no covers for moderate and high fever Use of a small fan, if necessary, to provide continuous supply of cool air	For radiation, conduction, convection, and evaporation mechanisms for lowering fever: 1. Avoid chilling 2. Evaluate methodology by monitoring body temperature every 15 min to 1 h until fever is lowered and by assessing skin temperature 3. Teach parents use of thermometer and methods of decreasing fever 4. Explain to parents rationale of various interventions to ensure and solicit cooperation
Evaporation: change of sweat from liquid to gas via thermal energy	Lightweight loose clothing, no covers for low-grade fever Minimal clothing, no covers for moderate and high fever Tepid-water sponge bath for fever of 39.5°C (103°F) which is not lower 1 h after administration of antipyretic and for high fever	Increase fluid intake to replace loss through perspiration
Antipyrogen: substance which lowers body temperature during febrile state	Acetaminophen 10-15 mg/kg/dose	Discuss with parents methods of giving antipyretics Discuss with parents side effects and overdosage Evaluate efficacy of medication by monitoring body temperature

result. The side effects of acetaminophen for normal children include anemia, pancytopenia, leukopenia, neutropenia, skin eruptions, and jaundice. Overdose can lead to hepatic failure and death.

Isolation

There are some sophisticated isolation methods in the hospital setting, especially at medical centers accustomed to dealing with children who have immune response deficiencies such as immunosuppression and neutropenia. The life island support system consists of a bed within a plastic tent. All the items used are presterilized, air moving through the unit is filtered, and contact with the child is accomplished with gloved sleeves which are part of the tent. However, this kind of isolation equipment is expensive to construct and maintain, and the effects of isolation and human deprivation are severe for the patient. Another type of isolation environment is the positive pressure laminar airflow room, with its filtered airflow unit which constantly removes room air, preventing contamination. Another advantage is that personnel wearing sterile attire (gowns, gloves, masks) can enter the room to care for a child. A portable laminar airflow unit is affordable for many institutions to purchase.

In most hospitals, however, isolation consists of placing the patient in a single room and having staff members and visitors wear gowns, gloves, and masks. The major purpose is to prevent transmission of pathogens from the patient to others, although on occasion protective (reverse) isolation is carried out to shield a child with compromised host defenses. Although not all-inclusive, some common types of isolation, reasons why isolation is required, and specific precautions to be taken are identified in Table 10-3.

The gowns worn in an isolation room should be used once and then discarded. They must be tied securely with the back edges overlapping. If a gown must be used again, concerted efforts should be made to ensure that the inside surface is kept "clean." After hand washing, the nurse removes the gown and hangs it on the inside of the door, with the edges of both sides folded together so that the inside surface of the gown (which contacts the wearer's clothing) does not become contaminated.

Whenever a disposable mask is used, both nose and mouth must be covered. It should be changed every 30 minutes or less, because a moist mask is not effective. *A mask should never be lowered to hang around the neck.* It is important not to touch the mask while in the room. Although an explanation of the type of isolation to be carried out is essential for both parent and child, a nurse needs to be conscious of the effects a mask may have on an imaginative patient. It is necessary to show one's face to the young patient before donning a mask.

Disposable single-use gloves are preferred for work in an isolation room. Others which can be sterilized and used again need special handling and should not be used.

Thorough hand washing after contact with a child or with any secretions which are potentially infectious is essential. When a nurse or other person prepares to leave an isolation room, after hand washing paper barriers need to be used to open the door or touch any equipment in the room.

Whenever linen or other articles are removed from isolation, a second person must be available to assist in their proper disposal. Every effort must be taken to decrease the possibility of contamination outside the confined area of the patient's room. For example, a linen bag is closed and tied by the nurse in isolation. A second person, outside, prepares another clean linen bag into which the contaminated bag is placed. Then the outer bag is tied and labeled before being put into the laundry chute. This double-bagging procedure is followed for the disposition of all equipment which leaves the room and is sent to the laundry, central supply, or any other destination. Even a single break in technique may cause contamination.

There are other basic principles which must be remembered. The amount of equipment in an isolation room is always kept to a minimum. Having adequate supplies, keeping clean and dirty supplies labeled properly, and ventilating the room are constant concerns. A nurse is responsible for coordinating diverse activities which range from asking the dietary department to send the isolated child's food on disposable dishes to instructing ancil-

TABLE 10-3 Types of Isolation

Condition	Specific Precautions	Special Considerations
Strict Isolation		
Rubeola, varicella, herpes zoster, extensive infected burns (staphylococcus), vaccinia, pneumonitis, meningococcemia, neonatal vesicular disease (herpes simplex), congenital rubella	Private room with door closed; gowns, gloves, and masks are discarded in proper receptacles in child's room; wash hands on entering and leaving room; any articles leaving room must be double-bagged and properly identified before being sent to laundry, central supply, etc.	Rubella titers of all nurses assigned to children with congenital rubella must be reviewed; since baby sheds virus for many months, all women of childbearing age are endangered, including nurses, ancillary personnel, and visitors

Continued.

TABLE 10-3 Types of Isolation—cont'd

Condition	Specific Precautions	Special Considerations
Respiratory Isolation		
Bacterial meningitis, tuberculosis, pertussis, staphylococcal pneumonia, mumps	Private room with door closed; masks should be worn by susceptible individuals; all persons must wash hands on entering and leaving room; gowns and gloves are not necessary; articles contaminated by secretions must be treated separately and cleaned as well as disinfected properly	Children with bacterial meningitis are isolated until 24 h after start of treatment
Protective Isolation		
Immunosuppression therapy, agranulocytosis, certain lymphomas and leukemias	Private room with door closed; gowns and masks worn; gloves used only by persons having direct contact with the child	No special handling of articles taken outside the room
Enteric Precautions		
Shigellosis, salmonellosis, *Escherichia coli,* gastroenteritis, intestinal parasites, hepatitis	Single room; gowns used when having direct contact with child; gloves worn when handling diapers or bedpans; all persons must wash hands when entering or leaving room	Children with hepatitis also are on needle and syringe precautions; gloves should be changed whenever contaminated by blood, excreta, or parasites
Wound and Skin Precautions		
Impetigo, streptococcal skin infection, extensive burns not infected with staphylococcus or group A streptococcus, any extensive wound infection, staphylococcal skin and wound infections	Single room desirable but not necessary; gowns worn by those who have contact with patient; gloves must be worn by those who will have contact with affected areas; masks are worn only during dressing changes	Care must be taken to dispose of all dressings properly; instruments used must be washed, dried, double-bagged, and labeled "contaminated" before being sent to central supply room

lary personnel about the specific isolation procedure instituted. Preventing transmission of the infectious process to health care providers, visitors, and other employees depends on rigid adherence to existing policies. Caring for a child in isolation requires a nurse to be organized so that the number of trips into and out of the room is kept to a minimum. A nurse faces no greater challenge in practice than keeping the door of an isolation room closed.

Specimen Collection

Samples from various body sites are collected from pediatric patients for many reasons. Some common types of specimen collection—blood, urine, spinal fluid, and throat cultures—will be covered in this chapter in tabular form (Table 10-4). Others are discussed in Part III.

In general, the same developmental principles that were described for the administration of medications are used for collecting specimens. If a child must be immobilized, the mummy restraint can be used in children up to 5 years of age.

The infant cannot easily avoid those who wish to collect specimens. Following the procedure, he needs to be held and comforted either by a parent or by a nurse. The toddler is approached positively and firmly prior to the procedure. He is given simple instructions and is told that it is permissible to cry. Opportunities to resolve feelings thoroughly are provided. The preschooler is approached in much the same way as the toddler. If possible, the preschooler is also allowed choices (e.g., which arm will be used for venipuncture). School-age children need to know what the procedure is and why it is being done.

Parents may remain with the child during specimen collection. They are not asked to help restrain the child. They may comfort the child during and after these procedures.

TABLE 10-4 Collection of Specimens

Name and Purpose	Procedure	Nursing Implications
Capillary puncture Obtain blood for wide variety of microdeterminations	Physician or lab technician prepares skin with alcohol; firm stab is made in finger pad, toe, or heel; blood is collected in pipette	Explain purpose and procedure to parent and/or child; help restrain child, if necessary, to assure that puncture site is stable; hold pressure over puncture site to stop bleeding; apply colorful strip bandage or one with happy face over puncture site
Venous puncture Obtain blood sample for wide variety of reasons	Blood may be drawn from a vein in an extremity, jugular vein, or femoral vein; type of restraint depends on site 1. Extremity: Physician or lab technician prepares skin with alcohol; tourniquet is applied to distend veins; a 20- to 22-gauge needle or scalp vein infusion needle is attached to syringe; vein is stabilized and punctured; plunger is pulled back (negative pressure allows blood to flow into syringe); tourniquet is released, and needle is removed; dry sponge is placed over site and pressure is applied until bleeding stops 2. Jugular vein: After infant is restrained, skin is washed with alcohol; a 20- to 22-gauge needle or scalp infusion needle is attached to syringe; vein is punctured by physician; blood is withdrawn, and dry sponge is placed over site as needle is withdrawn; infant is placed in sitting position; pressure is held over venipuncture site for 3 to 5 min 3. Femoral vein: After infant is positioned, artery is palpated by physician; skin is then prepared with iodine and alcohol; a 20- to 22-gauge needle is attached to a syringe; femoral vein is entered, and blood is withdrawn; dry sponge is placed over puncture site as needle is withdrawn; pressure is held for 3 to 5 min	Explain purpose and procedure to parent and/or child; help restrain child if necessary 1. Extremity: Stand on side opposite area to be used; lean over to restrain limb; may need to use modified mummy restraint, e.g., one limb kept free 2. Jugular vein: Mummy restraint is used; infant's head is turned to one side and extended over edge of table (45° angle); increase in intrathoracic pressure from crying distends vein; infant's head must be kept absolutely still (see Fig. 10-25) 3. For femoral vein: Infant is restrained in frog-leg position; person who restrains him leans over his trunk from one side and positions his legs; restrainer's body blocks infant's view of procedure (see Fig. 10-26); child needs comforting after blood specimens are taken
Urinalysis Determine pH, specific gravity, and presence of glucose, protein, ketones, casts, cells, crystals, and bacteria Normal: pH: 4.0-8.2 Specific gravity: 01.024-1.030	Child is asked to void into bedpan or urinal, and specimen (correctly labeled) is sent to laboratory	Purpose and procedure are explained to parents and/or child; an early morning specimen is best because formed elements are preserved in concentrated acidic urine; *fluids should not be forced because dilute urine may obscure abnormalities and give false results*
Clean voided specimens Collect urine for culture and to determine presence of an infection	1. Neonates: Suprapubic bladder taps are done to ensure a sterile specimen; skin is cleansed with iodine and alcohol; after bladder percussion, a 22-gauge needle with a syringe is inserted and urine is removed; when adequate amount is obtained, dry dressing is applied; this is considered a sterile procedure	Both purpose and procedure are explained to parents, and any questions they have are answered; this tape should be done about 1 h after baby has voided; it is necessary for nurse to restrain neonate supine in frog-leg position for procedure

Continued.

TABLE 10-4 Collection of Specimens—cont'd

Name and Purpose	Procedure	Nursing Implications
	2. Infants: After proper cleansing and drying (described below), a plastic collecting bag is applied (see Figs. 10-28 and 10-29); proper adhesion is key to obtaining a urine sample; bag must firmly adhere to perineum, but care must be taken so that the adhesive backing is not placed over anal opening (stool contaminates the specimen); cutting a slit in disposable diaper and placing collecting bag through to outside allows nurse to observe receptacle and remove it immediately after infant has voided	In each instance, purpose and procedure are described to parents and/or child; older infants or toddlers may need to be restrained; if parents are present, this need can be eliminated
	3. Girls: When a girl has assumed sitting position on the toilet, labia are spread with a sterile gloved hand and vulva and meatus are cleansed with benzalkonium chloride (1:750) using cotton or gauze with single strokes front to back; area is dried, and patient is encouraged to void; after stream has started, catch the sample in a wide-mouth container	In addition to discussing procedure, it is important for nurse to respect modesty and privacy of school-age children; cleansing anatomic area properly is a critical action because it is easy to contaminate a clean voided specimen; after collection and labeling, specimen should be sent to laboratory as soon as possible
	4. Boys: Ask him to assume voiding position, then cleanse glans penis and meatus as previously described; in uncircumcised male, foreskin must be retracted for thorough cleansing; with foreskin retracted, boy is asked to void and midstream urine is obtained	Same as for girls
"Plant" clean voided specimen on screening media which identify the presence of bacteria and allow for colony counts	5. Patient with an ileal conduit: Area around stoma is cleansed and dried as described, and then nurse expresses urine which is in conduit; a sterile catheter is gently inserted, and urine is collected into a sterile basin; after the specimen is obtained, a filter paper dipstick is used to inoculate an agar plate, which is placed in an incubator (37°C) overnight	While these media are handy screening tests for urinary tract infections, the type of organism present cannot be identified; after a colony count has been made (e.g., 0-2 colonies, negative; 3-23 colonies, suspicious; 24 colonies, positive), plates of positive results should be sent to lab for identification of organism and sensitivity tests
Throat culture Determine presence of group A beta-hemolytic streptococcus in pharynx	Under sterile conditions, remove cotton plug from mouth of sterile test tube; remove sterile swab from tube; ask child to open mouth; depress tongue with metal or wooden tongue depressor; swab pharynx in circular motion, making sure to cover entire pharyngeal area; replace swab in sterile test tube and reinsert cotton plug; label tube; send to lab (usually not done before 2-3 yr of age unless there are older siblings)	Explain to child, if old enough to understand, that you will "tickle" back of throat with swab; asking child to breathe in and out through mouth may prevent gagging; if necessary, parents can be asked to help restrain child; call lab in 24 h for preliminary results; if further scrutiny of culture by laboratory personnel is needed, call again in another 24 h; if culture is positive, child will need appropriate antibiotics

*CSF = cerebrospinal fluid.

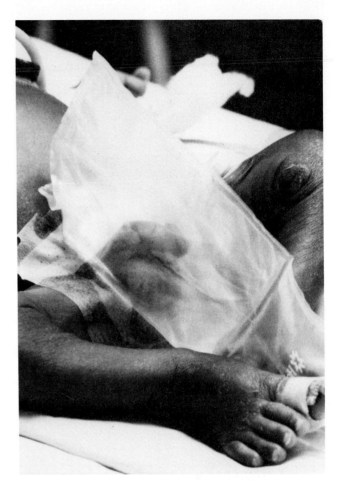

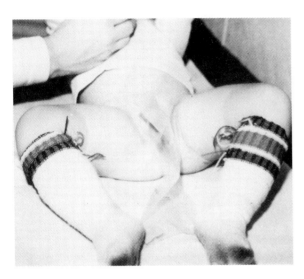

FIGURE 10-28   Collecting a urine specimen from a female infant. *(Photo courtesy of David Stewart, M.D.)*

FIGURE 10-29   Collecting a urine specimen from a male infant. *(Photo courtesy of Bob Thiefels.)*

Learning Activities

1. Design a teaching plan for parents to give oral medications to their toddlers.
2. Design a protocol for explaining to parents the restraints used for:
   (a) Jugular venipuncture
   (b) Femoral venipuncture
   (c) Lumbar venipunture

References

Committee on Infectious Diseases: "Aspirin and Reye's Syndrome," *Pediatrics,* **69:**810-812, 1982.

Curran, C., and M. Kachoyeanos: "The Effects on Neonates of Two Methods of Chest Physical Therapy," *MCN: American Journal of Maternal Child Nursing,* **4**(5):309-313, 1979.

Hazinski, M.F.: *Nursing Care of the Critically Ill CHild,* Mosby, St. Louis, 1984.

Russell, H.: *Pediatric Drugs and Nursing Interventions,* McGraw-Hill, New York, 1980.

Shirkey, H.C.: *Pediatric Dosage Handbook,* American Pharmaceutical Association, Washington, D.C, 1973.

Younger, J.B., and B.S. Brown: "Fever Management: Rational or Ritual?" *Pediatric Nursing,* **11**(11):26-29, 1985.

11

Fluid and Electrolyte Problems in Childhood

Objectives

After reading this chapter, the student will be able to:
1. Discuss the movement of body fluids, solutes, and waste in the body.
2. Describe the functions of the major cations and anions in the body.
3. Identify the differences between metabolic acidosis and alkalosis.
4. Describe the role of the gastrointestinal system in fluid and electrolyte balance.
5. List the purposes of fluid and electrolyte therapy.
6. Identify three nursing diagnoses for children who are experiencing fluid and electrolyte deviations.
7. Discuss five critical nursing assessments which are essential in caring for a child who is in fluid and electrolyte imbalance.

Water is essential to the human body. It is the medium which circulates blood cells and nutrients to the body and excretes the waste products of metabolism. The complex chemical and physiological processes which sustain life and maintain homeostasis cannot occur without this liquid. A pediatric nurse must understand fluid, electrolyte, and acid-base balance because disturbances in these areas occur more frequently in newborns, infants, and children, affecting the course of their illnesses.

Fluid Compartments

Total body fluid (TBF) can be divided into intracellular fluid (ICF) and extracellular fluid (ECF). Potassium, phosphate, sulfate, and protein are found in large amounts in the ICF. The ECF, which consists of interstitial fluid, plasma volume, and transcellular fluid, contains large amounts of sodium, chloride, and bicarbonate.

The distribution of TBF changes with age. For example, a preterm neonate's body is approximately 90 percent water, a newborn's body is 70 to 80 percent water, and an adult's body is 60 percent water (Metheny and Snively, 1983). Even more important, 40 percent of a neonate's TBF is extracellular, while the ICF compartment accounts for 35 percent of TBF. In essence, the smaller the infant, the greater the extracellular compartment volume, which is why a newborn's susceptibility to fluid loss increases. At the end of the first year TBF decreases to approximately 64 percent of body weight, with the ECF constituting 30 percent and the ICF 34 percent. The decrease in ECF is related to the growth of solid anatomic structures during infancy. Although differences in body fluid distribution decrease over the first 2 years of life, adult distribution norms are not achieved until adolescence.

The smaller percentage of ICF in an infant is due to the amount of adipose tissue present. Fat contains very little water, and infants have relatively more adipose tissue than do adults. After 2 years of age the fat difference is minimal.

Movement of Body Fluids, Solutes, and Waste

Water distribution in the body is affected by the solutes present and either the membranes present or the osmotic pressure which develops. A *solute* is a substance which is dissolved in solution. In the human body there are three kinds: (1) electrolytes, such as sodium, calcium, and potassium, (2) nonelectrolytes, such as glucose, creatinine, and urea, and (3) large molecules, such as the plasma proteins.

The constant movement of body fluids and solutes between the ICF and ECF compartments depends on mechanisms such as osmosis, diffusion, colloid osmotic pressure, capillary dynamics, and active as well as passive transport. *Osmosis* is the movement of water across a semipermeable membrane from a more dilute solution to one with a greater concentration. The process ceases once the concentrations are equal. When the pressures on both sides of a membrane are equal, a solute moves from an area of greater concentration to one of lower concentration; this phenomenon is called *diffusion*. Protein solutes which have high molecular weights need to exert *colloid osmotic pressure*, or oncotic pressure. *Crystalloid osmotic pressure* refers to the osmotic pressure of nonprotein solutes.

The transport of water, nutrients, and cellular waste from the blood to interstitial fluids and their return to the bloodstream is called *capillary dynamics*. Several factors affect this exchange, including (1) capillary blood pressure, (2) capillary membrane permeability, and (3) protein in the blood and interstitial fluid. The second and third factors are relatively stable except under abnormal conditions, but capillary blood pressure fluctuates with changes in the fluid pressure of the blood. Therefore, capillary blood pressure is a major factor in adequate capillary-interstitial exchange. In areas of the body where capillary blood pressure is elevated, fluid is forced into the interstitium. Fluid enters the capillaries when capillary blood pressure is decreased.

A physiological process known as *active transport* involves the movement of electrolytes from areas of lesser concentration to areas of greater concentration. It is an energy-producing process in which electrolytes are pumped into or out of cells. This mechanism is involved in pumping sodium out of cells and potassium into cells. The energy source is adenosine triphosphate (ATP), which is produced in the mitochondria of cells. While sodium and potassium are carried to all cells by means of active transport, ions such as chloride, hydrogen, phosphate, and calcium are capable of moving through only some cell membranes. *Passive transport* refers to the movement of water and solutes from areas of greater concentration to areas of lower concentration. Water and many metabolites move into and out of cells by this mechanism.

Large molecules, such as fats and proteins, need to be distributed to various parts of the body; however, they are not able to cross cell membranes by means of diffusion or active transport. As a result, the cell wall forms a vesicle, engulfs the large molecule, and absorbs it into the cell. This process, called *pinocytosis*, is used in certain instances to gain access to a cell.

Internal Exchanges

The internal redistribution of body water occurs as a result of the loss or gain of water or the loss or gain of sodium. Normally, the osmotic pressures of the ECF and ICF are equal. However, if a large amount of sodium moves to the extracellular compartment, the osmolarity (tonicity) of the ECF increases. Following this occurrence, water from the ICF enters the ECF to equalize the osmolarity. Although TBF remains the same, ECF is increased and ICF is decreased. If sodium chloride is removed from ECF, its osmolarity decreases and water from the ECF moves into the ICF to maintain the critical osmotic equilibrium. In this instance, the ECF volume decreases while the ICF volume increases.

A gain of water initially affects the ECF because it dilutes all solutes and decreases the osmolarity. Similarly, a loss of water from the ECF results in the movement of water from the ICF to the ECF in an attempt to adjust the imbalance which occurs.

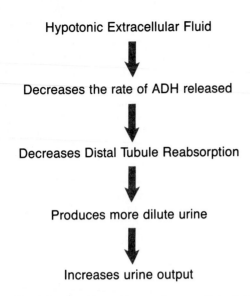

Hypotonic Extracellular Fluid

↓

Decreases the rate of ADH released

↓

Decreases Distal Tubule Reabsorption

↓

Produces more dilute urine

↓

Increases urine output

FIGURE 11-1   The effects of hypotonic extracellular fluid.

External Regulation of Fluid

Other factors which affect the regulation and maintenance of fluid are thirst and antidiuretic hormone (ADH). Thirst is regulated by receptor cells in the hypothalamus and determines water intake in a healthy individual. If the level of electrolytes in the ECF rises or if dehydration is present, an increased intake of water occurs.

Supraoptic nuclei cells in the hypothalamus are responsible for the continuous secretion and regulation of ADH. The osmolarity of ECF determines the rate of release of ADH. With *hypertonic* ECF, ADH increases, stimulating the distal tubules of the kidneys to increase water reabsorption, leading to a concentrated urine output and a decrease in urine output. Hypotonic ECF results in a decreased rate of ADH release. The distal tubules of the kidneys reabsorb less water, the output of urine increases, and the concentration of urine decreases (Fig. 11-1). Thus equilibrium between ECF and ICF is restored.

Fluid and Electrolyte Balance

The regulation of fluid and electrolyte balance is an extremely complex physiological process. In addition to the factors described above, other variables affect this extremely delicate equilibrium. The adrenal cortex continuously secretes *aldosterone,* a hormone which affects the retention and excretion of sodium and potassium by the renal tubule cells. The plasma level of sodium is the major determinant of aldosterone secretion. Hydrogen and potassium compete for sodium. The retention of sodium by the renal tubules through the action of aldosterone results in water retention, hydrogen retention, and potassium excretion.

Chloride and bicarbonate also are affected by aldosterone. These electrolytes are anions (negatively charged); sodium, potassium, and hydrogen are cations (positively charged). As a result of their electrical activity, either chloride (Cl^-) or bicarbonate (HCO_3^-) binds to the sodium as it enters the ECF. Therefore, electrolyte excretion (sodium, potassium, hydrogen chloride, and bicarbonate) is regulated by aldosterone. Other variables which produce or result in the increased aldosterone secretion include physical or psychological stress, trauma, elevated extracellular potassium levels, decreased plasma sodium, and decreased extracellular volume.

The intravascular volume also affects fluid and electrolyte balance. Renal perfusion and glomerular filtrate formation are increased or decreased by changes in blood volume. This mechanism in turn affects the secretion rate of aldosterone and ADH.

The renal system also plays a vital role in maintaining fluid and electrolyte equilibrium. Body fluid and its solute particles are filtered continuously through the glomerular capillaries of the kidneys. This material is referred to as the *glomerular filtrate.* Each minute approximately 125 ml of filtrate is formed by the renal system. Eventually reabsorption of amino acids, glucose, water, electrolytes, and other substances occurs so that approximately 1 ml of urine results from the original filtrate. The kidneys are responsible for the excretion of hydrogen ions.

Electrolytes

Electrolytes control the formation and retention of water in the ICF and ECF. They are charged substances which exert electrical activity and break up (dissociate) into ions in solutions in all body fluids. Potassium, sodium, magnesium, and calcium are positively charged (cations) while chloride, sulfate, phosphate, and bicarbonate are negatively charged (anions). Equal numbers of cations and anions result in electroneutrality. Each electrolyte has the potential to combine with an oppositely charged one. They are measured in milliequivalents (meg) per liter, which expresses the electrochemical combining power of an electrolyte for each 1000 ml of body fluids.

Sodium (Na^+) is the major cation found in the extracellular compartment and is responsible for the osmolarity of ECF. Active transport constantly removes this electrolyte from inside the cell. Water also accompanies sodium out of the cell. This electrolyte is responsible for maintaining intravascular and interstitial volumes within the body.

Potassium (K^+) is the major cation found in the intracellular compartment, although a small amount is found in the ECF. The concentration differences between the sodium extracellularly and the potassium intracellularly are responsible for the effectiveness of muscle contraction and nerve impulse transmission. Extracellular (serum) potassium critically affects cardiac muscle function; for example, an elevated serum potassium can result in ventricular fibrillation. Potassium also is necessary for the entry of glucose into cells. An excess of hydrogen forces potassium out of body cells and into the bloodstream, whereas a deficit of hydrogen forces potassium out of the plasma and into body cells.

Calcium (Ca^{2+}) influences the movement of sodium into cells, thereby affecting the rate of muscle contraction. The degree of contraction is a result of the release of calcium intracellularly during the transmission of a nerve impulse.

Magnesium (Mg^{2+}) is primarily an intracellular ion, with a small fraction found extracellularly. It plays a major role in glucolysis and other intracellular processes. Large amounts of magnesium are combined with phosphorus and calcium in bone. An inverse relationship exists between calcium and magnesium. Hypomagnesemia is found with hypercalcemia, and high levels of magnesium accompany hypocalcemia.

Chloride (Cl^-) is the primary extracellular anion. It acts to maintain electroneutrality between the total number of anions and cations in the ECF (Burgess, 1979). It is passively transported toward cations. Chloride excretion or reabsorption by the renal system depends on the extracellular increase or decrease in bicarbonate.

Bicarbonate (HCO_3^-) is found primarily in the ECF and acts as a buffer to maintain acid-base balance. Phosphate serves the same purpose and also aids in bone formation.

Acid-Base Balance

Acid-base balance refers to the precarious equilibrium which is essential for optimal functioning of the human system. Hydrogen ion concentration, or blood pH, must be maintained within a limited range (7.35 to 7.45) to be compatible with life. *Acids* are substances which either donate or contain hydrogen ions. *Bases* are substances which accept hydrogen ions. *Buffers* reduce the free hydrogen ion concentration of body fluids and play a critical role in maintaining the balance between acids and bases. The renal and respiratory systems regulate acid-base balance.

The respiratory system controls acid-base balance through the retention or release of carbon dioxide (CO_2). Carbonic acid (H_2CO_3) is formed when carbon dioxide reacts with water (H_2O). This compound in turn dissociates into bicarbonate and water ($HCO_3 + H_2O$). The level of carbon dioxide in the blood is measured as dissolved carbon dioxide, or PCO_2, and ranges from 35 to 45 mm Hg.

Bicarbonate forms from the dissociation of carbonic acid; normally there are 20 parts HCO_3 to 1 part dissolved CO_2. This ratio is critical to acid-base equilibrium. The ability of the renal system to excrete hydrogen ions and bicarbonate can be inferred from the blood bicarbonate level.

Acidosis indicates a high hydrogen ion (H^+) concentration, and the blood pH is less than 7.35. The elevated H^+ and PCO_2 stimulate the respiratory system to increase the rate of respirations, leading to elimination of excess H^+ and CO_2. *Alkalosis* indicates a decreased hydrogen ion concentration, and blood pH is greater than 7.45. The decreased H^+ and PCO_2 affect the respiratory center, leading to a decreased respiratory rate and retention of carbon dioxide and hydrogen. This reaction is known as the *respiratory buffering mechanism*.

The renal system controls hydrogen ion concentration through the excretion or retention of hydrogen and bicarbonate. When H^+ is elevated, the renal tubule cells excrete hydrogen and conserve bicarbonate. In alkalosis, hydrogen is conserved and bicarbonate is excreted. This mechanism is called *renal buffering*.

Extracellular, or blood, buffer systems act instantaneously and continuously. The blood bicarbonate buffer system is of major importance because both the renal and respiratory systems eliminate the chemical constituents. Carbonic acid (H_2CO_3) and a sodium bicarbonate salt ($NaHCO_3$) are the elements of the blood buffering system. This bicarbonate–carbonic acid system stimulates the respiratory system to increase CO_2 elimination when a hydrogen ion load is given, while the renal system conserves bicarbonate. When the hydrogen ion concentration is decreased, the renal system retains hydrogen and excretes bicarbonate, the respiratory system retains CO_2, and the normal pH value is maintained. The 20:1 ratio must exist in the bicarbonate–carbonic acid system for extracellular buffering to function optimally in maintaining acid-base balance.

Intracellular buffering is the process which occurs in the presence of persistent acidosis or alkalosis. When the hydrogen ion concentration is *excessive*, potassium moves from the ICF to ECF in exchange for hydrogen. Thus, hyperkalemia accompanies acidotic conditions. Hydrogen ion *deficits* force the movement of potassium into cells while hydrogen moves extracellularly, resulting in hypokalemia. Therefore, electrolyte balance is affected by these changes in hydrogen ion concentrations. Over a period of time ranging from hours to several days, the renal system acts to restore the normal pH. In acidosis, hydrogen is excreted either as H_2PO_4 or as water and carbon dioxide. Hydrogen also may be eliminated in the urine as ammonium chloride. Alkalosis leads to hydrogen retention by the renal tubules and the excretion of bicarbonate. The 20:1 ratio of bicarbonate to carbonic acid is of primary importance in acid-base equilibrium. *Blood pH values lower than 6.8 or higher than 7.8 are incompatible with life.*

Metabolic Acidosis

Metabolic alterations are the result of excess bicarbonate reabsorption or excretion or increased production or retention of hydrogen ions (Table 11-1). Metabolic acidosis occurs when the HCO_3/H_2CO_3 ratio is less than 20:1:

$$\left(\frac{HCO_3}{H_2CO_3} < \frac{20}{1}\right)$$

It may be precipitated by multiple variables. Chronic renal insufficiency results in decreased hydrogen excretion and may hinder bicarbonate reabsorption.

Neonates have a decreased ability to excrete hydrogen ions as a result of their low glomerular filtration rate. They

TABLE 11-1 Acid-Base Problems

Problem	Laboratory Value	Causes	Clinical Signs	Nursing Management
Respiratory alkalosis	Plasma pH above 7.45; PCO_2 below 40 mm Hg; bicarbonate below 24 meq/liter	Develops as a result of other primary problems such as the ingestion of salicylates, hyperirritability of respiratory system with meningitis or encephalitis, hyperventilation in an anxiety attack, or improperly set ventilators	Rapid respirations, paresthesia, light-headedness, twitching or seizures	The initial problem needs to be treated; having the child breathe into a paper bag raises the CO_2 level; support, reassurance, and encouragement are essential in lowering the rapid respirations, which are anxiety-provoking
Respiratory acidosis	Plasma pH below 7.35; PCO_2 above 40 mm Hg; bicarbonate above 24 meq/liter	Occurs in situations where there is CO_2 retention which results in alveolar hypotension *Acute:* Respiratory distress syndrome, upper airway obstruction, respiratory failure, cardiac arrest *Chronic:* asthma, cystic fibrosis, advanced muscular dystrophy	Dyspnea, confusion, tachycardia, air hunger, cyanosis	All efforts are directed toward improving oxygenation; these children are observed closely and positioned frequently; breath sounds need to be evaluated before and after nebulizer treatments and chest physical therapy; blood gases are done frequently, so children need to be comforted and reassured; at times $NaHCO_3$ may be ordered intravenously, and the flow rate is monitored at least hourly and must be given slowly
Metabolic alkalosis	Plasma pH above 7.45; PCO_2 above 40 mm Hg; bicarbonate above 24 meq/liter	Constant nasogastic tube suctioning; persistent vomiting as in pyloric stenosis	Slow, shallow respirations; nausea, vomiting, twitching; seizures; confusion and disorientation; cardiac arrhythmias	It is most important to prevent further losses, so intravenous chloride-containing solutions with potassium are monitored and recorded hourly; safety measures, especially in the presence of seizures, are important; it is essential to estimate vomitus as diligently as possible and maintain an accurate intake and output; confusion and disorientation are perplexing to the child, and so the presence of a parent or nurse is reassuring; comfort measures such as mouth care also are essential
Metabolic acidosis	Plasma pH below 7.35; PCO_2 below 40 mm Hg; bicarbonate below 24 meq/liter	Starvation, diarrhea, vomiting, salicylate ingestions, impaired renal function, diabetes mellitus, hypoxia	Hyperventilation, confusion or disorientation, acetone odor to breath, weakness, muscle twitching, coma	Efforts are directed toward treating initial problem; when sodium is infused, rate of flow is monitored hourly; mouth and skin care are given in presence of vomiting or diarrhea

Source: Adapted from: N. M. Metheny and W. D. Snively: *Nurses' Handbook of Fluid Balance,* 4th ed., Lippincott, Philadelphia, 1983; P. M. Meservey, "Fluid and Electrolyte Balance," in M. Smith et al., *Child and Family: Concepts of Nursing Practice,* McGraw-Hill, New York, 1982, pp. 586-613.

are susceptible particularly to metabolic acidosis. Poor pulmonary perfusion leads to anaerobic metabolism at the cellular level, and thus hydrogen ion production increases. The immaturity of the renal system perpetuates the problem of acidosis. Neonates subjected to cold stress respond with an increased metabolic rate. If carbohydrate supplies are inadequate to meet energy requirements, fats are utilized to meet metabolic demands. The increase in organic acids leads to metabolic acidosis.

Severe diarrhea leads to a loss of bicarbonate in the stool. Oxidation of fats for energy leads to increased organic acids and excess hydrogen ions. Fluid volume loss from diarrhea or other causes can produce a decrease in circulating blood volume leading to shock and acidosis. Diabetes, salicylate poisoning, and excessive ammonium chloride ingestion can produce metabolic acidosis.

The respiratory system partially compensates for the decreased numerator in the ratio by stimulating hyperventilation. The elimination of carbon dioxide is increased; therefore, less carbonic acid is formed and the denominator is reduced. Even though the absolute values may not be within normal limits, the ratio is critical in acid-base regulation.

Metabolic Alkalosis

Metabolic alkalosis results from significant hydrogen loss or excess intake of sodium bicarbonate. Hydrogen ions may be lost because of vomiting (loss of HCl) or gastric suctioning. The HCO_3/H_2CO_3 ratio is greater than 20:1:

$$\left(\frac{HCO_3}{H_2CO_3} < \frac{20}{1} \right)$$

TABLE 11-2 Fluid and Electrolyte Problems

Problem	Causes	Clinical Signs	Nursing Management
Hyponatremia Mild: Na 120-130 meq/liter Moderate: Na 114-120 meq/liter Severe: Na below 114 meq/liter Specific gravity below 1.010	Inadequate Na intake; loss through perspiration with excessive sweating (fever); Na loss which occurs in use of soap suds enemas; burns; wounds; GI losses from vomiting, diarrhea, or nasogastric suction; decreased ADH secretion; receiving electrolyte-free infusions; impaired kidney function or a salt-losing problem	Slow sodium loss: nausea, vomiting, dizziness, tachycardia, hypotension, decreasing urinary output, poor skin turgor, abdominal cramping Rapid sodium loss: headache, confusion, lethargy, twitching, convulsions	Fluid intake is restricted, and intake and output are monitored and recorded carefully; these children should be placed on seizure precautions and observed closely; seizure precautions (padded siderails, working suction, oxygen, and a rubber airway) need to be taken; adequate explanations, support, and reassurance are important interventions
Hypernatremia Na greater than 147 meq/liter Specific gravity above 1.030	Diabetes insipidus; children unable to ask for fluids when thirsty (those in coma, retarded, too young to talk, etc.), excessive water loss as in diarrhea; neurological problems which affect thirst center of hypothalamus; high-protein feedings given without adequate water intake	Nausea and vomiting, dry and sticky mucous membranes, flushed skin, lethargy, irritability, muscle rigidity, disorientation, tremors or seizures, coma, edema, anuria or oliguria	With treatment aimed at diluting sodium without affecting other electrolytes, intravenous therapy needs to be monitored closely and recorded at least hourly; if a diuretic is ordered, child's response must be observed carefully, especially in regard to weight loss or increased urine output; accurate intake and output recording is important; seizure precautions must be instituted; neurological assessments need to be done when child is confused or disoriented
Hypocalcemia Ca below 4.5 meq/liter	Inadequate intake of foods rich in calcium and vitamin D, excessive wound drainage, poor GI absorption, poor renal tubule reabsorption, excessive losses in diarrhea, decreased secretion of parathyroid hormones	Neuromuscular irritability from tingling in fingers or twitching to seizures, hyperactive reflexes, cardiac arrhythmias, or respiratory involvement which affects breathing	Planning a dietary intake which is calcium-rich or administering calcium preparations which are ordered by physician; vitamin D preparations are given; if calcium preparations are given IV, they should be administered within the parameters ordered by physician; infiltration of calcium causes tissue sloughing; seizure precautions need to be taken; parent and patient teaching focuses on consuming adequate amounts of calcium as well as eating foods from four basic categories
Hypercalcemia Ca above 5.8 meq/liter	Excessive intake of milk, bone tumors, prolonged immobilization, increased secretion of the parathyroid hormone	Hypotonic skeletal muscles, anorexia, nausea and vomiting, pathological fractures, abdominal pain, deep bone pain, and flank pain (from kidney stones); in an acute crisis, dehydration, delirium, coma, and cardiac arrest may occur	A child's calcium intake is restricted, and IV saline solutions are ordered to enhance the excretion of excessive Ca; intake and output are monitored closely, as is infusion; child is in pain, and interventions are directed toward alleviation of discomfort, especially in diversional activities, quiet surroundings, medications as ordered, and rest; parental presence is always encouraged; observations of child and his responses to treatment and careful recording of intake and output as well as infusing solution are very important notations
Hypokalemia K below 4 meq/liter	The use of diuretics without K supplements, nasogastric suctioning, wound drainage, diarrhea, vomiting, poor food intake, burns, heat stress, excessive sweating, metabolic alkalosis, NPO for a prolonged period	Muscle weakness, diminished or absent reflexes, hypotension, nausea, anorexia, decreased bowel sounds, abdominal distention, shallow respirations, weak or irregular pulse; in severe cases, can result in variety of arrhythmias, and heart block	Replacing K occurs over several days and may be done by child eating potassium-rich foods (bananas, oranges) and taking K supplements; supplements are taken best when very cold and disguised in small amount of juice; when KCl is added to an IV solution, it must be mixed thoroughly afterward; when infusing KCl, rate cannot be rapid because it irritates the vein and may cause cardiac arrest; rate should be less than 20 meq/h in correct dilution; in many facilities, children have their

Source: Adapted from N. M. Metheny and W. D. Snively, *Nurses' Handbook of Fluid Balance,* 4th ed., Lippincott, Philadelphia, 1983; P. M. Meservey, "Fluid and Electrolyte Balance," in M. Smith et al. (eds.), *Child and Family: Concepts of Nursing Practice,* McGraw-Hill, New York, 1982, pp. 586-613.

Continued.

TABLE 11-2 Fluid and Electrolyte Problems—cont'd

Problem	Causes	Clinical Signs	Nursing Management
			ECGs monitored when receiving KCl by infusion; vital signs should be taken frequently (including blood pressure readings); urinary output needs to be established before such treatment is started, because presence of renal failure may result in hyperkalemia
Hyperkalemia K above 5.6 meq/ liter *Cardiac toxicity is imminent when K is 8 meq/liter*	Burns: too much oral or parenteral K, adrenal insufficiency, renal failure, metabolic acidosis	Irritability, diarrhea, nausea, muscle weakness and cramping, paresthesia, a variety of arrhythmias and cardiac arrest	All potassium is withheld (oral or parenteral); calcium gluconate may be ordered to protect myocardium from effects of the hyperkalemia; a variety of substances such as sodium bicarbonate, glucose, and insulin may be ordered in an effort to force K into cells; these infusions must be monitored very closely, and accurate recording is critical; these children need to be observed for the signs and symptoms of metabolic acidosis which may be associated with hyperkalemia; K levels need to be monitored diligently, because cardiac arrest can occur; if ECG is being monitored, rationale for its use should be explained to child and parent; while infusions described above lower plasma potassium levels by forcing K into cells, dialysis may be necessary to remove K from the body

The respiratory system attempts to compensate through hypoventilation, increasing carbonic acid formation as demonstrated by an increase in the denominator of the equation. However, the oxygen demands of the body limit this compensatory mechanism. Sodium and chloride losses as well as hypokalemia may be associated with metabolic alkalosis.

In pediatric clients acidosis is much more common than alkalosis. However, it is necessary for nurses to be knowledgeable about conditions which precipitate both. Other fluid and electrolyte problems are described in Table 11-2.

Replacement and Maintenance of Body Fluids

In the maintenance and replacement of body fluids, the nurse must take into account the physiological variables found in the pediatric client as well as the pathophysiological problems. Infants and small children have a greater volume than do older children and adolescents. The daily turnover rate of water is higher in children under 2 years of age. The ratio of total body surface area to body weight is greater in the infant than in the adult. Thus, the infant's heat production per kilogram of body weight is twice that of the adult (Burke, 1976). Insensible water losses are also increased as a result of greater body surface area. The

TABLE 11-3 Normal Physiological Fluid Losses

Area of Loss	Amount, ml/100 cal
Insensible	
Lungs	15
Skin	30
Sensible	
Sweat	20
Stool	5
Urine	30-80

metabolic rates of neonates, infants, and children are higher than that of an adult. An adult expends approximately 40 cal/kg body weight; an infant expends 100 cal/kg. With each 100 cal expended, 100 ml of water is lost, and this deficiency makes infants extremely susceptible to fluid imbalances. The immature renal system contributes further to this vulnerability. Insensible and sensible fluid losses occur normally through elimination and evaporation (Table 11-3).

Gastrointestinal disease and/or alterations can produce fluid and electrolyte imbalances. Diarrhea and vomiting, which are primary clinical manifestations of gastrointestinal disease, lead directly and commonly to dehydration and electrolyte imbalance. Intraabdominal surgery complicates these problems. In addition to a malfunction

TABLE 11-4 Electrolyte Composition of Gastrointestinal Secretions

Location	Na^+, meq/liter	K^+, meq/liter	Cl^-, meq/liter	HCO_3^-, meq/liter
Gastric secretions	20-80	5-20	100-150	—
Pancreatic secretions	120-140	5-15	40-80	70-100
Bile secretions	120-140	5-15	80-120	30-50
Small intestine	100-140	5-15	90-130	20-40
Ileostomy	45-135	3-15	20-115	—
Diarrhea	10-90	10-80	10-110	5-20

caused by a gastrointestinal tract abnormality, increased loss of water and electrolytes may occur following anorexia, starvation, poor or improper feeding practices, malabsorption due to a systemic disease, or the administration of chemicals or medications for other reasons. Vomiting and diarrhea are common in conditions such as infectious diarrhea, diabetic ketosis, adrenal crisis, infections, and disturbances of the intestinal mucosa.

Because gastrointestinal intake and output of water account for a large exchange of water, water loss and the subsequent dehydration occur rapidly. When oral intake is inadequate to balance the loss, further dehydration results. Loss of body water is more rapid in an infant than in an older child. In the presence of diarrhea, fluid requirements may be as much as three times the normal daily requirement. Symptoms occur when there is an acute loss of 5 percent of body weight as water. It is considered severe at 10 percent, with peripheral vascular collapse occurring at 15 percent. It may take 36 to 48 hours to reverse dehydration, and the volume administered is the sum of the daily maintenance requirement plus the dehydration factor.

The degree of imbalance depends on the composition of the gastrointestinal fluids being lost (Table 11-4). Gastric fluid loss occurs through vomiting, gastric suction, fistulas, ostomies, and diarrhea. The most common modes of loss must be measured accurately and adequately for monitoring and replacement. However, loss from fistulas is not measurable, and accurate estimation of severe vomiting is difficult. Fluid loss is replaced volume for volume.

All gastrointestinal losses, particularly those from diarrhea, contain moderate to large amounts of sodium. The large intestine reabsorbs water as well as salt (as sodium and chloride) and exchanges potassium and bicarbonate. The small intestine fluid (containing digestive secretions) is high in bicarbonate and sodium and relatively lower in chloride and potassium. Sodium loss is high in the presence of vomiting because gastric mucus contains high concentrations of sodium, and production of the mucus is stimulated by vomiting, adding to sodium loss.

Sodium replacement in parenteral fluid therapy depends on the degree of sodium loss in comparison with water loss and the size of the patient, which determines the speed with which the loss is replaced. Therapy aimed at correcting dehydration is based on average deficits for water, sodium, and chloride. The degree of sodium loss in proportion to water loss is determined by serum sodium

and indicates the type of dehydration being treated. Deficits of water and electrolytes are estimated as mild, moderate, or severe and are treated in combination with maintenance therapy.

Loss of some potassium occurs in almost all states of dehydration. Potassium deficiency, or hypokalemia, may result from a greatly reduced intake as in fasting due to the body's subsequent breakdown of body fat and protein. Diarrhea, particularly when prolonged, produces high potassium loss. Hypokalemia may cause, as well as be the result of, vomiting, creating a vicious circle. Increased amounts of potassium are excreted in the urine because of early renal response to an acid-base imbalance. Administration of potassium after 24 hours of parenteral fluid therapy is a common practice. Initially, during therapy for diarrhea and/or vomiting, potassium is not administered for the first 12 to 24 hours until urine excretion is established as normal.

Diarrhea is the foremost cause of water and electrolyte loss in pediatric patients. There are three main physiological disturbances in diarrhea: dehydration, metabolic acidosis, and shock, which occur when dehydration is severe enough to produce circulatory disturbances. The two important variables to be considered in initiating therapy are the volume of body fluids and their osmolality. Since the composition of intestinal fluids resembles the composition of ECF, diarrheal dehydration is a loss of extracellular water and electrolytes, resulting in the clinical signs of thirst, cold extremities, poor skin turgor, and weight loss. Weight loss is useful in assessing water loss and replacement for short periods of time. In addition, fluid replacement must include estimates of normal body needs and ongoing losses (such as continued diarrhea). Because the sodium content of the body and its accompanying chloride determine the distribution of body water, an increase or decrease in sodium in the plasma or serum reflects changes in the ECF. These proportions (or the osmolarity of body fluids solute concentration) are important in determining the extent of dehydration and shock. In about two-thirds of diarrheal dehydration, loss of salt is in proportion to loss of water (isotonic dehydration). *Hypernatremic dehydration* may be seen when any factor (such as fever, hyperventilation, or a dry hot environment) increases water loss. Very small and very young infants are prone to hypernatremic dehydration. In situations where water intake has been stopped suddenly while loss continues, this form of dehydration may develop. A small number of patients may develop *hyponatremic dehydration* in diarrheal disease when given sugar water, weak tea, or another fluid which contains no appreciable amount of salt (electrolytes).

Potassium losses in diarrheal stool are great, and when diarrhea has been present for over 24 hours, they can be significant. Replacement is usually made on the basis of an average because deficits are hard to measure, even with a serum potassium blood level. Lowered calcium levels may occur in the presence of potassium losses.

Abnormal postoperative fluid losses usually occur through the gastrointestinal tract in the form of diarrhea or vomiting. These losses must be monitored closely. After an extensive resection of the gastrointestinal tract, there may be partial or complete failure of carbohydrate, fat, amino acid, water, electrolyte, vitamin, and mineral absorption in varying degrees. Peritonitis causes additional fluid and electrolyte loss (internal or "third space" loss), which can be particularly difficult to manage. An abnormal leak of plasma proteins into the abdominal cavity occurs because of the large inflamed area. Water and extracellular electrolytes are lost secondarily to this leak. Most patients show a mild to moderate respiratory alkalosis; thus sodium chloride rather than sodium bicarbonate should be used in replacement. If losses are severe, overt circulatory collapse may occur. Replacement is based on the degree of clinical dehydration, calculation of loss in relation to body weight, and monitoring of the circulatory status.

The most common cause of metabolic alkalosis in pediatric patients is *protracted vomiting* of gastric juices, predominantly hydrochloric acid, as in pyloric stenosis. In addition to the hydrochloric acid, there are small amounts of sodium and potassium in gastric juice, both as chloride salts. Loss of gastric juice causes a large loss of hydrogen and chloride as well as small losses of sodium and potassium, resulting in metabolic alkalosis and hypochloremia. Infants who vomit from causes other than pyloric stenosis may have a blood pH which is alkaline, normal, or acidic. When a child vomits with an open pylorus, the vomitus is a mixture of gastric acid and alkaline small intestine fluids (pancreatic juice, succus entericus, and bile). It is possible that the simultaneous losses of these two fluids will balance each other. When metabolic alkalosis does occur, further potassium and sodium losses result as the kidney attempts to restore balance. These losses come from body stores, since vomiting negates dietary replenishment. Changes in body composition also occur which reflect the

TABLE 11-6 Fluid Maintenance Requirements

Body weight, kg	Requirement
0-10	100 ml/kg
10-20	1000 ml + 50 ml/kg for each kg over 10 kg
> 20	1500 ml + 20 ml/kg for each kg over 20 kg

metabolic alkalosis, potassium depletion, and variable degrees of dehydration.

Body compensation to metabolic alkalosis is respiratory, but it is often unpredictable, irregular, or absent. It is necessary to rehydrate the infant and correct the alkalosis and hypocalcemia. Withholding of oral feeding and elimination of vomiting control the primary cause of alkalosis. Intravenous fluid therapy must include maintenance requirements, restoration of fluid losses, chloride (to expand the fluid lost extracellularly), and potassium.

Assessing Alterations in Fluids and Electrolytes

The purposes of fluid and electrolyte therapy are to (1) meet maintenance needs, (2) remedy prior deficits, and (3) correct ongoing losses. Maintenance therapy refers to fluid and electrolytes necessary to replace the physiological losses that result from normal metabolism. Prior or preexisting deficits refer to losses occurring before the institution of parenteral therapy. The amount and nature of the fluid loss must be estimated, and the fluid must be replaced. Ongoing losses are those which occur concurrently with existing therapy (e.g., diarrhea). All these patients require maintenance therapy by either oral or intravenous methods. If a deficit is present, it will continue unless adequate deficit therapy is also given. The replacement of any deficit may take several days.

Assessment

Maintenance needs can be calculated by estimating caloric expenditure. An accurate estimate of caloric expenditure can be done using body weight in relationship to known average calories expended over a 24-hour period. It is important to remember that 1 cal expended also requires the expenditure of 1 ml of water. Fluid maintenance requirements can be calculated by using the information in Tables 11-5 and 11-6.

The younger the client, the higher the metabolic rate and thus the need for higher maintenance and electrolyte requirements. Certain conditions, such as a febrile state and hypothermia, increase or decrease the metabolic rate, respectively, necessitating changes in the estimated caloric expenditure.

Body surface area (BSA) can also be used to calculate maintenance requirements. BSA is calculated through the use of a nomogram employing height and weight measurement (see Fig. 10-1). However, BSA calculations can

TABLE 11-5 Caloric Expenditure

Body Weight, kg	Expenditure
0-10	100 cal/kg
10-20	1000 cal + 50 cal/kg for each kg over 10 kg
> 20	1500 cal + 20 cal/kg for each kg over 20 kg

TABLE 11-7 Average Fluid and Electrolyte Requirements

	H_2O, ml/kg	Na^+, meq/kg	K^+, meq/kg
Newborn	40-60	0.8-1.0	0.8-1.0
4-10 kg	120-100	2.5-2.0	2.5-2.0
10-20 kg	100-80	2.0-1.6	2.0-1.6
20-40 kg	80-60	1.6-1.2	1.6-1.2

be difficult to use, particularly in emergency situations. The caloric expenditure method is the one most commonly used.

Management of Alterations in Fluids, Nutrients, and Electrolytes

Normal maintenance water requirements replace fluids which are lost through the skin, lungs, urine, sweat, and stool. Insensible losses normally amount to approximately 45 ml/100 kcal expended (Table 11-7). Urine output reflects water loss and the amount of exogenous solute (electrolyte) readied for excretion by the body. Generally, the amount of water lost through sweating is unremarkable while minimal water is lost in solid excreta in healthy states. In usual conditions the average normal water requirement totals approximately 100 ml per 100 kcal expended (Table 11-7).

Normal maintenance electrolyte requirements are not defined precisely since the renal system exerts great latitude in the conservation and excretion of electrolytes. Sodium (Na) and potassium (K) are usually provided in the form of chloride salt for maintenance therapy. These salts serve to replenish the chloride, sodium, and potassium lost during daily body functioning. The requirements for Na and K are given in Table 11-7. Another approximation of electrolyte requirements on the basis of caloric expenditure and metabolic turnover also can be carried out. With this alternative method, Na, K, and Cl are calculated as 3 meq, 2 meq, and 2 meq/100 ml per 24 hours, respectively.

Deficit replacement therapy refers to deficiencies in water, sodium, or potassium which develop as a result of (1) a poor or absent oral intake and (2) an abnormal loss which was not replaced. When present, such a deficiency always indicates that the total output has exceeded the total intake at a previous time period.

The calculation of a deficit is based on body weight. The loss of any body stores of water leads to a dehydrated state with its concomitant weight loss. The types of dehydration are related to plasma sodium levels and include (1) isotonic dehydration (normal sodium level), (2) hypertonic dehydration (elevated sodium), and (3) hypotonic dehydration (sodium level below 130 meq/liter). The sodium deficit often is in equal balance with the potassium deficiency. These losses are matched by a combination of bicarbonate and chloride loss. The health problems present determines the type of loss, which in turn determines the nature of the acid-base imbalance.

The osmolarity of the remaining body fluids is directly related to the type of dehydration (loss of electrolytes) which occurs and to its extent. Osmotic readjustment or redistribution of ECF and ICF takes place, and often it drastically affects the distribution of water in the body. A reduction in plasma volume (ECF) may have a serious effect on the circulation of the blood and cause a curtailment in the circulation to skin, muscle, and kidneys. Shock, which is often fatal in dehydrated patients, may develop. The changes which occur in ICF differ with each type of dehydration. A sudden change, as in the institution of replacement therapy, may cause shrinkage or swelling of tissue cells; therefore, *slow* replacement of deficits with a gradual return to a normal hydrated state is imperative.

Calculation of the replacement for any patient must be based on (1) the severity of the dehydration, (2) the type of dehydration, (3) the deficiency of potassium, and (4) the nature of the acid-base disturbance. The first phase of replacement therapy is aimed at restoring circulation. If shock is present or imminent, blood or a colloid solution is administered. An isotonic saline solution or one to which bicarbonate has been added is generally used in the initial therapy. Bicarbonate is not administered in the presence of metabolic or respiratory alkalosis. This phase is accomplished over the first few hours of intravenous therapy.

The second phase is aimed at restoring ECF volume and correcting sodium deficits. The specific fluids used during this phase depend on the type of dehydration (isotonic, hypotonic, or hypertonic) and the acid-base imbalance. The nature of the dehydration also dictates the length of this phase of replacement therapy.

During the third phase of treatment, potassium deficits are corrected after sodium chloride and water deficits have been remedied. No more than 3 meq/kg per 24-hour period is used for replacement therapy because of the potential danger of intracellular potassium overload. Several days may be required to repair potassium deficits, as intravenous potassium administration must proceed slowly.

The fourth phase of deficit therapy is aimed at restoring the body fats and proteins. Usually resumption of a normal diet accomplishes this objective. In some disease states oral intake may be contraindicated or may result in exacerbation of gastrointestinal malfunction (e.g., diarrhea). Parenteral hyperalimentation may be necessary.

Ongoing losses are replaced as they occur. The solutions used to replace ongoing losses should be similar to the fluid being lost. If possible, the electrolyte composition of the loss should be determined. For each 1 ml of fluid lost, 1 ml of appropriate solution is administered. Concurrent losses are estimated (both fluid and electrolyte content) every 4 to 8 hours, and replacement solutions are given in amounts equal to the losses of the previous 4- to 8-hour period. The electrolyte composition of gastrointestinal secretions is shown in Table 11-4. Losses are highly variable in individual pediatric patients.

Nursing Management

Nursing Diagnosis

Caring for children who have an alteration in fluid and electrolyte balance requires sharp observational skills in addition to a sound knowledge of developmental norms because of the vast differences which occur in the various stages of childhood. While a nurse needs to know what to look for, she also must record the data meticulously.

Nursing diagnoses serve to summarize the relevant data meaningfully. They are the basis for planning care because they describe actual or potential patient problems. Human beings are unique individuals, and so nursing diagnoses need to be highly individualized. The examples below are *not* all-inclusive; they are nursing diagnoses for children who are experiencing fluid and electrolyte deviations.

Fluid volume deficit related to an active loss

Altered oral mucous membranes related to dehydration

Fluid volume excess related to excess fluid intake

Altered tissue perfusion related to fluid and electrolyte imbalance

Potential fluid volume deficit related to the loss of body fluids

Potential electrolyte imbalance related to vomiting

A major nursing responsibility for all these nursing diagnoses involves identifying the minuscule changes which occur and typify the presence of fluid and electrolyte deficits or imbalance. The process of correcting these types of fluid problems is slow and involves total body responses to the treatment initiated. This complex replenishment takes time. A nurse constantly uses assessment skills to determine the improvement or deterioration of a child. The ongoing evaluation of a child's response to treatment is critical. It includes all the indicators which play a role in fluid and electrolyte balance and provide a nurse with invaluable data on which to base subsequent interventions. Thus, ongoing assessments and evaluations include the determination of intake and output, body weight, condition of the skin and mucous membranes, presence or absence of tears, depressed or flat fontanels, status of the eyeballs, and the child's general behavior.

TABLE 11-8 Urine Excretion

Age	Volume
Preterm neonate	1-3 ml/kg/h
Full-term neonate	3/4 ml/kg/h
6 months old	12 ml/h
1 year old	22 ml/h
5 years old	28 ml/h
12 years old	33-35 ml/h

Source: Meservey "Fluid and Electrolyte Balance," in M. Smith et al., *Child and Family: Concepts of Nursing Practice*, McGraw-Hill, New York, 1982, p. 608; J. R. Ingelfinger, "Renal Conditions in the Newborn Period," in J. P. Cloherty and A. R. Stark, *Manual of Neonatal Care*, Little, Brown, Boston, 1985, p. 379.

Intake and Output

In a child who is hydrated adequately, the intake and output totals for a 24-hour period are reasonably equal. This is not the case for a child who has a deficit or an electrolyte imbalance. Hence, it is important for a nurse to monitor closely and record accurately everything that is taken in or given off by the child. While all fluids given by mouth or by intravenous therapy are measured, fluids lost through nasogastric suction, vomitus, extensive wound drainage, urine, and stool also must be determined. Although the fluids taken in can be identified precisely, measuring the output can be a problem. For example, when a child is vomiting, it is important to record the number of times, the amount, and the nature of the vomitus. In this situation volume varies, and if the measurement is not accurate, the replacement of lost fluids and electrolytes will be much more difficult.

While the contents of nasogastric suctioning can be determined easily, a problem arises when the tube needs to be irrigated frequently for patency. The amount of saline instilled and the total amount withdrawn should be recorded meticulously. Obviously, a child with a nasogastric tube in place requires frequent mouth care. A child with a draining wound may need to have dressings weighed in order to identify more precisely the total fluids lost through drainage.

A significant amount of water can be lost in the stool, especially if the child is having diarrhea. It is essential to identify changes in the consistency, amount, or color of the stools.

Measuring urinary output in an infant or toddler who is not toilet trained can be a challenge. Many facilities have implemented policies which require routine weighing of the diapers (before and after) of all young children who are not toilet trained. The weight in grams equals the milliliters voided, or 1 gr = 1 ml. The weight of a dry disposable diaper is subtracted from the weight of the wet diaper to determine the volume voided. Normal urine volume for different age groups is identified in Table 11-8. This effective method of measuring urine output is much less traumatic than using 24-hour urine collecting bags, which do not adhere well, confine the infant to a crib, and can result in skin breakdown at the application site. Urine samples can be obtained easily by using a syringe (without a needle) to siphon urine from a wet diaper for use with a refractometer to obtain a specific gravity reading. It is important to examine the urine for odor, color, concentration (specific gravity), and amount voided. A rising specific gravity, infrequent voiding, and lesser amounts voided are all indications for concern.

Intravenous therapy is an important component of treatment; hence, careful monitoring is imperative. The type of solution running and the rate of flow should be determined as soon as a nurse becomes responsible for the child's care. The rate of flow is checked at 15- to 30-minute intervals and recorded on the flow sheet at least hourly. The use of calibrated burettes facilitates the administration of the prescribed hourly amount (Fig. 11-2).

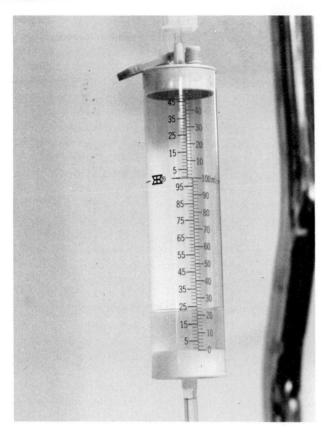

FIGURE 11-2   A calibrated burette for use in administering intravenous fluids. *(Photo courtesy of Bob Thiefels.)*

The meniscus must be read precisely. No more than a *2-hour* supply should be run into the burette; this limit decreases the likelihood of fluid overload. In some instances no more than an hour's supply of intravenous fluid is permitted. In many facilities a variety of infusion pumps are available. The use of such pumps does not free the nurse of responsibility for monitoring the rate of flow. Unfortunately, machines malfunction. Therefore, despite the use of an infusion pump, a nurse needs to monitor the level of fluid in a burette to ensure that the patient is receiving the hourly rate ordered and that the infusion pump is functioning correctly.

While intravenous fluids are being given to an infant or child, the site must be checked frequently for infiltration or infection. Infiltration can be extensive if the nurse relies solely on an infusion pump, especially when it malfunctions suddenly. Some pumps allow the fluid to run into tissue despite the presence of infiltration. If restraints are necessary to prevent dislodgement of a needle, they should be removed one at a time every 2 to 3 hours to exercise the extremity. Intravenous tubing also needs to be changed every 24 to 48 hours, depending on hospital policy. Once it is completed, a label should be placed on the tubing identifying the date, the time, and the person doing the replacement.

Body Weight

Since body weight is an extremely sensitive indicator of fluid loss or gain, accurate weighing of a child is an extremely important nursing action. A fluid volume loss is reflected quickly in weight loss. There are three significant categories in weight loss. A 3 to 5 percent weight loss indicates a mild fluid deficit, a 5 to 9 percent loss is considered a moderate deficit, while a loss of 10 percent or more is severe. A 15 percent loss in body weight can result in hypovolemia, a life-threatening situation. An accurate body weight is thus a critical factor in fluid and electrolyte replacement.

The child needs to be weighed without clothing at the same time every day and on the same scale. The presence of an arm board or a protective device such as a cup over the site should be noted when the weight is recorded. The removal of these items can result in drastic changes from previous weights. When children need to be weighed more frequently, it is done on every shift, with the same precautions. Balancing a scale properly, weighing the child accurately, and recording of the results are imperative. Any significant differences (loss or gain) should be reported promptly to a physician.

Vital Signs

The temperature, apical pulse, respiratory rate, and blood pressure readings provide vital information. These measurements are done every 4 hours, but any variation, such as a rapid apical pulse, necessitates more frequent monitoring and recording.

Generally, a child's temperature is elevated or subnormal. It is important to realize that an elevated temperature increases a body's fluid expenditure, thereby increasing the insensible water losses. The extent of such loss depends on how high the temperature rises and how long it remains elevated. Fluid deficits which result in body temperatures lower than normal occur because of decreased energy production. Since fluid loss is a major concern, an infant or toddler admitted with diarrhea should have axillary temperatures taken. The insertion of a thermometer stimulates the rectal sphincters, increasing stool excretion and causing additional water loss.

An apical pulse needs to be taken for a full minute to detect irregularities. For example, a child with hypokalemia may have an irregular rhythm. The rate usually increases as the fluid volume decreases. It is compensatory in nature: With a decrease in fluid volume, cardiac activity intensifies in an effort to continue providing essential nutrients to the body.

The respiratory rate, depth, character, and pattern are essential observations for a nurse. It is best to assess the respiratory status before disturbing a sleeping child, because it is free of factors (crying, irritability, agitation, etc.) which can contribute to obtaining less reliable data. Generally, as the respiratory rate increases, the depth of respirations decreases. There are variations and side effects. For example, in the presence of hyperpnea (increased rate, increased depth), there is a subsequent in-

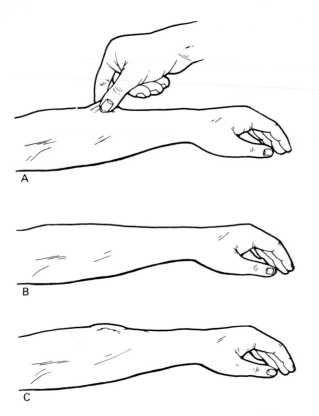

FIGURE 11-3   Assessment of skin turgor. When normal skin is pinched *(a)* it assumes its previous shape within seconds *(b)*. If the skin remains wrinkled for 20 to 30 seconds, the client has poor skin turgor *(c)*. *(From S.M. Lewis and I.C. Collier, Medical-Surgical Nursing, McGraw-Hill, New York, 1987, p. 242.)*

crease in insensible water loss from the lungs. Kussmaul's respirations, which are gasping respirations, or episodes of "air hunger," may be observed in children with metabolic acidosis. In this breathing pattern the respiratory system attempts to blow off both the excessive CO_2 and hydrogen. Slower, more shallow respirations are seen in children with metabolic acidosis. The success of the treatment protocol implemented is reflected in the return to a respiratory rate more appropriate for a child's age.

Skin

In assessing skin turgor, a nurse determines a client's state of hydration, because a simple maneuver elevates the elasticity of the body's largest organ system. By grasping a fold of skin between the thumb and index finger and then releasing it, the nurse observes the manner in which the skin returns to its previous state (Fig. 11-3). In dehydration, once the skin is grasped, it remains elevated for fractions of a second or longer. The skin remains in a raised position even when there is a mild dehydration. One differentiating feature must be considered in assessing skin turgor. If the nurse is examining a malnourished infant or child, the loose skin (and apparently poor skin turgor) may be due to a lack of subcutaneous tissue and not necessarily to dehydration.

With substantial fluid losses, the skin may be cool to the touch even when the child is febrile. In addition, its color may be gray. Both of these clinical manifestations are due to the decreased peripheral circulation which occurs when blood is shunted to vital organs in the body. These are important observations.

With fluid overload, edema occurs and puffiness is seen in the hands, feet, and faces and occasionally the scrotal sacs of male children. When finger pressure is applied to a puffy area and then released, an indentation occurs. It disappears *slowly* as fluid returns to the tissue tested. With this excess, other signs are evident, including an increase in body weight and urine output, falling specific gravity of urine, an increase in pulse and respiratory rates, and the development of rales on auscultation. Fluid overload can be avoided by means of an accurate determination of the child's specific needs and the conscientious monitoring and recording of intravenous fluids.

Mucous Membranes and Other Assessments

When a child becomes dehydrated, it is important for the nurse to evaluate the extent by looking for other indicators. For example, the mucous membranes of the mouth become dry. By placing a finger in the mouth and determining the moisture present in the area between the gum and cheek, one can quickly draw a conclusion. If it is dry, a fluid deficit is present. However, it is necessary to differentiate between mouth breathing and dehydration. In a child who is a mouth breather, the mucous membranes in this area remain moist, whereas they feel dry in a dehydrated child. Certainly diligent mouth care is an important intervention which increases a child's comfort level.

Another valuable observation is the presence or absence of tears. In a crying child with a fluid deficit, tears are absent and saliva is absent too. These signs can be observed in mild dehydration. The open fontanels of very young infants become depressed, and cranial suture lines also may be evident. The eyes of children with fluid deficits become sunken, and when the eyeballs are touched, they feel soft. These symptoms resolve slowly as a child's fluid and electrolyte status improves.

General Behavior

In working with a child who has a fluid or electrolyte imbalance, it is extremely important to assess the child as a whole. This is a difficult task when one considers the many stages of childhood. When the nurse meets a child for the first time, preexisting data are nil and parental input is absolutely essential. Parents know their children and can be extremely helpful in identifying deviations from a child's normal behavior. The observations of a nurse are enhanced when parents are involved.

When questions are posed by a nurse, the appropriateness of the responses must be evaluated, a task which is difficult with a child who has not mastered speaking. If tremors or lethargy is present, the increase, decrease, or duration must be identified. Irritability may be present, especially when the child is disturbed, and its progression requires careful examination. Deviations in levels of consciousness may necessitate a thorough neurological assessment in addition to notification of a physician.

The cries of infants and young toddlers are particularly informative. In the presence of fluid deficits and electrolyte imbalance, the cry may be weak, high-pitched, and of short duration. As fluids are replenished, the cry becomes more normal; e.g., it is lusty and of longer duration. Overall, the behaviors return to more normal levels as the body fluids and electrolytes are replenished.

Children with fluid and electrolyte problems pose many challenges to a pediatric nurse. Professional responsibilities encompass monitoring the administration of parenteral fluids, identifying changes which signify deterioration or improvement, utilizing observational skills in data collection, and processing the pathophysiological and developmental knowledge essential in providing high-quality nursing care. Recording this information accurately and identifying the many clues which children generate are critical nursing interventions.

Learning Activities

1. Determine the fluid maintenance requirements of a toddler who weighs 10.1 kg.
2. Develop one day's meal plan for an adolescent whose calcium intake is very poor.
3. Identify four nursing diagnoses for an infant who has just been admitted for diarrhea.

Study Questions

1. Normally, the osmotic pressures of extracellular fluid (ECF) and intracellular (ICF) are:
    A. Equal.
    B. Unequal, with ICF being higher.
    C. Unequal, with ECF being higher.
    D. Redistributed when potassium enters the system.
2. The major cause of water and electrolyte loss in children is:
    A. Vomiting.
    B. Polyuria.
    C. Excessive perspiration.
    D. Diarrhea.
3. An excess of hydrogen ions:
    A. Forces potassium from the plasma and into body cells.
    B. Moves calcium into bone.
    C. Influences the movement of sodium into body cells.
    D. Forces potassium from body cells into the bloodstream.

4. A weight loss of 5 to 9 percent in an older dehydrated infant is considered to be:
    A. An insignificant weight loss.
    B. A mild weight loss.
    C. A moderate weight loss.
    D. A severe weight loss.
5. The major intracellular cation is:
    A. Potassium.   C. Calcium.
    B. Sodium.   D. Chloride.
6. The excretion of hydrogen ions is the responsibility of the:
    A. Respiratory system.
    B. Sweat glands.
    C. Renal system.
    D. Gastrointestinal system.
7. The cation responsible for the osmolarity of extracellular fluid is:
    A. Potassium.   C. Calcium.
    B. Sodium.   D. Chloride.
8. Many pediatric units use infusion pumps in administering intravenous fluids to children; this:
    A. Ensures a free-flowing intravenous site.
    B. Allows the nurse to participate in other patient care activities.
    C. Does not free the nurse of responsibility for monitoring the rate of flow.
    D. Releases the nurse from any obligation regarding the rate of flow.
9. The most accurate respiratory rate a nurse can obtain:
    A. Includes the depth and character of respirations.
    B. Is assessed after developing a relationship with the child.
    C. Precedes the recording of an apical rate.
    D. Is done before disturbing a sleeping child.
10. When a nasogastric tube is in place, the nurse does not need to:
    A. Change the tube every 48 hours.
    B. Record the output at the end of a shift.
    C. Monitor the amount of saline used in irrigations.
    D. Administer mouth care frequently.

References

Adams, N.R., and S.M. Mantick: "Fluid and Electrolyte Imbalance," in S.M. Lewis and I.C. Collier (eds.), *Medical-Surgical Nursing: Assessment and Management of Clinical Problems*, McGraw-Hill, New York, 1983.

Burke, S.: *The Composition and Function of Body Fluids*, Mosby, St. Louis, 1976.

Ingelfinger, J.R.: "Renal Conditions in the Newborn Period," in J.P. Cloherty and A.R. Stark (eds.), *Manual of Neonatal Care*, 2d ed., Little, Brown, Boston, 1985.

Meservey, P.G.: "Fluid and Electrolyte Balance," in M.J. Smith et al., (eds.), *Child and Family: Concepts of Nursing Practice*, McGraw-Hill, New York, 1982.

Metheny, N.M., and W.D. Snively: *Nurses' Handbook of Fluid Balance*, 4th ed., Lippincott, Philadelphia, 1983.

Emergencies in Childhood

Objectives

After reading this chapter, the student will be able to:

1. Understand the ABCs of cardiopulmonary resuscitation in infants and children.
2. Describe the management of airway obstruction in infants under 1 year of age and children over 1 year of age.
3. Understand the emergent nature of shock and the need for prompt intervention.
4. Recognize the need to counsel parents about ingestions and ensure that parents have telephone numbers for the local poison control center and for emergency services.

Situations that may necessitate cardiopulmonary resuscitation (CPR) in infants and children include injuries, suffocation (aspiration of foreign bodies), smoke inhalation, infantile apnea, infections, and ingestion of toxic substances. Injuries account for approximately 44 percent of deaths in children from 1 to 14 years of age. Forty-five percent of these deaths involve motor vehicles, 17 percent are attributed to drowning, and 21 percent are related to burns, firearms, and poisonings. In infants less than 1 year of age, poison ingestion, suffocation, and motor vehicle accidents account for 41 percent of accidental deaths (Statistics Resources Branch, 1984).

In 1983 more than 130,000 children under 5 years of age were brought to emergency rooms for ingestions; 13.9 percent were admitted to the hospital. Only 55 died, a marked decrease from the 450 who died in 1961. Pharmaceutical products accounted for the highest percentage of ingestions in 1981 (40 percent), followed by cleansers and polishes (14.3 percent), plants (12.8 percent), cosmetics (12.0 percent), pesticides (5.5 percent), paints and solvents (4.0 percent), petroleum products (2.8 percent), and gases and fumes (0.2 percent) (Massachusetts Medical Society, 1984).

Cardiopulmonary Resuscitation (Basic Life Support)

In general, if CPR is begun within 4 minutes of respiratory and cardiac arrest and followed quickly by advanced life support, the victim will have an excellent chance for recovery. Infants and children who are victims of drowning and exposure to cold, however, may recover fully after a longer time period. There are three basic rescue skills, the ABCs of CPR. Each includes an assessment which must be followed by appropriate action.

Establishing an Airway (A)

The rescuer first must determine whether the infant or child is conscious. The victim's shoulder is tapped or shaken gently. The rescuer calls loudly for help. If the victim is unresponsive, he is turned as a unit, without twisting the head, neck, and torso, to a flat, supine position on a hard surface. Firm support must be supplied to the head and neck when turning, especially if there is evidence of head and neck injury (National Conference on CPR, Part IV, 1986).

Since cardiac arrest in infants and children rarely is of cardiac origin but usually is secondary to respiratory difficulty or arrest, it is imperative to open the airway in order to prevent cardiac arrest. Two methods of opening the airway are the head tilt/chin lift maneuver and the jaw thrust maneuver; the latter is used when a neck injury is suspected (e.g., drowning or automobile accidents) (National Conference on CPR, 1986).

Head Tilt/Chin Lift

The palm of the hand closest to the head is placed on the forehead, and the head is tilted back gently to a "sniffing"

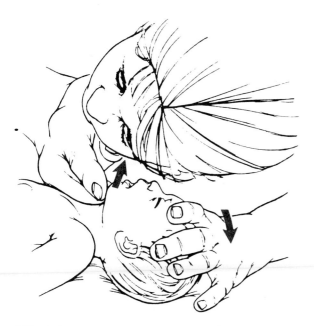

FIGURE 12-1 Head tilt/chin lift. (From *JAMA*, June 6, 1986, Vol. 255, p. 2956. Copyright 1986, American Medical Association.)

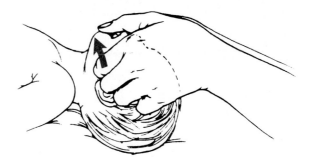

FIGURE 12-2 Jawthrust. (From JAMA, June 6, 1986, Vol. 255, p. 2956. Copyright 1986, American Medical Association.)

or neutral position in infants under 1 year of age. For older children, the head is extended slightly (Fig. 12-1); while the head tilt is maintained with one hand, the chin lift is performed with the other hand. The fingers are hooked under the bony part of the lower jaw nearest the rescuer. The chin is lifted upward (Fig. 12-1). The lips must remain open for free passage of air. The rescuer must have her fingers (not thumb) along the jawbone, *not* on the soft parts of the underchin.

Jaw Thrust

With elbows resting on the hard surface, the rescuer places one hand on either side of the victim's head. Two or three fingers of the hand are placed behind the angle of the lower jaw, and the jaw is displaced forward (Fig. 12-2).

Determination of Breathlessness

To determine if the child is breathing, the rescuer must use the senses of sight, touch, and hearing. The rescuer places her ear within an inch of the victim's mouth and nose and listens for exhaled air, looks for chest and abdominal movement, and feels for exhaled air across her cheek and ear. If the child is not breathing, rescue breathing must be begun (National Conference on CPR, Part IV, 1986).

Rescue Breathing (B)

While maintaining a patent airway, the rescuer takes a breath and leans over the victim to deliver the first breath. In an infant, a seal is formed with the rescuer's mouth over the victim's nose and mouth (Fig. 12-3). In children over 1 year, the victim's nose is pinched to seal the nostrils and the mouth is sealed with the rescuer's mouth fully covering the victim's mouth (Fig. 12-4). The breath is delivered slowly in 1 to 1.5 seconds with sufficient force to allow the chest to rise normally. As the victim is exhaling, the rescuer takes a breath in preparation for delivering the second slow breath to the victim (National Conference on CPR, Part IV, 1986).

If the chest does not rise, there is airway obstruction. Since the tongue is the most common cause of airway obstruction, the rescuer can assume that the head tilt/chin lift or jaw thrust has been performed incorrectly. The

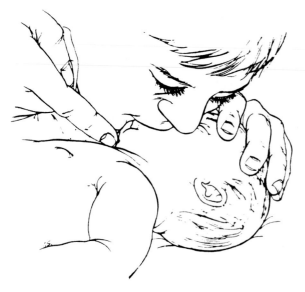

FIGURE 12-3 Mouth-to-mouth rescue breathing and nose seal. (From *JAMA,* June 6, 1986, Vol. 255, p. 2956. Copyright 1986, American Medical Association.)

Circulation(C)

Assessment of the Pulse

To determine whether cardiac arrest has occurred, the pulse in a large central artery must be assessed, using *gentle* pressure (not compression). In children over 1 year of age, the carotid artery is used (Fig. 12-5). The rescuer maintains the head tilt with one hand on the forehead and locates the Adam's apple with the first two fingers of the other hand. The two fingers are then moved sideways, toward the rescuer, to the groove between the trachea and the neck muscles. The artery is palpated gently for 5 to 10 seconds. In infants, either the brachial pulse (Fig. 12-6) or the femoral pulse is used (National Conference on CPR, Part IV, 1986).

If the pulse is present but the child is not breathing, rescue breathing is continued until spontaneous respirations occur. For infants the rate is once every 3 seconds (20 times a minute), and for children it is once every 4 seconds (15 times a minute). If the child is pulseless, chest compressions must be performed. If a second person arrives, the emergency medical system (EMS) must be activated. If not, CPR must continue until someone else

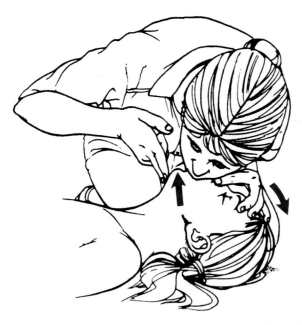

FIGURE 12-4 Mouth-to-mouth seal. (From *JAMA,* June 6, 1986, Vo 255, p. 2967. Copyright 1986, American Medical Association.)

head is repositioned to assure proper opening of the airway, and two slow breaths are delivered as described above. If the chest still does not rise, the obstruction may be from a foreign body (see Accidental Airway Obstruction below). Once two successful ventilations have been completed, the pulse is assessed (National Conference on CPR, Part IV, 1986).

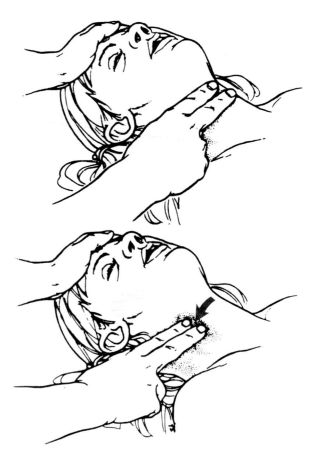

FIGURE 12-5 Locating and palpating the carotid artery pulse. (From *JAMA,* June 6, 1986, Vol. 255, p. 2967. Copyright 1986, American Medical Association.)

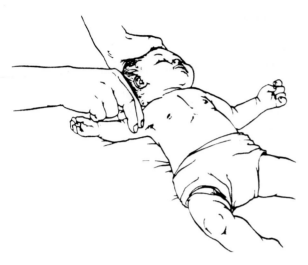

FIGURE 12-6 Locating and palpating the brachial pulse. (From *JAMA,* June 6, 1986, Vol. 255, p. 2968. Copyright 1986, American Medical Association.)

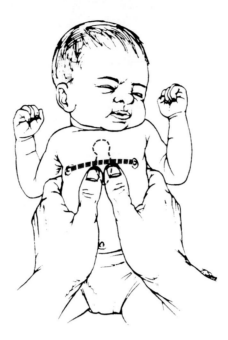

FIGURE 12-8 Side-by-side thumb placement for chest compressions in small neonates. (From *JAMA,* June 6, 1986, Vol. 255, p. 2972. Copyright 1986, American Medical Association.)

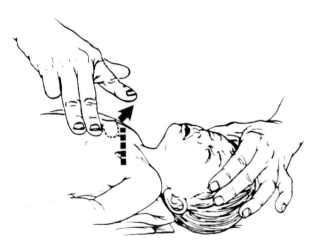

FIGURE 12-7 Locating the finger position for chest compressions in an infant. (From *JAMA,* June 6, 1986, Vol. 255, p. 2968. Copyright 1986, American Medical Association.)

comes to relieve the rescuer or the rescuer is exhausted (National Conference on CPR, Part IV, 1986).

External Chest Compressions

Chest compressions and rescue breathing must be coordinated. The site for compressions is different in infants and in children up to 8 years of age from that in adults. To locate the area of compression in neonates and infants, the rescuer first draws an imaginary line between the nipples. One finger width below the spot where this line intersects is the top of the area of compression (Fig. 12-7). The tips of two or three fingers are placed on the sternum, and the sternum is compressed to a depth of 1.3 to 2.5 cm (1/2 to 1 in). Pressure is then released without removing the fin-

gers from the sternum, and the sternum returns to its normal position. There should be at least 100 compressions per minute (National Conference on CPR, Part IV, 1986).

An alternative technique for performing chest compressions in small neonates involves the use of the thumbs. Both thumbs are placed on the middle third of the sternum just below the imaginary line. The fingers of both hands support the neonate's back (Fig. 12-8). In neonates, the depth of compression is 1.3 to 1.9 cm (1/2 to 3/4 in) and the rate is 120 per minute. No data exist to support a recommendation for compression/ventilation cycles in neonates (National Conference on CPR, Part VI, 1986); however, in infants beyond the neonatal period the recommended ratio is 5:1 (National Conference on CPR, Part IV, 1986).

For children 1 to 8 years of age, the rescuer first locates the lower margin of the child's rib cage using her index and middle fingers. With the middle finger, the rescuer follows the rib cage margin to the notch where the sternum and ribs meet. The index finger is then placed next to the middle finger. The heel of the other hand is placed along the sternum next to the index finger (Fig. 12-9). Using the heel of the other hand now in position (with fingers off the chest), the rescuer compresses the child's chest 2.5 to 3.8 cm (1 to 1 1/2 in). As the sternum returns to its normal position after each compression, the heel of the rescuer's hand remains in position. The rate of compression is 80 to 100 per minute. The compression/ventilation ratio is 5:1. Thus, for infants and children, at the end of every fifth compression a rescue breath is given (National Conference on CPR, Part IV, 1986).

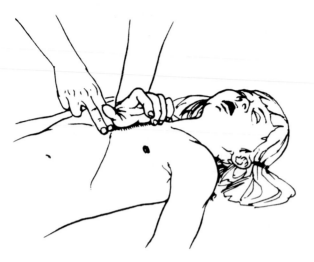

FIGURE 12-9   Locating the hand position for chest compressions in a child. (From *JAMA*, June 6, 1986, Vol. 255, p. 2958. Copyright 1986, American Medical Association.)

After 10 cycles have been completed, the pulse is palpated (brachial for infants, carotid for children). If the pulse is present, breathing is assessed. If the victim is still breathless, rescue breathing is continued. If the victim is pulseless, one slow ventilation is performed followed by five to one cycles of compressions and ventilations. This reassessment of circulation and breathing is repeated every few minutes until the victim is transferred to an advanced life-support facility.

Two-Rescuer CPR

When two rescuers are present, one rescuer assesses responsiveness, places the victim in the correct position, opens the airway, assesses respiratory status, ventilates, and checks the pulse. The second rescuer prepares to begin compressions if there is no pulse. After each fifth compression, the second person pauses to allow the first person to deliver a slow breath. The rate of compression and the ratio of compression to ventilation are the same as described above.

Accidental Airway Obstruction

If airway obstruction is due to infections such as croup or epiglottis, the infant or child must be transferred to an advanced life-support facility without delay. Such obstruction is not accidental. The use of back blows, chest thrusts, and the Heimlich maneuver would be ineffective and possibly dangerous.

If an infant or child is dyspneic, coughing, gagging, or stridorous (is making high-pitched crowing sounds), foreign-body aspiration should be suspected. When an aspiration is witnessed or strongly probable (e.g., if a toddler was playing with a toy that has small, detachable parts), the child is encouraged to continue with coughing and breathing efforts if the cough is effective (forceful). If the cough is or becomes ineffective, the child is increasingly

dyspneic, and stridor is present, attempts to relieve the obstruction are instituted. Relief also is attempted in unconscious infants and children who are not breathing (National Conference on CPR, Part IV, 1986).

Back Blows and Chest Thrusts

In infants under 1 year of age, back blows and chest thrusts are used to relieve foreign-body obstruction. The infant first is placed facedown over the rescuer's arm, legs straddling the elbow. The infant's head is lower than the trunk, and the rescuer supports the head and neck by holding the infant's jaw between the thumb and index finger. The rescuer provides additional stability by resting her forearm on her thigh. With the heel of the free hand, four back blows are delivered forcefully between the infant's shoulder blades (Fig. 12-10).

Head and neck support are provided while the infant is positioned on his back for chest thrusts. The rescuer places the free hand behind the infant's head and neck. The infant is now sandwiched between the rescuer's two hands and arms and is turned. The infant is lying on the rescuer's arm, and his head and neck are supported by the rescuer's hand. The head is lower than the trunk, and the rescuer's arm rests on his thigh. Four chest thrusts are applied in the same area as the chest compressions (Fig. 12-7).

Heimlich Maneuver

In children over 1 year of age the Heimlich maneuver is used. It may be delivered in conscious victims who are standing, sitting, or lying. If the victim is unconscious, he is always placed in a lying position.

To perform the Heimlich maneuver when the victim is standing or sitting, the rescuer stands behind the child. One foot is placed beside and the other foot behind the victim so that the rescuer can support the child and is in position to perform abdominal thrusts. If the victim is sitting in a chair, the chair back will provide support. The

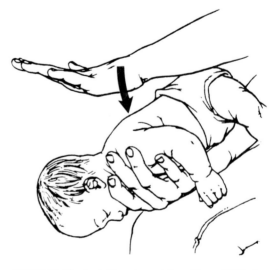

FIGURE 12-10   Back blow in an infant. (From *JAMA*, June 6, 1986, Vol. 255, p. 2959. Copyright 1986, American Medical Association.)

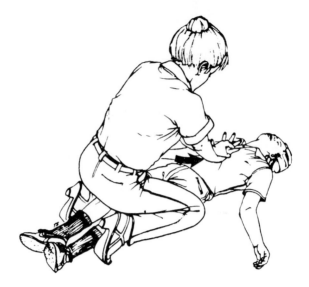

FIGURE 12-12 Heimlich maneuver with the child lying. (From *JAMA,* June 6, 1986, Vol. 255, p. 2959. Copyright 1986, American Medical Association.)

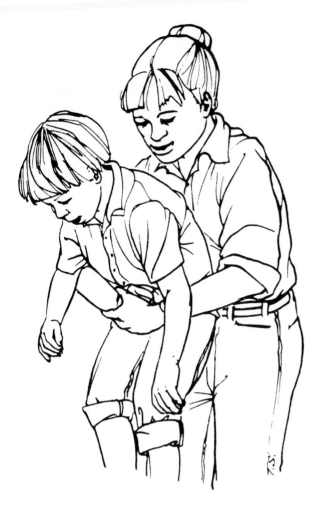

FIGURE 12-11 Heimlich maneuver with the child standing. (From *JAMA,* June 6, 1986, Vol. 255, p. 2959. Copyright 1986, American Medical Association.)

rescuer then wraps her arms around the victim's waist and makes a fist with one hand. The thumb side of the fist is placed midline on the abdomen, slightly above the umbilicus and below the xiphoid process. The fist is grasped with the other hand. Without exerting pressure against the rib cage with the arms, the rescuer presses her fist into the child's abdomen, using a quick inward and upward thrust (Fig. 12-11). To prevent damage to internal organs, the rescuer's hands do not touch or press on the rib cage or the xiphoid process. A rapid sequence of 6 to 10 thrusts is repeated until expulsion of the foreign body occurs (National Conference on CPR, Part IV, 1986).

A child who is lying is placed on his back, faceup. If the child is on the floor, the rescuer kneels at the child's feet, or if the child is large, the rescuer kneels astride the child (Fig. 12-12). For a child who is on a table, the rescuer stands at the child's feet. The heel of one hand is placed midline on the abdomen, slightly above the umbilicus and below the xiphoid process. The fingers should not touch the child's abdomen, xiphoid process, or rib cage. The other hand is placed on the first hand, and the heel of the bottom hand is pressed quickly inward and up-

ward in midline (not to either side). Only one thrust may expel the object but a series of 6 to 10 may be necessary. The thrusts are more gentle in small children than in larger children.

To check for a foreign body in the mouth, blind finger sweeps must never be used in infants and children. Such an action may cause further obstruction by pushing the object into the airway. Instead, the tongue-jaw lift is employed. When the rescuer grasps the lower jaw between the thumb and index finger and lifts, the victim's mouth is opened. The thumb is then pressed on the victim's tongue. The rescuer looks into the victim's mouth. If a foreign object is seen, it is removed with the fingers of the other hand (National Conference on CPR, Part IV, 1986).

Assessment of Respirations

Once efforts to remove the foreign body have been completed, the head tilt/chin lift is performed to open the airway and the rescuer assesses the victim's respiratory status. If the child is not breathing, rescue breathing is begun. If the chest does not rise, attempts to relieve the foreign-body obstruction are repeated. Throughout the process of relieving the obstruction, if attempts are unsuccessful, the emergency medical system must be activated once a second person arrives on the scene. Until that time the rescuer must continue with attempts to relieve the obstruction, rescue breathe, or do chest compressions and ventilations based on assessment.

All health care professionals, regardless of the setting, should be trained in basic life support. Advanced life-support training is necessary for those working in emergency rooms and intensive care units.

Shock

Shock is a secondary syndrome that can result from a variety of causes; however, its presence is so emergent that it commands immediate attention. There are three types of shock:

1. *Hypovolemic shock:* caused by hemorrhage and extracellular fluid losses (burns, fistulas, severe dehydration, intestinal obstructions, crushing injuries) and characterized by marked peripheral vasoconstriction
2. *Cardiogenic shock:* poor cardiac output which accompanies a variety of cardiac pathological conditions including myocardial infarction, arrhythmias, premature ventricular contractions, and impaired mechanical function, as in tamponade
3. *Vasogenic (neurovasogenic) shock:* peripheral circulatory failure due to arteriolar and capillary vasodilatation; seen in septic shock, patients who faint, anaphylaxis, and insulin shock

Although the mechanisms of these different types vary, basically shock is a defective venous return to the heart with a commensurate reduction in cardiac output. This circulatory inadequacy leads to very poor tissue perfusion and oxygenation. Failure to reverse this process leads to the death of tissue, organ, and ultimately the child.

While hypovolemic shock can occur in a child who has sustained a severe abdominal injury which results in significant blood loss (lacerated liver or spleen or torn pelvic blood vessels), more often it is a complication which is anticipated, as in a burn patient. It can also occur in a child who has ingested lethal amounts of iron, in a child who has had surgery (postoperative), or as a severe complication of sepsis (endotoxic shock).

The most common types of shock seen in the pediatric population are hypovolemic and septic (Corse and Lambert, 1983). Regardless of its cause, shock must be diagnosed accurately and treated aggressively if an adequate circulatory blood volume is to be maintained.

Signs of Shock

The signs of shock include a rapid, feeble, thready pulse; subnormal temperature; restlessness; hypotension; shallow, increasingly rapid respirations; pallor; cool, clammy skin; and diminished urinary output. A child's mental status varies from anxiety or apprehension to a comatose condition. Infants and young children in septic shock may be apneic, bradycardic (ineffective response to hypotension), and dehydrated (more sensitive to fluid loss due to greater proportion of body fluid to weight). Bradycardia is present in infants if the heart rate is below 80 and in children if the heart rate is below 60.

Treatment

Treatment of shock consists of checking airway patency to rule out obstruction; instituting the ABCs of CPR, as needed; stopping external bleeding, if present, through direct pressure; and restoring blood, fluid, and electrolyte equilibrium. The cause of the shock must be treated. Sometimes signs and symptoms of shock persist until the treatment is effective. Close observation and monitoring of physiologic and mental states are crucial in determining the efficacy of treatment.

If the infant or child is in cardiac arrest, ventilation and intubation are instituted to correct acidosis and hypoxemia. Epinephrine is given intravenously and repeated every 5 minutes as needed. The resultant vasoconstriction will increase perfusion pressure during chest compression. If cardiac arrest is prolonged or if the patient is hemodynamically unstable with concomitant metabolic acidosis, sodium bicarbonate is given. Epinephrine and sodium bicarbonate are never mixed because sodium bicarbonate inactivates epinephrine (National Conference on CPR, Part V, 1986).

To provide volume expansion and keep an intravenous line open for the administration of medications (e.g., lidocaine and atropine sulfate), Ringer's lactate or normal saline solution is begun. If the patient is in shock without cardiac arrest, volume expanders that will prevent progression to this state include blood, fresh-frozen plasma, colloid solutions (e.g., 5% albumin), and crystalloid solutions (e.g., Ringer's lactate solution or 5% dextrose in normal saline) (National Conference on CPR, Part V, 1986). For example, if shock is present, a bolus of Ringer's lactate solution is given intravenously (IV). If the blood pressure returns to normal, Ringer's lactate is given at 5 ml/kg/h. If the child is still hypotensive, the bolus is repeated. The blood pressure (BP) is checked; if it is low, the child receives a blood transfusion. During this time, the child is placed in Trendelenburg's position and heat loss is prevented. Both a nasogastric tube and a urinary catheter are put in place (Matlak et al., 1984). The child is then evaluated for regional trauma if history or signs so warrant.

The use of MAST (antishock) trousers, a pneumatic counter-pressure device, for children in hypovolemic shock is controversial. They *never* are used in the presence of cardiac arrest. If they are used for children in shock who are not in cardiac arrest, the abdominal compartment *is not inflated.* Such inflation can cause compression of abdominal organs against the diaphragm, impeding ventilation (National Conference on CPR, Part V, 1986).

Baseline laboratory tests which are important include blood culture and sensitivities; complete blood count (CBC); platelet count; electrolytes; blood urea nitrogen (BUN); creatinine; blood sugar; blood typing and cross matching; arterial blood for pH, PCO_2, and PO_2; coagulation screen; fibrinogen index and fibrin split products (FSPs); and urine culture and analysis. Results are compared over time with repeat tests to determine the physiologic and biochemical response to treatment.

Nursing Care

In caring for a patient in shock, time, organizational ability, technical skill, and expertise are crucial qualifications of the health team members who provide advanced life support. Use of a flow sheet after the recording of baseline data enables everyone to know a child's physiologic and biochemical determinations at a glance, provides a means of identifying changes quickly, and facilitates making necessary adjustments in the treatment regimen. Observing the child, assessing the child's status, and monitoring the response to therapy are the responsibility of the nurse. The child's level of consciousness should be assessed whenever he is approached.

Adequate tissue perfusion and oxygenation are the main aims of treatment. If tissue perfusion is inadequate, the nursing diagnosis is tissue perfusion: alteration in. To determination perfusion, the nurse can make several observations:

1. Blood pressure: hypotension or normotension (cardiopulmonary)
2. Central venous pressure (reliable guide to rate of fluid volume needed): if less than 15 mm Hg, need for more fluid (cardiopulmonary)
3. Capillary refill (skin over hand or foot is blanched through pressure and released; baseline color should return within 2 seconds): if prolonged, diminished peripheral perfusion (peripheral)
4. Urinary output (2 ml/kg/h up to 2 years and 1 ml/kg/h beyond 2 years): decreased or normal amount (renal)
5. Level of consciousness (alert, lethargic, stuporous, semicomatose, comatose): any evidence of dulled sensorium (cerebral)

   The listings which follow identify nursing actions which must occur at specific intervals to ensure the complete assessment of a child.

   15-minute intervals: BP, pulse, respirations, CVP (central venous pressure)

   30-minute intervals: IV rate (identification of fluid being infused), urinary output, specific gravity

   60-minute intervals: arterial blood gases, percentage oxygen given

Medications other than those noted under Treatment above depend on the cause of the shock. For example, in hypovolemic shock due to trauma, pain medications are given; in endotoxic (septic) shock, appropriate antibiotics are given.

When calculating intake and output, it is important to include urine, nasogastric (NG) suctioning, diarrhea, and vomitus. Also, a patient who is in shock must be kept warm. Overheating should not occur. Rest is important, but it may also be difficult to achieve. A nurse should coordinate all patient-related activities so that, when possible, all health care providers perform their functions at one time.

Complications

Some complications must be considered when a patient in shock does not respond satisfactorily or improves but then deteriorates instead of maintaining the initial progress. *Fluid overload,* or overinfusion, which occurs as a result of too much fluid received too quickly, can precipitate the development of acute pulmonary edema. Thus, nurses must be precise in making adjustments to the rate of flow. Judicious monitoring of CVP can prevent this occurrence.

Oliguria may indicate *acute renal failure,* which can result from prolonged impairment of renal perfusion. This problem is especially noteworthy in a burn patient whose thermal injury involves muscle and in a child who has sustained crushing injuries. Both types of patients are at risk because of increased amounts of hemochromogens in the blood. Decreased output, elevated BUN, hyperkalemia, and azotemia are consistent findings.

Disseminated intravascular coagulation (DIC) can occur in an infant with sepsis. Fibrinogen index and FSPs are the most accurate indexes of this coagulopathy. Whenever a patient appears to bleed excessively after a heel stick or venipuncture, DIC should be suspected.

The respiratory effects of septic shock can include *adult respiratory syndrome,* an insult to the alveolar-capillary unit. In this syndrome fluid accumulates between the alveoli and the capillaries. As the affected alveoli collapse, decreased gas exchange and severe hypoxia occur.

Ingestions

The American Association of Poison Control Centers (AAPCC) has estimated that there were over 1.9 million human poison exposures nationwide in 1985 (Litovitz, Normann, and Veltri, 1986). During 1985, 56 poison control centers participated in the AAPCC National Data Collection System. Children under 6 years of age accounted for 63.3 percent of the center contacts; 39.1 percent of all contacts were 1- and 2-year-old children. Gender distribution was predominantly male under 13 years of age and predominantly female thereafter (Litovitz, Normann, and Veltri, 1986).

Among those under 6 years of age, the most common nonpharmaceutical ingestions in descending order of frequency were plants, cleaning substances, cosmetics and personal care products, chemicals, and hydrocarbons. The most frequent pharmaceutical ingestions were analgesics, cold and cough preparations, vitamins, and topical medications. For both pharmaceutical and nonpharmaceutical ingestions, the order was plants, cleaning substances, analgesics, cosmetics, cold and cough preparations (Table 12-1). Acetaminophen ingestion occurred nearly five times more frequently than salicylate ingestion in children under 6, and the "preferred" acetaminophen was the pediatric formulation (Litovitz, Normann, and Veltri, 1986). Neither of these analgesics accounted for any fatalities in the pediatric population.

Forty-two fatalities in children 17 years of age or younger were reported to the AAPCC in 1985. Of that number, 21 occurred in children over 6 years of age: 13 were intentional suicides, 5 involved intentional abuse (e.g., sodium nitrate, freon, street drugs), 2 were accidents (carbon monoxide), and 1 was unknown. In the younger group ($n = 21$) 15 deaths occurred in children 9 to 26 months, and 6 children were 3 to 6 years of age. Thirteen of these 21 fatalities involved nonpharmaceuticals (fumes, gases, or vapors; insecticides; alcohols; gunbluing; hydrocarbons; and plants). Pharmaceuticals included among the remaining eight fatalities were sedatives, analgesics, anesthetics, antidepressants, cardiovascular drugs, electrolytes, and minerals. Several of these 42 children presented with cardiopulmonary arrest.

It would appear from the AAPCC data that young chil-

TABLE 12-1 Nine Most Common Categories of Substances and Products Ingested by Children Under 6 Years of Age*

Category	Number	Percent
Plants	64,616	11.3
Cleaning substances	55,108	9.7
Analgesics	46,810	8.2
Cosmetics and personal care products	45,726	8.0
Cold and cough preparations	30,415	5.3
Vitamins	26,167	4.6
Chemicals	26,109	4.6
Hydrocarbons	25,775	4.5
Topical preparations	22,003	3.8
Total	342,729	60.0

*Total contacts, all categories, reported to the AAPCC for this age group = 566,843.

Source: Adapted from T. Litovitz et al., "1985 Annual Report of the American Association of Poison Control Centers National Data Collection System," *American Journal of Emergency Medicine,* 4(5):427-458, 1986.

dren are at risk for ingestions and that parents would be wise to keep the regional poison control center's telephone number taped to the home phone. These centers can be contacted 24 hours a day to determine immediate treatment for known ingestions. Information that center personnel need includes the following:

1. Name and telephone number of caller
2. Name and age of child
3. Substance or product and amount ingested
4. Condition of child (e.g., alert, awake, convulsing)
5. Signs and symptoms (e.g., nausea, vomiting, choking, dizziness, drowsiness, clammy skin, rash)
6. Whether there is syrup of ipecac and activated charcoal in the home

Once the poison is identified, immediate treatment is begun. Depending on the poison, signs and symptoms and condition of the child, the parent may be advised to begin treatment, call the emergency medical service, or go immediately to the emergency room. Parents may also be asked to take the container, the clothing the child was wearing at the time of ingestion, and specimens of vomitus, urine (e.g., wet diapers), and stools to the emergency room, particularly if the product has not been identified. In the majority of cases reported by the AAPCC, treatment for poisoning occurred in the home (Litovitz, Normann, and Veltri, 1986).

When vomiting must be induced as immediate treatment, the parent is advised to give 5 to 10 ml of syrup of ipecac for children under 1 year of age and 15 ml for children over 1 year of age, followed by 100 to 300 ml of water. If vomiting does not occur within 20 minutes, the dosage is repeated once. If the child still does not vomit, he is transported to a hospital for gastric lavage. Depending on the material ingested (e.g., plants), 1 oz of activated charcoal in water may be given to absorb the poi-

son, following administration of ipecac syrup, *after vomiting has ceased* (Keim, 1983). Syrup of ipecac is not given for strychnine, corrosives (e.g., alkalis and strong acids), and petroleum distillates (e.g., gasoline, oil, cleaning fluid) or if the child is unconscious. In the AAPCC report, 68 percent of children 17 years of age and younger who received syrup of ipecac were treated at home (Litovitz, Normann, and Veltri, 1986).

Conclusions

Many lives can be saved through the prompt application of CPR, relief of airway obstruction, treatment for shock, and treatment for ingestions. A recommendation from the National Conference on Cardiopulmonary Resuscitation and Emergency Cardiac Care (Part IV, 1986) is that basic life-support skills be taught to the parents of young children. This group also noted that over "90% of deaths from foreign-body aspiration in the pediatric age group occur in children younger than 5 years of age, and 65% are in infants" (p. 2959). Thus parents need to know how to manage airway obstruction due to foreign bodies such as food (e.g., hot dogs, round candies, nuts) and other small objects (e.g., buttons, marbles, removable parts of toys). All parents should be given the local poison control number and the emergency medical number (in many communities 911) so that prompt attention can be given to children who are experiencing emergencies.

Learning Activities

1. Ask your instructor to arrange a laboratory experience for you to practice CPR on infant- and child-sized teaching models and practice positioning and placement of the hands for chest thrusts and back blows on infant-sized models and the Heimlich maneuver on child-sized models.
2. Develop a teaching plan to discuss prevention of childhood poisoning.

Study Questions

1. Assessment for cardiopulmonary resuscitation in infants and children begins with:
   A. Opening the airway.
   B. Determining if the victim is conscious.
   C. Placing the head in a neutral position.
   D. Determining whether the infant is breathing.
2. The most common cause of airway obstruction is:
   A. The tongue.
   B. A foreign body.
   C. Accumulation of mucus.
   D. Distended abdomen.

3. In performing rescue breathing in children:
   A. Quick breaths are delivered.
   B. The rate is once every 4 seconds.
   C. Chest compressions must always be performed.
   D. The pulse in the carotid artery is compressed for 5 to 10 seconds.
4. The main aims of treatment for children in shock are:
   A. Ruling out obstruction and treating the cause.
   B. Correcting acidosis and hypoxemia.
   C. Ensuring adequate tissue perfusion and oxygenation.
   D. Removing poison and providing rest.
5. If a poisonous substance has been ingested by a child, the parent first should:
   A. Notify the pediatrician.
   B. Give syrup of ipecac 5 to 10 ml to induce vomiting.
   C. Call the local poison control center.
   D. Talk to a nurse.

References

Corse, K.M., and L.E. Lambert: "Multisystem Disorders: Shock and Trauma," in J.B. Smith (ed.), *Pediatric Critical Care,* Wiley, New York, 1983.

Keim, K.A.: "Preventing and Treating Plant Poisoning," *MCN: The American Journal of Maternal Child Nursing,* 8(4):287-289, 1983.

Litovitz, T.L., S.A. Normann, and J.C. Veltri: "1985 Annual Report of the American Association of Poison Control Centers National Data Collection System," *American Journal of Emergency Medicine,* 4(5):427-458, 1986.

Massachusetts Medical Society: "Perspectives in Disease Prevention and Health Promotion, Poisoning among Young Children—US," *MMWR,* 33(10):129-130, 1984.

Matlak, M.E., D.G. Johnson, M.L. Walker, W.M. Palmer, and P.M. Stevens: "Initial Management of the Injured Child," in M.F. Hazinski (ed.), *Nursing Care of the Critically-Ill Child,* Mosby, St. Louis, 1984.

National Conference on Cardiopulmonary Resuscitation (CPR) and Emergency Cardiac Care (ECC): "Standards and Guidelines for Cardiopulmonary Resuscitation (CPR) and Emergency Cardiac Care, Part IV: Pediatric Basic Life Support; Part V: Pediatric Advanced Life Support; Part VI: Neonatal Advanced Life Support," *JAMA,* 255(21):2954-2973, 1986.

Statistics Resources Branch, Division of Vital Statistics: *Final Mortality Statistics, 1981,* National Center for Health Statistics, Hyattsville, Md., 1984.

Bibliography

Gildea, J.: "A Crisis Plan for Pediatric Code," *American Journal of Nursing,* 86(5):557-565, 1986.

Rimar, J.M.: "Sodium Bicarbonate During CPR," *MCN: The American Journal of Maternal Child Nursing,* 1(4):245, 1986.

Wagner, T.J., and M. Hindi-Alexander: "Hazards of Baby Powder?" *Pediatric Nursing,* 10(2):124-125, 1984.

13

The Abused or Neglected Child

Objectives

After reading this chapter, the student will be able to:
1. Describe the forms of child abuse and neglect.
2. List characteristics of victims and abusers.
3. Identify the responsibility of the nurse in reporting abuse and neglect.
4. Discuss nursing actions/interventions appropriate to the care of the child and family.
5. Describe the role of the nurse in primary and secondary prevention.

Violence within the family has emerged as a major concern of the decade. Gelles (1979) stated that "People are more likely to be hit, beat-up, physically injured, or even killed in their own home by another family member than anywhere else, and by anyone else, in our society (p. 11)." This sad, but true, comment describes the setting in which child abuse, spouse abuse, and elder abuse all take place. Within this setting, the roles of victim and aggressor are learned by the child as the victim of abuse or the observer of violence between parents or other family members. For several years, attention has focused on the effects of actual abuse and neglect on the child's subsequent development. Only recently (Westra, 1984; Davis, 1988) have health care professionals begun to examine the effects of interparental violence on children. As child abuse is discussed, nurses must keep in mind that in many cases other forms of abuse are also occurring and that violence is an accepted behavior in the family setting.

Significant Historical Facts

The first recorded case of child abuse in the United States was in 1874 in New York. A 9-year-old girl was found to be beaten, starved, and imprisoned by her adoptive parents. Concerned individuals could find no appropriate place to report the incidents and, in desperation, notified the American Society for the Prevention of Cruelty to Animals. These efforts led to the organization of the New York Society for the Prevention of Cruelty to Children. In 1877 the American Humane Association was established.

No additional cases were reported until 1946, when Dr. John Caffey cited six case studies in which the patients "exhibited 23 fractures and 4 contusions of the long bones. In not a single case was there a history of injury to which the skeletal lesions could reasonably be attributed and in no case was there clinical or roentgen evidence of generalized or localized skeletal disease which would predispose to pathological fracture" (p. 163). The next significant contribution to a growing field of literature occurred in 1961 when Dr. Henry Kempe coined the term "battered child syndrome." It was used to describe a "clinical condition in young children . . . (who) have received serious physical abuse, generally from a parent or foster parent" (Kempe and Helfer, 1962, p. 17). A more encompassing description of child abuse and neglect, the "maltreated child," was proposed by Fontana (1963).

Child abuse and neglect or child maltreatment now encompass physical abuse and neglect, emotional abuse or neglect, and sexual abuse. Medical care neglect, safety neglect, educational neglect, and abandonment are all encountered and inadequate parenting is the major issue. Fontana (1984) stated:

> Considering then the maltreatment of children in the context of these various signs of abuse and neglect, one can state that in the 1980s child maltreatment is a major problem confronting a large number of parents caught in the web of a multi-troubled family unit (p. 736).

Incidence

The abuse and neglect of children is a major pediatric problem. It has been increasing at a rate of 15% to 20% every year throughout the United States (Fontana, 1984). In 1985, 1.9 million cases were reported nationwide, a rate of more than 30 per 1000 children (Cupoli, 1987). Most experts believe that reported figures probably represent less than half of the cases that actually occur. The Department of Health and Human Services estimates that 68% of all cases are not reported (Cupoli, 1987). The National Center for the Prevention of Child Abuse and Neglect estimated that 4000 children die annually in the United States from abuse and neglect (Fontana, 1984).

Definitions

There are no definitions agreed to by all who come in contact with child abuse and neglect. There are, however, terms acceptable for the purposes of discussion.

Physical abuse is an action by a caretaker that results in non-accidental injury to a child. It may be intentional but often is not premeditated. The injuries can range from mild bruising to life-threatening trauma and death. More recently, intentional poisoning of children was identified as a form of physical abuse (Dine, 1982; Kunkel, 1984).

Physical neglect is commonly an act of omission and includes the failure to provide adequate food, shelter, clothing, medical care, and a safe environment.

Emotional abuse is the use by the caregiver of verbal expressions that are meant to dominate, belittle, reject, or instill fear in the child. Scapegoating, name calling, threatening, and continually telling the child he cannot do anything right are forms of emotional abuse.

Emotional neglect is the failure of the caregiver to provide nurturing, caring, affection, and developmental stimulation for the child.

Sexual abuse is defined by Kempe and Helfer (1980) as the involvement of dependent, developmentally immature children and adolescents in sexual activities that they do not fully comprehend, to which they are unable to give informed consent, or that violate the social taboos of family roles. Included in sexual abuse are incest, molestation, exhibitionism, rape, and the exploitation of children and adolescents in prostitution and pornography.

Identification and Assessment

Components of the identification and assessment process are considered separately, but it is important for the nurse to know that commonly more than one type of abuse occurs at the same time. All aspects appropriate to the particular situation must be assessed. The nurse must maintain a high index of suspicion. A knowledge of the physical and behavioral indicators of abuse and neglect, characteristics of the participants in an abusive situation, and precipitating factors is necessary. Careful history taking and observations of the interaction during the assessment process provide valuable information.

Characteristics of the Participants
Several characteristics are pertinent to this problem. The interacting variables most commonly considered in explaining child abuse and neglect are a special child, a parent with the potential to abuse, and stress or environmental factors that trigger the event.

Parents or Perpetrators
Researchers have found that abusive and neglecting adults come from all socioeconomic backgrounds, educational levels, and professions and occupations. Most often the perpetrator of the abuse is a parent, but other relatives, siblings, foster parents, babysitters, daycare personnel, friends, and neighbors have been involved. Some authors indicated that the 20- to 40-year old mother is most often the abuser (Justice and Justice, 1976). The neglectful parent is most often the young, single mother (Polansky et

al., 1981). The father is most often the perpetrator in reported cases of sexual abuse, but most authorities agree that underreporting is very high.

Bergman et al. (1986) suggested that child abuse, es-

pecially serious and fatal cases, may be occurring more frequently at the hands of men. This finding represents a change and may be explained at least in part by the greater social acceptance of varying "living together" ar-

TABLE 13-1 Indicators of Physical Abuse

Physical Indicators	Behavioral Indicators in Child	Parental Behaviors/Characteristics
Bruises and welts	Believe they deserve punishment	Offers illogical, contradicting, or chang-
On face, lips, mouth	May be wary of adult contacts	ing explanation of injury
On torso, back buttocks, thighs	Become apprehensive when other chil-	Seems unconcerned about child
In various stages of healing	dren cry	Blames injury on child or someone else
Red-purple 2-4 hours	Exhibit behavioral extremes	(e.g., sibling)
Green 5-7 days	Withdrawal	Does not respond to child's crying or
Yellow 8-14 days	Aggressiveness	needs
Brown/fading 2-4 weeks	Inappropriate maturity	Uses harsh discipline, inappropriate to
Clustered, forming regular patterns	Much manipulative behavior	child's age, condition, or behavior
Reflecting shape of article used to in-	Exhibit fear of parents or of going home	Is unable to supply history of child's de-
flict injury (e.g., electric cord, belt	May report injury by parent	velopment, milestones, etc.
buckle, hand)	Do not cry when approached by exam-	Delays bringing child in for treatment
On several surfaces	iner or during painful procedures	Refuses to consent to diagnostic studies
Burns	Form only superficial relationships	"Hospital shops"
Circular burns (i.e., cigarette) espe-	Engage in indiscriminate displays of af-	Is emotionally immature
cially on soles, palms, back, or but-	fection	Has low self-esteem
tocks	Respond to questions in monosyllables	Is isolated—no support system
Immersion burns (socklike, glovelike,	Demonstrate poor self-concept	Has unrealistic expectations of children
perineal) symmetrical, absence of		Expects children to meet their
"splash" marks		emotional needs (role reversal)
Patterned object used (iron, radiator,		Sees the child as "bad," or "different"
stove burner)		
Rope burns on arms, legs, neck, or		
torso		
Infected burns indicating a delay in		
seeking treatment		
Fractures/Dislocations		
To skull, nose, facial structures, ribs,		
clavicle		
Femur fractures in the nonambulatory		
child		
Multiple, in various stages of healing		
Spiral fractures indicative of twisting of		
extremity		
Lacerations and abrasions		
To face, torso, back of arms or legs,		
external genitalia		
Bite mark appearance		
Abdominal injuries		
External bruises		
Internal injuries		
Renal		
Pancreatic		
Ruptured liver, spleen, intestinal perfo-		
ration		
Head injuries		
Subdural hematomas		
Skull fractures		
Scalp swelling		
Bald patches on scalp		
Retinal hemorrhages		
Black eyes		
Chemical		
Unexplained repeat poisoning, drug		
overdose, or other unsuual substance		

rangements and the fact that larger numbers of women work, so men are spending more time caring for children.

While investigators cannot reliably predict who will abuse children, some common characteristics have emerged over the years of study. Abusive individuals exhibit low self-esteem and a low tolerance for frustration, often acting on impulse. They are socially isolated, with few friends or relatives nearby, and tend not to trust, which increases the isolation and inability to use resources. They have frequently been abused themselves and have many unmet needs for love, affection, and nurturing. The child is expected to meet these needs (role reversal) and, when unable to do so, is viewed as rejecting the abuser. The abuser lacks parenting skills and knowledge, resulting in unrealistic expectations of the child.

Abused Children

The victims of child abuse and neglect are viewed as "different" by the abuser. The child may be "special" for real or imagined characteristics. The infant who is preterm or of low birth weight may lack responsiveness to the parents, create financial stresses, and generally not meet the

expectations of the parents. If temperament, sex, physical appearance, or other characteristics are not congruent with parental expectations, the child may be at risk for abuse. Children who are handicapped or developmentally delayed have also been found to be at greater risk.

Boys and girls are at nearly equal risk for abuse, and it occurs in all ages through age 18. The infant and young child are at greater risk for more severe injury, permanent physical disability, and death because of their inability to escape or defend themselves. Girls are at significantly greater risk for sexual abuse.

The nurse should note the behavior of the child. Role reversal in which the child takes on parenting tasks and cares for the parent is common. Withdrawal, hostility and aggression, overcompliance, detachment, and depression are all behavioral characteristics of the abused and neglected child. Additional indicators are listed in Tables 13-1 to 13-4.

Environmental Factors

The third variable to be assessed is that of stresses or crises and the potential effect on the abusive or neglecting situation. Are there problems or unemployment, lack of

TABLE 13-2 Indicators of Physical Neglect

Physical Indicators	Behavioral Indicators in the Child	Parental Behaviors/Characteristics
Underweight, poor growth patterns, failure-to-thrive	Begs, steals food	Has chaotic home life
Hunger, poor hygiene, inappropriate clothing	Arrives early and stays late at school or is frequently absent from school	Has inadequate, unsafe living conditions
Abdominal distention	Is fatigued and listless, falls asleep in class	Lacks knowledge of child's needs
Wasting of subcutaneous tissue	Inappropriately seeks affection	Has low self-esteem
Unattended physical problems or medical needs	States he has no caretaker	Is passive, has little motivation to effect change in lives
Abandonment	Assumes adult responsibilities and concerns	Lives isolated from friends, neighbors, and relatives
	Is delinquent	
	Abuses alcohol and drugs	

TABLE 13-3 Indicators of Emotional Abuse and Neglect

Physical Indicators	Behavioral Indicators in the Child	Parental Behaviors/Characteristics
Failure-to-thrive	Infant—lack of social smile and stranger anxiety	Blame and belittle the child
Feeding disorders	Withdrawal	Withhold love
Speech disorders	Self-stimulating behaviors such as sucking, biting, rocking	Are cold and rejecting
Sleep disorders	Antisocial behaviors—destructiveness, cruelty, stealing	Have unrealistic expectations
Enuresis	Lags in emotional and intellectual development	Verbally abuse (name calling, constant criticism)
Lags in physical development	Behavior extremes: passive and compliant to aggressive and demanding	Treat children in home unequally
	Unusual fearfulness	Minimize child's problems
	Psychoneurotic reactions—phobias, obsession, compulsions	Have personality disorders
	Suicide attempts	

TABLE 13-4 Indicators of Sexual Abuse

Physical Indicators	Behavioral Indicators in the Child	Parental Behaviors/Characteristics
Difficulty in walking or sitting	Infant-Toddler	Has low self-esteem
Torn, stained, or bloody underclothing	Irritability	Has unmet emotional needs
Pain on urination	Sleep disturbances	Lacks social and emotional contacts out-
Bruises or lacerations of external genita-	Altered level of activity	side the family—isolated
lia, vagina, or anal areas	Preschool child	May have marital problems with spouse
Pain, swelling, or itching in genital area	Nightmares	and seek affection from child
Mouth and throat injuries	Regression in development	May have experienced loss of spouse
Sexually transmitted disease in the child	Explicit knowledge of sexual acts	through death or divorce
under 12 years	Clinging/whining to nonabusive parent	
	Fear of places, persons, or situations of	
	which not previously afraid	
	School-Age Child	
	Behavioral problems	
	Frightening dreams, sleep disturbances	
	Withdrawal, regression, fantasy	
	Unwilling to change for or participate	
	in physical education	
	Poor peer relationships	
	Decreased school performance	
	Truancy, running away	
	Bizarre sexual knowledge and behavior	
	Adolescent	
	Fright, confusion	
	Anger, acting out	
	Truancy, running away, promiscuity,	
	prostitution	
	Depression	
	Drug and alcohol abuse	
	Poor peer relationships	
	Suicide	

adequate housing, financial deficits, alcoholism or drug addiction, divorce or desertion, or other chronic stresses? Has there been a recent move, loss of support systems, the birth of another child? Are substitute caretakers involved?

Additional Observations

While assessing the above factors, some additional information may be obtained by observing the interactions between parent and child.

1. How does the parent talk to the child? Always a demand?
2. Are the parents' verbalizations about the child always negative?
3. How does the parent respond to the child's crying? Are needs ignored?
4. Does the child seek comfort from the parent during medical procedures?
5. Does the parent seem to have fun with the child?
6. Does the parent strike the child in the nurse's presence?
7. Is the parent able to provide a knowledgeable history of the child's milestones, nutritional patterns, and daily activities?
8. Does the parent readily relinquish care of the infant or child to the nurse? Is the care too much for the parent?

Physical Abuse

As can be seen in Table 13-1, physical abuse can present with one or more of a variety of injuries, ranging from mild to severe and life-threatening. Bruises, welts, abrasions, lacerations, burns, fractures, head injuries, abdominal injuries, and chemical abuse are indicators of possible abuse (Figs. 13-1 to 13-5). The location, shape, size, pattern, and color of injuries should be documented. Body diagrams are useful for this documentation. The circumstances surrounding the injury should be determined, since incompatibility between injury and history is a common indicator of abuse. For example, a fall from a bed or sofa onto a carpeted floor does not usually result in skull fractures and subdural hematomas.

It is uncommon for the child to betray the parent and confess to the abuse received. In spite of the abuse, victims are loyal to the perpetrator. The child may fear losing whatever security and affection the parent provides between episodes of abuse. He also believes that the abuse is his fault. The child may also fear more abuse if he does not support the parent's story.

The nurse should consider the injury in relation to the developmental capabilities of the child. Accidents do happen to children, but bruises from accidental falls are typically on knees or elbows, not on backs and buttocks. Immersion burns to the perineal area can be inflicted when a

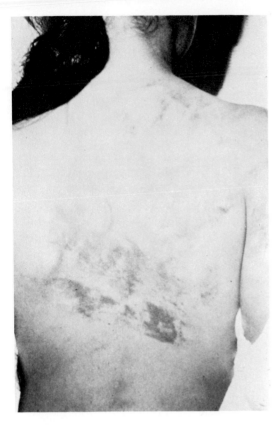

FIGURE 13-1 Multiple bruises on the back.

parent has unrealistic expectations in toilet training the toddler. Accidental contact with hot water will result in "splash marks" as the child tries to avoid the hot water. In accidental injuries, parents tend to blame themselves, show concern for the child, and provide comfort to the child. Abusive parents may show no concern for the child and his injury but focus instead on some other personal concern or problem. They may voice anger toward the child and blame him for the injury. The parent does not offer comfort, and the child may not seek it from the parent.

Documentation includes colored, dated photographs. Additional evaluation involves:

1. A skeletal survey when there is any serious injury and in any child under 2 years of age.
2. Coagulation studies to rule out abnormalities.
3. A developmental assessment.
4. A neurologic examination.
5. Other tests as indicated by the injury.

The nurse or other health care provider interviewing the parents should be nonjudgmental and accept them as worthy individuals while not condoning the behavior. Recognition of one's own feelings and the feelings and needs of the parents and the child are necessary if one is to begin developing the relationship needed for continuing assessment and intervention.

Physical Neglect

The physically neglected child may be underweight, with poor growth patterns, hunger, poor hygiene, abdominal distention, and wasting of subcutaneous tissue (Table 13-2). The failure-to-thrive infant or child is usually a victim of both physical and emotional neglect. Failure-to-thrive is a condition found in infants and young chil-

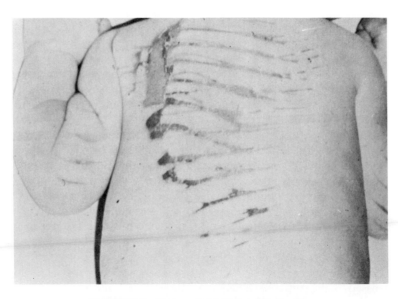

FIGURE 13-2 Lines probably infliced by burning.

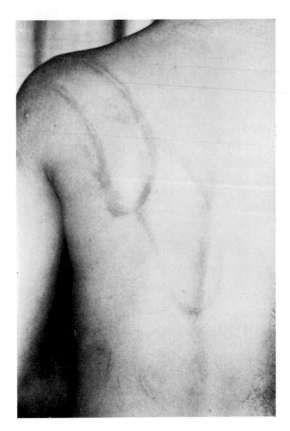

FIGURE 13-3   Loop cord marks.

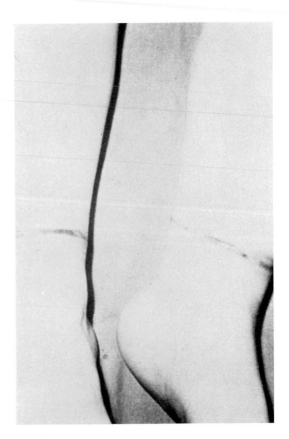

FIGURE 13-4   Lines secondary to cord restraint.

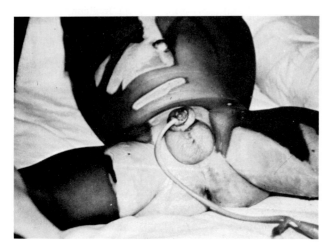

FIGURE 13-5   Immersion burns in a 15-month-old child.

dren from birth to 3 years of age, manifested by weight and usually length or stature below the fifth percentile on the growth charts. It is estimated that nearly 80 percent of these cases are nonorganic, and the most common cause is environmental deprivation. Some parents do not possess the necessary resources, some do not have the knowledge, some just forget to feed the child, and a few may intentionally starve the child. The emotional relationship between the child and caregiver is also a factor.

Intervention must be based on the particular situation. Assessment includes a health history, developmental history, nutritional assessment, general appearance, sequen-

tial length/stature and weight measurements, and observation of the child's levels of understanding, alertness, and interactions with the parent and the environment. For the failure-to-thrive infant or young child, it is necessary to assess the feeding abilities of the parent, the eating abilities of the child, and the emotional relationship of the parent and child. Hospitalization is usually required for the failure-to-thrive infant and is often diagnostic, since the child will gain weight rapidly when removed from the depriving and neglecting environment. The public health nurse should be involved to carry out an assessment of the home environment for additional intervention, planning, and implementation.

Emotional Abuse and Neglect

While emotional abuse has been suspected for some time, it is only now being focused on by the media and the public. Definitions are not as specific and it is less reported than other types of abuse. The child is belittled, teased, blamed, called names, and criticized, leading to loss of self-worth and identity. The child sees himself as incompetent and unworthy. Extremes of behavior (e.g., withdrawal or acting out and antisocial behavior) may be manifestations of emotional abuse (Table 13-3). Emotional neglect may be manifested as failure-to-thrive or lags in emotional and intellectual development. A developmental assessment and home evaluation are necessary to determine appropriate intervention.

Sexual Abuse

Sexual abuse is thought to be one of the most common but underreported crimes against children. According to Fore and Holmes (1984) statistics indicate that 330,000 sexual offenses are committed against boys and girls each year, with 90 percent of the children being female and 10 percent male. While girls are most often the victims in reported cases, some experts believe boys are victims more often than indicated. Incidence rates for boys range from 5 to 6 per 1000 to a high of 1 in 10 (Zaphiris, 1986).

Many cases are not reported at the time of occurrence and are only discovered several years later as adolescent delinquency, pregnancy, and psychiatric illnesses are encountered. Kempe (1980) indicated that half of the adolescent runaways in his patient population were victims of sexual abuse and frequent physical abuse as well.

Sexual abuse is differentiated according to whether it occurs within or outside the family. In either case, the perpetrator is known to the child an estimated 75 to 80 percent of the time. Nonfamilial abuse accounts for 20 percent of the cases and includes both violent and nonviolent abuse. The offender is often known to the victim or family and may be a friend, neighbor, or someone in a position of authority to the child. While the abuse may be a single event, it often goes on for weeks or months.

Familial abuse accounts for 80 percent of the reported cases. Incest is defined as "any form of sexual activity between a child and a parent or a child and a stepparent or extended family member (e.g., grandparent, aunt, uncle)" (Sgroi, 1982). In reported cases of incest, about three-fourths of the time the father or stepfather and daughter are involved. Mother-son, mother-daughter, and sibling incest account for most of the remaining cases. The incestuous relationship is usually prolonged, with a duration of 1 to 14 years in nearly 70 percent of the cases. The usual age of the victim is 10 to 14 years.

As outlined in Table 13-4, sexual abuse may present with clear physical findings, but most often there are few or no physical indicators. A thorough physical examination should be done to determine the presence or absence of such findings. Since behavioral manifestations are often the only indicators, it is extremely important that the health professional listen and observe. Many of these children are seen in the clinic or emergency room, and the nurse may be involved in the initial assessment. Sensitive questioning is necessary, and the child should be allowed to describe the events in his own words. The use of drawings or anatomically correct dolls may be helpful when the victim is a young child. In nonfamilial sexual abuse, the parents are usually present and supportive of the child. Anger, guilt, and concern may be verbalized. When the child is a victim of incest, it is more common for the parent not to believe the child or even to blame the child. The nurse may need to be the support person for the child during the examination and questioning.

As listed in Table 13-4, behavioral indicators vary with age. To identify potential sexual abuse, the nurse must be alert to clues. In addition, some children may have symptoms not suggestive of sexual abuse, such as complaints of headaches, abdominal pain, or hysterical symptoms of paralysis or paresthesia. When no physiologic cause can be determined, one must consider the possibility of "masked sexual abuse." It is permissible for the school-age child or adolescent to have these symptoms. It is very difficult to admit to ongoing sexual abuse by known and trusted adults, even family members.

Reporting and Legal Implications

All 50 states have statutes that relate to child abuse, neglect, or maltreatment. Definitions and the reporting process may vary, and the nurse should be familiar with the specific state laws. In most if not all states, nurses are required to report suspicions of child abuse and neglect. Failure to report is usually a misdemeanor. Immunity from liability is provided when reports are made in good faith. In addition to health care providers, educators, licensed child care providers, law enforcement officers, and others may be mandated reporters. Any agency providing health care for children should have a procedure for reporting and intervening in child abuse. The American Hospital Association (1986) has issued guidelines for management in the hospital setting.

The nurse may, at times, suspect abuse though others in the administrative structure do not want to report it. As an advocate for the child and from a legal standpoint, the nurse must report. Though the nurse may be harassed for superceding the decision of one in authority, the nurse cannot be legally terminated for carrying out the law. Continued education of all persons in positions requiring identification and reporting of child abuse and neglect may eventually decrease the misconceptions and obstacles encountered in the process of protecting the child.

Intervention

The overall goals of intervention are to protect the child from further injury, to provide assistance and support for family members, and eventually to reintegrate the family as a functional unit. The nurse may be involved in the hospital setting or in the community as a public health nurse providing ongoing services to the family. While seriously injured and young children are admitted to the hospital, probably the vast majority of abused and neglected children remain in the home or are placed in foster care. The parents and the child are the clients in either setting, and both must receive help. Treatment is directed toward four separate but interrelated facets: (1) the family's need for help in understanding child growth and development; (2) the family's need to become a part of the world around them; (3) the parents' need for help in strengthening interspouse relationships; and (4) the child's need for treatment and support.

Selected Nursing Diagnoses and Planning for Needs

Nursing diagnoses are numerous and vary with the type of abuse or neglect. Some applicable diagnoses are:

Potential for violence
Pain related to the injuries
Altered nutrition: less than body requirements
Altered parenting
Ineffective individual/family coping
Social isolation
Altered family processes

Some general needs of parents and children can be identified and included in the planning and implementation of nursing care. The parents need:

A reduction of stress
Someone they can trust and someone who will listen
To feel good about themselves—an increase in self-esteem
Someone to help them develop problem solving skills and learn to use resources
To develop realistic expectations of children and to be able to allow their children to be dependent on them
Someone who will not criticize them, even when they ask for it
Someone who will not try to tell them how to manage their lives but help them learn how

Abused and neglected children need:

Consistent routines allowing predictability and testing of feelings and actions
Reasonable and clear expectations
Positive attention and positive reinforcement
Success in their endeavors
Time to establish trust
Opportunities to make choices and to have a sense of control
Opportunities to express emotions and know that it is alright to do so
Predictable adult behavior

Intervention in the Hospital Setting

The nurse who works with the abused child and his family must first deal with personal feelings, which may involve anger and disgust toward the parents and a need to rescue the child. To be nonjudgmental is difficult. It is important that the nurse not take over the parenting role and exclude the parents. It is helpful to realize that most parents do love and want their children, however ambivalent their feelings.

When the child is admitted, the parents may be expressing hostility or they may be relieved that the problem has been detected and they may be asking for help. Even in the latter situation, the problems of lack of trust, suspiciousness, and defensiveness must be dealt with as the nurse attempts to establish rapport with the parents. Recognizing and focusing on the needs of the parents will facilitate establishing a relationship that will allow for continuing support and intervention. Nursing care approaches should emphasize the shared concern of the parents and the nurse for the child.

As with any child entering the hospital, it is important to obtain a nursing history. The data base should include information about the child's eating, sleeping, play, and toilet habits; siblings; developmental levels; previous hospitalization experiences; and security objects. History tak-ing gives the nurse an opportunity to communicate to the parents some recognition of their frustration with parental roles and to assess parental knowledge, expectations, and perceptions of their child. The nurse must use judgment in determining the best method and timing for obtaining the information. The parents also need orientation to the pediatric unit and encouragement to participate in the care of their child.

Presenting a warm and helpful attitude to the parents rather than a punitive one forms the basis for working with them. Looking for strengths and acknowledging positive factors, no matter how serious the family dysfunction, will help to promote a sense of parental adequacy and increased self-esteem. Encouraging the family to visit and being available during the visits will allow the nurse opportunities for role modeling and demonstration of alternative ways of dealing with the child's behavior and may help the parent and child express feelings.

Keeping the family informed of what is happening and what to expect is important. Silence will only increase suspiciousness. The parents need to know that the reporting is legally required, that they are not being accused but that many factors must be considered if they are to be helped with the problems that led to the injury, and that several people will be talking with them.

Continued observation during hospitalization provides data vital to planning the care and making the ultimate decision for placement of the child back in the home or in foster care. It is important to evaluate the parent-child relationship, the parent's response to the child's behavior, and the child's response to adults in the hospital setting. While nurses should communicate concern for and be supportive of the parents, it is important that they convey the seriousness of the situation. Documentation of observations must be objective and factual. In written notes, specific behaviors and actions of the parent or child are documented, specific statements are cited, frequency and length of visits are recorded, and actual intervention and plans are indicated.

The child needs consistency among those providing nursing care, appropriate preparation for procedures, and inclusion of the parent in his care. Management of the child's behavior may present some special problems. A wide range of behaviors may be exhibited. The child may be described as fearful, withdrawn, lacking trust, testing limits, provocative, clinging, indiscriminate in relationships, or normal. The child who is fearful of all adults, who clings to any adult in the setting, or who seems to invite punishment with his behavior needs intervention specifically planned to his needs. The pattern and duration of behaviors are more significant than is a single episode.

Limit-setting and discipline are needed but should be carried out in a nonpunitive manner. Meaningful interactions and relationships with a limited number of persons are necessary, and continuity in caregivers should be planned. Expression of feelings and mastery of the situation can be enhanced through the use of play. A well-developed and written care plan along with well-documented nursing notes provide guidance and promote consistency in the care of the child and family.

Planning and preparation for discharge may involve additional factors when the patient is an abused or neglected child. While the ultimate goal is the return of the child to a family capable of providing adequate care, it is often necessary to separate the child and family temporarily. The child has a need and a right to be prepared for placement in a foster home or other setting. Parents may be able to help the child in the transition but often are so stressed themselves that they cannot be supportive. The person who has the most positive relationship with the child can best prepare the child. Early involvement of the community agency and community health nurse and education of the new caregiver about the needs of the individual child are part of the planning.

Since most hospitalizations are relatively short, only minimal progress can realistically be expected. The environmental stresses may be the initial priority need in crisis intervention. The parental needs for nurturing and emotional growth may limit their ability to benefit from role modeling and information on parenting skills. Intervention is long term and needs to involve a number of community services during the process of rehabilitation. Coordination of and communication between those involved is essential. Referral to a community health nurse for additional assessment of the home and ongoing long-term intervention is indicated, and such a nurse may be the best person to coordinate the services to the child and family.

Prevention

Children who are abused or neglected are far more likely than other children to act out in society, to become violent toward themselves or others, and, later, to populate juvenile and adult correctional facilities in higher proportions than children from the general population (Alfaro, 1984). While tertiary prevention in the form of long-term intervention after abuse occurs is vital in preventing further abuse, efforts in primary and secondary prevention need to be increased.

Can families at risk for abnormal parenting practices be identified early? Can effective intervention be provided to prevent abuse and neglect? Can community programs be developed that will enhance parenting skills and family interaction? In the lives of individuals whose past history indicated a potential to abuse, can positive events that allowed them to break the cycle of abuse be identified? Several authors proposed that such indicators can be identified and effective interventions developed (Gray et al., 1979; Hunter et al., 1978; Hunter, 1980; Josten, 1981; Christiansen et al., 1984; Velasquez, 1984; Anderson, 1987).

Primary Prevention

Primary prevention refers to actions that are taken to promote adequate family function and that advocate changes in social and environmental conditions leading to dysfunction. Education and advocacy programs at agency, community, and state levels are necessary. Communication and cooperation among professionals, educational institutions, and interested community agencies and groups can result in positive effort. Educational programs aimed at primary prevention could include (1) perinatal education and coaching programs to assist new and young parents in learning how to interact with their newborn infants and solve day-to-day problems; (2) expanded well-baby care to provide more anticipatory guidance and comprehensive assistance to parents; (3) home visitor programs; (4) preschool and primary school education to help children develop interpersonal problem-solving skills; (5) junior and senior high school programs that focus on interpersonal skills, family life responsibility, and parenting skills; and (6) parenting classes.

The prevention of sexual abuse has been receiving increased attention. The focus of many community and school programs is on teaching children an awareness of dangerous and uncomfortable situations, the importance of saying "no," and telling parents or other trusted adults. Parents are also being given information on how they can protect their children against possible molestation.

Community development of support programs and services could include (1) mother's-day-out programs; (2) parent-relief and respite care services; (3) day care and nursery school accessibility; and (4) self-help groups. Advocacy activities might include legislative efforts to provide programs to enhance parenting and family life and to decrease the sanctioning of violence in society. Nurses as health care professionals and members of groups and of a community are in a position to assess needs and initiate action to develop programs that promote primary prevention.

Secondary Prevention

Secondary prevention is focused on the identification of individuals and families at risk for abnormal parenting practices and the development of intervention programs to prevent abuse and neglect. Much data have been collected about the variables that, in combination, result in abuse and neglect of children. These components can be summarized under three major areas: (1) unusual child-rearing practices, (2) disturbed family relationships, and (3) environmental stress. Unusual child-rearing practices and disturbed family relationships are present not only in overt abuse and neglect but in many less obvious situations that may be damaging to the child and family. The common findings of "poor parenting as children," low self-esteem, high dependency needs, isolation, and a view of the child as being "special or different" by the parent provide a base on which to begin identifying parents and children at risk. Environmental stresses related to living conditions, finances, marital discord, or other variables can also be assessed. No one factor singles out a parent or caregiver as a potential abuser, but a combination of factors and the resulting interplay between a child's factors and an adult's factors may lead one to identify a high-risk situation.

Screening programs for the population at risk are being developed and used in a variety of prenatal, obstetric, and pediatric settings. Criteria for inclusion in the population at risk may include infants who are of low birth weight, who have congenital defects or medical problems, who have feeding problems or failure-to-thrive diagnoses, or who have multiple developmental delays. Parental factors might include a teenage mother, one who does not return to the nursery or pediatric unit for instruction in infant care, or one who demonstrates inappropriate interaction with her infant or child. Families in which the use of drugs or alcohol is suspected; in which there is a past history of abuse, neglect, or unusual sibling death; or in which there are several stresses such as marital problems or financial difficulties would also be included.

Several investigators (Hunter, 1978; Gray, 1979; Josten, 1981) have studied factors that can be identified in prenatal, perinatal, and postpartum situations as indicators of a potential for abuse. Intrapartum and postpartum observations have been found to be the most predictive. Risk factors in the prenatal period include unrealistic expectations for the baby, denial of pregnancy, depression, lack of support systems, lack of preparation for the baby, and inadequate parenting as a child in the background of the mother. Risk factors in labor and delivery center around rejection behaviors, negative comments about the baby's appearance or sex, and refusal to look at or hold the infant. Length of labor and degree of discomfort must be considered when evaluating the mother's reaction to the baby. In the postpartum period, observations related to support systems, family reaction to the baby, mother's reaction to the baby's crying, feeding, and need for diaper changing can provide clues as to risk. The way the mother holds the baby, talks to the baby, and verbalizes about him may also demonstrate negative factors. The teaching of skills in feeding, diapering, and holding; assistance in interpreting the infant's behavior; and listening to concerns are vital functions of the nurse in the postpartum setting.

When the mother and infant are separated during the postpartum period due to illness of the mother or intensive care nursing needs of the infant, additional intervention is needed to promote the parent-infant attachment process. Policies to allow the involvement of parents in all neonatal intensive care nurseries and sick infant nurseries should be promoted by all health professionals.

Other studies have added additional information helpful in prediction and prevention. Hunter (1980), in asking why some parents who had been abused as children went on to abuse their children and some did not, found that those who did not had been able as children to rebuild a trusting relationship with a parenting figure. As adults they had been able to build support systems within and outside the family. Other researchers have found other family background indicators and environmental stress factors to be predictive of the potential to abuse. Christiansen et al. (1984) used adolescent experiences of the mother, such as foster care, alcohol and drug abuse, police involvements, and attempted suicide, to identify at-risk families with whom to implement prevention strategies. Anderson (1987) found the five factors of education, income, number of police involvement by family members, life change unit scores, and mother's perception of harsh discipline to children to distinguish between abus-

ing and nonabusing families. Nurses and other must continue to research predictive measures and implement programs in all settings to prevent the problems of child abuse and neglect and promote positive family function.

Learning Activities

1. Discuss probable reasons why no child abuse was reported in the United States from 1877 to 1946. What was occurring politically, culturally, and economically during that time period?
2. Review case studies of children who have been abused. What were the child's characteristics? What were the perpetrator's characteristics?

Independent Study Activities

1. Obtain the child abuse statutes in your state. How do the definitions in the state law compare to the definitions in this chapter? Who is responsible for reporting child abuse? What are the penalties for not reporting child abuse?
2. Obtain the procedure for reporting and documenting child abuse in your hospital. How does it compare to the content in this chapter? What is the role of the Child Protective Team?

Study Questions

1. Mandated reporting of suspected child abuse is included in the law of all states.
   A. True   B. False
2. Abusive and neglecting adults come from
   A. A low socioeconomic background.
   B. A home where education is not stressed.
   C. Blue-collar families.
   D. All socioeconomic, educational, and occupational levels.
3. Indicate whether the definitions below identify primary or secondary prevention:
   1. The identification of individuals and families at risk for abnormal parenting practices and the development of intervention programs to prevent child abuse and neglect.
   2. Actions that are taken to promote adequate family function and that advocate changes in social and environmental conditions leading to dysfunction.
   A. 1 is primary prevention; 2 is secondary prevention.
   B. 2 is primary prevention; 1 is secondary prevention.
   C. Both are primary prevention.
   D. Both are secondary prevention.

4. There are three variables that, in combination, can result in abuse and neglect of children. They are (1) unusual childrearing practices, (2) disturbed family relationships, and (3) environmental stress.
   A. True   B. False

5. When assessing a family for potential abuse, it is important to identify positive factors and strengths as well as risk factors.
   A. True   B. False

6. Child abuse is not usually associated with other forms of family violence.
   A. True   B. False

7. Some common needs of the abusive parent are:
   A. Low self-esteem.
   B. Low tolerance for frustration.
   C. High needs for love and nurturing.
   D. All of the above.

8. The abused child may exhibit behaviors of withdrawal, hostility, detachment, and depression.
   A. True   B. False

9. Toddlers may be at risk for abuse related to unrealistic toilet training expectations on the part of the parent.
   A. True   B. False

10. If questioned, the child will usually tell the authorities who abused him.
    A. True   B. False

11. The parents of a suspected abused child should
    A. Be kept informed as to what is happening.
    B. Be allowed to help in the care of their child.
    C. Be informed as to what reporting means for them.
    D. All of the above.

12. Prevention of child abuse and neglect is important. One approach that might be taken is:
    A. Parenting classes during the prenatal period.
    B. Education and anticipatory guidance for each developmental level.
    C. Counseling for families at risk.
    D. All of the above.

13. Abusive or potentially abusive parents tend to make many demands on their children, expecting them to satisfy many unmet parental needs and to act in a manner beyond their developmental levels.
    A. True   B. False

14. Solving problems of housing, food, and transportation may be a prerequisite for motivating parents to move ahead and to cope with the needs and problems of human interaction, self-esteem, and realistic, positive child-rearing practices.
    A. True   B. False

15. Which of the following is *not* considered a risk factor for identifying potentially abusive parents in the labor and delivery situation?
    A. Mother and/or father not looking at the newborn.
    B. Father not present during the delivery.
    C. Negative comments about the baby's sex and/or appearance.
    D. Refusal to hold the baby.

References

Alfaro, J.D.: "Helping Children Overcome the Effects of Abuse and Neglect," *Pediatric Annals*, 13(10): 778-787, 1984.

American Hospital Association: "Management of Child Abuse and Neglect Cases," AHA, 840 North Shore Drive, Chicago, Illinois 60611, 1986.

Anderson, C.L.: "Assessing Parenting Potential of Child Abuse Risk," *Pediatric Nursing*, 13(5): 323-327, 1987.

Bergman, A.B., R.M. Larsen, and B.A. Mueller, "Changing Spectrum of Serious Child Abuse," *Pediatrics*, 77(1):113-116, 1986.

Caffey, J.: "Multiple Fractures in the Long Bones of Infants Suffering From Chronic Subdural Hematomas," *American Journal of Roentgenology*, 56:163-173, 1946.

Christiansen, M.L., B.L. Schommer, and J. Velasquez: "An Interdisciplinary Approach to Preventing Child Abuse," *MCN: The American Journal of Maternal Child Nursing*, 9(2):108-112, 1984.

Cupoli, J.M.: "Piecing Together the Pattern of Child Abuse," *Comtemporary Pediatrics*, 4(12):12-30, 1987.

Davis, K.E.: "Interparental Violence: The Children as Victims," *Issues in Comprehensive Pediatric Nursing*, 11(5-6):291-302, 1988.

Dine, M.S., and M.E. McGovern: "Intentional Poisoning of Children: An Overlooked Category of Child Abuse: Report of Seven Cases and Review of the Literature," *Pediatrics*, 70(1):32-35, 1982.

Fontana, V.J.: "The Maltreatment Syndrome in Children," *New England Journal of Medicine*, 269:1389, 1963.

Fontana, V.J.: "The Maltreatment Syndrome of Children," *Pediatric Annals*, 13(10):736-744, 1984.

Fore, C.V., and S.S. Holmes: "Sexual Abuse of Children," *Nursing Clinics of North America*, 19(2):329-340, 1984.

Gelles, R.J.: *Family Violence*, Sage Publications, California, 1979.

Gray, J.D., et al.: "Prediction and Prevention of Child Abuse," *Seminars in Perinatology*, 3(1):85-90, 1979.

Hunter, R.S.: "Parents Who Break With an Abusive Past: Lessons for Prevention," *Caring*, 6(4):1,4,6, 1980.

Hunter, R.S., et al.: "Antecedents of Child Abuse and Neglect in Premature Infants: A Prospective Study in a Newborn Intensive Care Unit," *Pediatrics*, 61(4):629-635, 1978.

Josten, L: "Prenatal Assessment Guide for Illuminating Possible Problems with Parenting," *MCN: The American Journal of Maternal Child Nursing*, 6(2):113-117, 1981.

Justice, B., and R. Justice: *The Abusing Family*, Human Science Press, New York, 1976.

Kempe, C.H., and R.E. Helfer: "The Battered Child Syndrome," *The Journal of the American Medical Association*, 181:17-24, 1962.

Kempe, C.H., and R.E. Helfer: *The Battered Child* (3rd ed.), University of Chicago Press, Chicago, 1980.

Kunkel, D.B.: "The Toxic Emergency: The Chemically Abused Child," *Emergency Medicine*, 16(5):181-190, 1984.

Polansky, N., et al.: *Damaged Parents: An Anatomy of Child Neglect*, University of Chicago Press, Chicago, 1981.

Sgroi, S.: *Handbook of Clinical Intervention in Child Sexual Abuse*, Lexington Books, D.C. Heath and Company, 1982.

Velasquez, J., M.I. Christiansen, and B.L. Schommer: "Intensive Services Help Prevent Child Abuse," *MCN: The American Journal of Maternal Child Nursing*, 9(2):113-117, 1984.

Westra, B.: "Nursing Care of Children of Violent Families," in J. Campbell and J. Humphries (Eds.) *Nursing Care of Victims of Family Violence*, Reston, Virginia, Reston, 1984.

Zaphiris, A.G.: "The Sexually Abused Boy," *Preventing Abuse*, 1(1):1-4, 1986.

Bibliography

Campbell, J., and J. Humphreys: *Nursing Care of Victims of Family Violence*, Reston, Virginia, Reston, 1984.

Helberg, J.L.: "Documentation in Child Abuse," *American Journal of Nursing*, 83(2):236-239, 1983.

Kelley, S.J.: "Interviewing the Sexually Abused Child: Principles and Techniques," *Journal of Emergency Nursing*, 11(5):234-241, 1985.

Robertson, K.E., and J.A. Wilson-Walker: "A Program for Preventing Sexual Abuse of Children," *MCN: The American Journal of Maternal Child Nursing*, 10(2):100-102, 1985.

Ryan, M.T.: "Identifying the Sexually Abused Child," *Pediatric Nursing*, 10(6):419-421, 1984.

Sisney, K.F.: "Breaking the Link: Nursing Intervention in the Incestuous Family," *Issues in Comprehensive Pediatric Nursing*, 4(4):51-59, 1980.

14

Emotional Disorders of Childhood and Adolescence

Objectives

After reading this chapter, the student will be able to:
1. List four factors that may contribute to the development of emotional disorders in children and adolescents.
2. Describe pathological communication patterns in families with disturbed children.
3. Describe the major characteristics of infantile autism, pervasive developmental disorder, attention deficit disorder, conduct disorder, substance abuse disorder, anxiety disorder, depression, suicidal tendency, schizophrenia, and eating disorder.
4. List nursing approaches suitable in the general hospital or clinic setting for the care of children or adolescents with the emotional disorders listed in Objective 3.

The primary focus of this chapter is emotionally disturbed children and adolescents with physical illnesses or injuries who enter community and general hospitals or clinics. The intent is not to provide the reader with the knowledge necessary to function as a child psychiatric nurse but to supply the information needed to deliver appropriate nursing care for an emotionally disturbed child in the general setting.

Child and Family Responses to Illness and Hospitalization

It is important to be aware that the child does not exist alone but is part of a group—the family. The family provides the child with opportunities for learning and for developing interpersonal relationships as well as coping abilities. Although physiological and metabolic defects may be responsible in part for psychological disturbances, it is vital to recognize the impact of the family and environment as well.

Children's Feelings

A child who is emotionally disturbed has more difficulty coping with life situations and stress, including physical illness, than does a normal child. While the prospect of surgery or hospitalization is frightening to most children, it causes greater distress to a child who is emotionally disturbed. As the child is part of a family, this additional stress has an impact on a family's functioning and ability to cope, which affects the family's ability to assist the child during this crisis period.

Adults' Feelings: Parents and Nurses

Emotional disorders of childhood are caused by a multitude of factors, including physiological, biochemical, genetic, social, psychological, and environmental causes. This lack of definitive causation often leads to confusion and frustration on the part of both families and health care providers. Nurses may find that they need to assist families in dealing with feelings of guilt concerning the child's illness.

Nurses and other health care providers may need assistance in dealing with their own feelings of confusion, anger, frustration, and despair about a profoundly disturbed child. Acknowledgment of the difficulties of working with such a child and peer consultation on the part of staff members (e.g., team conferences) can supply much needed support.

Role of the Nurse

An important aspect of the nursing care of the emotionally disturbed child is the nurse-client relationship. *All* nursing interventions, psychological and physical, and the child's subsequent response are based on the quality of the relationship. In working with emotionally disturbed children in general settings, the nurse intervenes not only with the ill child but with family members too. This contact may occur in the hospital setting or in the home. The nurse thus must feel competent and confident in helping family members cope with an ill child.

One of the most vital factors in the nursing care of an emotionally disturbed child is the need to focus on the child's behaviors rather than on his diagnosis. In short, intervention should be planned according to the way in which the child behaves, not his diagnostic label. Accordingly, the nurse must know what constitutes normal growth and development in order to accurately assess the child and provide the appropriate intervention.

Nurse-Client Relationship

In the nurse-client relationship the child and his needs are the primary focus of all interactions. Such a relationship is characterized by the nurse's ability to win the child's trust and to be accepting, caring, honest, and empathic. The value of the relationship is measured by the quality of each encounter with the child rather than by the amount of time spent with the child. A minimal amount of time spent in an unhurried manner is more beneficial than a longer period spent rapidly doing treatments and moving quickly to complete tasks. The nurse's ability to establish a trusting relationship with the child in a general hospital or community setting may be somewhat hampered by the brevity of contact. However, development of an effective relationship is still feasible.

Acceptance

Perhaps the most important aspect of the nurse-child relationship is the nurse's demonstration of acceptance of the child and the way he behaves. Some behaviors are not strictly "acceptable" because they need to be modified to enhance growth and development and allow for maximum functioning and adaptation. However, in view of the added stress placed on the child during hospitalization or treatment for physical problems, it is generally not recommended that new or additional demands be made at this time in relation to his emotional disorder. An exception to this strategy is a child who engages in behavior which is destructive to himself (suicide attempts or self-mutilatory behavior such as biting, burning, or cutting himself).

Trust

In order to demonstrate an attitude of acceptance, the nurse must behave in a manner which the child can trust. Verbal and nonverbal communication with the child must be honest, straightforward, and appropriate to the child's age and developmental capabilities. Nonverbal behavior is especially important since disturbed children take in a great deal of meaning in this manner. For example, the nurse conveys acceptance to the child if she comes close to him and uses language he can understand in a soft tone of voice. Acceptance can also be demonstrated by staying with the child even though he may be exhibiting bizarre or undesirable behavior. For example, the nurse who remains with an autistic child while he flaps his arms and picks his nose demonstrates acceptance of his behavior and self.

Empathy

Another crucial aspect of the nurse-client relationship is *empathy,* which can be defined as the attempt by the nurse to understand the feelings and experience of the child and to communicate this understanding to the child.

The ability to empathize requires close observation of the child's verbal and nonverbal behaviors to assess the child's feelings and emotional state. Although empathy is more readily accomplished with an older child who has mastered verbal communication, it is also possible with a younger client. In the process of empathic understanding, the nurse first must identify and assess her own feelings and deal with them. Then the feelings of the child need to be assessed and reflected back to the child to determine whether the assessment is correct. The nurse then assists the child in coping with his feelings. It is important to note that a correct assessment and verbalization of the child's feelings demonstrates to the child that the nurse is attempting to understand him. This in turn indicates to the child that the nurse is paying attention to him and cares about him.

The following examples demonstrate two attempts by the nurse to utilize empathy with a child who is able to communicate verbally. Norman, a 12-year-old, is hospitalized with acute appendicitis and is scheduled for an appendectomy. As the nurse enters the room, Norman is crying and is lying curled up in his bed, clutching his right side.

Example 1: Incorrect Use of Empathy
  NURSE: "Norman, you're crying. You'll feel better if you don't stay curled up in bed." Nurse remains at the foot of the bed.
  NORMAN: "Go away and leave me alone." Norman continues to cry.
  NURSE: "Okay, I'll come back to see you later." Nurse leaves the room.

Example II: Correct Use of Empathy
  NURSE: "Norman, I see you're crying. You look like it really hurts." Nurse stands at head of bed, bends over, and attempts to establish eye contact with Norman.
  NORMAN: "Yes, I wish it would go away. I'm afraid." Norman stops crying and looks at nurse.
  NURSE: "I'll stay with you for a while." Nurse sits at Norman's bedside and holds his hand.

In Example I the nurse begins the process of empathic understanding by observing Norman's behavior and pointing it out to him. However, there is no clear demonstration of caring or concern. The nurse's telling Norman how to relieve his pain is an *indirect* expression of caring. However, it is likely that the child receives the "advice" message rather than the caring one. In Example II the nurse conveys concern and caring both verbally and nonverbally. She tells him that she sees his distress, his crying, and states what she perceives—his pain. The nurse demonstrates concern nonverbally by standing at the head of the bed and attempting to establish eye contact and later by sitting with him and holding his hand. Both verbal and nonverbal behaviors show the child that the nurse is taking the time to pay attention to him and to his needs.

For a younger child who has not mastered verbal communication, nonverbal communication, including touch, may be the only way to demonstrate caring and acceptance. Holding a small child may help allay some of his fears. However, the child must trust the nurse before this type of intervention is initiated. Trust can be facilitated by the nurse's initially making brief, frequent contacts with the child in an unhurried manner, especially when no treatments are necessary. Consistency contributes to the development of a trusting relationship.

The emotionally disturbed child will most likely have difficulty trusting the nurse. Therefore, it is important for the nurse to administer nursing care accordingly. For example, when caring for a child who can understand verbal communication, the nurse must be honest. The nurse should refrain from telling the child that a painful procedure will not hurt. Although it may initially relieve some of the nurse's own anxiety, it will cause unnecessary anxiety in the child when he finds out through experience that the procedure does hurt and that the nurse whom he was beginning to trust lied to him. Clearly, it is more beneficial to the nurse-client relationship (and therefore to the child) for a nurse to tell the truth initially and then assist the child in dealing with it. This action is important in caring for an emotionally disturbed child since the child's ability to trust is often severely impaired.

When carrying out the procedure, the nurse should tell the child what is going to happen beforehand. It is important to move slowly and speak with a soft, calm voice. This relaxed manner assists the child in feeling comfortable and safe. Quick movements and rapid speech can increase the child's feelings of discomfort and lead to unnecessary anxiety. Honesty, consistency, and calmness enhance the effectiveness of the relationship between child and nurse.

The Influence of the Family

Although the causes of most emotional disorders are multiple, it is important for a nurse to be aware of the function of the family and its role in the emotional development of the child. According to systems theory (Chap. 3), the family unit functions as a whole. The members of the family are emotionally tied together—what affects one person affects them all. This factor is especially crucial when considering the emotionally disturbed child because he cannot be considered apart from his family. Although parents may identify a child as being "sick" and causing distress to the family, the child's behavior is more accurately understood as a "symptom" of family dysfunction rather than the cause. Accordingly, from a systems theory perspective, a dysfunctional family is likely to *produce* children with emotional or behavioral disturbances rather than the child causing the dysfunction. Communication patterns in the family are a major factor in emotional disturbance.

Communication Patterns within the Family

All interaction that occurs in the family is accomplished by means of communication, both verbal and nonverbal.

Stated simply, the clearer the communication patterns among family members, the healthier the family system. It is particularly important when one considers that the child learns how to communicate and relate to others from experiences in the family.

In dysfunctional communication, the messages sent are unclear, vague, or inconsistent. The receiver of the messages does not seek to clarify or validate what he has heard. Consequently, the meaning of the message may be misinterpreted, resulting in confusion. This confusion hinders the relationships among those involved in the communication. Consistently unclear or ambiguous communication can be considered both a symptom and a cause of dysfunction in the family. A child who persistently has received unclear, inconsistent messages has difficulty in relationships with others. He has not learned to accept communication at its face value because he has always received confusing messages. This experience adversely affects his ability to trust others and establish relationships with them.

Double-Level Messages

The adverse influence of unclear communication on emotional development can be understood by examining one type of such communication, the *double-level message.* Here the child receives two conflicting messages which lead to confusion and provide no acceptable way for the child to respond. An example is a mother telling her child that she loves him while pushing him away. The verbal message "I love you" is incongruent with the nonverbal message of pushing the child away. The child does not know how to behave in a manner which elicits the mother's approval (i.e., should he hug his mother or should he remain distant?).

Another example of a double-level message is a parent giving a child two toys for his birthday and then, when the child plays with one, saying, "Don't you like the other toy I gave you?" The child is left with no acceptable way to behave because he cannot play with both toys at the same time. Clearly, double-level messages occur frequently in families and between individuals.

Double-Bind Communication

A type of double-level message which is particularly unhealthful and can lead to severe emotional dysfunction is called *double-bind communication.* Three factors must be present for communication to be double-bind in addition to double-level:

1. Double-level messages must be given repeatedly and over an extended period of time.
2. The messages must come from persons who have survival significance (i.e., the child cannot survive without them) for the child, usually his parents.
3. The child learns over time that he cannot ask his parents how they would like him to act. It leaves the child with no acceptable way to behave and thus invites rejection from the parents.

Double-bind communication leads the child to mistrust others and causes a poor self-image due to parental rejec-

tion as well as lack of positive feedback from significant others. These factors contribute to emotional disturbance.

In summary, since the family is the initial interpersonal situation, it can have a profound effect on the child's ability to communicate and relate to others. A child who frequently experiences inconsistent and misleading communication from his family develops impaired relationships with others outside the family. Of course, other factors also affect the child's emotional health. These variables—genetic, chemical, and biological—will be discussed briefly as they relate to specific disorders.

Emotional Disorders of Childhood and Adolescence

Pervasive Developmental Disorders

Before 1980, when the American Psychiatric Association revised its diagnostic nomenclature, children in this diagnostic classification were referred to as schizophrenic or psychotic. The term *pervasive developmental disorder* was adopted to provide greater diagnostic specificity and clarity. These disorders are characterized by severe behavioral disturbance that affects *numerous* aspects of psychological functioning, including language, interpersonal interaction, attention, perception, and motor activity. The pervasive developmental disorders, discussed below and in Table 14-1, are *infantile autism* and *childhood-onset pervasive developmental disorder.*

Infantile Autism

This devastating disorder is fortunately rare, affecting only 2 to 4 children per 10,000. It appears to be more common in the upper socioeconomic classes and is three times more common in boys than in girls. It is considered to be a neuropsychophysiological disorder rather than a disturbance caused by inadequate interpersonal relationships in the family.

At one time it was thought that autistic children are highly intelligent but that their intellectual abilities are overshadowed by the interpersonal impairment. Our current understanding is that only 30 percent of children with autism have IQs of 70 or higher. Epileptic seizures are a major medical complication of infantile autism and often occur in children with IQs below 50 (APA, 1980).

There is no cure for autism. Practically every treatment modality has been tried, including family therapy, child psychotherapy, behavior modification therapy, sensory stimulation, isolation, and several drugs including hallucinogens. None of these treatments alters the course of the syndrome, but it is possible to increase the level of most children's functioning and to provide assistance for the family. Nursing management is described in Table 14-1.

Childhood-Onset Pervasive Developmental Disorder

This disorder is extremely disabling (Table 14-1). More boys than girls are afflicted. No predisposing factors have been identified, and there is no familial pattern. Although

TABLE 14-1 Pervasive Developmental Disorders

Characteristics of the Disorder*	Nursing Interventions
Infantile autism Chronic, incapacitating Appears before age 30 months Child lacks responiveness to people: Does not make eye contact Does not ackowledge others Resists touch, affection Language is frequently absent Nonverbal communication is inappropriate Resists change in environment or daily routine; e.g., may become extremely upset if toys or furniture is moved Uses objects in idiosyncratic, odd ways; e.g., may sniff toy truck rather than push it along table or floor Demonstrates bizarre facial expressions and repetitive, ritualistic body movements: spinning, rocking, arm flapping, hand clapping, etc.	Consistency both in caregiver and in manner of providing care; perform treatments at same time of day and in same way, preferably by same person Invite parents to participate in care; communicate with child in a manner consistent with parents' usual way Although child may not make eye contact or respond to touch, administer care in humanistic, warm, accepting way: Introduce yourself and call child by name Keep voice gentle and speech slow and calm Explain to child what you are doing Assume child is aware of environment and events even though his response may not indicate it Provide as much stimulation as child will tolerate during the day to prevent boredom that contributes to ritualistic, repetitious behavior (may include self-destructive activity such as head banging or arm biting); spend short periods of time with child when not giving him care; offer toys without expecting him to respond as children usually do
Childhood-onset pervasive developmental disorder Begins after 30 months of age but before 12 years; has many of the same characteristics as infantile autism; severe disturbance in interpersonal relationships and bizarre behavior in other areas of functioning; child may have sudden mood swings, including severe anxiety and panic; bizarre motor activity resembles that in infantile autism; self-mutilating behavior may be present; voice tone may be peculiar	Consistent and humane approach as described for infantile autism

*Distortions occur in *multiple* areas of psychological functioning: language, social skills, attention, perception, and motor coordination.

this condition probably has a more favorable outcome than does infantile autism, it is a chronic disorder requiring long-term special education and lifelong supervision. Nursing approaches for the care of a child with childhood-onset pervasive developmental disorder in a general hospital are listed in Table 14-1.

Attention Deficit Disorder with Hyperactivity

Children with this disorder were previously described as minimally brain damaged, hyperkinetic, or hyperactive. This discussion will focus on children who exhibit hyperactivity along with inattention.

Although the disorder is probably present by the age of 3, it often goes undiagnosed until the child enters school, where his behavior is noticeably disruptive (Table 14-2). Not all children who have attention deficit disorder with hyperactivity exhibit all the behaviors listed in the table. Behavior varies from child to child and also depends on the situation; it is commonly exacerbated in a setting in which the child is expected to perform (such as school) and more moderate in a new situation or when the child is interacting with one other person.

Attention deficit disorder with hyperactivity is 10 times more common in boys than in girls (APA, 1980). Mental retardation, epilepsy, and other neurological disorders may predispose its development. The symptoms of the disorder have been treated with varying success by medication, psychotherapy, and special education. In

some children symptoms disappear completely, while other children are left with residual effects. Nursing management is described in Table 14-2.

Conduct Disorders

There are several types of conduct disorders (APA, 1980). The common behavioral manifestations are shown in Table 14-3.

Conduct disorders occur more often in boys than in girls and are more common in children whose parents have antisocial personality disorders or abuse alcohol. Family and interpersonal factors as well as harsh, unfair methods of discipline and inconsistent parenting also may encourage the development of a conduct disorder. Parental rejection and inconsistency, with subsequent mistrust and low self-esteem on the part of the child, can lead to the development of the unsocialized behavior displayed by young people with these disorders. Parenting, including discipline, is discussed in Chap. 3.

Outcomes for children and adolescents with conduct disorders vary. Frequently persons with mild disorders demonstrate improved functioning as adults. Individuals with severe undersocialized and aggressive behavior are likely to experience difficulties as adults.

Nursing Management

Treatment for conduct disorders varies in success depending on the severity of the disorder. Family therapy of-

TABLE 14-2 Attention Deficit Disorder

Characteristics of the Disorder	Nursing Interventions

Child is impulsive:
  Acts before thinking
  Switches from one activity to another
  Has difficulty organizing work
  Requires excessive supervision
  Has difficulty taking turns
Hyperactivity may or may not be present:
  Leaves tasks unfinished
  Seems not to listen
  Is easily distracted
  Cannot concentrate for long
  Demonstrates excessive gross motor activity (running, climbing, wiggling, fidgeting) and "can't sit still"; may move excessively during sleep
	Do not expect sustained attention to any one activity; do not expect to prevent hyperactivity; set limits on activity only as necessary to prevent danger to child or others; provide setting for active play but do not overstimulate child (e.g., with roughhousing) or permit child to become overly tired (fatigue leads to pronounced lack of self-control); be calm; be patient when working with child and allow him to move about the room if necessary while giving care; provide various activities for short periods (e.g., alternate a few minutes of TV with game playing and walking in the hall); visit and interact with child frequently and briefly

TABLE 14-3 Conduct Disorders

Characteristics of the Disorder	Nursing Interventions

Begins around puberty
Behavior is persistently inappropriate to social setting for child's age and impinges on the rights of others:
  Destruction of property
  Stealing
  Running away from home
  Physical violence
  Persistent lying
  Persistent irritability or tantrums
  Precocious sexual behavior
Child does not form close interpersonal relationships; appears to lack empathy and affection
Experiences repeated conflict with parents, school, and other authorities; is suspended from school and has legal difficulties; blames others for troubles
Projects outwardly "tough" attitude to cover up low self-esteem
Early smoking, drinking, and other forms of drug abuse are common
	See Table 14-4

ten is helpful in providing support for parents in dealing with the child's behavior. Parents are encouraged to set firm limits, which demonstrates that they care, in order to help the child alter his behavior. In attempting to alter behavior, a therapist helps the child recognize the consequences of his actions. In instances where behavior change is minimal and the behaviors are extremely antisocial, institutionalization is sometimes required.

Many of the behaviors exhibited by the adolescent with a conduct disorder are similar to those demonstrated by the client who abuses substances. Although the behavior of the child with a conduct disorder often is inappropriate and offensive, the nurse must learn to deal with her own personal feelings and demonstrate acceptance of the child. The "tough-guy" exterior put forward by the child is his way of dealing with feelings of inadequacy resulting from an environment which lacks consistency, caring, and emotional support.

Substance Use Disorders

Substance use disorders include the abuse of alcohol, hypnotics, cocaine and other stimulants, and hallucinogens. Alcohol abuse and alcohol dependency are infrequently diagnosed before age 20, although many adolescents and a sizable number (though a small percentage) of children abuse alcohol. Abuse of other substances is frequently diagnosed in late adolescence but often begins considerably earlier. Alcohol abuse and dependence occur more often when other family members abuse alcohol, and genetic factors have been implicated in its cause ("Summary," 1984).

Heavy use of alcohol and other mind-altering drugs in childhood or adolescence carries many risks, including an increased likelihood of accidents, interpersonal violence, and entanglements with legal authorities. Substance abuse can significantly impair development by disturbing social, educational, and occupational activities and interests in ways that may have lifelong effects. Substance abuse in adolescence is often associated with conduct disorders.

The use and abuse of substances is related to poor self-concept and low self-esteem. An individual may drink to excess in order to cope with feelings of inadequacy. Adolescents, because of their need to belong, often succumb to peer group pressure and drink, smoke, or take drugs because "everybody else is doing it." The behavior is a manifestation of the person's feelings and the individual needs assistance with these feelings.

Substance use disorders may be treated on an outpatient basis at mental health centers and community clinics. Although individual psychotherapy may be of some use, it is important for the entire family to be involved in the treatment. Nursing management is described in Table 14-4.

TABLE 14-4 Substance Abuse Disorders

Characteristics of the Disorder	Nursing Interventions

Impulsiveness
  Seeks prompt gratification of wishes without considering probable consequences
  Speaks and acts abruptly
  Readily displays anger when frustrated
	Recognize and deal with your own responses to impulsive, manipulative, or hostile behavior
	Encourage child to *talk about his feelings rather than act on them*

Manipulation Attempts to influence others in order to have his own wishes fulfilled without regard to effect this has on others	In an objective, nonaccusatory, nonpunitive way point out to the child his provocative or unwise behavior and help him recognize its negative consequences

Hostility, physical aggressiveness
  Makes sarcastic or belligerent remarks or threats
  Tense, angry facial expression and posture
  Throws, hits, or breaks things when thwarted
	Encourage client to communicate needs and wishes directly rather than translating them into manipulative, impulsive, or aggressive actions; be aware that client's undesirable behavior is motivated by feelings of inadequacy and expectations of rejection; rather than falling into the trap of reinforcing his negative feelings and expectations, help him break the pattern by experiencing success and self-esteem
	Anticipate (and help client anticipate) situations that are likely to "set him off"; help him discuss his feelings and identify alternative courses of action before acting
	Limit setting is essential:
	  Establishing rules can be helpful; define expectations clearly and communicate them firmly in a nonaccusatory, nonthreatening way
	  Set limits on inappropriate behaviors only; do not say no to everything
	  Do not make rules that cannot be enforced; be realistic; be consistent; follow through
	  Maintain communication among staff members to ensure consistency

Anxiety Disorders

Anxiety disorders of childhood may begin as early as preschool age and are fairly common in both sexes (APA, 1980). The main characteristic is anxiety, which may focus on a specific situation, as in separation anxiety disorder, or be generalized, as in overanxious disorder. Treatment for the anxiety disorder involves psychotherapy for the child and family. Sometimes psychotropic drugs are used to relieve excessive anxiety. Nursing management is described in Table 14-5.

Affective Disorders: Depression and Suicidal Intention

The affect or mood disorder nurses encounter most often is depression. School-age children and adolescents sometimes become severely depressed in response to a loss or a seemingly insurmountable problem or intolerable situation, either actual or imagined. They may conceive of suicide as the most suitable solution to their problems, and there is little doubt that some "accidental" injuries and deaths of children and youths are actually unrecognized or unreported suicide attempts or self-inflicted deaths. Suicide is the third leading cause of death during adolescence, after accidents and homicide. While a youngster may not verbalize depressed feelings, the behavior described in Table 14-6 is observable and the recent history may reveal a marked change from previous patterns of

mood and activity. Medical treatment often includes mood-elevating drugs and individual and family psychotherapy.

Nursing Management

It is important to recognize depression and suicidal intention in order to take appropriate measures to preserve life and reduce suffering. Injuries, particularly repeated ones and suspicious ones such as unlikely falls, drug or toxin ingestion by school-age children or adolescents, and driver-only one-car accidents, may not be accidental. At the time the young person is treated, he may not disclose that his health problems are self-inflicted. Suicidal depression does not always follow a particular pattern, but a number of common predisposing factors have been identified (Table 14-7).

The top priority in nursing care for a client who is depressed is to maintain his safety by preventing self-injury. It is perfectly appropriate—obligatory, in fact—for a nurse simply to ask the client directly whether he is considering suicide: "Are you thinking of killing yourself?" While this kind of questioning is unsavory for many nurses because of their feelings about suicide and death of the young, it is important to realize that there is no danger of causing a suicide by "suggesting" it. Being asked whether he is considering suicide will not induce a non-suicidal person to attempt to kill himself. This is especially

TABLE 14-5 Anxiety Disorders

Characteristics of the Disorder	Nursing Interventions

Overanxious disorder
  Child worries about past and future
  Is excessively concerned about performance, self-consciousness, physical symptoms, and inability to relax
  Somatic complaints for which no physical cause can be found are common; child may have history of extensive but unproductive diagnostic workups
  Parents may be dissatisfied and concerned about child's achievements even when he functions at above-average level
	Parent or close family member should stay with child, especially during anxiety-generating procedures
	Be honest and provide age-appropriate information; encourage family members to be truthful and avoid misleading child
	Reassure child who fears dark that a light will always be on

Separation anxiety disorder
  Excessive anxiety occurs when child is separated from family and familiar environment: cries, pleads, is apathetic and sad, is unable to concentrate on school or play
  Child refuses to stay overnight at a friend's house, may be unable to stay alone in a room
  Clings and complains of physical symptoms in anticipation of (or in response to) separation from parents
  May have sleep problems, fear of the dark, preoccupation with morbid thoughts concerning well-being of family members
  Separation anxiety disorder often begins after loss of a loved one or change of residence
  May refuse to attend school ("school phobia") in order to remain with parent or in the home environment
	Accept the anxious, sad feelings child expresses since they are real and he is suffering; do not use glib or belitting remarks ("Don't be a baby"; "There is nothing to worry about"); offer objective, emphatic statements which demonstrate respect for the child's feelings and concern about his discomfort ("It must be hard for you to be away from home," "You seem very worried about your family")
	Be calm and speak softly; a nurse who appears to be anxious increases the child's level of anxiety

TABLE 14-6 Depression

Characteristics of the Disorder	Nursing Interventions
Sad facial expression Loss of interest in previously enjoyed activities Withdrawal from friends and family; spends more time alone Decrease in appetite, weight loss Difficulty sleeping or excessive sleeping Increased difficulty with schoolwork, dropping grades Comments on own guilt and worthlessness History of injuries or "accidents" that may not be truly accidental Increased interest in or inquiry about death and lethality (e.g., guns, overdoses) Particulary in school-age children, early signs of depression may be a paradoxical, defensive increase in activity and overt anger and antisocial behavior (destructiveness, cruelty to animals, aggression)	Assess mood frequently by observing body language and asking open-ended questions ("What's on your mind right now?" "How have things been going for you lately?"); avoid asking for explanations (reasons) why client feels or acts as he does Depressed persons may think slowly and take a long time to answer or carry out activities; be prepared to spend extra time Support self-esteem: without overdoing it or seeming insincere, provide honest praise and recognition of child where possible (comment on his good points, recognize his having managed well during a difficult situation, etc.) Listen with real interest when client speaks, accepting his feelings and attitudes and helping him explore how *he* feels; avoid temptation to cut off his expressions that are uncomfortable for *you,* and do not attempt an "easy fix" for his negative views; remarks to the effect that client is mistaken or exaggerating how bad things are remain unconvincing and teach him only that he cannot count on you Spend periods of time with the child when not giving him care; voluntarily being with him, even in silence, lets him know that he is accepted and cared about, and this fosters trust and self-esteem If you think the client may be suicidal, ask With potentially suicidal persons the first priority of care is safety; outpatients must be referred to a mental health professional or pediatrician for immediate intervention, and parents or other responsible persons must be counseled about the seriousness of the child's situation; inpatients must not be left alone; make environment as safe as possible: place client in room near nurses' station, be sure bathroom door does not lock, remove dangerous items such as razors and pills

important to remember in order to avoid extreme feelings of guilt if a suicide does occur.

In addition to promoting the safety of depressed clients, the nurse undertakes to alleviate feelings of worthlessness, low self-esteem, and despondency. It is inappropriate to attempt to "cheer up" depressed persons of any age by approaching them in an overly cheerful manner. Such behavior demonstrates to a client either that his feelings are unimportant or that his pain is not recognized; in either case he may feel uncared for and more isolated and will be less likely to enter into a therapeutic relationship with the nurse (Table 14-6).

Schizophrenic Disorders

Schizophrenic disorders are rarely seen in childhood; the onset of these disorders usually occurs during adolescence or early adulthood (APA, 1980). While there are

TABLE 14-7 Risk Factors for Suicide*

Long-term (years) feeling of rejection or inability to please significant others
Impulsiveness
Abuse of alcohol or other drug that impairs perception and judgment
Disrupted family relationships
Feelings of guilt and anger
Previous suicide by close family member, friend, or admired person
Males: adolescent males exceed females in suicide by about 3 to 1, *but* many more females than males *attempt* suicide; attempting suicide must always be regarded as life-threatening, since death can result even if unintended
Recent breakdown of meaningful social relationship
Other recent crisis: school failure, pregnancy, family quarrel, etc.
Social isolation: "loner," feeling of being unnoticed, unimportant, or misunderstood
Feeling of "nothing to live for"

*See also Table 14-6.

many types of such disorders, several factors are characteristic of all forms, as shown in Table 14-8. Schizophrenic disorders are treated most often with the major tranquilizers and psychotherapy. It is helpful for the entire family to be involved in treatment, especially since interaction within the family appears to influence the development of this disorder. A nursing management is outlined in Table 14-8.

Eating Disorders

There are four classifications of eating disorders which occur in infancy, childhood, and adolescence: *rumination disorder* of infancy (repeated self-induced vomiting), *pica* (repeated eating of nonfoods such as dirt, laundry starch, or paint chips), *anorexia nervosa,* and *bulimia* (binge eating) (APA, 1980). This section discusses anorexia nervosa since it is the disorder in which a nurse intervenes most frequently (Table 14-9).

Nursing Management

Severe anorexia nervosa constitutes a medical and psychiatric emergency. Hospitalization frequently is required in order to prevent starvation, and death occurs in 15 to 21 percent of cases (APA, 1980).

Treatment first focuses on preventing death from malnutrition caused by starvation. An adequate diet must be established and maintained. It is most often accomplished in the general hospital setting through the use of a behavior modification program. This type of program rewards weight gain with pleasurable activities such as watching television or having visitors. After the immediate life-threatening situation is resolved, maintaining nutrition is still a priority. The behavior modification program can be continued on an inpatient or outpatient basis. Emphasis is placed on involving the entire family in treatment, with the focus on family communication patterns as well as relationships among family members.

TABLE 14-8 Schizophrenic Disorders

Characteristics of the Disorder	Nursing Interventions
Altered perception of reality: *Hallucinations* (sensory perceptions that are not in agreement with reality), particularly hearing instructions from voices that are not real *Delusions* (fixed, often bizarre beliefs that have no basis in fact); client may believe that he has special powers or that evil forces are after him Inappropriate mood or affect, e.g., laughing at serious situations Blunted, flat affect (lack of emotional response) with immobile facial expression and monotone voice Withdrawal from others Detachment from the environment Preoccupation with self Suspicion and mistrust	Work toward establishing a degree of trust; proceed slowly and be trustworthy—give accurate information, keep promises, and when possible avoid alarming the child (e.g., if he has an unrealistic fear of being touched, do not touch him without explanation or unnecessarily) Describe ahead of time what you or other staff personnel are going to do, in words the child understands Avoid generating or supporting fantasies, hallucinations, or delusions but do not argue with child about what is real or true and what is not; restate your own view of the situation in an "I" statement Provide reality orientation and build trust by talking about noncontroversial issues (who came to visit, what was served on the lunch tray, etc.)

TABLE 14-9 Anorexia Nervosa

Characteristics of the Disorder	Nursing Interventions
Usually begins in early to late adolescence	Promote nutrition according to psychotherapist's treatment plan; one approach frequently used is behavior modification program, in which client earns desired activities (watching TV, having visitors) as reward for gaining prespecified amount of weight
Rare in males	
Client has great dread of becoming obese; body image is distorted so that client considers self overweight in spite of clear evidence to the contrary (weight chart, scales, mirror, photo)	
Thin, gaunt, losing weight	If client is inpatient, observe and record food intake and eating behavior; discourage or prevent vomiting (e.g., do not permit client to use bathroom alone after meals); do not nag or cajole client to eat
Onset sometimes preceded by a stressful life event and usually by history of mild or moderate overweight and reduction diet	
Amenorrhea with no other cause except malnutrition	
Client is devious about avoiding food intake: pretends to eat when being observed but may actually hide food in clothing or napkin for later disposal	Encourage client to verbalize feelings and thoughts; encourage open, honest communication with family members (e.g., if client expresses dissatisfaction with parents, say, "I'm wondering if you've shared that with them"
Diets secretly	
Induces vomiting after eating, may use laxatives or enemas to prevent food absorption	Encourage family discussion of matters not related to food, such as family and school activities (avoids conflict and increases communication)
May be overactive; excessive exercise may be used to burn calories	
May demonstrate anxiety, crying, sleep disturbances	Adhere to psychotherapist's plan of care; e.g., if reward is to follow specified weight gain, do not reinforce unless that gain is achieved
Rejects adult sex role; dresses childishly, avoids mature sexual behavior in any form	Help client identify areas of her life in which *she* is in control and for which she is responsible; provide feedback when she has achieved a goal
Often has exceptionally high level of achievement in school or other activities and feels pushed by parents to do well	Provide accurate information and teaching about sex-related matters; correct misinformation and inaccurate fantasies

Learning Activities

Self-Assessment

Working effectively with emotionally disturbed children requires self-awareness and an understanding of one's response to the child and his behavior. In this exercise you are to think about the behaviors listed below and write how you feel about each behavior. Spend some time considering what factors (your own beliefs and values, past experience, events in your family) may influence your response.

Child's behavior

Bites self	Throws toys
Sets fires	Smiles at nurse
Cries often	Hits nurse
Laughs at nurse	Stares at wall
Sits alone	Flaps arms
Hugs nurse	Pulls own hair
Refuses food	Screams loudly
Bangs head	

Demonstrating Acceptance

The demonstration of acceptance of the child is a necessary component of all interactions. For each of the following situations, list both verbal and nonverbal behaviors that the nurse may exhibit which may indicate to the child that she accepts him. Discuss your results with your classmates.

Situations

1. A 6-year-old boy has been admitted for observation after falling out of a tree house. Although he has been told to stay in bed, the nurse finds him running down the hall, entering other rooms, and playing with the elevator doors.
2. A 12-year-old girl has been admitted for corrective orthopedic surgery. When the nurse enters her room, she observes that the child is picking her nose, staring into space, and mumbling to herself. She also laughs periodically for no apparent reason.
3. A 15-year-old boy has been admitted following a suicide attempt. He does not talk and avoids looking at the nurse.
4. A 16-year-old girl has been admitted for exploratory abdominal surgery. When entering her room, the nurse finds her smoking in bed. When the nurse tell her that this not allowed, the client uses foul language and tosses a cup of water in the nurse's face.
5. A 3-year-old boy has been admitted for a tonsillectomy. When given toys by the nurse, he ignores them. He does not look at the nurse, and will not eat unless he has a certain spoon. The nurse observes that he flaps his arms and wiggles his fingers directly in front of his eyes.

Study Questions

1. The nurse's most important therapeutic tool in caring for a disturbed child is:
   A. Knowledge about the child's medications.
   B. Understanding of the family background.
   C. Knowledge about the child's medical (psychiatric) diagnosis.
   D. The nurse-client relationship.

2. Emotional disturbance of a child is best described as:
   A. Caused by faulty parenting.
   B. Symptomatic of family disturbance.
   C. A cause of adjustment problems for the siblings.
   D. Self-induced.

3. Double-level communication is:
   A. Verbal communication accompanied by nonverbal communication.
   B. Conflicting instructions from both parents.
   C. A message with two conflicting meanings.
   D. Socially unacceptable nonverbal communication.

4. An example of a double-level message is:
   A. Picking up a child and saying, "I love you."
   B. A parent giving a child two toys and then asking which he likes better.
   C. Hugging a child and saying, "You're cute."
   D. Saying "I love you" while pushing the child away.

5. Nursing actions appropriate for a child with autism or pervasive developmental disorder in the general hospital include:
   1. Respect and support for the family's methods of providing care for the child.
   2. Talking calmly to the child and explaining what the nurse is doing even though he may not seem to hear or understand.
   3. Introducing new approaches in order to help the child become more flexible.
   4. Reminding the child to use toys in ways typical of normal children his age.
   A. 1 and 2   C.1 and 4
   B. 2 and 3   D.1, 2, 3, and 4

6. Hyperactive children with attention deficit disorder:
   1. Should be encouraged to engage in active play and "roughhousing" so that they will become tired enough to sleep well.
   2. Can be disciplined into sitting still and behaving.
   3. May impulsively do things that endanger themselves or others.
   4. Should be left alone as much as possible to eliminate unnecessary stimulation.
   A. 1, 2, 3, and 4   C.3
   B. 1, 2, and 3   D.2 and 4

7. Conduct disorders are characterized by:
   1. Antisocial, "delinquent" behavior.
   2. Abuse of alcohol, tobacco, and other drugs.
   3. High achievement in school.
   4. Running away from home.
   A. 1, 2, 3, and 4   C.3 and 4
   B. 1 and 2   D.2 and 4

8. Indications of depression commonly include:
   1. Lack of interest in things that formerly seemed important.
   2. Sleep disorders.
   3. Decrease in the level of school achievement.
   4. "Macho" or "tough" behavior to compensate for low self-esteem.
   A. 1, 2, 3, and 4   C.3 and 4
   B. 1, 2, and 3   D.1 and 2

9. Nursing intervention for a depressed child or adolescent includes:
   1. Asking, "Do you ever think about killing yourself?"
   2. Describing others' problems so that the client will get a perspective on the relative importance or unimportance of his problem.
   3. Listening without interruption even though what is said may be unpleasant or unwelcome.
   4. Returning the client to the home setting as soon as possible.
   A. 1, 2, 3, and 4   C.1 and 3
   B. 2 and 3   D.2 and 4

10. Anorexia nervosa is:
    1. Life-threatening.
    2. Most common in adolescent females.
    3. Usually treated with a behavior modification approach.
    4. Associated with a sincere belief that one is too fat.
    A. 1, 2, 3, and 4   C.2 and 4
    B. 2   D.1 and 3

References

American Psychiatric Association: *Diagnostic and Statistical Manual of Mental Disorders,* 3d ed., American Psychiatric Association, Washington, D.C., 1980.
"A Summary: The Fifth Special Report to the U.S. Congress on Alcohol and Health," *Alcohol, Health, and Research World,* 9:40, 1984.

Bibliography

Carino, C.M., and P. Chmelko: "Disorders of Eating in Adolescence: Anorexia Nervosa and Bulimia," *Nursing Clinics of North America,* 18(2):343-352, 1983.
Edwards, B.J., and J.K. Brilhart: *Communication in Nursing Practice,* Mosby, St. Louis, 1981.
Keidel, G.C.: "Adolescent Suicide," *Nursing Clinics of North America,* 18(2):323-332, 1983.
Knopf, I.J.: *Childhood Psychopathology,* 2d ed., Prentice-Hall, Englewood Cliffs, N.J., 1984.
Mein, E.C.: *Communication in Nursing Practice,* Little, Brown, Boston, 1980.
Miller, S., and P. Winstead-Fry: *Family Systems Theory and Nursing Practice,* Reston, Reston, Va., 1982.
Moore, J.A., and M.U. Coulonon: "Anorexia Nervosa: The Patient, Her Family and Key Family Intervention," *Journal of Psychiatric Nursing and Mental Health Services,* 19(5):9-14, 1981.
Pallikkathayil, L., and S. Tweed: "Substance Abuse: Alcohol and Drugs in Adolescence," *Nursing Clinics of North America,* 18(2):313-321, 1983.

15

Chronic Illnesses in Children

Objectives

After reading this chapter, the student will be able to:
1. Identify three causes of chronic problems in children.
2. Discuss parental responses to having a child with a chronic illness or disability.
3. Explain five factors which influence the presence of chronic illness.
4. Define the reactions of siblings to a brother or sister who is chronically ill.
5. List at least five nursing interventions which are used in working with chronically ill children and families.
6. Describe the role of the nurse on an interdisciplinary team.

The Concept of Chronicity

Chronic illness is a substantial health problem in children. The number of individuals who must live with a variety of long-term problems is on the increase. As a result of the decrease in infectious diseases of childhood, aggressive drug treatment, innovative surgical techniques, and advances in technology, there is an ever-increasing capability to sustain life, even when it is not possible to restore health. It is extremely important for nurses to have insight into and an understanding of the effects of chronic illness on children and their families. Although each chronic illness is unique and has a different impact on the child and family, physical and dietary limitations, stress, monetary problems, retarded growth, hospitalizations, pain, medications, dependence, and feelings of being different pervade most of these illnesses. It is important to remember too that each child is a developing person with different

271

needs, abilities, and responses, depending on his stage of development, so that the nature and extent of disruption vary according to the stage at which the disease occurs.

Since most of these children are cared for by their families, it is important for nurses to understand the extent of this health problem. A prime nursing responsibility is to provide families with information and demonstrate attitudes which will enable them to function more effectively in their roles as decision makers, caregivers, advocates, and teachers (Horner, 1987).

Definitions

Mattson's definition of long-term or chronic illness is used frequently as a frame of reference. Mattson defined a chronically ill patient as "a person who has any disorder with a protracted course which is progressive and fatal *or* associated with a relatively normal life-span despite impaired physical or mental functioning. Such a condition is handicapping and disabling and it has periods of acute exacerbation requiring intensive medical care" (Mattson, 1972, p. 801).

Hobbs defined a chronic health problem as "a condition which interferes with daily functioning for greater than three months in a year, causes hospitalization for more than one month in a year, or (at a time of diagnosis) is likely to do so" (Hobbs, 1984, p. 206). It should be noted that the words *disability, illness, disease, condition, impairment,* and *handicap* are used interchangeably in discussing chronic illness.

Incidence

The true incidence of chronic illness is unknown, primarily because of differences in nomenclature, classification, and methodology. Some researchers list the multiply handicapped according to *each* condition present, which overestimates their frequency, while others group the conditions together, which underestimates their numbers.

It is estimated that 30 to 40 percent of children under 18 years have one or more long-term disorders. Even when these percentages are corrected to include only children with chronic *physical* disorders, Mattson (1972) estimated that 7 to 10 percent of all children are affected. It is known that the rate increases with age, that school-age children and adolescents are the most commonly affected, and that the visual and hearing impairments; speech, learning, and behavioral disorders; and developmental disabilities and other conditions add up to staggering numbers. For example, in the United States about 2 million handicapped children require special care, about 1.5 million have asthma, 50,000 have sickle cell anemia (Bracht, 1979), and according to the National Foundation, about 240,000 newborns annually have birth defects.

Causes and Types

There are numerous childhood conditions which result in chronic illness, including the following:

1. Congenital disorders which occur during fetal development and can result from drugs, radiation, maternal in-

fections (rubella, cytomegalovirus), combinations of these causes, or unknown causes
2. Genetic disorders which have been expressed in previous generations (sickle cell anemia, Tay-Sachs disease), but also new mutations which will affect future generations, such as cystic fibrosis and muscular dystrophy
3. Acquired disorders such as leukemia, respiratory problems, renal disease, acute infections such as meningitis, and the sequelae of accidents including severe head injuries and burns

Regardless of the specific condition or its cause, these long-term disorders are characterized by one or more of the following: permanence, residual disability, nonreversible pathological alterations, and the need for lengthy periods of supervision, observation, care, and/or rehabilitation.

Costs

The financial costs of caring for these children and adolescents are astronomical. Closing a ventricular septal defect may cost $40,000, including cardiac catheterization and 12 to 14 days of hospitalization but not counting the surgeon's fees. The actual cost of a bone marrow transplantation exceeds $50,000, excluding prior workup, immunosuppressive treatment, and hospitalization.

Each year children with birth defects spend more than 6 million days in the hospital. Enormous monetary and health personnel expenditures are involved in innumerable diagnostic measures, surgical procedures, hospitalizations, and habilitative or rehabilitative services.

No statistics can express the emotional costs of chronic illness or describe the extent of the physical or mental handicaps with which some children are afflicted. The demands and challenges for nurses are overwhelming at times; however, the overall rewards and satisfactions of working with these children and their families can be most gratifying.

Factors that Influence Chronic Illness

The presence of chronic illness stresses and drains all the members of a family over an indefinite period of time. There are several variables that have a direct effect on the overall presence of chronicity.

The uncertain prognosis is an important factor. Advances have been made in correcting a variety of birth defects, and life expectancies have improved greatly. However, acute exacerbations and the potential for considerable variations leave both parents and children in a state of uncertainty and anxiety. The degree of disability or the limitation of normal function can have profound implications on the extent to which a disease affects a family's life-style (Fig. 15-1). Finally, the visibility of the defect or disease, for example, the facial scars from a burn, can subject the child to attention from everyone. Less visible conditions can spare a child the unwanted attention, but other problems may develop; for instance, a deaf child may be perceived as hostile, a behavior problem, or dumb.

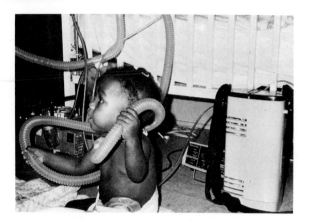

FIGURE 15-1 This child is confined to her room most of the day because of oxygen dependence. Her mobility is impaired by decreased activity tolerance related to lung disease following a premature birth. (*From M. Smith, J. Goodman, and N.L. Ramsey, Child and Family: Concepts of Nursing Practice, McGraw-Hill, New York, 1987, p. 1200.*)

Chronic illness does not always presume a handicap. In the presence of end-stage renal disease with dialysis, fluid and dietary restrictions, pain, growth retardation, and frequent hospitalizations present major obstacles to the child even with optimum emotional adjustment. Even a child with a correctable, repaired congenital heart who is free of physical handicaps may be psychologically crippled.

Impact on Families

Several variables influence the response of a family to chronic illness. The more debilitating the illness, the poorer the prognosis; the more complicated the treatments, the greater the stress which family members experience. If the course is progressively deteriorating or unpredictable, they must face the constant threat of death, as in congenital heart disease or severe asthma. If the disease has a genetic base, as in muscular dystrophy and Tay-Sachs disease, there is parental guilt about transmission.

Age is a critical factor. If the diagnosis is made during the neonatal period, the parents never experience the child as normal, and so their expectations are altered from birth. If it occurs later, after the child's personality has developed and he has been normal and healthy, the sense of loss is even greater. The earlier the diagnosis is made, the more likely it is that parents will view the child as handicapped, fragile, and limited and the more likely they are to be overprotective and overindulgent, distorting the parent-child relationship and inhibiting normal growth and development.

The type of deformity or disease influences its effect on the family. In the case of a visible, congenital defect, burn scars, or severe developmental disability, family members are continually confronted by the discomfort of the sick child. The respiratory care, medications, injections, and special diets may be resisted or resented, in-

creasing the amount of work and the emotional strain.

The presence or absence of other children makes a difference in regard to the effects of chronicity on a family. If there are healthy, able-bodied siblings, they will lessen parental feelings of inadequacy. However, if one child has already been lost to the disease, the parents will have more difficulty adjusting to the currently affected child.

The repeated hospitalizations and surgical procedures intensify guilt feelings, especially in the case of infants or toddlers who are unable to understand. Sometimes parents are forced to make life-or-death decisions without any assurance that they are making the correct choice. Although each family places a different value on physical ability, appearance, and cognitive function, every family's life-style is forced to change. There are disruptions in eating patterns and the carrying out of normal activities, financial burdens, the loss of school or work, and interruptions in personal plans or goals. A family living with chronic illness does not choose to follow a particular life-style; their life-style gradually evolves as a result of pressures with which they are not prepared to deal, and they may not have the strength, support, or knowledge to improve it.

Initial Parental Responses

Reactions differ markedly from family to family and vary within a particular family from one time to another. Problems emerge as the family members attempt to cope with the presence of chronicity. There is shock and disbelief. It is a crisis, a period of disorganization, a time when the family is overwhelmed by a problem which cannot be solved quickly by the usual coping mechanisms, which have been rendered inadequate. Support systems and previous skills in coping with difficult situations will affect the outcome. If this crisis is managed well, it can be a growth-producing experience. If not, the family will emerge as a much weaker unit.

The initial emotional reaction is denial, which may decrease as the family comes to grips with reality. If the initial reaction persists, however, it will interfere with learning to live with the situation and meet the child's needs, perpetuating the crisis and prolonging the adjustment. Anxiety also should subside in time; otherwise, it may lead to overprotection, overindulgence, and a myriad of psychosocial problems.

Many families also experience feelings of guilt and self-blame. Some parents view the child's condition as proof of their inadequacy and inability to produce a normal, healthy child.

Some parents direct their anger inwardly and become depressed. This emotion stems from their deep mourning for the child who "might have been." Occasionally there is resentment and rejection as well as disappointment. Covert rejection is evidenced by inadequate, inconsistent care, unnecessary demands in the hospital setting, or complete avoidance of the child by working. There is shame and embarrassment, withdrawal from community activities, and alienation from and bitterness toward relatives, neighbors, and friends at a time when they are needed most for support.

Mourning is an ongoing process, and it may persist for many years. However, denial, anger, and feelings of helplessness should decrease in intensity as parental psychic energy is mobilized to deal with the problem. Olshansky's (1966) concept of "chronic sorrow," although initially used with families of retarded children, is appropriate in discussing chronic illness because there too a family experiences the loss of a "normal" child. It is most evident when the chronically ill child is unable to achieve the expected developmental milestones, regardless of the cause. All the members of a family will always feel this loss.

On occasion, in spite of all efforts to facilitate adaptation, some parents are unable to achieve it. Although overt rejection (using the child as a scapegoat) sometimes occurs, overprotection is more prevalent. Its presence needs to be understood because it not only serves to deny reality but also impedes normal development of the child. Overprotection can be a form of covert rejection. For example, when parents fail to discipline a child, causing further misbehavior, they can use the experience to rationalize the rejection.

The repeated hospitalizations, the surgical procedures, the difficulties parents experience in providing physical care—especially feeding and toileting—and the uncertain future contribute to the stress, tension, and anxiety which perpetuate the overprotective tendencies. In turn, the child is unable to experiment; he is fearful of exposing himself to frustration and unable to experience successful ventures. This phenomenon can lead to problem behaviors and inhibit normal personality development. Although he may resist initially, eventually the child will succumb. Such dependency has long-range social and developmental implications.

Parenthood, one of the most complex responsibilities of adulthood, is made even more difficult by the presence of chronic illness. The physical demands of caring for a child at home, the emotional drain of day-to-day activities, and the financial burdens can affect any marriage, but in one which is already strained it may seem that the chronically ill child is "the last straw." Of course, this problem occurs at a time when the child's dependence emphasizes his need for two parents.

When they are anxious about finances, fathers may get second jobs, and mothers may also seek employment, returning home in the evening to care for the child. A promotion may not be accepted because the physical move would not place the parents near a comparable medical center. They do not go out because they are tired, cannot afford it, or cannot find a baby-sitter. Sexual intercourse may be avoided because they fear producing another defective baby. They spend less and less time together until the social unit simply disintegrates. Suicides are higher in families with chronically ill children (Lawson, 1977), and divorces are much more common (Bracht, 1979).

Impact on Well Siblings

Siblings are affected by the chronic illness of a brother or sister. Some feel guilty about being healthy. They may resent the time the parents spend with the sick brother or sister and interpret differential treatment as preferential treatment. It is not unusual for able-bodied siblings to have to arrange their schedules to meet the needs of a sick child. Repeatedly they are told to be considerate or to select the TV programs the sick child wants to watch. They resent the sick child for not adhering to the standards of behavior which apply to them. There are no more outings or vacations because the family would be too far away from the medical center. They may be embarrassed by the sick sibling's physical features or behavior. There are separations from their parents whenever a hospitalization occurs. Invariably, it means physical displacement, being lodged at the home of friends or relatives. Thus it is understandable that they demonstrate adjustment problems such as nausea, vomiting, diarrhea, headaches, and other vague complaints as well as changes in academic performance such as truancy or the development of school phobias. They may be irritable, impatient, and withdrawn. Sometimes they display antisocial, attention-getting behaviors, regressive tendencies, or anxiety-related activities such as stuttering and nail biting (Breslau, Weitzman, and Messenger, 1981).

Every child has special needs at particular times. The loss of peer group activities or the assumption of responsibilities which involve physical care may damage these parent-child relationships and affect sibling relationships as well. Parents who are trying to find blood donors, seeing physicians, or checking on the extent of insurance coverage often forget about the children at home. However, parents must be reminded that the well children are there and that they too need time with the mother and father. Nursing assessments of siblings and their adjustments to the presence of a chronically ill child are not completed as consistently as they should be.

Effects of Chronic Illness on a Child

The effects of chronic illness vary tremendously from one youngster to another. However, one fact does not change: Each young patient is a child first and chronically ill second. Every child has needs and the right to optimal care. He is part of a family, in need of love, discipline, and independence. The psyche and soma are inseparable, and it is critical for a child to be treated holistically. In an era when lives are being prolonged extensively, understanding of the emotional aspects of prolongation has not kept pace with technological advances. Although there may not be cures for many of these diseases, the quality of these children's lives can be improved with more coordinated interdisciplinary management and more humanistic health care.

The psychological impact of chronicity is determined by the child's level of development, experiences with illness, type of health problem, and relationship with his family, his peers, and the community. The ability to understand the ramifications of an illness is not necessarily accompanied by an ability to accept them. Thus the experience of the disease and the restrictions imposed can interfere with the successful achievement of normal developmental tasks and a healthy sense of self-esteem.

Self-Esteem

The evaluation which a child makes of himself expresses an attitude of approval or disapproval—the extent to which he considers himself capable, significant, and worthy. Self-esteem develops as a result of how children feel they are loved and approved of by those who are significant to them, how good they are at performing tasks, and the extent to which they can influence their own and others' lives. It is a key to both success and happiness. Although self-esteem develops over time, it emerges when a child enters school and fluctuates dramatically as he interacts with peers. In a school setting, then, teachers, classmates, and academic achievement affect self-esteem.

At home a deformity is incorporated into one's self-image gradually, but the self-image is threatened on contact with peers when comparisons occur and especially when a "difference" is clearly visible. If a child has accepted his self-image, he can cope with peer acceptance, which is important to all children but absolutely crucial to adolescents, who are also dealing with autonomy and sexuality. Conversely, if a child is embarrassed and ashamed about his deformity or illness, these feelings may contribute to alienation from his peer group.

Among the stigmatizing characteristics to which a chronically ill child is desensitized are the irritating cough, the loss of hair from chemotherapy, the foul flatulence of cystic fibrosis, and the smell of urine that envelops a child with spina bifida. A child desires friends and wants to be like his friends. He is eager to be a member of the group, but he must risk the possibility of devastating his self-esteem because of the problems which characterize his chronic illness.

Dependence, Restrictions, and Isolation

An acute exacerbation forces a child into a dependent state, perhaps after he has struggled to achieve a level of independence. This enforced dependence can be a source of conflict. There are times when a child with cystic fibrosis needs to be "clapped" and must depend on an adult to perform this task or when a hemophiliac who is bleeding actively needs to be hospitalized. In the active phase of any disease, the client needs the security provided by parents or nurses. These are situations in which parents and providers see immature, regressive behavior and accept the dependence. It seems that adults tend to reward the dependence in an effort to help the child feel secure and comfort him. If dependence becomes excessive and sustained, it may prove to be so satisfying that the child may strenuously resist relinquishing it. Then it can impede the process of acquiring independence, which is important to the child's self-confidence and initiative. It can affect rehabilitative endeavors and interfere with maxi-

mum functioning. The goal is to maintain a delicate balance, allowing for dependence when it is appropriate, in the acute phase, but encouraging independence whenever possible. Achieving this tenuous balance can be extremely difficult.

Chronically disabled children have physical limitations which curb their motor activity, as a result of spina bifida, muscular dystrophy, and spinal cord injuries. These limitations prevent them from taking part in many activities which facilitate the normal discharge of energy and aggression. Children with certain conditions also experience sensory restrictions, for example, children who are hearing-impaired, those who are blind, and those with decreased tactile stimulation, such as a child whose hands have been burned.

The progressive or sudden curtailment of activities can result in frustration along with feelings of helplessness and anger. The immobility or sensory impairment interferes with a child's physical ability to "let off steam." If a child has mastered language, he can verbally communicate his displeasure, but it is not possible for some chronically ill children.

Isolation occurs as a result of these limitations. It may be more physically difficult to seek out friends, and so chronically ill children *must* rely on the children who come to visit them. Some chronically ill children may be restricted in the degree to which they can participate in games. Fatigue often prevents children with heart disease, renal failure, leukemia, or cystic fibrosis from taking part in activities. Children with dietary restrictions also are affected. Those with asthma may not be able to play outdoors at times or even visit friends who have pets. Social ties can be severed when a child who is hospitalized is transferred to another unit or a roommate is discharged.

Hospitalization

Unfortunately, chronically ill children have acute exacerbations which necessitate hospitalization. In this situation they bring with them their fears and coping mechanisms (good and bad) as well as their physical, psychological, social, financial, and educational problems. Despite positive measures to prevent or minimize the negative effects of hospitalization, many children experience this confinement in less than optimum circumstances. The intrusions, fantasies, helplessness, crying, and screaming of others as well as the frightening equipment make it difficult to endure, especially for children up to about 4 years of age. If they have been hospitalized before, they know how bad some of their experiences are going to be. It means being away from home, from school, and from friends. If there is surgery, it means pain. Anna Freud stated that the experience of surgery does not depend on the type or seriousness of the procedure but on the type and depth of fantasies aroused by it. Nurses must make a conscious effort to improve the hospital stays of these children. Joint teaching by nurses in schools, the community, and hospitals with abundant appropriate explanations, handling of equipment, and arranging for rooming-in may improve the quality of such confinements.

Pain

Pain is an emotional experience which may be constant in the presence of some long-term diseases, although it may be mild, intermittent, or rare in others. Younger children are said to feel less pain than older children or adolescents because they have had less experience with it. Pain from within or outside the body is indistinguishable to the infant or toddler, and so it is just frightening. Pain is usually easily forgotten, except when it is augmented by anxiety, in which case it is intensified and remembered. Since young children perceive adults as powerful and capable of removing all pain, failure to do so is interpreted as an expression of anger or hostility toward the child. This concept is reinforced if the adult becomes angry with a child's complaints or apprehension about a procedure.

Fears of surgery are greatest in toddlers and adolescents. Toddlers view it as punishment, while adolescents are concerned about deformities and mutilation because of concern about body image. Teenagers need to be the same as their peers. If they are different in some way, they feel inadequate. For older children, the existence of pain also indicates loss of control over both the disease and the treatment.

While an acutely ill child expects rapid pain relief, a child who is chronically ill expects it to continue and may have disturbances in sleep patterns, lose his appetite, become irritable, withdraw, or demonstrate depression. What is usually realized is a compromise between pain diminution and patient function, or learning to live with pain, modified just enough to "take the edge off" by medication.

Medications, Treatment Plans, and Compliance

Following a particular treatment regime is difficult and trying for everyone involved. Certain drugs affect a child's alertness (barbiturates) or behavior (corticosteroids). Potent medications with a variety of side effects (chemotherapeutic drugs) can cause tremendous anxiety as a result of disturbances in body image. Timed regimens (q 3 h, q 6 h) can alter the family's schedule of activities. In addition, prolonged and regular use of drugs such as insulin and anticonvulsants may be accepted when children are young but rebelled against in adolescence. Acceptance too is seen as a sign of weakness, a constant reminder of the disease, and evidence of dependence and inadequacy the child would like to forget.

Sometimes parents or children are viewed as noncompliant, uncooperative, or rebellious for refusing to follow a certain plan. It is important to remember that they must continue to manage their daily lives in the context of the regimens developed by providers. At times it is difficult.

The problems associated with performing procedures not only involve complexity or the anxieties which are generated but they may have an impact on personal identity. It is very disturbing to a child to be told that he must

stay on insulin for life, smear his entire body with disgusting topical ointments, or be a slave to the dialysis machine. It takes time to do a treatment two to four times a day; at times everything in the household must stop to do so. These children become the focal point of a family's existence. Sometimes parents need increased levels of energy to perform certain procedures on terribly verbal and physically resistant toddlers. Parents are less apt to follow management plans which are expensive, whose efficacy is not speedily demonstrated, and which cause discomfort to the child.

School and Lack of Peer Contact

Absences from school can amount to 6 to 8 weeks a year for the average chronically ill child. Lawson (1977) found that 26 percent of these children were below their expected grade levels, with educational lags increasing as years in school increased. These absences not only contribute to falling behind academically, but also interfere with peers relationships and socialization. Some children exhibit increased truancy, get into trouble in school, and become socially isolated from their classmates. As a result, they develop changed perceptions of themselves and a decreased sense of self-worth with concomitant lower levels of self-esteem and self-confidence.

Teachers encounter families in which no one is allowed to talk about the handicap or disease and any attempts by a teacher to discuss the problem openly in the classroom with peers are vehemently resisted. There are parents who insist that a child succeed in a task he simply cannot accomplish, such as expecting a child with a spastic arm to write.

A common situation involves teachers who use a different set of standards for the handicapped. While disciplining an able-bodied student presents no problem, there is insecurity where a disabled child is concerned. Certainly both should be judged by the same disciplinary standards. The emphasis should be on the act *itself,* not on the child who commits it. This approach should prevail in any disciplinary action at home, at school, or in the hospital. Allowances must be made for physical limitations, but chronically ill or disabled children must learn to develop a positive self-image. They need to learn how to tolerate frustrations as their able-bodied classmates do.

The passage of Public Law 94-142, in 1975 mandated an equal education for all children and special attention to the individualized needs of a child. "Mainstreaming" placed handicapped children in community schools with nonhandicapped students. There have been some difficulties. Even teachers with training in special education may be unfamiliar with the educational and emotional problems of these children. The uniqueness of each situation makes it imperative for educators to combine their knowledge of growth and development with greater understanding of the chronically ill child and his family. Although schools have been forced to make major shifts in allocating their revenues and resources, the social attitudes of the communities in which these children live need to change too if these youngsters are to experience maximum development of their potential as productive adults.

Nursing Management of Children with Chronic Health Problems

The Nurse on an Interdisciplinary Team

There are many types of health problems which can result in a chronically ill child. Hence, an interdisciplinary team approach is essential if the child and family are to receive the quality of care that supports maximum habilitation or rehabilitation and optimum health maintenance. Each member of the team serves the family as an expert from a particular discipline. For example, a team may consist of a nurse, a physical therapist, a nutritionist, a social worker, a prosthetist, and a pediatrician. A number of physicians from different specialties may become involved in the medical or surgical care as a particular need arises.

It is the responsibility of the team to assess the needs of the child and family members and to provide for those needs as thoroughly as the resources available permit. Effective communication is important both among members of the team and between the health providers and the family. The team members need to be sensitive to what the family is experiencing and to one another's needs. There are situations in which one team member receives support from others as they all work to help the family.

The nurse remains a constant member of the team, despite the fact that team membership changes as the needs of the child and family change. It is the nurse who gives direct care to the child and has extensive contact with the child and parents in addition to collaborating with other health care providers. However, in order to maximize her effectiveness and utilize her unique skills, the nurse must be an *active* interdisciplinary team member. The knowledge gained from working closely with the child and family makes it appropriate for the nurse to coordinate all of the team's activities. There is no provider who is more informed or in a better position to ensure the highest caliber of health care.

Nursing Diagnosis

Nurses play a vital role in helping children and their families cope with disease or disability, thereby enhancing their adaptation to the presence of a chronic health problem regardless of its origin. In order to maximize each child's potential, it is important to develop nursing diagnoses which provide direction for effective interventions.

The nursing diagnoses below are not all-inclusive. They are common, appropriate diagnoses for planning the nursing care of chronically ill children and their families.

   Body image disturbance
   Self-esteem disturbance
   Personal identity disturbance
   Altered role performance
   Social isolation
   Anxiety
   Fear
   Ineffective airway clearance
   Activity intolerance
   Pain
   Ineffective family coping: compromised
   Altered parenting (actual and potential)
   Impaired verbal communication
   Potential impaired skin integrity

Nursing Interventions

Adaptation is critical in retaining family integrity. Many times this social unit is totally unaware of its strengths because they have not been tested before. Although chronic illness has an impact on everyone involved, there are some strategies which may facilitate the adaptive mechanisms of the family members.

How well a child adjusts to his disability is influenced by his parents because attitudes are learned from parents first and from peers second. There are stages that the parents of handicapped children move through before coming to terms with the defect, deformity, or disease. They include denial, shock, anger, anxiety, and ultimately adaptation and reorganization. Some families adapt more quickly than others; unfortunately, some never adapt. However, many parents adapt by the time a child starts school. In accepting the reality of the situation, parents can emphasize the child's strengths.

It is important for nurses to be available and to listen, for both actions serve to reduce the isolation and stress experienced by these children and families. When obtaining an accurate, thorough history, a nurse should not simply collect data which pertain to the illness. It is important to solicit information about each family member, especially in relation to how he or she is adjusting to the problem. It is necessary to do an ongoing assessment of the family's current knowledge, status, and difficulties. There are no quick solutions to the problems of these children and their families; however, by providing continuity of care, anticipatory guidance, and support, the nurse can help potentiate the quality of their lives. The feelings of parents (anger, hostility, and guilt) are natural and justified. They tend to snowball unless they are dealt with openly, honestly, and nonjudgmentally.

Parents have a need to vent their feelings, which will facilitate acceptance, living with the child, and becoming realistic in their expectations for him. They need anticipatory guidance, especially in regard to the child's pattern of development. Counseling them about realistic limit setting is important because the relaxation of disciplinary measures reinforces the sick role, making normally unacceptable behavior routine. When parents are consistent in disapproving the act committed rather than focusing on the child who committed it, they can avoid a number of subsequent problems.

In a hospital or clinic setting parents should be involved in any treatments that are done. This activity increases their competence, but more important, it gives them a sense of the time and energy involved in doing the necessary procedures. Children should be encouraged to give themselves insulin, apply their own braces, and test their own urine. These types of activities nurture their independence.

Parents need to talk, to support each other, and to include all members of the family in the decisions which have to be made. Since fathers have more difficulty adjusting to the realities of child's limitations, they need more professional support and more thorough explanations (McKeever, 1981). Both parents need to cultivate support networks. They also should be encouraged to go out together and to get away for a day alone. These support systems which play a vital role in the family's adjustment usually include family members, health care providers, neighbors, friends, and the community at large. Through a variety of activities which include both practical assistance and emotional support, the family is better able to cope with the ongoing problems associated with caring for the child.

Parent groups are especially helpful because they provide concrete assistance and because their discussions examine parental feelings about children's disabilities. They share methods of dealing with common problems. Their own practical experiences and the experiences of others increase parental understanding of the child's illness, improve case management, and clarify any misconceptions which may exist. This parent-to-parent interaction is a successful method of helping parents cope with their problems (Holaday, 1984). These groups also lobby for research, legislation, and improved facilities for the disabled.

Families can adjust to the presence of chronic illness if they are provided with information and involved in devising a management plan based on the priorities as they perceive them. The lives of all family members can be enriched if they understand and anticipate the child's developmental needs, learn to set age-appropriate expectations and limits, and appreciate the constructive nature of stress in promoting both growth and mastery.

If siblings are to adapt successfully, they must be allowed to express their hostility and resentment openly. They need to be provided with age-appropriate explanations and be taught about changes in the treatment of their brother or sister. Parents can demonstrate their interest in and support for their well children by attending school functions, encouraging peer groups activities, and talking with teachers and peers about the sibling's illness. When well children become involved in physically caring for a disabled child, they can increase their level of self-esteem, share in the crisis affecting the family, and develop a strong appreciation for their own good health and abilities.

The chronically ill child needs to be allowed to express his thoughts and feelings about the disability. He should be asked how he sees himself so that his parents can better understand his emotions. Such positive reinforcement can enhance the child's self-esteem and establish healthy, honest, and open parent-child relationships. By allowing chronically ill children to participate in a variety of realistic activities, parents can identify and encourage the development of intellectual, creative, and manual activities which foster independence but acknowledge the limitations of the child.

School and peers are very important to children, and so explanations to teachers, the school nurse, and peers are essential. In meeting with these individuals, parents get an opportunity to identify the child's physical limitations, the need for taking medications, and the need for rest periods or scheduled absences. When informed, everyone strives for the same goal, which is to maximize the normalization of the child.

Adaptation and acceptance come in time. They are facilitated by nurses who understand and care enough to invest significant amounts of energy in assisting families with children who are chronically ill. McKeever (1981, p. 128) stated that for parents, "acceptance is finding whatever pleasure they can in caring for their child every day. It means looking at other children without wishing it was their son or daughter. It means looking at the situation—identifying what can be done to enhance the child's potential. It means letting him progress at his own rate. It means being proud of him and wanting others to know him too."

Parents want their children to participate in the mainstream of society and to have access to the full range of opportunities available to all citizens. Nurses have a formidable task in educating the able-bodied to understand and accept those with chronic disorders and disabilities as well as in helping to destroy the prevalent stereotypes about handicapped people.

Learning Activities

1. Conduct nursing rounds in the hospital and focus attention on the placement of children with chronic illnesses on a particular unit.
2. Assign students to the lounge areas of long-term facilities, where they may take note of the conversations of family members.
3. Invite parents of children with chronic problems to come to class and share their experiences with students.
4. Invite children with chronic health problems to class so that they may share their personal experiences of living with a disease or disability.
5. Assign children of different ages who have chronic illnesses to students in the clinical area.

Independent Study Activities

1. Select a child with a chronic illness and act as an advocate during his hospitalization.
2. Make an appointment with a community agency that serves children with chronic illnesses or disabilities and spend more time observing the care provided to these children.
3. Attend a local support group for the parents of children with chronic problems.
4. Evaluate the community to determine the facilities and services available to children with a chronic illness.
5. Simulate a disability and spend 24 hours living with it.
6. Read articles in newspapers and magazines which pertain to chronic illness and examine them for accurate portrayals of the condition.

Study Questions

1. An effective method of alleviating guilt in parents who have a child with a disability is to:
   A. Increase the community support systems available.
   B. Teach them how to care for the child.
   C. Schedule a visit with the psychiatric nurse clinician.
   D. Involve them in a parent support group.
2. Positive peer interactions at school can be realized for chronically ill children if a nurse:
   A. Meets with children in the class the child is entering.
   B. Knows the psychosocial aspects of chronic illness.
   C. Shares information with all the adults at the school.
   D. Prepares his peers for the health problem the child is experiencing.
3. In the presence of a disability evident at birth, it is more difficult for parents to demonstrate early attachment behaviors; hence, a nurse needs to:
   A. Provide anticipatory guidance.
   B. Spend more time with these parents.
   C. Focus attention on accomplishing this task.
   D. Teach parents how to care for the newborn.
4. A major breakthrough in providing equal education for all children and special attention to the specific needs of disabled children was the passage of:
   A. Public Law 94-142.
   B. Public Law 93-247.
   C. Public Law 92-143.
   D. Public Law 91-159.
5. A child's ability to cope with his chronic health problem is very important if he is to:
   A. Attain peer acceptance.
   B. Achieve self-esteem.
   C. Accept the chronic health problem.
   D. Be successful in his endeavors.

6. Olshansky's concept of "chronic sorrow" may be demonstrated by parents of a chronically ill or disabled child when the child:
   A. Is hospitalized for surgery.
   B. Is having problems interacting with peers.
   C. Is unable to achieve expected developmental milestones.
   D. Is unable to participate in peer group activities.
7. A nurse needs to recognize the fact that within a family, the person who has more difficulty in adjusting to the realities of a chronically ill child's limitations is the:
   A. Mother   C. Sibling
   B. Father   D. Affected child

References

Bracht, N.F.: "The Social Nature of Chronic Illness and Disability," *Social Work in Health Care,* 5(2):129-143, 1979.

Breslau, N., M. Weitzman, and K. Messenger: "Psychologic Functioning of Siblings of Disabled Children," *Pediatrics,* 64:344-351, 1981.

Hobbs, N., et al.: "Chronically Ill Children in America," *Rehabilitation Literature,* 45:206-213, 1984.

Holaday, B.: "Challenges of Rearing a Chronically Ill Child: Caring and Coping," *Nursing Clinics of North America,* 19(2):361-368, 1984.

Horner, M.M., P. Rawlins, and K. Giles: "How Parents of Children with Chronic Conditions Perceive Their Own Needs," *MCN,* 12(1):40-43, 1987.

Lawson, B.A.: "Chronic Illness in the School-Age Child: Effects on the Total Family," *MCN,* 2(1):49-56, 1977.

Mattson, A.: "Long-Term Physical Illness in Childhood: A Challenge to Psychosocial Adaptation," *Pediatrics,* 50:801-811, 1972.

McKeever, P.T.: "Fathering the Chronically Ill Child," *MCN,* 6(2):124-128, 1981.

Olshansky, S.: "Parental Responses to a Mentally Defective Child," *Mental Retardation,* 4:21-23, 1966.

Bibliography

Featherstone, H.: *A Difference in the Family: Life with a Disabled Child,* Basic Books, New York, 1980.

Fife, B.L., M. Huhman, and J. Keck: "Development of a Clinical Assessment Scale: Evaluation of the Psychosocial Impact of Childhood Illness on the Family," *Issues in Comprehensive Pediatric Nursing,* 9(1):11-32, 1986.

Pollock. S.E.: "Human Responses to Chronic Illness: Physiological and Psychosocial Adaptation," *Nursing Research,* 35(2):90-95, 1986.

Rapoff, M.: "Helping Parents to Help Their Children Comply with Treatment Regimens for Chronic Diseases," *Issues in Comprehensive Pediatric Nursing,* 9(3):147-156, 1986.

Robinson, C.A.: "Double Bind: A Dilemma for Parents of Chronically Ill Children," *Pediatric Nursing,* 11(2):112-115, 1985.

Rose, M.H., and R.B. Thomas: *Children with Chronic Conditions: Nursing in a Family and Community Context,* Grune & Stratton, Orlando, Fla., 1987.

Sabbeth, B.: "Understanding the Impact of Chronic Childhood Illness on Families," *Pediatric Clinics of North America,* 31(1):47-57, 1984.

Siemon, M.: "Siblings of the Chronically Ill or Disabled Child: Meeting Their Needs," *Nursing Clinics of North America,* 19(2):295-305, 1984.

Stullenbarger, B. et al.: "Family Adaptation to Cystic Fibrosis," *Pediatric Nursing,* 13(1):29-31, 1987.

Tamlyn, D., and M.M. Arklie: "A Theoretical Framework for Standard Care Plans: A Nursing Approach for Working with Chronically Ill Children and Their Families," *Issues in Comprehensive Pediatric Nursing,* 9(1):39-46, 1986.

Yoos, L.: "Chronic Childhood Illnesses: Developmental Issues," *Pediatric Nursing,* 13(1):29-31, 1987.

16

Terminal Illnesses in Children

Objectives

After reading this chapter, the student will be able to:
1. Understand the influence of religious and other beliefs on a society's definition of life and death.
2. Analyze the technological progress that has changed the character of living and dying in western countries.
3. Trace the concept of death from early childhood through adolescence.
4. Examine the effects of two death-related crises on children and their families.
5. Suggest several preventive counseling techniques which teach children positive ways of coping with death.
6. Explore three major ways in which nurses play a vital role in helping families face terminal illness.

The extent to which death and dying have affected the lives of children is probably not appreciated by many adults today. Evidence is mounting that children are especially vulnerable to the immediate and long-term effects of deaths that remove significant persons from their lives and to life experiences that expose them to their own existential vulnerabilities. Experiences with death are important contributors to the development of personality and the capacity to cope with adversity and change. The outcomes of children's experiences with death are heavily dependent on parental behaviors and family environments which in turn have their origins in cultural values and societal practices. This chapter considers the multiple and complex meanings of death and dying in childhood as a basis for examining the implications for nursing practice of what is currently known about children's experiences with death.

Social and Cultural Meanings of Death

Since the beginning of human life, birth and death have existed as moments of significance in the ongoing life of social groups. These important events serve as markers of transition and change, and social rituals and special practices are used by groups to identify the rites of passage associated with the gain or loss of a member. Customarily, special functionaries such as priests or healers are designated to officiate at the ceremonies and assist the other members of the group through the period of transition. All human societies have developed one or more cultural systems—combinations of words and actions—which serve to help the members come to terms with and adapt to the personal and social meanings of death.

Human beings learn to interpret death on the basis of the cultural and social values of the society in which they live. The values that dominate in the society determine to a great extent the settings in which people die, the events which take place when a person is defined as dying, and the behaviors which are expected of the various people who are involved. In a real sense, the orientations toward death in a society are expressions of the general character of the culture of that society.

Death Systems and Societal Needs
Functions of Death Systems
The meaning of death at the level of society is multiple and complex. In Kastenbaum's (1977) view, each society has a death system through which the group's relationship to mortality is mediated and expressed. This system provides social mechanisms through which death-related functions are performed for society as a whole and collective meanings of death are established. Just as certain people and places—such as coroners and funeral homes—come to be associated with death, so also do certain times, objects, and symbols. The Days of the Dead in Mexico, for instance, take place on the Catholic holy days of All Saints and All Souls (November 1 and 2); the festivities at this time include candies shaped like skulls and coffins, visits to the cemetery to decorate graves and offer prayers for the dead, and rituals at home with special foods and gifts (*muertos*) for visiting friends and relatives (Green, 1980). In Israel a special site in Jerusalem serves as a memorial to the millions of Jews who were killed in the Holocaust in Europe during World War II. The point is that all societies have symbols, objects, and special occasions that carry death meanings tied to unique historical and cultural circumstances.

The death system for society is a complex social network that serves many functions. It provides mechanisms for warning people of danger and predicting the possibility of death. It offers techniques for preventing death. It prescribes norms and rules governing care for the dying, disposal of the dead, and social consolidation for survivors after death. It offers explanations for making sense out of death. It creates rationales for justifying the killing of animals and humans.

People's expectations about death and their behaviors in response to death are reflections of the values and practices of their societies in combination with the circumstances at hand. In other words, norms, and expectations are likely to be different in a disaster, on a battlefield, and at a funeral.

Cultural Values and Death Expectations
Although human beings share some common experiences in this area (e.g., the death of family members), their actions in relation to death and their beliefs about its meanings can vary greatly. Religion and other belief systems influence people in two interrelated ways. They provide a basis for explaining the meaning of life and death. They prescribe rituals and ceremonies to be practiced in relation to significant events and transitions: birth, attainment of puberty, marriage, death, and occasions of importance to the followers of a particular faith. There are wide variations in beliefs about death and afterlife among the many religions of the world and, not surprisingly, variations in burial practices and other activities before and after someone has died. These practices include disposal of the body (e.g., cremation or burial); characteristics of the funeral ceremony, including the uses of sound, color, and prayer; and special gifts or memorials in honor of the deceased.

Religion alone cannot account for human variations in beliefs and customs pertaining to death. Such beliefs and customs derive also from an intermingling of cultural values and kinship structures and relationships. In a cross-cultural study of grief and mourning, Rosenblatt et al. (1976) found evidence that sadness, fear, and anger commonly are experienced during bereavement with a great deal of similarity among men and women. In societies with sex differences in regard to the expression of emotion, women tended to cry and self-mutilate more than men and men tended to express anger and aggression away from themselves. Some societies use ritual specialists, such as priests, to help curtail the expression of aggression; in other societies control of aggression is achieved through the use of marking or isolation of the bereaved. In general, the rites of passage associated with death include (1) rituals of separation providing individuals with opportunities for grief and mourning and (2) rituals of reintegration ensuring the ongoing continuity of the family and society. In societies which encourage remarriage of widows, tie-breaking customs are commonly used to facilitate separation from attachments to the deceased. These customs include giving away the deceased person's property, abandoning the dwelling in which living together was shared, or practicing a taboo on the name of the deceased.

Although religious tradition often prescribes specific rituals to assist families with mourning, the ways by which the tradition is expressed reflect ethnic customs and practices as well. Jewish law, for example, provides 7 days after the funeral (the *shiva*) for unrestrained weeping and withdrawal from the usual activities of living, 30 days (the *shloshim*) for a gradual return to social relationships, and a full calendar year of mourning during which the mourner is expected to abstain from participation in public entertainment. Yet the mourning practices observed by Palgi (1973) in Jewish families in Israel following the Yom Kippur war in 1973 showed the variable influences of many countries of origin, with European families demonstrating little external display of emotion in contrast to middle eastern families, in which lamentation and wailing, feasting, and ceremonial dancing were commonplace. Even in societies that share a common heritage, differences in bereavement customs and familial practices can lead to tension among generations and difficulties for individuals in postbereavement adaptations.

Death Expectations in the Twentieth Century

Despite ethnic variations, the meaning of death to people across the world has been affected by significant social and technological changes in the twentieth century. Particularly in western societies, the character of living and dying has been changed by the application of new technologies to many facets of everyday life: food production, communication, modes of travel, and delivery of services (Benoliel, 1978). Changes that have contributed to new attitudes and practices include low mortality rates, increased division of labor in work related to death, and a secularization of society under the influence of the norms of science. In contrast, patterns of living in third world countries continue to be influenced by high mortality rates, extended family systems, and religious traditions that include magical-mystical beliefs (Corr, 1979).

Medical Technology and Caretaking

One important change affecting attitudes toward death came with the medicalization of human death leading eventually to an institutionalization of the lifesaving ethic (Benoliel, 1978). The industrialization of death control introduced profound changes into the caretaking systems in western societies. One important feature of the modern death system is a division of labor among various specialists, some of whom offer services to the dying, some to the dead, and still others to the survivors. Heavily influenced by the high value attached to science and technology in western society, the education of these many specialists (funeral directors, members of the clergy, physicians, nurses, social workers, and others) has emphasized the technical aspects of their work. Relatively less attention has been given to preparing these many specialists for the task of providing psychosocial care to patients and families faced with life-threatening illness or with the emergency of sudden and unexpected death.

For health care workers, education for terminal care has stressed the application of medical technology to the prevention of death and encouraged the attitudes of "lifesaving at all costs." Thus, the importance attached to science and technology has led to educational practices which emphasize the *cure goal* of practice at the expense of the *care goal.*

The influence of technology on caretaking in the twentieth century is epitomized in the development of life-prolonging machinery and techniques. Since World War II new surgical techniques, antibiotics and chemotherapy, advances in parenteral medication and treatment, and life-assisting mechanical devices have made possible the prolongation of living—and the prolongation of dying. Useful as these discoveries may be, the new technologies have added to the complexity of medical decisions when the threat of death is present (Glaser, 1970; Cassem, 1980).

Medical specialization and applied technology have contributed to the development of a variety of special-purpose hospital wards, a number of which are designed specifically to offer intensive treatment through the application of highly specialized techniques and lifesaving procedures. There has been an increase in specialization among physicians and a tremendous growth in both numbers and types of paramedical workers. These two outcomes of medical specialization have combined to create problems in the delivery of *personalized services* not only to patients who are facing death but to patients in general.

The great increase in the numbers of different types of health care workers and the development of special-purpose wards in hospitals have had important consequences for both patients and staff. The organizational structures of hospitals have become extremely complex, resulting in barriers to effective patient care. For example, communication between and among the many different health care workers employed in the hospital is difficult to achieve. The heavy focus on lifesaving at all costs and the development of intensive care wards in which large numbers of patients are facing the threat of death have increased the psychological stresses and strains of hospital work when patients are thought to be dying. These problems are exceptionally acute in settings where nurses are faced with life and death choices at frequent intervals; reports have described the situational and psychological stresses and strains experienced by nurses on intensive care wards (Hay and Oken, 1972; Huckabay and Jagla, 1979).

Clearly, the problems associated with death in the hospital have increased in intensity. More and more people are being sent to hospitals to die. Reflecting the primary values of society, the hospital system places a high priority on the delivery of life-prolonging services. Such a system serves to perpetuate the general societal pattern of denying the reality of forthcoming death and facilitates a depersonalization of experience during the final period of living.

A major characteristic of modern society is the social isolation of the person who is dying. This isolation takes two forms: placement in special settings remote from home and family and limitations of opportunity to talk about the reality of forthcoming death. The removal of those who are dying into hospitals and other special institutions means that increasingly nurses and other health care personnel are involved in social affairs that once belonged primarily to the family, the extended kinship group, or both. Nurses are faced with many situations in which the goals of care and cure come into conflict.

Death Customs in the United States

As far as each individual is concerned, the personal meanings of death are influenced by cultural and social conditions: the amount of direct exposure a person has to death and dying, membership in an ethnic subgroup with values and beliefs at variance with the dominant system, and membership in a particular religious denomination. The death expectations and attitudes of people in the United States have been affected by four important conditions. First, with the increase in longevity there is a tendency for people to transpose death from an immediate and always present menace to a distant and remote prospect. It is no longer natural to die at an early age, and death has come to be equated with being old. Second, Americans in general are insulated from perceptions of death and direct experience with persons who are dying because the ill and elderly tend to be removed to special institutions and communities. Third, the growth in scientific knowledge and applied technology in the twentieth century has created the expectation that death, too, can be defeated if enough time, energy, and money are invested to solve the problem. Fourth, people no longer participate in a society which is dominated by tradition, by lineage and kinship ties, or by accepted dogma. The old systems of social control once clearly provided by church, state, and family have given way to the concept of individual freedom, accompanied by a sense of personal responsibility and increased levels of anxiety.

As these changes took place in the United States, a sociocultural system evolved which has led to a depersonalization and fragmentation of the experience of human death. From the perspective of sociology, such a system serves to protect society from the disruptive influences of death by separating the dying from the living and by developing bureaucratic procedures for managing death and dying as routine social matters. Psychologically, however, persons who are facing death—whether as patients with incurable illness, as members of families, or as caretakers—are not provided with easy answers for the problems they encounter; nor have they been prepared for effective performance in the new roles and role relationships which the event of death brings into being.

The Family as the Mediator of the Culture

Children are socialized to the norms and expectations of society through membership in families. Although child rearing is a universal human activity, the techniques and strategies used by parents and other adults vary depending on the values, beliefs, and practices of the group. Janosik (1980) found that attitudes and patterns related to such activities as eating styles, child training, and care of the elderly persist in various ethnic and subcultural groups even though people migrate to new countries and are exposed to modern life. It follows that there are variations among families in regard to how children are socialized to the meaning of death and dying. In modern nuclear families parents generally have the major responsibility for determining how much and what kind of contact children have with death and dying and whether and in what circumstances death is discussed openly with them. Out of experiences in the family, children are socialized to what is expected in times of bereavement.

Cultural Patterns of Bereavement

Although the conceptual understanding of death can be shown to follow a definite developmental sequence that is roughly the same in children in all societies, attitudes and expectations associated with death are not necessarily the same and are learned from experiences in particular cultures. Through a combination of direct and indirect practices of adults, children are socialized to behave toward death in patterned ways that are typical for the society in which they live. Not only do children learn particular sets of ideas about death, they also learn particular ways of acting and reacting when someone dies. Bereavement behaviors derive from patterned systems of family and kinship relationships, and these relationships influence the range, frequency, intimacy, and quality of interaction among the persons who compose the system.

Patterns of emotional attachment are not the same in all societies, and different bereavement behaviors are observed in societies with different kinship structures and customs. In western societies of the northern European traditions, for example, the open expression of grief is not encouraged, and controlled behavior in public is expected during the period immediately following a death. By comparison, in traditional Arab communities, the open expression of grief is anticipated and mourning among family and friends is demonstrated loudly and obviously immediately following a death. Knowledge about cultural and ethnic differences is essential if effective services for psychosocial care are to be made available.

The development of emotional responses to death is critically influenced by the attitudes and actions of the family members who socialize the child into the customs of his society. Not only do they introduce him to the roles he will be expected to play, they also provide him with ways of conceptualizing the meaning of life, generally through a form of religious training. In particular, religious upbringing influences what a child will learn about death and afterlife, and religions differ in what they teach about life, death, and the existence of an afterlife. Schowalter (1972) is of the opinion that children exposed to death in a nonfrightening way tend to be less fearful than those without such exposure and that belief in a benevolent God and reunion after death may be more hopeful than belief to the contrary. By comparison, religions that espouse severe punishment after death do not provide much consolation, and children socialized into such systems of belief may respond to serious illness with intense fear—even terror. The point is that religion per se cannot be viewed as a safeguard against fears about death; thus, to be effective in interaction, the nurse needs to understand the patient's responses in terms of his religious beliefs rather than her own.

Death Experience and Identity Development

Although experiences with death and dying are often perceived as tragic events with negative consequences for people, they can also be viewed as maturational crises through which individuals learn to cope with themselves in times of adversity and change. In a sense, experiences with death can be conceptualized as developmental tasks which influence human development throughout the life span but which may be highly disruptive in childhood when an individual's basic identity is in the process of formation (Benoliel, 1981). There is growing evidence that death has multiple meanings in the lives of children. Nurses who work with children and their families can be most effective when they understand and appreciate the complex circumstances that influence the meaning of death to young people.

Cognitive Meanings of Death

The development of a concept of death takes place by stages that are directly related to the normal developmental sequence of biological and psychological growth. The age of the child influences his ideas about death, and these ideas in turn influence the way he responds when he is faced with death as part of his personal situation. Movement toward comprehension of death from an adult perspective is a steplike process through which a child passes as he comes to understand death both as an abstract entity and as a universal human experience. How the process takes place is determined in great measure by the adults who are responsible for socializing the child. Whether adult comprehension is eventually attainable does, of course, depend on the child's having an intact and functioning neuroendocrine system.

Reviewing the work of other investigators, Kastenbaum (1977) proposed that children's concepts about death are probably more closely related to their mental development than to chronological age per se and are undoubtedly influenced by their personal experiences with death, including exposure to television, deaths of insects and animals, and stories recounted by adults. The classical studies showing that concepts of death are developmentally tied to age require modification to make a fit with newer naturalistic observations showing that even very young children can sometimes recognize the essence of death. Yet an understanding of the broad, general stages by which concepts of death are formed is useful for comprehending children's responses to the experience of life-threatening illness and hospitalization.

Because the child under 3 years has not yet learned to separate life and death, he thinks of death as a reversible fact. Not surprisingly, when he is informed that someone has died, he continues to talk about the dead person from his own frame of reference—as a living being. The young child's pattern of thinking is not the same as that used by an adult, and fantasy and reality are not sharply separated from each other.

Between 3 and 6 years the majority of children begin to understand death as something that happens to others. Children at this age are better able to tolerate short separations than are younger children, but their ideas about death are strongly affected by their feelings in response to relations with their parents. For example, the child's aggressive impulses and actions as he strives for autonomy are often thwarted by his parents, and he in turn develops hostile death wishes toward them. During this period of developmental conflict the child tends to personify death, and often the concept becomes confused in his mind with magical thoughts, mystery, and punishment. The diagnosis of serious illness in the child at this time in his development can easily be experienced as a retribution for "bad thoughts" or actions.

The child of 6 to 11 years moves closer to identifying death as a personal event. According to several studies, children in this age group conceive of death as being caused by an external agent. Also during these years, children are prone to associate injury and mutilation with death itself. Children are unable to differentiate between the *wish* and the *deed;* hence they easily feel remorse and guilt even though those reactions are not at all consonant with the realities of the situation. It is useful to be aware that children in preadolescence are vulnerable to intense feelings of guilt in association with death because of patterns of thinking and reacting that are characteristic of development during these years.

By the time of early adolescence most children intellectually understand the universality and permanence of death. Although in a general and abstract sense these young people conceptualize death as an inevitable process, in the personal sense they may not truly comprehend death as an event occurring to persons close to them (Portz, 1972). Applying the concept of death to themselves is a devastating experience for young people in adolescence. Physical illness in and of itself is hard to bear during this time when physical beauty and physical activity are important standards of personal esteem and social worth. To know that life is being cut short by fatal illness means *death before fulfillment*—a fate which few if any can face with equanimity.

According to Lonetto (1980), between early childhood and adolescence the child's view of death shifts from a circular pattern in which birth and death flow into each other to a linear model in which birth and death lie at opposite ends of a straight line. This shift in perspective is a result of educational processing in which causal explanations are emphasized, and the shift is accompanied by a change in the meaning of time. Gradually there is an awareness that both past and future are different from the present and that being human includes learning to hope for things to come. Knowledge about measured time serves as an indicator of movement toward the use of logical rather than magical models in the child's thinking about the meaning of events in the world.

Emotional and Existential Meanings of Death

The meaning of death to children involves more than cognitive understanding of a concept. It also involves emotional responses to a phenomenon which is awesome because it implies an end to the self. The emotional meanings of death to children are related to their experiences with other people and a gradual awareness of the finiteness of personal existence. The psychoanalytic tradition views death anxiety in infants as arising from the baby's utter helplessness and complete dependence on significant others; thus fear of loss of the mother and fear of helplessness come to be equated with fear of death (McCarthy, 1980). Using a psychosymbolic perspective, Lifton (1980) stated that both death imagery and death anxiety have their origin in three basic polarities: connection versus separation, integrity versus disintegration, and movement versus stasis.

The child who is 3 years of age or younger does not distinguish between death and absence, and for this reason the departure of the mother (or other significant person) is experienced as abandonment. When these young children must be hospitalized, they generally respond to the departure of parents with expressions of anger and loud protest. In his studies of young children's reactions to the experience of hospitalization, Bowlby (1960) described three phases of response to separation: protest, despair, and detachment, during which phase the parents may be completely ignored by the child. Studies have shown clearly that children under the age of 5 years respond with *separation anxiety* long before they are able to consider the possibility of their own deaths.

Initially children's fears about death exist as a kind of undifferentiated anxiety. As their thinking develops conceptually, these fears about death begin to focus on specific dimensions: the dark, monsters, ghosts, and burglars (McCarthy, 1980). Developmentally the focus of a child's fear of death is tied to its conceptual meanings. For the very young child, fear of separation is central. For the older child, fear of personal attacks and violence to the body is of prime concern. In adolescence fear is associated with death (Lonetto, 1980). It is important to recognize that children are not always consciously aware of their fears and anxieties in relation to death, and often their efforts at achieving mastery over them take place through dreams, fantasy, and childhood play (McCarthy, 1980).

As older children become aware of the certainty of death, they also begin an inner search for affirmation of the meaning of personal existence. This search for purpose in life means grappling with ideas about the relationship of self to the larger world and ways of explaining the existence of suffering and human tragedy. Existential concerns and questions about adult values are particularly acute during adolescence as the young person struggles for automony and certainty of self. In McCarthy's (1980) view, depression and increased death anxiety are normal occurrences during this period of change. The problem of establishing a positive identity appears to go hand in hand with the effort to find a sense of purpose in life. According to Hancock (1975), the adolescent's movement toward personal autonomy is aided by a family atmosphere in which parental behaviors and values are consistent and, conversely, is inhibited by exposure to an atmosphere of inconsistency in parental attitudes.

The quest for existential answers can take many directions, including involvement in religion, political action, and special groups; it can also take the form of withdrawal from other people. When threats to self-esteem are high, movement into authoritarian movements or cult religions can provide a built-in sense of identity and purpose and can thereby counteract the anxiety and depression associated with the adolescent's struggle for independence (McCarthy, 1980).

Direct Exposure to Death

The amount of direct exposure a child has to death has been found to influence the way the child conceptualizes its meanings and causes. In western societies death and dying in the twentieth century moved from the public domain of human existence into a hidden place remote from daily living. As a result, many young people found little opportunity to learn about the circumstances of human dying, except for those portrayed on the ever-present television set. Open conversation about the personal meanings of death and dying are generally avoided, and many children learn not to talk about such matters with their parents. Yet not all young people in western societies have been protected from direct experience with death, and in some countries children are exposed to death on a regular basis.

A study of death conceptualization in midwestern children and youths in the United States revealed that death due to violence was found more frequently among children of lower socioeconomic status than in those of a higher socioeconomic level (McIntire et al., 1972). Black children who grow up in the inner cities, unlike their counterparts in the white suburbs, are exposed to the fact of death early—sometimes in brutal ways, as Rose (1972) pointed out. So also are children who are born and reared in countries ravaged by war and constant internal strife, and their adaptations to the process of living are strongly influenced by these experiences.

Children who undergo catastrophic life experiences have been found to show signs of severe psychic trauma including fears about personal death. Opportunity for understanding the impact of such experience occurred in 1976 when 26 children (ages 5 to 14 years) were kidnapped on a school bus by three masked men, driven about for 11 hours in two blacked-out vans, and finally transferred into a buried truck trailer (a "hole" in the ground) for 16 hours before they managed to escape. The effects on the children were not recognized immediately, and Terre (1981) was consulted 5 months after the incident when some of the parents became concerned about their children's emotional reactions. Interviews with 23 of the children and their parents showed that the experience led to immediate and delayed emotional outcomes. The immediate emotional sequelae for the children included fears of additional trauma, hallucinations, misperceptions about what had happened, and the formation of omens to "explain" the kidnapping. Somewhat later the children experienced other posttraumatic symptoms: reenactments of fantasies and behaviors that occurred during the kidnapping, play that repeated the experiences they had undergone, traumatic dreams involving death and terror, and fears of another kidnapping as well as fears of many ordinary life experiences (being alone, being in the dark, sounds, confined spaces, strangers, and vehicles).

The analysis by Terre (1981, p. 19) clarified some important differences between child and adult responses to catastrophic trauma:

1. Unlike adults, the children had no periods of amnesia or haziness.
2. Unlike adults, the children did not use denial.
3. The children reported no sudden involuntary flashbacks, as has been reported by adults.
4. The major indicators of ego dysfunction were cognitive malfunctions: misperceptions, overgeneralizations, and time distortions.

The children's use of reenactment in an effort to achieve mastery appears to be different from responses used by adults, and parents may need help in understanding the normality of this behavior. Perhaps the most important outcome of this research was the finding that the children had lost a sense of trust in the world. Despite much parental reassurance, they continued to remain on guard against the "dangers" that exist "out there." Like adults in similar circumstances, the children showed a shattering of the illusion of personal invulnerability (Lifton and Olson, 1976).

Even a death-denying society cannot completely protect its children from the painful realities of death. Children, just like adults, can find themselves having to cope with such difficult life experiences as the sudden death of a parent or the prolonged dying of someone near and dear. According to Furman (1974), the unexpected death of a parent is a unique experience for a child for three reasons. It suddenly takes away a special relationship, one that can never be completely replaced. It leads to some impoverishment of personality development because the child's personality is enmeshed to some degree with the personality of the parent. It removes the person who under ordinary circumstances would help the child through the mourning process.

Loss, Death, and Identity Development

Developmentally, losses of many kinds occur as part of the normal process of growth and change. Indeed, for every gain in human development there is a loss to be experienced. For example, the child's capacity to crawl and walk increases the ability for independent action, but at the same time it means moving away from the security of the mother's lap. Since loss produces anxiety, a great deal of human behavior is devoted to counteracting that anxiety while reaching for new gains. The development of identity is an ongoing process of balancing gains against losses and of achieving mastery over a series of basic conflicts. Erikson (1963) defined these conflicts as the challenges to be met in moving toward a sense of personal unity. Bowlby (1973) stated that healthy human development is closely tied to affectional attachments to other people and that growth of self-reliance is directly tied to family experiences providing respect for personal aspirations and consistent support. Similarly, Seligman's (1975) research provided evidence that the development of a sense of mastery depends on responsive mothering and that helplessness and depression are facilitated by the absence of the mother, stimulus deprivation, and nonresponsive mothering.

Children are very vulnerable to the loss of persons important in their lives. Recent evidence suggests that loss of a significant person during childhood not only influences ideas about death but may also seriously interfere with personality development and may even contribute to behavior disorders in later life (Bowlby, 1980). In a very real sense, the defense mechanisms developed by a child for coping with death are dependent on the child-rearing practices used by the adults who socialize him in combination with direct experiences that are perceived by the child as threatening to existence.

The major crises of identity center on three aspects of human experience: the loss or threat of loss of someone important, the introduction of new and threatening relationships, and changes in significant relationships. Children are particularly vulnerable to these crises because their concepts of self and strategies for coping with life are in process of creation (Benoliel, 1981). According to Bowlby (1973), personality structure is very sensitive to family environmental influences during the early years of life, and experiences of loss and separation from attachment figures can divert optimal development toward a maladaptive course. Even short separations can stimulate anxiety in children and reactivate conflicts about connection and separation. A mother's hospitalization for serious illness can be such an experience. The opportunity to visit the mother in the hospital can be very important for the young child who, as Fig. 16-1 shows, may need to maintain some distance from the familiar person who looks somewhat strange.

There is considerable evidence that loss may be a major contributor to suicidal inclinations in young people and that vulnerability to suicide is associated with feelings of worthlessness and low self-esteem (Klagsbrun, 1976; Grueling and DeBlassie, 1980). This vulnerability is directly related to life experiences that stimulate negative views of self, world, and future. Circumstances contributing to these directions in personality development include disturbed family relationships, alienation from others, and loss of significant persons through death or separation (Tishler et al., 1981).

The sudden and unexpected death of a parent can create special problems for a child's development because it simultaneously removes a significant person and leaves the remaining parent in difficult circumstances for offering patience and understanding to the child. The difficulties the child experiences are directly related to the effect of the loss on the surviving parent's behavior in relation to the child. Although many parents in such circumstances are able to maintain supportive relationships with their children, others respond in ways that interfere with optimal personality development. Children may be sent away from home, expected to "replace" the departed spouse, exposed to inconsistent or harsh discipline, or left on their own to cope with the loss (Bowlby, 1980). Without access to a supporting environment, those who lose a parent by death in childhood or adolescence are at

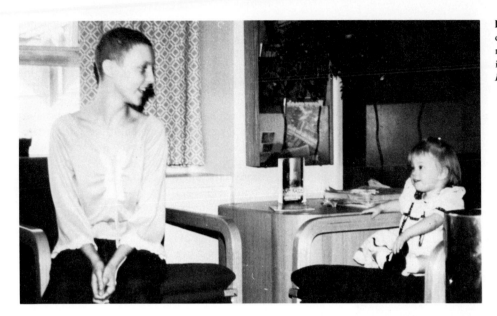

FIGURE 16-1 The child's need for distance from a mother whose illness causes her to look "different" is a normal reaction. *(Courtesy of Ruth McCorkle.)*

greater risk than others for developing depression and other psychological impairments.

The prolonged dying of a member of the family can also introduce children to the rough realities of death, but at a slower pace and in a different manner. When the dying person is a parent, children generally must adjust to a reorganization of the household to meet the needs of the sick adult. Their personal wishes and wants easily become secondary or lost, and living in general changes its character and flavor. When a parent is dying at home, children are sometimes expected to remain at home to help care for the sick parent. If carried to extremes, these demands can interfere with normal contacts with peers and opportunities for social activity. One way to counterbalance these expectations is to encourage the child's friends to visit in the home. Children in the home may also help the dying parent to be part of the ongoing process of living (Fig. 16-2). Depending on the adults around them, children may be active participants in family efforts to cope with the dying transition or left to their own devices to cope with their confusions, fantasies, and tensions (Benoliel and McCorkle, 1978). Usual roles and role relationships within the family are often altered by prolonged dying, and these changes usually impinge on many aspects of children's daily living. The dying of a parent is a stressful experience, and children's behavior often reflects the tensions they feel.

Bereavement and Resolution

Despite the trauma of losing a parent in this unexpected way, some children resolve the loss successfully while others do not. The difference appears to rest with the circumstances surrounding the death, the child's stage of development, and the behaviors of various adults during the periods of crisis and bereavement. Problems in successful mourning have been associated with the child's being present during a difficult death, the dead parent's inability to fulfill a final promise, or the removal of a child from ac-

tive participation in the funeral and other rituals of transition. In general, the younger the child, the more difficult the adjustment, yet the vulnerability of age can be countered by the attitudes and behaviors of adults. Furman (1974) believed that children must understand what caused the death of a parent in order to come to terms with it and that their opportunities to know about and discuss the death depend almost entirely on the adults who constitute their worlds. Children need the comfort of daily routines, regular meals and care, and concerned adults around them in order to mourn successfully.

Following the death, children as well as adults need the opportunity to participate actively in the grieving process but often need help in going through the mourning process. Children often express their tensions by "acting out" their thoughts and feelings at this time. Adults may need help in recognizing these behaviors not as "problems" but rather as manifestations of the need to mourn. To add to the complexity, adults may be caught up in their own reactions and concerns, thereby having limited resources for giving support and guidance to others. Children's opportunities to adapt successfully to the aftermath of prolonged dying require a social environment responsive to their personal needs. They need adults willing and able to communicate at the level of their basic concerns.

Death-Related Crises and Transitions

Experiences with death and dying are not isolated events in the ongoing lives of individuals and families. Rather, they are episodes which provide opportunities for the growth and maturation of family relationships as well as personal development.

Life-Threatening Disease: A Psychosocial Transition

Probably the ultimate introduction to personal awareness of death comes with the experience of being a dying per-

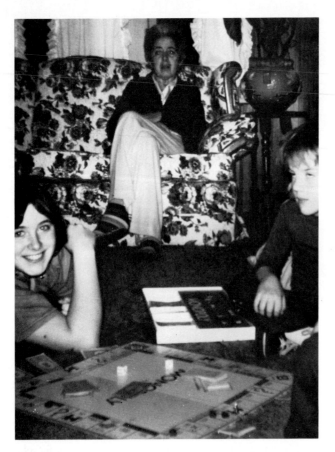

FIGURE 16-2   Play activity in the home can normalize living for children and the dying parent. *(Courtesy of Ruth McCorkle.)*

son. Although fatal disease brings problems in living not associated with age alone, terminal illness in a child is unique in the sense that death is coming before its anticipated time. Neither child nor family is prepared for the impact of living with life-threatening illness or for the effects of this change on their relationships with each other.

Temporal Phases and Markers of Change

To think about death in the abstract is one thing; direct experience with the psychological impact of death as a personal threat is quite another. For both the child and his family, the process of living with life-threatening disease requires psychological adjustments that take place by stages. The process begins with the announcement of the diagnosis.

Crisis of Discovery

For parents, the crisis of discovery begins when they are told the diagnosis of fatal illness, although they are often aware that "something is wrong" prior to this event. Typically, parents respond to the announcement with feelings of "shock," sometimes disbelief. During this critical period of initiation, emotional reactions of guilt and self-blame are frequent. So is a persistent effort to seek information about the disease by asking questions, reading newspapers and magazines, and actively seeking data that will refute the negative prognosis.

The child's reaction at the time of diagnosis depends on a combination of circumstances. His age, what he is told about what is happening, and whether he is hospitalized all influence the child's behavior in response to his illness. If the crisis begins with an acute episode of physical illness, the child may display little psychological response or open expression of emotions simply because his energies are taken up in combating the disease process. For example, fever and dehydration are physically depleting experiences; under these conditions the child is prone to be both lethargic and apathetic.

Children tend to be sensitive to the covert as well as the overt reactions of their parents. They respond to the tensions they sense in their parents even though they do not understand the name of the disease and the prognosis. They know something is wrong, but the extent to which they associate what is happening at this point with their own death at some time in the future varies widely.

Course of Illness

The process of discovery marks the beginning of a social experience which has been termed the *dying trajectory* (Glaser and Strauss, 1965). There are several types of dying trajectories, and the social characteristics of each are directly tied to the course of the physical illness. In some cases, the crisis of discovery is followed rapidly by the child's death after an accident or an acute fulminating illness. In such circumstances the family has little opportunity for *anticipatory grief* and must abruptly find ways of adapting to the sudden loss of a child.

Death may not always take place immediately, however, and the time interval prior to the end may extend for a few days to several weeks. This relatively short-term pattern of dying can be precipitated by accidents and other injuries, serious burns, acute communicable diseases, and infections that do not respond to treatment. When the course of illness is extended and death is delayed, the persons involved have time to begin the adjustment to forthcoming death by anticipatory grieving. The extent to which they can do so depends on whether they are able to face the reality that the child is dying and are allowed or encouraged by others to enter into mourning.

Facing the prospect of the loss of a child may be especially difficult when the anticipated death is due to an accident, and markedly so if the parents see themselves as having caused the injuries sustained by the child. Severe reactions of guilt can be expected under these conditions, often effectively interfering with initiation of the process of grieving. (Similar reactions can also appear in siblings, though the hospital staff is not always aware that other children in the family are caught up in these feelings of guilt and blame.)

A somewhat different situation occurs when a child is born with a life-threatening disability such as a congenital defect of the heart. Such a child essentially begins the dying trajectory at the moment of birth, and families find themselves living with a "dying" child from the very beginning. In such situations the change in the child's status may come about only through surgical intervention which, if successful, can result in "cure" for the life-threatening situation. At times, such intervention terminates the trajectory, with the child's death in the operating room or during the early postoperative period.

Another pattern of dying is one in which the course of disease spreads across a number of years. Leukemia is a disorder marked by exacerbations and remissions of physical illness. It persists for an uncertain number of years before death finally comes. Under these conditions, the child and his family find themselves having to learn to live with the ambiguities of an uncertain future. The adaptational tasks required of these families have been described as follows: The parents must maintain an investment in the welfare and future of the sick child while preparing for his death through anticipatory mourning. Parents face the dilemma of maintaining a sense of mastery while coming to terms with the terminal nature of the child's illness. The child himself faces the equally problematic dilemma of integrating the losses and changes produced by his illness while still fulfilling his personal potential for life to the extent that he is able (Hoffman and Futterman, 1971).

A similar pattern of living with uncertainty exists when a child is diagnosed as having cystic fibrosis. Although generally labeled as chronic rather than fatal, cystic fibrosis (especially when the respiratory system is involved) introduces families to a cyclic pattern of acute exacerbations of respiratory infection and a progressive tendency for multiple complications to develop. Because of its genetic origins, cystic fibrosis is also likely to appear in more than one child in a family. The psychosocial difficulties of daily living can be compounded tremendously when a family finds itself having to cope continuously with the special needs of several children with a chronic disease.

Parents of children with cystic fibrosis undergo the same intrapsychic reactions that have been reported in parents of leukemic children. They are faced with a time-consuming set of treatment procedures that openly impinge on other types of family activities. The life-threatening nature of cystic fibrosis produces another set of stresses reported by parents to include the following: extreme stress when the diagnosed child asks questions about the prognosis of his illness, the presence of siblings who are aware of the prognosis, and a feeling of anticipatory anxiety about a living cystic fibrotic child when there has been a prior death of a child from cystic fibrosis (Meyerowitz and Kaplan, 1967). The extent to which the "death concerns" associated with cystic fibrosis produce a social context of chronic stress has not been fully appreciated.

Phases of Psychological Adjustment

The process of learning to live with life-threatening illness takes place by phases. Everyone involved—family members, health care personnel, the child himself—goes through a series of psychological steps through which each assimilates the change in status into a personal concept of reality. The process of psychological adaptation to forthcoming death takes place through five phases: shock and disbelief during which denial is a commonly observed pattern of behavior, gradual awareness of the reality of the change in condition accompanied generally by expressions of anger and guilt, reorganization of relationships with other people, resolution of the loss through active grieving, and a reorganization of identity incorporating the changes that take place.

Concerning preparation for death, the third phase may include efforts to strike a bargain (usually with God but sometimes with the doctor) to have death postponed. Once the person begins to assimilate the reality of what is happening, he or she moves into depression and active grief. If enough time and energy can be given to mourning and preparation for death, the point of acceptance can finally be reached (Kübler-Ross, 1969).

These psychological phases of dying do not necessarily take place in a straightforward and easy manner. Rather, people generally have to repeat the reactions each time they go through a serious episode of physical regression and/or hospitalization. Those who work with dying children and their families need to recognize that the psychological responses can repeat themselves over and over again.

People vary in their capacities to experience the full impact of anger, frustration, guilt, sadness, and grief and to display these emotions openly. Persons who have been taught from early childhood that the open expression of feelings is legitimate will move through the stages of psychological adaptation with greater ease than those who identify overt expression of emotion as a sign of weakness or loss of control. Lindemann's (1944) well-known study of the processes of grief showed that resolution of grief requires some capacity to come to grips with guilt and mourning and that unresolved grief leads to pathological outcomes. Respect for individual differences in background and life experience is a necessary characteristic for nurses who seek to help dying children and their families come to terms with forthcoming death.

During the course of fatal illness in childhood, the child will commonly be in and out of the hospital several times before he dies. Each episode of acute illness can serve as the triggering mechanism for renewed concerns about death, but hospitalization per se can in and of itself contribute to difficulties. Very young children view separation from their parents as a form of abandonment, and repeated hospitalizations can lead to high levels of anxiety and a tendency to cling fearfully to the mother. The child who is somewhat older can come to associate hospitalization with active rejection by his family, and his concerns about separation are generally compounded by his fears about shots and other painful procedures. Caught up in emotions of fear and anger, a child can easily respond to reentry into the hospital by openly rejecting his parents through direct verbal attacks or by complete withdrawal from interaction with them. Either of these reactions is difficult for the majority of parents to bear and adds to the problems faced by nurses when the disease is known to be fatal.

Because hospitalization often entails painful procedures and difficult treatments for the child, readmission to the hospital is a difficult experience for the parents as well as for him. But during periods of remission of the disease, the parents and the child can easily deny the reality of the life-threatening situation. When hospitalization is again required, both are reminded once more of the terminal disease which affects their daily lives.

Psychosocial Problems and Adaptations

Life-threatening illness introduces changes of many kinds and impinges heavily on established patterns of family living. These new demands affect each member of the household as well as the family as a group.

The Child's Experience

The onset of a life-threatening illness in a child marks the beginning of a time interval during which major psychological and emotional adaptations are required of all persons involved. For the young person, the diagnosis serves as the marker initiating a major change in identity. Facing the prospect of a shortened life is especially difficult for adolescents, who understand more than do younger children that their lives are being cut short. Young people of this age feel bitter and resentful and express these reactions quite freely and openly to those around them. Other young people turn these reactions inward and respond by withdrawing from social contacts and social relationships.

A number of important changes are initiated by the diagnosis of fatal disease. In the first place, the child is faced with "being different," and this phenomenon contributes to changes in self-perception and role performance. If the physical changes produced by the illness are severe, these visible signs of "being different" add further to alterations in self-concept, in performance of roles, and in role relationships with significant persons.

The young person finds himself having to cope with and adapt to the changed reactions of other people toward him. Withdrawal by his friends may be extremely difficult to endure, and these actions by other people can add to the feelings of anger and futility produced by the illness. The process of disease is bound to interfere with the normal sequence of events associated with growing up and to alter the new roles and role relationships which are important to the social development of the child becoming an adult. The loss of peer relationships can be notably traumatic for young people who already feel isolated by the disease itself. The experience of being cut off from such important peer activities as dating, competitive sports, overnight slumber parties, and other social events is a cogent reminder that fate has dealt an unfair hand in the game of life.

The Family's Experience

The members of the family are also faced with the emotional impingement of this new experience on their roles and activities. The parents may react by becoming overly protective of the child with the illness, and the "favorite child" syndrome can result in all manner difficulties among the siblings in the family. Overprotection by the parents can also prevent the child from leading a normal existence, even when he is physically capable of doing so.

Members of the families find themselves caught up in complex emotional reactions that include sorrow, anger, and guilt. Feelings of sadness may cause them to feel physically tired much of the time and unable to function effectively in their ordinary tasks. Anger and irritation may lead to family arguments, or, not uncommonly, the members of the health care team become targets for the expression of irritation. Evidence from a number of studies shows that the presence of a child with fatal or chronic illness serves as a stressor on the marriage relationship (Mann et al., 1980; Johnson-Soderberg, 1981). Marital ties are put to the test when parents are faced with the problem of fatal illness in one of their children. Not all families are able to survive the strain.

Changes in the child's physical appearance can be extremely upsetting and especially difficult for the parents to see. Sometimes one or more members of the family cannot cope with the tensions produced by the situation and withdraw from active involvement in the ongoing social affairs of the family. This withdrawal by a family member adds yet another dimension of strain to the already burdened social system of human relationships.

There is growing evidence that life-threatening illness in a child can contribute to emotional difficulties and behavioral changes in the other children in the family. Sources of stress for the siblings rest as much with the effects of the terminal illness on the behaviors of others, especially parents, as with their personal responses to the ill child. Among the difficulties reported by siblings are problems in sleeping, concerns about health, feelings of resentment, and problems of adjustment in school (Kruger et al., 1980).

The introduction of life-threatening disease adds to whatever stresses and strains already exist within that family circle—and often the extended kinship group as well. In a profound sense the fatal illness can never be completely forgotten. The experience of living with fatal illness can serve as a mechanism for drawing people together, or where strain already exists among the members, it can add to their problems in daily living. The adaptational task of living with uncertainty over a period of years is an energy-depleting experience. People may reach the point of "wishing the child were dead," an emotional response that often triggers secondary reactions of guilt and self-blame. If the child takes a long time to die once he reaches the terminal stage, the parents and other relatives may have completed most of the mourning process long before the point of biological death. When circumstances of this nature arise, the child is treated as though already dead. The family members withdraw from their emotional attachments to him, and the delivery of personalized care often becomes a difficult nursing problem.

Social Adaptations to Treatment Regimen

The psychological reactions precipitated by terminal illness are difficult indeed. They are not the only outcomes of fatal illness, however, and often the treatment regimen can require major adaptations by the family in its style of living. Two examples can illustrate these problems of adaptation.

Although diabetes mellitus is generally not considered a fatal disease (at least in the same sense as leukemia), it is life-threatening when a proper treatment plan is not followed. In the case of juvenile-onset diabetes, insulin must be taken at the proper times and food eaten at proper intervals to avoid hypoglycemia and prevent the onset of ketoacidosis. The implementation of an effective diabetic regimen in insulin-dependent diabetes requires a time-bound kind of existence, and the diagnosis of diabetes in childhood has been found to require major adaptations in living by all members of the family. The parental style of behavior as the agent of delegated treatment is a factor of great importance in family adaptations to diabetes. Empirical evidence obtained in a study of young diabetics and their families showed that the patterns of adaptation varied depending on whether the parental style was protective, adaptive, manipulative, or abdicative (Benoliel, 1970).

In the situation of cystic fibrosis, prevention of pulmonary complications requires several time-consuming and arduous activities: use of a mist tent at night, postural drainage at specified intervals each day, and regular exercise to facilitate respiration and proper ventilation. Implementation of this rigorous regimen is an enterprise which impinges heavily on the parents' time and energy. Cystic fibrosis can make the parents—especially mothers—captives in their own homes (Kruger et al., 1980). Guided by middle-class norms of the health care system, parents of these children are expected to modify their personal activities to accommodate to the demands and requirements of the medical treatment. Families, however, may not be able to survive as intact social systems under these arrangements, and parental separations are not uncommon occurrences following the appearance of chronic illness in childhood.

The Awareness Dilemma

A problem of singular concern for the parents of a child with fatal disease centers on the question of how much the child knows, or should know, about the diagnosis and prognosis. In the case of diabetes mellitus, talk about the disease, its treatment, and its prognosis tends to be open. In the case of leukemia and cystic fibrosis, conversations about prognosis tend to be marked by ambiguity and evasiveness. The difficulty of talking directly with the child about his life-threatening situation has a direct relation to the perceived "lack of cure" for the disease. Health care personnel as well as the public are prone to avoid conversation about the future outcomes of these conditions and to focus attention on medical treatments and other cure-related matters.

In general, there are two viewpoints about what the child with a fatal illness should be told. Those who take the protective approach suggest that the ill child's (and often his siblings') emotional well-being is dependent on shielding him from the meaning of his illness and on maintaining a "normal" family life. The protective viewpoint includes a belief that the ill child should be shielded from knowledge about the disease, diagnosis, and prognosis. In contrast, those who advocate the open approach argue that a child with a fatal illness and his siblings need an environment in which they can ask questions and can know what is happening. The open approach advocates giving the child information about his illness and his future.

The general tendency for parents to shield their children from hearing the diagnosis and prognosis may well be tied to a general parental tendency to protect their children. There is also reason to think, however, that parents' inability to deal openly with the reality of fatal illness is tied more to their own concerns about the loss of a child than to concerns about helping the child cope with it.

Despite parental efforts to protect them from knowledge about the prognosis, children with fatal disease are aware of more than other people seem to recognize. Very young children, although they do not directly verbalize a fear about death, do demonstrate in their behavior a high degree of concern about separation, disfigurement, or pain. A number of reports provide evidence that children 4 years of age or older, even when not told directly about the prognosis, show in other ways that they are aware of the seriousness of their condition.

Terminally ill children have different conceptual orientations toward death than do other children. Their ideas about dying are directly learned out of their own experiences.

The extent to which other people (notably adults) are unaware of how much the child with fatal illness knows about his condition rests with the fact that they are for the most part unwilling to talk with him about it. A second reason, however, derives from the fact that children, especially very young ones, speak in symbolic language—a sort of language all their own in which words and phrases have cryptic and personal meanings, with messages often conveyed by action rather than through talk. Becoming aware of how much a child knows and understands about his life-threatening situation means learning to listen carefully to children at play and observe with an open mind what they say and do. Observation of the child as he is drawing or playing with his toys can provide useful clues to the thoughtful observer about the child's state of mind and state of feeling. The nurse in Fig. 16-3 has asked the child who is waiting to see the doctor to describe his drawing, and she anticipates learning something about his underlying concerns from the story that he tells.

Efforts of adults to protect children with fatal illness from knowledge about the disease may in fact do just the opposite by causing them to worry about that which is unknown. Children can cope with far more than adults

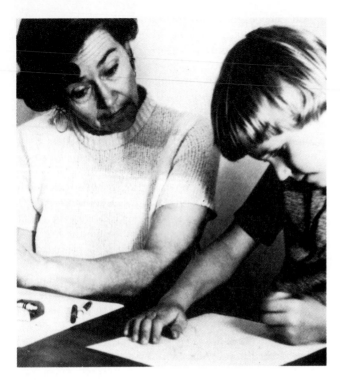

FIGURE 16-3   The nurse observes as a child draws a self-portrait and talks about it.

will allow and children appreciate the opportunity to know and understand what is happening to them.

Differences in Families

Nurses need to recognize that families are social systems with different capabilities and capacities for adapting to the impact of life-threatening illness, sudden death, and bereavement. Families defined as low in risk are those with plentiful resources to assist them in living through the experience of losing a child through death. At the other extreme are high-risk families, those with few resources for coping with the multiple stresses produced by life-threatening disease.

Nurses should be aware that family systems have differential abilities to adapt constructively to the stresses and strains of living with fatal illness of a member. These strains are particularly acute when the member happens to be a child. Any family or other social group that is deprived in social, psychologic, or economic resources can be defined as "high-risk" in vulnerability to the consequences of life-threatening situations.

Some years ago City of Hope Medical Center in California initiated a Parent Participation Program to help families of children with leukemia or cancer deal in a constructive way with the catastrophic consequences of fatal illness. Despite the overall success of the program, some families did not benefit from the service, and efforts were made to identify the reasons. The conditions associated with diminished capacity of families to cope adequately with the fatal illness included low capacity for coping with life's tasks in general, a history of prior marriages in

one or both parents, a diagnosis (such as nonoperable sarcoma) with few if any remissions, and a child 10 years of age or older (Hamovitch, 1964). Judging from these findings, families with one or more of the characteristics can be expected to encounter serious difficulties in adapting to the multiple strains imposed by terminal illness. If help is to be made available to such families, the services offered to them—including that provided by nurses—may need special modifications and additions in order for a usable support system to evolve.

Nursing interventions with a family faced with a life-threatening situation can be most effective when the nurses are knowledgeable about the social and cultural features of the particular family system. Nursing activities need also to take account of the stage in which the family finds itself, the family's previous experience with death and dying, the resources available to them, and any other circumstances that critically influence the meaning of the death of the child.

Terminal Stages of Illness

A common problem in nursing is that of providing care during the terminal stages of illness. Although the child who has cancer or other fatal illness often has several hospitalizations, there comes a time when the "nothing-more-to-do phase" appears. At this point, curative treatment of the disease is no longer effective, and only palliation is left. The nothing-more-to-do phase represents the end point of the dying trajectory; several serious nursing problems are likely to be present during the final period of the child's life.

Nursing Problems in Care Delivery

A nursing problem that is markedly difficult to manage takes place when the family and physician decide that the child is not to be told what is happening. For the nursing staff, the psychological difficulties can be intensified when curative life-prolonging treatments are continued and the child clearly does not want them. The difficulties can also be exacerbated if the child indicates that he no longer has trust in them or in anyone else. The youngster may respond to the context of closed awareness which others impose by withdrawing into himself. When a child turns his face to the wall, both the family and the staff are likely to be very upset because they feel that the child has rejected them.

When parents are unable to face the reality of the child's forthcoming death, it is the child who suffers—in the pain of social isolation and in the lack of opportunity to make his wishes known. Sometimes this suffering includes the indignity of dying in the intensive care unit (ICU) surrounded by strangers and with no chance to say good-bye and to share the final moments with those who are dear to him. Prevention of this latter form of suffering requires that the parents be helped to recognize the reality of their situation and to allow the child to be moved into a quiet, caring environment as his life draws to a close. In a very profound way, the major task that nurses face during the final phase of the child's illness may be the provision of support and care to the parents so that they in turn can support and care for the child.

A second type of difficult problem is that of the child in a coma. If the unconscious child dies in only a matter of hours or days, the problem for the nurses soon resolves itself. When the child exists for weeks or months in such a state, the problems for the family and the staff are multiplied. Sometimes the family can precipitate this difficult situation by not being able to "let go" of the patient and by insisting on the continuation of heroic treatments. Sometimes it is the staff members who cannot let the patient go and may perpetuate the use of intensive treatments even though the treatments have little to offer except additional expense.

The setting into which the child is placed has a definite influence on the services that are provided. The continuation of heroic lifesaving interventions is bound to continue if the child is hospitalized and placed in an intensive care unit. They are least likely to be used if the child is permitted to remain at home to die.

Another difficult situation for staff and family occurs when the child's terminal illness is marked by extensive pain and discomfort. In these circumstances the other feelings of distress precipitated by the child's forthcoming death are compounded by a disquieting sense of helplessness associated with the inability to offer him comfort and relief from suffering. A related problem that is equally difficult occurs when the child is clearly frightened by what is happening to him. Once again the staff members can experience strong feelings of helplessness, but they can also be forcefully and uncomfortably reminded of their own unresolved fears about the prospect of death.

Teamwork and the Caretaking Process

Finding solutions for these difficult problems requires a willingness to recognize that they exist and depends on teamwork and open communication among the many disciplines involved. Facing up to the reality that death is about to happen is not an easy matter, and there are many difficulties to be overcome in obtaining open and effective communication. Without effective communication, however, the child is likely to end his days in social isolation, and decisions are likely to be made without consensus among the persons involved.

This terminal period of illness is a time when choices are available and decisions must be made. This is a time when the family must decide whether to leave the child in the hospital or take him home to spend his final days. Members of the medical staff must decide about the continuation or cessation of heroic life-sustaining interventions and make decisions about what to tell the child.

The final period of living for the child is a time when the staff members who are providing care have their own needs for support. There is a need for regular meetings at which problems can be discussed and decisions made about steps to be taken. The achievement of death with dignity for the child is a process which takes place by helping the parents and key members of the family (and the staff) come to terms with what is happening. Only as they can face the reality of the child's death can they be willing to permit the cessation of lifesaving measures.

Often the family and staff members are so caught up in their own problems that they forget about the child's need to talk about what is happening to him. There is a tendency for both parents and health care personnel to be overly protective toward the child. One of the ways by which overprotection is manifested is avoidance of conversation about what is happening. Avoidance of talk can also be accompanied by avoidance of contact. Because the child is sensitive to the behavior of others, these patterns of withdrawal by others can add to his deep-seated fear of abandonment.

Nurses are in a position to offer the child outlets for talking about his concerns. The extent to which he will have realized his forthcoming death and be able to talk about it depends on how much his parents have permitted him to do so in the past. If the parents have been open and able to talk with the child about the reality of his death, it is unlikely that there will be a need for another person to be his listener. When the parents themselves have been unable to face the situation, the child is most in need of someone to serve as his confidant.

Nurses who wish to assume the caretaking role need to be aware that children frequently use symbolic language to talk about their own deaths. Learning the individual's symbolic language means paying special attention to the words that he uses and observing carefully what he does. Nurses who assume this special caretaking role with children need especially to learn how to handle their own anxieties about death. There is perhaps no greater tragedy in human experience than that of losing one's life before it has scarcely begun. The meaning of the time available to the child or adolescent whose life has been cut short by a life-threatening disease is determined in great measure by the other people around him. He can be placed in social isolation; at the other extreme, he can be involved in finding meaning out of each day that he has until he is ready to let go. Gadow (1980) makes a case that caregivers have an ethical obligation to engage in existential advocacy, by which she means helping the dying person find meaning in dying.

Implications for Nursing Practice

The multiple meanings of death in the lives of children have important implications for nursing and nurses. The health needs of children and families in relation to these multiple meanings support the importance of preventive counseling and death education, family-centered nursing services, and nursing care in terminal illness.

Preventive Counseling, Education, and Health Promotion

The past decade has seen the emergence of a counterculture against impersonal death, and this change has influenced public as well as professional attitudes toward death (Benoliel, 1978). One of the breakthroughs for children came by means of public television when *Mister Rogers' Neighborhood* presented a program in which the intellectual, emotional, and social aspects of death were considered in relation to children's needs to communicate about their experiences with death (Sharapan, 1977).

Death Education for Parents and Children

There is growing evidence that children who live in a death-denying society may have limited opportunities to learn positive ways of coping with death because of general tendencies to "protect" them by not talking openly about the topic and/or by keeping them removed from death-reminding experiences. Because parents occupy such pivotal positions for influencing children's experiences and personal development, their choices in these matters are critically important. However, many parents may not realize that children have a natural curiosity about death and would like to talk about the dead bird on the path or the cowboy who was killed on television. Efforts to protect children from the painful emotions associated with loss and death function as obstacles to the development of a sense of mastery over painful life experiences. Nurses who have ongoing contacts with families for purposes of health counseling are in an opportune position to educate parents about the importance of death to children and to help them find ways of communicating more openly with their own children.

One effective way of initiating communication about death can be through reading to the child or making available suitable books to those old enough to read on their own. Children's literature contains a variety of books and games that can be used to increase awareness of feelings and to understand life cycles in nature, body changes in death, and expressions of grief.

Counseling parents about the importance of death education for children can be done in conjunction with regular health services. Education for parents can also be developed as a group effort in collaboration with schools, churches, and other community organizations. Corr (1980) proposed specific guidelines for workshops to assist parents, teachers, counselors, and caregivers to learn together about children and their relationship to death. Nurses interested in developing death education for children can find direction from Bertman (1979-1980), who proposed the use of various art forms to help children articulate sentiments they may have previously kept to themselves.

A number of materials have been created explicitly to help parents and children focus their thoughts and feelings about an important loss in their own situation. Nurses at one medical center developed a coloring book about a frog family to help parents talk with their children about the death of a newborn (Oehler, 1981). Hammond (1980b) created an illustrated book, *When My Mommy Died,* to be read to young children by a surviving parent as a way of initiating talk about death. These resources and many others are available to assist nurses in helping families and children to understand the impact and aftermath of death for themselves and others.

Case Finding: Children and Families at Risk

Nurses who work in the community have many opportunities to identify children who are highly vulnerable to the possibility of suicide, the impact of loss of a parent, and the immediate and delayed effects of traumatic death-related experiences. Knowledge about the factors that increase the likelihood of suicide is essential for making assessments about the risk for particular children. For instance, the suicide attempt does not often take place precipitately and generally follows a developmental sequence (Grueling and DeBlassie, 1980):

1. A long-standing history of problems, from childhood to adolescence
2. A period of escalation during which new problems associated with adolescence appear
3. A final period of weeks or days during which there is a chain-reaction dissolution of the adolescent's few remaining associations

Identification of children and adolescents at risk for suicide also requires knowledge about the signs of extreme clinical depression: sleeplessness, loss of appetite, loneliness, and withdrawal from others.

Often the depressed adolescent cries out for help through silence, crying, and complaints of helplessness. However, the depression can also be masked by covering symptoms of despair with actions such as delinquent behavior, use of drugs and alcohol, and promiscuous sexual activity. In addition to depressive symptomatology, adolescents with impulsive character disorders are also considered possible candidates for suicide attempts (Grueling and DeBlassie, 1980).

Nurses in schools are in a position to collaborate with teachers in recognizing children involved in death-related crises that make them highly vulnerable to psychological impairments. Reports provide strong evidence that children are extremely vulnerable to the sudden and unexpected loss of one or both parents (Furman, 1974), to the prolonged dying of a significant member of the family (Silverman and Silverman, 1975), and to continuous living with a parent who could die at any time from a serious heart disorder (Bermann, 1973). The psychosocial demands and tensions of these situations impinge heavily on social relationships and family dynamics and result in stressful outcomes for each person involved.

In addition to these personal reactions, the family as a functioning unit is faced with a major crisis of adaptation. Life-threatening illness introduces many different kinds of stress and strain into the social system of family relationships. In the case of sudden death, the family faces adjustment to an unexpected and unforeseen loss, and young families in particular have had little or no experience to prepare them for coping with such events. When the crisis extends over long periods of time, as is true with certain chronic diseases, the adjustments required of the family vary and change depending on the stage of illness. The stresses and strains for families will be different at the time of diagnosis, during periods of exacerbation of illness, at the point when death occurs, and during the post-death period of bereavement (Wiener, 1970; Giacquinta, 1977).

Nurses in the community are often in a position to counsel parents about children's needs when someone close to them has died. Based on experience as a school counselor, Hammond (1980a) identified eight guidelines for working with families under these circumstances:

1. As soon as possible after the death, time should be set aside for telling the child what has happened, gently and truthfully.
2. Parents should be truthful with children and should answer questions without burdening them with more detail than they can handle.
3. Children should be encouraged to express their feelings, and it is helpful for them if the parents show feelings as well.
4. Families should be advised to take the children to the funeral and to encourage them to share in the mourning.
5. It is helpful for children to be present if a parent is buried.
6. After the death, it is helpful to provide an atmosphere in which children feel free to talk about the missing parent, to reminisce, and to hear others talk about their memories.
7. Children need to know that it is permissible to tell others about the death, that it is not something to be hidden.
8. Parents need to be encouraged to be themselves and to share their thoughts and feelings, thereby providing children with a model to follow.

Children and families who are involved in disasters are especially vulnerable to psychological sequelae. Terre (1979) stated that community help in these circumstances should take the following form:

1. During the waiting period, mental health workers should be available to families to form a relationship before the outcomes—whether positive or negative—are known.
2. Evaluation of the victims once released or found should include psychological evaluation by trained mental health workers as routinely as physical evaluation.
3. Continued individual contact with the children and families is encouraged as a mechanism for discharging hostility and anxiety as well as dealing with other reactions to the situation.
4. The long-term traumatic effects on children may not be recognized by parents for 6 to 12 months, and opportunities for counseling must be available when the parents are ready.

Family-Centered Nursing Services

Death-related problems in practice require assessment and intervention at both the individual level and the family level of function and adaptation. Assessment must identify coping resources and adaptive strengths as well as

problems that the children and their families face. Nursing interventions require more than activities of "doing to" and "for" people. For optimal effectiveness these interventions should assist the persons involved in mobilizing their resources and problem-solving skills in order to cope with the changes that death has introduced.

The Goals of Care and Cure

Nurses and doctors have always been caught between the two somewhat conflicting goals of practice: to do everything possible to keep the patient alive *but* to do nothing to prolong pain and suffering uselessly. The availability of life-prolonging machines, organ transplants, and other extreme treatments has contributed to the development of hospital environments in which *care of the person* has become secondary to prevention of death. For nurses, two matters that are of serious concern today: the difficult choices and decisions faced by them when the conflicting goals of recovery care and comfort-until-death care converge and the management of the social and psychological aspects of care when patients are dying.

The basic dilemma for nurses centers on the problem of delivering personalized care in the context which attaches prime value to cure. Whereas the cure goal deals with the objective aspects of the case, the care goal deals with the subjective meaning of the disease experience. In essence, personalized care requires practitioners to be concerned with the subjective elements of the situation and to treat the patient as a human being, not as a "case." In addition, personalized care means facing the reality that patient care today is provided by groups of practitioners who together provide services to patients. Personalized care for each patient can be thought of as having three components: *continuity of contact* with at least one person who is interested in him as a human being, *opportunity for active involvement* in social living to the extent that he is able—including participation in decisions affecting how he will die, and *confidence and trust* in those who are providing his care (Benoliel, 1972).

The delivery of care for patients facing death requires the efforts of many disciplines. The provision of personalized services requires a systems-oriented approach to planning based on the assumption that *continuity* as well as care must be built into the system when multiple numbers of people are involved. Persons holding key positions in the system must be willing to assume leadership in the direction and management of the social and psychological components of care.

Within the organized system of health care services, nurses hold key positions in the communication networks which influence what happens to children and families faced with life-threatening situations. Nurses in doctors' offices, in clinics, and in schools can often play a vital role in the ongoing daily experiences of children living with shortened life spans or the aftermath of significant deaths. To assist these children, nurses must be willing to accept responsibility for the difficult task of helping people cope with the multiple changes associated with terminal illness.

Teamwork is especially critical in matters of psychosocial care where the "expert" who is needed by the patient and/or family may or may not be a physician. Children with fatal illnesses as well as their families need different kinds of assistance at different points in time, and they face many problems that are nonmedical in nature. The child's need for help may be quite different from that of the members of the family, and often more than one helping person is needed if effective family-centered care is to be implemented. Thus, the goal of personalized, family-centered services can be achieved only when communication, collaboration, and cooperation among the different health care professional and nonprofessional workers are valued and encouraged.

In today's complex health care system the goal of personalized care cannot be achieved by any one discipline alone. Achievement of the goal requires that teamwork be recognized as a necessary commodity by *all* members of the health care team. Practice at teamwork needs to take place if persons in different disciplines are to learn how to solve difficult problems of patient care together. Each member of the team must be willing to accept responsibility for specific contributions to the overall plan and program of care and accountability for the outcomes. Nurses must be wiling to accept responsibility for their choices and actions in the provision of terminal care if the human needs of patients are to receive attention comparable with that currently given to lifesaving activities and procedures (Benoliel, 1976).

Nursing Services and Care Delivery
Because of the positions they occupy in the health care system nurses can offer assistance with two major types of death-related situations: crises associated with sudden death, disasters, and other unexpected occurrences in which threats to life are present and transitions produced by the experience of living with various life-threatening and long-term diseases and injuries. It follows that nursing services should be designed to offer two kinds of help to children and their families: crisis intervention and transition care.

Crisis Intervention
The goal of crisis intervention is to assist people in coping with a sudden situation that overwhelms their abilities to cope effectively. To be maximally effective this intervention should be started as soon as possible. It requires interpersonal skills and strategies for several purposes (Aguilera and Messick, 1981):
1. To help the participants gain intellectual understanding of the crisis
2. To provide an opportunity for the expression of feelings and concerns
3. To help people identify and use available resources and supports
4. To consider with them their usual coping mechanisms and the effectiveness of these approaches

Crisis intervention is a short-term service to provide support during a period of high stress and to encourage the use of problem-solving skills in responding to the crisis (Aguilera and Messick, 1981). It is a form of service that can be offered by one nurse or more depending on the intensity of the crisis and the number of people involved.

Transition Care
Transition care is a form of nursing care organized to provide long-term personalized services through activities designed to coordinate the goals of care and cure. It is a family-centered community service that was originally created to facilitate the dying person's opportunities for social control over living and dying and the achievement of personal goals (Benoliel and McCorkle, 1978). Transition care is a service by nurses to make available *coordination of care and problem-focused support* to families living with the changing demands of life-threatening illness. It depends on clinical skills and communication strategies for the following purposes (Benoliel, 1979):
1. Increasing the dying person's opportunities for achievement of personal goals by facilitating open communication among the persons involved
2. Improving the family's coping capacity by supplementing their support system and guiding them to effective use of their resources
3. Assisting the various participants to face and deal with the strong feelings and conflicting demands they experience
4. Counseling individual and family about physical changes, symptoms, and symptom management
5. Communicating directly with key providers to facilitate collaboration and coordination of services
6. Socializing the dying person and the family to the expected and unexpected occurrences associated with dying

Transition care is an ongoing service oriented to the changing needs of the child and the family. It is a form of service that depends on a network of nurses who can collaborate effectively in the delivery of personalized care.

Innovations in Care
The opportunities for nurses to help children and families cope with various death-related crises and transitions exist wherever nurses work. A nurse in one hospital for children took leadership in the creation of guidelines for offering comprehensive and coordinated care for families when children were dying; these guidelines offered direction for initial assessment of the family, identification of situations at risk, activities at the time of death, and follow-up care (Williams et al., 1981). Nurses in a clinic for children with life-threatening diseases introduced play therapy as a method for helping the children develop a sense of mastery over the events in their lives (Taylor and Williams, 1980). Nurses and other providers in a large medical center developed a family-centered weekend retreat to assist families in living with cancer by providing a broad selection of educational activities for adults and children of all ages (Johnson and Norby, 1981).

Community-Based Services for Terminal Care

Part of the counterculture against impersonal death has been a growing public and professional interest in opportunities to die at home. This interest has been manifested in the creation of hospices and humanistically oriented standards of care for the terminally ill person and family (Kastenbaum, 1977), family-centered counseling services to assist people in coping with the stresses and strains of terminal illness (Kopel and Mock, 1978; Krieger and Bascue, 1975), and bereavement services and follow-up care for survivors (Walker et al., 1977). Nurses have played a major part in the development and implementation of these community services, including home care programs for children who are dying (Lauer and Camitta, 1980).

Nursing Care in Terminal Illness

Because illness with fatal outcome is psychologically and socially depleting to a child who bears the disease, the child and the family need several kinds of assistance as they move from the point of diagnosis to the point of death—and even beyond, for the family. Nurses are often in contact with these children and their families at critical points along the way; therefore, they are in a position to play a singularly important part in providing assistance to them and can do so through supporting, teaching, coordinating, and caring functions.

The Supporting Function

The child with fatal illness and his family undergo a series of critical experiences including the final interval which ends in death. These critical experiences include the point of diagnosis, periods of hospitalization, and family crises which overlap with the many problems posed by the illness. Because nurses frequently are with the child and the family at points of psychological stress, they are clearly in a position to offer emotional support and other kinds of assistance during these critical moments.

The supporting function begins with the ability to listen with sensitivity and genuine concern. This ability is facilitated when the nurse understands the stages of psychological adaptation to terminal illness and at the same time can recognize when the person shows readiness to move to another stage. The most difficult periods for any listener are those during which the other person (whether child, parent, or staff member) is expressing anger or experiencing depression. Yet often it is at these times that people most clearly need to be able to express how they truly feel in order to move psychologically toward the point of acceptance.

Although listening is clearly important, the supporting function also includes helping the child and his family find other resources as needed. The types of assistance can vary a good deal. The family members may need help in financial matters. They may need day care services or help in finding someone to assist them at home. When the illness worsens, they may need referral to a visiting-nurse association. Families may be unaware of the many services available through voluntary agencies until these matters

are brought to their attention. Families also find support through contacts with parents' groups, such as the Candlelighters, families who have themselves lost a child through death and who want to help other families faced with the same experience.

A third way by which the supporting function is implemented is through competent performance of the technical tasks of nursing care. There is a special kind of support provided by physical ministrations which are deftly given. The nurse who can relieve the child's pain by the skilled administration of an injection provides an additional element of support. As the child becomes weak and dependent on others for his physical well-being, the supporting function demonstrated in good physical care looms high in importance to him (and to his family).

Whenever children are seriously ill or psychologically disturbed, they tend to regress to earlier patterns of behavior. To the consternation of parents, for example, old habits such as thumb sucking or bed-wetting may reappear in an 8- or 9-year-old child as the disease process continues. The physical regression so commonly observed as the illness progresses probably reflects a need for attention and care at a very primitive level of existence.

When the illness reaches the point of producing a state of complete physical dependency, the child's needs for care are much the same as they were during his infancy, and communication by means of touch becomes extremely important. No matter what his chronological age may be, the child who is approaching death wants to be held in his mother's arms. In fact, physical contact with someone who cares may be the primary source of comfort at this time, yet hospitals are often effectively organized to prevent this kind of care from being offered. For the child, nothing can replace the comfort of being held in his mother's arms. As Fig. 16-4 suggests, a special kind of relaxation takes place in the child who is permitted to experience communion of touch with the person who gave him birth.

Caught up in her own needs, however, the child's mother may not be able to recognize his wishes, or she may be afraid to touch him for fear of causing pain or other discomfort. Sometimes mothers (and fathers, too) need help in being able to share this important experience with their children. Nurses can do a great deal to provide support for children facing death by allowing this kind of parental caretaking activity to take place in the hospital and by encouraging parents to participate actively in the provision of physical care. Martinson (1976) demonstrated the effectiveness of the supporting function for helping dying children end their lives at home. Subsequent models of home care programs for children have validated the singular contributions of nurses to the support of families during the process of terminal care (Lauer and Camitta, 1980).

The Teaching Function

A second important way by which nurses can contribute in their ongoing contacts with terminally ill children and

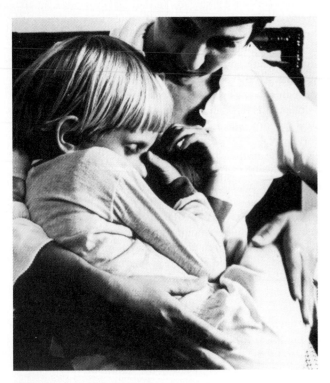

FIGURE 16-4   A special kind of relaxation occurs when a child is held by his mother.

their families is through the teaching function. This function is implemented through the provision of information and guidance to assist them directly in learning to live with the life-threatening disease and the treatment regimen that has been recommended.

A major segment of instructional assistance is the teaching of self-care activities and medical treatment procedures to be done at home, and effective teaching includes periodic follow-up sessions by the nurse to ascertain whether the child and his parents have a clear understanding of what they are doing. One key to the success of this component of teaching is the provision of information necessary to clarify their knowledge and understanding of the treatment, procedures, and routines to be done. The nurse also needs to be aware that a certain amount of repetition and reexplanation may be necessary along the way. Reexplanations may be particularly essential during the early stages of illness, when the parents are caught up in the immobilizing effects of psychological shock.

The teaching function also means answering questions about the disease, its treatment, and related matters at the time that these loom as important to the child and his parents. One explanation is often not sufficient for true understanding to take place, and sensitivity to the instructional needs of the patient and family is an important attribute for nurses to develop.

An important component of the teaching function is interpretation of the physician's orders and explanations. This component may be especially important when the family has had contact with a variety of different medical

specialists who use technical language and perform intricate procedures as they engage in consultation at the request of the primary physician. It can also be important, however, after any kind of contact with medical authority. To assist families in understanding special tests and unusual therapies, the nurse can identify misunderstandings and misinterpretations only by taking the time to talk with the families. Opportunity for discussion with the nurse *directly after* contacts with the doctor must be built into the plan of care or, as otherwise can happen, the parents' needs for explanation will be lost along the way.

A final point about nurse-physician communication seems in order here. To be highly effective in helping the child and his parents to understand the physician's orders and explanations, the nurse needs an effective, mutually respectful working relation with physicians. Only by having a clear understanding of the physician's plan of treatment can the nurse provide explanations which the child and the parent will find useful. When nurses are not informed about the physician's approach to therapy, they can easily add to a family's confusion instead of helping the family achieve understanding.

The Coordinating Function

Because patient care today is offered by multiple numbers of health care workers, the child and his family often find themselves involved with many different caretakers without clear direction as to the management of their situation. One of the important contributions that nurses can offer is the facilitating and coordinating function (i.e., the team concept in action). Activities central to implementing this function are the arrangement of regular conferences as needed to plan the care for and with the patient and his family and referrals to other facilities and services as needed, with adequate follow-up to ensure that the services desired were in fact given.

The facilitating and coordinating function is centrally concerned with the goal of *continuity of care.* In this regard, the facilitating and coordinating function often breaks down unless there is clear designation as to which nurse is to be the primary caretaker for the child and his family. Very often the nurse who works in a cancer clinic or physician's office occupies a key position as leader in the task of coordination, but the nurse must be willing to assume responsibility for these activities and not expect the physician to do so. If a goal of nursing is to help children with fatal illness and their families to cope with the *situationally derived* needs which result from the terminal situation and their reactions to it, the coordinating function may be a singularly important contribution that nurses can make to the ongoing services available for children faced with terminal illness.

The Caring Function

The caring function consists of activities that assist the child with the subjective experience of his terminal illness *on his own terms.* It has the goal of personalizing care for the child by providing continuity of contact with

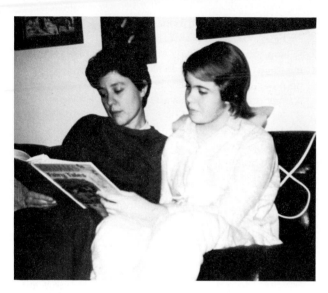

FIGURE 16-5   A nurse supports the child's personal needs for care by providing that which the child cannot do alone—in this instance, by reading to a child whose complications include blindness. *(Courtesy of Ruth McCorkle.)*

someone who is concerned about him and encouraging his participation in social living as long as he is able.

The caring function allows the child an opportunity to direct activities and to let his wishes be known (the principle of control over his own dying). The caring function is implemented by setting realistic limits for the child when in an authority relationship with him and by adhering to these limits with regularity (the principle of consistency) while providing nursing services. Another way by which the nurse can implement the caring function is to intervene on behalf of the child with members of his family, physicians, and others who are involved when the child's wishes and desires are not being heard (the principle of advocacy).

In addition to helping the child maintain some measure of control over his life, the nurse can also help to find simple enjoyments, for example, by having fun together to the extent that his physical condition permits and he so desires (Fig. 16-5). Perhaps most of all, the caring function means a willingness to hear the child when he indicates that he wants to talk about something important to him. When the child mentions death, either directly or indirectly, he is letting the nurse know that he is concerned about himself and is reaching out for human contact.

When he begins to cry, to ask questions about death, or to review his past, the child is indicating a desire to cope with his forthcoming death by approaching it directly instead of using avoidance behaviors. He is reaching out for a relationship now. The nurse who postpones the opportunity to share these moments with him will probably not have another chance. People who are dying initiate conversations about death when they are ready to do so. The caring function depends on nurses who have flexibility in their approaches to the planning of nursing care

and the ability to make rapid shifts in priorities when the human needs of the terminally ill child are in jeopardy.

Independent Study Activities

1. Over a week's time observe the media (newspapers, magazines, television) for what is reported about death and dying. Compare and contrast what is presented about the deaths of children and adults and relate your observations to what has been reported about the characteristics of death in modern society.

2. To broaden your understanding of the relationship of cultural values and beliefs to the "death expectations" of members of different subcultural and ethnic groups, investigate one subgroup living within the local community (preferably one quite different from your own). Learn something about this group's religious orientations and practices, time orientations (past, present, future), people orientations and person-to-person relationships (individualism, group, ancestors), and special rituals and social practices used prior to and following the death of a member. Obtain information through reading, direct contact with members of the selected group, and other means determined by you. Consider the following questions: How are the "death expectations" of the group related to the religious beliefs and past experiences of the group? How do individual adaptations to death seem to be influenced by the group's practices and beliefs? How much do children participate in the social activities related to the death of a member?

3. Review three books designed to present ideas about death to children of different age levels (e.g., preschool, 6 to 8 years, 11 to 12 years). Analyze the content and approach used in each case in relationship to what is currently known about the cognitive and emotional meanings of death to children of these ages.

Learning Activities

1. Invite the religious leader of the predominant local ethnic group to class to discuss the meaning of death to that community.

2. Use films such as *How Could I Not Be Among You?* and *Walk Me to the Water* to stimulate a classroom discussion about death from an individual's perspective.

3. To expand student understanding of the responsibilities of other providers involved in the death process, act as the moderator of a round-table discussion which includes a hospice nurse, social worker, pastoral counselor, and funeral director.

Study Questions

1. When considering cultural values and death expectations, the nurse must remember that:
   A. Religion alone accounts for human variations in beliefs and customs.
   B. There are wide variations in beliefs about death and afterlife among different religions and cultures.
   C. Activities and burial practices before and after death are essentially the same in all religions.
   D. Death has the same meaning in all cultures.

2. In the United States, technology has affected the dying person, family members, and caregivers by:
   A. Providing them with easy answers for all the problems encountered.
   B. Preparing them for effective performances in new roles and role relationships.
   C. Personalizing the experience.
   D. Institutionalizing the lifesaving ethic.

3. Most 3- and 6-year-old children:
   A. Begin to think of death as happening to others.
   B. Can tolerate long separations.
   C. Are sure that death is reversible.
   D. Understand the permanence of death.

4. Death of a person significant to a child:
   A. Has no influence on the child's ideas about death.
   B. Has no relationship to later behavior disorders.
   C. May seriously interfere with personality development.
   D. Enhances the child's sense of mastery.

5. The child's reaction at the time of a fatal diagnosis is influenced by a combination of which of the following factors?
   A. Age, information given, physical condition, and parental tensions.
   B. Physical condition, time of day, age, and parental tensions.
   C. Age, information given, time of year, and physical condition.
   D. Parental tensions, age, and time of year.

6. The third phase of psychological adaptation to death may include:
   A. Denial.   C. Guilt.
   B. Bargaining.   D. Active grieving

7. Facing the prospect of a shortened life is especially difficult for:
   A. Toddlers.
   B. Preschool-age children.
   C. School-age children.
   D. Adolescents.

8. Terminally ill children:
   A. Have the same conceptual orientation toward death as do well children.
   B. Have a conceptual orientation toward death different from that of well children.
   C. Are reassured by parents' protective efforts.

   D. Cannot cope with honest answers about their illness.

9. Persons observed to have the most difficulty in resolving their grief when a loved one dies suddenly and unexpectedly are those who:
   A. Are unable to discuss the death.
   B. Never see the dead body of the loved one.
   C. Are dazed and immobile.
   D. Are hysterical.

10. In helping families cope with death-related problems, the most effective nursing interventions are those which:
    A. Help family members mobilize resources and problem-solving skills.
    B. Identify resources and adaptive skills.
    C. Assess the problems the family is facing.
    D. Identify the changes that death has introduced.

11. Nursing care for terminally ill children and their families includes supporting, teaching, coordinating, and caring functions. The central concern of the coordinating function is:
    A. Listening to parents' concerns.
    B. Preparing parents for the child's care at home.
    C. Providing continuity of care.
    D. Arranging regular conferences to plan and evaluate care.

References

Aguilera, D.C., and J.M. Messick: *Crisis Intervention: Theory and Methodology,* 6th ed., Mosby, St. Louis, 1990.

Benoliel, J.Q.: "The Developing Diabetic Identity: A Study of Family Influence," *Communicating Nursing Research: Methodological Issues,* Western Interstate Commission for Higher Education, Boulder, Colo., 1970.

———: "Assessments of Loss and Grief," *Journal of Thanatology,* 1:190-191, 1971.

———: "Nursing Care for the Terminal Patient: A Psychosocial Approach," in B. Schoenberg et al. (eds.), *Psychosocial Aspects of Terminal Care,* Columbia University Press, New York, 1972.

———: "Overview: Care, Cure and the Challenge of Choice," in A.M. Earle et al. (eds.), *The Nurse as Caregiver for the Terminal Patient and His Family,* Columbia University Press, New York, 1976.

———: "The Changing Social Context for Life and Death Decisions," *Essence,* 2:5-14, 1978.

———: "Dying Is a Family Affair," in E.R. Prichard et al. (eds.), *Home Care—Living with Dying,* Columbia University Press, New York, 1979.

———: "Death Counseling and Human Development: Issues and Intricacies," *Death Education,* 4:337-353, 1981.

——— and R. McCorkle: "A Holistic Approach to Terminal Illness," *Cancer Nursing,* 1(2):143-149, 1978.

Bermann, E.: Scapegoat: *The Impact of Death Fear on an American Family,* University of Michigan Press, Ann Arbor, 1973.

Bertman, S.L.: "The Arts: A Source of Comfort and Insight for Children Who Are Learning about Death," *Omega,* 10(2):147-162, 1979-1980.

Bowlby, J.: "Grief and Mourning in Infancy and Early Childhood," *Psychoanalytic Study of the Child,* 15:9, 1960.

———: *Attachment and Loss,* vol. 2, *Separation, Anxiety and Anger,* Basic Books, New York, 1973.

———: *Attachment and Loss,* vol. 3, *Loss,* Basic Books, New York, 1980.

Cassem, N.: "When Illness Is Judged Irreversible: Imperative and Elective Treatments," *Man and Medicine,* 5:154-166, 1980.

Corr, C.A.: "Reconstructing the Changing Face of Death," in H. Wass (ed.), *Dying—Facing the Facts,* Hemisphere, Washington, D.C., 1979.

——: "Workshops on Children and Death," *Essence,* 4:5-18, 1980.

Erikson, E.: *Childhood and Society,* 2d ed., Norton, New York, 1963.

Furman, E.: *A Child's Parent Dies,* Yale University Press, New Haven, 1974.

Gadow, S.: "Caring for the Dying: Advocacy and Paternalism," *Death Education,* 3:387-398, 1980.

Giacquinta, B.: "Helping Families Face the Crisis of Cancer," *American Journal of Nursing,* 77:1585-1588, 1977.

Glaser, B., and A.L. Strauss: *Awareness of Dying,* Aldine, Chicago, 1965.

——: *Time for Dying,* Aldine, Chicago, 1968.

Glaser, R.J.: "Innovations and Heroic Acts in Prolonging Life," in O. Brim et al. (eds.), *The Dying Patient,* Russell Sage, New York, 1970.

Green, J.S.: "The Days of the Dead in Oaxaco, Mexico: An Historical Inquiry," in R.A. Kalish (ed.), *Death & Dying: Views from Many Cultures,* Baywood, Farmingdale, N.Y., 1980.

Grueling, J.W., and R.E. DeBlassie: "Adolescent Suicide," *Adolescence,* 15:589-601, 1980.

Hammond, J.M.: "A Parent's Suicide: Counseling for Children," *The School Counselor,* 27:385-388, 1980a.

——: *When My Mommy Died,* Cranbrook, Ann Arbor, Mich., 1980b.

Hamovitch, M.B.: *The Parent and the Fatally Ill Child,* City of Hope Medical Center, Duarte, Calif., 1964.

Hancock, L.D.: "Adolescence and the Crisis of Dying," Adolescence, 10:373-389, 1975.

Hay, D., and D. Oken: "The Psychological Stresses of Intensive Care Unit Nursing," *Psychosomatic Medicine,* 34(2):109-118, 1972.

Hoffman, I., and E.H. Futterman: "Coping with Waiting: Psychiatric Intervention and Study in the Waiting Room of a Pediatric Oncology Clinic," *Comprehensive Psychiatry,* 12(1):68-69, 1971.

Huckabay, L.M.D., and B. Jagla: "Nurses' Stress Factors in the Intensive Care Unit," *Journal of Nursing Administration,* 9:21-26, 1979.

Janosik, E.H.: "Variations in Ethnic Families," in J.R. Miller and E.H. Janosik (eds.), *Family-Focused Care,* McGraw-Hill, New York, 1980.

Johnson, J.L., and P.A. Norby: "We Can Weekend: A Program for Cancer Families," *Cancer Nursing,* 4:23-28, 1981.

Johnson-Soderberg, S.: "Grief Themes," *Advances in Nursing Science,* 3(4):15-26, 1981.

Kastenbaum, R.J.: *Death, Society, and Human Experience,* Mosby, St. Louis, 1977.

Kopel, K., and L.A. Mock: "The Use of Group Sessions for the Emotional Support of Families of Terminal Patients," *Death Education,* 1:409-422, 1978.

Krieger, G.W., and L.O. Bascue: "Terminal Illness: Counseling with a Family Perspective," *The Family Coordinator,* 24:351-355, 1975.

Kruger, S., et al., "Reactions of Families to the Child with Cystic Fibrosis," *Image,* 12(3):67-72, 1980.

Kübler-Ross, E.: *On Death and Dying,* Macmillan, New York, 1969.

Lauer, M.E., and B.M. Camitta: "Home Care for Dying Children: A Nursing Model," *Journal of Pediatrics,* 97:1032-1035, 1980.

Lifton, R.J.: "On Death and the Continuity of Life: A Psychohistorical Perspective," in R.A. Kalish (ed.), *Death, Dying, Transcending,* Baywood, Farmingdale, N.Y., 1980.

—— and E. Olson: "The Human Meaning of Total Disaster," *Psychiatry,* 39:1-18, 1976.

Lindemann, E.: "Symptomatology and Management of Acute Grief," *American Journal of Psychiatry,* 72:141-148, 1944.

Lonetto, R.: *Children's Conceptions of Death,* Springer, New York, 1980.

McCarthy, J.B.: *Death Anxiety: The Loss of the Self,* Gardner Press, New York, 1980.

McIntire, M.S., et al.: "The Concept of Death in Midwestern Children and Youth," *American Journal of Diseases of Children,* 123:527-532, 1972.

Mann, G.M., et al.: "The Effects on the Family of Life-Threatening Childhood Disease," *Essence,* 4:87-94, 1980.

Martinson, I.: "Why Don't We Let Them Die at Home?" *RN,* 39(1):58-65, 1976.

Meyerowitz, J.H., and H.B. Kaplan: "Family Responses to Stress: The Case of Cystic Fibrosis," *Social Science and Medicine,* 1:249-266, 1967.

Oehler, J.: "The Frog Family Books: Color the Pictures 'Sad' or 'Glad,'" *MCN: American Journal of Maternal Child Nursing,* 6:281-283, 1981.

Palgi, P.: "Sociocultural Expressions and Implications of Death, Mourning, and Bereavement Arising Out of the War Situation," *Israel Annals of Psychiatry and Related Disciplines,* 2:301-329, 1973.

Portz, A.: "The Child's Sense of Death," in A. Godin (ed.), *Death and Presence,* Lumen Vitae, Brussels, 1972.

Rose, B.: "Death is Alive and Well in the Ghetto," in E. Shneidman (ed.), *Death and the College Student,* Behavioral Publications, New York, 1972.

Rosenblatt, P.C., et al.: *Grief and Mourning in Cross-Cultural Perspective,* H.R.A.F. Press, New Haven, 1976.

Schowalter, J.E.: "The Child's Reaction to His Own Terminal Illness," in B. Schoenberg et al. (eds.), *Psychosocial Aspects of Terminal Care,* Columbia University Press, New York, 1972.

Seligman, M.E.P.: *Helplessness: On Depression, Development and Death,* Freeman, San Francisco, 1975.

Sharapan, H.: "'Mister Rogers' Neighborhood': Dealing with Death on a Children's Television Series," *Death Education,* 1:131-136, 1977.

Silverman, P.R., and S.M. Silverman: "Withdrawal in Bereaved Children," in B. Schoenberg et al. (eds.), *Bereavement: Its Psychosocial Aspects,* Columbia University Press, New York, 1975.

Taylor, M.A., and H.A. Williams: "Use of Therapeutic Play in the Ambulatory Pediatric Hematology Clinic," *Cancer Nursing,* 3:433-437, 1980.

Terre, L.C.: "Children of Chowchilla: A Study of Psychic Trauma," *Psychoanalytic Study of the Child,* 34:547-623, 1979.

——: "Psychic Trauma in Children: Observations Following the Chowchilla School-Bus Kidnapping," *American Journal of Psychiatry,* 138:14-19, 1981.

Tishler, C.L., et al.: "Adolescent Suicide Attempts: Some Significant Factors," *Suicide and Life Threatening Behavior,* 11:86-92, 1981.

Walker, K.N., et al.: "Social Support Networks and the Crisis of Bereavement," *Social Science in Medicine,* 11:35-41, 1977.

Wiener, J.: "Reactions of the Family to the Fatal Illness of a Child," in B. Schoenberg et al. (eds.), *Loss and Grief: Psychological Management in Medical Practice,* Columbia University Press, New York, 1970.

Williams, H.A., et al.: "The Child Is Dying: Who Helps the Family," *MCN: American Journal of Maternal Child Nursing,* 6:261-265, 1981.

Bibliography

Benoliel, J.Q.: "Loss and Adaptation: Circumstances, Contingencies, and Consequences," *Death Studies,* 9(304):217-233, 1985.

Betz, C.L., and E.C. Poster: "Children's Concepts of Death," *Nursing Clinics of North America,* 19(2):341-349, 1984.

Florian, V.: "Children's Concepts of Death: An Empirical Study of a Cognitive and Environmental Approach," Death Studies, 9(2):133-141, 1985.

Gyulay, J.: *The Dying Child,* McGraw-Hill, New York, 1978.

Martinson, I.M.: "Home Care for Children Dying of Cancer," *Research in Nursing and Health,* 9:11-16, 1986.

McClowry, S.G., et al.: "The Empty Space Phenomenon: The Process of Grief in the Bereaved Family," *Death Studies,* 11(5):361-374, 1987.

17

High-Risk Neonates and Their Families

Objectives

After reading this chapter, the student will be able to:

1. Have a fuller understanding of methods used to assess neonates.
2. Identify common problems of high-risk neonates.
3. Describe nursing care of high-risk neonates related to:
   (a) Thermal support
   (b) Ventilatory support
   (c) Nutritional support
   (d) Monitoring the neonate
   (e) Regionalization of care
   (f) Promoting parent-infant interaction
   (g) Stimulating the high-risk neonate
   (h) Parent support groups

A high-risk newborn is one whose life or quality of life may be in jeopardy. The hazards which place a baby in the high-risk category may be present long before the child is conceived, for example, chronic illness of the mother or hereditary defects in either parent's family. Other risk factors may arise during pregnancy, such as maternal infection, and still others may occur during labor and delivery, e.g., cesarean section. The nursing care of high-risk babies consists of identifying them as early as possible and intervening to maximize the well-being of the infants and their families.

Contributors to High-Risk Status

Many factors can alert members of the health care team to the possibility of the birth of a high-risk neonate, including the mother's previous obstetric history and health practices, social factors, paternal factors, and labor and delivery factors. In Table 17-1 various risk factors and possible outcomes are listed.

Assessment of the Neonate

Apgar Scoring

Apgar scoring has been described in Chap. 2 (Table 2-1). In this chapter methods of assessing the neonate to determine the score are presented.

As soon as the baby is completely delivered, the Apgar timer should be started. When the 1-minute signal is heard, Apgar observations should begin. The first and most important diagnostic and prognostic sign is the heart rate, which can be determined by means of auscultation of the precordium or palpation of the umbilical cord pulse at the junction between the cord clamp and the abdominal wall. Only the spontaneous heart rate is scored.

Respiratory effort is the second most important indicator of the infant's status. It may be assessed by means of auscultation of the chest wall or observation of chest wall excursions. Only the neonate's unassisted respirations are scored. The respiratory rate should be counted during the inspiratory phase of the respiratory cycle in order to identify delays in inspiratory effort.

Reflex irritability refers to the newborn's response to any form of stimulation. Suctioning of the neonate's nares and flicking of the newborn's heel are examples of stimulation that can be applied to evoke a response.

Muscle tone is assessed by observing the newborn's spontaneous flexion of the extremities. The observer should also attempt to extend the neonate's extremities, noting the baby's resistance to this maneuver.

The final observation is the neonate's color. This observation is, according to Apgar, the least satisfactory of the five. All newborns are cyanotic immediately upon delivery. The body then becomes pink, but the extremities may remain cyanotic. Within the first hour of life, this cyanosis of the extremities, termed *acrocyanosis,* should largely disappear. Persistence of cyanosis or acrocyanosis is a sign of oxygen lack.

The sheet used to score the neonate according to the Apgar method is reproduced in Table 2-1. Each of the above observations can be graded with one of three scores: 0, 1, or 2; the Apgar score is the sum of the five observations. The highest score a newborn can receive is 10, and the lowest is 0. A baby who receives a score of 0, 1, or 2 is considered severely depressed and requires immediate ventilatory assistance and intensive care. A moderately depressed neonate has a score of 3 to 6; this baby definitely requires close monitoring during the first day of life and may also require ventilatory assistance. Newborns

scoring 7 to 10 are in good condition and generally require routine observations and care.

A high-risk neonate is one whose Apgar score is less than 7. In the care of these babies, three areas of concern should be uppermost: thermal, ventilatory, and nutritional support. The method by which these supports are provided depends on the status of the newborn, his biological maturity, and the appropriateness of his size for gestational age.

Estimation of Gestational Age

Within the first 24 hours of life a complete physical examination, clinical estimation of gestational age, and determination of appropriateness of size in relation to gestational age are performed. The initial method used to determine gestational age was developed by Dubowitz, Dubowitz, and Goldberg (1970) (Chap. 2). This assessment takes 10 to 15 minutes to complete. Ballard, Novak, and Driver (1979) modified the Dubowitz procedure for use with well and ill neonates. It can be completed within 3 to 4 minutes and thus is less stressful to the newborn (Fig. 17-1). The Ballard method is used more commonly in newborn nurseries than is the Dubowitz instrument. Both methods provide an estimate which is accurate within 2 weeks of the actual gestational age. The Ballard assessment is described in this chapter.

Ballard, Novak, and, Driver (1979) selected six signs of neuromuscular maturity and seven signs of physical maturity. The method of scoring neuromuscular maturity is as follows (Fig. 17-1).

Posture The neonate is observed while supine and quiet. Scoring is as folllows:

Extended arms and legs = 0
Slightly or moderately flexed hips and knees = 1
Moderately to strongly flexed hips and knees = 2
Flexed and abducted legs, slightly flexed arms = 3
Fully flexed arms and legs = 4

Square Window (Wrist) The neonate's hand is flexed at the wrist. Sufficient pressure is exerted to obtain maximum flexion. The wrist is *not* rotated. The examiner measures the angle between the fleshy eminence on the ulnar side of the palm of the hand and the anterior aspect of the forearm. The angle of flexion is scored according to Fig. 17-1.

Arm Recoil The neonate is supine. The examiner fully flexes the forearms for 5 seconds and then extends them fully by pulling the hands and rapidly releasing them. If the arms remain extended (180°), the score is zero. If they flex to between 100° and 180°, the score is 2. Flexion between 90 and 100° is scored 3, and flexion less than 90° is scored 4.

Popliteal Angle The neonate is supine, and the pelvis is flat. The thigh is placed in the knee-chest position. The examiner uses the thumb and index finger of one hand to support the knee. With gentle pressure from the index finger of the other hand behind the newborn's ankle, the leg is extended toward the head. The angle attained is then scored (Fig. 17-1).

TABLE 17-1 Factors Associated with Fetal-Neonatal Risk

Risk Factors	Possible Outcomes
Previous obstetrical complications	
Fetal or neonatal loss, particularly SGA* neonate	Fetal growth retardation in successive pregnancies, sometimes in association with maternal hypertension
Multiple pregnancies (twins, etc.)	SGA, preterm neonate
Genetic defects	Recurrence in subsequent pregnancies
Toxemia	Preterm neonate
Diabetes mellitus or gestational diabetes	LGA* neonate with decreased blood sugar and increased bilirubin
Abnormalities of labor and delivery	Recurrence in subsequent pregnancies
Birth of preterm or postterm neonate	Recurrence in subsequent pregnancies
Health practices and social factors	
Lack of early, regular prenatal care	Fetal loss or damage
Maternal age	
Under 16 years	SGA and/or preterm neonate
Over 40 years	SGA neonate
Maternal nutrition	
Deficiencies in iron and protein	Infection, preterm, and/or SGA neonate
Folate deficiency	Decreased fetal oxygen, spontaneous abortion, stillbirth, malformations, preterm and/or SGA neonate
Maternal emotional health	Interference with fetal growth and development
Possible correlation between severe, prolonged tension from various causes (e.g., unplanned or unwanted pregnancy, divorce, illegitimacy, family rejection, loss, grief, enforced bed rest due to complications) and altered fetal environment or hormone balance	
Smoking	SGA neonate
Toxemia	Fetal death, preterm neonate, SGA neonate, hypoglycemia, aspiration syndrome, polycythemia and asphyxia
Maternal diabetes	Polyhydramnios, often associated with gastrointestinal and nervous system malformations and with premature rupture of the membranes, which predisposes fetus to infection or premature delivery
	LGA and/or preterm neonate, hypoglycemia, hypocalcemia, congenital abnormalities, hyperbilirubinemia, respiratory distress syndrome, infection
Maternal heart and lung disease	Fetal asphyxia, SGA neonate, preterm neonate
Maternal urinary disease	Polycystic kidney, SGA neonate, asphyxia, preterm neonate
Vaginal bleeding (placenta previa, abruptio placentae)	Asphyxia, preterm neonate
Multiple pregnancy	Preterm and/or SGA neonate, congenital anomalies, bacterial infection, hypoglycemia, asphyxia

*SGA = small for gestational age; LGA = large for gestational age; MR = mental retardation; DIC = disseminated intravascular coagulation; AIDS = acuired immune deficiency syndrome.

Source: Adapted from B. S. Rothbarth and C. Pedigo. "High-risk Infants and Their Families," in G. M. Scipien et al. (eds.), *Comprehensive Pediatric Nursing,* 3d ed., McGraw-Hill, New York, 1986, pp. 567-581.

Scarf Sign The neonate is supine. The neonate's hand is drawn across the neck and then across the opposite shoulder as far as possible. To assist in this maneuver, the elbow is lifted across the body. The score is attained as follows:

Elbow beyond opposite anterior axillary line = 0
Elbow at opposite anterior axillary line = 1
Elbow between opposite anterior axillary line and midline of thorax = 2
Elbow at midline of thorax = 3
Elbow not to midline of thorax = 4

Heel to Ear The neonate is supine, and the pelvis is flat. The examiner holds the newborn's foot in one hand and moves it as near as possible to the head without using force. The knee is not supported. The examiner measures the distance between the foot and the head and the degree of knee extension. The score is attained as shown in Fig. 17-1.

By adding the assigned scores for each observation, one attains the total score for neuromuscular maturity. The physical maturity score is attained by using the physical maturity scale shown in Fig. 17-1. The description in the scale that best agrees with the examiner's observations is used as the score for each of the seven physical maturity categories. The total physical maturity score and the total neurological maturity score determine the neo-

TABLE 17-1 Factors Associated with Fetal-Neonatal Risk—cont'd

Risk Factors	Possible Outcomes
Maternofetal blood type incompatibility	LGA due to edema, jaundice within 24 h
Rh	Petechiae and purpura due to thrombocytopenia and disturbance in coagulation, varying degrees of anemia
ABO	Less severe consequences than Rh
Maternal substance abuse	
Alcohol	Fetal alcohol syndrome
Drugs	Chromosomal abnormalities, SGA neonate, withdrawal symptoms
Maternal infections	
Rubella in first trimester	Preterm and/or SGA neonate, stillbirth, hearing loss, brain abnormalities, cataracts, heart defects, MR*
Cytomegalovirus	Preterm and/or SGA neonate, hydrocephaly, microcephaly, DIC*, focal/cerebral dysfunctions, MR, visceral and skeletal malformations
Syphilis	Anemia, hepatosplenomegaly, pseudoparalysis, painful extremities, jaundice, rhinitis
Herpes simplex II	Spontaneous abortion; after 20 weeks' gestation, preterm neonate or neonatal death 24-48 h after birth
Group B beta-hemolytic streptococci	Fetal infection, preterm neonate, neonatal sepsis
Candida albicans (moniliasis) vaginitis	Neonatal thrush
Toxoplasmosis	Hydrocephalus, microcephaly, MR, cerebral calcification, hepatosplenomegaly with jaundice, lethargy, convulsions
AIDS*	Infant AIDS at 4-6 mo of age
Paternal factors (speculative)	
Older fathers	Stillbirth, congenital anomalies
Inheritance of Rh+ genes from father if mother is Rh−	Erythroblastosis fetalis
Chronic alcoholism or diabetes mellitus	Impaired fetal development
Labor and delivery factors	
Uterine dysfunction: prolonged labor	Neonatal asphyxia, trauma, bacterial infection
Abnormal fetal presentation	
Breech delivery	Neonatal asphyxia, intracranial hemorrhage, visceral hemorrhage, spinal cord trauma, brachial plexus injury, fractures, edema
Face, brow, or transverse presentation	Neonatal edema, trauma, asphyxia
Premature labor (prior to 38 weeks' gestation)	Respiratory distress syndrome, preterm neonate, intracranial hemorrhage, trauma
Premature spontaneous rupture of membranes (especially if birth does not occur within 24 h)	Neonatal infection, neonatal sepsis
Late decelerations during contractions (as noted with fetal monitor), fetal scalp pH less than 7.25, and meconium-stained amniotic fluid	Neonatal hypoxia

nate's estimated gestational age as depicted in the maturity rating scale shown in Fig. 17-1.

Estimation of Growth

Lubchenco, Hansman, and Boyd (1966) developed the Classification of Newborns Based on Maturity and Intrauterine Growth. Their classification system is shown in Fig. 17-2. The birth weight, length, and head circumference of the neonate are plotted according to the neonate's estimated gestational age. From the results, the examiner can arrive at approximate definitions of newborns who are small for gestational age (SGA), appropriate for gestational (AGA), or large for gestational age (LGA).

Discrepancies in intrauterine growth are reflected first in the fetal weight, then in the length, and finally in the head circumference. Thus, at many centers growth esti-

mation is based on weight alone. In such instances a neonate whose birth weight is at or below the 10th percentile for newborns of the same gestational age is SGA. The LGA neonate has a birth weight at or above the 90th percentile. The AGA neonate's birth weight falls between the 10th percentile and the 90th percentile.

As diagrammed in Fig. 17-2, neonates from 37 weeks' gestation and below are *preterm,* neonates from 42 to 44 weeks' gestation are *postterm,* and neonates born after 37 weeks and before 42 weeks are *term.* Neonates who are preterm, those who are postterm, and those who have growth discrepancies are considered to be at risk.

Preterm Neonates at Risk

Approximately 25 percent of all newborns are preterm babies. Preterm newborns are physically less mature than

ESTIMATION OF GESTATIONAL AGE BY MATURITY RATING
Symbols: X - 1st Exam   O - 2nd Exam

NEUROMUSCULAR MATURITY

	0	1	2	3	4	5
Posture	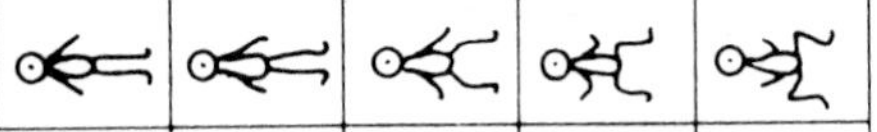					
Square Window (Wrist)	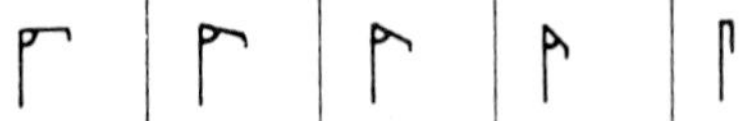 90°	60°	45°	30°	0°	
Arm Recoil	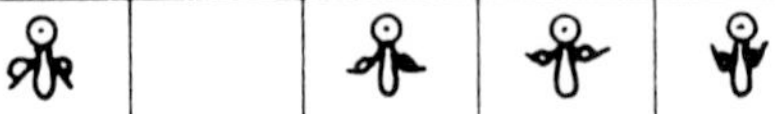 180°	100°-180°	90°-100°	< 90°		
Popliteal Angle	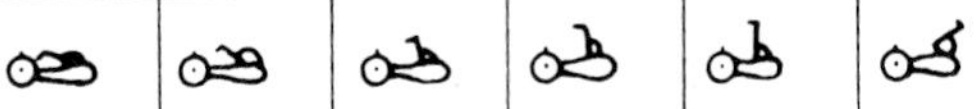 180°	160°	130°	110°	90°	< 90°
Scarf Sign	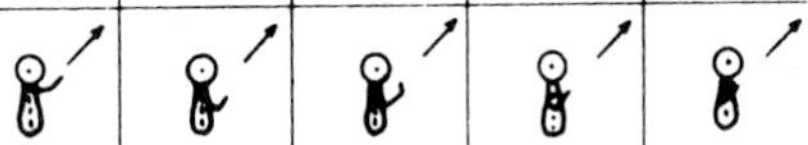					
Heel to Ear	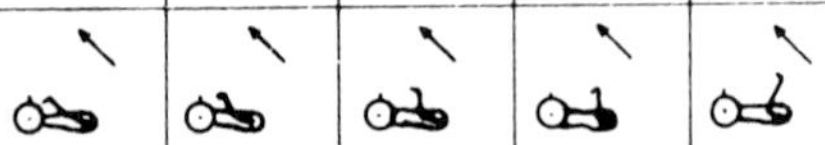					

Gestation by Dates _____ wks

Birth Date _____ Hour _____ am / pm

APGAR _____ 1 min _____ 5 min

MATURITY RATING

Score	Wks
5	26
10	28
15	30
20	32
25	34
30	36
35	38
40	40
45	42
50	44

PHYSICAL MATURITY

	0	1	2	3	4	5
SKIN	gelatinous red, transparent	smooth pink, visible veins	superficial peeling &/or rash, few veins	cracking pale area, rare veins	parchment, deep cracking, no vessels	leathery, cracked, wrinkled
LANUGO	none	abundant	thinning	bald areas	mostly bald	
PLANTAR CREASES	no crease	faint red marks	anterior transverse crease only	creases ant. 2/3	creases cover entire sole	
BREAST	barely percept.	flat areola, no bud	stippled areola, 1–2 mm bud	raised areola, 3–4 mm bud	full areola, 5–10 mm bud	
EAR	pinna flat, stays folded	sl. curved pinna, soft with slow recoil	well-curv. pinna, soft but ready recoil	formed & firm with instant recoil	thick cartilage, ear stiff	
GENITALS Male	scrotum empty, no rugae		testes descending, few rugae	testes down, good rugae	testes pendulous, deep rugae	
GENITALS Female	prominent clitoris & labia minora		majora & minora equally prominent	majora large, minora small	clitoris & minora completely covered	

SCORING SECTION

	1st Exam=X	2nd Exam=O
Estimating Gest Age by Maturity Rating	_____ Weeks	_____ Weeks
Time of Exam	Date _____ Hour _____ am/pm	Date _____ Hour _____ am/pm
Age at Exam	_____ Hours	_____ Hours
Signature of Examiner	_____ M.D.	_____ M.D.

FIGURE 17-1 The Ballard (Ballard, Novak, and Driver, 1979) adaptation of the Dubowitz method of estimating gestational age.

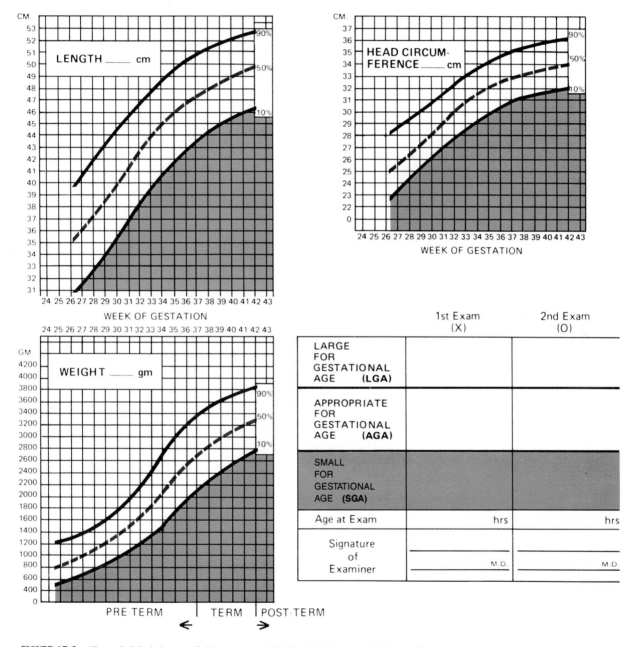

FIGURE 17-2   *(From L.C. Lubchenco, C. Hansman, and E. Boyd, Pediatrics 37:403, 1966; and F.C. Battaglia and L.C. Lubchenco, Journal of Pediatrics, 1:159, 1967.)*

FIGURE 17-3 Preterm black female. Birth weight was 1300 g (2 lb, 14 oz) at an estimated gestational age of 32 weeks. This photograph was taken at 38 days of age; weight was 1415 g (3 lb, 1½ oz). Thinness of the skin is evident. Absence of subcutaneous fat is especially noticeable in the thigh folds, in the labia majora, and over the ribs. The open hands and scarflike, draped position denote the diminished muscle tone of the preterm neonate.

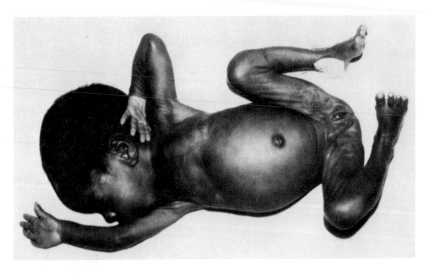

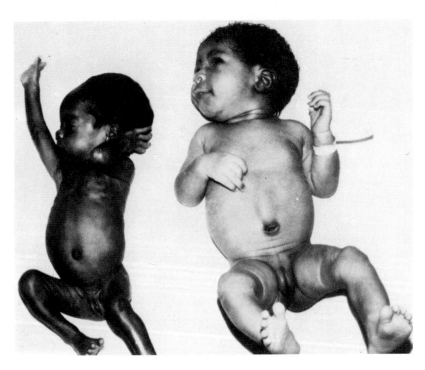

FIGURE 17-4 The preterm neonate pictured in Fig. 17-3 is shown with a 2-day-old black female born at 40 weeks' gestation and weighing 314 g (6 lb, 14 oz) at birth. This comparison demonstrates the full-term neonate's characteristically greater muscle tone, darker genital pigmentation, curlier hair, more abundant subcutaneous fat (including the genital region, where the labia majora cover the clitoris), sole creases, and open, mature eyes (in contrast to the birdlike eyelids of the preterm neonate).

term neonates (Figs. 17-3 and 17-4). Preterm babies have fewer sole creases, more lanugo, less cartilage formation (especially of the ears), less breast tissue, and underdeveloped genitalia. Neurologically they are less developed, and so there is decreased muscle tone and less flexion of the extremities than in term infants. The normal vital signs of neonates are shown in Table 17-2. Because of immaturity of all systems, the preterm neonate is at risk for problems that the term newborn seldom encounters. These problems involve instability of body temperature, hypoglycemia, infections, the respiratory system, the hemopoietic system, the nervous system, inborn errors of metabolism, and substance abuse.

Preterm neonates may be SGA, AGA, or LGA. In a Colorado study of babies born between 1974 and 1980, mortality was greatest in infants of less than 35 weeks' gestational age. Among this group the mortality rate was significantly higher in SGA newborns than in either AGA or LGA neonates. Among the LGA babies born at and after 35 weeks' gestation there were no deaths. The same was not true among those who were AGA and SGA, and the SGA group continued to have a higher mortality rate. All LGA babies born after 35 weeks' gestation weighed more than 2500 g (Koops, Morgan, and Battaglia, 1982).

Postterm Neonates at Risk

The postterm neonate is usually the product of a first pregnancy. Postmaturity occurs in approximately 12 percent of all pregnancies. Typically, postterm neonates are identified clinically by their characteristic appearance.

TABLE 17-2 Vital Signs of the Preterm Neonate

	Normal Range	Changes Accompanying Infection
Temperature (rectal or axillary)	36.5-37.2°C (97.7-99°F)	Usually decreases; may increase
Heart rate	100-120 beats/min (sleeping) 120-160 beats/min (awake but quiet) 160+ beats/min (active)	Usually normal
Respiratory rate	30-60 breaths/min	Usually increases; apneic episodes may also occur
Blood pressure	40-60 mm Hg systolic, 16-36 mm Hg diastolic	Usually normal; as sepsis progresses, systolic may fall below 50 mm Hg and diastolic may drop below 25, possibly to 0

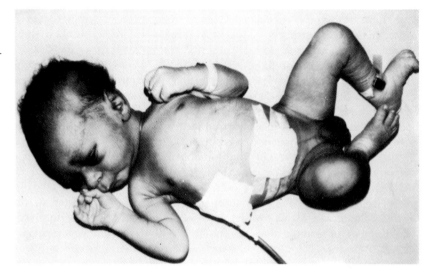

FIGURE 17-5 Postterm black male born at 43 weeks' gestation and weighing 2840 g (6 lb, 4 oz), 2 days old when photographed. Diminished subcutaneous fat, cracked skin (especially noticeable over the upper abdomen and hands), long nails which extend beyond the ends of the fingers, heavy genital pigment, sole creases, and curly hair, which distinguish the postterm neonate from the preterm baby, are evident.

Vernix caseosa (cheeselike material) normally serves to lubricate and protect the unborn neonate's skin. The absence of vernix in a postterm neonate, except in the deepest skin folds, produces a dry, cracked, parchmentlike appearance of the skin. The nails are longer than those of a term neonate. The body has wasted appearance as subcutaneous tissue has been depleted, leaving the skin loose, with almost nonexistent fat layers. The body is usually thin and long. Meconium staining may have occurred, leaving a green to golden-yellow staining of the nails, cord, and skin. Postterm neonates appear to be alert and wide-eyed (Fig. 17-5).

Postterm neonates are at risk for neonatal asphyxia and meconium aspiration. These problems are produced by degeneration of the postterm placenta as it ages. As placental function decreases, the neonate experiences inadequate oxygenation and may pass meconium as a result of this stress. Meconium aspiration occurs as a result of the neonate's gasping in utero during fetal stress and thus aspirating amniotic fluid that contains meconium into the lungs. Because of body wasting that occurs in utero, the postterm neonate may also be at risk for hypoglycemia resulting from insufficient glycogen stores for the increased metabolic activity necessary to produce an increase in body heat.

Postterm neonates may be SGA, AGA, or LGA. In the Colorado study cited above the mortality rate was greater in those who were SGA (2 percent) and those who were AGA (0.4 percent). No deaths occurred in the LGA group.

Neonates with Inappropriate Size for Gestational Age

As noted above, at many centers appropriate size for gestational age is estimated by weight alone (Fig. 17-2, weight chart). Thus, length and head circumference may be appropriate for gestational age, while weight is not.

SGA neonates appear thin and wasted. The skin is often loose because of a lack of subcutaneous tissue and may be dry, parchmentlike, and peeling. Meconium staining of the nails, cord, and skin is common. Their size is usually appropriate for length and head circumference but inappropriate for body weight related to gestational age. They appear alert, wide-eyed, and more active than infants of similar weight but younger gestational age.

SGA neonates are usually chronically stressed in utero and consequently are at risk for intrauterine hypoxia. Hypoxic episodes are accompanied by the passage of meconium, placing SGA neonates at risk for meconium aspiration, aspiration pneumonia, and possibly pulmonary hemorrhage. Because of IUGR, these neonates have very limited oxygen, fat, and glycogen reserves. They are therefore at risk for hypoglycemia because of their decreased glycogen reserves and increased metabolic activity.

SGA infants are at risk for hypothermia because of the discrepancy between body surface and body mass. Intrauterine growth retardation is most likely due to placental insufficiency. Therefore, the SGA neonate is at risk for problems similar to those of the postterm neonate. SGA neonates occasionally show an increase in blood viscosity manifested as polycythemia, which places them at risk for respiratory distress, cardiac problems, and circulatory problems.

The LGA neonate is similar in appearance to any infant of the same gestational age. The only difference may be the LGA baby's greater weight. Because LGA neonates are large, most of the problems for which they are at risk involve the delivery process and furthermore are more likely to arise during a vaginal delivery than during a cesarean section. Some of these risk factors are cranial trauma, phrenic nerve damage possibly leading to paralysis of the diaphragm, brachial plexus palsy, and fractured clavicle. The LGA neonate can also be at risk for asphyxia because of the prolonged time involved in delivery or to respiratory distress secondary to birth trauma.

Walther and Raemaekers (1982) questioned the use of weight alone and gestational age as an index of intrauterine growth. They suggested that Rohrer's ponderal index (Miller and Hassanein, 1971) is more informative. Frisancho, Compton, and Matos (1986), however, found that measurement of skinfold thickness more accurately describes a newborn's nutritional state (undernourished, normal, overnourished) than does the length/weight ratio (ponderal index) or the weight alone. To date, methods of estimating the neonate's size are imprecise, and further research is needed.

Common Problems of High-Risk Neonates
Instability of Body Temperature
Newborns who are at risk can maintain their own body temperatures without additional stress only if environmental temperatures are kept within a relatively narrow range. A *neutral thermal environment* is one in which the newborn maintains his body temperature at 36.5°C (97.8 to 99°F) without expending calories or utilizing additional oxygen, extra fat, or glycogen stores. Without the support of a thermal environment, such as an overhead radiant warmer or an incubator, a high-risk neonate loses heat and his body temperature drops as he experiences *cold stress.* If the change in temperature occurs in response to being in a cold environment, it is *hypothermia,* while a hot environment results in *hyperthermia.*

Shivering, with its subsequent increase in muscular activity, is a common method of producing body heat in an adult; however, it is seen very rarely in a newborn. Brown adipose fat, which usually is utilized within the first few weeks after birth, is found deposited between the scapulas, around the neck, in the axillas, and around the esophagus and trachea as well as the kidneys and adrenal glands.

It plays a vital role in production of body heat by the neonate.

A method of generating heat which is unique to the newborn is known as chemical, or *nonshivering, thermogenesis.* This process occurs during episodes of cold stress when receptors in the skin identify a change in the environmental temperature. These sensations are transmitted to the central and sympathetic nervous systems, which trigger the release of norepinephrine by the adrenal glands and at the nerve endings in the brown adipose fat. The fatty metabolism which occurs there generates internal heat which then is distributed by the blood throughout the body.

SGA and preterm newborns have significant differences between body surface area and mass; therefore, they require more heat than their bodies can produce. In addition, the very thin layer of subcutaneous fat is an extremely poor insulator, and so these babies cannot conserve body heat efficiently. As they attempt to generate more body heat to reach a desirable stable temperature, these neonates increase their metabolism, increase their oxygen consumption, use their fat and glycogen stores, and expend precious calories. When cold stress is not corrected, it may result in hypoxemia, hypoglycemia, and metabolic acidosis.

Hypoglycemia
During the last trimester a fetus converts maternal glucose to glycogen, which is stored in the liver, heart, and skeletal muscle for use after birth. After delivery the preterm or SGA newborn relies on these stores and external sources of glucose for a variety of physiological functions, such as respiration, muscular activity, and thermoregulation. However, the amount stored is inadequate; with the initiation of breathing in combination with cold stress or any respiratory difficulty, these glycogen stores are depleted rapidly and the neonate becomes hypoglycemic.

Generally, hypoglycemia is considered to be any deviation below the lower limits of normal for two consecutive blood sugar samples. A level under 40 mg/100 ml constitutes cause for concern. The signs and symptoms of hypoglycemia include any or all of the following: lethargy, irritability, tremors, weak or high-pitched cry, cyanosis, seizures, apnea, and poor feeding.

The range of normal blood sugar concentration differs between term newborns weighing more than 2500 g and low-birth-weight neonates. From 30 to 125 mg/100 ml is the normal range for term newborns; from 20 to 100 mg/100 ml is the normal range for low-birth-weight newborns. When the initial low blood sugar level is confirmed by a second low blood sugar, intravenous glucose infusion therapy is started. Initially a 10% glucose solution at 8 ml/kg of body weight per hour is administered. Further alterations in percentage concentration and rate of flow depend on subsequent blood sugar levels as determined by Dextrostix. The previous practice of adminstering a glucose solution greater than 10% is no longer recommended because of the potential to incur rebound hypoglycemia in the neonate.

If high-risk newborns are allowed to remain in a hypoglycemic and/or hypothermic state for any period of time, their ability to withstand thermal or respiratory distress is limited and the risk of morbidity or mortality is increased.

Infections

Preterm neonates are at risk for developing a variety of infections. As a result of their shortened gestational periods, they have acquired lesser concentrations of maternal antibodies, and those they have provide limited protection for a limited time period. The ability of these newborns to produce antibodies develops slowly. Neonates who spend time in the neonatal intensive care unit (NICU) also risk being infected with the resistant hospital flora which may be found in such units (Baron and Tafuro, 1985).

TORCH

TORCH is an acronym for several agents that are capable of infecting fetuses and causing a variety of congenital malformations or developmental problems. Generally, *T* stands for *Toxoplasma,* *O* for others, *R* for rubella, *C* for cytomegalovirus, and *H* for herpesvirus type 2. The "other" infections include syphilis and hepatitis (Table 17-3).

It is important to draw a blood sample from the newborn for a TORCH screening test as soon as possible. While an accurate maternal history is critical, if the mother is a nurse, the possibility of occupational exposure through work in an NICU or a dialysis unit also needs to be explored. Cultures are taken of vesicles if they are present, and viral cultures are done on the blood, nose, throat, and eye. A histological study of the placenta is done too. Determination of the liver enzymes [serum glutamic oxaloacetic transaminase (SGOT) and serum glutamic pyruvic transaminase (SGPT)], a platelet count, and clotting times complete the workup.

As soon as the presence of any of these infections is confirmed, treatment is started. A number of antiprotozoal medications are available for a neonate with toxoplasmosis; however, their use varies and depends on the degree of severity. No specific treatment is available for congenital rubella. These neonates are isolated because live virus continues to be found in secretions and excreta for months after delivery. There is also no specific treatment for infants with cytomegalovirus. It is important to note that these newborns may infect others. The neonate with a herpes infection is isolated, and antiviral drug treatment is started promptly.

Sepsis

Sepsis is a systemic infection, usually bacterial in origin, which because of its subtle, nonspecific nature is one of the most challenging pediatric health problems. Although early detection is very important, the symptoms are so vague and nondescript that the diagnosis is not made readily. For example, despite the presence of a generalized infection, there is no inflammatory process evident on examining the neonate, nor is the newborn's body temperature elevated significantly.

One factor which increases susceptibility is a shortened gestational period. Other factors which contribute to sepsis in the newborn include intrapartal maternal infections (amnionitis, those resulting from prematurely ruptured membranes, or a precipitous delivery), passage through the birth canal, and exposure to diverse vaginal flora, all of which provide exposure to an incredible number of sources. After delivery, infections can be acquired through cross-contamination from other infants, health

TABLE 17-3 TORCH Infections

Disease	Causative Agent	Mode of Transmission	Common Problems in the Neonate
Toxoplasmosis	*Toxoplasma gondii*	Consuming oocytes in raw or poorly cooked meat and contact with cat feces, which ultimately cross placenta	Microcephaly, hydrocephalus, intracranial calcifications, jaundice, chorioretinitis convulsions, ecchymosis, pallor, hepatosplenomegaly
Rubella	Rubella virus	After exposure to the rubella virus during pregnancy, crosses placenta and infects developing embryo/fetus (results are most severe in first trimester)	Mental retardation, congenital cataracts, retinopathy, variety of congenital heart anomalies (especially patent ductus arteriosus, and pulmonary artery stenosis), deafness, thrombocytopenia; these infants continue to shed active rubella virus up to 18 mo after delivery
Cytomegalic inclusion disease (CID)	Cytomegalovirus (CMV)	Exposure to virus which has been isolated from breast milk, saliva, urine, feces, and upper respiratory tract as well as from blood-borne infections transferred to infants who are receiving multiple transfusions	Although asymptomatic at birth, various problems become evident several months later, including hepatosplenomegaly, microcephaly, purpura, jaundice, and cerebral calcifications as well as deafness and blindness; while spastic quadriplegia and hypotonia are common in those who are severely affected, developmental delays extend from minimal involvement to a vegetative state
Herpes simplex virus (HSV)	Herpesvirus	Direct contact with infected maternal genital secretions during delivery	Skin lesions, hypoglycemia, lethargy, irritability followed by focal or generalized seizures, disseminated intravascular coagulation

care providers, or equipment used in invasive procedures, in resuscitation, and in the course of ventilator support. There are innumerable opportunities for infection to occur in a high-risk neonate.

Invariably it is the nurse who suspects something is wrong because the newborn is "not doing well." The clinical manifestations, which are similar to those of a large number of other, more specific conditions, include lethargy, irritability, hypotonia, tremors, and convulsions as well as a variety of color changes such as cyanosis, pallor, and mottling. Sometimes the skin is cool and clammy. There may be thermal instability, hyperbilirubinemia, and various respiratory symptoms such as apnea, grunting, and retractions. In addition, these neonates do not eat well, their oral intake is less, and their sucking reflexes are poor. Abdominal distention is present, and these neonates have diarrhea.

Isolating the causative agent is critical. A variety of cultures are obtained, including blood, urine, spinal fluid, nasopharyngeal secretions, and skin lesions if they are present. They are all collected *before* broad-spectrum antibiotics are started. Intravenous fluids, frequent recording of vital signs, and supportive measures are started. After the organism is identified and its sensitivities are determined, antibiotics may have to be changed to more specific and hence more effective drugs. The course of antibiotic therapy usually lasts 10 to 14 days.

Group B Streptococcus Infections

This organism is the major cause of septicemia in the newborn and deserves special attention. When signs of infection occur hours after delivery, neonatal morbidity and mortality rates are high. Frequently these newborns demonstrate symptoms of respiratory distress such as grunting, cyanosis, tachypnea, periods of apnea, and even shock.

A variety of cultures, including blood, urine, spinal fluid, and gastric contents as well as skin, are done immediately. Antibiotics are started as soon as the cultures are collected. These neonates deteriorate rapidly; therefore, a prompt diagnosis and especially the careful administration of drugs affect the ultimate outcome.

Respiratory Problems
Idiopathic Respiratory Distress Syndrome

Idiopathic respiratory distress syndrome (IRDS), a respiratory disease which affects preterm neonates primarily, is responsible for 12,000 to 25,000 neonatal deaths a year (Olds, London, and Ladewig, 1984). Its cause is a deficiency in *surfactant,* a phospholipid protein complex which lines the alveoli of the lungs.

Normally, after delivery, a newborn whose lungs are mature requires high distending pressures to snap open the alveoli during the first few breaths. Surfactant then is able to stabilize or maintain the alveoli, and subsequent breaths require significantly lower distending pressures. In a preterm infant who has immature lungs and develops IRDS, every breath is as difficult as the first. Without surfactant, the alveoli collapse on each respiratory cycle.

The signs of IRDS are evident within hours after delivery. Initially there are increased respirations and slight subcostal retractions. As breathing becomes more rapid and labored (exceeding 80 to 100 breaths per minute) there are xiphoid and intercostal retractions, nasal flaring, expiratory grunting, cyanosis, and frothing at the lips. The grunting is an effort by the infant to continue distention of the alveoli and to oppose their tendency to collapse from the lack of surfactant (Fig. 17-6). The newborn's temperature often is low. Dyspnea, pallor, and cyanosis increase as the neonate's condition worsens. Hypotension, edema, ileus, and oliguria also may be present.

As the neonate struggles to open the collapsed alveoli, it is necessary to use accessory muscles or respiration and expiratory grunting. Atelectasis occurs in areas of focal emphysema which increase the risk of spontaneous pneumothorax. In addition, blood is shunted from right to left, around the areas of atelectasis, with a resultant accumulation of CO_2. The acidosis that develops can be both metabolic, from the hypoxia, and respiratory, from the accumulation of CO_2. The acidosis also causes vasoconstriction, which decreases pulmonary circulation further. If the preterm neonate is to survive, oxygenation must improve and all these pathophysiological events must be reversed.

In treating mild IRDS, oxygen which is warmed and

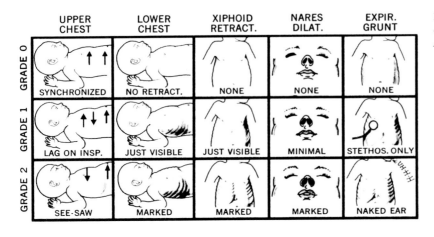

	UPPER CHEST	LOWER CHEST	XIPHOID RETRACT.	NARES DILAT.	EXPIR. GRUNT
GRADE 0	SYNCHRONIZED	NO RETRACT.	NONE	NONE	NONE
GRADE 1	LAG ON INSP.	JUST VISIBLE	JUST VISIBLE	MINIMAL	STETHOS. ONLY
GRADE 2	SEE-SAW	MARKED	MARKED	MARKED	NAKED EAR

FIGURE 17-6   Silverman's scoring of respiratory difficulty. *(Courtesy of Mead Johnson and Co., Evansville, Ind.)*

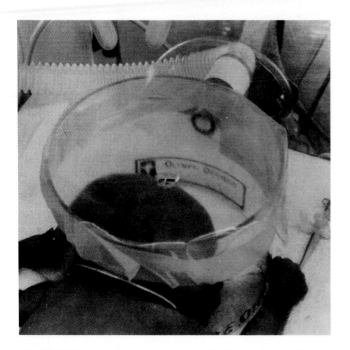

FIGURE 17-7 A preterm neonate whose head is enclosed with a plastic circular hood that maintains a constant humidified and oxygenated environment.

humidified is administered into a plastic hood or incubator (Fig. 17-7). Its concentration must be monitored very carefully so that it is not excessive for the developing retina. Maintaining adequate oxygenation is critical. If the newborn's condition continues to deteriorate, some neonatologists order the use of continuous distending airway pressure (CDAP), which can be applied through nasal prongs, a face mask, or a nasopharyngeal or endotracheal tube to maintain the alveoli in an expanded position. CDAP may decrease the time a neonate spends in high O_2 concentrations and sometimes decreases the need for mechanical ventilation. However, when an infant is not able to maintain an acceptable oxygen saturation level and CO_2 level continue to rise, mechanical ventilation through the use of a positive end expiratory pressure (PEEP) respirator may be necessary. In some medical centers surfactant is being given to these neonates. The success rate in preventing IRDS is promising.

It is important for the newborn to maintain body temperature within a normal range, because hypothermia increases the metabolic need for oxygen and the production of CO_2. The use of an abdominal probe, radiant warmer, hood, and the administration of warm humidified oxygen are critical measures.

Oral feedings are not given because of the respiratory distress, and intravenous feedings supply needed nutrients. Sodium bicarbonate may be ordered if the metabolic acidosis continues; however, it is extremely important for the infant to be ventilated adequately before $NaHCO_3$ is given. Plasma, plasma expanders, whole blood, and packed cells are administered as necessary.

The length of time required for recovery depends on many factors, including the severity of respiratory distress and the amount of oxygen required in the course of treatment. Neonates who are in mild or moderate respiratory difficulty usually improve in 3 to 5 days; newborns who are in severe distress may be ill for several weeks.

Apnea

Apnea is present when breathing is absent for more than 20 seconds. When bradycardia and cyanosis occur in conjunction with apnea, it is called an *apneic spell* or episode. The immaturity of a preterm infant makes him particularly vulnerable to these episodes.

Many factors contribute to the cessation of respirations, including hypoglycemia, hypocalcemia, sepsis, intracranial bleeding, anemia, hypo- or hyperthermia, respiratory distress syndrome, congenital heart disease, and hypo- or hypernatremia.

Preterm newborns and those who demonstrate apneic episodes are placed on cardiorespiratory monitors. When the alarm sounds, the neonate should be assessed for airway obstruction, cyanosis, and bradycardia. Although the average newborn responds to diffuse tactile stimulation, such as flicking of the feet, which reestablishes respirations, there are situations in which the infant may need to be bagged during the apneic episode. Apneic episodes which last more than 20 seconds can result in hypoxic brain damage; therefore, efforts always are directed toward reestablishing a breathing pattern. For frequent, prolonged spells it may be necessary to choose an alternative method. For example, a rocker bed or an oscillating water mattress may be used to increase afferent stimulation. It is important for all providers to avoid stimuli which can trigger apnea, such as suctioning and PO feedings. If the apneic episodes continue despite these interventions, neonatologists may resort to the use of mechanical ventilation, at least until the infant matures.

Complications of Oxygen Administration

Although the administration of oxygen often is perceived as a lifesaving measure, it can be harmful, especially when given in high concentrations and under pressure. Preterm neonates who are mechanically ventilated for prolonged periods are particularly vulnerable to some of the adverse effects.

Bronchopulmonary Dysplasia

Bronchopulmonary dysplasia (BPD) is a chronic pulmonary problem which can follow an acute episode of IRDS. Its cause is related to the prolonged mechanical ventilation which is necessary in treating that disease. Although the clinical manifestations depend on the severity of BPD, the preterm neonate usually is hypoxemic because of hypertrophied peribronchiolar smooth muscles, with air trapping and emphysema. The hyperaeration and atelectasis become chronic conditions.

If BPD is mild, the infant may be weaned from oxygen in a few weeks. Infants who are more severely affected have persistent pulmonary problems, especially chronic respiratory insufficiency, which may require the continuous use of oxygen at home. Right-sided heart failure is not uncommon and may require the use of digoxin and diuretics. The wheezing and hyperexpansion of the chest which are characteristic of reactive airway disease may necessitate the use of theophylline preparations, which are effective. Although this chronic condition may last 2 to 3 years, these infants may need to be hospitalized several times, especially during the first year of life, for lower respiratory tract infections. While the long-term implications of BPD are not known, some data indicate that abnormal pulmonary findings continue into late childhood (Nickerson, 1985).

Retrolental Fibroplasia

Retrolental fibroplasia (RLF) involves abnormal changes in the retina of preterm neonates, especially those who weigh less than 1200 g and are born before the 34th week of gestation. It is seen most commonly in neonates who have received oxygen at concentrations above 40% and hence have elevated blood levels for a prolonged period early in life. High concentrations of oxygen *are* toxic to the retina. Excessive amounts of oxygen result in the constriction of arterioles followed by dilatation and a twisting of retinal vessels. There is hemorrhage, edema, and ultimately retinal detachment which results in blindness. RLF is irreversible.

Preventing this eye problem is problematic. The duration and oxygen concentrations required to produce RLF are not known. Until additional data are available, O_2 concentrations should not exceed 40% unless specifically ordered by a physician.

Hemopoietic Problems
Anemia

A preterm neonate who has a slightly lower hemoglobin concentration than a neonate delivered at term is at greater risk of developing an anemia that is more severe and whose onset is earlier. The tendency to become anemic also may be attributed to a drop in the production of fetal hemoglobin and a shorter survival rate of red blood cells. *Anemia* is present in a newborn when the hemoglobin is less than 14 g/dl.

There are several causes, including blood loss (birth trauma, intrauterine placental bleeding), hemolysis in the presence of blood group incompatibilities, and a variety of infections which result in the development of hemolytic anemia. Normally there is a *physiological anemia* in all newborns which develops gradually over the first 3 months of life, but the bone marrow slowly begins to produce red cells and these infants do not require a transfusion or any other treatment. The hemoglobin of a preterm neonate drops more quickly. The red blood cells have shorter life spans, and there is reduced bone marrow activity. All these events contribute to the development of anemia. Another cause of anemia in a critically ill preterm newborn is the frequent blood sampling necessary to monitor his status.

Clinically, anemic newborns appear to be very pale, and a low red blood cell count confirms the presence of anemia. When the blood loss is acute, the neonate demonstrates all the signs of shock, including low arterial blood pressure, pallor, and a falling hematocrit.

A complete hematology workup is done, usually including a direct Coombs' test, enzyme tests, and tests for the presence of infection. While treatment is based on the cause and the severity, the infant's cardiorespiratory efforts are always monitored often. Frequent hemoglobin and hematocrit samples are also taken. Usually these newborns respond to iron supplements or improve after they begin to receive iron-fortified formulas. Transfusions are given to preterm neonates whose anemia is severe.

Hyperbilirubinemia

When there is an excessive accumulation of bilirubin in the blood of a newborn who also appears to be jaundiced, the condition is called *hyperbilirubinemia.* It is usually seen within 24 to 36 hours of birth. Although *physiological jaundice,* which is a comparable problem, is seen in healthy full-term newborns, the change in skin color appears later on or after the third day of life. This mild, self-limiting jaundice usually subsides by the tenth or twelfth day.

Hyperbilirubinemia is a very common problem in neonates. While preterm neonates are susceptible, other causes which contribute to its development include biliary duct atresia, a variety of intrauterine infections, breast-feeding, certain drugs, and sepsis. However, the more common reason for the jaundice relates to a blood group incompatibility.

The hemolysis that develops in the presence of an ABO incompatibility has its beginnings in utero, when a mother with a type O blood group is carrying a fetus whose blood type is either A or B. The antibodies present in the maternal blood cross the placenta and begin to destroy the red blood cells of the fetus. This process continues after delivery. Another form of blood incompatibility which used to be a common cause of severe jaundice in a newborn is related to the Rh factor. An Rh-negative mother, previously sensitized and currently carrying an Rh-positive fetus, responds to fetal red blood cells crossing the placenta by producing anti-Rh antibodies which then begin to destroy fetal red blood cells. The subsequent health problem, sometimes fatal, was known as *erythroblastosis fetalis.* It is an extremely rare occurrence now because Rh_o (D) immune globulin (RhoGAM) is given to a woman after birth or an abortion is performed to prevent the sensitization process from occurring.

Regardless of its cause, the high levels of bilirubin result in a jaundice which is evident in the skin, the sclera, and the mucous membranes. This condition is due to the presence of unconjugated bilirubin, conjugated bilirubin, or both.

On delivery, the neonate must conjugate bilirubin, or convert it from a lipid-soluble pigment to a water-soluble one. When red blood cells are destroyed in the process of hemolysis, hemoglobin breaks down into heme and globin. The globin, which is soluble in water, is used by the body. However, the heme fraction forms unconjugated bilirubin, an insoluble substance which binds to albumin. Ultimately, the major portion of unconjugated bilirubin is transported to the liver for conjugation; however, a very small fraction remains unbound. The conjugated or converted bilirubin then is secreted into the bile.

While both conjugated and unconjugated bilirubin can cause jaundice, the conjugated form is water-soluble, is nontoxic, and can be excreted in urine. The unconjugated form of bilirubin is not water-soluble and, more important, can be toxic to nerve tissue. With the blood-brain barrier immature and the infant's brain not fully developed, deposits of unconjugated bilirubin, especially in the presence of high serum levels (greater than 15-20 mg/dl), can be devastating. *Kernicterus* is severe irreversible brain damage due to these deposits of unconjugated bilirubin in the brain. Obviously, efforts are always directed toward avoiding levels that can have such dire consequences.

A preterm neonate's liver is immature and inefficient in conjugating and excreting bilirubin. These newborns have limited stores of oxygen and glycogen, both of which are critical to conjugation; therefore, they are at increased risk for developing hyperbilirubinemia.

Jaundice is evident in a neonate whose serum bilirubin level is greater than 6 mg/100 ml. It is important to acknowledge the unpredictable uniqueness of the individual. One neonate may have a serum bilirubin level of 15, continue to be active, suck well, etc., while another infant with the same level may be critically ill, i.e., severely jaundiced, with little spontaneous movement and a poor sucking reflex. Blood levels are parameters for managing these infants; however, the behavioral responses of newborns to the hyperbilirubinemia also are important.

Two methods of treating hyperbilirubinemia are phototherapy and exchange transfusions. Infants who have blood exchanges receive phototherapy afterward. The goals of treatment are to control or prevent hyperbilirubinemia, especially the development of kernicterus, and to control or prevent the development of cardiac failure, which is related to the severe anemia which results from hemolysis of the red blood cells.

The phototherapy consists of exposing the newborn to a source of alternating blue and white lights (wavelength 450 to 500 nm) placed 12 to 18 in above the neonate. The naked neonate is continuously exposed to this light source in order to reduce the serum levels of unconjugated bilirubin (Fig. 17-8). Phototherapy photooxidizes bilirubin to biliverdin, then to secondary yellow pigments, and finally to colorless and presumably nontoxic compounds. The newborn's eyes must be covered with patches of soft material during phototherapy to prevent retinal damage. (The reason for the eye patches should be explained thoroughly to parents.) Bilirubin and hemoglobin levels must be monitored often because the changes in skin color may not give a true reading of the neonate's status. Some of the common side effects of phototherapy are loose stools, skin rashes, alteration in the newborn's previous activity pattern, and overheating due to the heat produced by the phototherapy lights. Neonates receiving phototherapy should have fluid intake increased by 25 to 30 percent because of the insensible water losses which occur "under the lights."

In an exchange transfusion, a cannula is placed in the newborn's umbilical vein, and depending on the neonate's weight, from 5 to 20 ml of blood is alternately removed and replaced with warmed fresh whole blood. In Rh incompatibility, Rh-negative blood is used. In ABO incompatibility, type O blood is given. This procedure removes sensitized red blood cells, lowers the bilirubin levels by 20 to 30 percent, improves the anemia, and decreases the likelihood of congestive failure.

Hemorrhagic Disease of the Newborn

This bleeding disorder occurs in the first few days of life because of a deficiency of factors II, VII, IX, and X, the so-

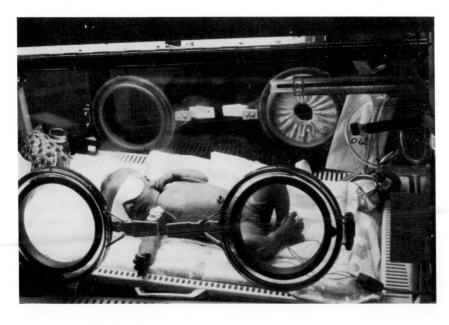

FIGURE 17-8 A jaundiced newborn undergoing phototherapy for hyperbilirubinemia. The newborn's eyes are covered to prevent the development of acute conjunctivitis. The newborn's entire skin area is exposed to provide maximum therapy from the light.

called vitamin K-dependent factors. The preterm newborn is not receiving or is not able to utilize vitamin K, upon which prothrombin and other coagulation factors are dependent for their production in the liver.

The neonate, especially in the second to fifth day of life, has oozing from the cord, hematuria, and gastrointestinal bleeding which may be extensive enough to result in bright red emesis. Stools may be tarry. Petechiae and ecchymosis are evident on the body. Anemia can result from the continued bleeding. The small amount of blood volume in a newborn is a prime concern.

Although the administration of vitamin K intramuscularly results in an increase of clotting factors, severe bleeding may necessitate a transfusion with fresh-frozen plasma and packed red cells. Anemia develops fairly quickly in small preterm neonates; therefore, a transfusion may be essential.

Disseminated Intravascular Coagulation

A problem in coagulation which appears in newborns who have a severe systemic disease such as sepsis, hypoxia, necrotizing enterocolitis, or acidosis is known as *disseminated intravascular coagulation* (DIC). It is not a primary problem but occurs after another pathological condition develops. The exact nature of the stimulation which results in the chaotic coagulation process is not known. However, massive deposits of fibrin in the small blood vessels lead to obstruction, thrombosis, and necrosis. Coagulation studies are changed drastically.

The signs and symptoms of DIC include hemorrhage, petechiae, and ecchymosis; prolonged bleeding episodes from puncture sites; and hypotension. Other organ systems may demonstrate ischemia or bleeding. The DIC can last for several days, or death can follow as a result of obvious hemorrhage and/or damage to vital organs.

Since DIC develops secondarily to another disease, it is important for physicians to treat the primary disease aggressively if the newborn is to survive. Fresh-frozen plasma and platelet transfusions are administered to control and stop bleeding. In neonates who have a major problem with thrombosis, physicians may elect to infuse heparin continuously in an effort to reverse fibrin deposits.

Neurological Problems
Seizures

The newborn has an immature nervous system which makes him susceptible to responding neurologically whenever physiological alterations occur. There are many causes of seizures in the neonatal period, all of which indicate the presence of a serious problem. A metabolic disturbance such as hypoglycemia, hyponatremia, hypocalcemia, or glycogen storage disease results in seizure activity. Birth trauma or hypoxia and the presence of infection in the form of sepsis, cytomegalovirus, or meningitis can cause seizures. The newborn of a substance-abusing mother also may demonstrate this neurological response. Its cause must be determined rapidly in order to decrease

the likelihood of irreversible brain damage, which can occur if the seizure activity continues.

Seizure activity in a newborn is not as evident as the tonic-clonic seizures with a loss of consciousness that typify such activity in an older child or an adult. It is far more subtle, involving side-to-side nystagmus, repetitive blinking, eye rolling, a rhythmic opening and closing of the fists, rigid extension of the extremities, or lip-smacking activities. Many of these activities can go unnoticed, or they may be dismissed as normal responses. Newborns should always be observed for these symptoms.

Treatment involves identifying the underlying cause and treating it. The range of possible causes necessitates a complete hematology workup including electrolytes, a variety of cultures, and spinal fluid analysis. Once a diagnosis is made, treatment is instituted and the seizures should cease. For example, once a low blood sugar value confirms the presence of hypoglycemia as the cause, intravenous glucose corrects the deficiency and seizure activity stops. If seizures persist, it may be necessary to give the newborn an anticonvulsant such as phenobarbital.

Intracranial Trauma

A difficult delivery may rersult in a number of complications for the preterm neonate. The most devastating trauma possible is a periventricular-intraventricular hemorrhage (PV-IVH), which occurs during the first 3 days in 30 to 40 percent of preterm infants who weigh less than 1500 g (Graef and Cone, 1985). Other examples of trauma include subdural hematoma, subarachnoid hemorrhage, and cephalhematoma. While some of these injuries may not be serious, others may be life-threatening or result in significant neurological sequelae. It is important to identify neurological symptoms early, especially in regard to an apparent increase in seizure activity.

In preterm neonates who have a severe PV-IVH, abnormal neurological signs begin to appear within hours after delivery. Initially there is hypotonia, diminished reflexes, lethargy, and irregular respirations. The deterioration is rapid thereafter, with apneic episodes, a high-pitched cry, pallor, cyanosis, a bulging anterior fontanel, seizure activity, decerebrate activity, bradycardia, and dilated pupils evident by the third day. The prognosis is grave. Among neonates who survive, some develop hydrocephalus; others may demonstrate a variety of neurological impairments. The ultimate outcome depends on the severity and extent of the ischemia as well as the supportive measures which are instituted to treat the acidosis, hypothermia, seizures, and other pathophysiological responses.

The neonate's status is precarious, and so he is handled very gently as efforts are made to improve his overall status. These newborns are placed in incubators or warmers; oxygen is administered, anticonvulsants may be given, and they may need ventilator assistance with continuous positive airway pressure (CPAP) to prevent additional hypoxia. Intravenous fluids are given to maintain cerebral perfusion; however, the rate of administration is adjusted carefully so that it is not excessive, which could worsen the cerebral hemorrhage. Spinal taps are done in severe cases to decrease the intracranial pressure and remove blood from the cerebrospinal fluid. If hydrocephalus develops, a shunt may be performed at a later date.

Inborn Errors of Metabolism
Glucose-6-Phosphate Dehydrogenase Deficiency

Glucose-6-phosphate dehydrogenase (G6PD) deficiency is a disorder of cellular metabolism in which an enzyme that normally regulates glucose metabolism in red blood cells is absent. A newborn with G6PD is more prone to acute hemolysis and jaundice due to hyperbilirubinemia. Although this deficiency does not always produce hyperbilirubinemia in a newborn, a hemolytic episode may occur more easily in the presence of a certain triggering agents, and the hyperbilirubinemia may be more severe.

The most common problem of this type in a newborn is an acute acquired hemolytic anemia which develops after exposure to certain drugs, chemicals, or infections. Drugs which begin this hemolytic response include aspirin, some sulfonamides, antimalarials, ascorbic acid, and chloramphenicol.

In a newborn with sickle cell anemia, G6PD deficiency can result in chronic hemolysis because of the increase in immature red cells and the fragile nature of the more mature red cells. A neonate who is in sickle cell crisis because of an infection is more likely to be exposed to drugs that may act as triggering agents, or the infection itself may precipitate an acute hemolytic episode.

The symptoms are similar to those present in anemia and include jaundice with hyperbilirubinemia, intermittent pyrexia, hypoglycemia, seizures, pallor, and ketonuria. Clinical signs appear within hours after a particular drug has been administered or a couple of days after exposure to an infectious process. The severity of the hemolytic episode varies and depends on the development of other symptoms and complications. The anemia that develops may be severe enough to require a transfusion. Normally, discontinuing the medication or treating the infection which is present relieves the acute hemolytic episodes.

Phenylketonuria

Infants with *phenylketonuria* (PKU) have a deficiency in the liver enzyme phenylalanine hydroxylase, which is essential in converting phenylalanine to tyrosine. Phenylalanine is an amino acid which is necessary for growth, and normally any excess in the body is converted to tyrosine. A neonate with PKU is unable to convert the excess. The accumulation of phenylalanine and its metabolites in the brain results in severe developmental delays as well as other neurological sequelae. Although there are several variations of PKU which pertain to lower blood phenylalanine levels, this discussion focuses on the "classic" form of PKU.

At birth, these preterm and full-term neonates appear to be normal, with blond hair, blue eyes, and fair skin. They have a predisposition to developing eczema. By 6 months of age they demonstrate a range of developmental delays, seizure activity, failure to thrive, and persistent vomiting. As they grow older, their general behavior worsens. A characteristic of the disease is the musty odor of the urine excreted, which is due to one of the metabolites of phenylalanine, phenylpyruvic acid.

The Guthrie test is required for all newborns in all states in an effort to screen newborns for PKU. An important aspect of this screening test involves proper timing. *The Guthrie test should not be done until after the neonate has received formula or breast feedings for at least 24 hours.* After oral feedings have been taken, phenylalanine and its metabolites begin to accumulate in the body and brain. In many states routine follow-up testing for PKU is performed about 6 weeks after birth to ensure identification of all those with the deficiency. When both tests are positive with plasma phenylalanine levels of 20 mg/dl, these infants are placed on a formula low in phenylalanine, such as Lofenalac. In the case of PKU, severe neurological impairment is preventable as long as the individual remains on a low-phenylalanine diet.

Since phenylalanine is essential for growth, it is important to include it in the diet. Therefore, long-term follow-up, especially nutritional counseling, is an important aspect of health care. Initially these infants are seen weekly as providers attempt to maintain phenylalanine levels between 4 and 8 mg/dl. Solids are introduced at the usual age (4½ to 6 months); however, these foods are added according to their calculated phenylalanine content.

There is no agreement about how long the diet should be continued. Although some suggest that this dietary control should continue through the sixth year of life, when maximum brain development occurs, others at conservative centers believe that the diet should be continued for life.

Substance Abuse
Fetal Alcohol Syndrome

The effects of alcohol use in pregnancy was first described in 1973, when investigators identified certain characteristics among newborns delivered to women who had consumed alcohol regularly during pregnancy. It is not known whether alcohol or the breakdown products of alcohol are responsible for the anomalies. Researchers also do not know how much alcohol needs to be ingested for its effects to be evident in the newborn; however, for mothers who consume 90 ml (3 oz) a day, the risk of fetal alcohol syndrome (FAS) can be as high as 30 to 50 percent (Cloherty and Stark, 1985).

These neonates have growth deficiencies in length and height, microcephaly, and a variety of facial abnormalities including micrognathia, maxillary hypoplasia, and epicanthal folds. Cardiac problems, especially septal defects, and a number of joint and limb abnormalities also are evident in physical assessments of these newborns. However, the organ that seems to be most vulnerable to damage from alcohol is the brain because of the range of developmental delay, which extends from mild to very severe cases of impairment. Later in childhood there is a higher frequency of failure to thrive, feeding problems, hyperactivity, and speech and language problems. In addition to these physical characteristics, the newborn has all the withdrawal symptoms of his alcohol-dependent mother, which usually occur in the first 24 hours of life, including tremors, abdominal distention, sweating, irritability, opisthotonos, lethargy, and seizures.

Treatment is symptomatic and supportive, since the problems are not life-threatening. Maintaining a quiet environment and preventing excessive stimulation decrease the likelihood of seizure activity in these infants. Long-term management includes infant stimulation programs and anticonvulsant therapy.

Narcotic Abstinence Syndrome

A narcotic-addicted mother gives birth to a neonate who suffers from *narcotic abstinence syndrome* (NAS) because almost all narcotic drugs cross the placenta, affect the developing embryo or fetus, and result in a passive type of addiction. Intrauterine problems such as fetal distress, anoxia, and asphyxia can result in stillbirth, preeclampsia, or placenta previa; abruptio placentae may cause a number of antenatal problems. Maternal infections, especially hepatitis or one of the sexually transmitted diseases, also may affect the fetus.

The neonate born to a narcotic-addicted mother can be preterm or SGA and/or suffer from IUGR. However, the most significant clinical findings are the signs of narcotic withdrawal, which are seen in 80 to 90 percent of these newborns (Merker, Higgins, and Kinnard, 1985). Usually they are evident in the first 24 hours. Hyperreflexia, clonus, hypertonia, a high-pitched cry, and hyperirritability as well as tremors, yawning, and sneezing demonstrate central nervous system involvement. Although the new-

born seems to have a ravenous appetite and a strong sucking reflex, feedings are not taken well and there is excessive drooling, vomiting, and diarrhea. Tachypnea, mottling, a "stuffy" nose, elevated temperature, profuse sweating, and erratic sleep patterns also are evident.

Swaddling helps decrease the irritability in some NAS infants. Others, however, may need to be given medications such as paregoric, phenobarbital, diazepam, chlorpromazine, or tincture of opium. The drug selected depends on the symptoms demonstrated.

The Neonatal Abstinence Scoring Tool is used to assess the overall status of the passively addicted newborn and especially to identify the progression or regression of withdrawal. Initially the neonate is observed hourly for the first 24 hours in order to collect baseline data and identify the beginning of withdrawal. The same characteristics are evaluated every 2 hours during the second 24-hour period and every 4 hours after 48 hours. The behaviors observed include some of the following: tremors, sleep patterns, stools, feedings, yawning, sneezing, respiratory rate, hyperreflexia, vomiting or regurgitation, and hypertonicity. The dosage of the drug is determined by the average daily score on this assessment tool and by the infant's body weight. If there is an increase in the score, the dose is increased; however, if the score decreases, it must remain low for 2 consecutive days before the dose is decreased. Thus the pharmacological management is related to the symptoms evident in the newborn; treatment otherwise is supportive.

Care of the High-Risk Newborn

Preterm infants account for about 22 percent of all births in the United States (Olds, London, and Ladewig, 1984); the majority of those in a high-risk intensive care setting

TABLE 17-4 Heat Loss and Gain in High-Risk Neonates

Type	Effect	Nursing Intervention
Conduction	Heat transferred to colder or warmer surfaces when objects are placed in *direct contact* with neonate's body; loss or gain increases with temperature differences and thermal conductivity of the object	Place neonate on covered table; dress in shirt, diaper if possible; stocking cap on head to prevent significant heat loss from head; dress warmly and wrap in prewarmed cotton blankets when removing from thermal environment; warm stethoscope before applying to body surface: place blanket over x-ray cassette
Convection	Heat loss or gain as a result of temperature of air surrounding neonate; velocity of circulating air also has adverse effect	Place neonate away from drafts in the nursery, especially fan or air-conditioning; neonate under radiant warmer particularly susceptible; a bassinet with the deep position of mattress protects the newborn during transport
Radiation	Heat transferred from baby to nearby solid objects which are *not* in direct contact with baby's body regardless of surrounding air temperature	Place warmer/bassinet away from outside walls, windows, drafts from air-conditioning
Evaporation	Loss of heat through evaporation of moisture, especially after delivery; moisture from skin and lungs which is converted from liquid to vapor	After birth, neonate is dried thoroughly with warm towels and placed in prewarmed radiant warmer or incubator; a humidified incubator decreases the heat loss, but water in the reservoir needs to be changed at least once a day, and silver nitrate should be added to decrease likelihood of bacterial colonization within water reservoir

require thermal, ventilatory, and nutritional support. If these support systems are not available, the preterm infants develop hypoglycemia, hypothermia, a number of metabolic problems, and an increase in existing respiratory distress or insufficiency. They fail to grow and deteriorate to the point where no support systems can ensure survival or safeguard the subsequent quality of life.

Providing Thermal Support

High-risk infants can maintain body temperature without additional stress only if environmental temperatures are kept within a relatively narrow range. The nurse's constant observations and assessments of the newborn's immediate environment and body temperature help ensure the delivery of safe and effective thermal support measures. Although the neutral thermal environment for any neonate depends on his weight, age, and maturity, it is usually well above the normal room temperature.

These particular newborns lose or gain body heat by conduction, convection, radiation, or evaporation. In Table 17-4 the mechanisms and some effective nursing interventions are reviewed. High-risk infants often are placed in overhead radiant warmers or incubators to achieve and maintain a body temperature of 36.5°C; however, it is important for a nurse to be aware of certain problems. For example, if the newborn is in a closed incubator, connective and conductive heat losses are less; however, evaporative losses continue, since some medical centers do not utilize humidified air because of the ever-present threat of bacterial colonization of the water reservoir in the incubator. A nurse also should realize that an infant in an incubator may still lose heat through radiation if the incubator itself is placed in a cold environment or may gain heat if it is in a very warm environment. Although the neonate may be in an overhead radiant warmer, the nurse needs to know that convective heat loss is possible with air circulating in the nursery; therefore, the warmer must be kept away from drafty areas. Evaporative water loss may be significant for a newborn who is maintained under a warmer for an extended period; thus in addition to monitoring the body temperature, it is necessary to maintain an accurate intake and output.

Whether the infant is housed under a radiant warmer or in an incubator, the use of an abdominal probe regulating system is recommended. This is a feedback system which regulates the infant's environmental temperature according to his skin temperature. A probe is attached to the neonate's abdomen over the liver, which is the point of maximum body temperature (Fig. 17-9). If the infant is under a warmer, the probe must be shielded so that it monitors the neonate's skin temperature, not the temperature of the radiant heat being produced by the overhead warmer. This precaution is not necessary when the baby is in an incubator.

When the baby's skin temperature begins to drop, the probe registers the fall in temperature and signals the heat production unit, through the feedback mechanism, to increase heat production as necessary to maintain the newborn's temperature at a preset point of 37.5°C (99.6°F). When the skin probe detects a rise in the neonate's temperature, the feedback system alerts the heat production unit so that heat production decreases in order to maintain the desired skin temperature. A major problem with this type of regulating unit is that it may mask the symptoms of hypothermia and hyperthermia. Therefore, it is most important for the nurse to monitor both the incubator hood temperature and the neonate's body temperature serially.

To maintain a constant, desirable environment, a newborn who is kept in an incubator should not be removed from it. When lengthy procedures warrant removal from the incubator, a radiant heater should be placed over the

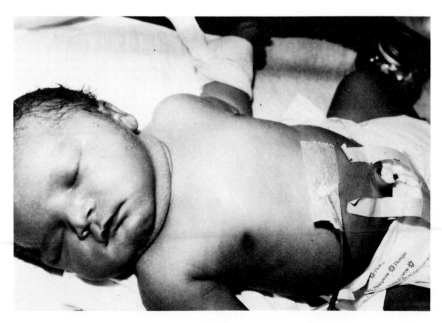

FIGURE 17-9 A neonate whose temperature is being monitored with a skin temperature probe. An umbilical arterial line for monitoring PO$_2$ is in place. *(Photo courtesy of David Stewart, M.D.)*

newborn to provide external heat and prevent heat stress. A nurse who has to transport the newborn should set up a battery-operated or prewarmed incubator in order to continue these thermal support measures.

It is critical for a nurse to make certain that any equipment which comes into direct contact with the infant is warmed beforehand. Body heat is lost quickly through conduction when a cold stethoscope is used on the chest or the newborn is placed on a cold x-ray cassette. It is important for the nurse to provide an environment in which heat loss or gain is minimal. Such interventions decrease the amount of additional stress placed on an already compromised neonate.

Providing Ventilatory Support

Providing ventilatory support to the high-risk newborn is another crucial aspect of care. Ventilators are used for several problems in the newborn, including hypoxia, hypercapnia, apnea, respiratory acidosis, and respiratory failure (Graef and Cone, 1985). The method by which this support is provided depends on the status of the infant. The high-risk neonate may quickly deteriorate to respiratory failure or death if deviations in the respiratory pattern are not recognized immediately. Therefore, the ability to identify respiratory distress is of utmost importance in caring for a high-risk newborn.

The respiratory cycle consists of an inspiratory phase and an expiratory phase. The clinically observed deviations in the inspiratory phase of a neonate in respiratory distress are retractions, seesaw breathing, and nasal flaring. The clinical manifestation of respiratory distress in the expiratory phase of the cycle is an expiratory grunt. Another symptom of respiratory distress is cyanosis, which is a sign of oxygen lack. Any of these signs is an indication that immediate ventilatory support needs to be provided.

If cyanosis is the only clinical sign of inadequate respiratory exchange, whiffs of low percentage concentrations of oxygen may alleviate the condition. If the blood gases and clinical appearance of the neonate indicate a need for continued oxygen therapy, the oxygen should be provided by means of (1) an oxygen hood, (2) CPAP, or (3) an infant respirator. Whichever method is chosen, *warmed humidified* oxygen should be administered in sufficient concentrations to maintain a PaO_2 between 50 and 80 mm Hg (normal PaO_2 is 80 to 100 mm Hg). These levels are considered adequate to meet the neonate's metabolic needs without affecting the developing retina.

A newborn who can ventilate adequately can be maintained in an oxygen hood if his oxygen concentration requirements can be met in this way. The oxygen hood is a plastic bubble into which the neonate's head is placed and through which warm humidified oxygen is delivered.

For a neonate who has respiratory distress syndrome and needs a positive pressure breathing apparatus to prevent the alveoli from becoming atelectatic (collapsed), CPAP or CDAP can be used (Fig. 17-10). This method involves attaching a newborn who is breathing spontaneously to a system that supplies oxygen under a constant distending pressure to the airway by means of a head box, face mask, or nasal prongs and to the lower airway by means of an endotracheal tube. The baby's blood gases must be monitored as frequently as every 3 to 4 hours. In addition, the concentration of oxygen the neonate is receiving and the respiratory pattern of the neonate must be monitored continually.

Frequent suctioning of the endotracheal tube, nasal passages, or oropharynx, depending on the CPAP or CDAP delivery system being used, is important to prevent airway obstruction due to mucus in the posterior pharynx, glottis, trachea, or bronchi. Also, when done carefully,

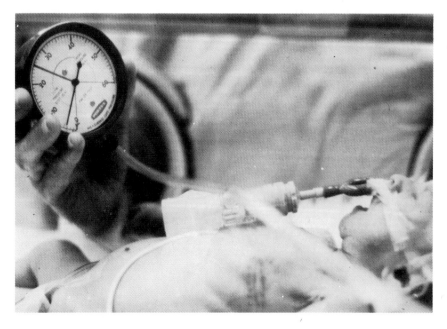

FIGURE 17-10 A neonate receiving continuous positive airway pressure. (*Courtesy of Howard A. Fox, M.D.*)

chest physical therapy mobilizes secretions and aids in their removal.

Newborns with respiratory distress syndrome who are unable to breathe independently or who are repeatedly apneic for prolonged periods and do not respond to CPAP should be placed on a respirator. Mechanical ventilation is the only effective treatment for severe hypercarbia ($PaCO_2$ of 70 mm Hg or more). There are two basic types of mechanical ventilators: positive pressure and negative pressure.

Positive pressure respirators are of two types. In one type, the volume of administered gas is controlled by limiting the inspiratory pressure created in the respiratory tract during its delivery. The second type can be pressure-restricted and can also limit the volume of gas delivered. It can ensure that preset pressure limits are not exceeded and provide a calculated volume of tidal air. The negative pressure respirator encloses the body from the neck down and moves gas into and out of the lungs by intermittently creating negative pressure around the trunk. It is rarely used nowadays except in newborns who have neuromuscular problems, primarily because their lungs are normal; however, their respirations are diminished.

By whatever means oxygen is delivered to an infant in respiratory distress, it is important that it be ordered by percentage concentration and not only by liter flow. Frequent clinical observations, the recording of vital signs, and documentation of the neonate's respiratory pattern are essential in providing the necessary ventilatory support. *Any time* oxygen is administered to a high-risk neonate, it *must* be warmed and humidified.

Providing Nutritional Support

Once a thermal environment and ventilatory support have been provided for a high-risk neonate, the next area of concern is nutritional support. High-risk neonates cannot tolerate nutritional deprivation because their caloric reserves are limited. If deprivation goes unchecked, these newborns fail to grow, metabolic and respiratory symptoms develop secondary to this deprivation, they suffer long-term effects in organ systems (especially the brain), and they eventually die. If the neonate is less than 33 weeks of gestational age, is in distress, and weighs less than 1500 g (3 lb, 5 oz), nutritional support must be provided by means of intravenous therapy.

Intravenous therapy is used to provide partial or complete maintenance of fluids and electrolytes because the preterm neonate's gastrointestinal tract is too immature to tolerate the fluid volume necessary for adequate nutrition. It is also used to supply adequate calories through a glucose solution to prevent hypoglycemia and provide protein-sparing calories until the gastrointestinal tract can tolerate nutrients. During the first 24 hours, 10% dextrose in water should be administered at a rate of 80 to 100 ml/kg/d, or 3 to 4 ml/kg/h. This amount of intravenous fluid provides for insensible fluid losses and adequate urine output, supplies 40 to 50 kcal/kg/d of carbohydrate, and is partially protein sparing. The total volume of fluids should

be increased if the infant is under a radiant warmer or phototherapy light.

Current literature suggests that total parenteral nutrition (TPN; hyperalimentation), which provides a highly concentrated solution of protein, glucose, and other nutrients, may be the most suitable way to provide the nutritional support that will facilitate weight gain in a sick low-birth-weight newborn. Emulsified fat also can be administered to promote weight gain. However, it cannot be mixed with glucose solutions and therefore must be administered in a separate intravenous line from the hyperalimentation solution.

Neonates who are not in distress but are of less than 33 weeks of gestation and therefore probably do not have a coordinated suck-swallow reflex, a gag reflex, and a fully developed esophageal sphincter can be fed by the gavage method. Newborns are obligatory nasal breathers, i.e., do not breathe through their mouths even if the nares are obstructed. It is recommended that feeding tubes be inserted through the mouth rather than through the nose, especially if the neonate is in respiratory distress. If the neonate is not showing any signs of respiratory distress and there is no danger of occluding the nares and thereby hampering ventilation, the neonate can be fed by the nasogastric (NG) route. Further information on gavage feeding is presented in Chap. 10.

Irritation of the nares and oral cavity can be prevented through the use of proper oral hygiene and cleansing of the nares. Antibiotic ointments sometimes are applied to the outside portion of the nares to prevent infection, and lemon-glycerine swabs can be used to cleanse the mouth to prevent drying and cracking. Neonates on CPAP or respiratory therapy should have an orogastric catheter inserted to prevent gastrointestinal tract distention.

Sometimes continuous NG feedings are ordered for very small newborns (less than 1000 to 1200 g) who cannot tolerate the passage of a gavage tube every 3 hours (Cloherty and Stark, 1985). In these instances a pump is used to deliver the prescribed hourly rate.

No matter which method of feeding is ultimately selected for a specific infant, it is important to provide nutritional support to every high-risk infant as soon after birth as possible. The first gavage feeding should begin within 4 to 6 hours after birth, and feedings should be given at least every 2 to 3 hours. If an infant is not able to tolerate gavage feeding owing to illness or immaturity, intravenous nutritional support can be begun almost immediately after birth.

High-risk neonates require 80 to 100 ml/kg of fluid intake during the first 24 hours and 100 to 150 ml/kg/d thereafter. It is important to monitor the infant's urinary output and to check the specific gravity, pH, and glucose of the urine every 8 hours. An increase in the concentration and a decrease in the volume of urinary output indicate the need to increase fluid intake. Alterations in the pH and glucose signal the need to alter the type of fluid being administered.

The caloric requirements of newborn infants are between 90 and 130 kcal/kg/d. High-risk newborns may eventually require more than 130 kcal/kg/d to achieve a satisfactory growth rate. Most standard formulas provide the required caloric balance of 10 to 15 percent protein, 45 to 55 percent carbohydrate, and 30 to 45 percent fat. If the mother chooses to breast-feed the newborn, her milk may be expressed and given to the neonate by gavage or bottle until the infant's condition permits breast-feeding.

Monitoring the Neonate

Nurses who work with critically ill newborns have highly refined observational abilities, have an extensive knowledge base, and possess the technical competencies to deliver care as needs arise. Certainly the sophisticated monitoring devices which are available in neonatal intensive care units enable nurses to perform many tasks very efficiently. Unfortunately, machines break down, and it is extremely important not to become too reliant on space-age technological advancements. Eyes and ears remain the most important tools available to a nurse who is assessing the overall status of a neonate.

When daily weights are ordered, they should be done on the *same scale,* at the *same time,* with the same attachments, and ideally by the same nurse. It is very important to pay particular attention to the presence or absence of arm boards, dressings, and intravenous lines, all of which affect the result. A loss in weight from the previous day may not be due to dehydration; it can be the result of a smaller dressing applied the day before. Even the smallest weight fluctuations are significant in a vulnerable neonate.

Nursing interventions which need to be implemented when working with these neonates include monitoring all vital signs, maintaining a neutral thermal environment, monitoring the administration of the proper percentage of oxygen and humidity, ensuring an adequate caloric intake, and observing the infant for signs of complications such as hyperbilirubinemia, hypo- or hyperglycemia, acidosis, hyponatremia, hypocalcemia, meningitis, and shock.

A newborn sometimes needs to be isolated and placed on precautions. It is the nurse's responsibility to ensure that all providers adhere to those measures, and the task is an enormous one. The nurse is in charge of controlling infections, enforcing meticulous hand washing by everyone, disposing of equipment properly, and teaching parents how they too play a vital part in controlling the infectious process. A nurse is charged also with overseeing individuals who have housekeeping responsibilities to ensure that they understand the need to be thorough in cleaning a private room, specific equipment, or an incubator so that there is no likelihood of future cross-contamination.

Newborns who are isolated for TORCH infections may necessitate changes in staffing patterns. For example, pregnant nurses should not care for neonates with cytomegalovirus. A newborn with rubella sheds active virus for more than a year after birth. Therefore, it is important to know the rubella titer levels of all nurses on the unit to be certain that only those with safe titer levels are assigned to care for the infant. Pregnant nurses and those who are attempting to become pregnant should refrain from any contact with these neonates. The devastating effects of rubella on a developing embryo necessitate an intensive educational effort to inform all female personnel and female visitors.

Intravenous therapy is an important aspect of treating these critically ill newborns. It is essential that the infusion rates which are ordered be received by the baby. Burette fluid levels are monitored and recorded at least hourly and more frequently in some medical centers. The pump must be examined to be certain it is functioning properly, and changes in the rate of flow must be made as promptly as they are ordered. When a bottle or bag of solution is added to the setup, it is checked and double-checked. Whenever a neonate is returned to the unit, the solution, which is up and running, is verified along with the rate of flow.

The intake and output of a sick neonate need to be recorded meticulously. Special attention is directed toward weighing diapers before application and after use to identify precisely these very small amounts of urine and/or feces. With frequent blood sampling for electrolytes, glucose, or a hematocrit, it is necessary to identify the blood volumes removed.

Many of the problems discussed above involve seizure activity in the newborn. It is critical for the nurse to describe and record the entire sequence of events. The starting time, the duration, the parts of the body involved, the behavior before and after, and the time all seizure activity stopped must be entered on the seizure chart. This form of data collection is important in helping physicians determine the cause of seizure activity.

Antibiotic therapy plays a major role in successfully treating a neonate with sepsis or another type of infectious process. Therefore, a nurse who administers these drugs must know them and their actions, side effects, incompatibilities, toxic signs, and proper methods of administration. The correct dose, which is determined on the basis of weight or body surface area, must be calculated correctly and mixed with the manufacturer's suggested diluent. The intravenous antibiotics must be regulated carefully to ensure that they are delivered within time parameters that maximize their effectiveness. A nurse also needs to evaluate the infant's response to these drugs. With infants who are discharged on certain medications, teaching parents all about the drugs is a time-consuming but extremely important activity.

There is no doubt that the parents are apprehensive or frightened about the equipment which surrounds a very tiny newborn who is in this strange environment of perplexing noises and unfamiliar health care providers. The primary nurse must develop a meaningful relationship with the parents in stressful circumstances. Warmth, compassion, and understanding play a large part in teaching, explaining, counseling, and interpreting the events that are taking place. Phenomenal advancements have been made in caring for these neonates. However, it is the human element—the empathy, the expertise, the understanding, the concern about improving patient outcomes—that continues to be the most constant contribution by nurses to the progress that has occurred.

Regionalization of Care

For several years there has been a nationwide movement toward regionalization of perinatal care. Within each geographic region one specialized referral hospital is established, and high-risk newborns (or, ideally, high-risk pregnant women) are transferred there for intensive care. The need for such specialized care facilities is substantial. Between 3 and 6 percent of the babies born in community hospitals require specialized perinatal care; a third of this group needs to be placed in intensive care units. Approximately 80 percent of all high-risk infants born each year find their way into an intensive care nursery. Each state is responsible for setting up and implementing the criteria for regionalization. Regionalization is based on a concept of levels of care. The objective is to centralize the technology and expertise in order to reduce maternal and neonatal mortality and decrease infant morbidity. The care that can currently be provided to high-risk mothers and infants can be divided into three levels; level 1 is the least sophisticated, and level 3 is the most sophisticated (Table 17-5).

The timing of the referral to a perinatal intensive care center is as important as the benefits of this center to the mother and neonate. Delay in transporting the mother or neonate to a center offering specialized medical and surgical care may prove detrimental to the immediate or long-term survival of the patient. It is preferable for a high-risk pregnant woman to be transferred before labor begins and to be delivered in a facility where a continuum of specialized care can be provided throughout labor, delivery, and the neonatal period. The uterus is the ideal incubator.

If a high-risk neonate is delivered in a community hospital, stabilization of the infant must be initiated by the delivering hospital and continued until transport can be effected by the regional center. It is preferable that transpoation of neonates be provided by level 3 regional perinatal centers. These centers have the specialized equipment and medical staff with the expertise to identify risks and provide the care needed to stabilize the neonate before transport and continue stabilization throughout the transport procedure.

Indications for perinatal intensive care may occur at any time during the prenatal or perinatal period: during pregnancy, immediately before delivery, upon delivery, and after delivery. More than half of neonatal deaths (those occuring within 28 days after birth) occur during the first 24 hours of life. Therefore, early identification of risk and appropriately timed transport to a regional perinatal center form an essential part of the care of high-risk pregnant women and neonates.

Transfer of the Neonate

Skilled health team members at these centers have the knowledge and expertise essential for dealing with the very special problems of an acutely ill neonate. When a

TABLE 17-5 Regionalization: Levels of Care

Level 1 Hospital

Care to mothers and neonates without complications
Staff members who can recognize maternal, fetal, and neonatal complications and make appropriate referrals
Facilities to perform an emergency cesarean section, resuscitate the newborn, and stabilize and observe the at-risk newborn
A 24-hour on-call blood bank
Anesthesiology service and radiology and laboratory facilities

Level 2 Hospital

Same as level 1 plus care of women who have complications of pregnancy
Capability of performing a cesarean section in 15 min
Staff members who observe and assess at-risk newborns and are prepared to provide short-term ventilation, external cardiac massage, IV therapy for infusion of sodium bicarbonate and blood volume expanders
Board-certified obstetricians and pediatricians
Nurses specially trained in high-risk maternity and neonatal care

Level 3 Hospital

Provision of full-range of maternal, fetal, and neonatal services including education and community outreach programs
Obstetric intensive care unit
Neonatal intensive care unit
Transportation from and consultation to level 1 and level 2 units

newborn needs to be transferred, consideration of the baby's physical status, the equipment of the transporting vehicle, and the coordination of administrative details between the hospitals contributes to the safety and efficiency of the transfer. Transfer has become relatively common, and some states now support programs designed to transfer neonates safely in specially equipped helicopters, airplanes, or ambulances.

Some regional perinatal centers have a transport team consisting of a physician, a nurse, and a respiratory therapist who are involved in transferring a critically ill neonate (Fig. 17-11). After an initial examination is done at the referral hospital, impending treatments or procedures are explained to parents and the necessary consent forms are signed. Admission forms also are completed at this time. These experienced personnel provide intensive care during the actual transport. Extensive specialized training qualifies these health care providers to deal with any emergencies which arise en route.

Physical Status of the Neonate

When an acutely ill neonate is to be transferred, provision should be made to ensure that the trip will be safe and that there will be no deterioration of the neonate's condition. It is especially important to prevent or immediately

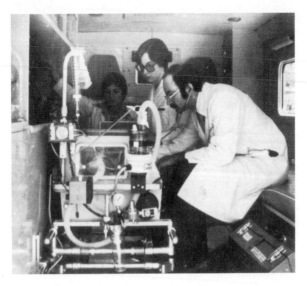

FIGURE 17-11 The transport team transferring a neonate to a perinatal center. The interior of the ambulance has been modified to accommodate essential equipment. *(Photo courtesy of I.J. Weinfeld, M.D., Toledo Hospital, Toledo, Ohio.)*

recognize and treat hypoxia, hypoglycemia, and hypothermia, and aspiration, since these conditions may contribute to the neonate's demise.

Because of their high metabolic rate, newborns are susceptible to hypoglycemia, especially if they are not fed by mouth during the first few hours of life. The symptoms of hypoglycemia are described above. Some physicians start a 10% glucose intravenous solution to prevent the occurrence of hypoglycemia during transport.

Hypoxia must be prevented. Oxygen, if necessary, should be administered by means of mask, an incubator, or assisted ventilation. Transporting a newborn with an endotracheal tube in place is particularly difficult; the tube may be dislodged in the course of moving, resulting in further distress. Adequate oxygenation decreases neonatal stress and prevents cerebral damage which may impair intellectual function.

Hypothermia is a major hazard to the neonate. The best means of ensuring temperature maintenance is a heated incubator with its own self-contained power pack or a warming unit for automotive currents. Blankets with an inner layer of aluminum foil are also effective in reducing heat loss.

Positioning remains an important measure for preventing aspiration. The baby should be kept on his side or abdomen while being transported. As always, the neonate's physical problem dictates the best position. A newborn who has a tracheoesophageal fistula, for example, must be kept in a sitting position to decrease the possibility of aspiration and the development of pneumonia, which would require postponement of surgery. Similarly, a neonate with an omphalocele is kept supine with the head to the side.

On occasion intravenous fluid therapy is begun before the newborn leaves the hospital. The infusion site should be chosen carefully. A scalp vein appears to be most suit-

able, for there is no interference when the body position is adjusted. The baby also is allowed freedom to move the head from side to side without the danger of infiltration, which is not the case if the infusion site is in an extremity.

The Transporting Vehicle

Several hours of travel may be required for interhospital transport when an ambulance is used; therefore, the ambulance must be adequately equipped for safe transfer, and all the equipment must be in working order. There must be an adequate supply of oxygen, including supplemental tanks if the vehicle is delayed by mechanical difficulty. No ambulance should be used unless it has adequate equipment to handle the routine and emergency situations which may arise during transport.

Many regional perinatal centers have their own ambulances and/or aircrft for transport. Personnel at other centers have persuaded ambulance personnel to modify one or two vehicles explicitly for neonatal transport. The interiors have been altered to accommodate a portable incubator, monitors, and heated aerosol, suction, and other apparatus. In addition, the electrical systems of these vehicles have been redesigned to permit the use of essential equipment.

Nursing Management

All pertinent information should accompany the infant as he goes from one hospital to another. A nurse who accompanies the baby tells the receiving health team members what has happened since the baby's birth. The report should include the maternal history, the infant's status at delivery (including the Apgar score), and his behavior in the nursery. The data accumulated up to the time the baby is received in the referral hospital will serve as a baseline against which to assess his subsequent status.

If it is not possible for a nurse to accompany the patient, a set of written notes, complete in every detail, should identify problems, report observations, and state the sequence of pertinent events. A more personal and more informative alternative is a telephone conversation with the head nurse of the neonatal intensive care unit to which the patient will be admitted. The nursing assessment with its observations and evaluations is usually graciously and gratefully accepted by those who will be responsible for caring for the baby. A report by telephone informs the nurses at the receiving station of the baby's status at the beginning of transport and gives them time to assemble the equipment they will need.

When an experienced transport team is involved, admitting sheets and consent forms accompany the newborn. However, when a community has no such arrangement and neonatal transfer is essential, legal consent forms and signatures for treatment may be overlooked. If the father accompanies the baby, there is no problem. However, when he elects to remain with his wife, arrangements may have to be made to send permissions or other legal forms acceptable to the receiving hospital by telegram.

The transfer of a critically ill newborn involves the

combined, coordinated efforts of many people in two health care facilities. Transfer must be done without delay and without needless administrative impediments. Although the ambulance or helicopter ride is traumatizing to any neonate, whether it contributes to a deteriorating health status depends on professional forethought in planning the move.

Parents whose newborns are moved to referral centers are forced to accept separation almost immediately after birth. Also, they may have to travel long distances to see their infants. Both factors preclude early or frequent contact with the baby. The personnel of obstetric units as well as those at the receiving hospitals need to be aware of the psychological and emotional impact on the parents of these children.

Promoting Parent-Infant Interaction

The birth of a high-risk neonate usually requires both physical separation of the neonate from the parents and emotional adjustment by the parents to the reality of the situation. Physical separation may be necessitated by the newborn's or mother's requirement for ongoing medical and nursing observations, the baby's need for a regulated thermal environment, required intervention to stabilize the baby immediately after birth, or transfer to a regional perinatal center.

Nursing staff members must be able to keep the parents informed of the status of the fetus or neonate as soon as a high-risk situation has been identified. Preparation for whatever is likely to happen next should be included in the information provided. It is important to make certain that the parents understand the information being given to them. The nurse should encourage the parents to repeat what they have been told, using their own terminology.

When the delivery of a high-risk neonate is anticipated, the expectant parents are encouraged to visit an intensive care nursery if this is at all feasible. A visit may help familiarize the parents with what to expect if the neonate is in need of such care. Every attempt should be made to have the parents see the newborn as soon after delivery as possible. Seeing rather than imagining is vital to acceptance, and physical separation for any length of time interferes with successful parent-newborn interaction. The incidence of infection in the nursery is not increased by parents' visiting as long as they adhere to proper hand-washing and gowning techniques (Fig. 17-12).

Visiting hours in the nursery should be flexible enough to meet the needs of the parents and the infant; they must also be compatible with nursery routines and emergencies. Therefore, parents should be informed that their visiting hours may be altered if an emergency situation arises. In many hospitals members of the extended family, such as grandparents, siblings, and significant others, are allowed to visit the newborn. This practice should be encouraged as long as hand washing, gowning, number of visitors, and time and length of stay are monitored.

Like grieving, the emotional adjustment of parents to the high-risk newborn involves three phases: initial shock, followed by an awareness of reality and, finally, acceptance of reality. During the shock phase, the parents' ability to cope with the situation may be limited. They should be encouraged to visit the infant as frequently as possible. The information given to them should be simple and honest since it may be difficult or impossible for them to deal with complex information at this time. It is important to establish a therapeutic rapport with the parents in which they will be able to express their feelings, whether positive or negative. They should be encouraged to interact both physically and emotionally with the newborn. Close contact with a neonate who subsequently dies does not intensify the grief reaction. It may actually help the parents experience grief in a more positive manner.

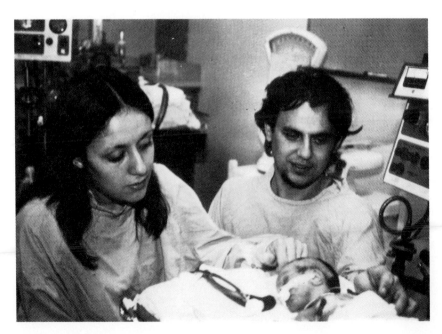

FIGURE 17-12   Visiting and early involvement with their tiny baby in spite of his apparent fragility and the surrounding equipment is now known to be extremely important to parents' well-being and the formation of the parent-infant bond. *(Photo courtesy of I.J. Weinfeld, M.D., Toledo Hospital, Toledo, Ohio.)*

Having a primary care nurse for each baby in intensive care is highly desirable. If each newborn has a nurse responsible for supervising his care and communicating with the parents, continuity of care and communication can be facilitated.

The second phase of parents' emotional adjustment is awareness of the reality of the baby's precarious situation. During this time staff members must be sensitive about recognizing, accepting, and helping parents with feelings of anger, guilt, and inability to take care of the baby. Realistic encouragement should be provided in assisting parents to achieve parenting behavior. It is important to teach parents to provide portions of the newborn's care and to facilitate the attachment process. Nurses should serve as role models to the parents, not as surrogate parents to the newborn.

Observing and documenting the parents' interaction with the infant is an essential part of nursing assessment and intervention with regard to the developing parent-infant relationship. The frequency of visits and phone calls should also be documented. When hospital visits are not possible, a letter to the mother from the neonate (as written by the baby's nurse) on a weekly basis may help create emotional closeness (Jenkins and Tock, 1986).

During visits, efforts should be made to provide parents with increasing periods of privacy with the baby. They should be observed intermittently to assess the progress they are making. Parents often feel inadequate about their ability to care for a baby compared with the skills of experienced nursery staff members. Continual attempts should be made to point out to the parents the positive aspects of their interaction with the baby, including their increasing skill in giving care.

Community resources can be extremely valuable in helping parents master parenting behavior. Parents may appreciate knowing about the availability of community resources to help them provide for the baby's special requirements. The appropriate resources should be identified and utilized as early as possible.

Acceptance of reality is the final stage of emotional adjustment. This stage may not occur during the time the baby remains hospitalized. Many centers have instituted outpatient clinics for follow-up of high-risk infants. Routine follow-up visits are set up to follow the health and development of the infant and to assess and support parenting. Community resources such as public health nurses also can be utilized for ongoing assessment of the infant's development.

Stimulating the High-Risk Neonate

It is important to meet not only the physical needs of high-risk neonates but also the developmental needs. To do so, the nurse must take into consideration the baby's basic needs, conceptual age (level of maturity), and state of alertness (Blackburn, 1983). For example, if neonates are hungry or are using energy to meet oxygen requirements (as in severe respiratory distress), they cannot attend to sensory stimuli very well. Newborns under 32 weeks of conceptual age may be overwhelmed by stimuli.

Once aroused, they may continue to respond until exhausted and disorganized. Babies at 34 to 35 weeks of conceptual age begin to respond to and seek social interactions. At 36 to 40 weeks they actively seek and respond to social stimulation (Gorski, Davidson, and Brazelton, 1979). They are more responsive in the quiet/alert state as opposed to the awake/drowsy and the active/alert states (Blackburn, 1983).

When interacting with ill and preterm neonates, nurses must realize that such babies may suffer sensory overload due to exhaustion. Preterm neonates generally can process only small amounts of sensory stimuli in one modality (touch, vision, or hearing). If the nurse or parent continues to subject the baby to either positive or negative stimuli, the newborn may show signs of sensory overload, including changes in color, respirations, heartbeat, and state (Blackburn, 1983; Hyde and McCown, 1986). When a state of sensory overload exists, the baby seems to recover more rapidly if left alone.

High-risk neonates need to be observed for their reactions to stimuli before an individualized program of stimulation can be developed. Types of stimulation are listed in Table 17-6. Rather than having planned interactions, the caregiver needs to take cues from the newborn and respond to the baby as an individual. Signs that the infant is attending to a stimulus include widening and brightening of the eyes, visual fixation, decreased motor activity, and turning to sound. Immature babies may not open their eyes and turn to sound, but they will decrease their activity with tactile stimulation (Blackburn, 1983). Also, neonates respond to auditory stimuli prior to visual stimuli.

TABLE 17-6 Types of Stimulation

Visual

En face position
Eye-to-eye contact with caregiver
Objects (black and white, brightly colored) that have pattern, contour, and slow movement

Auditory

Singing
Soft music from radio or piped-in music box
Talking at various pitches using different degrees of loudness

Tactile

Stroking
Bathing
Drying with soft cloth
Touching with variously textured materials
Soft roll or toy to lie against

Vestibular

Water bed incubator
Range of motion exercises (e.g., bicycling)
Change of position (e.g., holding upright, placing prone)

These newborns need various and novel types of stimulation (Table 17-6). Stimuli are presented over short periods of time. If signs of sensory overload are noted, the stimulis is discontinued and the baby is allowed to recover.

Nurses in neonatal intensive care nurseries should teach parents about the neonate and allow interaction between the parents and the baby. In this way parents can learn the cues presented by the neonate, the baby's actual abilities and reactions to parental stimuli, the maturity level and expected developmental course, the signs of overstimulation, and the need to allow the baby to recover alone if overstimulation occurs. When staff members are aware of both the neonate's and the parents' abilities, more positive parent-neonate interaction can become a reality.

Parent Support Groups

Parent support groups have been developed in several perinatal centers. Since some parents may not want to participate in a support group, the nurse should explain the purpose of the group and allow the parents to make the choice. MIles (1986) suggested that in centers where a parent support group is not available, a group can be established by the perinatal nurses and past high-risk parents. In these counseling groups parents who have had similar problems can help current parents of high-risk neonates deal with their emotions and problem solve. The current parents are allowed to discuss their feelings, concerns, and fears with veteran parents who understand what they are experiencing. These support groups do not take the place of intervention by health care personnel; their members, however, do supplement and enhance the information provided by the physicians and nurses.

Some parent support groups are available only while the neonate is hospitalized. Others continue through the first year of life.

Learning Activities

1. Form a small study group to practice the Ballard assessment technique for gestational age.
2. Compare the physical appearance (size, skin tones, subcutaneous fat, etc.) and behavior (crying, positioning, movement, etc.) of SGA, AGA, and LGA neonates and of preterm, term, and postterm neonates.
3. Practice visual, auditory, tactile, and vestibular stimulation of neonates. Note the babies' reactions and discuss a teaching plan for parents.

Study Questions

1. In Apgar scoring, heart rate is the first and most important diagnostic and prognostic sign of the five observations. The second most important is:
   A. Color.   C. Muscle tone.
   B. Respiratory rate.   D. Reflex irritability.
2. The Dubowitz and Ballard methods for estimating gestational age:
   A. Are used to assess the maturity and intrauterine growth of neonates.
   B. Are graded on a scale of 0 to 2.
   C. Also provide data related to respiratory effort and heart rate.
   D. Are accurate within 2 weeks of the actual gestational age.
3. A method of generating heat which is unique to the newborn is:
   A. Nonshivering thermogenesis.
   B. Shivering thermogenesis.
   C. Metabolic thermogenesis.
   D. Adrenal thermogenesis.
4. The major cause of septicemia in newborns is:
   A. TORCH.
   B. Group A beta-hemolytic streptococcus infections.
   C. Group B streptococcus infections.
   D. A shortened gestational period.
5. In preterm neonates, a deficiency in surfactant results in:
   A. Retrolental fibroplasia.
   B. Idiopathic respiratory distress syndrome.
   C. Anemia.
   D. Bronchopulmonary dysplasia.
6. To prevent heat loss by radiation in a high-risk neonate, the nurse should:
   A. Dress the baby warmly (shirt, diaper, stocking cap).
   B. Dry the baby with warm towels after bathing.
   C. Warm the stethoscope before applying it to the body surface.
   D. Place the baby's warmer/bassinet away from outside walls, windows, and drafts from air-conditioning.
7. Whenever oxygen is administered to a neonate, it must be:
   A. By positive or negative pressure.
   B. By liter flow only.
   C. Warmed and humidified.
   D. In sufficient concentration to maintain a PaO_2 between 30 and 70 mm Hg.
8. Neonates who are not in distress but are of less than 33 weeks' gestation can be fed:
   A. By the gavage method.
   B. By gastrostomy feedings.
   C. By bottle.
   D. By total parenteral nutrition.
9. It is important to know the rubella titer levels of all nurses working in neonatal intensive care units because:
   A. A nurse with rubella could infect the neonates.
   B. A newborn with rubella could infect the nurse.
   C. Pregnant nurses could be exposed to cytomegalovirus.
   D. If it is low, the nurse will have to stay home until the infected baby is discharged from the unit.

10. Newborns from 36 to 40 weeks' gestation are more responsive to social stimulation in:
    A. The active/alert state.
    B. The awake/drowsy state.
    C. The quiet/alert state.
    D. The initial state.

References

Ballard, J.L., K.K. Novak, and M. Driver: "A Simplified Score for Assessment of Fetal Maturation of Newly Born Infants," *Journal of Pediatrics,* **95**(5):769-774, 1979.

Baron, M., and P. Taforo: "The Extremes of Age: The Newborn and the Elderly," *Nursing Clinics of North America,* **20**(1):181-190, 1985.

Blackburn, S.: "Fostering Behavioral Development of High-Risk Infants," *JOGN Nursing,* **12**(Suppl):76-86, 1983.

Cloherty, J.P., and A.R. Stark: *Manual of Neonatal Care,* 2d ed., Little, Brown, Boston, 1985.

Dubowitz, L., V. Dubowitz, and C. Goldberg: "Clinical Assessment of Gestational Age in the Newborn Infant," *Journal of Pediatrics,* **77**:1-10, 1970.

Frisancho, A.R., A. Comptom, and J. Matos: "Ineffectiveness of Body Mass Indices for the Evaluation of Neonate Nutritional Status," *Journal of Pediatrics,* **108**:993-995, 1986.

Gorski, P.A., M.F. Davidson, and T.B. Brazelton: "Stages of Behavioral Organization in the High-Risk Neonate: Theoretical and Clinical Considerations," *Seminars in Perinatology,* **3**:61-72, 1979.

Graef, J.W., and T.E. Cone, Jr.: *Manual of Pedtriatric Therapeutics,* 3d ed., Little, Brown, Boston, 1985.

Hyde, B.B., and D.E. McCown: "Classical Conditioning in Neonatal Intensive Care Nurseries," *Pediatric Nursing,* **12**(1):11-13, 1986.

Jenkins, R.L., and M.K. Swatosh Tock: "Helping Parents Bond to Their Premature Infant," *MCN: The American Journal of Maternal Child Nursing,* **11**(1):32-34, 1986.

Koops, B.L., L.J. Morgan, and F.C. Battaglia: "Neonatal Mortality Risk in Relation to Birth Weight and Gestational Age; Update," *Journal of Pediatrics,* **101**:969-977, 1982.

Lubchenco, L.C., C. Hansman, and E. Boyd: "Intrauterine Growth in Length and Head Circumference as Estimated from Live Births at Gestational Ages from 26-42 Weeks," *Pediatrics,* **37**:403-408, 1966.

Merker, L., P. Higgins, and E. Kinnard: "Assessing Narcotic Addiction in Neonates," *Pediatric Nursing,* **11**(3):171-181, 1985.

Miles, M.S.: "Counseling Strategies," in S.H. Johnson (ed.), *Nursing Assessment and Strategies for the Family at Risk: High Risk Parenting,* 2d ed., Lippincott, Philadelphia, pp. 343-360, 1986.

Miller, H.C., and K. Hassanein: "Diagnosis of Impaired Fetal Growth in Newborn Infants," *Pediatrics,* **48**:511-522, 1971.

Nickerson, B.G.: "Bronchopulmonary Dysplasia," *Chest,* **87**(4):528, 533-534, 1985.

Olds, S.B., M.L. London, and P.A. Ladewig: *Maternal-Newborn Nursing,* 2d ed., Addison-Wesley, Menlo Park, Calif., 1984.

Walther, F.J., and L.H.J. Raemaekers: "The Ponderal Index as a Measure of the Nutritional Status at Birth and Its Relation to Some Aspects of Neonatal Morbidity," *Journal of Perinatal Medicine,* **10**:42-47, 1982.

Bibliography

Etzler, C: "Parents' Reactions to Pediatric Critical Care Settings: A Review of the Literature," *Issues in Comprehensive Pediatric Nursing,* **7**(6):319-331, 1984.

Haggerty, L.: "TORCH: A Literature Review and Implications for Practice," *JOGN Nursing,* **14**(2):124-129, 1985.

Miles, M., et al.: "Maternal and Paternal Stress Reactions When a Child Is Hospitalized in a Pediatric Intensive Care Setting," *Issues in Comprehensive Pediatric Nursing,* **7**(6):333-342, 1984.

18

Mental Retardation
in Children

Objectives

After reading this chapter, the student will be able to:
1. Understand better the scope of the problem of mental retardation in children.
2. Differentiate screening and assessment.
3. Discuss family reactions to the diagnosis.
4. Describe the role of a nurse caring for a child who is retarded and hospitalized in an acute care setting.
5. Discuss the different types of programs which are available in institutions where retarded children reside.

In the United States, an estimated 125,000 neonates who are mentally retarded are born each year. Although there is disagreement among published estimates of prevalence, a generally accepted figure is that 3 percent of the general population are considered to be mentally retarded, somewhat in excess of 6 million persons. In the past 30 years the philosophy of care has changed from one of isolation to one of normalization.

The *principle of normalization* was introduced in the mid-1950s but was not integrated into the delivery of services until the 1960s. The principle is based on the belief that persons who are mentally retarded are entitled to services which consider cultural norms so that the personal behaviors and characteristics to be established and/or maintained are as culturally normative as possible. These persons are kept in, or allowed admission to, the mainstream of life.

Children who are mentally retarded have the same basic needs as all other children. They are found in all segments of society. The multiple and complex problems they present demand the attention and services of providers in the health disciplines, education, and other helping professions. Each discipline contributes unique as well as shared knowledge and skills to the study and solution of these problems.

Nurses have major responsibilities in the areas of prevention, case finding, and management. Prevention is discussed last because one must understand what is to be prevented before considering methods of doing so.

Scope of the Problem

The methods of defining and categorizing mental retardation can determine the supportive services needed for children who are diagnosed as being mentally retarded. If these children are to reach their potential, a definition and a classification system which are consonant with the principle of normalization must be accepted. The American Association of Mental Deficiency (AAMD) worked with representatives of the World Health Organization and the American Psychiatric Association to provide a definition and classification scheme which can be used worldwide.

Definition

The AAMD (Grossman, 1983) defines *mental retardation* as "significantly subaverage general intellectual functioning existing concurrently with deficits in adaptive behavior and manifested during the developmental period." *General intellectual functioning* is reflected in the score(s) obtained in one or more standardized general intelligence test(s), such as the Stanford-Binet and the Wechsler Intelligence Scale for Children-Revised (WISC-R). Tests are administered individually, not in groups. *Significantly subaverage* refers to an IQ of approximately 70 or below. However, the upper limit can be extended to 75 or more, based on clinical assessment in relation to other factors such as behavior. *Impairments in adaptive behavior* include significant limitations in personal and social responsibility as defined by the individual's culture in relation to his or her age group. Assessment is based on clinical judgment and the results obtained on standardized scales such as the AAMD Adaptive Behavior Scales. The *developmental period* encompasses the period from conception to the eighteenth birthday. Developmental deficiencies may be evidenced as a result of central nervous system pathology or psychosocial factors.

Findings on both IQ and adaptive behavior measurements provide information related to *current functioning*. The definition of *developmental period* takes into consideration both clinical categories (about 25 percent of the identifiable mentally retarded population) and the psychosocially disadvantaged groups. In general, those in the clinical group are diagnosed from birth to early childhood and have an IQ in the profound, severe, or moderate range. Those in the psychosocial group may not be identified until school age and usually have an IQ in the mildly retarded range. However, the groups overlap (Grossman, 1983).

Classification

The AAMD classification system is based on "measures of intelligence and adaptive behavior, supplemented and reinforced by clinical judgment" (Grossman, 1983, p. 49). Intelligence tests measure achievement. Adaptive behavior scales are used to identify deficits which may be reflected in specific areas according to age group and culture.

Four levels of mental retardation based on the intelligence quotient (IQ) attained by an individual on a standardized test have been identified (Grossman, 1983):
1. *Mild retardation* IQ 50-55 to about 70
2. *Moderate retardation* IQ 35-40 to 50-55
3. *Severe retardation* IQ 20-25 to 35-40
4. *Profound retardation* IQ 20-25 or below

Clinicians have had less experience in using adaptive behavior scales than in using measures of intelligence. A number of scales are available. General areas of deficits in adaptive behavior follow. During infancy and early childhood, deficiencies in the development of sensorimotor, communication, self-help, and socialization skills may be noted. Expected basic academic skills, reasoning, judgment, social skills, communication, sensorimotor skills, and self-help skills may be adequate in school-age children and younger adolescents. Older adolescents may fail to develop anticipated skills as noted for children, interpersonal relationships, independent living skills, and vocational skills.

As the child's environment changes and/or expands, his intellectual functioning and adaptive behavior may also change and expand. Thus, the child may meet the criteria for a diagnosis of mental retardation at one time but not at another (Grossman, 1983).

Several classification systems for the causes of mental retardation can be found in the literature (Grossman, 1983; Crocker, 1983; Crocker and Nelson, 1983). The system used in this chapter is based on causation and the developmental period at which the condition can occur (Table 18-1). Selected examples of common conditions are listed. A specific etiology can be detected in only 25 percent of mentally retarded persons. Only 10 percent have the potential for cure or arrest through medical or surgical intervention. In the rest, inadequate prenatal and perinatal care, nutrition, child rearing, and social/environmental experiences are possible predisposing factors.

Rights of These Children

The National Association for Retarded Citizens (NARC), a voluntary organization, acts as a resource to local groups and lobbies for federal legislation which will protect the rights of persons who are retarded. Local branches, usually designated by county, provide information, offer support to families, and lobby for legislative changes on local and state levels. The national association for professionals and paraprofessionals is the AAMD. Its members lobby at the federal level.

TABLE 18-1 Causative Factors in Mental Retardation by Developmental Periods

1. Prenatal period
   (a) Chromosome anomalies
       (1) Down's syndrome (trisomy 21)
       (2) Klinefelter's syndrome
   (b) Errors of metabolism
       (1) Phenylketonuria
       (2) Hypothyroidism (cretinism)
       (3) Hurler's disease (gargoylism)
   (c) Malformation of the cranium
       (1) Microcephaly
       (2) Hydrocephaly
   (d) Maternal factors
       (1) Rubella (German measles)
       (2) Some other viral illnesses of the mother
       (3) Syphilis
       (4) Anoxia
       (5) Blood type incompatibility
       (6) Malnutrition
       (7) Toxemia
2. Neonatal or perinatal period
   (a) Anoxia
   (b) Intracranial hemorrhage
   (c) Birth injury
   (d) Kernicterus
   (e) Prematurity
3. Postnatal period
   (a) Infections
       (1) Meningitis
       (2) Encephalitis
   (b) Poisoning
       (1) Insecticides
       (2) Medications
       (3) Lead
   (c) Degenerative disease
       (1) Tay-Sachs disease
       (2) Huntington's chorea
       (3) Niemann-Pick disease
   (d) Physical injury
       (1) Head injury
       (2) Asphyxia
       (3) Hyperpyrexia
   (e) Brain tumors
   (f) Social and cultural factors
       (1) Deprivation
       (2) Emotional disturbance
       (3) Nutritional deficiency

Pertinent federal legislation enacted by Congress includes PL 91-230, the Education of Handicapped Act of 1967; PL 93-112, the Rehabilitation Act of 1973; and PL 94-142, the Education for all Handicapped Children Act of 1975. Section 504 of PL 93-112, the basic civil rights provision, states:

> No otherwise qualified handicapped individual in the United States shall, solely by reason of his handicap, be excluded from the participation in, be denied the benefits of, or be subject to discrimination under any program or activity receiving federal financial assistance.

This section is applicable to preschool, elementary, and secondary education programs receiving federal grants.

PL 94-142 applies to children and youths from 3 to 21 years of age. Handicapped children as defined by the act include those who are mentally retarded, have a hearing loss or are deaf, are orthopedically impaired, have other health impairments, have speech impairments, are visually handicapped, are emotionally disturbed, or have specific learning disabilities. Through this act, handicapped children are provided with special education and related services. Special education is defined as specially designed instruction, at no cost to parents or guardians, to meet the unique needs of a handicapped child, including classroom instruction, physical education, home instruction, and instruction in hospitals and institutions. Related services include transportation, developmental and corrective services, speech therapy and audiology, psychological services, physical and occupational therapy, recreation, and the diagnostic, evaluative, and counseling services required to help a handicapped child benefit from special education. Early identification and assessment of handicapping conditions in children are also provided. PL 94-142 requires that a child have an individualized written education program (IEP). The law specifically provides for

1. A free appropriate public education
2. Maintenance of an IEP
3. Complete due process procedures
4. Periodic consultation for the parent or guardian
5. Special education in the least restrictive environment
6. Nondiscriminatory testing and evaluation
7. Confidentiality of data and information
8. A surrogate to act for any child whose parents or guardian are unknown or for a child who is a legal ward of the state.

PL 91-230 was amended in 1983 as PL 98-199. Some provisions of PL 98-199 provide for state grants to plan, develop, and implement services for children from birth to 5 years and to enhance parent involvement through training projects. The 1986 amendments (PL 99-457) of PL 94-142 state in part that there must be competitive provision by states for resource centers to develop services for infants, toddlers, and families and for programs to serve them.

The rights of children who are mentally retarded and of their parents have been broadened by these acts. More funding has become available to enhance services and to train personnel to carry out the provisions of these acts. The lobbying efforts of NARC and AAMD have borne fruit over the past quarter century.

Screening and Assessment

Developmental screening of infants and children is performed in order to identify clients who have a high probability of significant developmental deficits. A screening test is not intended to be diagnostic. It can, however, provide a comparison of the child's behavior with that of the average child at that point in time. The purpose of assessment is to identify the nature and degree of the developmental problem and the child's current competencies so that appropriate interventions can be provided to the child and parents. Assessment is an ongoing process of observing, documenting, analyzing, and comparing findings with normal patterns of growth and development.

Screening

Children are screened in many ways. Techniques include a thorough history, physical examination, developmental evaluation, vision and hearing screening tests, and appropriate laboratory tests (Chap. 4). In many states additional screening for the newborn includes testing for phenylketonuria (PKU) and hypothyroidism.

Developmental evaluation is recommended during each well-child examination. It is also an integral part of the Early and Periodic Screening, Diagnosis, and Treatment (EPSDT) schedule. Through Title XIX of PL 74-271, the Social Security Act of 1935, Amended, financial assistance is provided to states for children who are receiving Medicaid. Thirteen EPSDT examinations at specified ages are authorized from birth to 21 years. The ages at which specific procedures may be appropriate are indicated on the schedule. Developmental assessment is recommended at each of the 13 visits. However, after 5 years of age, only observation is required. Despite various recommendations for screening, parents may be the first ones to voice concerns to the health care provider based on their observations at home.

Frankenburg (1983) suggested a two-step developmental screening protocol which is in concert with the American Academy of Pediatrics guidelines. He recommended that this process be initiated seven times in the first 6 years of life: at 3 to 6 months, 9 to 12 months, 18 to 24 months, and 3, 4, 5, and 6 years of age. The first step involves the use of a parent questionnaire to identify children who have a developmental problem. The second step is used to continue this identification but at the same time to decrease overreferrals.

The screening tools recommended by Frankenburg, Fandal, and Thornton (1987) are the Revised Denver Prescreening Questionnaire (R-DPQ) and the Denver Developmental Screening Test (DDST). The R-DPQ is a parent questionnaire and requires 10 minutes of the parent's time. The DDST is administered by the health care provider and requires 20 to 30 minutes to complete. In both instruments, personal-social, fine motor adaptive, language, and gross motor development are addressed. If there are no delays on the R-DPQ, no follow-up for that visit is necessary. With one delay, the R-DPQ is repeated after 1 month has passed. On rescreening, if one (or more) delay is found, the child is scheduled for a DDST. If two delays occur on the initial screening, the child should have a DDST as soon as possible. If the results are suspect, the child is referred for a further evaluation with follow-up to ensure that needed interventions are accomplished.

In addition to the two-step developmental screening process, Frankenburg (1983) discussed the use of the Home Screening Questionnaire (HSQ) developed by Coons et al. (1981). The HSQ is based on Caldwell's Home Observation for the Measurement of the Environ-

ment Scale. There are two forms: birth to 3 years and 3 to 6 years. It is recommended that selected parents complete the questionnaire at three points in time—9 to 18 months, 2 to 3 years, and 4 to 6 years—and that the HSQ be used only during the diagnostic phase, not the screening phase. However, Pidcock (1987) suggested a two-step screening of the child's home environment. The first step consists of asking the parents about the home environment when obtaining the history and paying particular attention to signs of malnutrition or neglect during the physical examination. If, in the examiner's clinical judgment, there is cause for concern, the parent is asked to complete the HSQ, which is the second step and which requires about 10 minutes. Based on the results, appropriate referrals may be made.

Nurses working in pediatric ambulatory settings will be involved in the developmental screening process. They should practice using and interpreting the R-DPQ, DDST, and HSQ with an experienced examiner in order to become familiar with these instruments. They can then clarify results with the parents and give them suggestions for promoting the child's development.

For school-age children and adolescents, Levine (1983) suggested that a questionnaire be used as a screening tool to identify children at risk. One such instrument is the ANSER system, which was developed at the Children's Hospital Medical Center in Boston. The ANSER system is a series of standardized health and developmental questionnaires that are completed by parents, teachers, school-age children, and adolescents. If the results are suspect, the child is referred for a neurodevelopmental examination.

Assessment

According to Grossman (1983), there are three components to assessment: intellectual functioning, adaptive behavior capabilties, and social environment. IQ and adaptive behavior levels reflect *current functioning*. An evaluation of the social environment provides information for understanding *why*. Assessment is conducted and interpreted by professionals who have had special training.

Several standardized intelligence scales are used commonly in assessment. During infancy and the preschool period, the Bayley Scales of Infant Development, the Gesell Developmental Schedules, the Stanford-Binet Intelligence Scale, and the Wechsler Preschool and Primary Scale of Intelligence may be employed. For older children, the Stanford-Binet and WISC-R may be used (Grossman, 1983).

Several standardized adaptive behavior scales are available for assessment. Two of the best known are the AAMD Adaptive Behavior Scale and the Vineland Social Maturity Scale (Grossman, 1983). Levine (1983) and his associates have utilized the neurodevelopmental examination for school-age children [e.g., the Pediatric Elementary Examination (PEEK) for grades 1 to 3]. It includes gross and fine motor function, visual spatial orientation, temporal-sequential organization, memory, language, and behavior style.

Environmental variables may hinder the child's development and diminish his adaptive behavior. Grossman (1983) noted that if the environment is not modified, "alterations in behavior are not likely to occur." Assessment of the environment may provide clues to the child's developmental progress or lack of progress. One widely used instrument for assessing the home environment is Caldwell's Home Observation for the Measurement of the Environment (HOME) (Bradley and Caldwell, 1977). There are two forms of this tool: one for children from birth to 3 years and the other for children from 3 to 6 years. Its use requires a home visit. It takes 1 to 3 hours to complete. As with assessment of intellectual functioning and adaptive behavior functioning, the persons who administer these scales and interpret the results have received special training in their use. At some diagnostic evaluation centers, the HSQ is completed first. If there is cause for concern, a home visit is planned for the administration of the HOME.

Interdisciplinary Centers

Screening for case finding is accomplished during routine health care visits. Pediatricians, family practitioners, nurse practitioners, and community health nurses are the health care providers who usually first suspect that an infant or young child is not progressing developmentally. Classroom teachers and school nurses may be the most likely case finders for older children and adolescents. When cognitive and/or adaptive behavior problems are suspected, plans must be made for future evaluation. Such services may be found in a university-affiliated facility, an evaluation center located at children's hospital medical centers, satellite centers with traveling consultants, and mobile clinics staffed by miniteams.

Regional programs can be located through the United Way and regional offices of the U.S. Department of Health and Human Services (DHHS). Head Start programs and Resource Access projects which help locate evaluation and treatment services for handicapped children are very useful. At the state level, institutions and state schools, Social and Rehabilitation Services (SRS), and the Developmental Disabilities Council can provide assistance. Crippled children commissions, the National Foundation-March of Dimes, the Easter Seal Society, the United Cerebral Palsy Association, and the Epilepsy Foundation often provide funds.

Since retarded children and their families have complex and varied needs and since in most cases these children will carry the disability into adult life, many professionals have found that an interdisciplinary approach to their care is extremely beneficial. This approach brings together individuals with expertise in their selected disciplines in an effort to provide delivery of complete, continuous, and coordinated service. Such a team may include a nurse, a physician, an audiologist, a speech pathologist, a special education teacher, a nutritionist, a dentist, a psychologist, a physical and/or occupational therapist, and a social worker. This systematic attempt at pooling professional resources and sharing knowledge and skills should result in more appropriate evaluation and less fragmented management for these children.

Family's Response to Diagnosis

Parents are encouraged to be participants throughout the initial assessment process, the various phases of intervention, and the periodic reassessments of the child. No conclusions or recommendations are made until all data have been analyzed. Results obtained from the standardized scales used, observations of the child, and interviews with people who know the child, coupled with clinical judgment, provide the necessary information for analysis.

In the past, there was a cultural tendency to value intellectual capacity and achievement and to feel threatened by persons who are defective in this area. Today, through acceptance of the principle of normalization, expectations regarding appropriate behavior and socialization of children who are mentally retarded have changed. Society is more accepting, and families are less isolated. Television portrayals of mentally retarded children by actors who themselves are mentally retarded have been helpful in bringing about this change in attitude.

Despite the wide range of parental reactions to a mentally retarded child described in the literature, some are more prevalent than others: guilt, ambivalence, disappointment, frustration, anger, shame, and sorrow. Specific responses and degrees of responses are governed by such varying factors as social class, marital relationships, attitudes toward deviance, past experiences, and parental aspirations.

For the majority of mentally retarded children, the diagnosis is not made at birth or in early infancy. Attachment between the baby and parents proceeds without knowledge that the new family member is retarded. As the infant exhibits developmental lags, some parents, in their eagerness to convince themselves of the child's normality, focus on one or two developmental tasks which he performs well and ignore the areas in which he displays limitations. Recognizing and admitting that the child has a problem can be a turning point in the parents' ability to adjust to the tasks of the present. Many may seek the cause in an effort to understand why this tragedy has occurred. Was it because of some past wrongdoing? Can it be cured? Can it be prevented in future children? The burdens with which some parents have to come to terms include misuse of drugs during the prenatal period, head trauma to the child following a negligent automobile accident or a beating, and failure to recognize the severity of an illness. Parents' ability to adjust is influenced by their personal strengths, economic circumstances, satisfaction with life apart from the reality of the child's problems, and the specific needs of the child.

Once parents accept the fact that a child is mentally retarded, they may alter their expectations. For example, they may expect the child to learn poorly, have minimal social experiences, and rely indefinitely on adults. Such perceptions may form the basis for protecting the child from experiencing many of the successes and failures encountered by other children. As a result, the child's development and self-image may be limited.

As greater numbers of mildly and moderately retarded children are being raised at home, nurses are recognizing the tremendous impact on other family members. Many parents who try to provide information and answer questions report difficulty with (1) putting the facts into understandable language based on the child's cognitive development, (2) updating their children's knowledge as their ability to understand increases with age, and (3) finding the time and patience to provide this information when the need is most acute.

The effect on siblings can be positive or negative according to the degree of family integration and the understanding of the child's needs. Most families experience ups and downs in the adjustment process of their children.

Siblings may become irritable, be withdrawn, and develop negative attitudes toward the child because parents pay less attention to them or expect them to take on care-giving tasks. They may be embarrassed or feel inferior because the child is "different." Adolescents may wonder about their own ability to have "normal children." However, siblings who have received adequate information, are involved in teaching a skill to the child, and are not pressured by their parents to excel in order to compensate for the child's deficit develop more positive attitudes. They are nurturing, cooperative, sensitive, and empathic.

Parents vary in their ability to accept and care for the child, and communities differ in regard to the resources available. Through community school programs, options for respite care, and varied social experiences available to the child, parents now have more time to devote to their other children and to the marital relationship. Local parent groups and health care providers can be of inestimable help in aiding families find resources which will enhance their ability to cope with stresses and to deal with the realistic demands of the child and his siblings. Parents can feel relief in knowing that they are not alone in facing the stresses and problems attendant to the discovery that a child is retarded.

Reactions to stress can take many forms. Parents may overprotect the retarded child by continuing to feed, dress, and bathe him even though the child has the potential to acquire these self-help skills, since the process is prolonged in relation to that of normal siblings. During the child's extended period of infancy and dependency, parents may fail to set limits. This pattern is ingrained by the time the child reaches a period when he can be reasoned with, and behavior problems may become evident. The overworked mother may become ill. Either parent may develop emotional problems, withdraw from social activities, or abuse the mentally retarded child. The father may become overly involved with the retarded child or may withdraw totally and expend his energies on the other siblings. Parents may require too much independent behavior of the siblings and/or may expect the siblings to assume too much responsibility for the care of the re-

tarded child. The siblings' resentment may be displayed through the development of behavioral problems.

From the time of diagnosis, health care professionals can help parents cope by giving them support in verbalizing their feelings, attempting to understand this crisis, and repeatedly seeing the reason for the child's retardation. Once the parents are able to come to terms with reality and are assured of assistance, they can assess the child's developmental level more accurately. Attention can then be focused on the child's current behavior and strengths, and plans can be made to help him reach his potential.

Retarded children experience stages of development similar to those of other children until they reach their developmental limits, but they progress at a slower rate and need more help in achieving developmental tasks. Health team members can explain the component behaviors of each task to parents. In this way, the child's progress becomes more visible and can be evaluated more accurately. Parents receive reinforcement for their efforts, and the child's progressive experiences help him advance along his continuum.

Nurses can help parents assess the child's developmental readiness for learning new tasks. As parents learn to read signs, they can provide the child with the necessary experiences and stimulation. Thus they can decrease their own feelings of frustration and disappointment and lessen the child's feelings of inadequacy and insecurity.

Interventions

The interventions discussed here include strategies which maximize the overall potential of the child and enhance the care-giving abilities of the family. They encompass the development of cognitive and sensorimotor skills and consider the psychosocial well-being of the retarded child as well as facilitate the adaptation of the family. Through the use of highly individualized methodologies, children are assisted in the development of skills which enable them to meet the demands of their physical and social environments. For the child, these goal-directed activities can increase self-worth, competence, and independence. Families also can be helped in developing the more effective coping skills which must evolve if they are to meet the challenges before them. When parents are the primary caregivers, they need to experience satisfaction in their roles and increase their competencies in managing the stressors experienced in the course of day to day living.

Early Intervention Strategies

Families of children who are mentally retarded now have a reasonable alternative to institutional care. Legislation has given impetus to the development of community-based health and educational services for children maintained in the home environment. Programs for all ages and all types and degrees of disabilities exist, providing for the continued development of the mentally retarded person throughout his life cycle.

The community services which are available are diverse and depend on the needs of children who are retarded and who reside there. The utilization of these programs is determined by their offerings. For example, if undesirable behaviors are present, parents may attend programs which teach them to decrease or eradicate such activities. Parents of young children can be counseled and taught a variety of methods which enhance their ability to care for the child and to provide stimulation to the infant. Adolescents attend programs which teach them skills, money management, and job application techniques. All efforts are directed toward maximizing a child's potential and capabilities.

Infant Stimulation at Home

The development of a self-concept begins in infancy and is a powerful factor in influencing what the child will become and how well he will be able to use the abilities he possesses. Through interactions with parents and others, a child learns what to expect of the world and what the world expects of him. At the same time, parents need experiences which enhance their feelings of satisfaction and adequacy as parents, which in turn promote more positive interactions with the infant. As a result, the child's self-concept evolves as one in which he is respected, wanted, valued, and loved.

Often parents assume that the infant draws sufficient stimuli from the environment and uses, assimilates, and integrates them automatically as he grows. While this may be the case in a developmentally normal child, the parents of a child who is retarded need to learn that the child requires a great deal of direction from birth because of his limited ability to learn on his own.

One of the best ways nurses can teach parents to interact more effectively with their children is through the use of modeling (i.e., demonstrating techniques with the child while the parents observe). Suggestions provided by the nurse for home stimulation should facilitate the parent-infant relationship. Activities should be mutually satisfying for the infant and his caregiver. Most of the time these activities can be implemented during routine caregiving (e.g., during bathing and dressing). Manipulation of the infant should be done slowly, giving the child the opportunity to react and accomodate himself to these new situations and experiences. The establishment of sequenced activities at set times of the day also assists the infant's adjustment. Tactile stimulation and passive range of motion exercises can be done with diaper changes and bathing. Parents should be encouraged to assume the *en face* position, especially during feeding. This position encourages mutual gazing and smiling responses. Brightly colored toys in the crib can also be used to encourage visual tracking.

Auditory stimulation is highly recommended. Mobiles and music boxes can be attached to cribs. Parents should be instructed to talk with and sing to the child during caretaking. Separate play times with each parent help the infant learn to distinguish voices and persons. He can be called by name from different directions to promote sound localization. Sounds made by the infant can be imitated by the parent to encourage vocalization.

Infants can be rocked or propped in swings for vestibular stimulation. Placing an infant on the floor in the prone position encourages exploration of the environment, head lifting, reaching, and grasping. Children learn best through activity, and what they learn is most likely to be reinforced if it is pleasurable. Involving siblings as helpers increases the infant's social experience and may facilitate an older child's acceptance of a new baby.

Nursing activities should focus on increasing parents' competence and confidence in child rearing by developing their problem-solving skills and coping modes. As parents' abilities to solve problems improve, they are more likely to adapt their behavior as the child's needs change and to devise their own creative solutions to new situations.

Early Intervention Programs

Technological advances have decreased the infant mortality rate; however, there are now larger numbers of preterm and low-birth-weight infants and children who are at risk and need special services. These early intervention programs (EIPs) developed as a result of the increasing numbers of survivors with identifiable problems, including those who are at risk developmentally because of biological or environmental factors. Their efforts are directed toward promoting more normal child development and helping families cope with the innumerable stresses they experience in caring for the child at home. While families are referred by hospitals, social workers, and nurses, they also find out about these programs through NICU parent support groups or meet parents who are in similar circumstances.

The EIPs are community-based agencies which provide an interdisciplinary approach to care. A wide variety of professionals are involved, including nurses, physicians, speech and language therapists, occupational therapists, physical therapists, social workers, nutritionists, psychologists, and special education teachers. The composition of a team depends solely on the child and family's needs. This type of health care delivery system facilitates the integration and contribution of all providers so that a comprehensive therapeutic care plan evolves for the child and family. Accessibility to this type of expertise and collaboration ensures the development of a cohesive plan of care which recognizes and incorporates the diverse needs of a family.

EIPs may provide services in the home, or families may choose to visit the center. They also can be provided with a combination of home and community center services. The decision is left to the family members after they have been informed fully about all the resources available to them. Certainly a parental decision to visit the center increases the likelihood of greater involvement in the support groups which are available. It also provides the parents with opportunities to meet other parents and children who are experiencing similar problems. It is imperative that these infants become enrolled in such programs early so that concerted efforts can be directed toward maximizing their potential.

Developmental Sequencing

One way nurses and other professionals can help parents increase their feelings of competence and confidence in child rearing is to teach them how to facilitate the child's development. Skills to be mastered are broken down into a series of successive steps.

Infants need to develop reach and grasp abilities in order to explore their environment. These skills are prerequisites for most self-help tasks that will be learned as the child progresses. A sequence of target behaviors or steps for the development of reach and grasp is presented in Table 18-2.

Toddlers and preschoolers learn through play to refine motor skills, develop communication, and assume independence in social and self-help abilities. However, it is important to understand that in play, the child who is retarded is less intense and has a shorter attention span; therefore, play is not as spontaneous as it is for the developmentally normal child. Providing opportunities for play and developmentally appropriate toys allows these children to practice new developmental skills.

Adults in the child's environment can help him to learn to manipulate toys and encourage his exploration of novel situations by their guidance and support. The mentally retarded child's development of imitative skills can also be utilized through group play with peers (Fig. 18-1). Preschools and day care centers teach preacademic and perceptual motor skills and often provide the retarded child with normal peer models. Head Start programs are now designed to handle handicapped children.

Teaching feeding skills begins with the introduction of solids into the infant's diet. Textures are presented gradually from fine to coarse in order to promote chewing. New foods should always be presented when the child is hungriest. Grimaces and spitting out are typical responses to new tastes or textures. Rather than assume he did not like it, the parent should offer the new food again in a few days. Infants generally advance from liquids to pureed foods, to mashed table foods, to semisolid foods, to chopped foods.

TABLE 18-2 Sequence for Reach and Grasp Skills

1. When a rattle is placed in his hand, the child will grasp it for 3 seconds.
2. The child will look at and play with his own hands.
3. The child will grasp a toy for 10 seconds.
4. When an object is held in front of him, the child reaches out and attempts to grasp it.
5. The child brings objects to his mouth.
6. The child explores objects with his hands.
7. From the crawling position, the child reaches with one hand.
8. The child can fling objects haphazardly.
9. The child transfers objects from hand to hand.

Dressing, a complex activity, requires the development and coordination of fine and gross motor skills. Although it is quicker and less frustrating for a parent to dress a child, the mentally retarded child needs many opportunities to learn to undress and dress himself. Learning these skills also facilitates toilet training (Fig. 18-3 and Table 18-3).

In the presence of other physical disabilities, some children who are retarded are unable to initiate mobility on their own. Physical therapists may become involved in devising methods which enhance the child's ability to ambulate. All children go through the same stages of sitting, standing, and cruising in order to achieve the goal of walking. However, retarded children proceed at a much slower rate and adapt accordingly to master this task.

Children exhibit many behaviors that indicate readiness for toilet training. The child should be urinating a moderate amount at one time rather than dribbling frequently. He should be staying dry for several hours throughout the day. Facial expressions or changes in posture may indicate that he knows he is about to urinate or defecate. Parents may need additional support or assistance during this period.

Later Intervention Strategies
School Age and Adolescence

Middle childhood and adolescence can be trying times for any child and his parents, but they can be particularly frustrating when mental retardation is a factor. Legislation guarantees appropriate public education for all children and should alleviate some of the difficulty in obtaining special services for this population. It is a difficult time because the child must deal with increased social expectations, academic goals, the onset of puberty, and preparation for employment.

Collaboration of school nurses, teachers, and special therapists is vital for consistent and individualized child programs. School nurses can interpret health and medical information to other school personnel, teach classes on nutrition and safety, consult in classrooms for individual programming or behavior management, help design adaptive methods or devices for physically handicapped children, and ensure that the environment is barrier-free. School nurses can also help these children correct unacceptable behavior.

At this time, the nurse's role with parents may include counseling, coordinating health and social services, directing them to recreational resources which provide social interactions for the child (e.g., Boy or Girl Scouts, church groups, and Special Olympics), and educating parents to be advocates for the child. The nurse may also be involved in assessing the child's abilities for various job skills during the decision-making process concerning the child's vocational training curriculum.

Sex education in the United States traditionally has been a parental responsibility. However, the parents of mentally retarded adolescents are often unsure of how to present such information and how to cope with questions

FIGURE 18-1   Developing imitative skills through group play. *(Courtesy of George Lazar.)*

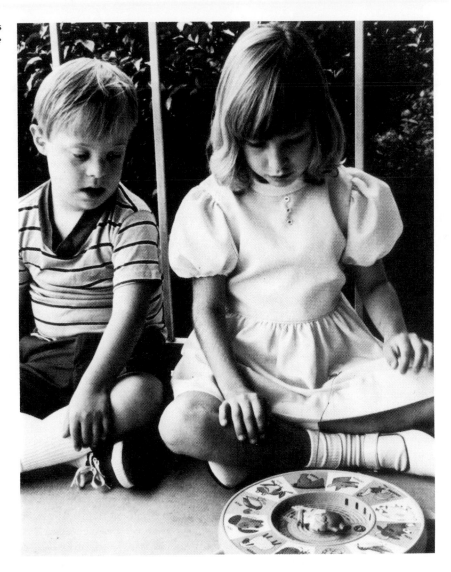

FIGURE 18-2   Trick-or-treat time provides an opportunity to practice language and social skills. *(Courtesy of Anne Ross Muir.)*

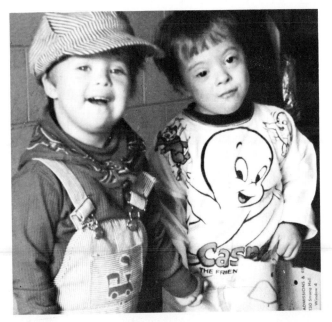

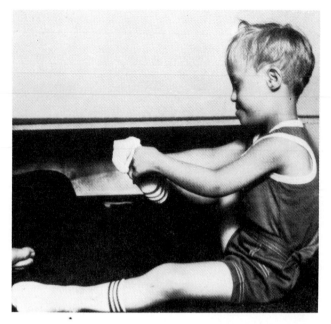

FIGURE 18-3   A 6-year-old child who enjoys being able to undress himself. *(Courtesy of Anne Ross Muir.)*

TABLE 18-3 Sequence for Dressing Skills

1. The child passively cooperates by lying still when dressed.
2. The child holds out his arms and legs while being dressed.
3. The child can remove a hat and place a hat on his head.
4. The child pulls off shoes and socks.
5. When they are unfastened, the child removes his coat and pants.
6. The child assists with pulling clothes down or lifting them up when dressing and undressing.
7. The child puts on oversized clothing.
8. The child undresses and dresses a doll.
9. With clothing off, the child pulls a string attached to a large zipper, moving it up and down.
10. With clothing on, the child pulls a string attached to a zipper, moving it up and down.
11. The child puts shoes on, not necessarily on the correct foot.
12. With arms or legs of an article of clothing held out, the child will put it on.
13. With verbal instructions, the child dresses independently except for buttoning.
14. The child initiates dressing himself.
15. With clothing off, the child unbuttons large buttons.
16. With clothing on, the child unbuttons large buttons.
17. With clothing off, the child buttons large buttons.
18. With clothing on, the child buttons large buttons.
19. The child can tighten laces on shoes.
20. The child completely dresses himself, zips, and buttons.
21. The child begins to tie his shoes by making the first knot.

---

and emerging sexual behavior. Frequently they seek advice from nurses. In some schools, nurses and classroom teachers together present biological facts and family planning information to groups of adolescents, depending on parental consent. Visual aids (e.g., pictures and models) make excellent instructional tools. However, information alone is incomplete, particularly when one considers that mentally retarded persons are often treated as asexual out of fear that they may harm others or display inappropriate public behavior.

A curriculum for sex education not only should correct misconceptions regarding body parts and functions but also needs to encourage questions, expression of feelings, exploration of ways to deal with sexual feelings, role playing to practice social interactions with the opposite sex, and acceptable alternatives for sexual fulfillment. By acknowledging these young adults' needs for intimacy, privacy, acceptance, and respect, nurses can aid mentally retarded adolescents in receiving normalized experiences.

Special Health Needs
Health professionals too often focus on the fact that a child is mentally retarded and then attribute any unusual symptoms or behavior to this fact, failing to look at the overall health status of the child. Retarded children often have lowered resistance to illness and need frequent medical and nursing care. Many also have congenital defects, such as a cleft palate or heart defects, which create special health needs.

These children are as varied and as individual in their health care requirements as any group of children, but there are generalizations which can be made. A child who has Down's syndrome may well have cardiac problems and will be more susceptible than most to upper respira-

tory tract infections. A child with cerebral palsy may have difficulty swallowing and may be susceptible to aspiration pneumonia. Children who are not active and who eat poorly may become constipated easily. A child who is in the inquisitive stage of exploration (regardless of chronological age) may put poisonous or other dangerous substances in his mouth or may injure himself in other ways.

Growth retardation is often seen in handicapped children. An assessment should include the community's nutritional characteristics as well as the child's nutritional status.

Dental care or its absence can affect the child's health and development. Poor dentition can be due to many factors, such as malformation of the jaw and dental structures, lack of stimulation from chewing inadequate cleaning of the teeth and gums, infrequent dental care, and the side effects of medications. The resulting unattractive mouth hampers not only the child's physical well-being but also his acceptance by others. As soon as deciduous teeth erupt, parents should begin cleaning them with cotton dipped in soda water or salt water. The child can be positioned supine with his head on the parent's lap and his mouth half open. If biting is a problem, a padded tongue blade or rubber door stopper can be placed between the biting surfaces of the upper and lower jaw. Around 2 years of age, the introduction of a child-size toothbrush and fluoride toothpaste is recommended. Using a circular motion inside and outside the teeth and gums is effective for cleansing. Flossing is necessary for plaque removal, particularly with permanent teeth. A commercial floss holder can be a valuable aid. Older children can be positioned either sitting on the floor with the head tipped back and the parent seated behind or sitting on a chair with the parent standing behind.

Once the child can get his hand to his mouth in a coordinated manner, independent tooth brushing may be taught. The inclusion of toothpaste application depends on the child's fine motor ability. Holding the brush can be facilitated by lengthening the handle with a piece of wood or enlarging the handle with foam or a bike handle grip. Electric toothbrushes may also be used. Disclosing tablets can be chewed to give feedback while the child is learning the skill. Parental supervision is recommended until the child has mastered this task.

Lack of exercise, sunshine, and fresh air can compound a child's physical problems. Contractures develop from positions maintained too long; vitamin D deficiency results from underexposure to sunshine. Poor appetite and general malaise also often result from these insufficiencies.

Impaired vision, hearing, or motor abilities may necessitate the use of glasses, hearing aids, or adaptive devices. These children often have allergies and/or seizures (Chap. 20) or may present with self-injurious behavior. Mentally and physically handicapped children are also at high risk for child abuse.

Additional Handicapping Problems

Some mentally retarded children also have a variety of other physically handicapping conditions, including sensory impairments (visual and/or auditory), motor deficits, and other structural anomalies. Each problem requires a special set of services, and these children with additional handicaps present a unique challenge to parents, professionals, and community resources. Coordinating all the health, educational, and social services they need is imperative if their complex needs are to be met. A nurse often is the best available provider for identifying, coordinating, and interpreting information for parents and for seeking out other health care providers as well as agencies that can provide family-focused services.

A child who is deaf or blind or both may become retarded as a result of limited learning experiences. Being born without hearing or vision does not mean that the intact senses are automatically more acute; therefore, parents and professionals need to teach these children to maximize their available avenues of sensory input. For example, reading aloud to a blind child can help sharpen his listening skills.

The child with a hearing impairment usually exhibits delayed language development. Nurses should be careful not to assume mistakenly that delayed language always means deficient intellectual ability. The nurse must also become familiar with the child's communication system, which may be oral (lipreading), manual (sign language),

or total (both oral and manual) or may involve the use of a communication board. The therapeutic goals for a hearing-impaired, mentally retarded child are to (1) amplify residual hearing, (2) teach a useful method of receptive and expressive communication, and (3) increase meaningful social experiences.

It is estimated that 80 percent of children who are multihandicapped and visually impaired are also mentally retarded. Among the most emotionally disturbed residents in institutions are those who are blind and retarded. The two main objectives of programs for these young children are to (1) prepare them for education at the appropriate age and (2) minimize the amount of educational retardation that often takes place in visually handicapped children as a result of sensory deprivation and lack of appropriate stimulation.

Nurses must remember that visually impaired children are not able to learn by imitation. Physical contact is an important teaching strategy for increasing their awareness of the environment, as is talking about activities and sounds taking place around them. Structuring their physical environment increases their familiarity and facilitates both orientation and mobility.

For the child who has orthopedic handicaps which restrict his gross motor and fine motor adaptive skills, the world is reduced to the immediate area unless someone helps him move about and explore and learn. Since much lifting and carrying of children is often involved, the nurse should review principles of body mechanics with the parents. Simple positioning techniques are useful for enabling the child to break out of obligatory reflex patterns to develop motor, self-help, and communication skills. The goal of exercises usually is to strengthen weaker muscles and maintain function. Meaningful skills are promoted when exercises are adapted for functional daily use. Factors influencing the child's progress are (1) the extent of brain damage, (2) the influence of maturation throughout childhood, often enhancing the effectiveness of therapy, and (3) the child's ability to learn to use an improved movement pattern effectively.

A child who has an unusual or unpleasant appearance is particularly handicapped in American society, where there is such a strong emphasis on physical beauty. He may be shunned by others who are shocked at his appearance and may be wrongly assumed to be mentally retarded. He may develop a negative self-concept and may not attempt to succeed in areas where he has to interact with others. Parents may be less inclined to include him in social family activities, sometimes out of their need to protect the child or his siblings. If his learning ability also is impaired, many more opportunities are closed to him.

Children with multiple handicaps need a great deal of individual attention and many special learning opportunities if they are to develop fully (Fig. 18-4). Interdisciplinary treatment and management, to whatever extent available, not only are beneficial to the child and his parents but also promote shared knowledge and skills among the professionals involved.

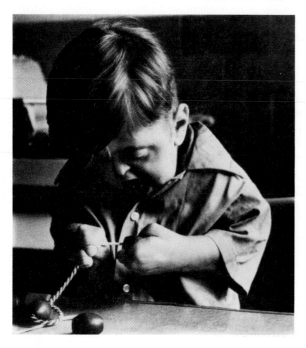

FIGURE 18-4 A multihandicapped preschooler learning fine motor skills. *(Courtesy of George Lazar.)*

The needs of parents with special children include understanding the meaning of the child's diagnoses (e.g., cerebral palsy, mental retardation), knowing the child's capabilities and limitations, accepting that he will be able to learn, and learning to use available community resources. Groups for parent education and for support of parents and siblings are useful. These families can often obtain needed time for themselves through respite care or temporary residential placement. If the nurse in the community proposes this alternative to a family, as with any intervention the approach and timing are critical. A nurse can facilitate the child's and family's adjustment by arranging a visit with them to the facility and including them in the preparation and program planning which occurs with the professionals who will be providing care in the institution. Upon the child's return home, the nurse can assist parents to maintain new skills learned by the child and can support them in dealing with any maladaptive behavior.

Hospitalization

Children and adolescents who are mentally retarded are admitted to acute care facilities from the community where they live with their families, from community residences, and from extended care facilities. While the most common causes are recurring health problems or chronic illnesses, neurological, metabolic, and nutritional disorders as well as cardiovascular problems also result in hospitalizations. The need for treatment is always a concern for families; however, if the child is retarded, the parents may be more anxious than usual. They fear regression in some of the self-help skills that have been mastered, isolation in "a room at the end of the hall," failure to meet the child's needs, and lack of understanding by the nurses or other providers.

Admission

When an admission is planned, a hospital tour and the other activities discussed in Chap. 9 should be scheduled, provided that they are available. These endeavors reduce the fears in a child and relieve the anxieties of the parents. On admission, one of the most important nursing responsibilities involves the taking of a nursing history. The data collected at this time can do a great deal to facilitate a smoother transition to the inpatient setting and to recognize skills which have been mastered. Chapters 5 and 9 provide additional information on history taking and orienting a child and family to the unit.

Most children who are retarded adhere to ritualistic behaviors, and so it is important to obtain information about their routines (feeding, toileting, bedtime). Outlining a typical day allows the nurse to utilize these data in planning care. If a behavioral management program (such as toileting or dressing) has been started at home, it is important to know the schedule, the terms family members use, the precise sequencing, etc. It is also important to continue them in a hospital setting. An adequate history also should identify skills the child has demonstrated, successful efforts in limit setting, and if self-stimulating activities are present, how parents manage them. It also is important to know how the child makes his needs known. The historians (parents and other adults) need to be as specific as possible in order to obtain information which will enhance the quality of the hospital experience. A list of favorite toys, drinks, and activities also should be compiled.

Children who live in community residences or extended care facilities usually are accompanied by staff members. Before the admitting date, these facilities should be asked to have the individual who best knows the child come to the hospital with him. If that request is made, the admitting nurse will be able to obtain the very specific information which is necessary.

In the course of obtaining the history, a nurse assesses the developmental level at which the child is functioning; this nursing function reinforces the need for a solid base of knowledge about growth and development. Once it has been identified, a primary nurse or other provider can approach the child knowing his cognitive level and thus be more effective in interacting with him.

Room assignment is important. A child who is retarded needs to be located in the mainstream of a pediatric unit, not in an isolated area, unless safety is an issue or his physical condition warrants separation from other children. Roommates should be at his developmental level; this can increase the likelihood of interacting socially. Roommate selection can be an issue, especially in the case of a retarded adolescent. Some children and adolescents who are developmentally normal may resent sharing a room and may demonstrate their dissatisfaction (Morrison, 1986). This kind of situation can be difficult; however, exploring the reluctant roommate's feelings may relieve some of the resentment. Time also diminishes the displeasure as roommates get to know each other. On occasion, a nurse is fortunate enough to identify a roommate who is understanding and sensitive, someone to whom the retarded adolescent can relate more easily. Certainly changing roommates should be avoided if at all possible, because the move can be devastating to the retarded adolescent, who probably has already experienced rejection.

The nursing history, the outline of a routine day, and any other appropriate information must be placed in the Kardex, where it is available to all nurses. It is imperative for everyone to be knowledgeable about the child's cognitive level and the skills mastered and for management programs to be continued so that a child who is retarded can maintain his independence despite hospitalization.

Preparation for Treatments and Procedures

Patient teaching is a major nursing function. When the child is retarded, it is important for the nurse to acknowledge that the teaching done is going to take more time and more patience. Any explanations given must be provided at the child's developmental level. This consideration is critical. Short, simple sentences, using a normal tone of voice, and appropriate terms are essential.

Controlling the environment is important too, because retarded children are distracted easily. A quiet room and curtains pulled around the bed are two ways to decrease external stimuli. The attention span of a retarded child is short, and efforts need to be directed toward maintaining his attention. Successful strategies include touching his shoulder or face, maintaining eye-to-eye contact, and calling him by name. When nurses anticipate the problems (distraction, short attention span), they can be dealt with more successfully.

It may be necessary to repeat instructions several times in the course of teaching or explaining. When the nurse asks a question, it is wise to ask one which requires a demonstration. This way it is very easy to determine whether the child understands what is being asked of him. Often a nurse who is demonstrating a dressing, for example, completes its application instead of allowing the child to do so. While the task is finished in a shorter period of time, the child has not done it, and that is the real issue. If independence in performing a skill is to be encouraged, it is necessary for *the child* to complete the task. When one considers the ritualism which typifies a retarded child's behavior, a nurse can rest assured that once something is learned, it will be done as the procedure has been taught.

Whenever possible, a demonstration or the use of visual aids is far more effective than explanations alone. Listening and seeing what is expected maximize the learning which occurs because one reinforces the other. As a result, an evaluation of one's effectiveness is accomplished more readily. If parents have elected to room in, they should be involved in any teaching plan. They know the child, and so they are especially helpful in selecting terms which may facilitate his understanding. Although teaching is a time-consuming aspect of caring for a child who is retarded, it can be an extremely rewarding experience for the nurse.

Any child appreciates being rewarded for following directions or demonstrating something, and acknowledg-

ment is even more significant to the retarded child. It is tangible evidence of his ability to perform, which should be recognized. If the task at hand is difficult, as each sequence is completed, the child may be rewarded with a candy, for example. Other rewards include playing an enjoyable game and receiving a special food at mealtime, a favorite drink, or, for the young child, a hug. Whatever the form of recognition, the child understands and enjoys his success.

Play Activities

Play is an integral component of any child's life in or outside the hospital. In selecting activities for a hospitalized child who is retarded, thought should be given to age-appropriate involvement—developmental age, *not* chronological age. Placing him in an activity in which he is incapable of succeeding only frustrates the child further. If the hospital has a very active play program, the adults who are involved in supervising activities in the playroom must be informed about the developmental level at which the child is functioning if they too are to be effective in their interactions with the child.

These children should be included in any group activities which occur on the pediatric unit or in the playroom. As usual, the playmates should be children at or close to their own developmental levels. With a little bit of thought, play activities can be utilized to generate new responses in new situations. It is important to realize that each sensory and motor experience to which a child is exposed serves as a foundation for acquiring additional competencies. In addition, by controlling this environment, it is possible to arrange positive social situations in which the child is accepted rather than teased, isolated, or ignored. When a nurse takes an active role in developing appropriate activities, the nurse becomes a role model for others. First, the nurse has assessed the child's developmental level and shared the information with other nurses as well as members of the health team. Second, by demonstrating acceptance of and respect for this child, the nurse can help other adults (parents of other children, extended family members, and providers) who do not "understand" the child or feel uneasy in his presence.

In an acute care facility, it is not unusual for a nurse to feel inadequate or insecure when caring for a child who is retarded. However, it is important to realize that these feelings may contribute to ignoring or isolating the child. If the retarded child is to be understood better, the first step should be a thorough assessment of his competencies. This information is critical to understanding him and making the hospital experience a rewarding, mutually satisfying one for the child and his nurse.

Institutional Programs

With normalization and improved community services available, the numbers of individuals confined to facilities for the retarded have decreased. Minimally and moderately retarded individuals have moved into community settings after being prepared for functioning in a mainstream environment. As a result, the largest percentage of those who reside in institutions are severely and profoundly retarded. These children also have a variety of additional problems such as seizure disorders and sensorimotor and speech impairments.

The decision to place a child or adolescent in a facility permanently is not made solely on the basis of the degree of retardation. It may occur as a result of difficulty in managing the child at home, total disorganization within a family, or parents who are no longer able to care for the child or adolescent. The services available vary among and within states. They may be purely custodial in nature or may include educational, vocational, and habilitative programs. It is hoped that each child's needs will be addressed according to the level at which he is functioning.

Extended Care Units

Children in an extended care unit require total and continuous nursing care. Usually these children and adolescents are severely and profoundly retarded and have serious physical disabilities as well as chronic or acute medical health problems. Some of these children can be taught self-help skills such as finger and spoon feeding. They may need assistance in learning how to play with toys or in developing personal and social skills. They are so debilitated that many are unable to participate in the various programs which are available.

Unit Living

Most children who are retarded and institutionalized live in individual units which are homelike environments. Unit assignment depends on a particular child's needs. For example, children in a basic skills of daily living group concentrate on learning activities associated with feeding, dressing, and toileting; however, they also are involved in physical, occupational, and recreational programs. Another group of children may be involved in preschool activities but concurrently increase their skills in recreational and socialization activities. Those who are candidates for community living focus on skills they need in that setting, such as vocational training, learning how to use money, and learning how to start a bank account.

A variety of special services are available to the residents, including physical therapy, speech and language programs, occupational therapy, psychological testing, and medical, dental, and nursing services. Access to the various programs depends on the child's needs. Each unit also has a team which consists of providers of these various services. It is the team members who develop individualized programs for each child in the unit.

Although parents and family members are encouraged to participate in the child's care, they may be unable to do so. For this reason, the Foster Grandparent Program fills a great need. These retired individuals who live in the community generously give time to individual children. While providing attention to different children, they freely give their love.

A great deal of progress in caring for these children has been made in the last two decades. Once the principle of normalization was implemented, a variety of new experiences became available. For example, it is not unusual for these children and adolescents to go to the circus, see Santa Claus, visit the zoo, or go out to dinner to celebrate someone's birthday. Some facilities have reciprocal arrangements with community schools in which retarded children from the community attend nursery school with those in the institution and vice versa. More and more communities and institutions have a mix of "normal" and retarded children in the same classroom.

Respite Care Programs

Gradually, facilities for the retarded developed temporary care programs which enabled children who lived in the community to be admitted on a shortterm basis. This admission process is called respite care. It is usually 1 month in length and is utilized during family crises such as the hospitalization of a parent or sibling, a death, or the birth of a sibling. Sometimes parents who are experiencing difficulty in teaching a child a self-help skill or in behavioral management may choose to admit the child for a short-term intensive training program. Regardless of the reason for choosing respite care, the time interval provides some relief from the awesome responsibilities these families have, and they are grateful for its availability.

Another important aspect of respite care is that it allows an extensive observational period, which may be an essential part of a comprehensive evaluation. It is not always possible to obtain such data in a doctor's office or outpatient department. Observing the child over time and in a variety of circumstances ensures a far more accurate, complete assessment.

Mental Retardation Nursing

The role of a nurse in a facility for the retarded is challenging and diverse. A nurse is involved in delivering comprehensive services which begin with preadmission planning and coordinating and continue through to discharge and referral to appropriate community agencies.

Although nurses are involved in developing and giving in-service programs to staff nurses and others who work with these children, they also are intimately involved in making decisions about the care these children receive, the activities in which they participate, and the programs which meet their individual needs. Health assessments, health education, and counseling also are within the realm of nursing practice in these facilities, and the opportunities to provide these services are innumerable.

Nurses expend a great deal of time, effort, and energy with a child and his family, whether in encouraging parental involvement in the child's care or supporting the parents as they make the decision to institutionalize the child. For the nurse who desires this type of consistent one-to-one involvement, the work can be rewarding and satisfying.

Case finding is another role of nursing, and these assessment and observational skills can be utilized in any setting. Nurses in newborn nurseries, inpatient and outpatient areas, doctors' offices, and schools as well as the community need to identify newborns and children who are demonstrating developmental delays. Case finding cannot be done without a thorough working knowledge of growth and developmental principles. Any infant or child who is observed with a delay must be referred to and evaluated by a skillful interdisciplinary team as soon as possible. Time is a critical factor.

Nurses play an integral part in providing emotional support to the child and family. Such support can be in the form of a hug for the child after accomplishing a task or just being there for family members who are trying to cope with the diagnosis. These parents need someone to clarify, reiterate, and interpret a great deal of information. Nurses are the most effective providers in these kinds of endeavors because they provide direct care and have extensive contact with the child and family.

In order to maximize one's effectiveness, it is essential for the nurse to be an active member of the interdisciplinary team. The knowledge gained from working so closely with a family makes it appropriate for a nurse to serve as coordinator of an interdisciplinary team. Many of these children have more than one problem, and so this approach is essential if they and their families are to have access to all available programs.

Although great strides have been made in educating the public, nurses need to continue participating in activities which clarify the misconceptions lay people have about mental retardation. Nurses need to be patient advocates, whether such involvement concerns the purchase of a home for community living, providing information to legislators, or giving public testimony at a hearing. Participation by nurses in such activities is imperative if the rights of the retarded are to be protected.

Prevention

Preventing the occurrence of mental retardation must be the goal of every nurse, regardless of the setting, if the numbers of children affected are to decrease. Once damage occurs, it is irreversible and the child's intellectual ability is altered forever; hence, concerted efforts must be made to lessen this possibility.

Before conception, genetic counseling may be appropriate for couples who have had a child with mental retardation, who have a family history of an inherited disease which causes intellectual impairment, or in which the female partner's age is 37 years or more. A women who has had multiple spontaneous abortions is also at risk. In seeking such counseling, potential parents can be provided with specific information identifying risk factors in order to reduce the numbers of children affected.

Once pregnancy occurs, it is critical for women to seek and receive prenatal care early. The teaching done at this time should include the need for a well-rounded dietary intake and the cessation of any alcohol consumption or smoking, with reasons why both should stop. When expectant mothers are informed of their harmful effects, the knowledge increases the likelihood of compliance. Nurses need to be involved in identifying maternal high-risk fac-

tors, initiating appropriate antenatal testing, and evaluating these expectant mothers on an ongoing basis, including careful monitoring during the birthing process.

Once a newborn is delivered, examined, and declared healthy, emphasis should be placed on parent teaching. In addition, the nurse needs to determine the extent of the learning which has taken place, because that evaluation is critical to the neonate's future welfare. There are so many opportunities for that one cerebral insult to occur, it is necessary to implement certain precautions at birth.

Nurses must know the specific causes of mental retardation and incorporate that information in the anticipatory guidance provided to parents during follow-up visits. For example, safety is an essential topic for discussion with parents. Head injuries, accidents, drownings, and accidental ingestions are potentially harmful events which can have devastating effects. Another necessary topic is a review of the immunization schedule with reasons why adherence to the schedule is so important.

With poverty a continuing problem, the contributions of sociocultural factors cannot be dismissed. As assessments are done and the presence of deprivation or malnutrition is identified, efforts must be directed toward improving the situation immediately. Infants and toddlers are especially prone to dire long-term consequences because their brains are growing at very rapid rates during these stages of development.

Nurses have an important role to play in preventing mental retardation. In addition to identifying its potential causes, counseling and teaching are major responsibilities. Another critical activity is increasing public awareness of the scope of the problem and the many variables which influence and affect the wellness of future generations.

Independent Study Activities

1. Perform a developmental screening test on a mentally retarded child and a normal child of the same chronological age. Compare the findings.
2. Visit a sheltered workshop in the community where retarded individuals participate in a "work-for-pay" program.
3. Request permission to attend a parent or sibling support group.

Learning Activities

1. Invite the mother of a child who is retarded to speak to students in the classroom about her reactions to the diagnosis and its effects on the family.
2. Make arrangements for students (individually or in pairs) to observe an interdisciplinary team meeting at a screening and evaluation center for retarded children.
3. Assign children who are retarded to students in the clinical area.

Study Questions

1. Among children who are mentally retarded, a specific etiology can be found in:
   A. 100 percent.   C. 50 percent.
   B. 75 percent.   D. 25 percent.
2. Developmental screening is performed:
   A. As part of the assessment of children who are suspected of being mentally retarded.
   B. To identify children who have a high probability of significant development deficits.
   C. To determine the intelligence level.
   D. To identify the nature and degree of a child's developmental problem.
3. When working with parents of children who are mentally retarded, it is important to focus attention on:
   A. The child's current behavior and strengths.
   B. The child's past behavior and strengths.
   C. The inability to determine a specific etiology in the majority of these children.
   D. The parents' feelings of frustration.
4. In instructing parents how to stimulate their infants, the most successful strategy a nurse can utilize is to:
   A. Direct parents step by step.
   B. Arrange for assistance from a community resource.
   C. Be a role model.
   D. Encourage their participation in a support group.
5. When teaching parents feeding skills to use with a retarded infant, it is important for a nurse to advise them to introduce solid foods:
   A. When the infant is hungriest.
   B. After giving the infant a bottle.
   C. Every other day.
   D. When the infant is very tired.
6. It is not unusual for a retarded child with a hearing impairment to demonstrate:
   A. Constant pulling on the ears.
   B. Evidence of delayed speech.
   C. Excessive smiling when spoken to.
   D. Decreased interest in participating in group activities.
7. In working with blind retarded children, it is important for a nurse to remember that:
   A. Their overall potentials are good.
   B. Intact senses become much keener.
   C. They cannot learn by imitation.
   D. Testing becomes a problem.
8. Mentally retarded children who become residents of long-term facilities usually are assigned to specific units on the basis of their:
   A. Sex.   C. Needs.
   B. Developmental age.   D. Physical problems.

References

Bradley, R., and B. Caldwell: "Home Observation for Measurement of the Environment: A Validation Study of Screening Efficiency," *American Journal of Mental Deficiency,* **81**:417-420, 1977.
Coons, C.E., et al.: *Home Screening Questionnaire Reference Manual,* JFK Child Development Center, Denver, Colo., 1981.
Crocker, A.C.: "Cerebral Palsy in a Spectrum of Developmental Disabilities," in G.H. Thompson, I.L. Rubin, and R.M. Bilenker (eds.), *Comprehensive Management of Cerebral Palsy,* Grune & Stratton, New York, 1983.
Crocker, A.C., and R.P. Nelson: "Major Handicapping Conditions," in M.D. Levine et al. (eds.), *Developmental Behavioral Pediatrics,* Saunders, Philadelphia, 1983.
Frankenburg, W.K.: "Infant and Preschool Developmental Screening," in M.D. Levine et al. (eds.), *Developmental Behavioral Pediatrics,* Saunders, Philadelphia, 1983.
Frankenburg, W.K., A.W. Fandal, and S.M. Thornton: "Revision of the Denver Prescreening Developmental Questionnaire," *Journal of Pediatrics,* **110**:653-657, 1987.
Grossman, H.J. (ed.): *Classification in Mental Retardation,* American Association on Mental Deficiency, Washington, D.C., 1983.
Levine, M.D.: "The Developmental Assessment of the School-Age Child," in M.D. Levine et al. (eds.), *Developmental Behavioral Pediatrics,* Saunders, Philadelphia, 1983.
Morrison, J.L.: "The Special Needs of the Special Patient," *RN,* July 1986, pp. 49-54.
Pidcock, F.S.: "Developmental Screening Techniques for Pediatricians," *Pediatric Basics,* **47**:5, 8-12, 1987.

Nursing Management of Children with Alterations in Body Systems

19

The Integumentary System

Objectives

After reading this chapter, the student will be able to:

1. Identify the basic subjective and objective data to be obtained in assessing the integumentary system of the child.
2. Describe general nursing measures appropriate for pediatric clients with problems of the integumentary system.
3. Identify common problems of the integumentary system.
4. Delineate specific nursing interventions appropriate to the care of children with a variety of integumentary system problems.
5. Identify factors related to the prevention of common problems of the integumentary system.

Anatomy and Physiology of the Skin

The skin consists of a superficial layer of stratified epithelium (epidermis) laid on a foundation of firm connective tissue of dermis (Fig. 19-1). Its major function is protection against the external environment. The skin forms a barrier to protect the body from trauma, radiation, penetration of foreign bodies, moisture and humidity, microorganisms, and macroorganisms. To perform these functions it has a highly integrated, efficient, and complex mechanism of keratinization, pigment production, sensory nerves, and circulatory regulation. The skin also maintains itself and efficiently and quickly repairs itself. The production of secretions from its surface glands maintains a buff-

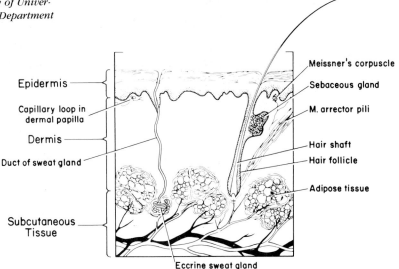

ered protective surface film which is said to be somewhat bacteriostatic. The skin functions as an important part of the body's defense system, recognizing foreign protein and setting in motion the immunologic response of the body. The internal fluid environment of the body is preserved by the skin, which prevents dissipation of the body fluids as long as the surface membrane is intact. When the surface membrane is injured or lost, as in extensive burns and severe skin diseases, large amounts of fluids, electrolytes, and proteins are lost from the body. The intact skin also serves in a minor way as an organ of elimination, excreting small amounts of sodium chloride and urea.

One of the most important functions of the skin is regulation of body temperature. The body must adjust to fluctuations in environmental temperatures as well as in the heat produced by its own metabolism. Adjustments in body temperature are made by adjusting the loss of heat from the body to the environment. Dilatation of the arterioles increases blood flow to the extensive capillary plexuses of the dermis when heat loss is needed. When heat must be conserved, large units of the capillary bed are shut off by direct arteriovenous anastomoses which shunt blood away from the surface. The adipose tissue functions as an insulating sheet against external temperature changes. Further cooling of the body can be provided when needed by an increase in sweat production. Perspiration on the skin surface provides cooling by evaporation.

Nursing Assessment

An adequate nursing assessment of the integumentary system is formulated from a nursing history and a physical examination. The complexity of the process depends on the child's health. The ill child requires additional assessment to provide proper teaching and treatment.

History

A well-child history is used to establish baseline data for the child. The history contains information regarding any previous skin diseases or other physical problems which may affect the integumentary system. A family history of skin problems is also included. In formulating an assessment of a healthy child, it is determined whether the present skin condition is usual for that child. Accurate documentation of the history is essential if the information is to be used as baseline data.

When a nursing history is being taken for an ill child, the child or the significant other is asked to describe the present condition. Solicited information contains the time elapsed since the initial appearance of the problem or condition, whether the lesions have spread, the area in which lesions have spread, the area in which lesions first appeared, and the pattern of spreading. The onset and duration of each symptom is noted and recorded. The child or significant other is asked about symptoms such as itching, scaling, and dryness. Information regarding symptomatology which may not appear to be related to the integumentary system initially is elicited. Whether anyone else in the family or within a group of friends has or had a similar problem is noted. If the problem is a recurring one, does it occur seasonally or with any type of pattern? Any factors which seem to aggravate the condition are also noted. The child or significant other is questioned about environmental factors such as recent trips, unusual leisure activities, emotional upsets, and increased stress.

It is important to determine the treatments or medications which have been tried by the parents in an attempt to resolve the problem. Successes and failures in treatment are documented. Medications, both systemic and topical, which are being used for other problems are recorded. At the conclusion of the interview, the child and parent can be asked if there is anything else important that they think the nurse should know. This question may uncover information which is helpful to the nurse in formulating her assessment.

Physical Examination

The physical examination of the integumentary system is very similar for both well and ill children. A good light source is essential. The best source is natural nonglare sunlight, although a low-wattage light bulb (such as a 60-watt bulb) on a stand may be substituted. The environmental temperature of the examining room should be moderate to prevent hyper- or hypothermia. Good hand-washing technique is mandatory for any physical examination. Privacy should be provided, and the child should be as relaxed as possible. The nurse examines and palpates all areas of the skin and inspects the hair, mucous membranes, and nails. Folds and creases are smoothed out so that all areas can be seen. Normal skin differs in appearance in various parts of the body. The integumentary system is viewed as a whole so that changes can be detected in the different areas of the body. It is helpful to stand a few feet away from the child so that large sections of the skin surface can be seen at one time.

Physical assessment begins with an examination of skin color, turgor, and texture. Skin color is affected by the color of the blood in the skin capillaries. The bluish hue of cyanosis may be caused by poorly oxygenated blood and/or by a cold environment which slows down the movement of oxygenated blood through the capillaries. In the latter, the slow movement allows the oxygen to be removed from the blood before it reaches all skin capillaries. Pallor is generally associated with skin capillary vasoconstriction. If most of the circulating blood is diverted to the internal parts of the body, paleness will occur. Color changes in black clients may be ascertained by examining mucous membranes or nail beds. It may also be possible to detect the absence of red undertones in black patients who are vasoconstricted. Jaundice and hypo- or hyperpigmented areas of the skin surface are assessed.

Good skin turgor indicates that the child is hydrated adequately. When dehydrated, the skin maintains position when pinched upward between the thumb and forefinger. Normally hydrated skin resumes its usual contours when released from the pinched position. Edema can be tested by pressing on the skin surface, usually the ankle. An indentation remains in edematous skin. Skin texture should be smooth, soft, and flexible. Dry and/or scalping skin is noted. Abnormal sweating and an increased sensitivity to touch is investigated; the latter may be difficult to determine if the child is irritable during the examination. Skin temperature is noted. Breaks in the skin, irritations, ecchymoses, or rashes are examined carefully. Normal lesions such as milia in the newborn are recorded.

The hair should be clean, shiny, and generally the same color. It should not be coarse, brittle, or dry. The hair growth is assessed for distribution and growth patterns. Nail color is observed and any lesions are examined and noted. Mucous membranes must also be visualized

and assessed. In a child, the primary (or earliest appearing) lesion must be identified, along with any secondary changes which may have occurred. A description of the color, arrangement, and distribution of lesions is also necessary. The lesion itself may be a variety of colors or even multicolored (Table 19-1).

Classification of Skin Lesions

All cutaneous lesions assume more or less distinct characteristics. Primary or secondary lesions may be: macules, papules, nodules, tubercles, tumors, wheals, vesicles, bullae, and pustules.

Macules are less than 1 cm in diameter; they are circumscribed alterations in the color of the skin, without elevation or depression. They may constitute the whole or a part of the eruption or may be an early phase or an associated symptom. Occasionally the spots become slightly raised and are desginated *maculopapules.* A patch is a macule greater than 1 cm in diameter.

Papules are less than 1 cm in diameter; they are circumscribed solid elevations with no visible fluid. They may be acuminate, rounded, conical, flat, or umbilicated and may appear white, red, yellow, yellowish brown, or black. Papules may be seated in the corium around sebaceous glands, at the orifices of the sweat glands, or at the hair follicles. Some papules persist as papules, whereas those of the inflammatory type may progress to vesicles, pustules, or eventually ulcers. A papule greater than 1 cm in diameter is termed a *plaque.*

Nodules are larger, solid forms of papules with a persistent character, perhaps midway between a papule and a small tumor. They differ from papules in that they are in close association with the corium or subcutaneous tissue and project both upward and downward.

Tumors may be soft or firm, freely movable or fixed, and are of various sizes and shapes. Consistency depends on the constituents of the lesion, which may be either inflammatory or neoplastic.

Wheals (urticaria) are evanescent, edematous flat elevations of various sizes. They are usually oval, white or pink, and surrounded by pink areolas. These lesions develop in seconds but disappear slowly; itching and tingling are almost always present.

Vesicles (blisters) are circumscribed epidermal elevations less than 1 cm in diameter and contain a clear fluid. They may be pale or yellow from seropurulent material or red from serum mixed with blood and occasionally have deep red areolas. Vesicles may arise directly from macules or papules and generally break spontaneously or develop into blebs or pustules within a short time.

Bullae (blebs) are rounded or irregularly shaped blisters containing serous or seropurulent fluid. They differ from vesicles only in size, being greater than 1 cm in diameter. They are usually single-chambered and located superficially in the epidermis so that their walls are thin and subject to rupture. With a lack of cohesion between the epidermis and the cutis, the epidermis can be rubbed off easily, leaving a raw, moist abrasion.

TABLE 19-1 Assessment of Pediatric Patient's Integument

I. Subjective data
  A. Presenting problem (e.g., "He has a rash"; "Her skin is dry.")
  B. History of presenting problem
    1. Onset—sudden or gradual
    2. Precipitating factors (e.g., emotional upsets, stress, season, food)
    3. Duration—length of time present
    4. Frequency—constant, intermittent, completely absent for a time, seasonal
    5. Type
      (a) Dryness
      (b) Scaling
      (c) Ecchymosis
      (d) Edema
      (e) Lesions (e.g., macule, papule)
    6. Progression
      (a) Area in which skin problem first appeared (e.g., anterior cheeks, collar region, chest, legs)
      (b) Appearance and any change (e.g., from macule, to papule, to vesicle)
      (c) Pattern of spreading (e.g., from chest, to face, to extremities)
    7. Current treatment—medications, over-the-counter drugs, home remedies; type of treatment, frequency, duration, and effect
    8. Associated symptoms (onset, duration, etc.) (e.g., itching and scaling of skin, rhinorrhea, conjunctivitis, sensitivity to light)
  C. Past history
    1. Skin problems
    2. Exposure to others who are ill (family, friends, schoolmates)
    3. Allergies
    4. Immunization status
  D. Family history
    1. Skin problems
    2. Allergies

II. Objective data
  A. Temperature, pulse, respirations, blood pressure
  B. Growth measurements
  C. General appearance (e.g., alert, irritable, lethargic; growth percentiles)
  D. Skin (see Classification of Skin Lesions and Table 6-4)
    1. Inspection—color of skin, mucosa; nail beds; dryness; scaling; hyper- or hypopigmentation; perspiration; breaks in skin; irritation; ecchymosis; exanthems
    2. Palpation—turgor, texture, pitting edema, elevation and size of lesions, sensitivity to touch, temperature
  E. Hair—inspection and palpation for coarseness, dryness, brittleness, distribution, nits, color
  F. Eyes—conjunctivitis, sensitivity to light, tearing (see also Chap. 21)
  G. Ears—otitis externa, otitis media
  H. Nose—exudate (color, consistency, etc.)
  I. Mouth—inspection and palpation of mucosa for enanthems (describe lesions); erythema
  J. Throat—inspection of mucosa for erythema, exudate, and enanthems; inspection of tonsils for size, erythema, exudate
  K. Chest—respiratory rate and rhythm, rhonchi, rales, wheezes (see Chap. 23)
  L. Heart—rate and rhythm, murmurs (see Chap. 24)
  M. Abdomen—organomegaly (see Chap. 26)
  N. Genitalia and urethral meatus—exudate (see Chaps. 27 and 29)
  O. Neurological system (see Chap. 20)
  P. Musculoskeletal system (see Chap. 22)

Pustules are small elevations of the skin which contain pus. They are similar to vesicles in shape, have an inflammatory areola, and may be unilobular or multilobular. They are usually white or yellow but may be red if they contain blood with the pus. They may originate as pustules or may develop as papules or vesicles, progressing through transitory early stages during which they are known as *papulopustules* or *vesicopustules.*

General Nursing Measures

Nursing Diagnoses

Examples of nursing diagnoses that may apply to a child with alteration in the integumentary system and the child's family are as follows:

Impaired skin integrity related to dermatitis, burns, or other alterations in the skin; the diagnosis may be actual or potential

Pain (or itching) related to burns, rash, or other lesion

Potential for infection related to impairment of skin integrity or scratching

Altered nutrition: less than body requirements, related to mouth lesions or metabolic demands of burns

Impaired physical mobility (actual or potential) related to burns, lesions, or bulky dressings

Self-esteem disturbance and body image disturbance related to dermatitis, psoriasis, burns, or other problems

With the multiple-system involvement of major burns, many additional diagnoses would be identified.

Nursing Measures

The skin responds constantly to both internal and external environmental changes. General nursing measures for the integumentary system focus on protecting the integrity of the skin through protection against the external environment.

The skin is protected from excessive heat and cold. The infant is particularly sensitive to changes in the environment because of the thinness of the epidermis and immaturity of the sebaceous glands. Many parents tend to overdress infants. They should be given guidelines for dressing as a part of the normal newborn teaching plan. Excessive sweating, a cooling mechanism for the body, will cause a loss of fluid and electrolytes and can be particularly dangerous in very hot environments.

Hygiene factors play an important role in protecting skin integrity. The skin must be kept clean and free from irritating substances. Excessive moisture is detrimental to the skin, and so skin surfaces must be kept dry and provided with good ventilation. Parents should be cautioned against excessive bathing, which can cause dryness, chapping, and itching. Oils and lotions can be recommended to the parents if the skin begins to appear dry. "Soapless" bathing may be used, since some soaps may cause dryness of the skin. Adequate fluid intake is also a necessity.

Prompt attention to skin problems is vital. Simple first aid measures, such as cleaning cuts and scrapes, are important in maintaining skin integrity. Special attention must be paid to a child who is immobilized. A reddened area, particularly over a bony prominence, indicates a lack of capillary blood flow. Redness is the first sign of a potential pressure sore and must be treated immediately. The best treatment, however, is prevention, which includes frequent turning, correct positioning, and an adequate diet. With proper nursing measures, pressure sores can be prevented.

Integumentary Diseases in the Infant and Toddler

Diaper Dermatitis

The diaper area of the neonate is exposed constantly to a wide variety of irritants, such as moisture, heat, and chemical substances. The contact dermatitis, or *diaper rash,* that develops is a troublesome, distressing problem. Erythema in the genital or perianal area usually signals the beginning of the rash. Left unattended, it quickly spreads throughout the diaper area as it progresses from macules and papules to eroded, moist, or crusted lesions.

Ammonia dermatitis, caused by the breakdown of urea in the urine to ammonia by fecal bacteria, presents a similar clinical picture. The areas of greatest involvement are the perianal and gluteal regions, where it appears as a diffuse erythema. As it spreads throughout the diaper area, the skin becomes shiny, red, and excoriated. Any infant with a diaper rash may be expected to voice pain and generalized discomfort, particularly when the diapers are wet or soiled. Ulceration of the urinary meatus in circumcised males sometimes develops with the diaper rash.

Chemical and physical insults such as ammonia and friction decrease the ability of the epidermis to maintain its integrity, resulting in the development of cutaneous lesions. Gluteal, inguinal, and neck folds are particularly sensitive. Maceration of any two skin surfaces in close opposition is termed *intertrigo.* Obese infants frequently develop intertrigo in the gluteal and neck folds. Poor ventilation, inadequate cleaning, and high humidity produce an irritating accumulation of sweat and sebum in the skinfolds. Erythema, maceration, chafing, and fissuring develop as the intertrigo progresses.

Nursing Management

Although it is difficult to pinpoint a single factor responsible for a particular diaper dermatitis and impossible to predict that any one treatment will both cure and prevent all diaper rashes, most of the principles for clearing diaper dermatitis also are used for prevention. The general principles of keeping the area dry, well ventilated, and free of irritating substances sound simple enough. Diaper rash is an annoying and embarrassing problem to mothers. It requires careful exploration of present care and a thorough explanation of these general principles.

Skin irritants include urine and fecal material, the increased amounts of organic substances in diarrheal stools; excessive perspiration, particularly in the intertriginous areas; and friction from the rubbing of rough diapers against the skin. Changing diapers as quickly as possible after soiling is of utmost importance. In a young infant, diapers are changed or at least checked for dampness every hour during the day and evening. Once the diapers are removed, the area is washed thoroughly with water or with bland soap and water if needed. Commercially available premoistened disposable towelettes also may be used. Careful attention is given to cleansing the intertriginous, genital, and anal areas, separating the skinfolds with one hand while washing with the other. All areas are patted dry with a soft cloth towel. Allowing the infant to go without diapers for short periods of time is healthful. Direct exposure to sunlight or artificial light is also beneficial. A gooseneck lamp with a 25-watt bulb placed approximately *1 ft from the infant's body* two to four times a day for 30 minutes promotes drying and healing. Intense heat to the raw areas, caused by the light being too close or too strong, may damage the epidermis. Ointments may increase the skin's sensitivity to the light; therefore, the areas should be clean and free of all ointments during lamp treatments. The lamp must be located securely where bedclothing and moving legs will not touch the bulb.

A variety of ointments, powders, and creams are used to prevent and treat diaper rash. The choice of agent depends on the condition of the skin. Ointments are useful in providing a protective barrier between the skin and moisture or irritants. However, since they limit aeration and keep moisture against the skin, they should be used only as a preventive measure on clear skin. Powders are used for their hydroscopic properties; they tend to cake and are never used on open lesions. Since powders are potentially harmful if inhaled, application should be directly into the diaper or onto a hand, away from the infant's face. Commercially available compounds for diaper rash are used for soothing and protecting minor rashes. Drying ointments and compresses of Burow's solution are indicated for acute weeping rashes. Steroid creams may be prescribed for their anti-inflammatory properties in stubborn or severe rashes but can be used safely for only short periods of time. Nurses should assume the responsibility for determining whether parents are using steroid creams as directed by the physician.

Rubber pants, occlusive plastic coverings, tightly pinned or double diapers, and heavy snug-fitting clothing increase the production and retention of body heat and moisture in the diaper area. Loose diapers and clothing provide better ventilation. Plastic pants are avoided. Disposable diapers may be replaced by loosely pinned, single cloth diapers, without occlusive coverings, until the rash improves. Legs of all pants should be checked and discarded if there is constriction of the thighs or legs. Overheating by room temperature, clothing, or blankets should be avoided.

Although infants may vary somewhat in their susceptibility to cutaneous irritants, substances left in improperly washed diapers are one of the main causes of diaper rashes. Diapers should be soft and free of soap, bacteria, and ammonia. Mothers are instructed to presoak soiled cloth diapers, wash them with a bland soap, and then thoroughly rinse them. The amount of residue left in water after swishing a clean, dry diaper in cool water determines the adequency of rinsing technique. A terminal antiseptic rinse with vinegar, Borax, or Diaperene neutralizes the ammonia produced by the urea-splitting bacteria. These diapers may be irritating to sensitive children. Generally, diapers are soaked for 20 minutes in the terminal rinse solution and then dried, preferably in the sun. Commercial diaper services function under strict regulations, and families using coin-operated laundries may find it more economical, efficient, and convenient to use such services.

Nurses and parents should see a noticeable improvement in the diaper dermatitis within a week if the previous general principles are followed. If the condition is not improving, an extensive area is involved, or weeping and oozing occur, a referral to the physician should be made. Secondary infections with bacteria and yeast frequently occur in the affected areas.

Diaper rashes are not without complications. A serious complication is stenosis of the urinary meatus as a result of ulceration and scarring. The possibility of permanent scarring and depigmentation in the diaper area is of concern to many mothers. They may be reassured that there is no permanent damage to the epidermis in most cases and that the skin returns to normal as the child gains bowel and bladder control.

Candidiasis (moniliasis) is a frequent primary or secondary form of diaper dermatitis. These lesions appear as red, scalding, sharply circumscribed moist patches. Flaccid, pustular satellite lesions surround the larger lesions. Because yeasts require high humidity for growth, they are found frequently in the diaper area, in the mouth, and as a part of the normal intestinal flora. An oral *Candida* infection (thrush) is often found in conjunction with *Candida* infection in the diaper area. Antibiotics may upset the normal balance and produce an overgrowth of *Candida.* Newborns are exposed to *Candida* from their mothers during birth. If diaper dermatitis has been present for some time prior to the development of the demarcated le-

sions, the moniliasis is most probably a secondary infection.

Nystatin (Mycostatin) cream or ointment applied to the affected areas is the treatment of choice. It may be used alone or in combination with compresses of Burow's solution three times a day. An oral preparation of nystatin is used if oral thrush is present. The general principles of preventing diaper dermatitis should be reviewed with the mother, and compliance should be encouraged. Careful hand washing is most important in preventing spread of the infection.

Bacterial dermatitis caused by other organisms, such as staphylococci, is unusual but may be found in conjunction with other low-grade infections. The distinctive lesions are papular, erosive, discrete, and deep with rolled edges. Antibiotics and steroids may be used in the treatment along with the general principles for care of the diaper area. Keeping the area dry is of particular importance. The nurse should observe for or instruct the parents to observe for signs of further infection and response to the therapy. If the infant does not appear to be responding to therapy within a couple of days, he should be reevaluated by the physician. During the acute stage of the bacterial dermatitis the bacteria may be recovered from the lesions. Therefore, in addition to the general principles referred to earlier, careful handling of linens and thorough hand washing are indicated.

Roseola Infantum

Roseola infantum (exanthem subitum) is a benign, self-limiting infection seen in children 6 months to 3 years of age. Transplacental passive immunity apparently protects infants under 6 months of age. Little is known about transmission, causative agent, or communicability. It is believed to be caused by a virus but does not have the contagious characteristics of the measles. Generally no known actual exposure to a child with roseola occurs; therefore, the incubation period is difficult to determine, but it is presumed to be between 10 and 15 days. Spring and fall are the seasons of greatest incidence; however, it is seen throughout the year. No specific diagnostic tests are available. The diagnosis is based mainly on symptoms and differential diagnoses.

The usual clinical course of roseola is diagrammed in Fig. 19-2. The temperature rises abruptly to 39.5 to 40.5°C (103 to 105°F) and remains at that level for 3 to 4 days. Temperature-controlling methods decrease the fever only for short periods before it returns to the same high levels. This prodromal period causes great anxiety in parents and medical people alike, as there are only very mild nonspecific symptoms other than the fever on which to base a diagnosis. The most striking characteristic is the contrast between the persistently high fever and a child who is alert, is playful, and does not look as ill as the fever would indicate. A mild pharyngitis, tonsillitis, otitis media, or lymphadenopathy may be present, but there are generally no signs of coryza, cough, or conjunctivitis. Leukopenia is present by the third day of the illness.

On the third or fourth day, the fever drops precipi-

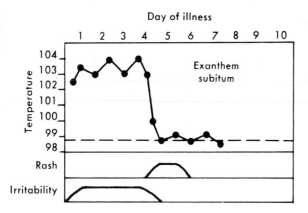

FIGURE 19-2   Typical clinical course of roseola infantum (exanthem subitum). The temperature drops to normal on the third or fourth day, and a maculopapular rash appears. *(From S. Krugman et al., Infectious Diseases of Children, 8th ed., The C.V. Mosby Company, St. Louis, 1985.)*

tously to normal and the rash appears. The rosy pink, discrete macules or maculopapules appear first on the trunk and then spread to the neck, the upper extremities, the face, and eventually the lower extremities. The lesions fade with pressure, rarely coalesce, and disappear without desquamation in about 2 days. Occasionally they may be evanescent and disappear in a matter of hours.

Nursing Management

During the prodromal period, control of the temperature with tepid sponge baths and antipyretics may be necessary around the clock. The nurse should outline the appropriate dosage and the schedule of antipyretics with the parents and give them a written copy of all treatments discussed. Acetaminophen (10 to 15 mg/kg per dose) every 4 to 6 hours is used during the febrile period. Sponge baths for 15 to 20 minutes several times a day may be used because tepid water and friction increase the amount of heat lost, thereby lowering the body temperature. Dressing the child in light cotton clothes, decreasing bedclothing, and keeping the room temperature normal all assist in controlling the child's temperature. These measures are in direct contrast to some of the older beliefs about treatment for chills and fever. Therefore, the nurse must make her explanations clear to parents in order to overcome their fears of making the child worse.

The child may be happier and more comfortable with quiet activities outside the bed. There are no indications for strict bed rest or for isolation. A diet high in fluids is preferable during the febrile period but may otherwise vary according to desire and tolerance. No immunization against roseola is available, and one episode is believed to confer permanent immunity.

Seborrheic Dermatitis

Seborrheic dermatitis is a common recurrent cutaneous disease of unknown cause and remarkable variation. It affects areas with a high level of sebum production and appears in the neonate as cradle cap, in the young infant as

dermatitis of the scalp and diaper area, and in the adolescent as dandruff or dermatitis of the midsternum, upper midback, and head. Hormonal stimulation of sebum is at a maximum during these ages, and the accumulation of sweat, sebum, and dirt is thought to be partially responsible for the scaly dermatitis. Seborrheic dermatitis often becomes a chronic inflammatory reaction that involves several areas of the body at one time. Complications include secondary infection of the involved areas with bacteria and yeasts.

Cradle cap in the infant and dandruff in the older child appear as mild inflammations of flat, adherent, greasy scales. Cradle cap is seen commonly in babies whose mothers are afraid to wash an infant's head. The scales continue to build and spread without adequate treatment and care. Eventually they cover the entire scalp and most of the skin surface as well. Another common site for the dermatitis is in the diaper area. At times these erythematous scales may be oozing. The abdomen and back may become involved as the process spreads. Affected areas may be pruritic. Scratching the lesions frequently leads to secondary bacterial infections. By the end of the first year the condition usually improves spontaneously, only to reappear at a later age as dandruff. Dandruff appears more often in the winter, when occlusive hats are worn. It may spread downward to the eyebrows, eyelids, neck, and external ear canal. In addition to redness and scaling, there may be weeping and crusting of the affected areas. Crusting usually indicates a secondary infection. After puberty the site continues to be the hair-bearing areas plus the midsternum and upper midback. The pale erythematous lesions differ from those in the young child by having sharply demarcated borders and a yellowish color of the greasy scales. Blepharitis is also a common finding in this age group.

Nursing Management

The areas involved by seborrheic dermatitis must be kept clean, dry, cool, and free of rubbing by clothes or scratching by fingers. The scalp may be cleansed in several ways. In mild cases, a vigorous shampooing may be sufficient. In more severe cases, commercially available shampoos containing tar (Sebultone), selenium sulfide (Selsun), or salicylic acid and sulfur (Sebulex) are used. They are left on the scalp approximately 10 minutes and then rinsed off thoroughly. The affected areas are dried. The use of hair dryers must be avoided, since flaking of the scalp may result. Warm mineral oil massaged into the scalp will soften thick adherent scales so that shampooing will be effective. Mothers need to be reassured that vigorous scrubbing of the infant's scalp and "soft spot" is not harmful. For stubborn, severe cases involving the scalp or for other areas of the body, topical corticosteroid creams applied two to four times a day are most effective. The temperature of the environment and the weight of the clothes should be controlled to decrease the amount of perspiration. Clothes should be soft, loose, and porous to prevent irritation from rubbing and to allow for adequate ventilation. Attempts should be made to prevent scratching of the affected areas and introduction of bacteria in the lesions. The nurse needs to review general principles of well-child care with the mother of a young child, particularly general hygiene, care of diapers, and care of the diaper area.

Atopic Dermatitis (Eczema)

Atopic dermatitis (eczema) is often the earliest manifestation of an allergic tendency. Usually a hereditary predisposition for the development of sensitization to common allergens is present. At various ages, children often develop the triad of atopic dermatitis, asthma, and hay fever. The primary "lesion" is the pruritus; the condition has been said to be an itch that rashes rather than a rash that itches. Secondary changes resulting from the trauma of itching and scratching account for most of the clinical manifestations of atopic dermatitis. The prognosis is good, although the course is prolonged and characterized by many exacerbations and remissions. The winter months show a worsening of the condition, followed by a general improvement in the summer. Secondary bacterial infections of the lesions commonly occur and are the complication most often associated with atopic dermatitis. The disease should be differentiated from contact dermatitis and seborrheic dermatitis.

Atopic dermatitis occurs in three stages with fairly distinct features. The *infantile stage* usually appears within the first year of life. This stage tends to be more exudative and inflammatory than are later stages. The cheeks are generally the area where the dermatitis is first evident. Initially, pruritus, erythema, and edema appear, caused by dilatation of blood vessels, followed quickly by the formation of papules and vesicles as fluid from the capillaries escapes into the tissues. The reaction often spreads to the forehead, scalp, and flexor surfaces of the extremities, particularly of the antecubital and popliteal fossae. Eventually it may cover most of the body surface. Because the pruritus is intense, the infant scratches the lesions, thus rupturing the vesicles and causing excoriation of the area. Weeping, oozing areas of thick yellow sticky exudate cover raw surfaces. As these areas dry, crusts form. Generalized lymphadenopathy, low-grade fever, and splenomegaly may also be found in this uncomfortable, fretful, and irritable infant. Eventually the acute process subsides and the crusts desquamate, leaving healthy new epithelium. Scarring may occur with secondary infections but is not a part of the eczematous process.

The *childhood stage* may occur after an apparent quiescent phase, typically during the ages of 3 to 5 years, or can follow the infantile stage without interruption. This phase is less inflammatory and is characterized more by pruritus, dryness, and the appearance over much of the truncal skin of tiny papules that look like "goose bumps" at the hair follicles. In some areas, particularly the flanks and dorsa of the upper arms, the papules become larger and harder and undergo follicular hyperkeratosis. As a consequence of scratching, irritation, and inflammation, the hard papules become confluent, thickened, and dark in color. The resultant lichenified plaques are the hallmark of chronic atopic dermatitis. Involvement of the face is less pronounced during this stage, and distribution favors the flexor creases, volar surfaces of the wrists, and extensor surfaces of the knees and elbows. As in the infantile stage, complete remission may occur at any time. The third, or *adult, stage* is characterized by further attenuation of dryness, lichenification, and pigment changes.

Nursing Management

Successful management of the child with atopic dermatitis requires a comprehensive approach on the part of the entire medical team. Parents must understand that atopic dermatitis is a chronic condition for which there is no cure. There are therapeutic regimens which are used to control the symptoms and define and alleviate the precipitating or aggravating factors of the scratch, itch, scratch cycle. *Control of the itching* is paramount. Specific antipruritic or antihistaminic drugs such as trimeprazine (Temaril), cyproheptadine (Periactin), and hydroxyzine hydrochloride (Atarax, Vistaril) may be administered orally several times a day. Since the worst scratching is often done at night, antipruritic sedation may be necessary at nighttime to ensure adequate rest. Diphenhydramine (Benadryl) is an effective antihistamine with sedative and antipruritic properties. Restraining a child may be necessary in order to prevent scratching and rubbing of the affected areas. Elbow, wrist, and ankle restraints and socks covering hands as well as affected parts are used as needed. Restraints should be applied loosely and carefully and only when absolutely necessary. They should be removed frequently to allow free movement and expressive play. The child's nails should be clipped and washed frequently to prevent scratching and introduction of bacteria into the lesions.

Dry skin due to a lack of sufficient water contributes significantly to the pruritus. Bathing with water, especially hot water, will remove water-soluble substances in the skin, thereby increasing dryness. During acute exacerbations, the use of warm water baths or soaks for 15 to 20 minutes followed immediately by an occlusive preparation to retain the absorbed water is advocated (Nicol, 1987). The occlusive lubricant or emollient applied to the damp skin seals in the moisture.

A careful, thorough past and present history may be most helpful in identifying allergens and external irritants. In children under 2 years of age dietary allergens are extremely common. Cow's milk, egg whites, wheat cereals, and fruits such as oranges commonly cause sensitivity. A diet eliminating possible allergens might be suggested. Most authorities now believe that diet modification is of value only when a food allergy can be definitely demonstrated. In older children foods seem to cause fewer reactions. Inhalants that produce reactions may sometimes be controlled by the elimination of dust-containing items in the child's bedroom. Rugs, drapes, stuffed fuzzy toys, and upholstered furniture all hold dust. The bedroom should be cool, well ventilated, and dusted frequently with a wet cloth.

Other common irritants include soaps and harsh fabrics. Soaps can be irritating either as residual in clothing or when used in bathing. Laundry soaps should have a neutral pH and should be rinsed thoroughly from the clothes. Body soaps should be mild and nonperfumed. Wool and other harsh fabrics aggravate atopic dermatitis as a result of contact irritation, overheating, and sweating. Furniture, rugs, blankets, toys, and even the mother's clothing may need to be free of irritating fabrics. Since sweating will increase pruritus, excessive clothing, high environmental temperatures, and overstrenuous activities should be avoided. Clothing should be soft and light-weight to decrease sweating and contact irritation.

Wet wraps can be used on severely affected or persistent areas of dermatitis. When they are used immediately after the occlusive preparation, hydration will be optimized and topical therapy will be enhanced. The total body, an extremity, or the face can be wrapped using combinations of Kerlix, tube socks, tubular bandaging, or other materials. The wet gauze wraps can be replaced two to three times daily or left in place overnight or up to 24 hours. They must never be allowed to dry out. Solutions should be at room temperature, and the room should be warm to prevent chilling.

Topical steroids may be needed to control acute flare-ups and reduce redness and inflammation. Coal tar products may be used, particularly in chronic maintenance control of the dermatitis. Systemic antibiotics are necessary for secondary infected lesions. The schedule of all treatments and medication should be outlined clearly with the parents and adhered to closely.

The medical team must be particularly aware of the mother's emotional state. Care of the child in the home is always preferable to care in the hospital, where exposure to a variety of bacteria is inevitable. Parents' feelings toward the child must be determined and discussed. Commonly a parent disgusted at the sight of weeping, oozing lesions; overwhelmed by the time-consuming treatments; and confronted by an impossible to satisfy, fussy, irritable, scratching child is overcome by guilt at producing the illness and has strong feelings of rejection toward the child. Nurses must be aware that these feelings are normal and should be expressed; they should offer constructive suggestions and explanations to decrease the burden and the anxiety. Maternal responses of anxiety, rejection, and overprotection are detected quickly by the child and may aggravate the condition. Continual reassurance, support, understanding, and praise will be needed by the mother over the years.

A child with eczema has the same needs for growth and development as any other child. Without a doubt his needs for love, attention, and expression of frustration are greater than those of the normal child. Mothers and other attending persons should be encouraged to use a gown or apron to cover their clothes and to handle and cuddle the child as much as possible. Visual and auditory stimulation should be provided while the child is restrained. Play should be provided with smooth, washable toys, stimulating the child's developmental level and satisfying his need for expression of frustrations.

Erythema Infectiosum, Fifth Disease

Erythema infectiosum is a mild, self-limiting disease that is thought to be caused by a virus. It appears to be mildly contagious and is seen in small outbreaks in the spring at intervals of several years. Children between the ages of 2 and 12 years are affected most commonly. The estimated incubation period is from 5 to 14 days. Erythema infectiosum is a benign disease with an excellent prognosis and with only rare complications of transient arthritis and arthralgia (more common in adults) and hemolytic anemia.

A prodromal period is usually absent but may include 1 to 2 days of low-grade fever and malaise. The exanthema erupts in three stages. In the first stage, a coalescent, erythematous, maculopapular rash appears on the cheeks. The affected areas are slightly raised, hot but not tender, nonpruritic, and with defined edges, giving the child a "slapped cheek" or sunburned appearance. The circumoral area is not involved and appears as pallor next to the intensely red, efflorescent cheeks. There may be discrete lesions on the forehead, chin, and posterior auricular area. This stage of the eruption lasts 1 to 4 days and then gradually fades. The second stage begins about 24 hours after the first stage with a symmetrical maculopapular rash on the proximal parts of the extremities, extending to the hands and feet and usually involving only the extensor surfaces. Within a day or two, the rash spreads distally to the hands, feet, buttocks, trunk, and flexor surfaces. It then assumes a lacelike pattern. The time required for resolution of all lesions varies from several days to a week or more. The third stage is said to begin after the rash has cleared. For a variable length of time, the rash may reappear when precipitating factors such as trauma, heat, cold, and sunlight irritate the skin. Throughout the illness the child usually remains afebrile and asymptomatic.

Nursing Management

The child with erythema infectiosum may be kept home from school, but isolation is not considered necessary. The child generally feels well, and no treatments are indicated. Parents should be given anticipatory guidance concerning the stages of the rash. They may be reassured particularly that the third stage is normal and that the problem will disappear in time. Aspirin may be given for arthralgia.

Scarlet Fever

Scarlet fever is an infection caused by the group A beta-hemolytic streptococci. The primary site of the infection is usually the pharynx. Scarlet fever is seen most often in children between the ages of 2 and 8 years, in the winter and spring, and in temperate and cold climates. The mode of transmission is usually direct contact, but it may be indirect or by contaminated foods. The incubation period ranges from 1 to 7 days. The most severe complications of scarlet fever are acute glomerulonephritis and rheumatic fever.

The typical clinical course of scarlet fever is shown

schematically in Fig. 19-3. The disease generally begins abruptly with fever, vomiting, a sore throat, headache, chills, and general malaise. The fever reaches a peak by the second day and returns to normal within 5 to 6 days. If penicillin is administered, the fever returns to normal within 24 hours. The pulse rate increases and is characteristically out of proportion to the fever. The tonsils are edematous, enlarged, and covered with patches of exudate, while the pharynx is edematous and beefy red in appearance. During the first day or two the dorsum of the tongue has a white furry coat with reddened papillae projecting through, giving the appearance of a white straw-

berry. By the fourth or fifth day "strawberry tongue" is noted as the white coat peels off and leaves the dorsum bright red. The enanthema consists of erythematous punctiform lesions and petechiae which cover the soft palate and uvula. The exanthema (Fig. 19-4a) appears 12 to 72 hours after the onset of the illness as a diffuse erythematous papular rash first on the base of the neck, axillas, groin, and trunk. Within 24 hours the entire body is covered with the diffuse lesions that blanch on pressure and feel like goose bumps. The face usually is spared of lesions. The cheeks are red and flushed, and the area around the mouth appears pale in contrast (circumoral pallor). In the flexor creases of the joints, the lesions form linear streaks or lines that do not blanch (Pastia's sign). The rash begins to desquamate at the end of the first week. Desquamation is first apparent on the face, becomes generalized by the third week, is characteristic of scarlet fever, and is directly proportional to the intensity of the rash. Cultures from the throat or portal of entry reveal group A beta-hemolytic streptococci. A significant rise in the antistreptolysin O titer is evident during convalescence, leukocytosis is present, and the Dick test reverts from positive to negative a few weeks later.

Nursing Management

Penicillin is the drug of choice and may be administered intramuscularly, orally, or both. Erythromycin may be used in patients who are allergic to penicillin. Adequate early treatment prevents complications of rheumatic fever and glomerulonephritis and eradicates the carrier state.

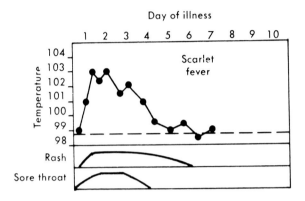

FIGURE 19-3 Typical clinical course of untreated, uncomplicated scarlet fever. Fever and a sore throat precede the rash by 24 hours. *(From S. Krugman et al., Infectious Diseases of Children, 8th ed., The C.V. Mosby Company, St. Louis, 1985.)*

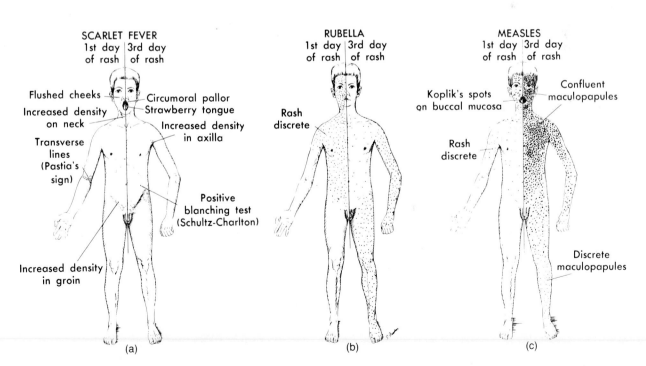

FIGURE 19-4 Differences in appearance, distribution, and progression of rashes of *(a)* scarlet fever, *(b)* rubella, and *(c)* measles. *(From S. Krugman et al., Infectious Diseases of Children, 8th ed., The C.V. Mosby Company, St. Louis, 1985.)*

NURSING CARE PLAN

19-1 The Child with Eczema

Clinical Problem/Nursing Diagnosis	Expected Outcome	Nursing Interventions

Skin irritation
  Weeping exudate lesions
  Redness
  Inflammation
  Dryness of skin
 	
Impaired skin integrity related to excoriated open lesions
	Child will experience no skin breakdown and will maintain optimal skin integrity, given appropriate treatment and supportive care	Assess and document location, type, and severity of lesions, especially over skinfold areas (popliteal, antecubital, and axillary surfaces); assess face, cheeks, and external surface of all extremities for skin breakdown and/or irritation
		Adequately control pruritus; prevent dryness of skin; preserve skin moisture
		Apply topical steroid creams as ordered (Kenalog, Valisone, Synlar cream); apply thin layers of cream several times during day as indicated
		Apply wet compresses saturated with room-temperature saline solution or solution as ordered for wet lesions (used for bacteriostatic drying and antipruritic effects)
		Avoid use of wet dressings at bedtime
		Apply topical creams ordered at bedtime
		Apply dressings with Kerlix for 25 to 30 min approximately 6 times a day; reapply and resoak dressings every 10 to 15 min during treatments
		For chronic and/or subacute lesions:
		Apply steroid cream, cover area with Saran wrap, seal with tape to create airtight environment; apply at bedtime and remove in morning
		Properly treat lesions as ordered
		For lichenified lesions:
		Apply coal tar preparation, ¼% 6 to 10 times a day as ordered
		Adhere to prescribed treatment plans that vary with child's specific needs and dermatologist's preference
		Assess and document effectiveness of prescribed treatment plan

Pruritus Pain related to itch-scratch cycle	Child will be able to rest and play in comfort and itch-scratch cycle will cease, given appropriate treatment and supportive care	Properly administer antipruritic and/or antihistaminic drugs as ordered Assess severity of itching during daytime compared with nighttime In presence of night scratching that is increased in severity, administer antipruritic sedation such as Benadryl elixir (diphenhydramine) (5 mg/kg/d), Phenergan Fortis (quinetolute) (25 mg/teaspoon ½ tsp hour of sleep), Trimeprazine, hydroxyzine hydrochloride (Atarax, Vistaril) which has been ordered PO [daytime antihistamines/antipruritics such as Periactin (cyproheptadine) 1 tsp tid and other drugs such as Actifed (guaifenesin), Chlor-Trimetron (chlorphenhydramine), or Pyribenzamine (tripelennamine), may be ordered] Assess child for effects of antipruritics and antihistamines on play activity and normal alert state Assure proper dose for age and weight; observe child for side effects; prevent oversedation or drowsiness during day to promote normal play and developmental growth Provide measures to maintain moisture of skin with application of lubricants and emollients such as skin softeners (Alpha Keri, Dormal, and Ar-Ex bath oil) Restrict bathing to once a week; encourage use of nonperfumed, bland, superfatted soaps Teach child and family that clothes need to be laundered with a neutral pH soap and must be well rinsed Teach child and family of need to avoid wearing irritating heavy clothing such as wool; encourage use of lightweight pajamas and cotton Minimize sweating which increases itching; prevent exposure to excessive environmental heat; discourage overstrenuous activity Support child and family during trial diets which may identify food allergens; provide teaching and written instructions regarding diet regimen Protect child from identified allergens and external irritants

Clinical Problem/Nursing Diagnosis	Expected Outcome	Nursing Interventions
Open skin areas Purulent erythematous lesions	Through early identification and prevention of infection, child will have negative wound cultures	Carefully assess child's skin lesions for signs of infection (increased erythema, draining purulent exudate from open skin areas, and elevated temperature) Properly obtain wound cultures as indicated
Potential for infection related to impaired skin integrity		Keep nails short and clean; mitt hands if necessary to protect child from introduction of bacterial organisms from scratching Protect open skin areas from urine and fecal contamination Ensure presence of clean, moisturized skin Properly administer systemic and/or topical antibiotics as ordered
Parents or child express anxiety, feelings of guilt, and frustration	Parents will verbalize and demonstrate an understanding of eczema and treatment and measures to control itching, dryness, and infection Child will achieve developmental milestones appropriate for age	Educate parents and child about eczema, required treatments, and comfort measures Teach parents and child proper application of topical steroid cream and about Burow's wet soaks for all required treatments as ordered Teach parents and child proper date, administration, and frequency of ordered medications and purpose of antihistamines and antipruritics Suggest measures to control itching (maintain skin moisture, prevent dryness and sweating, and avoid use of irritating soap, lotions, and clothing)
Ineffective individual coping and ineffective family coping related to long-term treatment and follow-up required for eczema Knowledge deficit related to care of child with eczema		Support parents and child through feelings of guilt, frustration, and anxiety related to chronicity of eczema as a skin condition; required treatments; and discomfort and irritability child experiences Encourage and support activities that promote the normal growth and development for child

The child is most comfortable in bed during the febrile period. After the temperature has returned to normal, quiet play activities should be provided in the home. During the acute phase, the upper respiratory tract symptoms probably cause the most discomfort. Acetaminophen, codeine, analgesic gargles, lozenges, and inhalation of cool mist may make the child feel better. A fluid diet is tolerated best during the febrile period. Parents should be informed about the natural course of the illness and should be instructed to observe for complications. Isolation of the child and his return to school depend on local regulations. Close contacts of the child should be watched for symptoms of a streptococcal infection; if symptoms occur, a throat culture should be done. A positive culture necessitates treatment with penicillin or erythromycin. Measures which prevent the spread of the bacteria at home include careful handling and thorough washing of the child's clothes, linens, and dishes; scrubbing dust-collecting surfaces; and cleaning and airing the child's room thoroughly after the illness.

Integumentary Diseases in the Preschool and School-Age Child

Varicella

Varicella (chickenpox) is a benign, self-limiting disease caused by the varicella-zoster (V-Z) virus. It is highly contagious and is seen year-round, with a predilection for late autumn, winter, and spring in temperate climates. Direct contact is the most common method of exposure, but indirect contact through a third person or contact with airborne droplets is also possible. A child with varicella may transmit the disease to susceptible children from 1 day prior to the eruption of his rash until all his lesions have become dry and crusted. The incubation period is from 10 to 21 days. Complications are not common, although secondary bacterial infection of the lesions, encephalitis, and pneumonia may occur. It is potentially fatal in a newborn and in children who are on corticosteroid therapy.

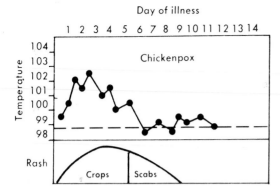

FIGURE 19-5 Clinical course of chickenpox. Crops of lesions appear with rapid progression from macules to vesicles to scabs. *(From S. Krugman et al., Infectious Diseases of Children, 8th ed., The C.V. Mosby Company, St. Louis, 1985.)*

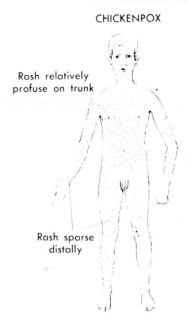

FIGURE 19-6 Typical distribution of rash of chickenpox. *(From S. Krugman et al., Infectious Diseases of Children, 8th ed., The C.V. Mosby Company, St. Louis, 1985.)*

The clinical course (Fig. 19-5) of chickenpox may be preceded by or occur with a prodromal period of anorexia, low-grade fever, and general malaise. In young children all symptoms usually occur on the same day, whereas the exanthema in adolescents and adults is more often preceded by a prodromal period of 24 to 48 hours. The lesions appear in crops, first on the trunk and then on the scalp, face, and extremities, with the heaviest concentration on the trunk and the lightest concentration on the forearms and lower legs (Fig. 19-6). Three successive crops over a 3-day period are the usual eruptive pattern. A most striking characteristic of the exanthema is the rapid transition from its beginning as a macule through stages of a papule, a vesicle, a ruptured vesicle, and finally a crust. This progression is accomplished approximately every 8 hours; therefore, any anatomic area will have lesions in all the stages of transition, and so recognition of chickenpox is relatively easy. The typical vesicle has the appearance of a thin fragile dewdrop on an erythematous base. It begins drying and forming crusts first in the center of the lesion, resulting in an umbilicated appearance. Scabs normally fall off in 5 to 20 days, leaving a shallow pink depression. Gradually, normal skin color returns without scar formation.

The mucous membranes also may be involved with lesions that rupture rapidly, leaving a white ulcer with an erythematous halo. The palate is most often affected; the palpebral conjunctiva, pharynx, larynx, trachea, and rectal and vaginal mucosa may be involved. The lesions are intensely pruritic until crusts form and cause extreme discomfort, particularly when located on the genitalia and in the vagina. Fever, anorexia, headache, and general malaise are common throughout the eruptive phase. The highest temperature is reached during the period of greatest eruption and is in proportion to the severity of the rash.

Nursing Management
Children with chickenpox are most concerned about the intense itching. Pruritus in the vesicular stage is the beginning of a cycle which may lead to scarring and septicemia

unless there is adequate treatment. Scratching causes rupture of the vesicles and the introduction of bacteria into the lesions. Normally they heal without residual effects, but those which are infected secondarily may leave permanent scars. A variety of treatments and preventive measures can decrease the possibility of infections. Calamine lotions, antipruritic ointments, antiseptic or starch baths, oral antihistamines, and sedatives are used in treatment, depending on the extent of the lesions and the response of the child. The hands, a source of infection, should be washed frequently, and the nails should be clipped short. In a young child or infant, mittens are used to decrease scratching. Clothing should be loose-fitting, cool, and lightweight and should be changed at least daily. Care should be taken never to break a vesicle deliberately. Gentle patting is preferable to rubbing when bathing the child or applying medication. Bed rest and antipyretics are indicated during the febrile period. Quiet play activities involving use of the hands should be provided. In addition to meeting the child's emotional needs, such activities serve as a substitute for scratching. Local regulations determine when the child may return to school. Generally, he is kept at home until all the vesicles have dried and the scabs are well formed. Parents should notify the physician if new symptoms develop. Neurological or respiratory symptoms are indicative of a complication. Lifelong immunity is provided by having the disease. No vaccine is available. Although varicella is usually a benign disease in childhood, it may be a severe and potentially fatal disease in adulthood. Consequently, attempts to prevent the normal child from exposure to varicella are not recommended. Conversely, exposed susceptible newborns, immunosuppressed individuals, and adults should be protected. High-titer zoster-immune globulin (ZIG) has been shown to be effective in preventing the disease in normal children and in modifying the course of illness in high-risk populations if given within 72 hours of exposure.

Rubella

The rubella virus produces a mild, self-limiting illness of major significance only because of the danger it presents to the developing embryo of susceptible women in the first trimester of pregnancy, when a variety of serious congenital abnormalities may occur. The virus is transmitted easily by airborne droplets, by direct contact, or by articles contaminated with secretions from infected individuals. An infected child frequently exposes others before his disease is suspected, as early as 7 days prior to the appearance of the rash, and as late as 14 days after the onset of the rash. The virus is found in nasopharyngeal secretions. First signs of the disease appear from 14 to 21 days after the initial exposure. One attack of rubella is thought to provide permanent immunity.

About 1 to 3 days prior to the development of the rubella rash, the child complains that the back of his neck is sore and stiff. Lymphadenopathy of the postauricular, posterior cervical, or suboccipital nodes is the reason for the complaints and is characteristic of the disease. A careful examination at this time usually reveals another sign— red spots, the size of a pinpoint, located on the soft palate. Named Forchheimer's spots, they are almost indistinguishable from the enanthemas of measles and scarlet fever and are not pathognomonic for rubella. In Fig. 19-7, the typical clinical course of rubella is diagrammed. A 1- to 5-day prodrome of malaise, anorexia, low-grade fever, sore throat, headache, cough, mild conjunctivitis, and coryza is seen in adolescents and adults but is only occasionally apparent in younger children. The exanthema (Fig. 19-4b) appears first on the face as a pinkish red discrete maculo-

papular eruption. Fever, rarely higher than 38.3°C (101°F), may be present. During the next 12 to 24 hours the rash spreads rapidly down the neck, arms, trunk, and extremities until the entire body is covered. On the second day, the temperature returns to normal and the majority of the symptoms subside. The rash begins fading on the face but remains on the extremities. The trunk becomes covered completely as the lesions coalesce and form a diffuse erythematous blush. In contrast, the lesions on the extremities do not coalesce and remain discrete. In most cases the rash disappears by the third day without desquamation. The duration of the exanthema varies from 1 to 5 days; rarely, the rash may be absent.

Lymph node tenderness usually subsides after the first day, but the nodes may be palpable for several weeks. Adolescents are prone to developing arthritis in one or more joints at about the same time the rash is fading. Fever may accompany the joint swelling and tenderness. Although the development of arthritis causes some anxiety in both parents and children, it usually clears spontaneously in 5 to 10 days.

Nursing Management

It is not unusual for a school nurse to find an older child attending classes with a rubella rash hidden under long sleeves. The child insists he is not ill enough to curtail his normal activities. The generally accepted feeling is, however, that it is more beneficial for the child, and others, to remain at home until the rash has disappeared. He need not stay in bed unless he has arthritis of the weight-bearing joints or other symptoms which make him feel quite ill. Acetaminophen controls the symptoms of fever and arthritis. Pruritus is not a problem. A persistent fever, continued malaise, abnormal neurological signs, purpura, or excessive joint involvement should alert the nurse to complications and the need for a physician to see the child.

Parents sometimes are confused about the differences between roseola, rubeola, and rubella and may report that their child is immune to measles. Careful questioning about the symptoms may reveal that a so-called rubella rash may in fact have been roseola, scarlet fever, or even a viral rash. Nurses should explain to parents that as a rule one attack of a particular disease, such as rubella, confers immunity for life.

In addition to immunity acquired by having the disease, a second form of active immunity is available through a single subcutaneous injection of rubella live attenuated virus vaccine (Chap. 4). Since the introduction of this vaccine in 1969 the incidence of rubella has declined to unprecedented low levels. Unfortunately, millions of children remain unimmunized, and rubella outbreaks have been reported.

Rubeola

Rubeola (measles, morbilli, red measles) is a highly contagious, self-limiting infection caused by the rubeola virus. It is a more severe disease in childhood than is rubella or

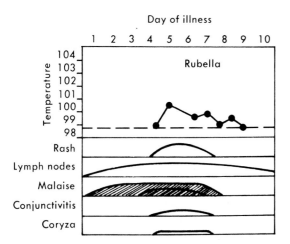

FIGURE 19-7 Clinical course of rubella. Three to 4 days before the rash, lymph nodes begin to enlarge. Prodromal symptoms are minimal in children (shaded area). Adults (hatched area) may have a 3- to 4-day prodrome. *(From S. Krugman et al., Infectious Diseases of Children, 8th ed., The C.V. Mosby Company, St. Louis, 1985.)*

roseola because of the intensity of the symptoms and the frequency of complications. Outbreaks occur in the winter and spring and reach epidemic proportions every 2 to 3 years. The incidence is greatest in children of school age, but rubeola may be seen at any age. The virus is transmitted directly by a cough or sneeze, directly by contaminated articles, or in the air by dust particles. The incubation period is from 10 to 12 days from the onset of the prodromal symptoms. Children are considered infective for a period of up to 2 weeks, from as early as the fifth day of the incubation period and up to a week after the onset of symptoms. The age of the child and the severity of the symptoms affect the prognosis. An infant with a severe case of measles has a greater probability of developing complications and therefore a poorer prognosis. Complications most often involve the respiratory tract, nervous system, eyes and ears, and occasionally the skin. Effective antibiotic therapy has decreased the mortality rate from secondary complications. The administration of gamma globulin after exposure to measles has improved the prognosis by causing the child to have only a mild or modified case of measles. The incidence of rubeola has decreased sharply in the United States with the use of live attenuated measles vaccine, but as with rubella, many children are still not immunized, and outbreaks of this preventable, potentially fatal disease have occurred. Children and adolescents who were immunized prior to 15 months of age are given a booster shot if a measles outbreak occurs in their school.

In the typical (Fig. 19-8) case of rubeola, a fever around 38.3°C (101°F) and general malaise are common on the first day. Within 24 hours the temperature increases and the child appears to have a severe cold. Sneezing, nasal congestion, brassy cough, and conjunctivitis are present. Generalized lymphadenopathy may occur. On the second or third day Koplik's spots appear on the buccal mucosa opposite the molars. These small, irregular, red-

dish spots with minute bluish white centers are diagnostic. On the third day an increase in the severity of all symptoms occurs. Usually by the third or fourth day the rash (Fig. 19-4c) becomes apparent. The erythematous maculopapules appear first around the hairline of the neck and forehead and spread downward to the feet over the next 2 days. By the time the rash reaches the feet as discrete maculopapules, those of the face and trunk may have become confluent. The child appears most ill when all symptoms reach a height on the fourth or fifth day of the illness or on the second or third day of the rash. The fever may be as high as 40.5°C (105°F); coryza is profuse; cough is harsh; the eyes are swollen, watery, and sensitive to light; the buccal mucosa is covered with Koplik's spots that are beginning to slough; and the rash is pruritic and almost covers the body. Within 24 hours, or around the fifth to sixth day, the temperature returns to normal and there is a noticeable improvement in the coryza, conjunctivitis, and cough. The rash begins fading in the same order in which it appeared and leaves a brownish staining on the skin and a fine, branny desquamation. The child coughs for a week or so, but there should be a steady improvement in his general condition during this time.

Nursing Management

A child with rubeola generally feels miserable and needs a good deal of supportive care. Bed rest is easy to enforce until the fever subsides. A variety of quiet play activities should be available to the child, but during the acute phase he probably will prefer to sleep. If photophobia is present, he will be most comfortable in a dimly lighted room. Watching television and reading may have to be postponed until sensitivity to light decreases. The eyes should be kept clean and free of crusts. They may be bathed with warm water to remove the matting associated with the conjunctivitis. Antipyretics are beneficial for fever and generalized discomfort. Medications for cough and coryza may be prescribed but are never too effective in rubeola. The nares may become excoriated by the continual nasal drainage and should be protected. Dressing the child in soft, lightweight cotton clothing provides maximum heat loss during the febrile periods and decreases the irritability of the rash. Calamine lotions may be used to control the pruritus if needed. Some parents become concerned about the brown staining of the skin as the rash fades (bathing in warm water makes this staining more apparent) but should be reassured that the staining will fade.

Antibiotics are not given or recommended routinely to prevent the bacterial complications of rubeola. Nurses must consider specific facts which influence complications when teaching parents about the disease. The more severe the illness, the greater the possibility of complications. The younger the child, the more prone he is to developing complications. Parents should be instructed to seek medical attention if there is not a noticeable improvement in the child after the third day of the exanthema, if there is prolonged fever or increased lethargy, or

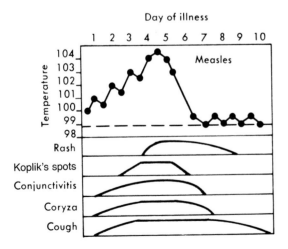

Day of illness

FIGURE 19-8 Clinical course of measles. The rash is preceded by 3 to 4 days of fever, conjunctivitis, coryza, and cough. Koplik's spots usually appear 2 days before the rash. *(From S. Krugman et al., Infectious Diseases of Children, 8th ed., The C.V. Mosby Company, St. Louis, 1985.)*

if the child has respiratory distress. Permanent immunity follows the disease whether it runs a full course or is a modified case. If a child has a chronic disease, is ill, or is very young at the time of exposure, the physician may believe that it is imperative for the child not to have rubeola. In this child, doses of immune serum are given to prevent the disease entirely. This passive immunity is, of course, temporary. Active immunity is also provided by a single subcutaneous injection of live attenuated measles vaccine (Chap. 4).

Impetigo

As a primary lesion, impetigo is an infectious disease of the superficial layers of the skin. There are two distinct clinical varieties. Nonbullous impetigo, the most common form, occurs in children and young adults and is caused by coagulase-positive streptococci and staphylococci. Both organisms can usually be cultured. In contrast, the bullous form is seen in infants and is primarily staphylococcal. Lesions may develop on any part of the body but are most common on exposed areas, especially the face, scalp, and extremities. Impetigo is contagious, spreads rapidly, and is rampant in the south, particularly during the summer months. It also is seen among children who are victims of poor hygiene, malnutrition, or crowded living conditions. The infection may be spread by direct contact with infected persons; it may be a complication of any skin condition in which there is a breakdown or irritation of the integumentary system, as in chickenpox, mosquito bites, pediculosis, or eczema; or it may be secondary to streptococcal infections of the upper respiratory tract.

In nonbullous impetigo, skin blisters develop from small reddish macules that fill with serum and rapidly become cloudy. Pustules form and then rupture, discharging serous and purulent fluid which forms straw-colored or brown, thick crusts on an erythematous base. Multiple lesions are common and may be present in all stages, sizes, and shapes. During this acute phase, chickenpox may be diagnosed erroneously. With proper intervention, healing usually occurs within a week or two, leaving a slightly reddened annular area that may be mistaken for ringworm. Bullous impetigo is characterized by large flaccid bullae that fill with a turbid fluid, collapse, and become crusted. The most serious complication of nonbullous impetigo is acute glomerulonephritis.

Nursing Management

Oral penicillin G (erythromycin for penicillin-sensitive children) is effective in eradicating streptococcal or penicillin-sensitive staphylococcal impetigo. Oral antibiotics are effective, however, only if given three to four times a day and for a full 10 to 14 days. A single injection of penicillin G benzathine (Bicillin) is just as effective as oral treatment and will eliminate failures due to poor patient compliance. Parenteral antibiotics and/or hospitalization are indicated in severe, extensive infections.

Local measures may be used as adjuncts to systemic antibiotics or as primary treatment in minor infections. The skin lesions are cleansed thoroughly with preparations such as hexachlorophene and Betadine one or more times a day, and then a topical antibacterial ointment is applied. Removal of crusts ensures a more rapid recovery. Soaks or compresses with normal saline or other solution softens thick, adherent scabs, making removal less painful. Once used extensively, local therapy is now considered to be of questionable value.

The lesions of impetigo are pruritic, and efforts should be made to prevent scratching, which can spread the infection. The fingernails should be clipped short and kept clean. Specific antipruritic therapy may be indicated. Since the disease is contagious, personal items such as towels and washcloths should not be interchanged among family members. In addition, all family members should be examined and treated at the first sign of infection. Cleanliness and adequate nutrition are of utmost importance.

Insect Bites

Bites and stings from insects should not be passed off as inconsequential. Serious hypersensitivity reactions may occur and are responsible for a significant number of deaths each year. Stings of Hymenoptera (bees, wasps, hornets, yellow jackets, and ants) account for the greatest number of deaths. The skin reaction to the bite of an insect results from hypersensitivity. A nonsensitized person will have little or no reaction, but a sensitized person may have an immediate, delayed, or combined reaction, evidenced by headache, fever, weakness, involuntary muscle spasms, and sometimes even convulsions.

With Hymenoptera stings, local hypersensitivity reactions vary from an evanescent, pruritic, erythematous urticarial papule to edema of an entire extremity. Generalized urticaria with symptoms of upper and lower airway obstruction, circulatory collapse, and anaphylactic shock may ensue as a systemic response. Serum sickness or nephrotic syndrome may be seen as a late sequela.

The venom of the scorpion can be both neurotoxic and hemotoxic, and death may occur, especially in children under 4 years of age. The hemotoxic venom causes painful swelling at the sting site; neurotoxic symptoms include numbness of the puncture site, convulsions with ascending motor paralysis, tachycardia, dysuria, and profuse sweating and salivation. Shock may ensue. The bite of a black widow spider may go unnoticed apart from the immediate sharp pain. Within a few minutes, severe pain develops and spreads throughout the extremities and trunk; the puncture site becomes inflamed and swollen and burns. In about 30 minutes, the venom enters the bloodstream, causing weakness, chills, vomiting, tremors, violent cramps, spastic contractions of the muscles, rapid shallow respiration, and tachycardia. Nephritis may occur. The black widow spider is endemic to nearly all areas of the United States and is responsible for most deaths due to spider bites.

Scabies is characterized by infestations with and sensitization to the tissue-invading mite *Sarcoptes scabiei.* (It is important to identify travel outside the country or camping trips during which the infestation might have occurred.) The mites copulate on the skin, and then the female burrows into the stratum corneum, depositing eggs and fecal material as she moves in a linear tunnel-like path. The eggs hatch and either make their own lateral tunnels or penetrate the roof of the burrow, beginning the cycle again. Severe itching, particularly at night, is characteristic and is a hypersensitivity response. Prolonged scratching may be associated with a scratch dermatitis and secondary infection. The characteristic lesion is the telltale burrow which appears as a dark, discrete papulovesicular linear scratch mark. The lesions usually appear between the fingers or on the hands, arms, axillas, nipples, lower abdomen, genitalia, and buttocks. In infants and young children, the scalp, face, and soles may be affected. The mite has adapted to living on humans and will not survive long if separated; transmission is by personal contact. Since the mite's life cycle is completed on humans, infestation will continue indefinitely unless treatment is instituted.

Nursing Management

Treatment of insect bites and stings is directed toward eradication of the symptoms and prevention. Application of ice to the site aids in slowing the reaction and in reducing swelling and discomfort. Corticosteroids may be used to reduce inflammation and combat urticaria and itching. Antihistamines minimize or counteract the allergic response. Ticks and stingers must be removed from the body for complete recovery. Attempts to detach a tick from the skin probably will result in the head being broken off and left in the skin. Instead, most ticks will withdraw when covered with volatile substances such as gasoline, acetone, alcohol, and fingernail polish. Excision is necessary for any portion of the head left in the skin. When the hypersensitive person goes into shock from an insect bite, epinephrine must be used immediately; tourniquets to affected extremities may be used to prevent further progression of the allergic reaction.

Specific antivenom is given for black widow spider bites and scorpion stings. Pain can be reduced by an intravenous infusion of 10% calcium gluconate either alone or in combination with morphine sulfate. Barbiturates may be needed to allay muscle spasms and pain. Neostigmine bromide may be used to reduce spasms of smooth muscles. Since no method of treatment is satisfactory for bites from mosquitoes, assassin bugs, and fleas, the hypersensitive person must learn to protect himself from these insects (Table 19-2). Awareness of the insects endemic to a particular region enhance the diagnosis and treatment of bites and stings.

Except in the case of a systemic hypersensitivity reaction, stings from Hymenoptera demand little attention other than removal of the stinger. The stinger and venom sac should be dislodged gently with a knife or other sharp object, taking care not to squeeze the venom sac. Pulling

TABLE 19-2 Ways to Decrease Outdoor Exposure to Stinging Insects

Avoid scented cosmetics, soaps, perfumes, etc.

Avoid areas known to attract insects (flowers, shrubs, wooded areas, swamps)

Avoid wearing floral-colored or dark clothing

Avoid loose-fitting garments which may allow insects to become trapped inside: wear long sleeves, hats, and socks; wear shoes at all times

Keep automobile windows closed when driving

Use insect repellents (helpful in some cases but of little benefit with Hymenoptera)

out the segments of the stinger or rupture of the venom sac cause dissemination of venom into the surrounding tissues. A paste of papain powder (meat tenderizer) and starch relieves pain quickly; topical antipruritic lotions and cool compresses provide additional symptomatic relief. In contrast, death may occur in a matter of minutes if immediate definitive treatment is not available to the hypersensitive individual. Aqueous epinephrine should be given immediately and repeated as often as indicated by the circumstances. Antihistamines, corticosteroids, cold compresses, and tourniquets are used as needed. The extremely hypersensitive person should know how to use and have available at all times a survival kit containing epinephrine, a tourniquet, and an antihistamine. In addition, desensitization, usually initiated with a very dilute solution of bee, wasp, hornet, and yellow jacket extract, should be undertaken. Although it is expensive, immunotherapy utilizing Hymenoptera venom conveys greater than 95 percent protection from subsequent sting reactions (Clausen, 1981).

Treatment of scabies includes thorough bathing followed by the application of scabicide to the entire skin surface from the neck down. Another bath is taken 24 hours later. Lindane (Kwell) is an inexpensive, effective scabicide. For complete cure, the bath-scabicide-bath regimen may need to be repeated in a few days. However, since the pruritic lesions represent a hypersensitivity response, slow resolution of pruritus and inflammation does not necessarily mean persistence of active infection. Application of topical steroids may speed resolution of the inflammatory changes. Clothing, including linens, should be washed in hot water with a strong detergent. Treatment of all family members or intimate contacts will help prevent the mite from spreading.

Poison Ivy

Poison ivy causes an allergic cutaneous contact dermatitis. It occurs as a delayed or cell-mediated response to direct contact with 3-pentadecylcatechol, a simple compound found in plant sap. Poison oak differs only slightly in structural detail. Children usually come in direct contact with the plant while playing, but highly sensitized persons may react to indirect contact with a pet carrying the allergen on its coat or to airborne ash from burning vegetation. Poison ivy is most common in school-age children in the spring and summer months. The eruption is self-limiting and clears in 2 to 4 weeks, although secondary bacterial infection of the lesions is a common complication.

Depending on the child's level of sensitivity, the vesicular lesions may appear at any time from a few hours to a few days after exposure. The lesions are seen most often on exposed parts of the body in linear tracks which coincide with scratch marks of the plant stem or brush marks of the leaves. It also may appear in areas in which the allergen has been spread by contaminated fingers, such as the face and genitalia. The vesicles rupture, crust, and normally heal without scarring.

Nursing Management

Pruritus is the common and constant complaint of children with poison ivy. Lotions containing calamine provide not only an antipruritic action but also lubrication, cooling, and drying, which are extremely beneficial. In more extensive cases in which control of infection is important, wet dressings, topical steroids, and antihistamines may be used. Oral steroids are reserved for very severe reactions with extensive involvement. The areas of involvement should be kept clean, dry, and well aerated, and the vesicles should be allowed to rupture spontaneously. Clothes should be lightweight and soft to decrease the irritation. Dressings generally are not needed, but if used, they should be loose and lightweight. Applications of lotion should be done with a patting motion rather than a rubbing motion. The child's hands should be washed frequently to prevent infecting the lesions, and he should be warned against scratching.

Parents should know that the more exposure to poison ivy the child has had, the more rapid and violent the reaction will be. Therefore, they should attempt to find and destroy plants in the immediate area and teach the child to recognize and avoid the plant. When exposure occurs, the child should learn to wash immediately with soap and water the areas that have been touched and possibly prevent the reaction if the antigen is washed off rapidly enough. Partial desensitization to 3-pentadecylcatechol is available, but it is not generally recommended except for highly sensitized children. The procedure takes at least 6 months and produces only a milder reaction to the plant.

Drug Eruptions

Adverse reactions to drugs are most often seen in the skin. They resemble other cutaneous diseases and are present in varying degrees of severity. Although the exact mechanism is not understood, there is good evidence for an allergic or hypersensitivity reaction in some drug eruptions. A variety of factors may influence or precipitate the development of a reaction to a drug. Age may be a factor in that adults have had greater exposure to drugs and an increased chance of developing allergies to them. Children

with serious diseases are more likely to have reactions. There is a high correlation between the number of drugs a person receives and the development of a reaction. In some cases the adverse interaction of drugs may be responsible. Toxic effects sometimes develop from an abnormal accumulation of the drug in the body. Some children metabolize drugs more slowly than normal because of inherited biochemical deviations. Illnesses affecting the renal filtration rate may decrease the normal urinary excretion time. Almost any drug, prescribed or proprietary, may produce a reaction when the circumstances in the child are conducive. The reaction itself depends on the particular drug and the child's individualized response. One child may respond to a specific drug with a single lesion, while another child may develop a life-threatening generalized epidermal necrosis. Drug reactions frequently involve other systems and organs in the body in addition to the skin. The prognosis depends on the identification and eradication of the causative agent, the extent of involvement, and the adequacy of treatment.

The most commonly seen drug eruption is urticaria, which is thought to be produced by the release of histamine in an allergic reaction. Urticaria, or wheals, begins with pruritus or numbness of a particular area which becomes erythematous and edematous; lesions with sharply demarcated elevated edges develop. If the lesions involve the lips, mucosa, or eyelids, there may be diffuse swelling rather than a recognizable lesion. The distribution of wheals varies. Some disappear in minutes, and others last for hours. Purpuric, maculopapular, and exanthematous eruptions are common. A fixed drug eruption, thought to be a delayed-type reaction, appears in the same location each time the causative agent is introduced. The single lesion appears as a purplish red, round, or oval plaque with sharp borders and is pruritic. It is most often located on an extremity but may be seen anywhere on the cutaneous surface. Cross sensitizations may occur in drug sensitivities, especially among the sulfonamides, barbiturates, and procaine anesthetics.

Nursing Management

Drug eruptions generally are self-limited and disappear in a short time when the offending agent is discontinued. Treatment is preventive and symptomatic. Through a detailed nursing history, the cause of the eruption can be identified. The offending drug is stopped as soon as possible. Epinephrine and antihistamines are antagonists of the histamine which is released in allergic responses and are used widely for symptomatic relief. Antihistamines are beneficial in relieving the burning and itching. Steroids are sometimes used with severe or widespread lesions or to speed the clearing process in less severe cases. After a drug reaction, even a small dose of the same medication will cause a recurrence. Parents should be informed of the drug or group of drugs responsible for the reaction and of the potential risk of giving the drug again. Children with sensitivities should wear a bracelet or necklace noting the allergy.

Integumentary Diseases in the Adolescent

Acne Vulgaris

Acne vulgaris, a chronic inflammatory disease of the sebaceous glands and hair follicles of the skin, afflicts 80 to 90 percent of all adolescents in varying degrees of severity. It develops during puberty and frequently lasts throughout adolescence and into early adulthood. Comedones, papules, and pustules are the characteristic lesions. Cysts and nodules may develop, and scarring is common. Regardless of the extent of the condition, it produces disfigurement, if only temporary, and anxiety. Even mild or inconspicuous lesions may be perceived by the adolescent as highly noticeable, causing him great worry and embarrassment. The type of lesions and their distribution, extent, and site of involvement vary. The basic cause of acne is still unknown; however, considerable knowledge of its pathogenesis does exist.

Acne begins with hormonal changes at puberty. Under androgenic stimulation, the sebaceous follicles begin to enlarge, secrete increased amounts of sebum, and become plugged by an altered keratinization of the sebaceous canal. As a result, normal flow of sebum onto the skin is obstructed, and the characteristic lesion of acne, the comedo, is formed. In an open comedo, which appears as a blackhead, the orifice is widely dilated and the contents easily escape to the skin surface. Although unsightly, open comedones are managed easily, and inflammation is rarely a problem. The closed comedo, or whitehead, is responsible for the inflammatory and severe lesions of acne. Because it has only a microscopic opening on the skin surface, sebum and keratin continue to accumulate within the closed follicle until the walls finally rupture. With the rupture, irritating free fatty acids, produced by bacterial lipases acting upon sebum, are released into the surrounding dermis, causing an inflammatory reaction. When the rupture is near the surface, a superficial pustule appears. These eruptions generally last only a short time and heal without permanent damage or scarring. If the rupture occurs deep in the dermis, a papule forms which heals more slowly and is more likely to develop into a cystic or abscesslike lesion. Destruction of the follicle and scar formation may be the end result.

During the course of acne, assessment of the adolescent's emotional state is as important as assessment of the lesions. His feelings about himself as a person, his peer relationships, his appearance, and his attitude toward the treatment regimen should be established. The distribution and extent of the lesions and the depth of tissue involvement should be assessed. The face, neck, chest, back, and arms, which are areas of large, active sebaceous glands, should all be examined for possible involvement. Scarring should be noted. If treatment has been in progress for some time, the effects of various medications should be evaluated.

Nursing Management

The long-range objective of therapy is to prevent permanent scarring and promote a healthy self-image in the patient. The adolescent must understand that although acne is a long-term condition, he does have some control over it. Periods of remission and exacerbation occur. A good understanding of the progression of the lesions and of the rationale of the various treatments recommended is essential. Since improvement sometimes takes up to 12 weeks, he should not be discouraged if improvement is not immediate. The adolescent should help plan his own skin care and should be encouraged to evaluate the results and assist in planning a new regimen if needed.

Specific therapeutic approaches are aimed at reducing free fatty acids, preventing follicular hyperkeratosis, and eliminating formation of comedones and other lesions. A variety of topical agents are used to attain these objectives. Systemic antibodies may be prescribed to decrease the population of *C. acnes.*

In females over 16 years of age, anovulatory drugs may be used to suppress androgenic stimulation of sebum production. The dosage required to suppress sebum production will cause feminizing effects if used in males and can inhibit bone growth in patients under 16 years of age.

Acne surgery or mechanical expression of comedones, pustules, and cysts is used by some dermatologists. Any squeezing of the lesions by the patient should be discouraged because it often causes rupture of the follicle and inflammation and scarring. The adolescent is encouraged to eat a balanced diet and to try to identify and eliminate from the diet specific foods that lead to the development of new lesions.

In patients not using tetracycline or vitamin A, sunshine is beneficial. Acne frequently clears during the summer months and flares up in the fall. Therapy with ultraviolet light produces a peeling effect and may be prescribed two to three times a week.

Adolescents should be cautioned that scrubbing or rubbing the skin too hard may damage it. An oil-base lotion may be prescribed if severe chapping occurs. Generally, however, adolescents are instructed not to use other creams or lotions on the face because the oil, grease, or wax contained in these applications plugs the follicles. Dry face powder, rouge, and eye makeup may be substituted. Oily or greasy suntan preparations should not be used on affected areas while sunbathing. Greasy hair preparations should be avoided. Seborrhea is often present as a result of marked oiliness of the scalp. To remove the excess oil, the scalp may need to be washed two to three times per week. Soapless shampoos are preferred to oily or superfatted ones. Many commercially available shampoos contain antiseborrheic agents. In severe cases, topical lotions or steroids may be used in addition to special shampoos.

Adolescents need support to cope with acne. They must be encouraged to find activities in which they can excel and in which they can increase their self-confidence and self-esteem. Expressing frustrations and feelings to an understanding person, such as a nurse, is also beneficial, particularly when contact can be maintained over a period of years. The scars left on the face and other areas generally show some improvement in a few years. If they are severe or create psychological problems,

NURSING CARE PLAN

19-2 *The Adolescent with Acne*

Clinical Problems/Nursing Diagnosis	Expected Outcome	Nursing Interventions
Comedones Papules Pustules Cysts Nodules Impaired skin integrity related to increased sebaceous activity, hormonal changes, and emotional stress	Adolescent will experience decrease in development of lesions, control excessive sebaceous gland activity, no permanent scarring, control of inflammatory process, and remain free of infection by following recommendations of nurse and physician	Assess distribution, extent, and type of lesions (inflamed and noninflamed) Assess depth of tissue involvement Examine areas with active sebaceous gland activity (face, neck, chest, back, and arms) Note presence of scarring Properly administer prescribed medication: topical keratolytic agents containing sulfur, resorcinol, or salicylic acid may be ordered for drying and peeling effects on skin in addition to desquamation, reduction in free fatty acids, and bacteriostatic effects; benzoyl peroxide and vitamin A acid may be prescribed in combination as their effects include fine desquamation of the skin and reduction of free fatty acids Administer systemic antibiotics, such as the tetracyclines, which inhibit growth of corynebacterium acne by decreasing fatty acids Administer corticosteroids for their anti-inflammatory actions and estrogen-progestins to suppress sebum production Promote use of cleansing agents and astringents that aid in superficial desquamation, opening plugged follicles 2 to 3 times a day Teach adolescent to avoid damaging skin with vigorous scrubbing and exposure to excessive warmth, heat, and humidity; using greasy oil-based cosmetics and leaving cosmetics on overnight; squeezing and picking lesions; using over-the-counter "fast" remedies; and overusing prescribed medications to speed desired effects Encourage meticulous and frequent cleansing of skin and hair with prescribed agents to decrease oiliness of skin; excessive dryness must be avoided Teach importance of taking medications exactly as prescribed; include adolescent in planning treatment regimen; encourage adequate rest and moderate activity and exercise; encourage a well-balanced diet and prevent constipation; preserve emotional health; reduce emotional stress Evaluate effectiveness of medications and prescribed treatments; assess adolescent's compliance; write treatment plan in clear, concise terms Facilitate adequate follow-ups with dermatology clinic
Adolescent verbalizes feeling "different," unpopular Body image disturbance related to inflamed skin lesions	Adolescent will be able to preserve self-esteem, participate in social activities appropriate for age, and comply with prescribed treatment plan following several teaching/education sessions with the nurse	Assess adolescent's perception of acne and how it has affected social interactions, dating, school and athletic activities Explore adolescent's feelings about himself as a person and about self in relation to family and peer relationships Explore adolescent's understanding of acne; educate adolescent about disease process, including possible causes and required treatments Assess adolescent's coping mechanisms and experiences in coping with stress and expressing feelings Identify and encourage activities that enhance the adolescent's strengths and feelings of self-confidence Assess adolescent's willingness to participate in planning treatment regimen and complying with prescribed care Facilitate consistent ongoing psychological and emotional support Carefully listen to expressed feelings, fears, and concerns; address them and provide reassurance

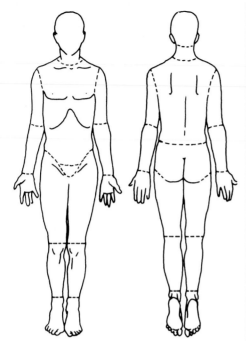

AREA	1 Yr.	1-4 Yrs.	5-9 Yrs.	10-14 Yrs.	15 Yrs.	Adult	2°	3°
Head	19	17	13	11	9	7		
Neck	2	2	2	2	2	2		
Ant. Trunk	13	13	13	13	13	13		
Post. Trunk	13	13	13	13	13	13		
R. Buttock	2½	2½	2½	2½	2½	2½		
L. Buttock	2½	2½	2½	2½	2½	2½		
Genitalia	1	1	1	1	1	1		
R.U. Arm	4	4	4	4	4	4		
L.U. Arm	4	4	4	4	4	4		
R.L. Arm	3	3	3	3	3	3		
L.L. Arm	3	3	3	3	3	3		
R. Hand	2½	2½	2½	2½	2½	2½		
L. Hand	2½	2½	2½	2½	2½	2½		
R. Thigh	5½	6½	8	8½	9	9½		
L. Thigh	5½	6½	8	8½	9	9½		
R. Leg	5	5	5½	6	6½	7		
L. Leg	5	5	5½	6	6½	7		
R. Foot	3½	3½	3½	3½	3½	3½		
L. Foot	3½	3½	3½	3½	3½	3½		
TOTAL								

FIGURE 19-9   Lund and Browder method of calculating burn size. *(From C.P. Artz and J.A. Moncrief, The Treatment of Burns, 2d ed., W.B. Saunders, Philadelphia, 1969.)*

several types of cosmetic treatments are available. They may provide the degree of attractiveness desired by the patient.

Thermal Injuries in Children

Burn injuries, the most severe form of trauma to the integumentary system, affect children of all ages. Burn injuries rank second only to automobile accidents as a chief cause of death due to accidents among children from birth to age 15 and some may be a result of child abuse. The causes and incidence of burn injuries in the pediatric population are as follows:

1. Scald burns account for 40 to 50 percent of burns.
2. Flame burns account for 20 to 30 percent of burns.
3. Chemical and electrical burns account for the remaining injuries.

Deitch and Staats (1982) found that 25 percent of pediatric patients admitted to their burn unit had inflicted burns. However, child abuse by burning often goes unrecognized because physicians and nurses are not aware of or do not observe for clues which would lead to such a diagnosis (Chap. 13).

The magnitude of the burn injury on the integumentary system of the body can be appraised by measuring the extent and depth of the injury, which usually is expressed as a percentage of total body surface area (TBSA) burned. A clinical method for calculating the percentage of burn in children is depicted in Fig. 19-9. This system takes into consideration the changes in percentage of body surface of various parts that occur during different

stages of development from infancy through childhood. It is particularly useful for children, since most fluid resuscitation formulas are based on this estimation.

Several classification systems to describe the depth of a burn injury are presented in Table 19-3. The actual depth of a burn injury is very difficult to assess, but the appearance of the wound, the way the injury occurred, the skin thickness over the parts of the body, and the variation in skin thickness in different age groups must be taken into account. In Table 19-4, different depths of injury and characteristics of each are described.

The depth of injury affects volume as well as composition of fluid lost from circulation. In a first-degree burn, which damages only the avascular epidermis, vasodilatation is the only major change and results in insignificant protein losses with little or no edema formation. Second- and third-degree burns are characterized by variable amounts of damage to the capillaries and account for the variability in the large amounts of fluid sequestered in and around the burn wound.

Damage to the integumentary system caused by the burn injury destroys the evaporative water barrier, thus increasing the insensible water loss from 4 to 15 times normal. Evaporative water losses are especially high in children since the ratio of body surface area to body weight is increased greatly. Very strict attention must be paid to fluid losses in an infant and young child. Physiological immaturity of renal-cardiovascular system prevents adequate response to hypervolemia or hypovolemia.

The burn injury also decreases the efficiency of the temperature control mechanism of the body. In the infant

TABLE 19-3 Classification of Burn Depth

Traditional Terminology	Anatomic Terminology	Depth of Involvement	Depth of Anatomic Involvement
First degree	Epidermal	Partial thickness	Stratum corneum of the epidermis
Second degree	Intradermal Superficial Deep dermal	Partial thickness	Dermis to a variable extent
Third degree	Subdermal	Full thickness	Subcutaneous adipose tissue, fascia, muscles, and bones

TABLE 19-4 Characteristics of Depth of Injury

Depth of Injury	Appearance	Pain Sensitivity	Edema Formation	Healing Time	Scarring	Cause
First degree	Pink to red	Painful	Very slight	3-5 days	None	Sunburn, flash, explosives
Second degree	Red to pale ivory and moist; may have vesicles and bullae	Extremely painful	Very edematous	21-28 days	Variable	Flash, scalds, flame, brief contact with hot objects
Third degree	White, cherry red, or black; may contain bullae and thrombosed veins; dry and leathery	Painless to touch	Marked edema (may require escharotomies)	Variable; requires grafting	Yes	Flame, high-intensity flash, electrical, chemical, hot object, scalds in infants and elderly

and young child hypothermia frequently occurs as a result of the increased caloric requirements, the labile heat regulatory system, and the high ratio of body surface area to body weight.

The destruction of skin by burning causes loss of the first line of defense against infection and produces an excellent culture medium for bacteria. Since the skin is so thin in children, conversion of deep dermal burns to full-thickness burns may result rapidly from bacterial, fungal, or viral invasions.

Local Treatment of Burn Wounds

Burn wound sepsis has long been a major problem of the burn patient. Streptococcal and staphylococcal sepsis have been brought under control with antibiotics only to have a new problem emerge, that of gram-negative bacteria (*Pseudomonas, Aerobacter, Klebsiella, Escherichia coli*, etc.). More recently, burn infections have been traced to such so-called nonpathogens as *Serratia, Providencia stuartii*, fungi such as *Candida* and *Mucor*, and even viruses. Numerous attempts have been made to control burn wound sepsis with multiple broad-spectrum systemic antibiotics, but they have usually failed because of lack of an effective blood supply to the burned area.

The most popular topical agent at present is 1% silver sulfadiazine (Silvadene), spread liberally over the wound. The treatment may be open, semiclosed, or closed. Some physicians prefer the semiclosed method, employing one

or two layers of fine mesh and light dressings to hold the mesh in place. These dressings may be changed once or twice a day. The advantages of silver sulfadazine are that it (1) is applied easily, (2) is soothing when applied, (3) softens the eschar, allowing less painful debridement and increased joint mobility, and (4) is absorbed more slowly, decreasing the chance of renal toxicity. This drug has been proved effective against a wide spectrum of gram-negative and gram-positive organisms as well as *Candida*. Researchers have failed to demonstrate the development of resistant strains. As with other sulfa drugs, a hypersensitive reaction occurs in approximately 5 percent of patients treated with silver sulfadiazine. This drug appears to have more of the characteristics sought in the ideal topical agent than others which have been developed to date.

Definitive Closure of the Wound

A discussion of wound care would not be complete without addressing debridement and closure of the wound—which is the overall long-term objective of burn therapy. Cleansing and debridement of the wound may be accomplished after initial fluid resuscitation and airway maintenance have been initiated. Debridement begins with the initial cleansing of the wound with a dilute iodine base solution and removal of all loose epidermis. It is carried out daily until all eschar is removed and the wound is healed by primary healing or secondary closure (as in skin grafting). Dead or dying tissue must either be removed or slough spontaneously before open wounds can heal. Early excision of deep dermal and full-thickness burns shortens the course of the illness by means of early closure, prevention of wound infection, and reduction of complications resulting from wound contracture and scarring. With the advent of improved infection control, the increased availability of homograft and heterograft, improved tissue typing techniques, and breakthroughs in transplant immunology, early staged excision has become the treatment of choice in most deep dermal and full-thickness injuries.

Tangential excision is a surgical technique of removing the burned eschar of deep dermal burns with a small freehand knife or dermatome. Thin layers of eschar are repeatedly shaved away until bleeding begins. Ideally, these wounds are then covered with autografts. When insufficient donor sites are available, homograft may be used as a temporary cover (2 to 6 weeks). This procedure must be performed early, preferably in the first 5 days, before significant wound colonization occurs. Its advantage is the early closure of the wound with increased joint function and less scarring. Fascial excision is a surgical technique of removing eschar from full-thickness burns. This technique involves the removal of not only the wound itself but also the underlying fat down to the level of the fascia. This procedure is chosen when large areas of full-thickness burn must be removed, since the fascia has a better vascular supply to support the take of the autograft. If small areas of full-thickness burns are to be excised in places other than a face, a tangential excision may be the procedure of choice because it conserves fat and normal body contours. These areas can then be covered on subsequent grafting procedures.

Advances in grafting techniques have improved mortality and morbidity. The *postage stamp* graft consists of small postage stamp-sized pieces of split-thickness skin placed on granulation tissue, allowing small intervening areas of granulation tissue to heal between grafts. With the *Tanner mesh graft* a strip of split-thickness skin is run through a special cutting machine. Multiple parallel rows of staggered small slits are cut in the skin, allowing it to expand and thus cover as much as nine times the area of the original donor skin. This technique and other advances have made it possible to cover burn areas of more than 50 percent in a relatively small amount of time, thus decreasing the morbidity and mortality.

Heterografts (animal skin) and homografts (human skin) also have decreased the overall morbidity and mortality of burns. The use of heterografts as a biologic dressing to protect the burn wound has increased as both fresh and lyophilized heterografts (porcine skin) have become commercially available. Homografts generally are preferred over heterografts, but the supply cannot meet the demand. Newer techniques of tissue typing have made the use of matched homografts for long-term "take" a possibility. In addition, experiments with artificial skin preparations are under way. Yannas and Burke (1980) developed an artificial dermis with a silicone covering that can be applied to the excised burn wound as a graft. Then, as donor skin becomes available, the outer covering is removed and the autograft is applied. Both homografts and heterografts are used in many ways to aid the recovery of the burn patient:

1. Immediate coverage of superficial second-degree wounds (hastens healing)
2. Debridement of "untidy" wounds as eschar separation nears completion
3. Promotion of healing of deep second-degree burns
4. Temporary, immediate coverage after excision
5. Coverage of granulation tissue between "crops" of autografts in the larger burn
6. "Test" material prior to autografting (adherence of homograft predicts success of autograft)
7. Coverage of other surgical wounds prior to secondary closure

Homographs and heterografts have several advantages, primarily the restoration of the function of the epidermis as a water vapor barrier and the virtual elimination of protein loss from the burn wound. This restoration of the water vapor barrier decreases the energy demands on the body, thus decreasing the massive caloric expenditures associated with large open wounds. Other major advantages include relief of pain, thus increasing joint mobility; reduction in the bacterial count of the burn wound as the grafts become adherent to the wound; and protection of exposed burns, tendons, vessels, and nerves from desiccation until a more definitive coverage can be obtained.

Response of the Cardiovascular System

In the immediate postburn period violent and dramatic changes in the dynamics of the whole circulation result in what is known clinically as burn shock. As plasma and blood volume begin to decrease rapidly, cardiac output drops even further. The striking decrease in cardiac output unexplained by any change in blood volume suggests a direct myocardial effect of thermal trauma. Although slower in onset than the decrease in cardiac output, the blood volume deficit after thermal injury can be profound and is proportional to the extent and depth of the burn. In burns of greater than 30 percent TBSA, increased vascular permeability exists throughout the vascular tree, although it is more pronounced in the burned area. Free loss of plasma protein, including fibrinogen, into the extravascular, extracellular space results in a concentration of protein in this area as high as 3 g/100 ml and probably acts later to perpetuate the holding of large volumes of fluid in the extravascular space.

The immediate red blood cell hemolysis does not exceed 10 percent; thus, the decrease in blood volume is due primarily to the loss of plasma volume. Measurements of the total functional extracellular fluid (ECF) volume indicate that the ECF volume deficit is considerably greater than even the plasma volume deficit. The greatest loss in both plasma and ECF volume takes place within the first 12 hours and continues at a much slower rate for only an additional 6 to 12 hours. This sequestering of fluids in the extracellular space may be accounted for by the avid uptake of sodium and water by injured tissue.

Replacement of fluids sequestered in the burn wound is the most important goal of the initial therapy of thermal injury. Lactate Ringer's solution is the solution of choice because it most closely approximates the composition of ECF. The total quantity of lactated Ringer's solution to be administered is based on the following formula: 4 ml Ringer's lactate per kilogram body weight per percentage of burned area. The total quantity of fluid is given during the first 24 hours, with one-half the amount given in the first 8 hours to coincide with the time of the losses of fluids from both the plasma and ECF spaces.

Approximately 20 to 30 hours after the burn the capillary integrity seems to be reestablished. The administration of colloid at this time in the form of plasma produces a substantial increase in cardiac output and plasma volume and maintains them at these levels without further administration of additional colloid. In the second 24 hours, a decreasing volume of administered fluids is required to maintain volume. Beginning approximately 24 hours after the burn, the increased evaporative water loss through burned skin is clinically apparent. Water must be supplied in an amount sufficient to maintain the serum sodium within a normal range (138 to 142 meq/liter). The increased daily water requirements vary according to the depth and extent of burn as well as age. Second-degree burns have a greater insensible water loss than do third-degree burns. Younger children (below the age of 3 years) require more proportionately since their normal insensible water losses may exceed 100 ml/lb/d. Occlusive dressings or burned surfaces in contact with the bed and not exposed to air and air velocity are other factors which may influence the amount of insensible water loss. Thus, replacement of daily water requirements must be based on frequent evaluations of serum sodium levels.

Beginning in the second 24 hours, potassium is excreted in large amounts and must be replaced. In children 40 to 100 meq potassium per day may be required to maintain a normal serum potassium concentration.

After 48 hours, mobilization of burn wound edema begins. The body weight begins to decrease and should reach preburn weight in about 10 days, at which time the majority of the burn wound edema should be mobilized. During this period there seems to be an expanded blood volume as evidenced by increased cardiac output, slight tachycardia, declining hemoglobin concentrations, and a notable diuresis; in reality a progressive profound anemia exists. Thus, fluid therapy after 48 hours should include water and electrolytes to maintain serum sodium and potassium within normal limits and packed red blood cells to maintain a normal hemoglobin concentration.

Pulmonary Response to Burn Injury

Pulmonary complications persist as a major cause of morbidity and mortality in the burn patient. The early (first week) complications include carbon monoxide poisoning; intrinsic and extrinsic obstruction due to edema of the face, neck, and upper airway; atelectasis resulting from restriction of the chest wall by the burn eschar; inhalation injury with resultant respiratory distress syndromes; and pneumonia. Late pulmonary complications include pneumonia, pulmonary edema, and atelectasis. During the early postburn period upper airway problems often present as edema and obstruction of the upper airway or bronchospasms due to chemical irritation of the upper airways from toxic products of combustion. Direct heat injury to the lower respiratory tract rarely occurs because of the remarkable ability of the moist air in the respiratory tract to cool entering hot air. Early recognition of potential respiratory complications is essential to successful treatment. Careful attention to history (preburn history as well as details of the burn injury), physical findings, and early baseline laboratory studies indicate predisposition to pulmonary complications. The history includes any previous respiratory condition such as asthma, bronchitis, chronic lung disease, or cardiac problems. It is important to have a complete history of the accident, including the burning agent, whether the accident occurred in a closed space, whether the patient had been unconscious or overcome by smoke, or in cases of chemical burns, if the patient aspirated any of the chemical. Any of the following physical findings should alert one to the possibility of respiratory burn: deep facial burns, singed nasal vibrissae, blistering of the mouth, oropharyngeal inflammation, soot in the oropharynx, progressive hoarseness, and labored or rapid breathing or hacking cough. Rales and rhonchi are not usually present for a number of hours but may occur at any time. Sudden high fever, extreme restlessness, and disorientation are early signs of hypoxia from respiratory complications. Circumferential eschar of the chest wall or neck; soft tissue injuries; obstructing edema of the lip, tongue, pharynx, or larynx; and fractures of the jaw or maxilla, larynx, or ribs are physical findings with important respiratory implications. Evaluating the patient's pulmonary status and noting his physical and laboratory findings are important for the prevention, diagnosis, and treatment of pulmonary difficulties.

Renal Response to Burn Injury

Burn-induced renal insufficiency during the early postburn period represents a reversible functional response to *hypovolemic shock*. With diminished cardiac output, renal blood flow is drastically reduced, resulting in impaired renal function and decreasing the effectiveness of the kidney in varying urine volume and concentration in response to homeostatic needs. Because of immature renal function in young children (under 2 years of age), they are more susceptible to impaired kidney function.

In burns covering more than 15 to 20 percent of body surface, reduced urinary output is immediately evident, and the essence of therapy is to establish adequate urine flow promptly. Large amounts of sodium-containing intravenous fluids must be administered early to prevent acute renal failure. Urine volumes in excess of 10 ml/h in the infant, 20 ml/h in the preschool child and older children up to puberty, are essential for the support of renal function.

Other renal complications beset the burn patient. Urinary tract infections, whether catheter-induced or systemic, occur frequently. Renal impairment may occur from the toxic products of systemic sepsis, low-flow states associated with sepsis, or drug toxicity. The nurse must always be aware of changes in kidney function and in renal function tests in order to detect renal complications early.

Gastrointestinal Complications

Two of the most common gastrointestinal complications associated with burns are acute gastric dilatation and paralytic ileus which occur early and are associated with burn shock. For this reason any child with a burn covering more than 30 percent of the TBSA should have a nasogastric tube inserted initially and gastric contents removed to prevent vomiting and aspiration. Usually, it may be removed in 18 to 24 hours when adequate resuscitation has been accomplished and bowel sounds have returned. In burns covering more than 60 to 70 percent of TBSA, bowel sounds may not return for 48 to 72 hours. Continued gastric decompression may be required to prevent vomiting and aspiration, which often have disastrous consequences.

Another common gastrointestinal complication of the early postburn period may be *hemorrhagic gastritis* resulting in coffee-grounds gastric aspirant. Frequently present during the first 24 hours to 48 hours, it represents bleeding from congested capillaries in the gastric mucosa and may be confused with Curling's ulcer. Hemorrhagic gastritis is characterized by small volumes of coffee-grounds fluid accompanied by large volumes of air in the stomach and may be relieved by decompression of the stomach with gastric suction via a nasogastric tube. Since acute hemorrhage from a Curling's ulcer often follows such findings, the patient must be watched carefully. Neutralization of gastric acids with drugs to control the gastric pH in the range of 5.5 to 6.5 prevents further erosion of the gastric mucosa.

The precise cause of Curling's ulcer remains obscure. In general, Curling's ulcer can be prevented with drugs to maintain the gastric pH in the normal range, the rapid restoration of nutritional intake through the gastrointestinal system, and the control of sepsis.

The initial treatment for Curling's ulcer should include decompression and evacuation of the stomach, gastric lavage with iced saline, blood transfusions as necessary, and general supportive care. Instillation of antacids through the nasogastric tube help maintain a neutral gastric pH. Although the use in children is still being established, histamine H_2 antagonists such as cimetidine and ranitidine are useful additives to antacid therapy in the presence of severe bleeding (Fuchs and Gleason, 1988). Since antacids impair the absorption of orally administered cimetidine or ranitidine when given simultaneously, a staggered dosing schedule is necessary.

Metabolic Response to Burn Injury

Weight loss accompanied by negative nitrogen balance characterizes the metabolic response in patients with extensive burns. This catabolic phase is followed by a prolonged period of anabolism with gradual restoration of body weight and lean tissue mass. The basal metabolic rate during the catabolic phase is increased markedly. Caloric intakes are predicted for children depending on age and percentage of burned area. A used formula with children is 60 kcal per kilogram of body weight plus 35 kcal per hundredth surface area burned equals daily caloric need.

The increased metabolic rates are a response to the trauma and are aggravated by exposure to cold, pain, anxiety, treatment-related factors, and complications, particularly associated infections (Souba et al., 1988). Hormonal alteration, altered glucose metabolism, and alterations in protein and fat metabolism all influence the nutritional needs of the burned child; the more severe the burn injury, the greater the physiological response.

The initial goal of nutritional therapy is to diminish the rate of weight loss and body protein breakdown. This goal is followed by maintenance of body weight and protein stores with eventual increase in body weight and protein mass. Enteral tube feedings or hyperalimentation intravenous infusions are required until the child is able to eat an adequate amount of food.

Neuromusculoskeletal Changes Secondary to Burn Injury

The physical impairments which accompany burns are the results of immobilization, infection, or metabolic changes and include contractures, dislocation of tendons, dislocation or fusion of joints, heterotopic bone formation, limb amputations, and weakness secondary to neuropathy. Since fibrosis is an unavoidable response to deep thermal injury, it would be unrealistic to expect to avoid all deformities, but simple preventive measures lessen the incidence and severity of these complications. Proper splinting and positioning can help prevent deformities (Fig. 19-10). Active and passive exercise and early ambulation are prophylactic measures which may be employed (Fig. 19-11). Adequate nutrition to prevent unnecessary wasting of lean muscle masses and other musculoskeletal changes is important to eventual recovery and rehabilitation. During all phases of burn care, concern is given to the prevention and treatment of deformities so that the patient can return to society as a functional member. Without adequate follow-up care, contractures as seen in Fig. 19-12 are not uncommon sequelae of thermal trauma. Results as seen in Fig. 19-13, however, are achievable with new techniques of early burn wound excision and with programs of exercise, splinting, and the use of pressure garments.

Psychological Sequelae of Burn Injuries

A burn injury is extremely stressful for a child and his parents. The injury itself is frightening, and during his prolonged hospitalization he and his family face both physical and emotional pain, helplessness, dependency, and the possibility of disfigurement, disability, and death. Medical personnel caring for these patients deal not only with shock, electrolyte imbalance, sepsis, nutrition, and wound healing but also with fear, depression, grief, and guilt in both the child and his family. Recent research, discussed by Knudson-Cooper and Thomas (1988), indicates better

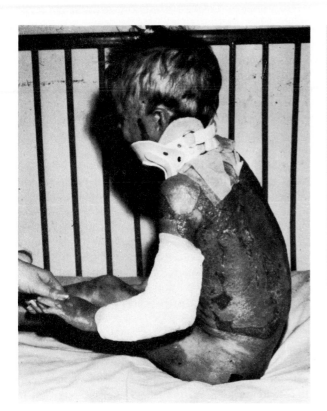

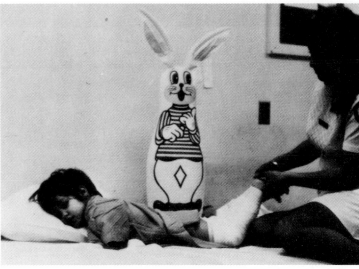

FIGURE 19-11   Physical therapist exercising patient to prevent new contractures in this child with a 10 percent burn to the legs.

FIGURE 19-10   Demonstrating the use of neck and elbow splints to prevent further contracture in a child with a 50 percent burn.

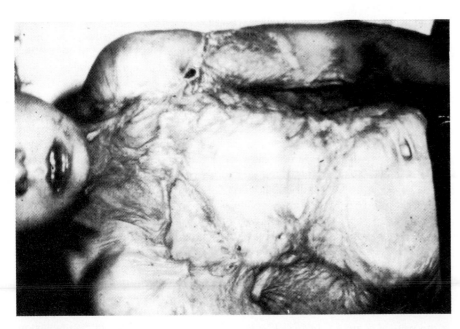

FIGURE 19-12   Contractures resulting from inadequate follow-up care after a 50 percent burn. This photograph was taken 2 years after the injury.

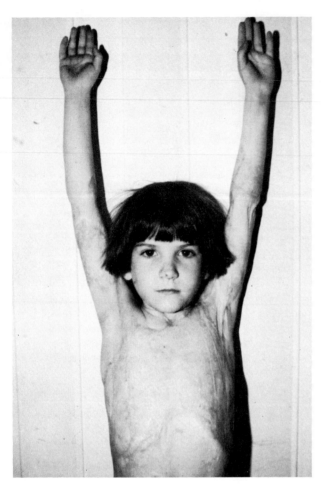

FIGURE 19-13   Results of a 40 percent full-thickness injury in a 4-year-old after early excision, grafting, and wearing of pressure garments for 13 months after the injury.

recovery and adjustment than was previously reported. In some studies, social support, especially family support, was the best predictor of adjustment. In others, preburn general functioning was closely related to postburn functioning. A high incidence of psychopathology in the family unit antedating the burn incident has been reported, suggesting that chronic relationship problems may become overtly manifest at the time of the child's injury.

An in-depth history of the psychosocial aspect of family life and the circumstances surrounding the burn accident should be a clue to the best approach to treating the potential psychological sequelae of the burn injury. The precise treatment of any individual must be based on the interactions of the patient, his family, and the medical, nursing, and paramedical personnel involved.

The burned child also experiences the anxieties of being removed from the care of his family and familiar surroundings and being placed in the care of total strangers in a strange environment. He may experience many other anxieties: the emotional trauma of the accident itself; the constant physical pain—the pain of movement, the pain of lying still, the pain of treatments, or the pain of someone trying to comfort or cuddle the child; the threat of

death and the wish to die; the threat of disfigurement and immobility; and the feeling of loneliness even when parents are present. All these emotional responses impinge on the child's response, both conscious and subconscious, and affect his ability to deal with the injury, treatment, and eventual rehabilitation. Obviously the age of the child determines which of these emotional responses is paramount in his adjustment to hospitalization and eventual disability and disfigurement.

Initially, in the preschool group, fear of strangers and strange surroundings and fear of painful procedures are major concerns. Children of this age group are frightened not only of strangers but also of people dressed in the isolation garb of the burn unit. The young child may fear his parents when they are attired in isolation mask, gown, and so forth. The frequent need to restrain the young child also adds to his fears. Many children this age experience fantasies about treatments and being restrained. Younger, preschool children (up to 3 years) usually will not express fears of death or disfigurement, but older preschoolers may ask such questions as "Am I going to die?" or "Will my skin grow back?" For the preschool child, frequent visits by parents and older siblings, familiar toys from home, and consistent care by a small number of nurses and paramedical personnel alleviate some of the early emotional stress. Where possible, it is important to limit painful procedures and the times when restraints are necessary. One of the most frequent coping mechanisms of this age group is withdrawal and regression. Attempts to change these coping behaviors rapidly may strip the child of his defenses. Patient acceptance and gradual replacement of these coping mechanisms with more appropriate ones are essential to the emotional support of the child. Continued support and education of the parents are essential to the care of the young child.

The school-age child presents a different challenge to those dealing with his emotional response to the burn injury. Although fearful of strangers and strange surroundings, he has learned that he can leave home and return and that his parents and familiar surroundings will be there. Therefore, his major concerns are what is happening to him, to his body, to his image of himself, and to his image as others see him. The child will want to know how did this happen, did I cause the accident, did someone else cause the accident, am I being punished for wrongdoing, why does it have to hurt so much? The school-age child often meets this emotional crisis with denial, withdrawal, and regression or open hostility. Initially the school-age child may deny that he is severely injured or that his burn wounds hurt. He may appear to accept completely what is happening to him. He often will be cooperative and say thank you to the person performing a painful procedure. Eventually this denial gives way to withdrawal. The child becomes more introspective, expressing concerns about death, disfigurement, and loss of self-worth. He may also become hyperactive or irritable during this phase. He may regress to more childish behaviors, whining, bedwetting, and crying for his mother. Usually this period is interspersed with periods of open hostility. Accusations of mistreatment by a trusted staff member or accusations that a parent does not care what happens to him or never visits him anymore may occur frequently. Sometimes the child is almost an adult with whom one can reason, and a moment later he is a small child having a temper tantrum. Just when the parent or nurse decides there is a way to relate to the child, he changes and no approach seems to work.

Loneliness is one of the major emotional hurdles of this age group. Even though the child's parents may visit frequently, he has lost all contact with his friends, his peer group. Initially his major concern is to return to his peer group. Later the realization that he will be different from his friends may increase his emotional stresses. "How will they relate to me?" may be the most pressing question on his mind as he begins to heal his wounds.

How to help the school-age child reduce these emotional stresses is a major concern of those caring for the patient. Accepting the child's behavior can be extremely frustrating. Understanding the child's coping mechanisms and his need for them may be easy on a cognitive level, but not when one must deal with this erratic behavior and accomplish the medical goals necessary for his optimum recovery. The merit of permissiveness versus a firm nonjudgmental approach is always the question. Unfortunately, neither approach is effective all the time, so that some mixture will usually produce the least stress for all involved. The child is often as confused by his own reactions as are his parents and the health care providers. An important aspect to remember about the school-age child is attachment to his peer group. Encouraging contact with his peers through letters, telephone calls, and, as he improves, visits may help ease the transition back to the peer group. Preparation of the peer group before the initial visit or the child's return to school often can prevent many problems between the child and his peer group. Also, planning for continuation of his schoolwork as soon as his condition permits helps keep him future-oriented and reduces the trauma of an eventual return to his school and peer group.

The adolescent approaches his initial injury and treatment phase with denial. Denial of the seriousness of the injury, of the loss of limb or disfigurement, or even of the threat of death is common in this age group. The teenager at first is cooperative and pleasant and complains very little. Sooner or later this coping defense gives way to withdrawal and/or open hostility. The identity crisis of the teenager never is felt more strongly. To be an adult and to face the responsibility of dealing with what life has dealt him or to be a child again and retreat into a protective environment is a major choice. Being an adult now has many more frightening concerns: How will others accept my disfigurement? How will I accept my disfigurement? The adolescent also may have to deal with guilt concerning the cause of the accident or anger against others who may have caused it.

Although caring for the adolescent may be met with withdrawal or open hostility, it is not usually as frustrating as dealing with the younger child. The adolescent usually can control these changes in mood, more or less. It is important to reassure the teenager that his reactions and moods are normal. He needs to be encouraged to talk about how he feels and often to express his intense anger. A typical response of the teenager is: Why did this happen to me? I was going to be captain of the football team next year. Why me? Why me?

Perhaps one of the most difficult problems in caring for the teenager is becoming involved with a disturbed parent-child relationship. Teenagers notoriously have difficulty coping with parents in their dependent/independent roles, and parents exhibit equal difficulties in these relationships. These same conflicts emerge in the sick adolescent. Parents tend to want to place the injured or ill adolescent in a dependent role, while the teenager tries to maintain independence. Hospital personnel can find themselves in the middle of this relationship like pawns in a chess game. Teenagers are masters at manipulation and often create tense situations between parents and hospital staff members as they relieve their own frustrations. Recognizing the dependence/independence crises of the adolescent and helping him move toward independence as he begins the long process of rehabilitation are most helpful in managing the emotional crises of the teenage burn victim.

Nursing Management

The nursing care of the burned child requires continued assessment, intervention, and evaluation of the numerous parameters of various phases of burn care. To simplify the multiplicity of nursing needs of these patients, they are discussed according to the phases of care: resuscitative phase (first 72 hours), acute phase (72 hours until healing or grafting occurs), and rehabilitative phase (postgraft).

Resuscitative Phase

Nursing care during the resuscitative phase is concerned with five major areas: fluid resuscitation, pulmonary care, prevention of infection, preservation of function, and psychological support. A detailed history including past medical record as well as a complete account of the burn injury should assist the nurse in planning nursing care and anticipating complications. For example, a history of asthma and the occurrence of the burn injury in a closed space indicate possible respiratory problems. A history of sickle cell disease suggests potential hematologic crisis with the hypercoagulability of burns added to the clotting difficulties associated with sickle cell disease. Also of extreme importance is a history of any drug or food allergies, since an allergic reaction may complicate the diagnosis and treatment of other supervening complications.

Early in the resuscitation period, diagnosis and treatment for pulmonary complications are of utmost importance. Upon initial examination, ascertaining that the patient has an adequate airway is paramount to his ultimate survival; it continues to be a major concern throughout the resuscitative and acute phases. The usual signs of acute respiratory distress (rales, dyspnea, increased respiratory rate, and bronchospasms) may be extremely rapid in onset in the burned child and are considered late signs of distress. The nursing management of a child with respiratory problems should include (1) observation of changes in rate and in character of respirations, (2) encouragement of coughing, deep breathing, and frequent changes of position to prevent atelectasis, (3) expertise in the management of patients on respirators, and (4) application of sterile technique and proper methods of suctioning when caring for patients with tracheostomies or endotracheal tubes.

Next in order of importance during the resuscitative phase is resuscitation for burn shock. Successful nursing management is dependent on the nurse's understanding of fluid therapy and the expected response to adequate resuscitation.

The expected signs of adequate resuscitation include: clear sensorium, urine output of 20 to 50 ml/h, a high normal pulse rate of 100 to 140 beats per minute, central venous pressure below 12 mmHg, and absence of acute gastric dilatation. An understanding of these signs enables the nurse to evaluate the patient's response to fluid therapy and anticipate complications arising from inadequate fluid therapy.

Infection control begins immediately and continues until spontaneous healing or grafting takes place. Extreme caution and superb aseptic technique must attend all procedures to protect the patient from infection. During the early postburn period (3 to 4 weeks) until granulation tissue is well established, patients with major burns (greater than 15 to 20 percent) should be afforded some type of isolation from the routine hospital environment. Isolation may range from a private room with reverse isolation precautions to specialized burn unit care.

Infection control of the burn wound begins with initial cleansing and debridement. Sterile technique should be used when cleaning all burned as well as nonburned areas with an iodine-containing solution to remove surface contaminants. Blisters that are intact should be left so unless they are in flexion creases (Carvajal and Parks, 1988; Kempe et al., 1987). All loose tissue should be removed. Immediately after debridement, definitive care with the selected mode of therapy should be initiated to prevent unnecessary contamination. Other early measures ordered by the physician to prevent burn wound infection are tetanus prophylaxis and the institution of preventive drug therapy, such as the use of a short course of prophylactic penicillin or other drugs to control an early streptococcal infection, which may occur during the first week.

Maintenance of function is also of utmost importance beginning in the resuscitation phase and continuing through the rehabilitation phase. During the resuscitation phase maximum joint function is maintained by proper positioning and slight elevation of burn extremities. The arms should be abducted from the body at 90-degree angles. The legs should be kept straight with the hips slightly flexed and the feet at 90-degree angles. Patients with burns of the neck should be positioned with the head slightly hyperextended. If the ears are involved, precautions should be taken so that pillows and other objects do not exert pressure on the ears, producing pressure necrosis. The patient should be turned frequently, and all joints should be exercised either actively or passively. Elevating burned extremities prevents further loss of tissue from increased edema and impaired circulation, resulting in progressive tissue necrosis. Frequently, elevation is not enough with circumferential, full-thickness burns of extremities, and escharotomies are necessary to prevent vascular occlusion and progressive necrosis. Proper positioning and elevation during this early postburn period prevent some of the later functional complications.

Psychological support for the burned child and his family also must begin with this initial phase. Pain, fear of the unknown, and fear of abandonment are all paramount in the child's thinking. As soon as resuscitation is begun and the patient is stable, analgesic medication should be administered so that debridement and other painful procedures can be accomplished without pain to the patient. Because parental support is extremely important for most children at this time, parents should be allowed to stay with the child as much as possible.

Parents also need support during this initial phase. They fear death, disfigurement, or deformity of the child and feel guilty for "letting" the accident occur or "causing" the accident. They need reassurance and simple explanations so that they can help the child cope with the situation.

Acute Phase
During the acute phase, infection control, maintenance of function, preservation of tissue, and psychological support continue to be primary nursing concerns. Careful observation for impending complications and adequate nutritional support become paramount.

Infection control during the acute phase continues to be a major concern. The fine balance between what to do and what not to do to protect the child becomes a problem. Absolute isolation severely limits many functions which seem to be important for the child's maximum physical and psychological rehabilitation. Some authorities believe that total isolation is imperative to infection control; others believe that with modern topical therapy, total isolation is not necessary. Resident skin flora and gastrointestinal tract flora are the most frequent colonizers of the burn. Therefore, total isolation systems may not provide the patient with the initially apparent safeguard. Careful reverse isolation technique in a "super" clean environment appears to offer the patient the environmental protection he needs without interfering with medical and nursing procedures and play activity which afford the patient both physical and emotional therapy.

Infection control centers on removal of eschar and necrotic tissue and protection of the developing granulation tissue. Painful debridement becomes an everyday encounter for the child and his nurse. Hydrotherapy, debride-

NURSING CARE PLAN

19-3 The Child with a Thermal Injury

Clinical Problem/Nursing Diagnosis	Expected Outcome	Nursing Interventions
Damaged integumentary tissue Destruction of skin surface and skin layers Impaired skin integrity and impaired tissue integrity related to thermal injury	Child will experience restoration of integumentary tissue, skin surface, and skin layers through prompt removal of eschar and necrotic tissue, rapid and thorough debridement of necrotic tissue, preservation of viable tissue, protection of developing granulation tissue, and healing of burn lesions without infection	Carefully assess and document type, location, extent, depth, and severity (total body surface area involved) of burn injury Assist with determination of percentage of total body surface area involved Assess appearance of all burn wounds: note presence of foreign material (glass); note color and pigmentation of wounds; assess presence of pigmentation and thickness of eschar; note degree of erythema and edema Continually assess for quality and progression of wound healing Assess quality of circulation and tissue perfusion: observe color and warmth of extremities, quality of pulses, and capillary refill Detect early signs of circulatory impairment from the burn wounds Support child and family through required surgical procedures, i.e., escharotomy and tangential excision Perform burn care recommended by health care team specified for type of burn presented; consult standards of burn care established for pediatric client as dictated by institutional policy Meticulously perform burn care with strict surgical aseptic technique Wash all burn wounds with warm sterile normal saline Support through hydrotherapy: regulate water temperature to 98 to 100°F; perform hydrotherapy 1 to 2 times daily; bathing in bed should be done systematically, exposing one extremity or area at a time to decrease heat loss Promptly debride eschar and necrotic tissue from burn wounds following hydrotherapy; remove loose tissue from wounds Avoid forcing removal of tissue (sterile scissors can be used to trim tissue edges) Note presence and degree of bleeding from burn wounds during burn care Consistently monitor complete blood count, hemoglobin, hematocrit, prothrombin time and partial prothrombin time, and platelet counts Properly apply topical antimicrobial creams as ordered over burn wounds: silver sulfadiazine (monitor child for leukopenia 5 to 7 days after treatment; does not penetrate deep eschar effectively) and Sulfamylon (mafenide) (effective for penetrating deep eschar; application of this antimicrobial is painful) Apply thin layers of antimicrobial cream over burn areas (antimicrobial cream may be aseptically applied to fine mesh gauze or aseptically applied by a gloved sterile hand using the butter technique) For occlusive dressings, secure with tubular netting: bandage fingers and toes separately, as these measures serve to keep antimicrobial cream and dressings in place and decrease evaporative fluid and heat loss while allowing skin to breathe For open wound treatment, provide warm environment, prevent evaporative fluid and heat losses, provide sterile sheets and bed linens, and use bed cradle to prevent friction and pressure of linens against child's skin Protect integrity of skin grafts: assess the grafts for hematoma or exudate formation; assess quality of tissue granulation with grafting Cleanse burn wounds; apply fresh antimicrobial cream and sterile dressings q 8 h as ordered by health care team and indicated by type of burn injury For discharge teaching in relation to burn care and follow-up treatments, develop teaching plan individualized to child and family's needs; determine need for visiting nurse support

Continued

Clinical Problem/Nursing Diagnosis	Expected Outcome	Nursing Interventions
Impaired skin integrity Altered immunoglobulin levels Presence of eschar and necrotic tissue Invasive catheters and invasive procedures required for treatment Increased protein loss through burn fluid	Given early detection and prevention of sepsis and burn wound infection, child will remain free of serious infection	Carefully monitor vital signs every hour (q 5-15 min during acute resuscitation phase) Assess heart rate for regularity, presence of arrhythmias, tachycardia, and bradycardia Auscultate lungs for equality of aeration; note rate, depth, and regularity of respirations Monitor temperature for hyperthermia or hypothermia (promptly report temperature of 38.5°C to physician); maintain normothermia; provide antipyretic measures Consistently assess child for early signs of sepsis: systemic vasodilation (extremities are warm with brisk capillary refill and bounding peripheral pulses) and for systemic pulmonary edema Monitor child for signs of an ileus: auscultate bowel sounds and measure abdominal girth
Potential for infection related to skin and tissue destruction		Assess patient for tachycardia, tachypnea, hypotension, and hypo/hyperthermia; note changes in child's behavior or feeding activity Carefully monitor burn wounds for color, increased erythema, drainage, change in appearance, microabscess formation, foul odor, and purulent exudate Ensure practice of strict protective isolation and meticulous hand washing techniques Properly administer tetanus antitoxin as ordered Perform meticulous burn care (see interventions under impaired skin integrity) with the proper application of antimicrobial ointment to wounds Optimize child's nutritional status and restore protein Properly dress and clean catheter sites; remove invasive catheters as soon as possible after acute resuscitation has been successful and child is stabilized Consistently assess quality and promotion of wound healing and granulation tissue formation; assess quality of circulation and tissue perfusion to burn wounds; assess all extremities Obtain routine serial surveillance cultures (urine, burn wounds, blood, tracheal secretions, and catheter sites)
Decreased intravascular volume Increased capillary permeability	Child will experience prompt correction of plasma and blood volume deficits and fluid, electrolyte, and acid-base homeostasis, given appropriate interventions	Carefully monitor vital signs; promptly report early signs of hypovolemic shock to physician for prompt intervention Auscultate apical pulse for rate regularity; monitor for arrhythmias and tachycardia/bradycardia Monitor blood pressure for hypotension, hypertension, and widened pulse pressure Assess child for changes in neurological status, behavior and sensorium Assess peripheral perfusion; note color and warmth of extremities, quality of peripheral pulses, and capillary refill
Fluid volume deficit related to loss of body fluid through injured skin tissue; fluid shifts from vascular compartments to burned tissue		Obtain accurate weight on admission (document scale used); monitor daily weights Monitor severity of burn wound edema Elevate burned extremities Document strict intake and output volumes hourly Insert Foley catheter as indicated by severity of burn wound (burns 20% of body surface area [BSA] require a Foley) Monitor urine output in response to fluid resuscitation; measure urine specific gravity, urine osmolarity, and electrolytes; note presence of protein, blood, ketones, and glucose in urine: obtain urinalysis for presence of hemoglobinuria/myoglobinuria Monitor blood urea nitrogen (BUN), creatinine, and 24-h urine collection; assess for signs of renal failure secondary to shock and decreased perfusion

Clinical Problem/Nursing Diagnosis	Expected Outcome	Nursing Interventions
		Ensure patency of intravenous catheters
		Administer volume replacement calculated for body weight and BSA of burn wound as dictated by child's hemodynamic stability (amount and type of fluids used in volume resuscitation vary with individual physicians and institutions)
		Monitor serum electrolytes, osmolarity, complete blood count, amylase, and liver enzymes; assess serum protein and nitrogen losses particularly 1 to 2 weeks after burn injury
		Assess for presence of metabolic acidosis related to renal failure, shock, and hypoxemia
		Monitor for presence of respiratory alkalosis related to hyperventilation
		Promptly correct electrolyte and acid-base imbalances as monitored by serum chemistries and lab values
		Avoid administration of potassium in presence of oliguria
		Prevent hypervolemia: with onset of diuresis, assess child for signs of fluid overload particularly 48 h after burn injury
		Avoid administration of intravascular injections to prevent risk of overdose from poor absorption of medications secondary to edema; avoid intramuscular injections to prevent infection and bleeding
		Closely monitor child's response to all medications administered (potential for impaired diffusion and absorption of medication)
Tachypnea Labored respirations Hoarseness and cough ─────────── Ineffective airway clearance related to thermal trauma of respiratory tract	Given early detection and prevention of airway obstruction and respiratory distress, child will maintain patent airway and adequate oxygenation	Obtain information relevant to history of burn: determine if child was in an enclosed space during thermal insult
		Identify inhalation of a chemical or burning agent
		Determine severity of smoke inhalation injury
		Carefully assess for presence of burns over face, neck, and chest wall; examine nose, tongue, lips, mucous membranes, larynx, pharynx, and glottis for presence of soot, blisters, edema, and erythema
		Note presence of black particulate matter in mucus or evidence of singed hair in nares or singed hair on child's head
		Carefully monitor child for signs of upper airway obstruction, laryngospasms, and bronchospasms; assess for presence of increased hoarseness in voice or cry, cough, stridor, or wheezing; promptly notify physician of signs of distress
		Assess for signs of respiratory distress: note rate, depth, regularity, and quality of respiration; observe child for labored respiration, nasal flaring, grunting, retracting, and increased respiratory rate
		Auscultate breath sounds for quality and equality of aeration in all lung fields: assess equality of chest wall expansion; assess for diminished breath sounds; note presence of wheezing and rales; monitor child's ability to clear secretions from respiratory tract; suction to maintain airway patency
		Monitor arterial blood gas values; obtain oxygen saturation values via pulse oximetry:
		Maintain $PO_2 > 90$ mmHg $PCO_2 < 40$ mmHg pH 7.35-7.45 O_2 saturation $> 95\%$
		Monitor carboxyhemoglobin values
		Properly administer humidified oxygen therapy; prepare for emergent endotracheal intubation or elective prophylactic intubation (secure endotracheal tube with cloth ties and avoid use of adhesive tape on burned face
		Perform pulmonary hygiene measures to prevent respiratory infection and atelectasis: elevate head of bed to promote maximum lung expansion, change positions frequently, and turn to mobilize secretions; administer nebulizers and/or medications for bronchodilation and antiinflammatory and mucolytic effects; monitor child's response and observe for side effects
		Perform chest physical therapy; encourage coughing and deep breathing; monitor results of chest x-rays to increase effectiveness of chest physical therapy

Clinical Problem/Nursing Diagnosis	Expected Outcome	Nursing Interventions
Tachycardia and hypotension Decreased peripheral perfusion Decreased cardiac output related to burn shock and reduction in circulating blood volume and direct myocardial effects from thermal injury	Child will experience correction of plasma and blood volume deficits, hemodynamic stability, and maintenance of optimal tissue perfusion, given appropriate nursing interventions	Assess child for signs of pulmonary edema related to increased capillary permeability; note amount, color, and consistency of pulmonary secretions Frequently monitor vital signs: auscultate apical pulse for rate and regularity; monitor for arrhythmias, tachycardia, and bradycardia; consistently monitor blood pressure for hypotension, hypertension, and widened pulse pressure Assess systemic perfusion: note color and warmth of extremities and quality and equality of peripheral pulses and capillary refill Monitor central venous pressure as available Type and cross-match blood for replacement needs: adequately warm blood and blood products prior to administration Properly administer crystalloid and/or colloid replacements on basis of weight, percentage of body surface area burned, insensible water losses, lab values, and clinical findings as ordered Monitor serum chemistry values, blood glucose, electrolytes, osmolality, protein, albumin, liver enzymes, complete blood count, and clotting factors Monitor strict input and output hourly Assess cardiovascular response to fluid resuscitative measures Prevent fluid overload; consult with physician regarding replacement, especially in first 24 to 48 h Maximize rest periods; eliminate environmental stressors; maintain normothermia (37°C) to decrease energy expenditure
Pain Inability to rest and sleep Anticipatory anxiety with burn care Pain related to thermal injury, burn care treatments, and dressing changes	Child will achieve: (a) adequate pain control as evidenced by child's ability to rest with comfort; (b) stable vital signs for age	Monitor vital signs for evidence of tachycardia and hypertension in presence of stabilized cardiac-respiratory function Observe child's emotional response to environment: assess appetite, interest in play, and ability to rest and sleep in comfort Understand child's difficulty and fear in verbalizing pain Properly administer intravenous analgesics as ordered; avoid use of intramuscular injections Administer analgesics prior to burn care (consider peak time of various analgesics prescribed): document and assess effectiveness of analgesia: observe child's cardiovascular tolerance to analgesics Monitor child's neurological status: pupillary responses, motor and sensory function, and changes in behavior Prepare child for dressing changes according to developmental level; encourage active participation Provide diversional activities (use of Walkmans and relaxation tapes) Provide comfort and support throughout all aspects of care

Hypothermia
 	
Ineffective thermoregulation related to destruction of protective skin barrier
	Child will attain normothermia: rectal temperature 37 to 37.5°C, given appropriate nursing interventions	Monitor temperature every 30 min to 1 h until stabilized
		Properly use warming blanket or overbed radiant warmer to achieve normothermia; avoid overheating; protect child from rapid decrease in body temperature to minimize stressors on cardiovascular system
		Administer warm humidified oxygen
		Administer warmed intravenous blood and volume solutions
		Prevent heat loss through evaporation of fluid
		  Expose areas on the body for cleansing burn wounds one small area at a time
		  Warm solutions to be used for burn care
		  Cover child to protect from drafts
		  Change bed linens often to keep them as dry as possible

Clinical Problem/Nursing Diagnosis	Expected Outcome	Nursing Interventions
Anorexia Pain Nausea and vomiting Hypermetabolic state<hr>Altered nutrition: less than body requirements related to increased metabolic demands	Child will learn to tolerate diet rich in calories and protein to promote adequate wound healing and will have positive nitrogen balance, given early detection of potential complications on the gastrointestinal system from thermal insult	Maintain NPO (nothing by mouth) for 48 h Insert nasogastric (NG) tube and aspirate gastric contents to prevent aspiration; maintain NG tube at low gravity drainage Measure NG tube output; check drainage for color, amount, consistency, and presence of coffee grounds or blood in drainage; maintain pH 5; administer prescribed antacids as appropriate Assess child for abdominal distention and tenderness; measure abdominal girths every 4 h Assess for presence and quality of bowel sounds; carefully monitor for presence of ileus (increased abdominal girth, distended abdomen, pain, and vomiting) Assess child for Curling's ulcer: hemetest stool and gastric secretions; note presence of nausea, vomiting, and pain (immediately notify the physician) Promptly institute nutritional therapy within 48 h of admission; assess child's ability to tolerate PO intake; supplement dietary needs with enteral feedings as needed; total parenteral nutrition may be considered as last resort if enteral feeds are not tolerated Consult dietitian and/or health care team to ensure accurate calculation of caloric requirements based on hypermetabolic state and increased needs (consider insensible losses and extent of burn injury); minimize environmental physiological stressors such as pain, temperature extremes, and anxiety Assess and document effectiveness of dietary plan; include parents in identifying favorite foods; provide small, frequent feedings; check residuals of child receiving enteral feedings; document daily calorie counts Monitor child's daily weight, using same scale, at same time every morning
Limited range of motion Decreased muscle strength Pain Scar and contracture formation<hr>Impaired physical mobility related to pain; burn trauma; scar and contracture formation	Given the necessary nursing interventions, child will not scar or form contractures and will maintain optimal joint and muscle function	Meticulously apply *constant* pressure over active, early scar formation; ensure proper application of pressure wraps or pressure garments at all times, except during bathing; pressure garments must be worn in presence of red, hypertrophied, active scar formation (possibly up to 1 year) Promptly consult physical therapist to measure child for splints and suggest positions that prevent contracture formation Remove splints q 4h for range of motion exercises Avoid positions that promote flexion in presence of neck burn (do not use pillows and keep head slightly hyperextended) Use cutout foam pillows to prevent pressure on burned ears Turn and position child to prevent contracture formation; avoid flexion
Anxiety Loss of control Disturbance in body image<hr>Body image disturbance Fear related to developmental stressors of hospitalization and required treatments	Given appropriate nursing interventions, child will preserve self-esteem, master hospitalization experiences, and maintain developmental milestones	Explore child's feelings about changes in body appearance through therapeutic play and art therapy Base preparation for procedures on child's cognitive and developmental level Facilitate opportunities for child to verbalize and express feelings and concerns in activity and talk, for example, story books that depict the fear of hospitalization and address specific experiences; carefully listen to reactions to story; provide opportunity for child to show his or her own illustrations in response to story Encourage child to write or draw pictures about hospital experiences or make his or her own story book Decrease effects of unfamiliar environment; give child favorite toy or security object; place pictures of family and friends on wall; encourage use of tape recordings with messages and stories from classmates; suggest that friends and siblings make cards and drawings Provide child with some control and choices; allow child to participate in burn dressings and care Arrange meetings with other children who have experienced pain from thermal injury Facilitate appropriate psychological intervention and ongoing support for child and family

ment, application of topical agents, and application of heterograft or homograft all evoke physical and emotional pain for the child and constitute a challenge for the nurse, who must cope with her own feelings as well as the behavior of the child. The ultimate goal of the acute phase is rapid debridement of dead tissue with preservation of viable tissue and definitive closure of the wound.

Exercise, splinting, and positioning to maintain function become a goal of physical therapy. Active and passive exercise to maintain joint function must be encouraged constantly if deformities are to be avoided. As long as the child is awake, is cooperative, and can be encouraged to move affected parts, splinting is not necessary. Splinting in a position of function is necessary during periods of inactivity, such as sleep, or when the patient is unwilling or unable to cooperate. Continuous splinting is recommended for any joint with an open capsule.

The child and his parents need continued reassurance and simple explanations. Procedures may have to be explained time and time again. This stage is extremely frustrating for health care personnel. Coping with the demanding behavior of the child, the antagonistic behavior of parents, and dealing with anxiety and frustration is very stressful for the nurse. Many of the acute emotional problems of the burned child and his parents can be managed best through psychological support for the nursing staff members so that they may help the patient and his family understand their coping behaviors.

An added concern in the acute phase is nutrition. The metabolic demands of the burned child are accentuated, and providing an adequate number of calories through conventional oral routes is frequently unsatisfactory for several reasons. The child may be unaccustomed to eating hospital food. His refusal to eat may be part of this reaction to the situation. He may be unable to tolerate oral alimentation because of gastric dilatation, paralytic ileus, or sepsis. His oral intake may be restricted because of surgical procedures. Ingenuity may be required to encourage oral intake. Careful planning among the nurse, the dietitian, and the mother can lead to a diet high in protein and calories which is acceptable to the child. Encouraging the family to bring favorite foods from home helps increase the child's appetite. If the child refuses to eat as part of his coping behavior, thus controlling at least one part of his new environment, hospital personnel must abandon conventional means of oral alimentation and use nasogastric feeding tubes or feeding jejunostomies to provide the necessary caloric support. These procedures never should be approached as punishment for the child's refusal to eat but as simple medical procedures to supplement care.

TABLE 19-5 Other Disorders of the Integumentary System

Disorder	Assessment	Intervention
Congenital lesions of the skin		
Pigmented nevi		
Mongolian spots	Flat grayish-blue areas usually in the lumbosacral area: commonly found in American Indian, black, and oriental infants	They tend to fade with time; no treatment
Moles	Pigmented (pale yellow to black or brown) macules or papules; small, round or oval, and smooth	Moles are removed if subject to trauma, for cosmetic reasons, or if they become dysplastic, indicating potential melanoma
Vascular nevi		
Capillary hemangioma (strawberry nevus)	Superficial soft bright red vascular macule that enlarges rapidly and becomes elevated, then slowly resolves	Most disappear by early school age
Cavernous hemangioma	Involvement of deeper, larger vessels—purple, soft, or moderately firm	Lesion tends to decrease in size but may require surgical excision
Portwine nevus	Flat, dark red, or purple; small or large	Nevus may fade; cosmetic surgery; possible laser therapy as young adult
Common fungal infections		
Tinea (ringworm)		
Tinea capitis (ringworm of scalp)	Thickened, broken hairs; erythema and scaling of the scalp	Griseofulvin is treatment of choice when hair and nails are involved
Tinea corporis (ringworm of body)	Annular marginated papules: enlarge peripherally and clear in center	Topical antifungals [tolnaftate (Tinactin)] are applied 2 or 3 times a day and continued for 1 wk after lesions clear
Tinea cruris (inguinal area)	Symmetrical sharply marginated lesions	Same as above
Tinea pedia (athlete's foot)	Erythema, scaling, maceration, peeling	Same as above
Pediculoses: skin, scalp, body, and pubic hair		
	Itching; macular erythematous rash possibly due to sensitization to parasite; lice and nits in hair and on clothing	Kwell lotion and shampoo; good hygiene; laundering of clothing and bedding important

The use of intravenous hyperalimentation has added a new dimension to providing the additional calories required by the burned child. However, this innovation should be approached with extreme caution in the case of a burned child because the infectious complications attending it are fierce even in a patient not already predisposed to infection.

The constant evaluation of the child's nutritional status requires accurate intake and output, daily calorie counts, and accurate daily weights. Without all three it is impossible to evaluate nutrition properly and plan measures to correct nutritional deficits. Careful consideration of the nutritional status of the patient should precede the planning of any surgical procedures, since an optimal level of nutrition improves wound healing postoperatively.

In the acute phase, which might also be named the "phase of complications," continued nursing assessment is vital. Patients need to be assessed for major complications such as burn wound sepsis, pneumonia, Curling's ulcer, suppurative thrombophlebitis, acute renal failure, and electrolyte imbalances. Others include throat and ear infections, urinary tract infections, childhood diseases (measles, mumps), and complications of preexisting conditions such as asthma, allergies, and cardiac disease. The complications of this period are often disastrous; if definitive therapy is to be instituted in time to salvage the patient, it is the diagnostic and assessment skills of the nurse which intervene and alter the eventual outcome.

Rehabilitative Phase

Preservation of new tissue and prevention of infection continue to be part of the rehabilitation phase. New tissue, whether the result of spontaneous healing or grafting, must be protected from breakdown and possible infection. Protective clothing, orthopedic equipment, and special skin care procedures may be required to prevent such occurrences. As scars mature and hypertrophic scarring and scar contracture take place, continued physical therapy is required to maintain joint function and minimize deformities. In time, further surgical procedures may be necessary. Cosmetic surgery to eliminate or improve disfigurement usually must wait until 18 months to several years after injury. Continued psychological support during this period becomes all-important. Parents and children become depressed, discouraged, and emotionally distraught as the ugly, disfiguring scars develop and function becomes more impaired. Realistic explanations and continued encouragement are necessary. Care should be taken to support the parent and child realistically so that they do not become too hopeful about the end result of reconstructive and cosmetic surgery and then suffer frustration and disappointment if the results are not spectacular. Psychological support for the child and his family during this period has a paramount effect on the eventual outcome of the illness and on whether the child will become a functional member of society or an emotional and physical cripple.

Other Integumentary Problems

Additional common disorders of the integumentary system seen in children are presented in Table 19-5.

Learning Activities

1. In caring for a child with atopic dermatitis, what parental concern could you anticipate?
2. Discuss the importance of early diagnosis in drug eruptions. How would you counsel parents regarding the cause and future preventive measures?
3. How would you counsel an adolescent whose friends are questioning the treatment of his severe acne?
4. Develop a nursing care plan for a 22-month-old female child (weight 14 kg) with 36 percent second- and third-degree burns from scald injury involving the lower extremities, abdomen, buttocks, and thighs. Focus on days 4 through 14 and include considerations for nutrition, infection control, maintenance of function, and emotional support of the toddler.

Independent Study Activities

1. Take a nursing history and perform a physical examination on a child with a skin disease. Formulate a nursing assessment and validate findings with the instructor.
2. Observe several infants with diaper dermatitis. What differences and similarities are evident?
3. Interview a school nurse. What role does she assume in counseling children with diseases of the integumentary system?
4. Develop a teaching booklet for 6-year-olds and focus on either nutritional needs of the burned child or exercises to be done when hands, arms, axilla, neck, or legs are involved.

Study Questions

1. The major function of the skin is:
   A. Protection against the external environment.
   B. Maintenance of a buffered protective surface film.
   C. Elimination of sodium chloride and urea.
   D. Regulation of body temperature.
2. Important historical information to elicit when assessing a skin rash is:
   A. The pattern of spread.
   B. The area in which lesions first appeared.
   C. The progression of the rash from first appearance to present status.
   D. The presence of itching, scaling, and dryness.
3. The presence of flat, adherent, greasy scales on a 2-week-old infant's scalp is termed:
   A. Dandruff.

B. Hormonal stimulation of sebum.

C. Cradle cap.

D. Atopic dermatitis.

4. In infantile atopic dermatitis, the area of skin where the dermatitis is first evident is:

A. The trunk.

B. The scalp.

C. The flexor surfaces of the extremities.

D. The cheeks.

5. The most important goal in the care of an infant with atopic dermatitis is:

A. Prevention of dry skin.

B. Control of pruritus.

C. Discovery of the causative allergens.

D. Skin hydration.

6. Koplik's spots, an enanthem of rubeola, are:

A. Erythematous maculopapules on the hard palate.

B. Small, irregular red spots with minute blue-white centers on the buccal mucosa.

C. Maculopapules seen on the skin.

D. Pinpoint red spots on the soft palate.

7. A teenager who has acne tells the nurse that he has squeezed out several blackheads. The nurse explains that:

A. Squeezing often causes rupture of the sebaceous follicle, inflammation, and scarring.

B. Squeezing causes keratinization of the sebaceous canal.

C. Squeezing causes oxidation of sebum.

D. It would be better to scrub or rub the skin vigorously.

8. A third-degree burn involves:

A. Epidermis and stratum corneum.

B. Stratum corneum and dermis.

C. Adipose tissue, fascia, and muscle.

D. Stratum corneum, dermis, adipose tissue, fascia, muscle, and bone.

9. Third-degree burns are:

A. Painless.   C. Painful.

B. Slightly painful.   D. Extremely painful.

10. Positioning after thermal injuries to the arms is as follows: The arms are slightly elevated and:

A. Adducted from the body at a 90-degree angle.

B. Flexed slightly at the elbow.

C. Extended and resting lengthwise.

D. Abducted from the body at a 90-degree angle.

11. A mother of a 2-year-old boy tells the nurse that her child has a mixture of small crops of flat red areas, raised red areas, small blisters, and broken blisters in the collar region and around the waist. There are isolated lesions on his right upper arm, left upper arm, and right upper eyelid. He has a slight fever and is lethargic. Which of the following conditions does he most likely have?

A. Varicella.   C. Impetigo.

B. Herpes zoster.   D. Variola.

References

Carvajal, H.F., and D.H. Parks (eds.): *Burns in Children,* Yearbook, Chicago, 1988.

Clausen, R.W.: "Diagnosis and Treatment of Stinging Insect Allergy," *Hospital Formulary,* September 1981, p. 1022.

Deitch, E.A., and M. Staats: "Child Abuse through Burning," *Journal of Burn Care and Rehabilitation,* 3:89-94, 1982.

Fuchs, G.J., and W.A. Gleason: "Gastrointestinal Complications in Burned Children," in H.F. Carvajal and D.H. Parks (eds.), *Burns in Children,* Yearbook, Chicago, 1988.

Kempe, H.C., et al.: *Current Pediatric Diagnosis and Treatment,* Lange, Los Angeles, 1987.

Knudson-Cooper, M., and C.M. Thomas: "Psychosocial Care of the Severely Burned Child," in H.F. Carvajal and D.H. Parks (eds.), *Burns in Children,* Yearbook, Chicago, 1988.

Nicol, N.H.: "Atopic Dermatitis: The (Wet) Wrap-up," *American Journal of Nursing,* 87:1560-1563, 1987.

Souba, W.W., et al.: "Nutrition and Metabolism," in H.F. Carvajal and D.H. Parks (eds.), *Burns in Children,* Yearbook, Chicago, 1988.

Yannas, I.V., and J. Burke: "Design of Artificial Skin: I. Basic Design Principle," *Journal of Biomedical Material Research,* 14:65-81, 1980.

Bibliography

Fleming, J.W.: "Common Dermatologic Conditions in Children," *MCN: The American Journal of Maternal Child Nursing,* 6(5):346-354, 1981.

Kempe, H.C., et al.: *Current Pediatric Diagnosis and Treatment,* Lange, Los Angeles, 1987.

Knudson-Cooper, M.S.: "Emotional Care of the Hospitalized Burned Child," *The Journal of Burn Care and Rehabilitation,* 3:109-116, 1982.

Krugman, S., et al.: *Infectious Diseases of Children,* 8th ed., Mosby, St. Louis, 1985.

Philbin, P., and J. Marvin: "Management of the Pedatric Patient With a Major Burn," *The Journal of Burn Care and Rehabilitation,* 3:118-125, 1982.

Weston, W.L.: *Practical Pediatric Dermatology,* Little, Brown, Boston, 1985.

20

The Nervous System

Objectives

After reading this chapter, the student will be able to:
1. Describe the functions of the neurological system.
2. Identify appropriate subjective and objective data to be elicited from the child and family.
3. Understand the purpose of diagnostic tests and medical treatment.
4. Explain general nursing measures appropriate for pediatric patients who have neurological problems.
5. Delineate specific nursing measures appropriate for pediatric patients who have various neurological problems.

Anatomy and Physiology of the Nervous System

The nervous system is the most highly organized system in the body and controls it in its adjustment to the environment. The system consists of two primary components, the central nervous system (CNS) and the peripheral nervous system. The central nervous system consists of the brain and the spinal cord (Figs. 20-1 to 20-3), and the peripheral nervous system consists of the cerebrospinal nerves and the autonomic nervous system which carry impulses to and from the central nervous system (Figs. 20-4 and 20-5). The purpose of the nervous system is ac-

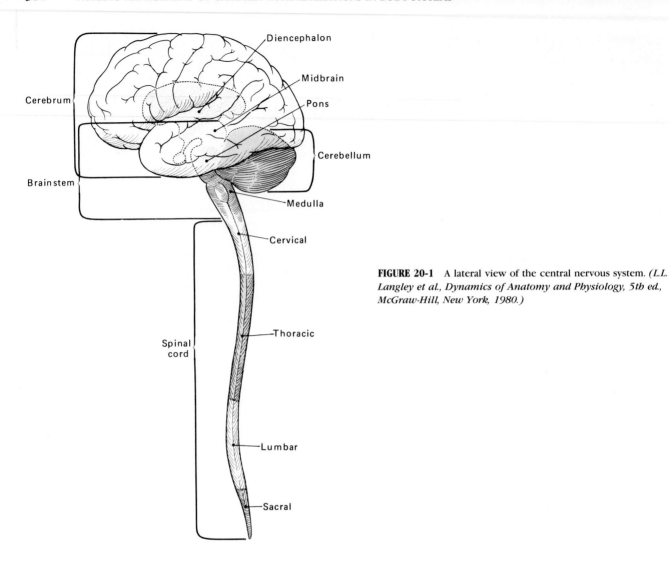

FIGURE 20-1   A lateral view of the central nervous system. (*L.L. Langley et al., Dynamics of Anatomy and Physiology, 5th ed., McGraw-Hill, New York, 1980.*)

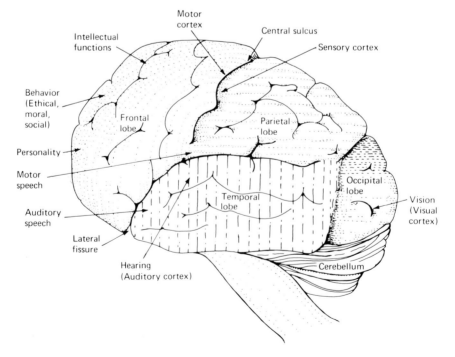

FIGURE 20-2   Lateral view of the cerebrum.

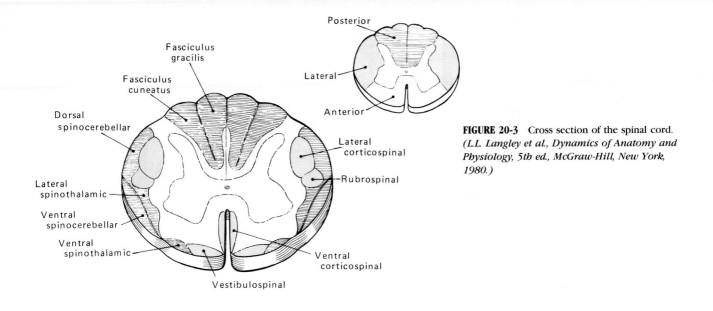

FIGURE 20-3 Cross section of the spinal cord. *(L.L. Langley et al., Dynamics of Anatomy and Physiology, 5th ed., McGraw-Hill, New York, 1980.)*

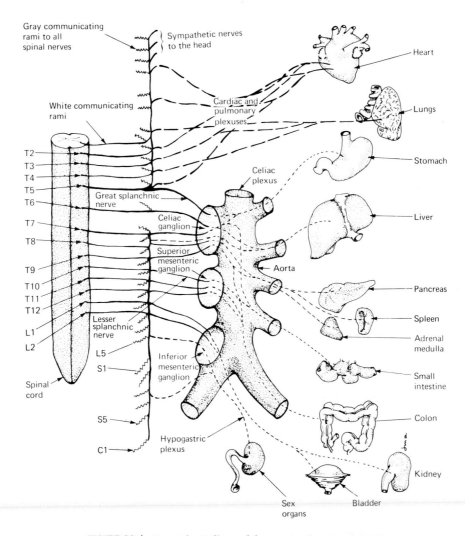

FIGURE 20-4 Sympathetic fibers of the autonomic nervous system.

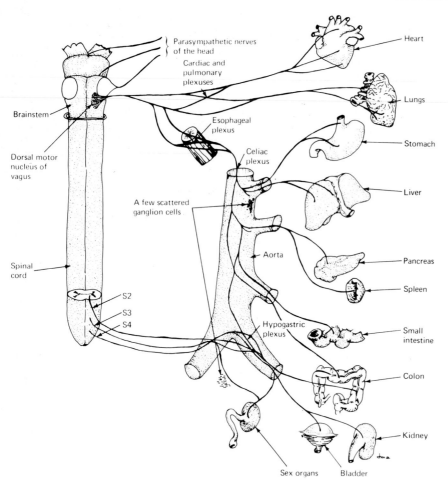

FIGURE 20-5 Parasympathetic fibers of the autonomic nervous system.

complished by an intricate conduction of impulses to and from specialized areas of control by electrical and metabolic means.

Properties of the Nervous System

Structure

The structural unit of the nervous system is the neuron, or nerve cell, which is composed of a cell body and one or more processes. All but one of the cell processes of the neuron are dendrites, which conduct impulses toward the cell body. Neurons have only one axon, which conducts impulses away from the cell body. A neuron is designated as afferent, efferent, or internuncial, according to its function. The afferent neurons are sensory, the efferent are motor, and the internuncial transmit impulses from one neuron to another within the spinal cord or the brain. The connections between axons and dendrites in a chain of neurons are called *synapses.*

Nerve tissue has two basic characteristics known as *excitability*—the ability to be affected by stimuli—and *conductivity*—the ability to transmit impulses from one area of the nervous system to another. A nerve impulse is self-propagating and travels at its own speed, depending on the thickness of the myelin sheath and the size of the nerve fibers, with large fibers being the most rapid in conduction. Appropriate levels of oxygen, glucose, sodium,

and potassium are necessary to support the property of conduction.

Regeneration

Healing of nerve tissue is dependent on the presence of centrosomes, or neurilemma, which are found in only two component parts of the nervous system. Neuroglial cells, the connective supportive tissue of the CNS, contain centrosomes and therefore can be replicated. The axons and dendrites of the peripheral nervous system contain neurilemma, which regenerate and allow for the continuation of nervous function. Regeneration within the peripheral nervous system is slow and may take up to 1 year for completion. Damage to the CNS creates permanent disability as the components of regeneration are not present.

Protective Mechanisms

Because the nervous system is so vital to the total body function, it is afforded much protection. The bony structure, meninges, cerebrospinal fluid, and blood-brain barrier all contribute to the maintenance of its integrity. The blood-brain barrier is a poorly understood phenomenon which protects the CNS by preventing specific substances from entering the brain tissue and the cerebrospinal fluid.

Vulnerability

The more specialized a tissue is within the body, the less it is able to adapt to deficits; thus, the nervous system is highly vulnerable to alterations in its metabolism. Of prime concern are the oxygen and glucose levels. The CNS requires 20 percent more oxygen than does the rest of the body, and its need for oxygen remains constant regardless of the stress or activity of the rest of the body. Insufficient oxygen to the CNS results in permanent brain damage in 4 to 5 minutes. Decreased glucose to the nerve tissue creates a buildup of acid substances within the CNS that interferes with the metabolic process. When appropriate glucose is not supplied, nerve tissue is destroyed.

Neurological Assessment

As Grundy so aptly stated, the "major goal of neurologic assessment in children is to monitor the maturation of the nervous system" (Grundy, 1978, p. 70). Such evaluation is accomplished by developmental assessment, which monitors behavior over time, and neurological assessment, which monitors physical neurological signs over time. Health care providers must keep in mind that the nervous system continues to develop after birth, at which time it has reached one-fourth its adult size. By 1 year of age it is one-half its adult size, at 3 years it has reached four-fifths, and by 7 years it has attained nine-tenths of its growth (Grundy, 1978). Therefore, neurological assessment assumes different forms according to age. The importance

of the health history, methods of developmental testing, and approaches at different ages are discussed in Chap. 6.

The neurological examination is composed of six major categories: cerebral function, cranial nerve intactness, cerebellar function, motor function, sensory integrity, and the reflexes (Table 20-1). For children up to 6 years of age, the Denver Developmental Screening Test (DDST) is one of the most effective means of testing cerebral, motor, and cerebellar function. Neurological assessment is a valuable tool for the establishment of subtle CNS changes in the child. However, because of its length, the nurse may delete aspects of the examination on the basis of the child's status.

Cerebral functions include behavioral, intellectual, and emotional activities; the level of consciousness; and thought content. The level of consciousness in children may be observed in their levels of motor activity. In the infant, alertness is determined by noting the recognition of mother and familiar objects and by general behavior. Immediate recall is tested in the child by asking him to repeat numbers in a series. Thought content is determined by eliciting statements which may indicate the presence or absence of delusions, illusions, or hallucinations. Memory is tested by having a child look at an object, telling him he will be asked about it later, and in 5 minutes or so asking him to describe what he saw.

Cranial nerve function is the next part of the examination (Table 20-2). By the age of 3 years most children will cooperate in the cranial nerve examination, particularly if

---

TABLE 20-1 Neurological Assessment of the Child and Infant

Child

I. Cerebral functions
  A. Level of consciousness
    1. General state: alert, lethargic, comatose
    2. Orientation to person, place, and time in older child
  B. Intellectual
    1. Language and clarity, reading and writing ability, counting and math ability
    2. Ability to draw a familiar object (e.g., family members)
    3. Special schooling or tutor
  C. Thought content: presence of any hallucinations, delusions
  D. Memory
    1. Immediate recall
    2. Recent and remote recall
II. Cranial nerve function (see Table 20-2)
  A. Olfactory (I)
  B. Optic (II)
    1. Snellen E or alphabet chart
    2. Peripheral visual fields by confrontation—eight positions using the clock
      Horizontally—9 and 3 o'clock
      Vertically—12 and 6 o'clock
      Diagonally—10:30 and 4:30, 1:30 and 7:30

  C. Oculomotor (III), trochlear (IV), and abducens (VI) (usually tested together)
    1. Movement of eyes in six cardinal positions of gaze
    2. Assessment of pupils and extraocular movements
      (a) PERRLA (cranial nerves II and III) (pupils equal, round, react to light, and accommodate)
        (1) Pupil size in mm

Pupil size, mm:

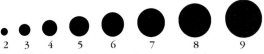

      2   3   4   5   6   7   8   9
        (2) Direct and consensual reaction to light
      (b) Eye movements
        (1) Nystagmus, strabismus
        (2) Position of pupils: midline or disconjugate gaze
        (3) Lids: ptosis, closed, open
  D. Trigeminal (V)
    1. Motor part
    2. Sensory

Continued.

TABLE 20-1 Neurological Assessment of the Child and Infant—cont'd

---

Child—cont'd

    E. Facial nerve (VII)
       1. Symmetry—"make a face"
       2. Tongue protrusion: presence of vacillations
       3. Taste ability: anterior tongue on right and left sides
    F. Statoacoustic (VIII)
       1. Vestibular portion—not routinely tested
       2. Cochlear
         (a) Weber
         (b) Rinne
         (c) Audiogram
    G. Glossopharyngeal (IX) and vagus (X) frequently tested together)
       1. Vital signs
       2. Movement of soft palate and uvula
       3. Gag and cough reflex
       4. Peristalsis
       5. Taste on posterior tongue
    H. Accessory (XI)
       1. Sternocleidomastoid—motion and muscle sense
       2. Trapezius—motion and muscle sense
    I. Hypoglossal (XII) tongue
       1. Any deviations on protrusion
       2. Ability to resist pressure (e.g., with tongue blade) on lateral tongue

III. Cerebellar function
    A. Activities of daily living and play
    B. Balance and coordination

IV. Motor function
    A. Assessment of size, symmetry, posture, movement, tone, and smoothness of muscles; spine, back
    B. Ability spontaneously to move extremities to verbal, tactile, and painful stimuli
    C. Muscle strength—graded from 0 to 6
       0—No movement
       1—Flicker of movement
       2—Movement when the part is free of gravity
       3—Normal movement against gravity but not against resistance
       4—Full normal movement which can be overcome by examiner
       5—Normal strength
       6—Greater than normal strength

*Infant**

I. Measurements
    A. Head, chest, and abdominal circumferences
    B. Weight and length
II. Reflexes
    A. Normal (see Table 20-3)
       1. Plantar
       2. Palmar
       3. Babinski—positive
       4. Tonic neck—asymmetrical and symmetrical
       5. Spontaneous crawling and Bauer's
       6. Rooting
       7. Sucking
       8. Moro
       9. Landau
       10. Bipedal, side-arm
       11. Parachute

V. Sensory system
    A. Primary
       1. Superficial tactile sensation
         (a) Face
         (b) Bilaterally of trunk and extremities
       2. Superficial and deep pressure pain
         (a) Pin on alternate sides of body and at different levels
         (b) Temperature perception—hot and cold test tubes—face, trunk, and extremities
       3. Vibration—tuning fork—sternum, elbows, knees, toes, and iliac crest
    B. Cortical and discriminatory
       1. Two-point discrimination
       2. Point localization
       3. Extinction phenomena

VI. Reflexes
    A. Superficial reflexes
       1. Plantar right and left
       2. Cremasteric right and left
       3. Lower and upper abdominal
    B. Deep tendon reflexes; bilateral assessment for symmetry and strength—graded from 0 to 4+:
       4+—Very brisk with clonus
       3+—Brisk
       2+—Normal
       1+—Low
       0—Absent
       1. Biceps
       2. Triceps
       3. Brachioradialis
       4. Patellar
       5. Achilles
    C. Normal reflextes
       1. Babinski
       2. Chaddock
       3. Oppenheim
       4. Gordon
       5. Chvostek

B. Abnormal
    1. Chaddock
    2. Oppenheim
III. Cranial nerves
    A. Olfactory (I)—not tested
    B. Optic (II)
       1. Visual fields—*six* positions (use bright object and use the clock method)
       Two diagonals—10:30 and 4:30; 1:30 and 7:30
       One horizontal—9:00 and 3:00
       2. Presence of extraocular movements—normal until around 3 months
         (a) Nystagmus, strabismus
         (b) Doll's eyes or oculocephalic reflex
         (c) Setting-sun eyes
    C. Hypoglossal (XII): assessment of strength of tongue movements and swallowing ability

---

*Addresses only specific aspects of neurological assessment which are different for infants.

TABLE 20-1 Neurological Assessment of the Child and Infant—cont'd

Infant—cont'd	
IV. Cerebellar function	V. Cortical and discriminatory sensations
A. Motor system	A. Superficial reflexes
1. Head control; head lag greater than 45° is abnormal	1. Upper and lower abdominal
2. Head, neck, and chest control	2. Cremasteric
3. Hand-to-mouth smoothness and range	B. Cry
B. Muscle tonus abnormalities	1. High-pitched
1. Asymmetric posturing	2. Strong and lusty
2. Overshooting	3. Weak
3. Clonus, tremors, startles	C. Response to stimuli (e.g., typical behavior when held and/or fed by significant other and/or staff)
4. Athetoid movements	
5. Resistance, hypotonus	

TABLE 20-2 Cranial Nerves

Number	Name	Function-Innervation	Testing Techniques
I	Olfactory	Sensory; smell	Assess patency of nares; have child identify familiar odors, such as peanut butter, with eyes closed; test each naris separately
II	Optic	Sensory; sight	Check for light perception, visual acuity, peripheral vision; assess optic disk
III	Oculomotor	Motor; movement for most of eye muscles; constriction of pupil and accommodation of the eye	Have child follow finger or object through six cardinal positions of gaze, using eyes only; do not turn head
IV	Trochlear	Motor; ability to turn eye outward and downward	Have child look downward
V	Trigeminal	Sensory and motor; sensations of touch, pain, heat, and cold to face, anterior one-half of scalp, and anterior two-thirds of tongue Mastication muscles Palate Corneal reflex Lacrimation	Have child clench teeth to assess muscle symmetry and strength; have child close eyes to assess ability to detect light touch on each side of forehead, cheeks, and jaw; test corneal reflex by touching a wisp of cotton to the edge of the cornea; blink is normal
VI	Abducens	Motor; movement of extrinsic eye muscles laterally	Have child look to each side; done at same time as check of III and IV
VII	Facial	Sensory and motor; taste buds of anterior two-thirds of tongue Muscles of facial expression Closing of lid to protect eye Secretions of lacrimal, submandibular, sublingual, nasal, and palatine glands	Test motor portion by having child smile, frown, raise eyebrows to assess symmetry; test sensory portion by having child close eyes and protrude tongue; have child identify sweet or salty taste when solution is placed on anterior portion of tongue—one side and then the other; give sips of water between tests
VIII	Statoacoustic	Sensory; hearing Equilibrium and orientation to space	Perform hearing test; note any vertigo or loss of equilibrium
IX	Glossopharyngeal	Sensory and motor; decrease in heart rate via *baroreceptors* which are sensitive to increased blood pressure Stimulation of the reticular formation to slow down heart rate Taste buds in posterior one-third of tongue; gag reflex Parotid gland secretions	Test IX and X together; have child say "ah" and observe movement of soft palate and uvula; assess gag and cough reflex and voice for hoarseness
X	Vagus	Sensory and motor; coughing, sneezing Respiratory rate—carotid body contains *chemoreceptors* which respond to alterations of carbon dioxide and oxygen content of the blood via the medulla	

Continued.

TABLE 20-2 Cranial Nerves—cont'd

Number	Name	Function-Innervation	Testing Techniques
		Reflex control of the lungs:	
		Stretch reflex—inflation of lungs stimulates medulla and inspiratory phase stops momentarily	
		Contraction of smooth muscles of trachea, bronchi, and bronchioles	
		Speech—muscles of the larynx	
		Peristalsis	
XI	Accessory	Motor; motion and muscle sense of sternocleidomastoid and trapezius	Have child shrug shoulders against pressure (trapezius) and press one cheek and then the other against pressure of examiner's hand (sternocleidomastoid); note strength and symmetry
XII	Hypoglossal	Motor; muscle sense and motion of the tongue	Have child stick out tongue as far as possible and observe for deviation to one side or tremors; test strength by having child push tongue against tongue blade

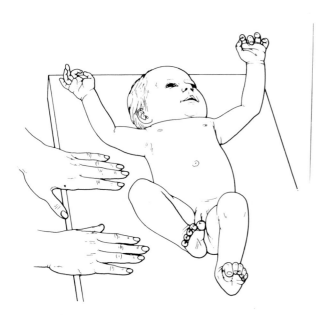

FIGURE 20-6 The Moro, or "startle," reflex. Note the position of the arms and the index finger and thumb.

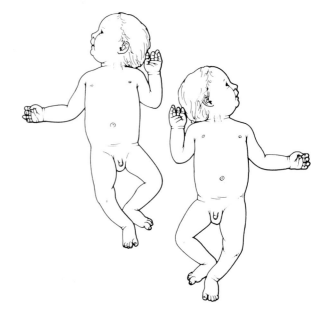

FIGURE 20-7 The tonic neck reflex demonstrating the typical asymmetrical fencer position.

the examiner first demonstrates what the child will be asked to do. The child may be unable to raise his eyebrows and frown, but he will try. The results of Weber's and Rinne's tests are questionable at this age. The audiogram is a more reliable tool at any age (Chap. 21).

The next aspect of the neurological examination is cerebellar function. The cerebellum is chiefly responsible for balance and coordination. Activities of daily living such as dressing, undressing, and play are excellent measures of cerebellar function. Assessment of motor function includes noting the size, symmetry, posture, and movement of muscles by both inspection and palpation. Muscle strength is then graded on a scale from zero to six (Table 20-1).

Assessment of the sensory system includes testing the child's perception of superficial tactile sensation, superficial and deep pressure pain, temperature discrimination, and vibration sense. Superficial tactile sensation is assessed by noting the symmetry of response to stroking the skin lightly with cotton. Superficial pain is tested with a pin on alternating sides of the body or at different levels on the same side. Temperature can easily be tested with test tubes filled with warm and cold water. Vibration is tested with a tuning fork.

Deep tendon reflexes (DTRs) are tested by briskly striking the biceps, the triceps, the brachioradialis, the patellar, and Achilles tendons with a reflex hammer. The response is graded from zero to four+ (Table 20-1). The

TABLE 20-3 Selected Infant Reflexes and Their Significance

Reflex	Expected Response of Infant	Clinical Significance
Birth to 3 or 4 Months		
Plantar grasp	Simultaneous flexion of all toes when examiner's index finger is placed at base of toes	Asymmetries are abnormal; reflex is absent in lower spinal column defects
Palmar grasp	Flexion of all fingers around examiner's finger as it is placed in baby's palm	Equality of strength of grasp is expected
Babinski	Dorsal flexion of big toe with fanning of smaller toes	Asymmetry is an indication of lower spinal cord defects
Chvostek's	Facial twitching elicited by briskly tapping the finger over the parotid gland, just in front of the ear	In tetany, in hypoglycemia, or among infants of diabetic mothers, a facial twitching may result
Tonic neck	Extension of face, arm, and leg on one side with flexion on the opposite side: "fencing position"	It is abnormal after 6 months; constant tonic neck reflex is sign of neurological defect
Spontaneous crawling and Bauer's response	Crawling movements forward; infant prone. If crawl not spontaneous, examiner's thumb is pressed gently on the soles to induce crawling	It is absent in weak or depressed infants
Rooting response	Directed turning of head toward stimulated side of the mouth or lips; mouth opens, jaw drops after stimulation of lower lip; baby attempts to suck stimulating finger	It is absent in depressed infants
Sucking response	After examiner inserts finger into infant's mouth, rhythmical sucking	Sucking is poor, weak, slow, for short periods only, or absent in weak or depressed infants, especially those affected by barbiturates
Moro	Abduction of upper limb at shoulder, forearm extension at elbow, finger extension, then adduction of arm at shoulder and flexion of forearm at elbow; baby is held horizontally in examiner's hands, with head supported; examiner's hands lowered rapidly and brought to abrupt halt	Asymmetry is indicative of Erb's paresis and clavicular fracture; Moro which is weak or absent indicates central nervous system deficit
Later Reflexes		
Landau (4-6 mo)	Lifting of head and extension of spine and legs when infant is placed on abdomen and lifted in examiner's hand	Transition to motor functioning; lack of response may indicate cerebral palsy
Bipedal (6 mo)	Bilateral extension of legs when infant is placed in sitting position and suddenly pushed backward	Transition to motor functioning; lack of response may indicate cerebral palsy
Side-arm (6-7 mo)	Outward extension of arm on side to which infant is pushed when he is placed in a sitting position and pushed first to one side and then to the other	Transition to motor functioning; lack of response may indicate cerebral palsy
Parachute (8-10 mo)	Extension of arms when infant is held under armpits and body is propelled downward, head first	Transition to motor functioning; lack of response may indicate cerbral palsy

Source: Adapted from M. L. Erickson, *Assessment and Management of Developmental Changes in Children,* Mosby, St. Louis, 1976, pp. 62-65.

DTRs are evaluated for symmetry and strength. The patellar, Achilles, and brachial reflexes are present at birth.

Some reflexes are age-specific. In Table 20-3 a list of representative infant reflexes is provided, and in Figures 20-6 to 20-8 some of the more important ones are illustrated. One of the most clinically useful abnormal reflexes in older children is the *Babinski*. The normal response is a curling of the toes, while an abnormal reaction is fanning of the toes and dorsiflexion of the great toe. The normal response may occur as early as 4 months of age but should definitely be present once the child is walking. Therefore, the normal response of the infant will be a fanning of the toes. An abnormal Babinski may indicate lesions of the pyramidal tract or the motor neurons. Reflexes may also indicate a metabolic dysfunction. For example, Trousseau's sign is a spasm of the muscles of the hand that causes flexion of the wrist and thumb with extension of the fingers and is a sign of hypocalcemic tetany. The *cremasteric,* a superficial reflex, is obtained in males by stroking the inner aspect of either thigh. The testis on the stroked side is drawn upward in the scrotal sac. The absence of this reflex may indicate a spinal cord lesion.

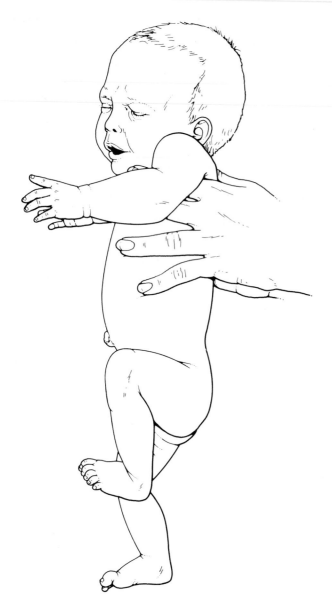

FIGURE 20-8   The stepping reflex.

Evaluative Tools

The appropriate use of evaluation tools in the clinical area can provide health professionals with data indicative of early developmental lags or regressions.

Children not only show individual differences in the rate of development but also require unique amounts of stimulation at specific times in their development. Part of the nursing milieu is taking responsibility for promoting optimum growth and development. Specific programs are provided for parents with developmentally delayed children which include the role of parenting, health promotion, prevention of additional deficits, feeding techniques, and teaching developmentally stimulating activities (Tudor, 1977).

A health crisis, family dysfunction, and other stresses may have a significant impact on the child's growth and development. Environmental factors which contribute to developmental lags or regressions include noise, crowded living conditions, inadequate nutrition, and learning and genetic abnormalities.

Neonatal evaluative tools such as the Brazelton Neonatal Behavioral Assessment Scale are essential. Utilization of the DDST provides normative data on the child's current development compared with average children. It does not supply information about projected future development.

While evaluative examinations are administered, consideration is given to the needs of the child or infant, and the parents are encouraged to express their fears and doubts regarding the development of the child. Helping parents observe and understand the role of their child's activities may enhance their parenting skills. Mothers are especially vulnerable to feelings of inadequacy. The nurse should take advantage of opportunities to reinforce appropriate maternal (and paternal) behavior (Powell, 1981).

Nursing Diagnoses

A variety of anomalies and disorders as well as disease processes can affect neurological function in the infant and child. The nursing diagnoses that can be delineated relate to presenting symptoms or actual or potential deficits in function. Some examples are

Sensory/perceptual alterations related to interrupted innervation

Pain

Impaired physical mobility related to lack of innervation

Altered levels of consciousness related to increasing intracranial pressure or seizure activity

Altered patterns of urinary elimination (incontinence)

Common Nursing Measures

Children manifest neurological disorders in a number of ways. Alterations in sensation, seizures, signs of increased intracranial pressure, and alteration in the level of consciousness are frequently seen as the presenting symptoms. Although these symptoms vary with the disease process and the age of the child, all require specific and knowledgeable nursing care.

Alterations in Sensation
Touch

Alterations in tactile sensation are manifested as paresthesia (the sensation of burning, crawling, tingling, or prickling), hyperesthesia (exaggerated sensitivity of the skin to touch), hypoesthesia (diminished sensation to touch), or anesthesia (absence of sensation to touch). Two forms of touch sensibility are recognized: (1) simple touch, which includes light touch, light pressure, and some tactile localization, and (2) tactile discrimination or proprioception, which includes the sense of deep pressure, spatial localization, and the perception of the size and shape of objects. The cause of altered sensations of touch may be a specific pathological condition, such as infection, trauma, tumors, toxins, and degenerative diseases, or medications which invade the nervous system. Diagnosis is based on the findings of a complete neurological assessment and specific diagnostic studies to identify any pathological condition (Table 20-4).

Nursing Management

The nursing goals for children with altered sensations of touch include prevention of atrophy and injury to the af-fected part and the maintenance of physical and psychological comfort. Frequent assessments are needed to evaluate the progress of the child and the effects of nursing interventions.

Altered sensations to touch create immobility in the affected area. Nursing intervention should be established

TABLE 20-4 Neurological Diagnostic Tests

Purpose	Procedure	Nursing Care (Before Test)	Nursing Care (After Test)
EEG *** To examine brain waves and electrical activity to: Identify damaged or nonfunctioning areas Identify seizure disorders Follow progress of child after encephalitis, encephalopathy, or head injury	Multiple electrodes are placed on various areas of head with adhesive Readings are taken sleeping, awake, and hyperventilating It may be done on an outpatient basis	Explain purpose to parents and child Explain placements of electrodes and that EEG is not painful May shampoo hair to remove oils that would interfere with electrode readings Do not give coffee, tea, Coca-Cola, or alcohol on the day of the examination (contain stimulants or depressants) Do not give medications unless specifically ordered Sleep-deprive 8-10 h prior to study if ordered	Wash electrode paste from hair Allow patient to rest Provide means of resolving feelings (e.g., therapeutic play)
Skull series To study bone configuration of skull to identify: Skull fractures Developmental disorders of bony growth (e.g., premature or postmature closing of fontanels) Tumors or hemorrhage Presence of old fractures to rule out child battering	X-ray is taken of head It may be done on an outpatient basis	Explain to parents and child x-ray equipment which may be frightening; explain that there is no pain and describe procedure Remove glasses, hearing aids, dentures, barrettes, hairpins, etc., from mouth or head	Allow child to express feelings created by this procedure
Pneumoencephalogram To demonstrate shape, size, symmetry, and position of ventricular system and subarachnoid spaces to identify: Space-filling abnormality of brain and meninges (except hydrocephalus) Tumors or masses	Air is injected into subarachnoid space from lumbar or cisternal site, and x-rays of head are taken General anesthetic is given Hospitalization is required	Explain to parents and child the procedure, NPO* for 6-8 h and prior to study, preoperative and postoperative occurrences	Keep flat, at rest, check neurological signs q ½ h × 4, then q 1-2 h as appropriate Observe and care for headache, vomiting, irritability, fever, meningeal irritation, intracranial pressure Encourage fluids if not contraindicated to assist in repletion of CSF Provide for means of resolving feelings when condition is satisfactory
Brain scan To identify brain tumors, some vascular lesions, and masses	Iodinated human serum (131I HSA) or Hq203 Neohydrin is given IV 2 h prior to scan X-rays are taken of head It may be done on an outpatient basis	Explain to parents and child the procedure, its purpose, that IV medication is given; describe x-ray equipment	Allow child to express feelings (e. g., therapeutic play)

*EEG = electroencephalogram; NPO = nothing by mouth; CSF = cerebrospinal fluid; prn = when necessary; CNS = central nervous sytem; CAT = computerized axial tomography; MRI = magnetic resonance imaging.

Continued.

TABLE 20-4 Neurological Diagnostic Tests—cont'd

Purpose	Procedure	Nursing Care (Before Test)	Nursing Care (After Test)
Ventriculogram To visualize ventricles of brain to identify: Hydrocephalus Masses, lesions	Air is injected into ventricles X-rays are taken during and after General anesthetic is given Hospitalization is required	Explain to parents and child the reasons for NPO 6-8 h prior to study, medication, preoperative and postoperative occurrences	Keep flat, at rest, check neurological signs q ½ h × 4, then as appropriate Severe headache likely for 12-48 h—provide comfort Encourage fluids to replenish CSF Observe for alteration in intracranial pressure Provide for therapeutic play when condition is improved
Myelogram To visualize subarachnoid space of spinal cord to identify: Tumors, masses Interference in flow of CSF Fractures, dislocations, foreign bodies	Air or iodinized contrast medium is injected into subarachnoid space via lumbar or cisternal puncture X-rays are taken Iodinized medium is removed Hospitalization is preferred	Explain to parents and child procedure, purpose, NPO for 6-8 h prior to study, sedative prn*	Keep flat, at rest Observe for headache, alterations in intracranial pressure, temperature for 24-48 h Comfort Encourage taking fluids
Subdural tap To identify: Subdural effusions Subdural or ventricular hemorrhage Bacteria in subdural or ventricular spaces To obtain fluid for laboratory analysis To relieve intracranial pressure To instill medication	Needle is inserted into subdural space or ventricle through open anterior fontanel or during craniotomy Hospitalization usually is required	Explain to parents and child procedure and need for consent concerning shaving area on head Shave hair over open anterior fontanel During procedure: Position child on back with head facing forward Hold head securely Observe child for tolerance of procedure Label tubes in order they were collected Tape tubes of fluid to child's bedside unit, label tubes according to day and time of collection	Keep flat, at rest Observe for alterations of intracranial pressure, leakage of fluid from tap site
Angiogram To identify: Vascular anomalies, lesions Hemorrhage Tumors, masses	Radiopaque substance is injected into carotid, brachial, vertebral, femoral artery or vein, or a dural sinus General anesthetic is given Surgical exposure of vessel to be injected may be necessary Hospitalization is required X-rays are taken	Explain to parents and child NPO for 6-8 h prior to procedure, sedative, preoperative and postoperative procedures	Observe for complications of: transient hemiplegia, seizures, petechiae, transient loss of vision, thrombus at injected site, hemorrhage, or hematoma at injected site (emergency tracheostomy may be needed if jugular was used), alterations in intracranial pressure and level of consciousness Provide for complications if they occur Comfort Help to resolve feelings with therapeutic play

TABLE 20-4 Neurological Diagnostic Tests—cont'd

Purpose	Procedure	Nursing Care (Before Test)	Nursing Care (After Test)
Lumbar puncture To identify: Intracranial hemorrhage in CNS* pressure To obtain: Culture, sensitivity, cell count, sugar, protein of CSF To reduce intracranial pressure	Needle is inserted into lumbar area of subarachnoid space Manometer is attached to determine pressure Queckenstedt test is performed CSF is collected in tubes which have to be numbered and labeled accurately It may be done on an outpatient or inpatient basis	Explain to parents and child procedure, purpose, need for sedation, and that some pain is encountered During procedure: Position child on side with knees flexed on abdomen and head flexed on chest to open lumbar space Hold child firmly Provide constant verbal support Observe child for tolerance of procedure Label and number tubes of CSF in order of their collection	Keep flat, at rest Observe and care for headache Encourage taking fluids Provide for therapeutic play
Ventricular tap	(procedure is same as for subdural tap)		
CAT* scan To identify by a combination of computer and x-ray techniques slight differences in density of tissue of intracranial structures: vascular anomalies, lesions, hemorrhage, tumors, masses, ventricular size	Patient is placed in a supine position on a special couch that moves into the scanning unit To facilitate study, area to be scanned is placed in a soft latex material, eliminating air between head and diaphragm of machine, permitting x-ray beams to penetrate more effectively The patient must remain motionless during procedure, which takes up to about an hour In some instances the physician may choose to inject a contrast medium into a vein and repeat scanning procedure to obtain additional information The procedure may be done on an outpatient basis	Explain to parents and child the procedure, its purpose, that IV medication may be given Describe the equipment Keep the child NPO if so ordered prior to the study Explain need for sedation, if patient is an infant or young child	Allow child to express feelings created by procedure If contrast material was injected, observe for thrombi at injection site
MRI* To delineate brain tumors, edema, hydrocephalus, vascular disorders, infectious lesions Better than CAT for studying posteior fossa contents	Noninvasive; patient is placed in supine position on examining table and moved into center of large metal cylinder Patient must remain motionless during procedure	Explain procedure to child and parents; describe equipment All materials which might be affected by magnetic fields must be removed Be sure technologist is informed of any metallic implants Patients with pacemakers, aneurysm clips cannot undergo MRI	Allow child to talk about procedure and express feelings

to prevent muscular atrophy, contracture of joints, and pressure areas. The decrease in circulation that accompanies immobility enhances the potential for tissue breakdown; therefore, active and passive range of motion exercises, proper positioning, frequent turning, and skin care are necessary to prevent further destruction of the affected area.

Children with altered sensations of touch are endangered because they cannot use this sense accurately to evaluate their environment. These children are not aware of pain, pressure areas, or extreme temperatures, all of which may be harmful. The nurse must teach the child and parents how to maintain a safe environment in the absence of a sense of touch in the affected parts (e.g., how to judge the temperature of bathwater, inspect the body area for lacerations or pressure at frequent intervals, and maintain appropriate body positions during sleep). It may be necessary to avoid excess handling of the affected area, use a bed cradle to reduce sensory stimuli, prevent injury by padding, alter the environmental temperature, or provide medication. It is frightening and distressing to the child when touch sensations are abnormal. Realistic support must be given to the child and the parents as changes occur and as plans for treatment are established.

Pain

Pain is a disagreeable, uncomfortable sensation caused by the stimulation of specialized nerve endings in the body. It is created by nerve impulses which travel to the posterior horn cells of the spinal column where they decussate to the anterolateral pathways, then to the brainstem, and on to the thalamus, where they are relayed to the somatesthetic area of the parietal lobe. Awareness of crude pain occurs when the impulse reaches the thalamus.

There are special nerve endings which receive specific stimuli from pressure, distention, inflammation, friction, contraction, or cell destruction and create the perception of pain. These special nerve endings respond to selected stimuli. Thus pain is *elicited* by cell destruction in the skin and external mucous membranes; pain is *caused* by friction, stretching, and inflammation of the arterial walls, dura mater, and pleural and peritoneal surfaces; and pain is *perceived* with contractions and distention in the hollow viscera. Pain may be described as severe, throbbing, dull, hot, searing, crushing, burning, or aching, depending on the location and degree of involvement to the nerve endings. *Referred pain* may be evident when pain is perceived in one area while the actual pain stimulus is in another area. Pain also may be experienced with emotional disorders in the absence of an organic pathological condition.

Pain may be a verbal description of the type and location or nonverbal communication, such as crying, restlessness, irritability, anorexia, insomnia, perspiration, pallor, shallow respirations, splinting, or rigidity of body movement. It is a significant symptom of the specific pathological condition and must be assessed as to its severity, location, type, and pattern to aid in revealing the condition.

Characteristic body language in children may indicate a pathological condition (e.g., pulling at the ears to indicate earache, exaggerated or frequent swallowing to indicate sore throat, or pulling of the knees up to the abdomen to indicate abdominal pain).

Nursing Management

Although each child has a personal threshold for pain, it varies according to age, fatigue level, anxiety, stress, and the degree of painful stimuli. Also, the method by which a child communicates pain is governed in part by his age, culture, family's expectations, and previous experience with pain.

Assessment is a critical nursing function since pain can be reduced by the application of either cold or heat. Cold constricts vessels, decreases metabolism, and reduces edema; heat dilates vessels, increases circulation, and promotes healing. Cold is most effective *immediately after* an injury; heat should be applied after edema and inflammation have developed. It is most important to evaluate the child's response to either cold or heat.

Splinting or immobilizing the affected area also may decrease pain. Although the child may initiate this action independently, the nurse may need to help the child achieve relief.

Analgesics, sedatives, narcotics, tranquilizers, and antispasmodics are types of medications used to control pain. Once the nurse has assessed the severity of pain and the physician has prescribed a particular drug, the nurse needs to determine its effectiveness in controlling the pain. This evaluation is done by questioning the child and observing his response to the medication.

Seizures

An insult to the CNS can result in a seizure, which is described as any abnormal, involuntary neuromuscular activity which encompasses a specific part or the total body and may create loss of consciousness and of bowel and bladder control. Normally, children have a convulsive threshold which is high enough to suppress excessive neuronal discharges. Seizures occur when certain factors precipitate a lowering of the convulsive threshold, temporarily or permanently.

The precise mechanism of seizures is not known. The neuromuscular activity of a seizure is described as *tonic* (rigid) or *clonic* (alternately rigid and relaxed). The cause of insult and the maturity of the child govern the specific seizure activity. Seizures are a common phenomenon in children and are most frequently encountered as sequelae to immaturity of the nervous system, brain damage, congenital defects, metabolic disorders, elevated temperatures, alterations in fluids and electrolytes, and invasions of the nervous system by infections, toxins, and drugs. Other precipitating factors include sleep, onset of menses, hyperventilation, and environmental variables, such as light patterns and music at certain frequencies (Sutherland and Eadie, 1980).

Seizure activity is diagnosed by the history and the observation of abnormal neuromuscular activity. An electro-encephalogram (EEG) confirms the diagnosis in the majority of children. Anoxia from seizures creates additional brain damage; therefore, seizures must be identified and treated rapidly. The primary means of treating seizures is to remove the causative factor or prevent it from occurring, but when the cause cannot be controlled, medications help prevent and regulate seizure activity. Barbiturates are the most frequently used drugs to control acute seizure activity.

Nursing Management

Nursing care is primarily directed toward providing safety and making astute observations of seizure activity. Measures should be taken to prevent seizures, but if they occur, the nurse must care for the child during the seizure.

Seizure precautions, designed to prevent injury to the child, consist of the following:

1. Placing the child in a quiet room to prevent additional stimuli and near a nursing unit where he can be easily observed
2. Providing a bed with siderails that are padded
3. Taping an oral airway to the head of the bed
4. Providing suction equipment, endotracheal tubes, oxygen, and emergency drugs at the bedside
5. Placing a seizure chart in the child's room

When a child demonstrates seizure activity, the first steps are to protect him from injury and to notify the physician. The nurse remains with the child and calls for help. If the child is in a semi-private room or a ward, the bedside curtain is drawn around his unit. Bystanders are asked to leave. Toys and other objects should be removed from his immediate environment. Once a seizure has started, the child should not be moved, but the head should be turned to the side to prevent aspiration of pooling secretions. A small, folded blanket placed under the head prevents head trauma if the seizure takes place when the child is on the floor. Neck flexion is avoided, since it may result in airway obstruction. Fitting clothing is loosened. No attempt should be made to restrain the child because the force of the tonic-clonic activity can cause fractures and dislocations if there is resistance to movement of the extremities. If the tonic-clonic activity is noted in the face and jaw, the airway may be placed between the teeth to prevent damage to the tongue and cheeks. The tonic-clonic muscular activity of the thoracic muscles may inhibit respirations, causing anoxia, and oxygen may be administered by mask. If adequate oxygen levels are not maintained, apnea may develop, and intubation will be required following the seizure. When the seizure activity has ceased, the child may appear very lethargic and sleepy and may have no recollection of the seizure activity. The nurse should return him to bed; assess the level of consciousness, motor response, pupil reaction, and vital signs; and allow him to sleep.

Necessary observations during and immediately after a seizure include noting the time of onset, the location of the neuromuscular activity, the type of activity (tonic, clonic, or both), the length and pattern of the seizure, the child's activity immediately preceding the seizure, the incidence of incontinence, and the child's level of consciousness. This information must be recorded on the seizure chart and in nursing notes.

When the child returns to clear sensorium after his seizure, vital signs should be checked and the neurological status should be evaluated frequently. The child may need readjustment to reality as he will have difficulty remembering the episode. Older children may feel guilt and embarrassment secondary to the incontinence and loss of body control.

Increased Intracranial Pressure

Increased intracranial pressure (ICP) occurs whenever the amount of tissue, cerebral spinal fluid (CSF) or blood increases within the cranium. The rapidity and severity of symptoms of increased ICP are determined by the maturity of the CNS and the stability of the cranium. The infant with open fontanels and an immature system does not develop evidence of increased ICP as rapidly as will the older child who has a closed skull.

The symptoms of increased ICP may occur in a matter of hours or days, depending on the cause of the increasing pressure (Table 20-5). As death and permanent brain damage may occur at any time, early diagnosis and institution of treatment are vital. X-ray and computerized axial tomography (CAT) scan studies are done; EEGs are used

---

TABLE 20-5 Symptoms of Increased Intracranial Pressure

Early Symptoms	Intermediate Symptoms	Late Symptoms
Irritability	Projectile vomiting	Decreased level of consciousness
Restlessness	Tense, bulging fontanel in child under 18 months of age	Decreased reflexes
Anorexia	Severe headache	Decreased respirations
Headache	Sluggish, unequal response of pupils to light	Elevated temperature
	Papilledema	Herniation of optic disk (creates blindness)
	Blurred vision	Absent doll's eye maneuver
	Diplopia	Sunset eyes
	Decrease in pulse and increase in blood pressure	Decerebrate rigidity
	Seizures	Death

NURSING CARE PLAN

20-1 The Child with a Seizure Disorder

Clinical Problem/Nursing Diagnosis	Expected Outcome	Nursing Interventions
Seizure activity characterized by uncontrollable onset of motor or behavioral activity with unpredictable occurrence in potentially unsafe environment Potential for injury related to involuntary neuromuscular activity Altered level of consciousness	Given a safe environment child will not experience injury	Remove hard, sharp, potentially dangerous objects from child's immediate environment Loosen clothing around child's neck and abdomen Protect child's head by providing soft, flat surface; encourage use of safety helmet as indicated Pad siderails of child's bed or crib Do not restrain movement of extremities Do not force tongue blade into oral cavity Provide oxygen and suction if necessary Prevent aspiration injury: promote side lying position or head to side; suction vomitus Provide quiet, calm environment; promote adequate rest periods; prevent overstimulation Assure proper placement and patency of the intravenous catheter Assist with proper administration of anticonvulsant drugs, emergency drugs, and all required medications; know proper date, route, and dilution required; carefully observe child for side effects and effectiveness of therapy Provide specific description of seizure with accurate documentation of neurological findings (keep bedside seizure record at all times) Note time of onset, location of neuromuscular activity, type of activity (tonic-clonic), and duration and pattern of the seizure; level of consciousness; airway management drugs and doses administered; interventions rquired; activity preceding seizure, presence of incontinence; vomiting; behavior after seizure *For postseizure activity:* Monitor vital signs and neurological status q ½-1 h Maintain seizure precautions
Drowsiness and/or altered gait Altered thought processes related to neurological pathological condition and seizure medications	Child will maintain developmental milestones through nursing interventions which fulfill optimal physical, emotional, and educational needs	Identify achieved developmental milestones; support and maintain developmental growth Provide resources and appropriate referrals for stimulation and intervention to support developmental, physical, and educational growth Support normal functioning in daily care as much as possible; encourage activities that promote self-esteem Assist in provision of an optional drug regimen for child that facilitates normal function; monitor anticonvulsant drug levels; document seizure activity and child's response to medications
Tachycardia/ bradycardia, hypotension, hypertension decreased tissue, perfusion, fluid and electrolyte imbalance Decreased cardiac output related to increased tissue and metabolic requirements	With appropriate nursing interventions, child will become normotensive for age, have adequate tissue perfusion, and experience decreased cerebral and tissue metabolic requirements	Monitor vital signs q 2 h Closely monitor child for alteration in vital signs (hypotension, bradycardia, and apnea) secondary to administration of drugs used in managing seizure activity Assess peripheral perfusion; note color and warmth of extremities and strength of peripheral pulses; capillary refill and urine output. Monitor electrolyte values; assist in correction of altered lab values Maintain potency of IV for fluid, electrolyte, and drug administration Provide antipyretic measures (Tylenol; tepid sponge bath) to decrease oxygen requirements and lower threshold for seizure activity

Clinical Problem/Nursing Diagnosis	Expected Outcome	Nursing Interventions
Irregular breathing pattern Shallow respirations Apneic episodes Ineffective breathing pattern related to thoracic muscular tonic-clonic activity; increased O₂ requirements; respiratory depressant effects of seizure medications	Child will achieve patent airway and adequate tissue oxygenation: O₂ saturation > 95 mmHg, given the proper nursing intervention	Position child to prevent upper airway obstruction; place roll under shoulders to extend neck; plan on using cardiac respiratory monitor as indicated Support maximal diaphragmatic excusion by elevating head of bed (HOB) 30° Properly administer oxygen therapy as indicated; suction airway to assure patency Assess quality of oxygenation; monitor O_2 saturation values and (ABG) values arterial blood gas Auscultate lungs for quality and equality of breath sounds; note color of lips and nailbeds Assist with intubation as indicated; place nasogastric tube to prevent aspiration Properly place (without force) oral airway in child who presents with biting tongue or cheek or active bleeding in oral cavity
Copious oral secretions Potential ineffective airway clearance related to altered level of consciousness	Child will not aspirate or experience insult to respiratory system	Position child with head turned, side lying to prevent aspiration of stomach contents Provide suction apparatus at bedside; suction oral cavity to assure airway patency
Family stress: anxiety related to coping with diagnosis requiring long-term medical care and follow-up care Parents communicate lack of knowledge about seizures and anticonvulsant therapy Potential ineffective family coping related to emergent need to accept responsibilities of long-term medical problem	Family and/or child will verbalize and demonstrate proper medication administration for anticonvulsant therapy, including dose and side effects Family and/or child will verbalize understanding of seizure	Teach child's family proper administration of anticonvulsants, accurate dose, and side effects of all medications Assess learning effectiveness by having parent or child redemonstrate medication preparation and administration Encourage use of a Medic Alert bracelet Teach child and family how to manage seizures safely at home (loosen clothing, avoid restraining movement or forcing any object into the oral cavity, protect head, and use safety helmet as needed)
Parents communicate difficulty in sleeping related to fear of child's having recurrent seizures	Child will learn to recognize an aura (if applicable) and to lie down in safe environment Family and child will feel support in coping with seizure disorder and daily medication regimen	Facilitate communication between health care facility and school nurse to reinforce information specific to child's needs Refer child and family to emotional support groups (self-help support groups for children with seizure disorders) Maintain developmental milestones with the provision of age-appropriate activity; use therapeutic play to support child's understanding of hospitalization experiences

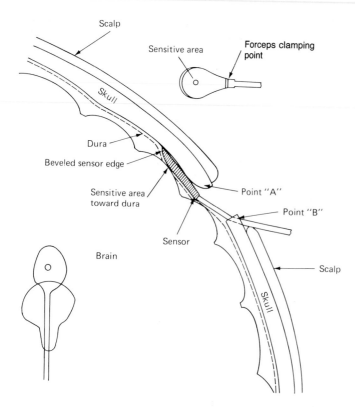

FIGURE 20-9 Ladd intracranial pressure (ICP) monitor demonstrating a sensor implant which provides ICP and mean arterial pressure readings. *(Redrawn form Ladd Research Industries Manual, pp. 3-13.)*

the opening can create herniation of the brainstem, resulting in a medical emergency.

ICP can be monitored directly and continuously by to diagnose and monitor the progression of brain damage; lumbar puncture is performed to measure the ICP and obtain CSF for laboratory analysis (Table 20-4). If lumbar punctures are done, the child must be observed carefully for signs of shock. The sudden release of pressure through means of a subarachnoid screw or an intraventricular catheter with sensors. Placement is through a burr hole, and the devices are connected to a pressure-monitoring system for a continuous readout of ICP levels (Fig. 20-9).

Treating increased ICP may involve removing masses or tumors by surgery and radiation, controlling hemorrhage and edema, and removing pooled secretions by tapping (subdural or lumbar puncture) or shunting. When the cause of the increased pressure cannot be alleviated, palliative measures, such as removal of skull plates, creation of burr holes, or decompression of masses, are instituted to reduce the effects of pressure. Barbiturates and tranquilizers are frequently ordered to control seizures and promote rest. To preserve brain tissue and reduce cerebral metabolism of glucose and oxygen, barbiturate coma may be induced in selected patients.

Cerebral edema may be controlled with diuretics, corticosteroids, such as dexamethasone, or hypertonic solutions, such as 50 glucose, glycerol which is administered orally, urea, mannitol, 10% sodium chloride, or salt-poor

serum albumen, which alter the osmotic effect of the cerebral tissue fluid. Antipyretics, analgesics, antiemetics, and stool softeners are instituted as necessary.

Evaluation of blood gases is necessary at frequent intervals when there is respiratory depression or the child is being maintained on respiratory equipment. Increased carbon dioxide levels cause dilatation of blood vessels and thus increase cerebral volume and pressure. Conversely, if the carbon dioxide level is low, the blood vessels constrict, resulting in decreased oxygen in the cells.

Administration of IV fluid is necessary for children with altered levels of consciousness. The fluid volume and electrolyte levels, particularly of potassium, sodium, and calcium, must be monitored carefully, because an imbalance creates increased ICP, edema, and nerve tissue irritability. Therefore, blood is drawn for electrolytes every 4 to 8 hours.

Nursing Management

The care of a child who has increased ICP requires a perceptive nurse who can quickly detect any change in status and institute proper nursing care. Frequent assessment is required to evaluate the degree of pressure and prevent unnecessary complications. It includes (1) level of consciousness, (2) eye movement, size, direction of gaze, and pupillary response, (3) vital signs, and (4) motor activity.

The level of consciousness indicates the highest level of cerebral activity and is evaluated by determining degree of alertness and orientation to person, place, and time. Ability to awaken, degree of lethargy, knowledge of being in the hospital, recognition of parents and staff, and ability to respond to visual, auditory, and somatosensory stimuli are a few of the signs by which the level of consciousness is assessed.

The eyes are evaluated by holding them open and noting movement, position, shape, and equality of pupils. Strabismus, nystagmus, absent doll's-head eye movement, sunset eyes, and inability to move the eyes through the six cardinal fields of gaze are examples of abnormality.

Next, pupillary reaction to light is assessed. Normal pupils have an equal, brisk constriction in response to light. The consensual response is also evaluated. When one holds both eyes open and shines a light in one pupil, the other pupil should also constrict. The mnemonic PERRLA is sometimes used to remind one of the ideal condition: *p*upils are *e*qual and *r*ound, *r*eact to *l*ight and *a*ccommodate. Corneal reflex is ascertained also. A blink is the normal response.

As ICP increases, the pupils will become sluggish to light, dilated, and eventually unresponsive. They can be fixed and dilated for no more than 5 minutes before irreversible brain damage occurs. The effect of increased ICP on the vital signs should be evaluated. A decrease in pulse and respiration accompanied by a widening pulse pressure is evidence of increasing ICP.

The pulse may become irregular as the ICP continues to rise. The child should be placed on a cardiac monitor for a minimum of 24 hours. Respirations will become rapid, shallow, and stertorous. As ICP continues to rise, hypoxia can develop, and intubation may be necessary. Pavulon (pancuronium bromide), a short-acting neuromuscular blocking agent which causes skeletal muscle relaxation, may be administered intravenously every 30 to 60 minutes to prevent the child from assisting the respirator on his own. The child who has received this drug may still hear, and the nurse as well as the family must reassure the child in order to maintain an orientation to the environment in this immobilized state. A frequent evaluation of lung fields is necessary also. Maintenance of a patent airway requires suctioning whenever necessary because of loss of the gag and cough reflexes. Frequent positional changes are also essential. Any change in neurological status is cause for close and frequent observation because even the slightest change is significant. Once the therapy is discontinued, the child is observed closely for signs of residual muscle weakness and respiratory distress from prolonged ventilator dependence.

Injury to any area of the nervous system generally will affect the child's ability to move. Therefore, motor activity is an important measure of CNS intactness. The quality and strength of motor activity are evaluated by having the child move all four extremities, grasp or squeeze the examiner's hand with both hands at once, and push against the examiner's hand with both feet. Extremities are tested for paralysis by raising the arms and letting them fall back to the bed. The affected arm drops more rapidly. The child's knees are flexed with his heels flat. The leg on the affected side falls outward, while the unaffected leg remains momentarily in position and then resumes its original position. The facial muscles are also observed by having the child smile, bare his teeth, and squeeze his eyes tightly shut. Facial asymmetry includes drooping of the eyes, ptosis, inability to close the eyes tightly, uneven wrinkling of the forehead, dropping of the corner of the mouth, and drooling. The tongue is evaluated for hemiparesis by asking the child to stick out his tongue. It deviates to the affected side (Table 20-1). Any inequality is noted in motor strength. Generalized weakness, tremors, ataxia, and altered sensation of position are significant indications of a nervous system pathological condition (Table 20-1).

To help control cerebral edema, fluid intake must be monitored. Children whose oral fluids are restricted should have their quota of oral fluids distributed over the 24-hour period. IV fluids are carefully monitored to prevent overhydration, which increases the production of CSF. Infusion pumps may be used to control the rate of flow of IV fluids. Elevating the child's head may decrease cerebral edema. Shock blocks at the head of the bed will both elevate the child's head and maintain straight body alignment, promoting comfort and adequate respiratory exchange.

A child with increased ICP may demonstrate an elevated temperature because of an inflammatory process, a systemic infection, or irritation or damage to the temperature-regulating mechanism in the brainstem. When a child's temperature is 37.7 to 38.9°C (100 to 102°F), the nursing treatment consists of cooling the environment by removing excess bed linen and clothing, opening the window, or turning on the air conditioner. Children with temperatures of 38.9 to 40°C (102 to 104°F) require more direct nursing interventions. Antipyretics, such as acetaminophen (Tylenol), may be administered orally or rectally. (Aspirin should be avoided as it interferes with the clotting time and creates gastric distress.) Tepid baths are effective cooling measures, but during the tepid bath care must be taken that the child does not become chilled. Shivering, the normal compensatory mechanism of the body to warm itself, counteracts the effects of this cooling measure. During the bath the child's temperature should be taken at 15-minute intervals, and the temperature should not be allowed to drop more than 0.5°C (1°F) per hour. Once the temperature has been reduced, it should be monitored at 1-hour intervals. If it rises again, the bath must be reinstituted. Ice baths, alcohol sponges, and ice enemas should be avoided with all children because the rapid reduction of temperature may lead to shock and possibly death. Children who have temperatures of 40 to 41.6°C (104 to 107°F) or who cannot maintain an appropriate temperature require the use of a hypothermia mattress. The mattress is usually discontinued once the child's temperature is within 1 to 2°C of the desired level to allow for the "drift phenomenon," in which the temperature will slowly decrease on its own if it is not hypothalamic in origin. The color of the lips, skin, and nailbeds is monitored for cyanosis, an indication of severe vasoconstriction.

Parents need to be involved in the child's care to help alleviate their concerns and fears. By observing the child's response to all nursing activities and parental stimuli, the nurse and the parents can identify patterns to the cycle of increased ICP, such as a particular position or talking to the child about siblings. The identified activities are avoided until the child's ICP returns to normal.

As the child improves, supportive equipment is gradually discontinued. Once bowel sounds and the cough and gag reflexes return, introduction of fluids and foods is begun following extubation. Active and passive range of motion exercises are continued in order to maintain musculoskeletal integrity.

Safety and comfort measures such as seizure precautions must be instituted. The child who is vomiting should be refed because vomiting is caused by neurological difficulties, not gastric irritation; however, if vomiting persists, feeding should be withheld to prevent the transient increased ICP encountered with vomiting. Headache may be reduced by maintaining head elevation, applying ice bags to the head and neck, and administering appropriate analgesics. The child with blurred or distorted vision requires additional communication with the nurse to alleviate anxiety and promote orientation to reality. Appropriate play and diversional activities should be provided. The child and family will continue to need much support from a wide range of health professionals in order to achieve optimum recovery from this life-threatening experience.

Alterations in Levels of Consciousness

The level of consciousness is the most important single indicator of cerebral function. Alterations in the level of consciousness may be slight or severe enough to render the child unable to respond to his environment. General anesthesia, intracranial pathological conditions, trauma, toxins, and metabolic disorders are the primary causes.

Alterations in levels of consciousness generally follow a sequential pattern. Initially the child is alert and knows who and where he is. He can readily engage in purposeful play and responds to his parents and surroundings as any child does according to the norms for his age. The progression of disorientation is usually time, place, and lastly person, which may be evaluated even in young children. With continued alterations in his level of consciousness, he becomes restless and irritable. His thrashing, restless behavior is not alleviated even with comfort from his parents. He becomes drowsy and may not be awakened from sleep, and if previously toilet trained, he may become incontinent. Although he is not able to waken totally, he can respond to direct commands, and painful stimuli elicit withdrawal of a part or facial grimaces. As the level of consciousness decreases, the following specific levels can be described:

1. Unconscious, purposeful response to pain
2. Unconscious, nonpurposeful response to pain
3. Unconscious, flexion to painful stimuli
4. Unconscious, extension to painful stimuli
5. Unconscious, decorticate posture—position of adducted, rigid flexion of arms and fingers with internal rotation of the hands
6. Unconscious, decerebrate posture—all extremities in rigid extension and adduction, back arched, and toes pointed inward
7. No response

Nursing Management

Observation at frequent intervals and maintenance of bodily functions are major nursing responsibilities. The nursing assessment must include a neurological check and appraisal of reflexes (e.g., gag, swallow, corneal) and neuromuscular abilities, including asymmetry of face and extremities.

Ineffectual gag and swallow reflexes require specific nursing interventions to provide for respiration and nutrition. Absence of these reflexes creates pooling of secretions; thus the child must be positioned on his side, and his mouth and nose must be suctioned at frequent intervals to prevent aspiration pneumonia and asphyxiation. Respiratory patterns are observed and recorded; the physician is notified of any change. Frequent turning, postural drainage, and mechanical respiratory assistance are necessary to prevent hypostatic pneumonia. Good oral hygiene is necessary to maintain the integrity of the oral cavity. Nutritional support is essential. Nasogastric or gastrostomy feedings are administered continuously by infusion pump or intermittently.

The corneal reflex must be checked frequently. When the eye does not close completely, the cornea becomes dry and ulcerated, and these ulcerations can result in permanent blindness. Saline eye drops, artificial tears, or lubricating agents, such as methyl-cellulose, can be used to keep the eye moist. Some physicians recommend the use of clear tape to hold the eye closed so that it will be quite obvious if the eye opens.

Children with decreased levels of consciousness are subjected to the hazards of immobility, and specific nursing care to maintain the integrity of the muscles, bones, skin, circulatory system, bowel, and bladder is required. Nursing interventions include frequent range of motion exercises to decrease atrophy and frequent turning and positioning to prevent contractures. A child who is able to do active range of motion exercises must be encouraged and helped to perform these exercises at least three times each day. Range of motion exercises incorporated into play activities increase their frequency and provide diversional activities. Passive range of motion is done three to four times a day for the child who is unable to perform active range of motion. The immobilized child should be turned and positioned every 1 to 2 hours to help prevent pressure or specific skin breakdown and contractures. The use of sheepskins, alternating-pressure mattresses, rubber pads, pillows, and splints can help maintain the proper body alignment and the integrity of his skin.

Maintenance of bowel and bladder function is essential for the child who is immobile and is best fostered by providing a diet that is well balanced with adequate amounts of fluids, fruit juices, and stool-softening medications. Rectal suppositories may be given to assist in the evacuation of feces in accordance with the bowel schedule.

These children are particularly susceptible to cystitis secondary to urinary retention and stasis. Incontinence and increased calculi development are additional problems. Medications, increased fluids, and cranberry juice maintain the urine in an acidic state, which decreases the possibility of infection and calculi formation. The specific gravity and pH of the urine should be measured at 8-hour intervals to determine concentration and acidity. A Foley catheter may be inserted to promote adequate drainage. The catheter should be clamped at all times and released every 3 to 4 hours for drainage to maintain the tone of the bladder.

Circulatory stasis in the immobilized patient may lead to phlebitis and thrombosis formation, and elastic stockings may be ordered by the physician. Postural hypotension occurs when the child's position is rapidly changed from horizontal to vertical and is evidenced by low blood pressure, pallor, circumoral, cyanosis, weakness, syncope, thready pulse, diaphoresis, or cool and clammy skin.

Sensory distortion due to sensory overload or deprivation easily occurs in children who have decreased levels of consciousness. People assume that these children are unable to comprehend or hear what is being said, although hearing is the last sense to be lost in an unconscious patient. Parents may sit by the bedside for hours without speaking to the child, and the nurse quietly hovers over him and does not say a word. The background

FIGURE 20-10 Normal circulation of the spinal fluid from the ventricles to the subarachnoid spaces around the brain and spinal cord and through the central canal.

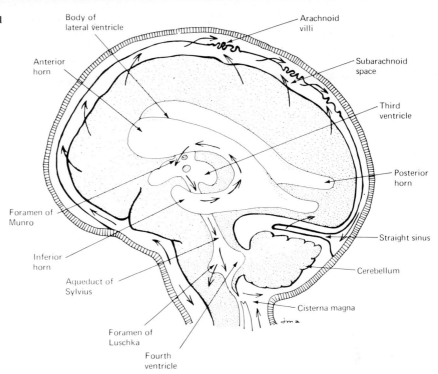

noise of machines beeping and humming and of people working is not meaningful to the child, and he sinks further into a world of oblivion. When hearing is the only contact with the real world available to the child, much can be done with the voice to bring about comfort, companionship, pleasure, knowledge of what is happening, trust, and understanding.

Neurological Disorders in the Newborn
Hydrocephaly

A neurological abnormality which may be present at birth or may become evident soon after is *hydrocephaly,* the abnormal increase in CSF volume within the intracranial cavity. Unless otherwise stipulated, hydrocephaly refers to internal hydrocephalus, a condition in which the fluid accumulates under pressure within the ventricles. Normal CSF circulation is depicted in Fig. 20-10.

Two forms of hydrocephaly should be noted for clinical clarity. *Noncommunicating,* or *obstructive,* internal hydrocephaly is caused by a blockage within the ventricles which prevents the CSF from entering the subarachnoid space. Dandy-Walker malformation is a congenital defect in which hydrocephaly results from atresia of the foramens of Luschka and Magendie. *Communicating* hydrocephaly occurs when the obstruction is located in the subarachnoid cistern at the base of the brain and/or within the subarachnoid space. Arnold-Chiari syndrome is an example of communicating hydrocephaly. It is caused by the downward displacement of the medulla and the cerebellum which blocks the circulation of CSF through the subarachnoid pathways around the brainstem (Behrman and Vaughan, 1983).

As the fluid begins to accumulate, the ICP increases, the cerebral cortex becomes thinner, the scalp becomes thin and shiny, veins dilate, and the cranial suture lines begin to separate. When the infant demonstrates a tense or bulging anterior fontanel and when cranial suture separation is apparent, hydrocephaly is suspected. Other clinical symptoms include vomiting, a wide bridge between the eyes, and bulging eyes in the classic "sunset" sign showing the upper scleras. In the severe form, head size increases rapidly, the infant's cry is shrill and high-pitched, and hyperirritability and restlessness are noted.

Optic atrophy resulting in severe visual deficits with increased pressure compresses the optic nerve and chiasm in chronic, untreated cases. When hydrocephalus occurs in late childhood as a result of an infectious process, subarachnoid hemorrhage, subdural hematoma, or a brain tumor, there is no head enlargement. The clinical manifestations include papilledema, spasticity, and ataxia affecting the extremities and a progressive decline in judgment and reasoning, with a charactertistic "empty chatter" type of speech pattern (Behrman and Vaughan, 1983).

Subsequent neurosurgical intervention offers the best prognosis for survival and intellectual functioning. The degree of neurological impairment cannot be predicted: Some children grow up to function normally, while others may be minimally or profoundly retarded. Their ultimate potential is difficult to forecast. CSF shunting procedures have become popular with the development of inert plastics which are well tolerated by the body (Fig. 20-11).

Nursing Management

Observation is essential, as is conscientious collection of data, including daily measurement of the head circumfer-

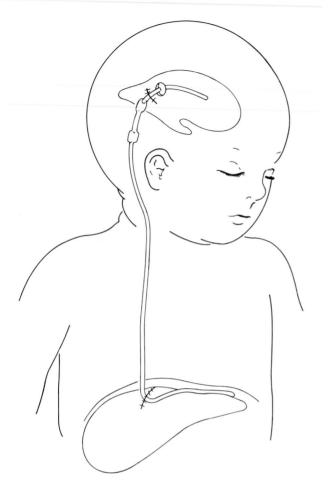

FIGURE 20-11 A ventriculoperitoneal (VP) shunt is one method of treating hydrocephaly. One catheter with a valve is inserted into a lateral ventricle and tunneled under the scalp and down the neck, while another one is inserted into the peritoneum via a small incision. It is then tunneled upward to a point where both are joined and sutured in place.

ence and a check of the size and fullness of the anterior fontanel. Noting any change in the infant's behavior is also important.

Nurses have a direct responsibility for the nutritional requirements of these newborns, but feeding may be a particularly time-consuming activity for the staff. When the infant is irritable or vomiting, various techniques should be attempted to provide adequate nutrients and fluids. Techniques that are successful for a particular infant should be shared with all persons involved in feeding him, including the parents. Feeding times should be flexible, and small feedings at frequent intervals may prove more successful.

The increased head size makes positioning a potential problem, especially when the head circumference is increasing rapidly. Hydrocephalic neonates may develop decubiti if they are not turned often. Frequent linen changes and the use of lamb's wool also help deter skin breakdown. The infant should be turned cautiously, for the increased head size places an additional strain on the neck.

The primary nursing goal for an infant after a shunting procedure for hydrocephaly is the promotion of CNS in-

tactness. The vital signs are frequently monitored, neurological assessments are performed, and the shunt pathways are closely examined.

The shunting of CSF extracranially has many technical problems. The sudden release of ICP with a shunt insertion may precipitate a seizure. The infant's immature system may not readily adapt to the rapid release of pressure. The shunt tubing may occlude or separate. Close attention is therefore given to vital signs, palpation of the anterior fontanel when the infant is quiet and in an upright position, feeding and behavioral patterns, and the signs and symptoms of increased ICP and cerebral irritability.

The physician may request that the infant be placed in semi-Fowler's position to assist in the draining of the ventricles through the shunt. The shunt pathways are observed for any infectious or inflammatory process. The insertion point of the shunt into the ventricles, the valve on the side of the head, and the extracranial shunt tubing paths are all examined for redness, swelling, or drainage. Tension on the tissue covering the shunt may cause skin erosion with the potential for a serious infection. With ventriculoperitoneal shunts, abdominal girths need to be measured. Pooling of CSF may occur because of the inability of the peritoneal cavity to absorb the relatively large volume of CSF. The physician or nurse may test the patency of the tube by pressing on the valve. The valve is functioning when it easily depresses and refills with CSF and returns to its original position. If the valve does not depress and refill easily, either the shunt is malfunctioning or the pressure of the CSF within the ventricles is inadequate.

These neonates also have emotional needs which should not be dismissed. They enjoy being held or cuddled. Although some nurses may be hesitant about handling the baby, it is important to remember that dexterity comes through experience. Such an endeavor on the part of one health team member may support and encourage others to do likewise.

Microcephaly

The presence of a head which is smaller then chest circumference is diagnosed as *microcephaly,* a condition secondary to microencephaly, or a small brain. It may be caused by maternal infections such as toxoplasmosis, irradiation, or any of a number of genetically or environmentally induced factors. Although the sutures close prematurely in microcephaly, they may be open at birth or in early infancy. With the arrest of brain growth, there is generally profound retardation which may be complicated by cerebral palsy or seizure activity. Therefore, a craniotomy is to no avail. In contrast, a condition known as *craniosynostosis,* in which brain size is normal but the fontanels and suture lines have closed at birth or in early infancy, necessitates surgical intervention which will allow the brain to continue to grow.

Nursing Management

Since microcephaly cannot be surgically corrected and mental retardation is a consequence, the problem of giving birth to a deformed infant is further complicated by knowledge of the infant's limited intellectual ability. Specific nursing interventions for these infants are not enumerated because the care given is routine from the standpoint of meeting their physical, emotional, and nutritional needs. The nurse should, however, offer a great deal of support to parents, for they are frequently faced with making difficult decisions which may include institutionalization. If these infants are cared for by parents, the community resources available should be identified for them (Chap. 18).

Neural Tube Malformations

Occasionally at delivery a neural tube malformation is identified. Although *spina bifida* refers to a congenital problem in which there is a defective closure of the vertebral column, whether this problem will be one of minimal involvement or whether the defect will have devastating consequences for the neonate depends entirely on the site and the extent of the anomaly. The cause of these malformations is unknown. The two major categories of spina bifida are occulta and cystica.

Spina bifida occulta is a commonly seen condition that is found in about 10 percent of the routine spinal x-rays of children and adults. Usually the 5th lumbar and 1st sacral vertebrae are affected with no protrusion of intraspinal contents. Many times it is discovered accidentally when other radiological studies are being performed. The skin over the defect may reveal a dimple, a small fatty mass, or a tuft of hair.

Spina bifida cystica is a more serious defect in which a cystic lesion develops in the midline of the vertebral column. Two common types of lesions are meningoceles and meningomyeloceles (myelomeningoceles). A *menin-gocele* is a protrusion through the spina bifida which forms a soft, saclike appearance along the spinal axis and contains spinal fluid and meninges within the sac. A more severe malformation is the *meningomyelocele,* which is also an external protrusion along the midline, but the contents of this mass include spinal fluid, meninges, spinal cord, and/or nerve roots.

Meningoceles and meningomyeloceles are covered by a thin, transparent membrane; a thicker, irregular epithelium; or normal skin. The neurological manifestations of a meningocele may be minimal; however, the symptoms manifested by the presence of a meningomyelocele vary and depend on the extent of the defect and the site of the protrusion (Fig. 20-12).

Parents' rights in the decision-making process regarding surgery for a neonate born with a major defect such as meningomyelocele are a highly controversial issue. However, if parents withhold permission for surgical intervention, nurses working with these infants and their parents must be aware of the differences in families' abilities to deal with deformed babies, the anguish experienced in arriving at a decision, and the needs of families to verbalize their feelings. While offering support to parents, these nurses must also identify and offer support to colleagues who grapple with their own reactions to denial of surgery.

When permission for surgery is granted, the protrusion is excised, the nerve tissue is placed into the spinal canal, and fascia and skin are sutured over the defect. With larger, more difficult repairs a neurosurgeon and a plastic surgeon may collaborate to close the malformation.

Nursing Management

These serious types of defects are usually identified at birth. In the special care nursery, before surgery, the neo-

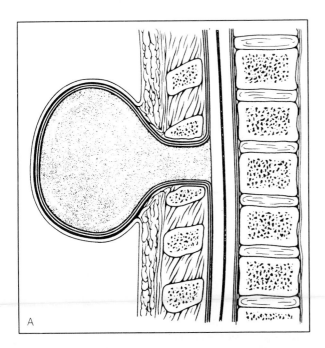
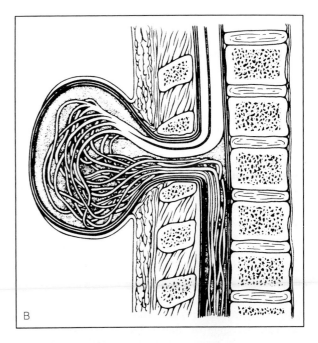

FIGURE 20-12   Congenital malformations: *(a)* meningocele, *(b)* meningomyelocele. *(B.A. Bowens, "The Nervous System," in J. Howe et al. [eds.], The Handbook of Clinical Nursing, Wiley, New York, 1984, pp. 311-343.)*

nate must be handled carefully. Rupture, infection, irritation, or leakage from the protruding mass may occur, placing the neonate's life in great jeopardy. Avoiding pressure over the meningocele, meticulous skin care, and positioning become important nursing measures. In observing the newborn, attention is also directed to the anterior fontanel; the nurse must note its tense, full, bulging, or normal status.

If the question of whether the patient has a meningocele or a meningomyelocele has not been answered, astute nursing observations and assessments may contribute to the final diagnosis. In a neonate with a meningomyelocele, the dribble of urine, the absence of anal sphincter control, and characteristic deformities of the feet emphasize extensive neurological involvement. The location of the lesion determines the extent of lower extremity involvement. There may be paralysis, flacidity, spasticity, or no impairment whatsoever.

Methods of protecting the meningocele or meningomyelocele vary and depend on the physician, the skin covering the protruding mass, and the time interval before surgery. Sterile dressings should always be utilized, but the decisions to apply topical ointments or antiseptic solutions depends entirely on the treatment selected by the physician. Generally, if surgery is not performed immediately, some method of protecting the mass must be devised.

Measures which will facilitate the drying and epithelialization of the sac are necessary if surgical closure is delayed. Prolonged use of moist dressings or ointments will result in maceration and skin breakdown. A doughnut-shaped device can be made from foam rubber or another soft spongy material and will provide protection for the sac.

Before surgery, the infant is kept in a prone position to prevent trauma to and tension on the sac. Postoperatively, the infant may be prone or sidelying, depending on physician choice and other associated problems in the infant. Though the infant is generally kept flat for 2 to 3 days with gradual elevation of the head, the neurosurgeon may determine that the infant should have the head of the crib elevated. As soon as permitted, the infant should be held by the nursing staff and parents for feeding and tactile stimulation. Positioning must also take into consideration the possible associated orthopedic problems and the need to keep the dressing free from soiling by urine and stool.

After a repair, nursing observations should focus on assessing the baby's neurological status, sphincter control, and movement of the lower extremities. Dressings are kept dry and clean. Many neurosurgeons utilize an elastic type of adhesive covering which facilitates keeping the wound clean and dry. Daily head circumference measurements are taken routinely because of the high incidence of hydrocephaly (80 to 90 percent) following neural tube closures. A bulging anterior fontanel, hyperirritability, a shrill high-pitched cry, and vomiting indicate increased ICP. Passive range of motion exercises should be done with impaired lower extremities (Chap. 22). Parents should be involved in caring for the infant as soon as they are emotionally ready to cope with his condition.

While these newborns face repeated hospitalizations, innumerable surgical procedures, and multiple, chronic problems, eventual habilitation depends on many factors. A nurse needs to become involved in teaching parents how to care for their newborn. An interdisciplinary team approach, early parental invovlement in the baby's care, a thorough knowledge of community resources, and parental understanding of the long-range implications greatly influence and affect this newborn's early years.

Neurological Disorders in the Infant
Febrile Seizures
Febrile seizures are convulsions which commonly occur during infancy and early childhood. They are frequently associated with an acute, benign febrile illness. However, an in-depth history and assessment may assist in eliminating other causative factors such as drugs, trauma, and recent illnesses. Children 6 months to 4 years of age with seizures lasting 10 minutes or longer are highly susceptible to nerve cell damage from cerebral hypoxia. These children are at high risk because their homeostatic mechanisms in a stressful situation deteriorate rapidly. Cerebral edema and cerebral hypoxia are the resultant sequelae.

The management of a febrile seizure includes the maintenance of a clear airway, ventilation, and the termination of the seizure. The drug of choice is diazepam (Valium) administered slowly intravenously over approximately 2 minutes. This drug may be repeated every 3 minutes for two or three doses. The child is monitored closely for respiratory depression.

The use of continuous anticonvulsant therapy after one febrile seizure remains controversial. Febrile seizures tend to follow a pattern. A short, benign seizure with one episode usually indicates that any following attacks will also be short and benign.

Nursing Management
The nursing management of children with a febrile seizure is directed toward lowering the temperature, maintaining fluid and electrolyte balance, providing for safety, and noting any further seizure activity. Close observation, assessment, and evaluation of nursing interventions are essential.

The child with a temperature of 38.9 to 40°C (102 to 104°F) requires the administration of antipyretics such as acetaminophen. Cooling the environment with an air conditioner or opening a window and removing excess clothing assists in lowering the child's temperature. Tepid baths are frequently effective, but care must be taken to ensure that the child does not become chilled. The temperature must be monitored every 15 minutes to ascertain the effectiveness of nursing interventions and to ensure that the temperature falls only 0.5°C (1°F) every hour. Close attention to the child's vital signs, behavior, and head circumference, especially in infants, permits the evaluation of the metabolic effects of the elevated temperature on the highly active cerebral nerve tissue. A 10 percent increase in metabolism is required for each degree rise in temperature (Celsius).

Maintenance of a patent IV line is essential as the intravenous fluids are frequently administered to hydrate the child and provide for metabolic activities. Seizure precautions are taken. The emotional support of the parents and child is essential because of the acute nature of this health problem, which is extremely frightening. Discharge planning includes instructing parents to administer acetaminophen and tepid baths whenever the infant is febrile.

Subdural Effusion

A collection of fluid in the subdural space, usually of 2 ml or more in volume, is termed a subdural effusion. The cause has not been clearly identified; however, head trauma and meningitis are known to increase the incidence. Subdural effusions are primarily found in infants, with a peak incidence at 4 to 6 months of age (Behrman and Vaughan, 1983).

The first sign of *acute* effusion is rapidly increasing ICP. The most frequent symptoms of *chronic* effusions are convulsions, irritability, stupor, and projectile vomiting. In addition, head enlargement, failure to thrive, and developmental lags have been reported to occur with chronic subdural effusions. Transillumination, subdural tap, and in some cases angiography are used in diagnosis. The fluid in the subdural space is characteristically found to have increased protein levels and may be accompanied by red blood cells.

If the infant has no evidence of neurological changes, he should be observed closely. No treatment is instituted because some children have had resolving effusions with no sequelae. Subdural taps are performed on those who evidence clinical signs of neurological dysfunction. Generally no more than 30 ml is removed at one time. Taps are usually done as needed every 1 to 4 days until fluid production in the subdural spaces has ceased. If fluid production continues more than 14 days, a craniotomy to remove the fluid-producing membrane may be performed. Repeated taps may still be necessary following surgery; if continuation of fluid development persists, shunting may be instituted.

Nursing Management

The nurse must be alert to any signs of increased ICP. A neurological check done at frequent intervals is particularly important after a subdural tap, as signs of increased pressure can develop suddenly following a period of decreased pressure. Close observation of the fontanels for signs of bulging and daily measurement of the head circumference are important nursing measures.

Since the infant may be subjected to repeated, painful subdural taps, the nurse should take time to hold and fondle him to help develop a trusting relationship. Allowing the parents to be with the infant as much as possible will decrease their anxiety and help overcome feelings of sep-

aration. The parents of these infants are very distressed because it may be many weeks or months before the full potential of their child can be identified.

Neurological Disorders in the Toddler
Cerebral Palsy

The term *cerebral palsy* (CP) is used to describe disorders created by damage to the motor centers of the brain before, during, or shortly after birth. Perinatal intrauterine deprivation of oxygen and nutrients causing fetal growth retardation is identified as the most significant risk factor. Preterm infants are also at high risk. Trauma at birth, infections, and kernicterus during the postnatal period may also cause brain damage. One infant in 1000 live births is born with this condition every year. Of the six out of seven who survive, some will be profoundly retarded and may be institutionalized; others will be so mildly affected that little or no treatment is necessary. The remaining children will have moderate to severe handicaps.

CP is characterized by various neuromuscular abnormalities such as weakness, paralysis, and incoordination of voluntary movements. Other disorders include emotional problems, hyperactivity, and cognitive dysfunctions of abstraction and reasoning. Fifty percent of these children experience visual deficits, such as strabismus, nystagmus, refractory errors, and visual field defects; 10 percent have high-frequency hearing loss; and 65 percent are mentally retarded. Seizures occur most commonly during the first year and may persist for life. Speech, articulation, and breath control difficulties may develop.

The clinical manifestations of CP are categorized by the type of motor disturbance: spasticity, athetosis, ataxia, rigidity, tremors, and atonia. *Athetosis* refers to constant, irregular, and involuntary slow movements which may affect the entire body and become more severe distally. Facial grimacing, drooling, swallowing, mastication, and dysarthria may occur as a result of involvement of the facial, laryngeal, and pharyngeal muscles. Athetoid movements decrease with fatigue, distraction, the prone position, and relaxation. *Spasticity* refers to exaggerated reflexes and jerky, uncertain movements. CP is suspected in the infant who fails to respond normally to a neurological examination and who demonstrates flaccidity; prolonged tonic neck, Moro, or fisting reflexes; and fixed positioning. Extensor postures with arching of the back and rigid extension, adduction, and internal rotation of the legs may be present. Severe hip adduction results in *scissoring*, or crossing over, of the legs. Deep tendon reflexes are usually brisk with sustained clonus, and the Babinski reflex remains positive after the age of 2. Severe, prolonged spasticity and rigidity may result in heel cord contractures, limitation in abduction with external rotation of the hips, and a reduction in supination and extension of the forearms.

Some infants may experience *hemiplegia*, or involvement of one side of the body, as evidenced by sensory deficits, asymmetrical postures, a stronger Babinski reflex on the affected side, and inequality of the Landau and parachute reflexes (Table 20-3). Older children demonstrate flaccidity and hypotonia (Levine, 1980).

A diagnosis is made as soon as possible. An in-depth family, prenatal, and perinatal history and neurological examination are necessary to rule out other disorders (e.g., brain tumor, spinal cord lesion, hydrocephalus, and neuromuscular disorders). Once the problem is identified, specific management guidelines are developed.

Parents may describe an infant who is quiet, sleeps for long periods, and cries little. Feeding difficulties, concerns about the infant's inability to suck and keep the nipple or food in his mouth, and difficulty diapering the baby because of scissoring may be the reasons cited for bringing the infant to the health care facility (Brown, 1979). Two simple screening tests for CP may easily be performed: (1) A clean diaper is placed over the infant's face. The normal response is removal with both hands, but the CP infant either will use only one hand or will not remove the diaper at all; (2) the infant's head is turned to one side. The examiner observes for persistence of the tonic neck reflex, an indication of CP.

Nursing Management

Early diagnosis helps the parents accept their child as an individual with basic needs for love and care. Parents who have accepted the child initially as a "normal" child, with "normal" potential, encounter greater difficulties in accepting their child with his handicaps at a later time. They may exhibit the following three emotional phases: hostility to the physician who has confirmed their fears that something is wrong with the child, the search for a physician who will reverse the first diagnosis, and acceptance. Until the period of acceptance has been reached, therapeutic interventions are not helpful.

Changes in neuromuscular status are monitored over time. The presence of abnormal posturing, flaccidity, or rigidity is noted. Spastic infants scissor when picked up, while ataxic infants assume a sitting position. Although CP is nonprogressive, infants who initially presented with hy-

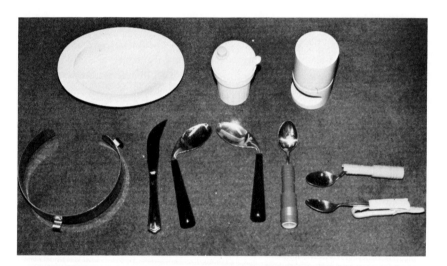

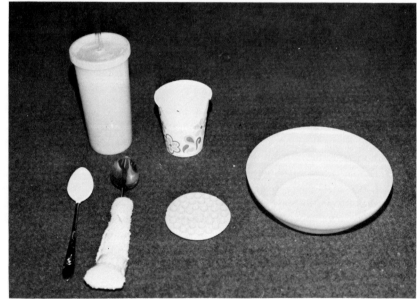

FIGURE 20-13 Adaptive feeding equipment. *(top)* Specialized utensils. Reading clockwise: Shallow Melmac bowl with sides to provide a scooping surface; plastic feeding cup with lid, spout, and gravity device to control the flow; Melmac cup with indentation to facilitate grasp; place guard, attached to plate to provide a scooping surface; curved knife to allow cutting with slight movement; right-handed and left-handed spoons for pronation or supination difficulties; spoon with built-up handle for easier grasp; spoon with strap, placed over the back of hand to allow self-feeding by an individual who cannot grasp a spoon; swivel spoon to help those without the arm flexion needed to change the direction of the spoon as it reaches the mouth. *(R.B. Howard et al., "The Nervous System and Handicapping Conditions," in R.B. Howard and N.H. Herbold [eds.], Nutrition in Clinical Care, McGraw-Hill, New York, 1978, p. 482.)*

TABLE 20-6 Promoting Independent Feeding Skills in the Handicapped Child

Problem	Desired Outcome	Techniques and Equipment
Poor head control, sitting balance, and/ or tendency to hyperextend back and neck	Child will maintain an erect, supported, flexed sitting posture with arms forward; swallowing will improve, and gagging will decrease	1. Chair to support those parts of body which child cannot control 2. Footrests to support feet 3. Headrest or hand support for head 4. Table and chair arranged to permit child easy access to food
Difficulty holding and controlling spoon and cup and getting them to mouth due to motor incoordination	Using adaptive equipment, child will be able to feed self with spoon and cup	1. Padded/built-up handles on forks, spoons, to facilitate grasp; reduced paddling as child increases skill 2. Training cups with covers, weighted bottoms 3. Plates with deep dish sides 4. Suction cups, clamps, or cutout board to hold plate in place
Abdominal muscle tone in jaw, lips, tongue due to hypertonicity or hypotonicity	Child will be able to: 1. Use lips (not teeth) to clean food from spoon 2. Chew food 3. Maintain mouth closure while eating	1. Give small amounts of food 2. Encourage child to use lips, not teeth to remove food from spoon 3. Provide adequate time for chewing 4. Begin with easily chewed foods 5. Encourage child to keep mouth closed while eating

potonia may gradually become hypertonic after 18 months of age (Brown, 1979). Assessment for vision, hearing, and speech deficits is essential. For example, the infant is observed for sensory responsiveness, early speech sounds, and the use of a few single words by 7 months of age. The 4-year-old is tested for vision with the Snellen E chart and for hearing via audiometry.

Nursing interventions include instruction in feeding and positioning techniques, sensory stimulation, and range of motion exercises. Feeding techniques include utilizing appropriate equipment (Fig. 20-13), closing the jaw by raising the mandible and stroking the throat gently upward, or tapping under the chin and exerting pressure on the mandibular joint (Table 20-6).

Range of motion exercises developed by the physical therapist are reviewed with the parents, and *slow and gentle manipulation* is emphasized. The importance of locomotion at an individual pace and provision of large toys that involve the use of both hands are discussed. Verbal interaction with the child using slow and distinct speech and involvement of the child in identifying objects, colors, people, and smells in the environment are encouraged.

A major nursing goal is to foster in the child with cerebral palsy a positive self-image—his motivation to learn, his development of independence, and his need to socialize and be accepted by his "normal" peers. This goal is difficult for the child to achieve because he is so often frustrated by his inability to coordinate the muscular activity required for speech, mobility, posture, and facial expression. The level of the acceptance and support offered to the child with CP from people significant to him and his degree of neuromuscular involvement determine his ability to function within society. It must be stressed that children with CP are like normal children in their need for love, independence, success, and acceptance by others; the only difference is that they cannot control their bodies with ease.

Once the parents have accepted the child, the remainder of the medical treatment is related to preventing deformities and promoting "normal" growth and development (Chap. 22). Training of the child who has CP is ideally managed by an interdisciplinary team and carried out in a relaxed setting. The sequence of training and the goals established are in accordance with the abilities and handicaps of the individual and should help him reach the highest level of functioning.

Head Trauma

Most head trauma is accidental. The most common types are concussions and fractures (linear, depressed, basilar), both of which may be accompanied by intracranial hemorrhage. A *concussion* is the jarring of the skull contents which may create a loss of consciousness. A *contracoup concussion* is created when the skull contents strike against the skull wall on the side opposite the blow. A *simple fracture,* in which there is no displacement of bone, is called a *linear fracture.* A fracture creating displacement of the skull is called a *depressed skull fracture.* A *basilar fracture* is one found in the base of the skull.

Concussion is the most frequent type of head trauma in children (Fig. 20-14). The shifting of skull contents during a blow to the head may result in a brief loss of consciousness. The child regains consciousness rapidly, may complain of pain, but quickly returns to play. Memory loss frequently occurs. *Retrograde amnesia* is memory loss

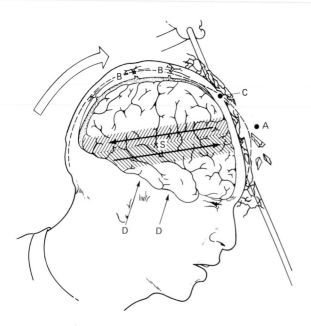

FIGURE 20-14 Closed blunt injury of the head. Skull molding occurs at site of impact. *(a)* Stippled line: preinjury contour. *(c)* Contour moments after impact with inbending at point A and outbending at vertex. *(b)* Subdural veins torn as brain rotates forward: S, shearing strains throughout brain. *(d)* Direct trauma to inferior temporal and frontal lobes over floors of middle and anterior fossa. *(S.G. Eliasson et al., Neurological Pathophysiology, Oxford University Press, New York, 1974, p. 293.)*

concerning events preceding the injury. *Antegrade amnesia* is memory loss about occurrences after the injury. Trauma to the brain may cause bleeding or edema which develops slowly, allowing the child to be asymptomatic for 6 to 18 hours following the injury. As the hemorrhage or edema increases, the child demonstrates symptoms of increased ICP, usually lethargy, irritability, nausea, and vomiting.

The diagnosis of skull fracture is confirmed by x-ray. Depressed fractures may be found by palpating and observing the contour of the head. The diagnosis of basilar skull fractures is further supported with evidence of drainage of CSF or serosanguineous fluid from the nose, mouth, or auditory canal.

Children with head trauma may display minor symptoms or may demonstrate severe neurological deficits. The symptoms of head trauma are not specific but appear with the development of cerebral irritation or increased pressure due to edema or hemorrhage. Hemorrhage is classified according to its location and may be found in the subdural, epidural, or subarachnoid spaces and within the cerebral tissues, (Fig. 20-15).

Subarachnoid hemorrhage occurs within the subarachnoid space from bleeding of damaged vessels on the surface of the brain. The onset of symptoms is gradual, within 24 to 48 hours after injury. Increased ICP and meningeal irritation are manifested by elevated temperature and alterations in level of consciousness. Laboratory

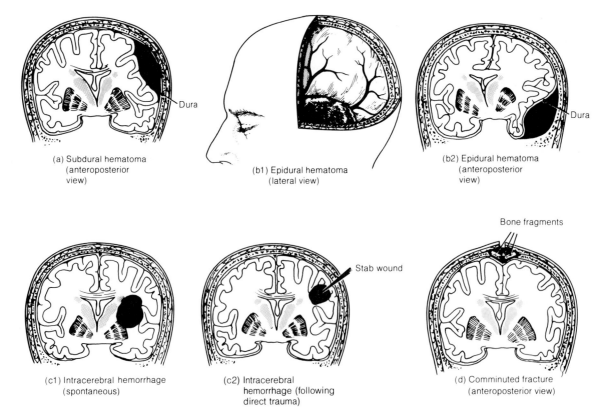

FIGURE 20-15 Cranial hemorrhages and fractures. *(A.E. Hinkhouse and N.A. Kirby, "Traumatic Disturbances in Perception and Coordination," in D.A. Jones et al. [eds.], Medical-Surgical Nursing: A Conceptual Approach, 2d ed., McGraw-Hill, New York, 1982, p. 1240.)*

findings demonstrate blood in the CSF. The treatment consists of rest and reduction of pressure. The prognosis depends on the degree of hemorrhage, with massive brain damage evident in the severe cases.

Subdural hematoma is a unilateral or bilateral collection of blood between the dura and the arachnoid mater. The *subdural hematoma* is classified as *acute* when it is associated with meningeal tears and severe head trauma which result in deep coma and increasing ICP. The highest incidence occurs in infants between 2 and 6 months of age with a history of birth trauma or a head injury. Subdural hematoma is the most serious sequela of the battered child syndrome in terms of mortality. The hematoma without a fracture is due to violent shaking which tears the subdural veins. Associated retinal hemorrhage confirms the diagnosis. A *chronic subdural hematoma* results from gradual leakage of blood from the frontal or parietal veins within the subdural space. The symptoms may not develop until 2 to 4 weeks after head trauma. Infants demonstrate tight or bulging fontanels, enlargement of the head, anorexia, irritability, vomiting, low-grade fever, hyperactive reflexes, retinal hemorrhage, and increased transillumination. Older children demonstrate signs of increasing ICP. The diagnosis is based on EEGs, CAT scan, carotid angiography, and subdural taps. Treatment consists of daily subdural taps to decrease the ICP. Surgical intervention is frequently required for infants with chronic subdural hematoma.

Extradural hematoma is bleeding into the space between the dura and the cranium from laceration of the middle meningeal artery. The onset of symptoms may be rapid, constituting a surgical emergency. The child shows evidence of concussion with lateralizing neurological signs, hyperactive deep tendon reflexes, positive Babinski sign, and increasing ICP. The lumbar puncture shows clear fluid and slightly increased pressure. Immediate surgery is imperative.

Treatment of head injuries is primarily supportive until the degree and location of the injury are identified. Children with no immediate evidence of CNS involvement may not require formal medical attention. Parents, however, should be instructed to observe the child for lethargy, vomiting, irritability, and muscular weakness. If these signs of increasing pressure occur, the child is hospitalized. Frequent, complete neurological assessments are necessary to identify rapidly the site of cerebral trauma and the correct treatment to prevent further brain damage.

Surgery is performed when there is massive hemorrhage and rapidly developing ICP. The primary purpose of surgery is to decompress (reduce pressure), control bleeding, or remove bone fragments and foreign bodies. Slow bleeding or edema formation may be best controlled by allowing the pressure developing within the skull to act as local pressure on the bleeding sites.

A child who has incurred severe head trauma may have permanent brain damage which cannot be evaluated fully until all cerebral edema has subsided. This process may take weeks or months. Seizure activity is found in about 10 percent of the children with severe head injury (Behrman and Vaughan, 1983). For this reason children with moderate to severe head injuries may be placed on seizure medications prophylactically for a minimum of 1 year.

Nursing Management

The primary goal in the care of the child with head trauma is to prevent further brain damage. The nurse must be alert at all times for the slightest change in the child's condition. Frequent assessment of the neurological status is important, including the level of consciousness, motor and sensory function, and pupillary response.

Close attention to the vital signs is important because the child may have a lucid period prior to marked neurological deterioration. Intracranial hypertension may also develop. The child is observed for behavioral changes, irritability, or drowsiness. Maintenance of strict intake and output is essential in order to prevent cerebral edema. IV fluids are given, and there is no attempt to compensate for fluid deficits because the ICP may rise. The ICP is monitored to determine its severity and the effectiveness of treatment. The patient is usually maintained in a supine position to decrease the risk of brainstem herniation.

The child with a head injury and his family need reassurance and support in a possibly life-threatening situation. Allowing a family member to stay with the child is helpful. The nurse should explain all procedures to the family to allay fears; her presence at frequent intervals is also reassuring.

In contrast to the child with brain surgery, who has a clean surgical incision draining small amounts of serosanguineous fluid, children with head trauma have increased drainage onto their dressings because of the deep traumatic nature of their injuries. The amount of fluid loss must be carefully measured by weighing the head dressing before its application and after removal and by circling the drainage area with a nonabsorbable pen. The chance of a child developing an infection is compounded in the traumatic open injury; therefore, it becomes vital to reinforce or change moist dressings to prevent capillary introduction of pathogens into the wound. A child with a basilar skull fracture may have serosanguineous drainage from the nose, mouth, or ears which could be cerebrospinal fluid. The drainage is tested for glucose by utilizing a Dextrostix. A positive result confirms a CSF leak. Because the presence of such drainage increases the chance of admitting pathogens directly to the CNS, sterile dressings may be applied loosely to the child's ears or nose to prevent contamination. The majority of head traumas are due to accidents. The nurse should stress to the family the safety measures that may prevent a similar accident in the future.

Lead Poisoning (Plumbism)

Lead poisoning, or *plumbism*, remains an extremely serious but preventable health problem worldwide. It persists despite the use of lead in only exterior house paint since the 1940s. Young children living in old buildings where

NURSING CARE PLAN

20-2 The Child with a Subdural Hematoma

Clinical Problem/Nursing Diagnosis	Expected Outcome	Nursing Interventions
Lethargy and drowsiness Increased irritability Change in behavior (decreased interest in play) Altered thought processes related to neurophysiological pathological condition	Child will be protected from further brain injury	Monitor vital signs qh for alterations Assess neurological status qh: sensorium, level of consciousness, and pupillary response (equality and reaction to light) Assess motor and sensory function, ability to focus and track objects, quality of cough and gag reflexes, response to environment and painful stimuli, and presence of retinal hemorrhage Monitor child for signs and symptoms of increased intracranial pressure (ICP) (increased irritability, drowsiness, and/or change in behavior and feeding pattern); widened pulse pressure; hypertension and bradycardia; increased head circumference; bulging fontanel in infants Assess child for presence of seizure activity; enforce seizure precautions as indicated
Shallow, irregular respirations Potential ineffective breathing pattern related to compromised neurological function	Child will maintain patent airway and adequate oxygenation: O_2 saturation > 95 mmHg	Assess child for signs of increased bleeding Frequently monitor heart rate respiratory rate, blood pressure, and temperature for changes from baseline Assess rate, rhythm, regularity, and depth of respirations Auscultate lungs for equality and quality of aeration Monitor child for presence of apnea and periodic breathing Note color of nailbeds and mucous membranes Monitor ABG, O_2 saturation, and hemoglobin and hematocrit values Properly administer oxygen therapy and protect child's airway
Decreased systemic perfusion Decreased cardiac output related to compromised neurological function	Child will demonstrate adequate systemic perfusion and normal vital signs for age	Assess child for presence of tachycardia/bradycardia and hypotension Note strength and quality of peripheral pulses bilaterally Assess warmth of extremities, capillary refill, and color of nailbeds and mucous membranes Monitor temperature; maintain normothermia
Polyuria: specific gravity > 1.006 Decreased urine osmolality Plasma hyperosmolality Hypernatremia Vomiting Potential fluid volume deficit and electrolyte imbalance related to compromised regulatory mechanisms (diabetes insipidus)	Child will maintain intravascular volume homeostasis and fluid and electrolyte balance	Monitor strict intake and output; assess urine output q 30 min Monitor serum and urine electrolyte lab values and acid-base; replace urinary, fluid, and electrolyte losses Assess hydration status; note presence of depressed fontanel and dry mucous membranes Administer vasopressin as ordered; note effect of medication on child
Fear and anxiety Anxiety related to strange environment and invasive procedures	Child will develop coping mechanisms appropriate to his or her age	Prepare child for surgical intervention focusing on developmental concerns Anticipate and manipulate stressors for child within developmental framework Maximize and support coping mechanisms used by child Utilize play therapy to support child's expression of hospital experiences

peeling exposes old lead paint are vulnerable because they may chew old, lead-painted wood, plaster, or paint flakes. This condition is frequently seen in a child with pica. Inhalation of airborne lead from industrial sources and gasoline contributes to the lead burden because the respiratory system quickly mobilizes lead. Other lead sources include dust from lead-painted ceilings and walls, cigarette smoke, drinking water from lead pipes, food cooked in water from lead pipes, food grown in urban plots, eating urban snow and ice, old newspapers with newsprint made from lead pigments, food and juices from lead cans, sucking a contaminated thumb, and eating with dirty, lead-dusted hands.

An estimated 4 percent of children in the United States have blood lead levels ≥25 mcg/dl. It is most prevalent in poor, inner-city black children and least prevalent in rural white children. Acute symptomatic episodes are seen most frequently during the six warmer months of the year (Chisolm, 1987). The peak age of occurrence is between 2 and 3 years. The age factor is probably related to the curiosity about the environment of the toddler and preschooler and to hand-mouth activity.

Lead absorption through the gastrointestinal tract is affected by increased motility, which decreases lead absorption; age, with younger children at higher risk; nutritional deficiencies, such as inadequate intake of protein, calcium, iron, zinc, magnesium, and copper; and a high-fat diet. Children are at risk because they absorb about 50 percent of the ingested lead, which is distributed to soft tissue, where it may remain for 1 month, and to the metaphyses of long bones, where it may remain for 25 years if untreated. The most vulnerable organs and tissues are the brain, kidney, and bone marrow.

There is no known "safe level" of lead for children. An association has been found between sustained levels of 40 mcg/dl or greater in young children with or without clinical symptoms, and persistent cognitive alterations are present even after levels have declined to an acceptable range. About 50 percent of children with lead encephalopathy suffer serious irreversible brain damage (e.g., mental retardation, hyperactivity, seizures) (Chisolm, 1987).

Lead poisoning is a chronic process, although acute episodes may occur. *Acute lead encephalopathy,* the most severe form of lead poisoning, usually is caused by the ingestion of lead salts. The onset of symptoms is rapid, and the child is critically ill. The acute symptoms of increased ICP include sudden persistent vomiting, encephalopathy, abdominal pain (*lead colic*), ataxia, inappropriate antidiuretic response, renal dysfunction, heart block, alterations in the level of consciousness, seizures, coma, and death in 1 to 2 days if untreated.

Chronic lead poisoning is the most common form of this health problem. The symptoms are insidious in onset, proceeding from mild to severe. Three to six months of lead ingestion is generally necessary before symptoms occur, because the body's lead burden accumulates slowly. Lead is excreted by the kidneys. It takes the body twice the ingestion time to mobilize and finally remove lead by normal physiological means. Early diagnosis and treatment are essential to prevent sequelae.

The child may be asymptomatic or exhibit the following early symptoms of CNS toxicity: weakness, irritability, vomiting, ataxia, loss of appetite, developmental regression, speech delay, anemia, and abdominal pain. Later symptoms of CNS toxicity are stupor, seizures, coma, and death. Children with chronic lead poisoning may develop an acute episode if lead levels suddenly peak.

Efforts to prevent undue lead absorption and lead poisoning require early detection and effective intervention. The Centers for Disease Control (CDC) (1985) has recommended a particular screening protocol and risk classification (Table 20-7) for asymptomatic children. The population to be screened is children between the ages of 9 months and 6 years who are known or suspected to have been unduly exposed to lead. Symptomatic children require immediate and thorough diagnostic evaluation, not screening, followed by prompt treatment as indicated by findings. The target population is screened at least once a year; children from 9 months to 3 years of age are screened every 2 to 3 months during the summer months. Negative results do not preclude subsequent exposure. The screening method recommended by the CDC is free erythrocyte protoporphyrin (FEP) determination followed by measurement of blood lead (Pb) levels if results are positive (i.e., FEP ≥ 35 μg/dl). Since a moderately elevated FEP (i.e., FEP ≥ 35 to 249 μg/dl) may be found in iron-deficiency anemia, iron-deficiency anemia must be ruled out. The CDC therefore suggests that (1) enough blood be collected to determine the Pb level (safe level < 25 μg/dl) and hemoglobin or hematocrit if the FEP is ≥ 35 μg/dl, or (2) the child remain at the screening site until the FEP level is known. The child is classified according to results (Table 20-7). This classification suggests relative risk, not a diagnostic classification. Class IV children must have a diagnostic evaluation within 48 hours and class III children within 3 working days.

If the Pb level was done on capillary blood, a venous Pb level must be determined, since the first specimen may have been contaminated with environmental Pb. A complete blood count, serum iron, total iron-binding capacity, and serum ferritin are determined to rule out iron-deficiency anemia. If the venous blood confirms an elevated Pb level, a detailed health history (including pica, possible Pb sources, and developmental regression) is taken and a thorough physical examination is done (Chap. 6).

All symptomatic and asymptomatic children with confirmed lead poisoning are at *urgent risk* for encephalopathy. If acute encephalopathy develops, 80 percent of these children may have permanent and severe brain damage. The need for chelation therapy rises in relation to the height of the Pb level. Chelating agents bind with lead and form a nontoxic compound, a *chelate,* which is then excreted by the kidneys.

TABLE 20-7 Classification of Lead Poisoning, Diagnostic Evaluation, and Follow-up

Classification			Diagnostic Evaluation		Follow-up		
Class	FEP*	Pb*	Evaluation	When	Age	When	Method
IV	110-249	70+	1. Detailed health history taken	Within 48 h			
	250+	50+	2. Physical examination				
			3. Nutrition status and hematologic evaluation for iron deficiency		9 mo-6 yr	At least once every month	Venous†
			4. Confirmatory tests (venous blood)				
			5. Additional confirmatory tests (disodium edetate provocative)				
III	110+	25-49		Within 3 working days			
	35-249	50-69					
II	35-109	25-49		Within 2 weeks	9 mo-6 yr	May-October—monthly November-April—every 2 mo	Fingerstick or venous
I	0-34	0-34	No diagnostic evaluation necessary—periodically rescreen (see Follow-up)		9 mo-3 yr	Once every 6 mo	Fingerstick or venous
	0-34	Not done					
Ia	35-249	0-24	Complete blood counts, serum iron, total iron binding capacity, and serum ferritin if available (see Follow-up)		3 yr-6 yr	Once every 12 mo	
Ib	0-35	25-49	No diagnostic evaluation necessary—repeat fingerstick to confirm (see Follow-up)				
EPP	250+	0-24	Erythropoietic protoporphyria				
	50-250+	NSQ	Blood lead necessary to estimate risk	Within 3 days			
	0-34	50+	Not generally observed—repeat with venous blood sample	Within 3 days			
	35-109	70+					

*FEP = free erythropoietic protoporphyrin; Pb = blood lead.
†A class III or IV child should never be followed via fingerstick until all lead hazards have been removed from the environment and FEP and Pb levels have continually declined for at least 6 months or have stabilized.

Source: Boston Childhood Lead Poisoning Prevention Program, Office of Environmental Affairs, Community Health Services Division, Department of Health and Hospitals, City of Boston.

The chelating medications most commonly used are Ca EDTA and dimercaprol or British antilewisite (BAL). The calcium salt of EDTA is administered to prevent hypocalcemia and tetany. It may be administered orally but is more effective parenterally. Ca EDTA is thought primarily to remove lead from bone. BAL removes lead from the soft tissues and the red cells and causes a marked decrease in the blood lead levels. These drugs are administered together to increase lead excretion and reduce mortality.

If the child has recently ingested lead, the intestinal tract may be emptied via enema or cathartic or gastric lavage to avoid a rapid rise in blood lead levels following BAL administration. In the critically ill child, IV chelating therapy may be initiated immediately. BAL is contraindi-

cated in hepatic disease and is nephrotoxic, and Ca EDTA is contraindicated in renal disease.

Oral D-penicillamine (Cuprimine) may be administered following a course of BAL and Ca EDTA. It is given on an empty stomach to avoid the binding of dietary metals. D-penicillamine (PCN) ensures the continued mobilization of lead from soft tissues and the bones.

In acute encephalopathy BAL and Ca EDTA are administered simultaneously by deep intramuscular injection with adherence to a preplanned site-rotation schedule: 500 mg of BAL and 1500 mg of Ca EDTA per square meter of body surface per 24 hours (Behrman and Vaughan, 1983). BAL is first administered alone as a priming dose. Then, every 4 hours, both drugs are injected simultaneously at separate, respective sites on the right and

NURSING CARE PLAN

20-3 The Child with Lead Poisoning

Clinical Problem/Nursing Diagnosis	Expected Outcome	Nursing Interventions
Weakness Irritability Delayed speech Loss of developmental milestones, headache	Child's blood lead levels will be reduced significantly	Monitor vital signs parameters for changes from "normal" or baseline values appropriate for age Assess heart rate for rhythm, regularity; assess peripheral perfusion for warmth of extremities, quality of capillary refill, quality of peripheral pulses, auscultate breath sounds for quality and equality of aeration Assess respirations for depth, regularity, and rate; observe child for signs of distress or irregular breathing patterns
Altered thought processes related to neurophysiological pathology secondary to lead poisoning	Child's neurological status will be evaluated and maintained at an optimal level	Monitor blood pressure using appropriate blood pressure cuff size; note presence of hypertension or hypotension, widened pulse pressure Assess neurological status every hour; note pupillary size, equality, and reactivity to light; note changes in mental status and feeding or behavior patterns Monitor for signs of increased intracranial pressure; observe for seizure activity; maintain seizure precautions; administer anticonvulsants diuretics as ordered Maintain accurate intake and output and record hourly Identify achieved developmental milestones; loss or absence of appropriate growth parameters for age Administer Denver Developmental Screening Tool Note clarity of speech and motor, and sensory functions
Anemia Fatigue	Child will be adequately oxygenated with the conservation of energy	Assess ability to tolerate play and routine acivity levels Conserve energy reserves; provide adequate rest periods, promote quiet play
Activity intolerance related to anemia, generalized weakness		Monitor complete blood count; oxygen saturation values; provide supplemental oxygen as needed
Decreased urine output Proteinuria Glucosuria Ketonuria	With the proper administration of chelating agent, the child's specific gravity, urine output, blood urea nitrogen, and creatinine will indicate the maintenance of normal renal function	Monitor strict intake and output volumes (voiding 1 ml/kg/h) Provide for adequate hydration Monitor specific gravity with (< 1.020) every void; check for protein, ketones, glucose, blood in urine with every voiding Notify physician and hold chelating therapy for a specific gravity > 1.020; and for the presence of protein, blood, and glucose in urine. Monitor renal function values (blood urea nitrogen, creatinine), urinalysis, electrolytes.
Altered patterns of urinary elimination related to renal dysfunction secondary to chelating agents; hypovolemia		Ensure proper administration of chelating agents; carefully observe child for drug side effects (hypertension, tachycardia, renal dysfunction, fever)
Anorexia Nausea, vomiting Constipation Abdominal pain	Child's intake of a diet high in protein, calcium, magnesium, and vitamins will ensure the provision of maximum nutrients	Maximize caloric value of intake with adequate vitamins and metabolites Optimize intake of protein, calcium, magnesium, phosphorus Promote fluid and electrolyte homeostatis Assess stooling pattern for regularity, consistency; observe for abdominal distension, abdominal pain
Altered nutrition: less than body requirements related to anorexia, nausea, vomiting		
Pain	With the use of a local anesthetic, child will have pain-free injections	Advocate the use of a local anesthetic, i.e., lidocaine to be administered with chelating agent to decrease the pain of the injection Rotate intravenous sites; prevent infiltration Provide warm baths, warm soaks, moist heat to injection sites
Pain related to multiple intramuscular injections, intravenous sites for chelating agents		

Continued.

NURSING CARE PLAN 20-3 The Child with Lead Poisoning—cont'd

Clinical Problem/Nursing Diagnosis	Expected Outcome	Nursing Interventions
Hardened or fibrosed muscle tissue	Child will be protected from infection and fibrotic areas	Rotate injection sites and carefully document the rotation schedule; palpate the appropriate muscle for hardened or fibrosed areas prior to the location of injection sites
Potential impaired tissue integrity related to multiple intramuscular injections with chelating agents		Monitor injection sites for signs and symptoms of infection or abscess formation (redness, induration, pain at sites) Encourage ambulation and range of motion of all extremities
High risk living environment with the potential recurrence of lead poisoning	Child will live in a lead-free environment Parents will understand required treatment and follow up for lead poisoning	Involve social work and public health services to aid in the identification of the source of poisoning Assess parental understanding regarding the importance of identifying and eliminating the source of lead poisoning. Support family with feelings of guilt; encourage verbalization of concerns
Potential for injury (recurrence of lead poisoning) Knowledge deficit		Provide family with teaching about lead poisoning, required therapy, prevention and need for follow-up care and developmental stimulation Facilitate follow-up care with lead clinic for medical treatment Faciitate follow-up of developmental assessmental stimulation programs as needed
Fear and anxiety Separation from parents	Child will receive parental support and comfort	Encourage the parents to participate in the child's daily care Provide the child with a familiar toy from home or a security object, i.e., favorite blanket
Anxiety related to stressors of hospitalization and treatments, separation anxiety	Child will master the stress of hospitalization and therapy	Encourage therapeutic medical play specific to developmental level to facilitate the expression of fear with IV therapy or IM injections Perform all painful procedures in the treatment room Provide choices, i.e., type and size of bandage

left sides, in six divided doses, for 5 to 7 days.

Children who demonstrate clinical improvement after the initiation of chelation therapy wil have BAL discontinued after 3 days and the total dose of Ca EDTA reduced by one-third after 72 hours, thereby decreasing risk of renal damage. If a repeat course is necessary, the reduced dosage is utilized. Additional management includes monitoring for the side effects of Ca EDTA: hypercalcemia, elevated blood urea nitrogen, lacrimation, nasal congestion, muscle pain, and hypotension. The side effects of BAL include vomiting, salivation, lacrimation, local pain, and paresthesias. Maintenance of renal function is essential. An IV of 10% dextrose and water, the insertion of a Foley catheter, and the administration of mannitol 20% is utilized if increased ICP is present. This approach initially increases urine output and reduces ICP by osmotic diuresis. Corticosteroids may also be administered. Calcium gluconate 10% may be helpful in controlling the colic that sometimes occurs.

Strict intake and output are essential, and IV fluids are administered via controlled infusion pump. Replacement of emesis and insensible water loss is minimal to limit fluid intake and avoid increased ICP.

Seizures may occur, and diazepam (Valium) administered intravenously usually assists in terminating the seizure. Paraldehyde is frequently administered and the dosage is reduced after the anticonvulsants phenobarbital and phenytoin sodium (Dilantin) reach adequate blood levels.

In children who do not have encephalopathy, the first course of BAL-Ca EDTA is for 5 days. If symptoms abate within 24 hours, BAL is discontinued. (If the initial venous Pb level is < 70, BAL may not be needed at all.

In asymptomatic children with blood Pb levels > 70 μg/dl, a BAL-Ca EDTA course is given. For blood Pb levels between 70 and 90 μg/dl, Ca EDTA is given for 5 days but BAL is given for only 48 hours. A blood Pb level of 50 to 69 μg/dl requires Ca EDTA for 3 to 5 days followed by D-penicillamine. Zinc supplements are administered because they may provide some protection against the sequelae of lead toxicity. Other minerals, including calcium, iron, and phosphorus, are replaced as necessary. A nutritious diet which addresses the child's cultural and individual food preferences is provided.

Nursing Management

Health education begins when the child is screened and is reinforced each time the child is seen. Discussion includes sources of lead; preventive measures (e.g., sweeping up and removing paint flakes and dust); the danger of ingestion of paint chips, soil, and dust; education of older siblings who may be involved in the child's care; and the need for rescreening until the child's sixth birthday. The same information is given to the community at large at every opportunity.

The child and family with lead poisoning require much emotional support. All procedures and treatments are explained thoroughly each time they are used. Therapeutic play, including needle play, is provided, since the child will receive many injections over a 5-day period. Because of the age group, it is essential to reassure the child and siblings that nothing they did caused the health problem and that the hospitalization and parenteral therapy are not a punishment. The use of a nurse/doctor kit, drawing, and toys the child may bang and throw to alleviate hostile feelings is encouraged. Alternate periods of quiet and active play related to the child's energy level and developmental needs are provided. The child may exhibit anger, regression, and withdrawal as coping patterns because of the pain and the intrusive nature of the therapy. Since body integrity is a prime concern, each puncture site is gently covered with a Band-Aid. Parents and significant others may have feelings of anger and guilt. The nurse encourages them to share their feeings and to visit the child regularly and often. Consistent caregivers are important to the development of trust for both child and family.

The nursing care during chelation therapy includes performing an in-depth history and collecting baseline data prior to the initiation of the therapy. The child's vital signs and weight are obtained. A urine specimen is collected to determine specifc gravity and the presence of sugar and acetone. A dipstick test is also done. The CNS is evaluated for the subtle and overt signs of lead poisoning and for an acute episode of encephalopathy.

After the initiation of therapy, the child is observed for the side effects of chelating agents, especially renal dysfunction. Strict intake and output records are maintained, the infusion rate is monitored closely, and any abnormality in fluids and electrolytes is reported immediately. Vital signs, including blood pressure, are obtained in the minutes following the injections and for approximately 2 hours afterward, because the development of hypertension and tachycardia is dose-related. A fever reaction is seen in approximately 30 percent of the children. Accurate collection of 24-hour urine samples is essential to evaluation of therapy.

The medications are injected into the large muscles of the right and left vastus lateralis, ventrogluteal, and glu-

teus medius muscles. The gluteus medius is utilized only in older children because younger children have poor muscle development. Warm compresses over the injection areas help relieve induration and pain, and warm baths are soothing. To avoid unnecessary strain on sensitive muscle areas and to allow the child to recuperate from the around-the-clock administration of chelating agents, periods of rest are essential. The child is awakened prior to the simultaneous injections. Otherwise, the child will quickly learn not to sleep soundly until exhausted because of the terror of being aroused by these painful injections.

Discharge planning, community involvement, close follow-up, and accurate and consistent health records as well as confirmed lead-free housing are necessary to prevent the recurrence of lead poisoning. Collaboration among health professionals is essential. The involvement of the child's school and other community resources provides further support. The education of the public, industrial managers and owners, and legislators about the continued existence of this frequently serious but preventable health problem is a prime concern for all who work with children. Successful treatment depends on treating the child and his environment; the relationship that develops among the child, his family, and health care providers; and nutritional counseling.

Neurological Disorders in the Preschooler
Meningitis

Meningitis is an inflammation of the meninges (Fig. 20-16). It can be caused by a number of organisms, both bacterial and nonbacterial. The most common organisms and symptoms and the age groups generally affected are listed in Table 20-8, and laboratory findings are compared in Table 20-9. Host factors which predispose the child to bacterial meningitis include preexisting CNS anomalies, neurosurgical procedures or injuries, immunoglobulin deficiencies, treatment with immunosuppressants, sickle cell disease, and primary infections elsewhere in the body. Inappropriate antimicrobial therapy for minor infections may be another factor.

The most common causes are gram negative bacilli in neonates. Between 2 months and 12 years of age the causative bacterial organisms include *Haemophilus influenzae* type B, *Streptococcus pneumoniae,* and *Neisseria meningitidis.* *H. influenzae* is generally seen in the fiirst 5 years of life. The bacteria causing meningitis in adolescents include *S. pneumoniae* and *N. meningitidis.* When the child's immune system is altered, other organisms such as *Pseudomonas,* staphylococci, salmonellae, or *Serratia* may be the infectious agent (Behrman and Vaughan, 1983).

The signs and symptoms of meningitis may be preceded by several days of upper respiratory or gastrointestinal symptoms or a purulent draining ear. In some children, and particularly in young infants, the specific signs of meningeal irritation may be minimal or absent. Irritability, restlessness, and poor feeding, with or without fever, may be the only signs.

The child acquires meningococcal meningitis from an adult carrier. Children who live in a crowded environment are at high risk. The mortality rate is below 10 percent (Gaddy, 1980). Fulminant septicemia is the most severe form of meningococcal meningitis with the development of endotoxic shock, disseminated intravascular coag-

ulation, and cutaneous and mucosal hemorrhages. Meningococcal meningitis may produce a purpuric or petechial rash, which is seen in about 50 percent of cases. The lesions result from inflammatory changes in superficial blood vessels and capillaries.

Classic signs of meningeal irritation include Kernig's sign, Brudzinski's sign, and nuchal rigidity. During infancy, Kernig's and Brudzinski's signs may not be positive.

The diagnosis of meningitis is based on symptoms and laboratory data, including cultures of the spinal fluid, nasopharynx, and blood. The CSF pressure is usually elevated, although crying will give a falsely high reading. Gram's stain usually identifies the organism. The cell count, appearance, glucose, and protein levels vary with the type of meningitis (Table 20-9). The blood culture is positive and the white blood cell count is elevated in about 50 percent of the cases. Other laboratory findings indicative of severe physiological stress include hyperglycemia, glycosuria, elevated uric acid, ketonuria, proteinuria, and an elevated urine sodium osmolality and specific gravity related to the syndrome of inappropriate antidiuretic hormone secretion (SIADH).

The child with meningitis requires emergency treatment with antibiotic therapy and isolation for 24 hours following the first dose of medication. Generally, the drug management is initiated with ampicillin every 4 hours and chloramphenicol every 6 hours IV to cover most of the common causative organisms. If the organism is a resistant strain or is more sensitive to other drugs, the appropriate antibiotic (e.g., penicillin, oxacillin, nafcillin, or methicillin) is administered. The medication is continued until the child is afebrile for 3 consecutive days (average time is 2 to 3 weeks).

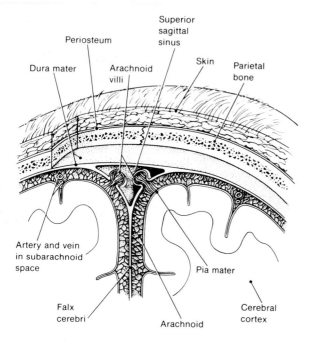

FIGURE 20-16   A section of the brain showing the meninges and associated structures.

TABLE 20-8 Types of Meningitis

Causative Organism	Symptoms	Age Group Affected	Need for Isolation
Bacterial			
Haemophilus influenzae, type B (H-flu)	Chills, fever, vomiting, headache, stupor, convulsions, nuchal rigidity; positive Kernig's and Brudzinski's signs	Infant to school age	None
Meningococcus	Same as above with sore throat, purpuric rash	Preschool age	Respiratory isolation
Streptococcus pneumoniae	Same as H-flu (following respiratory infection)	Preschool age	None
Streptococcus	Same as H-flu	Preschool age	None
Staphylococcus	Vomiting, irritability, high-pitched cry, convulsions, bulging fontanel	Infant	None
Enteric bacteria *(Escherichia coli)*	Same as *Staphylococcus*	Infant	None
Nonbacterial			
Coxsackie B virus	Fever, headache, vomiting, lethargy, stupor, stiff neck	Preschool age	Excretory precautions
Echovirus	Same as above	Preschool age	Excretory precautions
Rubella virus	Same as above	Preschool through school age	Excretory precautions
Mumps virus	Same as above	Preschool through school age	Excretory precautions
Herpesvirus	Rapid onset, severe and rapid deterioration; brain damage (death usually results)	Infant	

TABLE 20-9 Meningitis: Comparison of Laboratory Findings

Test/Normal Values	Bacterial	Viral	Encephalitis
Cerebrospinal fluid analysis Appearance	Cloudy, turbid, purulent	Clear	Clear or opalescent; exception in herpesvirus
Glucose Newborn: 20-40 mg/dl Infant/child: 70-90 mg/dl	0-15 mg/dl or less than one-half of blood glucose	Normal or elevated	Initially normal
Total protein Newborn-1 mo: 20-120 mg/dl Infant/child: 15-45 mg/dl	Elevated to 500 mg/dl	Normal or slightly elevated	Normal or moderately increased to 60-150 mg/dl
White blood cells (WBC)/mm³ Newborn: 0-15 Infant: 0-8 Child and others: 0-5	Elevated, 1000 or more cells/mm³, polymorphonuclear leukocytes predominate	Elevated but below 150 cells/mm³; lymphocytes predominate	Elevated, 200 cells/mm³; lymphocytes predominate

TABLE 20-10 Types of Brain Tumors

Name—Location	Age of Peak Incidence	Symptoms	Treatment	Prognosis
Astrocytoma—cerebellum (slow-growing) Staging: grade I least infiltration; Grade IV greatest	Any age; primarily between 3-8 yr	Insidious onset and a slow course; increased ICP* early in course; possible hypotonia; intention tremor on side of lesion; head tilt; gait ataxia with "drifting" toward side of lesion and other unilateral cerebellar dysfunctions "Cerebellar fits": loss of consciousness; rigid extremities, neck flexion, dilated pupils; abnormal breathing patterns	Tumor is removed surgically; radiation is used for recurrent tumors or when neoplasm is not resected completely	With complete excision, there is a 90 percent cure in grades I and II tumor Outlook is hopeful if there is no recurrence 18 mo after surgery Tumor regrowth is a poor prognostic sign Prognosis is poor in grades III and IV and when tumor is inaccessible or minimal amount of tumor is resected
Medulloblastoma—cerebellum with seeding along cerebrospinal axis (highly malignant, rapidly growing)	3-5 yr; boys affected twice as often as girls	Nonspecific, vomiting, anorexia, and cerebellar symptoms of gait disturbances; decreased deep tendon reflexes; headache, fine symmetrical nystagmus; as tumor enlarges, papilledema, drowsiness, and other ominous manifestations	Surgery relieves increased ICP; tumor is highly susceptible to radiation Chemotherapy may include vincristine, cyclophosphamide (Cytoxan)	A 20-30 percent cure rate has been achieved with surgery plus radiation (Behrman and Vaughan, 1983)

*ICP = intracranial pressure.

Continued.

TABLE 20-10 Types of Brain Tumors—cont'd

Name—Location	Age of Peak Incidence	Symptoms	Treatment	Prognosis
Brainstem gliomas— pons and medulla	7 yr through adolescence	Progressive, multiple bilateral cranial nerve palsies, including facial (VII), glossopharyngeal (IX), vagus (X), trigeminal (V), and abducens (VI) Gait disturbances; spastic hemiparesis and positive Babinski sign (increased ICP is a late symptom)	Surgery confirms diagnosis; cannot be excised because of location Radiation is done	Prognosis is poor, with death occurring within 18 mo
Ependymoma—lining of the floor of the fourth ventricle, extending upward obstructing cerebrospinal fluid flow (slow growing)	Birth through 3 yr	Increased ICP; nausea; vomiting; unsteady gait; headache Cranial nerve palsies and positive Babinski sign indicative of brainstem infiltration	Since tumor is attached to the floor of the fourth ventricle, it cannot be totally excised; bulk of tumor is removed, and shunting procedure is done to allow cerebrospinal fluid to circulate Tumor is radiosensitive, and radiation is done	Its location makes the prognosis poor; there are very few long-term survivors
Craniopharyngioma— within or outside sella turcica (congenital; benign)	Any point in childhood or adolescence	A variety of visual problems including bitemporal hemianopsia and gradual loss of visual acuity; asymmetrical field defects, unilateral blindness; an arrest in linear growth as well as various signs of hypothalamic and/or pituitary dysfunction; increased ICP; alterations in personality and memory; delayed sexual maturity in the adolescent	Tumor is removed surgically: either complete or subtotal excision; repeated surgical procedures may be necessary to control tumor size, since cells remaining after initial surgery proliferate Although radioresistant, future tumor growth can be controlled with radiation	Prognosis is good *if* tumor is totally resected and/or radiation is done; visual losses which occur are permanent Diabetes insipidus is a frequent postoperative problem; although hormonal replacement therapy is necessary, including antidiuretic hormone and corticosteroids, these children can live relatively normal lives for years

Preventing the spread of meningococcal infection is done by administering the appropriate oral antibiotic to people living in the same household and to peers in a day care center. Staff members are not routinely treated. Vaccines, such as serogroup A and C meningococcal polysaccharide, have recently been developed. They are FDA-approved and are given in one dose.

A single dose of serogroup C vaccine is about 70 percent effective for a period of 6 to 9 months in preventing meningococcal disease in children over 2 years of age. Serogroup A is effective in children over 3 months of age. The use of these vaccines is recommended in addition to antibiotic prophylaxis for children exposed within the household or day care nursery to confirmed cases of serogroup A or C meningococcal disease.

If meningitis is treated early, the prognosis is good, but there may be complications and long-term effects. Subdural effusion is frequently a result of *H. influenzae* meningitis, especially in neonates. Other sequelae may be hydrocephalus, impaired intelligence, seizure disorders, visual and hearing defects from damage to the cranial nerves, personality changes, and anemia.

Nursing Management

Whenever there is elevated temperature, nausea and vomiting, restlessness, or the possibility of seizures, the nurse must provide rest and quiet, prevent dehydration, institute safety measures, maintain a patent airway, and use an appropriate isolation technique. Medications, generally phenobarbital and Valium, are given to control restlessness and prevent or treat convulsions.

General comfort measures are important, and frequently the nurse must use ingenuity to provide comfort and adequate rest to the irritable, restless child. Fever, if present, is treated with antipyretics such as acetaminophen, tepid sponging, turning on the air conditioner, and hypothermia mattress as necessary. It is essential to reduce the temperature to decrease cerebral metabolic stress. Vital signs and neurological evaluation are done hourly at first or more frequently if necessary. When IV fluids are administered, the danger of increasing ICP is very real and the fluid volume must be monitored closely via buretrol and infusion pump. Fluids are maintained at two-thirds maintenance for several days or until the condition stabilizes. Strict intake and output measurements with hourly checks of specific gravity are done because severe CNS infection may result in an inappropriate antidiuretic hormone response with oliguria and low urine osmolarity. This syndrome results in water intoxication and cerebral edema.

A position flat in bed is generally more comfortable for the child with meningitis, especially when there is opisthotonic nuchal rigidity. Because sitting and movement of the head cause increased pain, care is taken to have as little movement as possible. If opisthotonos is present, the child is positioned on his side. Adequate hydration is important, and fluids are gradually increased with improvement in the child's clinical status. Fluids are administered preferably in ways that do not require sitting. Straws should be used, and gelatin desserts or Popsicles may be offered.

The child is observed for the development of subdural effusions and empyema. The signs include irritability, increasing ICP, temperature elevations, and transillumination. Head circumferences are measured, and palpations of the anterior fontanel are continued in infants. Serial CAT scans are performed. Medications are administered intravenously in high doses. These medications, toxic and irritating to the vein, tend to create phlebitis during prolonged administration. The use of IV filters may reduce the risk of phlebitis. Medication sites should be observed for evidence of infiltration or development of tissue irritation. If the nurse administers the medication slowly in a dilute form by IV piggyback, irritation can be prevented. The nurse must know the characteristics of the specific medication she is administering, including the proper dilution and the side effects. The child should be restrained in a functional position which safeguards the integrity of the IV infusion and still allows for mobility.

The child is observed for arthralgia and myalgia, muscle pains, and transient arthritis seen in bacterial meningitis. Acetaminophen may be administered for relief. The exudate of the meningococcal rash is treated carefully to avoid the spread of the organism. Warm normal-saline soaks will help remove any exudate.

Emotional support of the family includes an environment where parents express their concerns about the child. Assessment of the parents' knowledge and perception of their child's guarded prognosis permits the nurse to clarify misconceptions about any changes in the child's clinical course and to refer parents to the physician as necessary.

Developmental lags may occur; therefore, the utilization of the DDST and other assessment tools is essential. Therapeutic play activities can be initiated. Referrals to the community health nurse for emotional and developmental evaluations and follow-up care are also essential. Parents require education in drug therapy if the child is placed on anticonvulsants and if family members require antibiotic prophylaxis. The importance of contacting the physician if there is a temperature elevation, increased irritability, or the development of poor feeding patterns is stressed to parents. When able, the child should be allowed to ambulate and play.

Encephalitis

The term *encephalitis* describes an inflammatory process of the brain. The encephalitic process occurs in two phases. In the *nonneural phase,* the child exhibits an acute, febrile illness from the bite of an arthropod or ingestion of an enterovirus (the most common cause of encephalitis). If the organs propagate large numbers of causative organisms, secondary seeding (phase two, the *neuronal phase*) occurs with invasion of the CNS. Severe neurological dysfunction is the sequela (Behrman and Vaughan, 1983). Chickenpox, measles, mumps, Coxsackie virus A and B infections, and herpes simplex may cause encephalitis as a complication of the disease process, and encephalitis may occur as a complication following routine vaccinations for smallpox, poliomyelitis, diphtheria, pertussis, and influenza. Immunosuppressed children are at high risk.

The clinical features of encephalitis vary according to the invading organism and its prime location within the brain. Characteristically there is a sudden or insidious onset of headache and elevated temperature which may be followed by drowsiness, which can then progress to a deep coma. Symptoms of meningeal irritation may be present (see Meningitis above). Encephalitis carries a greater morbidity and mortality than does meningitis. Sometimes the onset is marked by changes in behavior and hyperactivity. Seizures are more likely to occur in the infant, whereas paresis of one or more of the cranial nerves, disorders of speech, ataxia, weakness of muscle groups, diplopia, alterations of reflexes, and disturbances of the autonomic nervous system may occur as single entities or in combinations in the preschool child with encephalitis.

Diagnosis is based on an in-depth history of the onset of symptoms and the result of laboratory studies. Historical data include the child's geographic location; illness contacts; exposure to arthropods (e.g., mosquitoes and ticks), horses, and other animals; ingestion of pesticides and toxic metals; and recent infections. The CSF is often within normal limits initially, but a moderate increase in leukocytes may be evidenced after 48 hours. The sugar content of the CSF is usually normal but may be low, and the protein count is either normal or slightly elevated. Vi-

20-4 *The Child with Meningitis*

Clinical Problem/Nursing Diagnosis	Expected Outcome	Nursing Interventions

Lethargic; altered level of consciousness; increased irritability; vomiting; nuchal rigidity; bulging fontanelle; pupillary dilation with decreased reactivity to light	Child will demonstrate progressive improvement in neurological status as evidenced by appropriate behavior for age: increased activity level	Monitor vital signs qh; note irregularities in heart rate or respiratory pattern; note hyper/hypotension (use proper size blood pressure cuff for consistency)
		Frequently assess neurological status (qh)
		Note
		  Level of consciousness (LOC)
		  Change in behavior
		  Increased lethargy or irritability
		  Change in feeding pattern

Altered thought processes related to neurophysiological pathology	Child will maintain developmental milestones	Nausea, vomiting, pupillary size, and reactivity to light
		  Increased bulging of fontanel; separation of suture lines
		  Baseline head circumference; then measure head circumference q 8 h
		  Response to pain reflex activity in all extremities bilaterally

	Child will demonstrate controlled progression of neurological sequelae secondary to meningitis as evidenced by controlled intracranial pressure (ICP) seizure activity; normal vital signs for age	Muscle strength; motor and sensory function in extremities bilaterally Presence of nuchal rigidity and positive Kernig's and Brudinski's signs Presence of decorticate or decerebrate posturing Presence of seizure activity Signs and symptoms of subdural effusion; subdural empyema (fever and signs of increasing ICP) Assure prompt and proper administration of IV antibiotics with required safe dose and dilution of medications; assess for side effects; monitor antibiotic drug levels Support child through auditory testing
	Child will demonstrate consistent improvement in neurological status	*To prevent and control increased intracranial pressure:* Promote cerebral venous return by elevating HOB; position head midline and prevent flexion Monitor oxygenation to maintain the PCO_2 at 25 to 30 mmHg $PO_2 >$ 100 mmHg; CO_2 saturation > 95 mmHg; mild respiratory alkalosis (clarify individual parameters with physician)
	Child will maintain normal hearing and visual acuity	Assess rate, depth, regularity, and quality of respirations and breath sounds Place child on cardiac-respiratory monitor as indicated Note color of nailbeds and mucous membranes; immediately report signs of hypoxia or hypoventilation to physician for emergent intervention Properly administer oxygen therapy as ordered Use sunctioning judiciously Maintain fluid restriction and strict input and output Properly administer anticonvulsants, and steroids as ordered Maintain fever and pain control Assess for seizure activity (note changes in pupillary response, nystagmus, and labile blood pressure) assure prompt intervention; enforce seizure precautions
Possible spread of infection Shallow, irregular respirations; periodic breathing; apnea	To prevent spread infection to others Child and family will strictly adhere to required isolation precautions	*For client with bacterial meningitis:* Maintain respiratory isolation precautions for 24 h after start of antibiotic therapy *For patient with aseptic (viral) meningitis:* Maintain on excretion/secretion precautions Teach child and family mode of transmission of meningitis with proper isolation precautions required
Potential for infection (transmission) Potential ineffective breathing pattern related to infection; increased ICP	Child will maintain patent airway and adequate oxygenation: $PaO_2 > 100$ mmHg, O_2 saturation > 75 mmHg, adequate CO_2 removal, and PCO_2 25-30 mmHg	Demonstrate strict hand washing Thoroughly monitor respiratory status for rate, depth, regularity, and effectiveness of respirations Auscultate lungs for quality and equality of breath sounds Constantly monitor color of nailbeds and mucous membranes Monitor for signs of respiratory distress (nasal flaring, grunting retracting, irregular breathing patterns, and cyanosis) Assess for signs of hypoxia (increased restlessness, irritability, and lethargy)

Clinical Problem/Nursing Diagnosis	Expected Outcome	Nursing Interventions
	Child will maintain adequate systemic perfusion and normal hemodynamic parameters for age (heart rate, respiratory rate, blood pressure)	Provide oxygen therapy as ordered; elevated HOB to promote maximal lung expansion Place child on cardiac-respiratory monitor as indicated by clinical status Monitor O_2 saturation with external oximeter or arterial blood gases for oxygenation assessment
Tachycardia/ bradycardia Hypotension/ hypertension Decreased systemic perfusion Potential decreased cardiac output related to infection, septic shock, and ICP	Child will maintain adequate systemic perfusion and normal hemodynamic parameters for age (heart rate, respiratory rate, blood pressure)	Frequently monitor child for stable vital signs Report significant changes to physician immediately *Assess for adequate systemic perfusion:* Assess stability of blood pressure; strength of peripheral pulses and warmth of extremities; brisk capillary refill (compare findings bilaterally); note pink color of nailbeds and mucous membranes Assess urine output for adequate volume for weight *Assess child for signs and symptoms of sepsis:* Alteration in vital signs: tachycardia/bradycardia, hypotension, fever, pallor, cyanosis, sluggish capillary refill, cool clammy skin, weak peripheral pulses, change in level of consciousness behavior Observe child for signs of disseminated intravascular coagulation Note presence of petechiae, ecchymotic areas, and hemorrhage Monitor lab values for evidence of coagulopathy (elevated prothrombin time and partial prothrombin time) Assess for seizure activity and signs of renal failure; notify physician immediately of abnormal findings Administer antibiotics as ordered; monitor for therapeutic levels
Decreased urine output (<1 cc/kq/h) Increased urine specific gravity >1.020 Decreased serum osmolality Increased urine osmolality Hyponatremia Weight gain Anorexia Nausea and vomiting Potential fluid voluem excess and electrolyte imbalance related to compromised regulatory mechanisms and syndrome of inappropriate antidiuretic hormone secretion	Child will maintain fluid and electrolyte balance as evidenced by: urine output ≥ 1 cc/kq/h; normal serum NA^+ (135 to 140 meg); normal serum and urine osmolality; prevention of H_2O intoxication elevated ICP	Monitor child for alterations in baseline vital signs Assess neurological status as outlined (note signs and symptoms of ICP seizure activity) Consistently monitor urine and serum electrolyte values Monitor urine and serum osmolality values Immediately report results indicating decreased serum NA and decreased serum osmolality; report electrolyte imbalance promptly to physician for treatment Document strict intake and output volumes; monitor and record urine specific gravity and dipstick results with every voiding Maintain fluid restrictions as ordered Administer NaCl/diuretics as ordered; document effectiveness Monitor weight bid (weigh child on same scale at same times)

Continued.

NURSING CARE PLAN 20-4 The Child with Meningitis—cont'd

Clinical Problem/Nursing Diagnosis	Expected Outcome	Nursing Interventions
Fever Hyperthermia related to infection	Child will achieve a rectal temperature of 37.5°C, given the necessary nursing interventions	Frequently monitor temperature for elevations (qh until afebrile); document temperature results to follow spike patterns Notify physician for temperature > 38.5°C; administer antipyretic measures as ordered (Tylenol and tepid sponge baths); utilize hypothermia blanket for temperature ≥ 39°C; assess effect of febrile state on hemodynamics (note degree of tachycardia and assess blood pressure) Assess neurological status for changes to increased oxygen needs; properly institute O₂ therapy as needed Assess for fluid and electrolyte imbalances secondary to febrile state Assess effectiveness of antipyretic measures on ability to decrease child's temperature gradually Provide age-appropriate play activities which support coping with hospitalization
Pain Nuchal rigidity Positive Kernig's and Brudzinski's signs Headache Arthalgia, myalgia, and generalized muscle pain Pain related to meningococcal signs secondary to infection	Child will be comfortable as evidenced by increased ability to rest and sleep, be consoled, and maintain acceptable vital signs for age	Monitor vital signs for tachycardia, hypo/hypertension, and respiratory effort Note changes in neurological status (signs of elevated ICP) Note presence of pallor and cyanosis Group activities to promote longer periods of rest Promote calm, quiet environment; avoid use of bright lights and loud noises Speak calmly, quietly, and softly to child; prevent overstimulation Support neck with position changes Position with HOB elevated with ICP; if ICP is absent, position side lying or supine to comfort Administer Tylenol as ordered for analgesic effects (may mask fever spikes; clarify order with physician)
Parents communicate fear, anxiety, and stress over child's sudden illness Child demonstrates fearful behavior Potential ineffective family coping related to knowledge deficit; situational crisis of emergent hospitalization	Family and child will feel supported by health care team Parents will understand illness, treatments, and prophylactic therapy required as ordered by physician Parents will mobilize support systems to optimize family coping mechanisms	Assess parent and child's understanding of illness and required treatments Identify teaching needs; clarify questions Enforce teaching related to prophylactic treatment for exposed siblings, classmates, and family members as ordered by physician; provide teaching for children requiring continued anticonvulsant therapy; provide teaching to family prior to discharge concerning signs and symptoms of infection to facilitate prompt medical intervention (elevated temperature, irritability, change in behavior or feeding pattern, and lethargy) Familiarize parents and child with the hospital unit if this service was omitted on admission

ral studies of CSF, blood, urine, feces, and secretions facilitate identifynig the causative agent. Although they take several weeks to complete, these results provide valuable information. Usually a serum specimen is sent 10 to 14 days later.

The prognosis is guarded. Recovery may be dramatically sudden within a few hours or may not occur for days, weeks, or months. Death may be the result. Infants are more likely to have permanent residual effects than are older children. While a brain biopsy may be necessary to identify the organism, antibiotics are not usually helpful, so treatment is symptomatic. However, Viar-A (vidarabine) is given for herpes encephalitis. Residual effects may be in the form of seizure disorders, hemiplegia or monoplegia, bizarre behavior patterns, and mental retardation. Evidence of residual damage may not be apparent until the child fails to meet developmental levels or has difficulty with learning.

Nursing Management

The symptoms dictate plans for nursing care. The child is placed on isolation in an area where he can be observed closely for evidence of seizures and increased ICP. Nursing assessments must be done continuously because a child with encephalitis may demonstrate signs of respiratory distress from paralysis of the respiratory muscles or involvement of the respiratory center of the brain. If the child has difficulty swallowing, pooled secretions may contribute to his respiratory difficulty. To maintain adequate respiratory function, the child may require intubation or a tracheostomy.

If the child is comatose, he may emerge rapidly or somewhat slowly from this state, often with some immediate residual effects such as ataxia, behavior changes, and general confusion. The child must be oriented to time and place and told what has happened. In evaluating a child's progress, the nurse may conclude that play should be incorporated into the care according to age and physical abilities to foster the return of neuromuscular function. Working with clay, stringing beads, and throwing balls are possible, enjoyable, and beneficial activities. Living with and accepting the unknown create anxieties for both the parents and the child during his convalescence, but the full potential for residual effects may not be known for many months. The nurse should assist the parents in their acceptance of their child with his current disabilities and project hope for the future that is based on reality. The family that must eventually accept the child with permanent disabilities needs additional support from the health team.

A schedule for routine evaluation of the development level should be established as part of the discharge plan. A referral to the public health agency provides necessary follow-up.

Brain Abscess

A *brain abscess* is a localized collection of purulent material in any section of the brain. Some causative organisms are *Staphylococcus aureus,* pneumococcus, *Proteus, H. influenzae,* and *H. aphrophilus* (Behrman and Vaughan, 1983).

Children with cyanotic heart disease (right to left shunts) are at greatest risk because of reduced blood filtration through the alveoli and the presence of a hypoxic brain which serves as a culture medium for anaerobic bacteria. Less than 50 percent of brain abscesses in children are related to infections elsewhere (mastoids, paranasal sinuses, skull) or to trauma (Wing, 1981).

The symptoms are focal in nature, determined by the structures involved. While epidural/subdural abscesses are rare, they can occur following frontal sinusitis or infection of the scalp and skull. If the abscess is in the cerebellum, there is nystagmus and ataxia.

Headache, vomiting, papilledema, increased ICP, and behavioral changes may be present, regardless of the structure involved, because of an increase in local pressure and a decrease in venous drainage. These symptoms can persist for several weeks without the child being acutely ill.

A diagnosis is confirmed by brain scan, CAT scan, and EEG. Lumbar punctures are not done because of risks associated with brainstem herniation, and unless the abscess has ruptured, a CSF culture is sterile. Some physicians advocate excision of the brain abscess if it is localized and the child is comatose from the increased ICP. High doses of wide-spectrum antibiotics are necessary in an effort to avoid rupture of the abscess, which could result in an overwhelming meningitis. The most common sequelae are seizures, which can be controlled by phenobarbital and Dilantin.

Nursing Management

The goal of caring for a child with a brain abscess is to provide physical and emotional support and to avoid an increase in ICP. Since the illness is lengthy with very gradual improvement, both parents and child need consistent attention from caregivers and a great deal of emotional support. Parents should be encouraged to visit and to become involved in the care being given. While the child can benefit from play therapy, opportunities need to be provided for parents to verbalize their feelings about the prolonged hospitalization as well as the potential long-term results (seizure activity).

The high doses of wide-spectrum antibiotics necessitate observing the child for the side effects which can develop. Teaching done by a nurse needs to focus on the child's special needs and on the medications which may have to be administered after discharge.

Brain Death

Brain death is the cessation of neurological function despite the fact that respirations and circulation may be maintained with the use of a ventilator. These children are usually flaccid, have fixed pupils, and are markedly hypothermic, although DTRs may still be present. Confirmation, which is achieved by taking two consecutive EEG readings for 30 minutes or longer at 24-hour intervals, reveals the complete absence of brain waves. While hospital policies differ, several physicians must agree that brain death has occurred and that the lack of brain wave activity is not secondary to hypothermia or drugs. Hence, all serum toxicology screening tests must be negative before brain death is identified.

Nursing Management

Providing care to these children can be difficult for the highly skilled professional nurse who works in an intensive care setting. While carrying out physicians' orders, the nurse is in an environment which has phenomenal capabilities to prolong life. In this type of practice the nurse confronts many moral, ethical, and legal issues which are without precedent. These topics are covered in Chapter 8.

Families who are coping with the financial and emotional aspects of maintaining respiratory and circulatory function in the child also need to be involved actively in any decision making which affects future care. They need a great deal of information which needs to be provided in an unhurried environment that allows them to raise questions and arrive at decisions. Permitting them to participate in caring for the child decreases parental feelings of helplessness and allows them to begin the grieving process. Parents also need time to ventilate their feelings of sorrow, guilt, and anger. While it is extremely difficult, nurses need to accept these emotions and support parents during this period. Data acquired by the nurse are critical elements in determining the cessation of life.

Neurological Disorders in the School-Age Child

Reye's Syndrome

Reye's syndrome is characterized by acute encephalopathy with a fatty degeneration of the viscera associated with elevated concentrations of blood ammonia and serum transaminase. Typically, there is severe vomiting, with a gastrointestinal disturbance or flulike symptoms a few days before the onset of the disease. These children are febrile and have white blood cell counts up to 40,000 to 50,000 cells per cubic millimeter, elevated serum amylase and blood urea nitrogen levels, a pH ranging from acidic to alkaline, and normal blood pressure. There is a rapid progression in the client's level of consciousness from drowsiness and lethargy to stupor and coma. It is a syndrome found more commonly in infants, in blacks, and in families where siblings develop its symptoms.

Its cause is unknown; however, some investigators theorize that it may be a toxin-viral reaction or pathological condition within lipid metabolism which results in an increased level of free fatty acids. The latter alters the metabolic processes within the CNS, leading to coma. Also, there may be a genetic metabolic predisposition to developing Reye's syndrome. The normal ammonia level is 48 to 80 μg/dl; however, in this disease the level may reach 150 to 750 μg/dl. There may be severe dysfunction of both liver and kidneys.

A CAT scan demonstrates cerebral edema, and a high-voltage EEG depicts a slow dysrhythmia. A liver biopsy may be done in atypical cases to confirm the diagnosis. Hypoglycemia is found in these young children.

Constant monitoring is essential because of the rapid deterioration of the child's neurological status. Death can occur following brainstem herniation from cerebral edema. Treatment is symptomatic. Neomycin and lactulose, given by nasogastric tube and by enema, reduce ammonia production. These clients have Foley catheters inserted to ensure careful output. Arterial and central venous pressure lines and a peripheral intravenous line are in place too. Intravenous solutions of hypertonic glucose decrease the metabolic and neurological effects of hypoglycemia. Since the child is dehydrated, fluid deficits are corrected in the first 24 hours, and fluid is then restricted to two-thirds of maintenance requirements. Dexamethasone, mannitol, or glycerol is administered to prevent cerebral edema. An ICP-monitoring device may be placed.

Mechanical ventilation is frequently necessary. The patient's condition can change very rapidly, and the following tests are done frequently: blood gases, serum electrolytes, blood urea nitrogen, hematocrit, glucose, and serum osmolality. In addition, coagulopathies are treated as necessary.

Nursing Management

The goal of nursing activities in Reye's syndrome is to prevent or minimize the metabolic and nervous system damage from encephalopathy and degeneration of the viscera. When hypertonic glucose solutions are used, urine is tested for sugar and acetone every 2 hours. The renal threshold is frequently altered, and rebound hyperglycemia with glucosuria may occur. Diarrhea stools from the lactulose administration cause skin excoriation and may potentially contaminate the Foley catheter. Diligent skin care is essential. Strict control and precise recording of intake and output are maintained to prevent fluid overload. Steroids cause ulceration of the gastrointestinal tract; therefore, stools and nasogastric drainage are evaluated for guaiac. Antacids are frequently administered prophylactically and as necessary.

Osmotic diuretics, when administered, require evaluation of the interval between administration of the drug and its effects on urinary output and a decrease in ICP. Good pulmonary care is essential if complications are to be avoided. If the patient is on a respirator, it must be checked to ensure that it is functioning properly. Since the child can deteriorate rapidly, neurological assessments are done hourly. Oximeters are used to assess the adequacy of ventilation. The nurse is responsible for minimizing the psychological effects of the intensive-care environment and assessing family support systems during this health crisis. The sights and sounds of a critical care area are frightening, and the nurse who takes the time to explain the equipment and allows the parents to become involved in caring for the child makes a significant contribution toward allaying their fears and anxieties. In talking with parents, a nurse facilitates the ventilation of intense emotions, identifies additional stressors, and assesses a family's support systems.

Guillain-Barré Syndrome

Guillain-Barré syndrome consists of an acute symmetrical polyneuropathy. The course is variable from *ascending* motor paralysis to a combination of signs and symptoms of cranial and peripheral nerve dysfunction. The onset usually occurs 3 to 4 weeks after a respiratory infection or as a complication of the receipt of tetanus antitoxin or a vaccine.

Myelin and axon alterations of the anterior and posterior rootlets of the spinal nerves, degeneration of the cranial and proximal portions of peripheral nerves, or both occur. Initial symptoms are weakness of the lower extremities seen in gait abnormalities or pain and paresthesia with decreased muscle tone. Weakness progresses to the arms, intercostal muscles, and facial muscles. Ventilatory assistance is frequently required. Paralysis usually reaches its height between 1 and 21 days. Bowel and bladder functions remain intact.

Speech becomes decreased in volume and clarity. There is a reduction in the strength of the voluntary cough and in the depth of respirations. Other clinical symptoms include transient mild stiff neck, orthostatic hypotension, intermittent hypertension, papilledema, and increased ICP.

Children with extensive involvement may be left with permanent disability and muscle atrophy. Progressive improvement over a year or more may occur in children with severe motor dysfunction.

Nursing Management

The nursing goals for children with Guillain-Barré syndrome include maintenance of a patent airway and sensory and motor system intactness. Neurological assessment with the close evaluation of bilateral sensory discrimination and motor strength provides data on the extent of the nerve involvement. Accurate assessment of the child's status depends on the cooperation given by the young client. Creativity on the part of the nurse may assist in making the evaluation process less anxiety-provoking.

Bilateral muscle strength is assessed by asking the child to squeeze the examiner's hands and then asking him to raise his arms and then his legs as high as he can. Deep tendon reflexes in all extremities are evaluated because they may be absent. The quality of respirations is observed. Tidal volumes are measured with a respirometer attached to the appropriate size Ambu-mask or other similar means. The child is encouraged to cough to assess the strength of his protective mechanism. The clarity and volume of speech are noted (in the case of an infant, the character of his cry). The presence or absence of facial paralysis is determined. It can be easily overlooked because the deficit is symmetrical in nature. The child is asked to squeeze his eyelids shut. The ease of opening the eyelid indicates facial nerve paralysis or weakness. Eye movements and pupillary responses are assessed for any additional nerve dysfunction.

An individualized rehabilitation program based on the assessment of sensory and motor function is immediately initiated in conjunction with a physical therapist, the family, the nursing and medical staff, and other appropriate health team members. Passive range of motion exercises, therapeutic play, environmental stimulation with television or radio, and reading to the child are examples of rehabilitation and stress-reducing modalities.

The recuperative process may last a year or more; therefore, ongoing physical therapy is frequently continued after discharge from the hospital. The effects of an altered body image on the child with a residual disability are evaluated by the nurse. Tutoring may be required for the school-age child in the hospital and home environment. The importance of maintaining peer relationships cannot be overemphasized.

Brain Tumors

Brain tumors, after leukemia, are the most common solid neoplasms seen in infancy and childhood. Seen most commonly in the 6- to 10-year age group, brain tumors are divided into two broad anatomic groups: (1) *infratentorial* and (2) *supratentorial*. The infratentorial group includes the cerebellum, the brainstem, the fourth ventricle, and

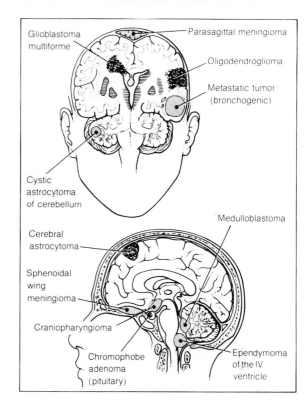

FIGURE 20-17   The anatomic relationship of the different types of brain tumors. (*A.H. Harvey, "Neoplastic Disturbances in Perception and Coordination," in D.A. Jones et al [eds.], Medical-Surgical Nursing: A Conceptual Approach, 2d ed., McGraw-Hill, New York, 1982, p. 1331; after H. Kryk et al., "Grand Rounds on Brain Tumors," Cancer Nurse, September 1975, p. 43*)

the optic chiasm, while the supratentorial group encompasses all other structures of the brain (Fig. 20-17).

About two-thirds of all tumors occur in the infratentorial region, and so the signs of increased ICP develop early because of obstruction in both the circulation and absorption of CSF (Fig. 20-10). About 75 percent of the brain tumors seen in children are gliomas. While primary prevention is not possible, early diagnosis may prevent irreparable damage.

The prognosis is related to the child's age and sex, the tumor type and location, and available treatment modalities. While female children have a greater survival rate, younger children have a poorer prognosis. The long-term prognosis of all children with brain tumors has improved with multimodal therapy (Table 20-10, pp. 419-420).

The *signs* and *symptoms* of brain tumors vary because of the child's developmental level, the location of the tumor, and the extent of damage done. For example, an unexplained enlarged head and bulging fontanels in an infant must be evaluated for a possible tumor. Later, in childhood, when the fontanels and suture lines are closed, symptoms of increased ICP may indicate compression of the brain, meninges, and cerebral arteries and veins.

Infants who have brain tumors have an increased head circumference and may have seizures, may vomit, and may be lethargic and lose some of their mastered developmental milestones. Unfortunately, older children have a variety of symptoms, which makes diagnosis more difficult.

An *alteration in the child's level of consciousness and cognitive ability* may be an early or late sign of a neoplasm. Frequently, over time, parents note changes in or deterioration of school performance, personality, affect, speech, and memory (recent and remote events). Bizarre behavior, school phobias, short attention spans, and impaired safety judgments concern both parents and teachers. The child may not be admitted for a neurological workup until other serious symptoms of increased ICP develop, such as lethargy or severe ataxia. Precious time has been lost because of these nonspecific manifestations.

The *headache,* which is a common complaint, results from the tumor's stretching the dura, blood vessels, and pain-sensitive cranial nerves. Typically, the child complains of severe headache on rising or when awakened during the night. At first the headache is dull, intermittent, and diffuse; then it becomes more severe and prolonged. Its pain is increased by coughing, straining, or stooping actions, which increase ICP.

Nausea and *vomiting* are common complaints and are due to a compression of the medullary emetic center either by the tumor or as a result of increased ICP. The vomiting may be projectile (forceful) without nausea. Parents frequently comment on the fact that the child eats immediately afterward, without difficulty. Infants may fail to thrive.

As a result of localized or generalized increased ICP, *seizures* can occur at any time. Grand mal seizures, with or without an aura, are seen most frequently. The Cushing reflex of a widening pulse pressure, bradycardia, and an altered respiratory pattern are late signs.

There are *visual disturbances* such as papilledema and hemianopsia. The former is not seen in infants, but it develops rapidly in young children. Obstruction of retinal blood flow causes severe engorgement. There is diminished visual acuity. Optic atrophy on the side of the tumor site and contralateral papilledema may occur.

Cranial nerve dysfunction develops as a result of susceptibility to the increased ICP and possible damage from the tumor. Any or all of the cranial nerves may be affected by the neoplasm's compression. *Head tilting,* which may result from IVth cranial nerve dysfunction, can be the first sign of reduced visual acuity. The VIth cranial nerve, the abducens, is frequently involved in nerve palsies, blurring of vision, or diplopia. Teachers identify a child's inability to read material on the blackboard. The optic, oculomotor, and trochlear nerves may be involved too.

The *ataxia* seen in children with brain tumors develops slowly. Initially, a child compensates for any disturbance in coordination. However, it persists; the child seems to trip or fall with increasing frequency, and performance in games or sports deteriorates. In time the child demonstrates the *cerebellar* symptoms of ipsilateral ataxia, loss of fine motor control, intention tremors, staggering or widebased gait, dysmetria, hypotonia, and nystagmus.

A child suspected of having a CNS lesion is admitted for a complete neurological workup which includes laboratory tests, a developmental assessment, and an ophthalmologic examination. Visual testing is done to determine the cause of blurring of vision or other eye problems. The child is also asked about *photopsia,* which is the sensation of sparks of light and optic hallucinations.

Many clinical studies are needed to confirm the diagnosis, including an EEG, skull x-rays, radio-isotope brain scanning, CAT scans, magnetic resonance imaging (MRI), and routine blood work. Other radiological studies, such as a cerebral angiogram or pneumoencephalogram, are done only when necessary.

Surgical intervention depends on the type and location of the lesion. Since a diagnosis is confirmed on biopsy, a craniotomy is necessary. While radical excision of the mass is most desirable, a tumor that is very deep or near vital centers of the dominant hemisphere, brainstem, or corpus callosum may not be removed completely. The prognosis is good for a child who has had a tumor removed in toto.

Another modality used in the treatment of brain tumors is *radiation therapy,* which reduces the lesion's size. Whole brain and spinal cord irradiation is frequently done in the presence of a medulloblastoma or ependymoma.

The institution of *chemotherapy* is an especially challenging treatment for the nurse in view of the myriad problems which can emerge. It is used in selected and/or recurring brain tumors. The effectiveness of a drug is dependent on a number of variables including tumor location, size, mitotic activity, growth rate, cell type, prior management of the tumor, and integrity of the blood-brain barrier. Many drugs are used in chemotherapy, alone or in combination. Some of them are vincristine, lomustine (CCNU), carmustine (BCNU), prednisone, procarbazine, cyclophosphamide (Cytoxan), nitrogen mustard (mechlorethamine), and intrathecal methotrexate.

Nursing Management

The nursing care of the child with a brain tumor may be divided into five phases: diagnostic, preoperative, postoperative (maintenance), radiation, and discharge. Throughout each of these phases the nurse must assess the child for evidence of alteration in neurological status and for response to the diagnostic or therapeutic measures.

Diagnostic Phase

When a brain tumor is suspected, the child and his family approach hospitalization and the diagnostic studies with great anxiety. Many parents feel guilty for not seeking help earlier because they thought the child had the flu or did not want to go to school. Many parents express the fear that their feelings will be confirmed, yet they also want an explanation for the changed behavior. The child also is concerned about what will happen to him. A trusting, therapeutic relationship with the parents and child must be established at the time of admission. An ideal time to do so is while taking a nursing history during the admission interview. A therapeutic relationship is very important since the nurse will provide primary care not only during hospitalization but also possibly for the life span of the child. A nursing assessment of the family unit and its coping mechanisms should be made at this time.

Collecting information which serves as baseline data is a crucial nursing activity. The child's previous health and developmental history, allergies, height and weight, and nutritional status, along with clinical and laboratory studies, provide the health team with valuable facts.

Neurological assessments are done at 2- to 4-hour intervals, including deep tendon reflexes. The child's motor strength and movement can be tested by grasp and release ability, "arm drifting," and observation of both coordination and balance. Asymmetrical responses are especially noteworthy. While pupil size and extraocular movement are significant, a nurse also needs to identify the presence of nystagmus and head tilting. Certainly, any deterioration (hypotonia, ataxia, uncoordinated movement) or any abnormal pattern (respirations) or posturing (decerebrate, decorticate) must be reported to a physician immediately.

During this period it is important for a nurse to make careful assessments of the child. By playing a game of "Simon says" the nurse can identify the patient's ability to follow simple commands. Speech and memory problems can be validated by asking the child, "What is the name of your dog?" or "Can you tell me your name?" Alterations in sleep-wake cycles, lack of response to significant others, a decrease in motor and verbal activity, and hyperirritability are significant observations to record.

Since the headache is a common complaint in a child suspected of having a lesion, it is critical for a nurse to note its quality, nature, location, duration, and frequency and the time it appears. If a medication has been ordered for the headache, it is important to record its effectiveness.

It is important for a nurse to ascertain the presence of a pattern for the child's nausea and vomiting. In examining and measuring the emesis, it should be guaiac tested for the presence of blood. Since ICP rises with vomiting, vital signs need to be monitored closely during these episodes.

In many facilities children suspected of having CNS lesions are placed on seizure precautions. If one occurs, it is essential to maintain a safe environment and to record the precise nature of the seizure as described under Seizures of Childhood and Adolescence below. In addition, cranial nerves must be assessed frequently.

Following diagnosis, a decision is made regarding the most appropriate treatment for the child. If no treatment is appropriate, the child is discharged with only supportive measures and the family must be taught to care for the child at home. A liaison within the community, such as a community health nurse, is essential to provide continuous support for the family.

Preoperative Phase

If surgery is a part of the treatment of the child with a brain tumor, the nurse must understand the purpose of the surgery and prepare the child and his parents for the craniotomy or craniectomy. The child and the parents need careful explanation and preparation for the change in appearance postoperatively. They need to know that the child's head is shaved and that massive head dressings will be in place. Some physicians advise that the entire head be shaved; others advocate cutting the hair short and shaving only the incision area; still other surgeons shave only the operative site and leave the rest of the hair intact. Regardless of the technique, the loss of hair can be very traumatic to the child and his parents. It may be possible for the child to pick out a wig prior to surgery, but specific preparation of the head should be planned in collaboration with the neurosurgeon and the child.

The parents must also be prepared for the appearance of facial edema and the possibility that the child will be in a comatose state immediately after surgery. The nurse must understand that parents have difficulty comprehending such possibilities as they watch the child preoperatively.

If the child is to be admitted to an intensive care unit after surgery, a preoperative tour of the facility, a basic explanation of the equipment, and an introduction to its nurses can lessen his anxiety. It also demonstrates the primary nurse's concern for the child and strengthens the child-family-nurse relationship. As usual, the questions raised must be answered honestly and in language that can be understood by all concerned.

Postoperative Phase

During surgery and postoperatively, the nurse who has assumed responsibility for continuity of care must be available to the parents for continued support. When the child has regained consciousness, the nurse who is providing primary care should visit with him several times a day in the intensive care unit. At this time of increased stress the total family benefits greatly from the therapeutic relationship established by the primary care nurse in the preoperative period.

Postoperative care of the child who has undergone brain surgery is critical. The postoperative care provided to a child who has had a neurosurgical procedure is time-consuming, precise, and demanding, with a number of unknown variables which need to be identified. Interoperative brainstem and cerebellar manipulation in the presence of an infratentorial lesion, for example, can affect respiratory integrity. Potential damage to the IXth and Xth cranial nerves, which affect swallowing, coughing, and innervating the muscles of the pharynx, larynx, and vocal cords, is an unknown until the child begins to recover.

A child usually remains intubated until adequate tidal and minute volumes are maintained, gag and cough reflexes are present, and normothermia is established. After extubation, the patient needs to be observed carefully to detect the presence of dysphagia and drooling, for an inability to handle secretions can complicate recovery. When the patient is awake, it is necessary to encourage deep-breathing exercises and to perform chest physical therapy every 2 hours if necessary. It is important for a nurse to auscultate lung fields every hour in order to assess the child's pulmonary status. Suctioning is usually done only to maintain a patent airway.

In the unit, neurological assessments are done hourly. Vital signs are monitored at 15- to 30-minute intervals until they are stable. Then they are done hourly for 72 hours because cerebral edema may develop during that period. Observing the child for either cerebral edema or an increasing ICP is imperative. In addition, a child who has had infratentorial surgery is at high risk to develop a tonsillar herniation, which can be detected by a sudden pupillary dilation.

Edema of the neck, face, and intracranial spaces is present, and its extent must be ascertained. While the child may not be able to open and close the eyes, which is a source of discomfort, intracranial edema can inhibit respirations and compromise the patient further. If ordered, the head of the bed can be raised 30° in an effort to reduce the edema. Cool compresses applied to the face and neck may help, however, care needs to be taken when they are applied to the head. Sterility of the dressing must be maintained. Methylcellulose eye drops can be soothing, and they lessen the possibility of corneal damage. Reducing the ambient light can decrease the eye discomfort.

Positioning the child after neurosurgery is an important nursing function, with the operative technique dictating the position to be assumed. Children who have had *infratentorial* lesions removed can be placed on either side, with the bed flat, thereby avoiding pressure on the site and decreasing the likelihood of aspiration. The head and neck should be in a midline position, with a slight neck extension, in order to maintain a patent airway. Head and neck alignment can be maintained by using a pillow or folded bath blanket. When turning the child, two nurses utilize the log-rolling technique, while the child's arms are folded on the chest and a pillow is secure between the legs. It is essential for one nurse to support the head and neck while the second nurse turns the child with a turning sheet. Once he is in the new position, it is necessary to examine the patient's total body alignment as well as to inquire about the child's comfort.

The child with a *supratentorial* lesion usually has the head of the bed elevated 30 to 45°. This angle facilitates venous return, reduces the excessive cerebral blood flow, and prevents hemorrhage.

Hyperthermia can develop early postoperatively. Its cause may be a wound, urinary tract infection, the presence of blood in the CSF, or the development of pneumonia. Blood cultures are drawn, and x-rays are taken. A nurse needs to observe the child for signs of meningitis, specifically for nuchal rigidity meningismus, photophobia, and the assuming of opisthotonic position. The febrile state may be hypothalamic in origin, as a result of tumor infiltration or of compression or manipulation during surgery. Symptoms of this cause are no sweating, diurnal (daytime) temperature fluctuations, and little response to antipyretics administered; however, there is a drop in the elevated body temperature when the child is placed on a hypothermia mattress. Therefore, hypothermia mattresses are usually on the bed of a child who has had a brain tumor removed.

The fluid requirements and electrolyte levels are monitored judiciously. Frequently, the intravenous fluids given are dextrose and balanced saline solutions, such as dextrose 5% and 0.25 NaCl. Initially, the volume is two-thirds to three-fourths of the child's maintenance requirement in an effort to decrease the development of cerebral edema. The protocol usually calls for the replacement of fluid lost in urine, and so hourly outputs are recorded. A Foley catheter is in place to ensure accuracy. While the symptoms of diabetes insipidus can develop postoperatively in a child who has had a subtotal excision of a craniopharyngioma, another problem, SIADH, can occur in other children who have had other types of brain tumors removed. In the former, fluid intake may be increased to compensate for the large urinary output with its low osmolality and for patient complaints of thirst; however, in SIADH, fluids are restricted and sodium replacement is done to relieve the hyponatremia.

With a nastogastric tube in place, patency must be checked frequently. Gastric contents should be guaiac tested for occult blood at least once a shift, because the vagus nerve (X) affects the gastrointestinal tract. Some complications which can develop are a paralytic ileus, gastric irritation and constipation. In addition to monitoring stools, bowel sounds should be evaluated routinely.

Children are usually kept NPO (nothing by mouth) for a minimum of 24 hours after surgery. Before clear liquids are started, gag, cough, and swallow reflexes must be intact. If the child's state of consciousness is in question or any of the reflexes are not present, fluids are withheld.

It is not unusual for these patients to complain of pain from the operative site, and a medication such as acetaminophen provides relief. They also complain of muscle aches, which are present as a result of positioning while lying on an operating room table for 6 to 8 hours. Narcotics such as morphine sulfate are not given for two reasons: They can affect respiratory function, and they mask signs of increased ICP.

Many drugs are given to these children following brain surgery, often including mannitol, glycerol, furosemide (Lasix), and steroids. Nurses must know the actions, side effects, and contraindications and must also compute the precise dosages and administer them properly.

The nurse should observe the head dressing carefully for signs of drainage. Some drainage may occur, and the color, amount, and odor should be reported immediately. The area of drainage should be circled with a pen or pencil and timed. Felt-tip pens are not used, as this ink is rapidly absorbed to the incision level. With a simple craniotomy, drainage should be slight and should consist primarily of serosanguineous fluid from the skin. If burr holes have been made or skull plates removed for decompression, the drainage is likely to be greater. If large amounts of drainage are noted, the nurse may reinforce the dressing with additional material and report the situation to the physician immediately.

Sometimes the Jackson-Pratt drain, a small, plastic, egg-shaped device, is inserted. When it is in place, the output needs to be measured at the end of every shift; this task is easily done because of the calibrated markings on the drain. If the neurosurgeon orders the drain emptied, diligent sterile technique must be carried out. The color and consistency should be recorded. The necessary negative pressure can be achieved by compressing the drain walls. It usually remains in place for 48 to 72 hours.

CSF leaks can occur following neurosurgery. They can result in a potentially fatal CNS infection. Otorrhea and rhinorrhea indicate a CSF leak. In using a sterile sponge to obtain a specimen and utilizing a dipstick to confirm the presence of glucose in the specimen, a nurse can identify the watery substance as CSF. Occasionally the CSF may mix with blood and mucus. In any instance the neurosurgeon must be contacted. CSF leaks are treated by elevating the head of the bed by 30°, inserting an external CSF drainage system, or performing a lumbar puncture and removing some CSF to lower the pressure. Antibiotics are started too. Nasal packing can serve as a reservoir for infection, so it is not done. In addition, suctioning, blowing the nose, and intermittent positive pressure breathing machines are avoided.

When the child's condition is stabilized, he is returned to his previous unit. During the recovery period he is allowed and encouraged to return to independence, although this task may be complicated for the child who has residual effects from his surgery. The child and parents need to be told that these residual effects are due in part to edema and the surgical trauma and thus may disappear as the healing process is completed. Many parents are so relieved that the surgery is over and have such concern for the child who experienced surgery that they tend to be overprotective and indulgent. Both the parents and the child must return to the "well role."

Play should be encouraged for fun as well as for its therapeutic results. Care must be taken, however, that the child does not hit his head or fall until he is completely healed. Stocking-knit and head dressings may provide enough protection, depending on the type of surgery and the child's age. For some children a football helmet or wig is necessary to prevent trauma should they fall.

Postoperatively, children do not usually have difficulties adjusting to their altered appearance from loss of hair as long as the dressing is in place. When the dressing is no longer needed, many children exhibit extreme difficulties in accepting their baldness and adjusting to their body self-image. Stocking-knit caps, head scarves, or hats may be enough to allow the child to cope with his baldness and once again interact with other children and resume active participation in his recovery phase. Some children do better if a wig is supplied until the hair has grown in. If the head has not been totally shaved, the creative nurse may be able to comb the child's hair so that the area of loss is not so evident.

Radiation Phase

Radiation therapy is an essential component of current singular or multimodal management of almost any type of cancer in children. Its goal is to destroy malignant cells or render them incapable of cell replication. Unfortunately, this treatment affects normal and abnormal proliferating cells in the body.

The type of equipment selected as the source of this energy varies and depends on a number of factors, including tumor depth. It is utilized for palliation or as a cure. As palliative therapy, it reduces the size of the tumor and thereby provides significant relief from the pain being experienced.

The *short-term effects* include nausea, vomiting, malaise, alopecia, diarrhea, mucositis, skin irritations, and bone marrow depression. In patients whose cranial vaults have been irradiated for brain tumors, the hair may never grow back. If the white blood cell count drops drastically, the therapy may be suspended temporarily. The child may not demonstrate any untoward effects until the second to fourth day; however, this outcome depends on the tumor site and the amount of radiation the patient is receiving.

Potential long-term effects consist of an increased susceptibility to developing cancer in the irradiated sites, genetic mutations, sterility, and in the case of total body irradiation, leukemia. Certainly the child's age, total radiation dose received, and location of the tumor are factors to consider in relation to some of these long-term consequences. However, it is also important to realize that young children's organs are more radiosensitive than those of adults.

Considering the possible sequelae, an informed consent for radiation must be obtained. Then a nurse can begin to prepare the child and family for this therapy. If a nurse is present as the physician discusses this approach with the family, it is easier to clarify and reiterate the information that is given.

A point which needs to be emphasized relates to the painlessness of the therapy; however, all family members must also realize that unpredictable side effects can occur. Advising them of comfort measures which can be instituted allays some of their concerns. Parents may need to be encouraged to send the child to school in spite of the therapy. Since fatigue should be expected, teachers can facilitate frequent rest periods without disrupting the classroom. If that strategy is not possible, perhaps a tutor can be provided by the local school district.

Nurses in some facilities have prepared brochures for distribution to children and parents which contain information about radiation therapy. Some other helpful methods of relieving the apprehension that this type of treatment generates include showing a model of the room in which the child is irradiated, showing photographs of the equipment and its operating personnel, and making a visit to radiology which permits the child to lie on the table,

TABLE 20-11 Nursing Management of the Side Effects of Radiation Therapy

Potential	Nursing Implications	Potential	Nursing Implications
	withdrawal; encourage verbalization of feelings and concerns by child and parents; encourage child's participation in therapeutic play, if appropriate; provide consistent caregivers	Bone marrow depression	Monitor results of all blood studies done as dictated by protocol, especially platelets, granulocytes, and white cells; observe for anemia, pallor, ecchymosis, petechiae, and decreased enegy levels; monitor vital signs q 4 h; notify a physician of any elevated temperature; assess lungs, urine, and skin for any signs of infection; do not take rectal temperatures because of possibility of mucosal irritation in presence of low platelet count
Pleural rub; pericarditis	Auscultate heart and lungs every 4 h; report any signs of friction rub, pericarditis, or pleural rub; observe for cough, dyspnea, weakness, or pain on inspiration		
Mucositis	Prophylactically, encourage mouth washes (2 qt water to which 1 tsp each of baking soda and salt have been added) 6 to 10 times per day; provide soft toothbrush; offer soothing, cool substances such as Popsicles, ice cream, and ices; provide fortified liquids such as milk shakes, eggnogs, and cream soups, and add powdered milk to breakfast mixes; avoid use of ginger ale, coffee, and alcohol and avoid cigarette smoking (mucosal irritants) as well as hot, spicy foods; avoid full-strength citrus fruits (these juices may be tolerated if diluted 1:1)	Crystalluria	Observe uric acid levels closely; encourage fluids to decrease the likelihood of renal damage; offer cranberry juice to increase urinary acidity
		Diarrhea	Assess quality of a patient's bowel sounds; check stools by guaiac test for occult blood; monitor weight daily; provide low-residue diet and consult with a nutritionist; give antidiarrheal drugs as prescribed
Headache	Assess quality, frequency, pattern, and associated verbal and nonverbal pain behavior; administer prescribed drugs such as acetaminophen; apply cool compresses to head and neck; provide rest and a quiet environment	Nausea and vomiting	Administer antiemetics prior to, throughout, and following therapy, as prescribed by a physician; wherever possible, schedule therapy in morning; provide diversional activities for both young children and adolescents; if necessary start small, frequent, bland feedings; routinely, monitor intake and output, measure specific gravity of urine, and guaiac test any emesis for the presence of blood
Alopecia	Discuss with children use of wigs, scarfs, or hat and use of very mild shampoo; examine scalp often (some physicians prescribe lotions or oils for excessive dryness; hair may start to grow back in 8-16 weeks, except in cases of cranial irradiation, when it may never return because of follicular destruction)	Sterility	Shield gonads; on counseling, discuss with male adolescents possibility of donating to a sperm bank prior to start of radiation therapy
Decreased energy levels	Provide frequent rest periods, especially following therapy; monitor child's nutritional intake and record fluid intake and output; provide well-balanced diet and nutritious snacks	Skin reactions	Examine both target and exit surfaces of skin for reactions (the presence of mild erythema is a normal response; a *dry desquamation* consists of a redenning of skin, associated with a dry appearance and an itchiness; in presence of a *wet desquamation,* skin blisters and may slough; while it is a more serious reaction, it is *not* indicative of too much radiation; this response may need to be treated further); during therapy, advise child and/or parents to avoid tight, constrictive clothing; inform them that skin may turn a dark tan 2 to 4 weeks after irradiation therapy is completed

Source: J. W. Riley Hospital for Children Radiation Therapy Manual, Indianapolis; Kelly and Tinsley, 1981; Luckmann and Sorensen, 1980.

use the intercommunication system, and meet the staff.

The nurse plays a vital role in this type of therapy, for it is this professional who reviews the purpose of radiation, discusses the equipment in depth, and elaborates on the first visit to this department. At that time, the radiation oncologist identifies anatomic structures to be irradiated and marks specific areas of the body with an indelible pen. This procedure takes about 1 hour, and it is important to emphasize that no irradiation is done at this time. These markings remain for the duration of therapy. It is significant for the nurse to review the radiation therapy schedule and additional information found in Table 20-11.

Discharge Phase

Although hospital staffing patterns and policies do not usually allow the primary nurse to maintain contact with the family in the community, the nurse may be able to see the child in the clinic and maintain contact by telephone. Whether or not these communications occur, a referral is made to a community health nurse to reinforce teaching and maintain therapeutic support for the family. The child's teacher and school nurse are contacted so that they are able to support the child on his return. They can prepare the child's classmates for his return and help them with their feelings of concern for the change in appearances and behavior. These explanations should include some information about the child's inability to engage in contact sports. Rest periods may need to be provided at school, and attendance should be on a part-time basis initially. Although school is fatiguing, it is a normal part of a child's life, and the satisfaction of learning and socializing with friends is important.

Seizures of Childhood and Adolescence

Recurrent Seizures

Recurrent seizure activity is a significant problem in pediatrics. Approximately 3 percent of American children experience one seizure in their early years. The negative connotations of epilepsy have resulted in the preferred use of more specific classifications of intermittent seizure activity experienced by children (see below).

The cause of this erratic electrical activity in the brain may be either idiopathic (cryptogenic) or organic (symptomatic). An idiopathic or cryptogenic cause means that the specific determinant is unknown, while in the case of an organic or symptomatic seizure, the precipitating factors are understood.

Two major categories of seizures are *partial* and *generalized. Partial* or focal seizures are limited to a circumscribed area of the cerebral cortex. *Generalized* seizures result from widespread, diffuse electrical discharges within a central portion of the brain which spread to the cortex and brainstem, thereby affecting other systems of the body. They are bilateral and symmetrical, because both hemispheres are stimulated by these excessive neuronal discharges. An alteration in or loss of consciousness may occur. These types of seizures may or may not have prodromal symptoms.

It is important to obtain as complete a history as possible, especially events surrounding birth (injury, infection, trauma, or metabolic stressors such as hypoglycemia). A child who exhibits any stereotypical behavior or complains of unusual, repeated sensory or motor activity should be suspected of having a neurological dysfunction. A familial seizure history is also significant.

An extensive physical and neurological examination is done. Diagnostic tests frequently include an EEG, CAT scan, skull x-rays, toxicology screening, and blood analyses. An EEG may not demonstrate a seizure unless one is occurring while this test is in progress. By the same token,

TABLE 20-12 Common Seizure Terms

Term	Definition
Aura (prodrome)	There is a peculiar feeling, sound, sight, smell, twitching, or spasm of small muscle groups which precede actual seizure; prodromal symptoms such as headache, irritability, or gastrointestinal upset may also herald onset of a seizure; they can occur several days or immediately prior to the seizure
Ictal period	Since ictal refers to seizure, it is the time during which children experience a wide variety of motor, sensory, and behavioral alterations related to specific seizure type
Postictal period	It is the time following a seizure when children experience alterations in levels of consciousness, are lethargic, or sleep; may be momentary or last for several hours
Interictal period	It is the time between seizures when children may be asymptomatic
Eye movements	Eyes deviate away from hemisphere with hyperexcitable neuronal activity; after a seizure, eyes "look toward" area involved; during a generalized seizure, with both hemispheres involved, eyes deviate upward, "roll back," or remain in midline

an EEG may be grossly abnormal without the child having had a documented seizure.

Grand mal seizures are generalized convulsions and are indicative of disturbance in brain function. The onset is abrupt, although many will have a warning known as an *aura.* Common seizure terms are listed in Table 20-12. The aura is described as peculiar feelings, sights, sounds, tastes, smells, or twitching or spasm of small muscle groups. The tonic phase may occur simultaneously with loss of consciousness and violent muscular contractions. The child falls to the ground, his color becomes pale, the pupils dilate, the conjunctivae are insensitive to touch, the eyes roll upward or to one side, the head is thrown backward or to one side, the abdominal and chest muscles are held rigidly, and the limbs are contracted irregularly or are rigid. As the air is forced out by the sudden contraction of the diaphragm against a closed glottis, a short startling cry may be heard. The tongue may be bitten by the contracting jaw. Involuntary urination and sometimes defecation occur with the contractions of the abdominal muscles. The pallor may change to cyanosis depending on the length and severity of this phase, for respiration is inhibited. The tonic phase may last 20 to 40 seconds or longer. It is followed by the clonic phase, which involves the entire body. There is jerking movement of the extremities and generalized twitching. Consciousness returns slowly during the postictal period.

The child sleeps after the seizure has stopped (postictal

period). On awakening, he appears drowsy and stuporous and accomplishes routine tasks in an automatic fashion. The child may also manifest headache, fever, diaphoresis, and hypertension. Occasionally a child has a seizure during sleep, evidenced by bitten areas in the mouth, blood on the pillow, or a wet bed. He awakens with no recollection or memory of the seizure. When seizures are so frequent that they appear to be constant, the child is said to have *status epilepticus,* a medical emergency which may result in brain damage because of a decreased oxygen supply to the cerebrum.

The most common reason for status epilepticus is noncompliance with anticonvulsant therapy, especially in the child who does not want to be "different" from peers. After a seizure-free period of time, either parents or the adolescent decide the problem is cured and do not adhere to the medication protocol. Some other reasons for this phenomenon are incorrect administration techniques, inadequate therapeutic drug levels, side effects of some drugs, and the failure to renew prescriptions enough in advance. The drugs used most frequently to control seizures are listed in Tables 20-13 and 20-14.

Petit mal seizures, or *absence spells,* are transient losses of consciousness. The patient may exhibit eye-rolling movements, drooping or fluttering of the eyelids, drooping of the head, or slight quivering of the limb and trunk muscles. These seizures develop between 4 and 8 years of age, may be inherited, and frequently disappear with adolescence. They are more common among females. The child who has petit mal seizures is frequently described by parents and teachers as having "dizzy spells," "absences," "lapses," or "daydreaming episodes." If he is in the middle of a task, he drops whatever is in his hand; on completion of the seizure, he immediately resumes the activity without knowledge of ever having stopped. Exposure to blinking lights or hyperventilation may initiate a petit mal seizure.

The seizure usually lasts for 5 to 10 seconds and rarely exceeds 30 seconds. There is no aura or postictal drowsiness. Data are obtained from parents, teachers, or other observers. Most cases resolve spontaneously by the third decade of life, while the remainder progress to recurrent tonic-clonic patterns.

The *ketogenic diet* has been useful in certain instances where drugs have not been successful in the control of seizures. Usually these children are under 5 years of age. Although the precise mechanism is unknown, it is thought that the sustained ketosis affects the seizure threshold. A 3:1 ratio of fat to carbohydrate and protein is utilized to induce ketosis. Hypoglycemia can occur in the first few days after the diet is started. Some children complain of gastrointestinal discomfort after being on this diet, espe-

---

TABLE 20-13 Drugs Commonly Used for Childhood Seizures

Drug	Indication	Side Effects
Carbamazepine (Tegretol)	Tonic-clonic seizures, partial complex	Nausea, vomiting, diplopia, drowsiness, ataxia, aplastic anemia
Clonazepam (Clonopin)	Myoclonic seizures, infantile spasms, petit mal seizures, akinetic seizures	Increased bronchial secretions, ataxia, drowsiness, irritability, nystagmus
Diazepam (Valium)	Minor motor, generalized tonic-clonic, grand mal seizures	Amnesia, drowsiness, ataxia, headache, aplastic anemia, hiccups, dysarthria
Phenobarbital	Generalized tonic-clonic, focal, psychomotor; neonatal seizures	Drowsiness, lethargy, stupor, coma, paradoxical hyperactivity, nystagmus, rash
Phenytoin (Dilantin)	Generalized tonic-clonic, focal, motor, psychomotor seizures	Gingival hyperplasia, nystagmus, ataxia, rash, liver damage, lymphadenopathy, hirsutism, blood dyscrasias
Primidone (Mysoline)	Focal motor, partial complex, minor motor, tonic-clonic seizures	Sedation, vertigo, ataxia, nausea and vomiting, diplopia, nystagmus, personality change, hyperkinesia, rash, macrocytic anemia
Trimethadione (Tridione)	Absence seizures	Ataxia, hiccups, photophobia, blood dyscrasias, kidney damage, personality change, rash, alopecia
Ethosuximide (Zarontin)	Absence, minor motor seizures	Drowsiness, abdominal pain, hiccups, anorexia, irritability, ataxia
Methsuximide (Celontin)	Absence, minor motor seizures	Bone marrow depression, gastrointestinal disturbances, drowsiness
Sodium valproate (Depakene)	Absence, partial complex, minor motor, multiple seizure types	Hepatic dysfunction, blood dyscrasias, central nervous system depression, gastrointestinal disturbances, muscle weakness, hyperactivity
Acetazolamide (Diamox)	Absence seizures	Anorexia, polyuria, paresthesias
Ketogenic diet	Minor motor seizures	Ketosis and acidosis of starvation; restriction in diet of protein and carbohydrate intake, supplying four-fifths of calories in the form of fats; most effective in children between 2 and 5 yr; successful in increasing seizure control, although mechanism is poorly understood

TABLE 20-14 Emergency Anticonvulsant Therapy

Drug	Route	Dosage	Rate	Special Considerations
Diazepam (Valium)	IV*	0.2-0.4 mg/kg	Give 0.03-0.5 mg/kg very slowly; may repeat two times at 10- to 15-min intervals	It is a short-acting drug with more than 50 percent metabolizing in 15 min; child is monitored closely for hypertension and respiratory depression
Phenytoin (Dilantin)	IV	Loading dose of 10 mg/kg	Administer at no greater than 50 mg/min in adolescents, but varies with age	The intravenous line must be flushed with saline before and after administration; it may be used concomitantly with Diazepam
Phenobarbital	IV	Loading dose of 5.0-7.5 mg/kg; then in 5 min, 2.5-3.0 mg/kg	Administer slowly	Emergency equipment should be available because of danger of hypotension after rapid administration; total dose *must not* exceed 20 mg/kg
Paraldehyde	IV	Addition of 4 ml paraldehyde to 100 ml normal saline for a 4% solution	Administer very slowly; up to 0.15 ml/kg may be necessary to control seizure; do not exceed 5 ml per dose	It is administered very slowly IV to avoid a circulatory collapse or pulmonary edema; emergency equipment should be at bedside
	Per rectum	0.15 ml/kg; diluted with a thin oil (peanut, olive) to minimize irritation		This medication should always be drawn up in a well-ventilated room; glass syringes and metal needles are always ued when working with paraldehyde because it reacts with plastic in disposable needles and syringes
	IM*	0.15 mg/kg q 4-6 h		It is extremely irritating to subcutaneous tissues

*IV = intravenously; IM = intramuscularly.

cially nausea and vomiting. The advent of medium-chain triglycerides (MCTs) has resulted in a greater ketogenic effect by providing at least 50 percent of the calories as MCT oil. Since compliance is critical, it is easier to initiate in young children. Parents need to be taught how to test urine for ketones, because it must be monitored closely. They also should be instructed in preparing and weighing foods to ensure that the correct proportions of fat, carbohydrates, protein, and MCT oil are being given to the child.

A *myoclonic seizure* is a common form of recurrent activity, prevalent in school-age children and adolescents, usually occurring after rising or going to sleep. Symptoms vary. These contractions may be mild or severe, occur singularly or with other seizures, and result in a loss of consciousness. They can lead to tonic-clonic seizure activity: Children are taught to identify the beginning of the seizure pattern to prevent injury.

Partial seizures can occur with elementary or complex symptomatology. With elementary partial seizures, consciousness is not altered; however, there may be a number of motor, sensory, autonomic, or combined symptoms related to the cortical area stimulated. Motor activities include localized or focal jerking motions. When

there is a progression of seizure activity with additional muscle groups becoming involved, other classification systems refer to it as a *Jacksonian march seizure.*

Focal or *Jacksonian seizures* are sensory or motor, depending on the location of disturbed neural discharges. Occasionally Jacksonian seizures have been identified in the absence of organic lesions, but they are primarily indicative of a CNS lesion. Focal seizures are preceded by a brief tonic phase; however, they are clonic in nature. They begin in one muscle group and proceed to other muscle groups in a fixed manner (e.g., finger to wrist to hand to arm to face and then to the leg of the same side). When the attacks are brief, there is no loss of consciousness, but if the spread is rapid and extensive, consciousness is lost, and it is followed by a generalized convulsion that is indistinguishable from a grand mal seizure. Other motor symptoms include a sharp turning of the head and eyes.

Nursing Management

The attitude of society as a whole is not supportive to the family that has a child with seizures. The term *epilepsy* has a stigma attached to it ("fits"). Throughout history people with epilepsy have been branded as "outcasts," "feebleminded," "beseeched with evil spirits," "witches" or "insane." Even today some of these attitudes prevail. Many children with seizures have been considered mentally retarded, although mental retardation is not found with this disease unless there are organic lesions or it results from status epilepticus.

The nurse must be cognizant of the fact that initially the parents often have the same misconceptions about the child's diagnosis. The nurse can help by teaching the family about the seizure type and about the specific needs of the child.

The parents must understand the purpose of the child's medication and be taught to observe for signs of toxicity and evidence that the dosage may need alteration. They should be instructed always to have the drug available, including on trips and vacations. The medication should be stored in a safe place, away from children who may accidentally ingest it. If the child must take the medication at school, an extra supply is often maintained by the school nurse or teacher who supervises its administration. If the school cannot support the child in this manner, only the exact dose of medication should be sent to school with him. The child must be taught that his medication is important to him but dangerous to other children.

A young child and family must be aware of safety factors. If frequent grand mal seizures occur, it may be necessary for the child to wear a football helmet at all times to prevent a head injury. Wearing a helmet can and usually does create social difficulties, and it should be utilized only when absolutely necessary. The child is not allowed to participate in activities that would be hazardous, such as swimming and horseback riding, unless accompanied by a responsible person. Children with seizures should wear Medic-Alert bracelets with all necessary information, such as diagnosis and drug regimen, so that appropriate assistance may be offered should they have seizures when they are not with their families or close friends.

The nurse can assist the child to develop a healthy self-concept. Children with seizures are frequently described as having personality disorders such as egocentricity, shallowness, religiosity, and chronic negativism. These personality disorders can be prevented if the parents accept the child. Care must be taken to discipline, to set limits, and to love. Some children may use their seizures to "control" their parents, and thus a circular effect of manipulation between the child and parents develops.

As adolescence approaches, the child may act out, much like the diabetic adolescent. He may stop taking his medication, engage in activities that have been forbidden, and subject himself to undue stress. This type of behavior causes parents great concern, but the understanding parent recognizes this behavior as essentially normal, allows for the testing, and supports the adolescent in the final resolution of acceptance.

Legal ramifications for adolescents with recurrent seizures have changed dramatically in the last 20 years as a result of improved seizure control, a more knowledgeable public, greater advocacy, and, in some instances, court

challenges. Adolescents who are seizure-free for varying periods of time can obtain driver's licenses. Getting insurance can be a problem, and when it is obtained, these adolescents are usually placed in assigned-risk categories.

Employment opportunities have improved. Many states have policies which encourage the employment of individuals with such a handicap, and more important, an employer's insurance rating is not altered if a seizure-related accident occurs. Adolescents who are well controlled may usually pursue any career except public transportation. The armed forces, however, still refuse these applicants, even those whose seizures are well controlled. Many special workshops are available, and they facilitate job training while considering an adolescent's health limitations.

Schooling and appropriate counseling are essential components in maximizing the potential of children and adolescents with seizure disorders. They can attend college and enroll in various vocational programs which enable them to seek employment in their areas of interest.

Adolescents need counseling about marriage and pregnancy also. If the seizure disorder is familial, specific information is imperative. Two people with seizure disorders are at a greater risk of having a child with a similar problem or with a number of congenital malformations.

Neurological Disorders in the Adolescent
Spinal Cord Injury
Spinal cord injury occurs when there is compression or destruction of the cord. Approximately 3 per 100,000 individuals are affected yearly in the United States, with males involved five times as often as females. Urban families experience significantly higher percentages of these types of injuries from major trauma. The peak ages among pediatric clients are those in middle and late adolescence. Accidents are the most common cause of spinal cord injury among children, and diving, boating, snowmobiling, skiing, surfing, and automobile accidents are frequent causes of trauma. Bullet wounds also are responsible for some cord injuries. Caring for these patients requires astute long-term management because of the acute and devastating nature of injuries which dramatically alter family life.

Compression is the most common cause of cord damage. Subluxation, crushed laminas, and dislocated fractures are most frequently responsible for pressure on the spinal cord, which results in the reduction of ascending and descending nerve transmission. Return of function below the level of injury may occur if there is prompt relief of the compression. The outcomes of a *cord contusion* include demyelination, degeneration, and necrosis of cord tissue, while a *cord laceration* causes a transection of nerve tracts and loss of function. *Cervical flexion fractures* occur from occipital blows, while *cervical extension injuries* result from facial blows or damage to the anterior longitudinal spinal ligaments, causing vertebral instability and cord pressure. In addition, fractures of the lower spine, most frequently T12, L1, and L2, sustained in falls can affect the spinal cord. Since the spinal cord is housed in a relatively small bony area without an extensive blood supply or a well-developed collateral circulation, minimum edema or hemorrhage compresses the cord.

A complete or partial severance of the cord is less frequently seen than is compression. Hence, an initial assessment of the injury, especially whether paralysis was immediate or slowly progressive, is critical. The prognosis is far better in a gradual paralysis than in one that is immediate and total. The degree of return depends on the severity of damage from compression and the rapidity with which the pressure was removed. When the cord is partially or completely severed, return of function is not possible.

The clinical manifestations of a spinal cord injury depend on the location, the extent, and the specific nature of the insult. The degree of paralysis is determined by the level of injury. When it is high, involving the 3d and 4th cervical vertebrae (C3 and C4), there is paralysis of both the intercostal muscles and the diaphragm, affecting respirations. At lower levels (C5 and C6) there is paralysis of all extremities and of the abdominal muscles. In either instance there is loss of voluntary motor function and bowel and bladder control.

Injury to thoracic vertebrae results in a paralysis of the lower extremities, abdominal muscles, bladder, and rectum. At first the paralysis is flaccid, but later it becomes spastic.

In the lumbar region, an injury affects the cauda equina, conus medullaris, and possibly segments of the lower cord. As a result, there are flaccid paralyses of the lower extremities and rectal muscles and an atonic bladder.

The emergency care of a patient with a suspected spinal cord injury requires an immediate evaluation of respiratory status and immobilization of the spine with sandbags, tape, a door, or other special devices. A cervical collar is not recommended because it may act as a tourniquet, hiding an expanding cervical hematoma, and in addition is an inadequate stabilizer. If the accident is water-related, allowing the child to float may be a lifesaving measure, especially since untrained individuals unknowingly may cause severe cord damage as they drag the adolescent out of the water. Should the patient vomit, the neck must be stabilized as the patient is log-rolled to the side with extreme caution. Any transferring activities *must* be performed utilizing a transport board and four individuals who move the patient as a unit. A person suspected of having a spinal cord injury should not be allowed to walk, sit, or have anything placed under the occipital area.

In the emergency room, a careful initial assessment includes a general physical and an extensive neurological examination. Periodic rectal examinations are performed because the lack of sphincter control may indicate a complete spinal cord insult or conversion from a partial to a complete cord injury.

Baseline laboratory data are compiled, and peripheral

intravenous therapy is started. A Foley catheter and nasogastric tube are inserted. Emergency skull, cervical, and spinal x-rays are done. A CAT scan and myelogram may also be performed. A lumbar puncture may be done if hemorrhage or blockage of CSF is suspected. Prophylactic antibiotics, steroids, and antacids are administered. Mannitol may be given to improve spinal cord perfusion.

Systemic shock is demonstrated soon after the injury is experienced. The suddenness of the loss of function requires the body to initiate massive compensatory actions, and the lack of movement and muscle support to the vascular system creates a variety of circulatory difficulties. An increase in the pulse and respirations with a decrease in blood pressure and a loss in temperature control in the involved area are noted. The shock response is intensified when the respiratory area is affected by the insult.

Sacral sparing is seen frequently in incomplete cord injuries where the perineal and anal areas respond to painful stimuli such as a pinprick. This phenomenon occurs because of damage to the central cord with the lateral sensory tracts remaining intact, and it is a positive prognostic sign for the return of some sensation to the lower extremities.

Spinal shock, resulting from a sudden injury to the cord, is an acute loss of motor, sensory, autonomic, and reflex activity below the level of the insult. It may persist for weeks or months and causes a disturbance of the reflex arc which leads to flaccid paralysis. As the reflex arc

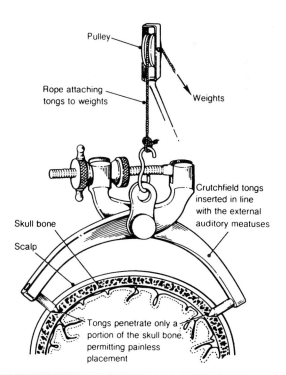

FIGURE 20-18 Cervical traction is attached to tongs inserted into the skull. *(A.E. Hinkhouse and N.A. Kirby, "Traumatic Disturbances in Perception and Coordination," in D.A. Jones et al. [eds.], Medical-Surgical Nursing: A Conceptual Approach, 2d ed., McGraw-Hill, New York, 1982, p. 1267.)*

FIGURE 20-19 Stryker turning frame comes with anterior and posterior frames. Once placed on the frame, a patient may be turned from abdomen to back to abdomen. Cervical traction may be applied. *(Courtesy of Stryker Corporation, Kalamazoo, Mich.)*

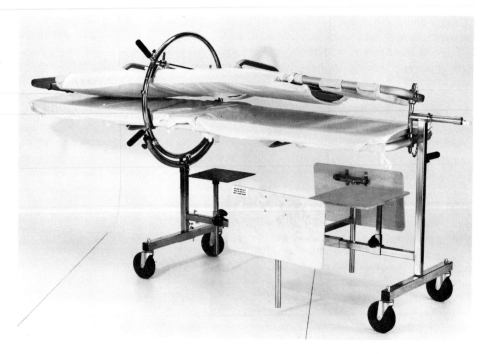

FIGURE 20-20 Circo-Electric bed provides a wide variety of potential positions. Turning is done as slowly as necessary to avoid vertigo. *(Courtesy of Stryker Corporation, Kalamazoo, Mich.)*

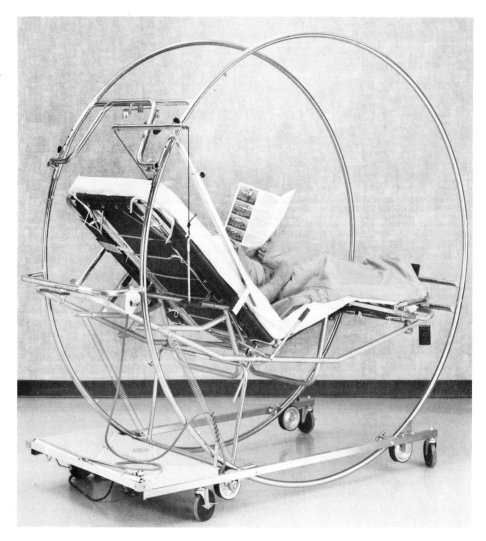

becomes adjusted to its current state or as the pressure is removed, paralysis becomes spastic. The reflex arc, once reactivated, has a tendency to become overactive, and subsequent spasticity becomes a serious problem for the adolescent.

Skeletal traction is applied frequently to (1) prevent damage from unstable bone fragments and (2) realign and promote healing of the vertebrae and spinal cord ligaments. Some methods of immobilization include bed rest, turning frames (Stryker, Foster), a Circo-Electric bed, traction, and braces (Figs. 20-18 to 20-20).

Currently, Gardner-Wells or Heifetz tongs are used for dislocations of C1 to T1 because of ease in insertion. The temporal area just above and in front of the ears is prepared by shaving the hair, applying an antiseptic, and anesthetizing the area. The neurosurgeon then inserts the tongs and applies necessary weights. The amount of weight is related to that needed to overcome muscle spasm and maintain adequate alignment, which is confirmed by x-ray. Elevating the head of the bed on shock blocks provides countertraction. Stabilization of the spine usually occurs in 2 to 6 weeks. Complications of cervical traction may include overreduction of the injury with an increase in neurological deficit, dislodgement of vertebrae, and cranial erosion from the tongs with perforation of the dura.

Following the removal of cervical traction, immobilization is continued with the use of various braces, such as the Halo or the Peterson, or a plastic body shell, casts, or jackets (Chap. 22) for 3 to 6 months. Surgical intervention also may be necessary to stabilize the vertebral column further.

A *surgical fusion* is the removal of bone or bone chips from one part of the body such as the iliac crest and grafting them onto selected vertebrae. After the graft has "taken," immobilization, increased stability of the spinal column, and loss of movement within the surgical area are accomplished. A *posterior fusion* is performed most frequently, with direct access obtained through an incision in the adolescent's back. Following a spinal fusion, the patient is fitted for a body brace or shell, which is worn for 6 more weeks. The degree of participation and the types of activities permitted afterward vary. There are certain types of *internal fixation* devices utilized for unstable thoracic or lumbar vertebrae, including Harrington rods or instrumentation, which provide excellent immobilization (Chap. 22).

As a result of such an injury, the adolescent is susceptible to a wide range of problems stemming from severe neuromuscular and cardiovascular alterations. *Autonomic hyperreflexia,* a pathological condition which occurs only in high cervical or thoracic insults, results from a severely altered response to stress stimuli such as bowel or bladder distention. Stimulation of the autonomic nervous system results in acute vascular constriction *below* the level of injury with marked hypertension, while *above* the level of injury there is marked vasodilatation with bradycardia. Treatment involves elevating the head of the bed, reliev-

ing the stressor (which may be, for example, a clogged Foley catheter), notifying the physician, monitoring vital signs, and administering diazoxide (Hyperstat) or sodium nitroprusside (Nipride) for the acute episode. Recurrent episodes are managed with alpha-adrenergic blockers such as phenoxybenzamine (Dibenzyline) at bedtime. If the condition is resistant to treatment, a cordotomy may be necessary; however, it may reduce the potential for successful bowel and bladder retraining.

Deep venous thrombosis related to immobility also may develop. Its symptoms include swelling, erythema, and increased warmth as well as an elevated pulse and temperature. Also, pulmonary emboli may occur. Treatment includes intravenous heparin therapy and oral anticoagulants.

Pain may become a chronic problem after a spinal cord injury. Phantom limb pain, which the adolescent describes as a burning or tingling, can occur. Causalgia-like pain, described as a sharp, shooting pain, develops in incomplete insults to the cauda equina. Severing the spinothalamic tract is done as a palliative procedure in chronic cases.

Nursing Management

Upon arrival in the emergency room, the adolescent must be evaluated immediately for the degree of shock and neurological function. Intravenous fluids are started to establish a route for emergency medications, and vital signs and neurological status are monitored every 15 to 30 minutes. Arterial blood gases are sampled and evaluated as necessary. Since cervical involvement inhibits respiratory function, respiratory assistance may be necessary in the form of an endotracheal tube, tracheostomy, or mechanical respirator. Although a patient is encouraged to cough and breathe deeply, suctioning may be necessary. It is important for a nurse to evaluate the patient's pulmonary status frequently because the development of pneumonia can be potentially life-threatening.

Respiratory care for the child or adolescent with quadriplegia is likely to be managed with a tracheostomy. This opening allows for easier clearing of secretions and is preferred to long-term respirator dependence. Vital capacity will be reduced greatly even in lower lesions (below C4). Intermittent positive pressure breathing treatments, percussion and vibration, and breathing exercises may be a part of the respiratory regimen.

Vital signs are taken on a regular basis, with careful attention given to temperature and blood pressure. Temperature elevation may indicate a need for environmental change (clothes, blankets, room temperature) or may indicate a respiratory or urinary tract infection. Prompt action is required if hypertension is due to the development of autonomic dysreflexia.

Skin integrity is maintained by diligently adhering to a turning schedule, using an alternating-pressure mattress or other device, and carefully checking for signs of pressure. Bony prominences are especially susceptible to skin breakdown. Keeping the skin clean and dry is also impor-

TABLE 20-15 Assessment Guide to Determine Approximate Level of Spinal Cord Lesion

Cord Level Associated with Motion	Movement to Be Requested of the Patient	Body Part to Be Observed	Cord Level Associated with Sensation in Each Listed Body Part*
S2-S4	Tighten the muscle around my finger (finger in anal sphincter)	Perineum	S5
L5, S1, and S2	Bend and straighten your toes	Toes	L5
L2-L4	Straighten your leg	Knees	L3
L1-L3	Bend (flex) your hip	Hips	L2
T5-T12	Tighten your abdomen	Abdomen	
		Pubis	L1
		Navel	T10
		Nipple line	T4
C8-T1	Appose your thumb to each fingertip; make a fist	Thumb, first two digits, little finger	C6
			C7
			T1
C6	Bend your wrist up (only the radial wrist extensor will contract)	Wrist	C6 (thumb side of wrist)
C5	Bend your elbow	Elbow	Radial side C6 Ulnar side T1
C3, C4, and C5	Shrug your shoulders; take a deep breath (diaphragm descends causing abdomen to bulge; upper chest does not move)	Shoulder, chest, and abdomen	C4

*Light touch, pinprick, position.

Source: A. E. Hinkhouse and N. A. Kirby, "Traumatic Disturbances in Perception and Coordination," in D. A. Jones et al. (eds.), *Medical-Surgical Nursing: A Conceptual Approach,* 2d ed., McGraw-Hill, New York, 1982, p. 1140.

tant. Since cervical tongs (Fig. 20-18) are in place, the entry sites need special care at least once every 24 hours; that is, cleansing the areas, examining sites for inflammation and/or infection, and applying an antibiotic ointment such as Betadine.

Physical therapy provided by therapists and the nursing staff involves maintainence of good body alignment using splints, footboards, and boots as necessary. Passive and active range of motion exercises aimed at maintaining or increasing strength in intact musculature and preventing contractures must be carried out on a regular basis. In Table 20-15 a guide to approximate levels of sensory and motor function is provided.

Neurogenic bladder and bowel problems require careful assessment and ongoing monitoring. A Foley catheter will initially be inserted to prevent urinary retention and monitor output. However, a bladder training and intermittent catheterization program will begin early in the convalescent period. Maintaining an acidic urine will decrease the potential for infection and stone formation. The goal of bowel training is to prevent constipation and accidents through the development of a regular evacuation time. A diet high in fiber, the use of suppositories, and the selection of a feasible time based on other activities form the basis of the program.

Rehabilitation efforts begin early, and an interdisciplinary team approach is utilized. Nurses, physicians, physical therapists, vocational and occupational therapists, and sexual counselors are among the providers involved in potentiating the adolescent's recovery. Since the physiological and psychosocial implications of such an injury are complex, rehabilitation usually occurs at a highly specialized center which is adapted to meet the specific and total needs of this particular population. Through the use of myriad mechanical devices, braces, and electronic wheelchairs, an adolescent with a spinal cord injury can be taught to maximize whatever function is present.

This type of injury is devastating, especially when one considers the age of most patients. It is important to be objective in providing care. While it is easy to be overly empathetic or oversolicitous to the spine-injured adolescent, feeling sorry for the patient does not help; in fact, it hinders his progress. Rehabilitation is a most rigorous, demanding, long-term effort. Therefore, the nurse's great challenge is to assist and encourage the adolescent in making those difficult, small strides which ultimately result in optimum rehabilitation.

Independent Study Activities

1. Observe two healthy children and then observe two children with cerebral palsy. Compare and contrast the different positions and activities in which both sets of children participate.
2. Arrange for a group visit to a rehabilitation facility. Identify the role of the nurse, other health care providers, and the client and family in the rehabilitative process.
3. Perform a community assessment on the utilization of lead by both homeowners and industries in a selected area. Identify the established environmental safeguards and improvements which could be made.

   What is the incidence of lead poisoning in this community?

   What is the projected rate of undetected cases?

   What are the specific roles of the health department and of other health care providers in identifying, preventing, and treating this serious health problem?
4. Carry out a discussion and education session with a class of sixth- to ninth-graders to determine and enhance their understanding of seizures.

Study Questions

1. For children up to 6 years of age, the most effective standardized method of testing cerebral, motor, and cerebellar function is the:
   A. Boyd Developmental Progress Scale.
   B. Developmental Attainment Form.
   C. Denver Developmental Screening Test.
   D. Guide to Normal Milestones of Development.
2. When the outer aspect of the sole of the foot is stroked with a fingernail, starting at the sole and moving to the small toe and then across to the great toe, the nurse is attempting to elicit the:
   A. Gordon's reflex.
   B. Chaddock reflex.
   C. Babinski reflex.
   D. Oppenheim reflex.
3. The rapidity and severity of the symptoms of increased intracranial pressure are slowest to appear in the child under the age of:
   A. 9 months.   C. 36 months.
   B. 18 months.   D. 48 months.
4. When a 2-year-old newly admitted for head trauma becomes very restless and irritable, the nurse concludes that these behavioral changes are due to the:
   A. Pain being experienced.
   B. Increased intracranial pressure.
   C. Separation from his parents.
   D. Strange hospital environment.
5. In children, the major cause of increased intracranial pressure is:
   A. Inadequate cerebral perfusion.
   B. Herniated cerebellum.
   C. Cerebral edema.
   D. Severe hypertension.
6. An inappropriate nursing intervention for a comatose child is:
   A. Frequent positioning.
   B. Range of motion exercises.
   C. Diligent mouth care.
   D. Decreased fluid intake.
7. An activity which must be included in a teaching plan for the parents of an infant who has had a shunting procedure for hydrocephaly is:
   A. Taking the temperature every day.
   B. Doing a dipstick test once a day.
   C. Monitoring the fluid intake.
   D. Palpating the anterior fontanel.
8. After a meningomyelocele has been repaired, it is critical for the nurse to:
   A. Monitor bowel and bladder patterns.
   B. Limit movement of the lower extremities.
   C. Assess for neurological deficit.
   D. Measure head circumference.
9. In doing a physical assessment on an infant with cerebral palsy, a common finding is:
   A. The presence of a congenital hip.
   B. An asymmetrical Landau.
   C. Bauer's response.
   D. Scissoring of the lower extremities.
10. When a nurse observes serosanguineous drainage from the nose of a child with a basilar skull fracture, the drainage needs to be tested immediately for:
    A. Glucose.   C. Sodium.
    B. Potassium.   D. Copper.
11. The principal function of administering Ca EDTA to a toddler with chronic lead poisoning is to remove the lead from the:
    A. Renal tubule.   C. Bones.
    B. Brain.   D. Soft tissues.
12. A unique characteristic of Guillain-Barré syndrome is its:
    A. Rapid onset.
    B. Hyperreflexus.
    C. Ascending paralysis.
    D. Hypertonicity.
13. A common complaint from a child with a brain tumor is a headache, which is most severe:
    A. After vigorous play.
    B. While doing close work.
    C. On getting up in the morning.
    D. On falling asleep at night.
14. The volume of intravenous fluids given after a craniotomy is usually two-thirds to three-quarters of a child's maintenance in an effort to:
    A. Increase renal perfusion.
    B. Compensate for the large urinary output.

C. Maintain a specific gravity of 1.020 to 1.030.

D. Decrease the development of cerebral edema.

15. In seizure terminology, the ictal period refers to the time:

A. Between seizures.   C. Of the seizure.

B. Following a seizure.   D. Before a seizure.

References

American Academy of Pediatrics, Committee on Environmental Hazards: "Statement on Childhood Lead Poisoning," *Pediatrics,* 79:457-465, 1987.

Behrman, R.E., and V.C. Vaughan (eds.): *Nelson Textbook of Pediatrics,* 12th ed., Saunders, Philadelphia, 1983.

Brown, M.S.: "How to Tell If a Baby Has Cerebral Palsy. . . And What to Tell His Parents When He Does," *Nursing '79,* May 1979, pp. 88-91.

Centers for Disease Control: *Preventing Lead Poisoning in Young Children,* U.S. Department of Health and Human Services, Atlanta, 1985.

Chisolm, J.J.: "Lead Poisoning," in A.M. Rudolph and J.I.E. Hoffman (eds), *Pediatrics,* 18th ed., Appleton-Lange, Norwalk, Conn., 1987.

Gaddy, D.S.: "Meningitis in the Pediatric Population," *Nursing Clinics of North America,* 15(1):83-97, 1980.

Govoni, L.E., and J.E. Hayes: *Drugs and Nursing Implications,* 4th ed., Appleton-Century-Crofts, New York, 1985.

Grundy, J.H.: "The Pediatric Physical Examination," in R.A. Hoekelman, et al. (eds.), *Principles of Health Care of the Young,* McGraw-Hill, New York, 1978.

Kelly, P.P., and C. Tinsley: "Planning Care for the Patient Receiving External Radiation," *American Journal of Nursing,* 81(2):338-341, 1981.

Luckmann, J., and K.C. Sorenson: *Medical Surgical Nursing,* 2d ed., Saunders, Philadelphia, 1980.

Powell, M.L.: *Assessment and Management of Developmental Changes and Problems in Children,* 2d ed., Mosby, St. Louis, 1981, pp. 169-182.

Tudor, M.: "Developmental Screening," *Issues in Comprehensive Pediatric Nursing,* 2:1-13, 1977.

Wing, S.: "Brain Abscess," *Journal of Neurosurgical Nursing,* 13(3):123-126, 1981.

Bibliography

Castiglia, P.T., and M.A. Petrini: "Selecting a Developmental Screening Tool," *Pediatric Nursing,* 11(1):8-17, 1985.

Dalgas, P.: "Reye's Syndrome Update," *MCN: American Journal of Maternal Child Nursing,* 8(5):345-349, 1983.

Griffiths, S.S.: "Changes in Body Image Caused by Antineoplastic Drugs," *Issues in Comprehensive Pediatric Nursing,* 4(1):17-27, 1980.

Jackson, P.L.: "When the Baby Isn't Perfect," *American Journal of Nursing,* 85(4):296-299, 1985.

Kempe, C.H., et al. (eds): *Current Pediatric Diagnosis and Treatment,* 9th ed., Appleton-Lange, Norwalk, Conn., 1987.

Killam, P.K., et al.: "Behavioral Pediatric Weight Rehabilitation for Children with Myelomeningocele," *MCN: American Journal of Maternal Child Nursing,* 8(4):280-286, 1983.

Klopovich, P.D., D. Suenram, and N. Cairnes: "A Common Sense Approach to Caring for Children with Cancer: The Community Health Nurse," *Cancer Nurse,* 3(3):201-208, 1980.

Kosowski, M.M., and D.L. Sopczyk: "Feeding Hospitalized Children with Developmental Disabilities," *MCN: American Journal of Maternal Child Nursing,* 10(3):190-194, 1985.

Macedo, A., and L.F. Posel: "Nursing the Family after the Birth of a Child with Spina Bifida," *Issues in Comprehensive Pediatric Nursing,* 10(1):55-65, 1987.

Maul, S.K.: "Childhood Brain Tumors: A Special Nursing Challenge," *MCN: American Journal of Maternal Child Nursing,* 9(2):123-131, 1984.

McGrath, D.M.: "Video Recording Seizure Activity in Children," *MCN: American Journal of Maternal Child Nursing,* 8(3):218-220, 1983.

Morray, J.P.: *Pediatric Intensive Care,* Appleton-Lange, Norwalk, Conn., 1987.

Parrish, M.A.: "A Comparison of Behavioral Side Effects Related to Commonly Used Anticonvulsants," *Pediatric Nursing,* 10(2):149-152, 1984.

Pellock, J.M., and E.C. Meyer: *Neurologic Emergencies in Infancy and Childhood,* Harper & Row, Philadelphia, 1984.

Percy, A.K., and P.O. Percy: "Acute Management of Seizures in Children," *Nurse Practitioner,* 11(2):15-28, 1986.

Reilly, A.N., et al.: "Head Trauma in Children: The Stages to Cognitive Recovery," *MCN: American Journal of Maternal Child Nursing,* 12(6):405-412, 1987.

Richardson, K., et al.: "Biofeedback Therapy for Managing Bowel Incontinence Caused by Myelomeningocele," *MCN: American Journal of Maternal Child Nursing,* 10(6):388-393, 1985.

Steele, S.: "Young Children with Cerebral Palsy: Practical Guidelines for Care," *Pediatric Nursing,* 11(4):259-267, 1985.

Strauss, S.S., and M. Munton: "Common Concerns of Parents with Disabled Children," *Pediatric Nursing,* 11(5):371-375, 1985.

Sullivan-Bolyai, S., et al.: "Toilet Training the Child with Neurogenic Impairment of Bowel and Bladder Function," *Issues in Comprehensive Pediatric Nursing,* 7(1):33-43, 1984.

Tse, A.M.: "Seizures and Societal Attitudes: A Teaching Tool for Children, Siblings, Classmates, Parents, and Classroom Teachers," *Issues in Comprehensive Pediatric Nursing,* 9(5):299-303, 1986.

21

The Special Senses

Objectives

After reading this chapter, the student will be able to:
1. Describe the functions of the special senses.
2. Identify the basic subjective and objective data to be obtained in assessing a child's special senses.
3. Understand the purpose of diagnostic tests and medical treatment.
4. Describe general nursing measures appropriate for pediatric clients who have problems involving the special senses.
5. Delineate specific nursing interventions appropriate for pediatric clients who have problems involving the special senses.

Anatomy and Physiology

Eye

The cornea is the transparent structure of the eye composed mainly of stroma, with regularly arranged epithelium on the outer surface and a single layer of endothelial cells lining the inner surface (Fig. 21-1). The anterior portion of the cornea is bathed in tears, and the posterior part is bathed with aqueous humor. The lens maintains a high intracellular potassium content and is bathed in a solution of relatively high sodium content. The aqueous humor contributes to maintenance of intraocular pressure, supports lens metabolism, and is partly responsible for nu-

443

FIGURE 21-1 *Anatomy of the eye. (From G.M. Scipien et al. [eds.], Comprehensive Pediatric Nursing, 3d ed., McGraw-Hill, New York, 1986, p. 1367.)*

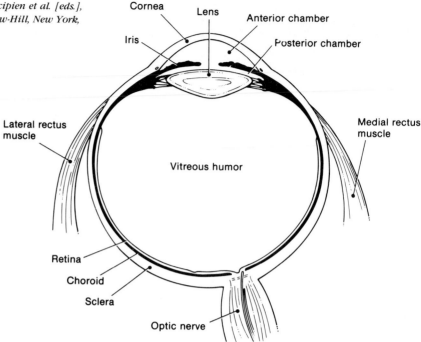

trition of the cornea. Tears, formed by accessory lacrimal glands along the lid margin and conjunctival fornices, are distributed over the eyeball by periodic involuntary blinking, which also causes a pumping action in the lacrimal drainage system. Tears are secreted in response to psychic stimuli and reflex stimuli.

The metabolism of the retina may be divided into a general metabolism required for cell integrity and a specialized metabolism related to photoreception and nerve impulse transmission. The general metabolism of the retina depends on a continuous supply of glucose from the bloodstream. Interruption in blood supply for 6 minutes results in irreversible retinal degeneration.

Some structures of the eye form an optical system which focuses the light rays from outside objects to form sharp images within the eye. Other structures react to light rays that compose the images and give rise to nerve impulses which result in various sensations of form, contrast, and color.

Photochemistry

Electromagnetic energy must be absorbed to exert an effect. To initiate a chemical change, that portion of the electromagnetic field known as light must be absorbed by the pigment molecule of the disks in the intersegment of the rods and cones. The chemical change gives rise to a nervous impulse that is amplified in the retina and relayed to the brain, where perception occurs.

The electromagnetic spectrum (EMS) contains many wavelengths that are reflected, absorbed, or transmitted. The portion of the EMS with wavelengths between 400 and 700 nm is visible light and passes through the cornea and lens. It is absorbed by the photosensitive pigment in

the rods and cones and initiates the chemical change that sets off the nerve impulse, which in turn is transmitted to the brain and causes subjective sensation.

The radiant energy of visible light is not colored. Color sensation is caused by absorption of energy by the photosensitive visual pigments of the retina, of which there are three types responding to red, green, and blue. The color perceived depends on the wavelength absorbed. Color blindness is believed to occur as a result of a deficiency or abnormality in the photosensitive pigments.

Neural Activity

The formation of minute images by the rods and cones of the retina is not conveyed to the brain by the optic nerve as a neat colored picture. Each ganglion cell receives its input from many receptors, but not all connections to the retina cause excitement. If this response were the case, vision would be blurred. By means of a complex code, the rate of firing of the ganglion cell is increased or decreased. Although the nature of the integration of neural activity of the human retina is unknown, experiments on lower animals suggest that the retina carries on a complex filtering of information before passing it on to the brain.

Refraction

When a ray of light passes through one transparent medium to another, its velocity increases if the medium through which it is passed is less dense; the velocity decreases in a more dense medium. If the medium is not perpendicular to the ray of light, the emerging ray has a different direction from that of the entering ray. This change in direction is called *refraction* and is measured in focal length or diopters. The refractive surfaces of the eye are the cornea, the aqueous humor, and the lens. The anterior cornea is the chief refracting surface because it separates media of such different optical density as air and corneal substances. The lens at its anterior and posterior surfaces is convex, but because it is immersed in liquid on both sides, it has less refractive power than does the cornea. Optically the lens behaves as if it were composed of a series of concentric lenses so that its total refractory index is greater than that of the individual portion of the lens. Errors in refraction occur when there is a failure of refractory power of the anterior segment to correlate with the length of the segment. Two factors are involved: (1) the refractory power of cornea and lens and (2) the length of the eye. Most persons have good correlations so that parallel rays of light fall on the retina.

Accommodation

The process by which the refractory power of the anterior segments increases in order that distant and near objects can be distinctively focused on the retina is termed *accommodation.* It is stimulated by a blurred image on the retina which gives rise to active contraction of the ciliary muscle, resulting in relaxation of the zonule, in turn freeing the lens from compression force. The elasticity of the lens capsule allows the lens to assume the shape of a sphere. The lens, which is soft and pliable in youth, becomes harder and less compressible with age; the capsule becomes less elastic. The result is less of a change in shape and therefore a gradual loss of accommodation. The lens itself continues to grow throughout life and does not shed any of its cells; therefore, its central portion becomes more compact and closed. There is a tendency toward myopia and eventual opacity. With age there is also increased weakness of the ciliary muscle. All these factors result in decreased accommodation.

Ear

The eustachian tube in the middle ear has three major functions. It protects the middle ear from nasopharyngeal secretions, serves as a pathway for drainage of middle ear secretions in to the nasopharynx, and provides ventilation of the middle ear in order to equalize middle ear air pressure with atmospheric pressure (Fig. 21-2). It protects the eardrum from being forced inward or outward when outside pressures increase or decrease, as happens with changes in altitude when flying.

The two muscles of the middle ear, the stapedius and the tensor tympani, have two opposing functions: (1) to increase the sensitivity of the eardrum and the ossicular chain to signals of weak intensity and (2) to mediate the action of the ossicular chain when the eardrum receives an unusually intense stimulation. The latter aspect is important because of the protection it affords the inner ear.

The *round window,* another connection between the middle and inner ears, is just below the *oval window.* It is covered with an elastic membrane and serves as a termination of the acoustic pathway of the inner ear. Both of these windows communicate with different parts of the inner ear. The inner ear is both the end organ for hearing and the sensory organ for balance.

Physiology of Hearing

Air Conduction

The majority of the sounds heard are airborne because air conduction is much more sensitive than the mechanism of bone conduction. Sound waves in the environment are picked up by the pinna of the external ear and then directed into the external acoustic meatus, where the sound waves exert a force on the eardrum. It in turn is set into vibration by the movements of the air particles. The handle of the malleus embedded in the eardrum sets the os-

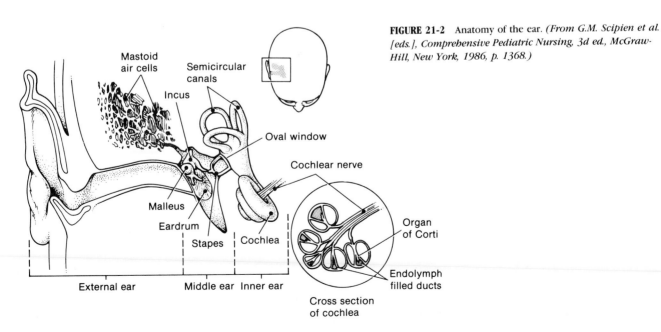

FIGURE 21-2   Anatomy of the ear. *(From G.M. Scipien et al. [eds.], Comprehensive Pediatric Nursing, 3d ed., McGraw-Hill, New York, 1986, p. 1368.)*

sicular chain into vibration. The in-and-out vibration of the eardrum results in a rocking motion of the stapes in the oval window which produces a pressure wave in the perilymph. The ossicular chain transforms the energy collected by the eardrum into a greater force but with less movement, thus matching the impedance of the sound waves in the ear to that in the fluid in the vestibule. The inward movement of the footplate of the stapes produces pressure on the fluid of the inner ear, which is incompressible, necessitating some provision for relief of the pressure. It is accomplished by the round window, whose membrane reacts to the movements of the footplate in the stapes of the oval window. As the footplate pushes inward on the oval window toward the inner ear, the membrane of the round window is pushed outward toward the middle ear cavity. The fluid motion from the oval window to the round window is transmitted through the cochlear duct, causing movement of the endolymph within it and also movement of the basilar membrane where the hair cells of the organ of Corti are located. the movement of the membrane results in its displacement, which in turn causes a shearing effect on the hair cells by the tectorial membrane above. The nerve impulse is thus initiated, is carried by the nerve fibers to the main trunk of the acoustic portion of the VIIIth cranial nerve, and finally is received by the brain.

Bone Conduction

The inner ear is encased in bone so that vibrations of the bone are transmitted directly to the inner ear, causing movement of the fluid. It is not necessary to produce vi-

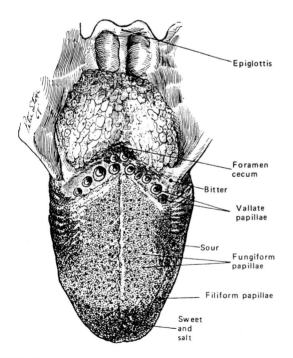

FIGURE 21-3 The dorsum of the tongue with primary taste buds. *(From L.L. Langley, I.R. Telford, and J.B. Christensen [eds.], Dynamic Anatomy and Physiology, 5th ed., McGraw-Hill, New York, 1980, p. 349.*

bration of the drum or ossicles. Bone conduction requires vibrations intense enough to set the bones of the skull in vibration. The sound waves must go through skin, soft tissue, and bones so that the wave often is distorted. However, the mechanism of bone conduction provides an alternative pathway for sound in people who have impairment of air conduction.

Gustatory and Olfactory Organs

Taste and smell have some effect on the appetite, the beginning of digestion, and the avoidance of harmful substances. *Gustation,* or the act of tasting, is present at birth, and salivation begins at about 3 months of age. Four primary sensations which are generally agreed on are sour, salty, sweet, and bitter. Acids cause a sour taste. Ionized salts elicit a salty taste. Many chemicals, such as sugars, glycols, alcohols, and ketones, are responsible for a sweet taste. A bitter taste is caused by alkaloids and long-chain organic substances. Many drugs, such as quinine, caffeine, strychnine, and nicotine, and many deadly toxins found in poisonous plants are alkaloids. The highly acute bitter taste sensation provides an important protective function in that if it is intense, a person rejects the substance offered.

Most taste buds are located on the anterior and lateral surfaces of the tongue, but a few are found around the nasopharynx (Fig. 21-3). Taste hairs (microvilli) in the taste buds, which are thought to provide the receptor surface for gustation, are found in three cranial nerves: facial (VII), glossopharyngeal (IX), and vagus (X). Taste activation, adaptation, discrimination, and preference are not clearly understood. Since taste buds are chemoreceptors, a substance must be in solution to cause activation, but the actual mechanism is not known. Taste buds exhibit some adaptation. Although they react quickly to a substance, within a few seconds impulse rates become slow and steady. Prolonged exposure to most substances results in almost complete loss of taste. Although taste buds are specific to the four primary sensations of taste, in reality any one bud will respond to all four, but perhaps more vigorously to a specific taste. Temperature, texture, and odor may play a role in discrimination. The food preference mechanism to bodily needs is not understood. Taste reflexes are called forth by a little-understood mechanism by which the secretion and consistency of saliva (dilute and watery versus thick and mucous) are controlled.

Olfaction, or the sense of smell, is slight in the newborn and develops slowly, although the neonate does smell milk. The primary sensations of smell have not been classified completely, but seven primary odors may be the following: camphorous, musky, floral, pepperminty, ethereal, pungent, and putrid. Only a minute quantity of the stimulus is required. Impulses proceed along the olfactory pathway to the central nervous system.

Olfactory cells are chemoreceptors. The exact mechanism of chemical stimulation is not known, but the substance causing stimulation must have three qualities: volatility, slight water solubility, and lipid solubility. Thus is can be sniffed, pass through the olfactory mucosa, and penetrate the olfactory hairs and outer tips of the olfactory cells. Olfactory responses may also vary with attentiveness, state of the olfactory membrane, hunger, status of neural mechanisms, and sex. Olfactory adaptation is more rapid than is the gustatory mechanism.

Assessment of the Special Senses

The baby's perception of the world is built upon and shaped by his initial tactile experiences. As the baby is cared for and handled, the special senses become organized neurologically into a pattern of behavior which is important in determining the child's subsequent development. A functional deviation in one of the senses, such as hearing, will affect the development of the other senses. For example, the deaf may manifest their handicap in defective speech. The blind infant relies upon his other senses to help him learn what the outside world looks like. The nurse can detect and assess potential or already present evidence of deviations in the special senses. Early detection of seemingly insignificant variations may influence subsequent development. Prompt treatment instituted properly is often the major difference between the elimination or modification of difficulties and the development of serious complications.

Touch

Touch is one of the most important avenues of learning. With it one can explore the environment, reach out, and become part of the world in all its dimensions. Without it one is physically isolated from the world. Touch, together with the rest of the senses, provides a complex system of communication and interaction, enabling a person to express to others his inner feelings and reactions and to perceive theirs. A handshake, a hug, a kiss—all have meaning to the giver and the receiver. All human beings have a desire to reach out, to touch, and to be touched.

The sense of touch is well developed in the neonate, particularly on the tongue, lips, forehead, and ears. He is sensitive to cutaneous pressure, ambient temperature change, and pain. The neonate exhibits a generalized behavioral response to environmental and internal stimuli. Selective responsivity improves with growth, maturation, and functional elaboration. As myelination and further maturation of sensory receptors progress, the infant demonstrated increased responses to cutaneous pressure and pain. As the toddler explores the environment, the sense of touch is important in developing gross and fine motor skills. The preschooler proceeds from global and passive to methodical tactile exploration. The progression to orderly search in the school-age child supplements visual input.

In assessing touch, then, it is important to ask parents the following questions:

1. Do the parents hold, cuddle, pat, and kiss the infant or child?
2. What does the infant or child do when he is touched?
3. How does he react to pressure on the skin, to pain, to ambient temperature change?
4. When exploring the environment, does he touch objects?
5. Is the act of touching passive and global or active and orderly?

The nurse can validate information gleaned from the parents by observing the infant or child's response to touch and his use of touch in exploring the environment. (Further information on touch and pain may be found in Chap. 20, Cranial Nerve V and Alterations in Sensations. Response to ambient temperature change is discussed in Chap. 10, Methods of Dealing with Increased Temperature.) Following the collection of pertinent subjective and objective data, nursing assessments are made.

Gustation (Taste) and Olfaction (Smell)

Little study has been done on taste and smell. The gustatory and olfactory senses are closely related in that they must interact for the infant or child to discriminate different flavors. Both senses are present at birth but are not highly developed. The exact developmental sequence is not known. The neonate does, however, respond to sweet, acid, sour, and bitter substances as determined by his acceptance of sweetened fluids and his turning away from the other three types.

The nasal cavities contain not only olfactory cells but also turbinates and septum. The surfaces of these structures warm, moisten, and filter air. Thus, exudate in the nasal cavities can compromise not only the gustatory and olfactory senses but also the respiratory system. Nasal inflammation may extend into the paranasal sinuses: frontal, ethmoid, sphenoid, and maxillary.

The ethmoid, maxillary, and sphenoid sinuses are small but present at birth. The frontal sinuses cannot be detected radiologically until 6 years of age, and the ethmoid, maxillary, and sphenoid sinuses are seen sometime between birth and 3 months. The maxillary sinus is developed completely by 7 years of age. The sphenoid and frontal sinuses mature slowly until 7 years of age and complete their growth after puberty (about 15 years of age). The anterior ethmoid attains nearly complete development by 7 years of age, and the posterior ethmoid by 12 to 14 years. Fluid secreted by the sinal mucosa drains into the lateral wall of the nasal cavity.

Exudate can accrue in the nares as a result of rhinitis, sinusitis, and a foreign body in the nose. Since the gustatory and olfactory senses are so intricately entwined, an infant or child who has exudate blocking his nares will have a decreased sense of taste and smell. Therefore, collection of data will address rhinorrhea (Table 21-1).

Since rhinorrhea is one of the prodromal symptoms of several communicable diseases, assessment for skin rashes is essential. Nasal inflammation may extend through the nasolacrimal duct to the conjunctiva of the eye. The mucosa lining the nares is continuous to the middle ear cleft, the throat, and the respiratory tree. Therefore, the tympanic membrane, throat, and chest are assessed. Following the collection of pertinent subjective and objective data, nursing assessments are made.

TABLE 21-1 Assessment of a Pediatric Patient with Rhinorrhea

I. Subjective data
  A. Presenting problem—"He has a runny nose."
  B. History of presenting problem
    1. Onset—sudden or gradual
    2. Duration—length of time present
    3. Frequency—constant, intermittent, completely absent for a time and then present
    4. Discharge—color, consistency, odor
    5. Progression—better or worse than when first noted
    6. Circumstances—present at night, during day, better or worse with change of position, exploratory behavior (e.g., putting small objects in nose)
    7. Current treatment—medications (e.g., antihistamines and decongestants); over-the-counter drugs (e.g., nose drops); home remedies (e.g., saline nose drops and nasal aspiration); vaporizer (plain water or medication); type, frequency, duration, and effect of current treatment
    8. Associated symptoms (onset, duration, etc.)—mouth breathing, ear pain, sore throat, respiratory distress, fever, cough, skin rash, conjunctivitis, decreased appetite, diarrhea
  C. Past history
    1. Respiratory problems (e.g., pneumonia, frequent colds)
    2. Otitis media
    3. Exposure to others who are ill (family, friends, schoolmates)
    4. Allergies (e.g., hay fever)
    5. Immunization status
  D. Family history
    1. Respiratory problems
    2. Allergy
II. Objective data
  A. Temperature, pulse, respirations
  B. Growth measurements and percentiles
  C. General appearance—alert, irritable, lethargic, etc.
  D. Skin—rashes (see Chap. 19)
  E. Eyes—exudate, redness, swelling, tearing, Dennie's sign, allergic shiners
  F. Ears—tympanic membrane (mobility, landmarks, light reflex, color)
  G. Nose—patency of nares; discharge (amount, color, odor, consistency); turbinates and mucosa (color, edema); foreign body
  H. Sinuses—transillumination of the frontal and maxillary sinuses after 7 years of age
  I. Throat—color, exudate, enlarged tonsils, cough, hoarseness, dysphagia
  J. Mouth—dryness of tongue, with or without coating (mouth breather)
  K. Lymph nodes—enlargement, tenderness
  L. Chest—(see Chap. 23)
  M. Heart—rate, rhythm
  N. Neurological system—(see Chap. 20, Neurological Assessment—cranial nerves I, VII, and IX)

Source: G. M. Scipien et al. (eds.), *Comprehensive Pediatric Nursing,* 3d ed., McGraw-Hill, New York, 1986, p. 1371.

Vision

The full-term neonate has eyebrows and lids. Eyebrows which are bushy, overly heavy, or joined over the bridge of the nose may indicate an abnormality. The lids should close completely over the orbit when the baby is asleep.

Usually, there is no epicanthal fold unless the infant is of Oriental parentage. Both eyes should open simultaneously and should be symmetrical and equidistant from the nose. Visual acuity is about 20/200.

The infant has well-developed peripheral vision at birth. In the early postnatal days the eyes are sensitive to light and are closed most of the time. By the end of 2 weeks the infant is able to look at large objects but does not follow them to any great extent. By 4 to 6 weeks he can follow to midline a large object or light held close to the face; this action can be achieved past midline by $2\frac{1}{2}$ to 3 months. Moving an object quickly toward the eyes elicits a blink response. Binocular fixation occurs at approximately 3 months. The infant at this age becomes fascinated by his moving hands. By 6 months of age, the infant is able to watch others move about the room. Small objects are observed easily by 9 months of age. Visual acuity at 1 year is approximately 20/50. By 3 years visual acuity is usually 20/30, and it advances to 20/20 by 5 to 6 years.

When assessing vision, the nurse must keep sequential development in mind. Appraisal involves the collection of subjective and objective data. Subjective information is gleaned from the parents and/or child (if age, vocabulary, and status permit). Objective information is obtained through physical examination and laboratory and diagnostic procedures. Assessments are made through synthesis of subjective and objective data. Subjective data include the child's presenting problem, history of the presenting problem, past history, and family history (Table 21-2). Objective data include examination of the various structures of the eye (Table 21-2), appropriate laboratory and diagnostic procedures (see various diseases and deviations throughout chapter), and vision screening.

Common Signs of Eye Problems

Certain characteristic actions are performed by children who are having difficulty seeing: frequent rubbing of the eyes, shutting or covering an eye when reading or looking at or playing with a toy, tilting the head or thrusting it forward, and holding objects to be examined close to the eyes. School-age children may have difficulty reading, looking at the blackboard, or doing close work. They also blink more frequently, squint the eyelids together, or frown constantly. Assessing the eyes is an important nursing responsibility. One should note strabismus and eyes which are red-rimmed, edematous, or encrusted. Watery, inflamed eyes are commonly seen in children with eye problems. Recurrent styes should prompt an ophthalmologic examination.

Young children may complain that their eyes itch, burn, or feel scratchy. All these symptoms should be investigated. Repeated complaints of a child's inability to see, especially in the classroom, should be followed up by the school nurse. After doing close work, some children with visual deficits state that they feel dizzy, have headaches, or are nauseated. Verbalizations regarding blurred vision or the presence of diplopia are serious clinical manifestations which should be thoroughly investigated immediately.

TABLE 21-2 Assessment of the Eye

I. Subjective data
  A. Presenting problem (alone or in combination)
    1. Excessive tearing ("He always has tears in his eyes.")
    2. Exudate ("He has sleep stuff in his eyes and on his lashes.")
    3. Erythema ("Her eye is all red.")
    4. Photophobia ("She squints in bright light, and her eyes tear.")
    5. Cat's-eye sign—white appearance of pupil ("The middle of her eye is white when light hits it.")
    6. Strabismus ["One eye turns in (out, up, down) when he looks at something."]
    7. Discomfort, pain ("He says his eye hurts.")
    8. Itching ("She says her eye itches.")
    9. Edema ("His eyelids are swollen.")
    10. Foreign body ("He got something in his eye.")
    11. Blurring of vision ["She says when she tried to read (or look in the distance), it gets fuzzy."]
    12. Diplopia ("She says she sees double.")
    13. Ptosis ("His eyelid droops.")
    14. Exophthalmos ("His eyes look pushed out.")
    15. Rubbing eyes, squinting, frowning, seeing "spots" before eyes
    16. Trauma ("He got hit in the eye.")
    17. Inability to distinguish colors ("He can't tell me the color of things.")
  B. History of presenting problem
    1. Onset—sudden or gradual
    2. Duration—length of time present
    3. Frequency—constant, intermittent, completely absent for a time and then present
    4. Type (some examples)
      (a) Exudate—color, consistency, odor, amount
      (b) Strabismus—inward, outward, downward, upward
      (c) Trauma—blunt, sharp
    5. Progression—better or worse than when first noted
    6. Circumstances—better or worse with activity, at night, during day, with change in position
    7. Current treatment—medications, over-the-counter drugs, home remedies; type, frequency, duration, and effect
    8. Associated symptoms
  C. Past history
    1. Prenatal history—trauma, anoxia, maternal systemic disease (e.g., cytomegalovirus, rubella, toxoplasmosis), maternal sexually transmitted disease (e.g., chlamydia, gonorrhea)
    2. Perinatal history—preterm infant in oxygen
    3. Trauma
    4. Any of the presenting problems noted above
  C. Family history
    1. Primary glaucoma
    2. Congenital cataracts
    3. Retinoblastoma
II. Objective data
  A. Temperature, pulse, respirations, blood pressure (3 years and above)
  B. Growth measurements
    1. Length or stature ⎫ for calculation of medication
    2. Weight ⎭
    3. Head circumference (particularly with exophthalmos)
  C. Eyes
    1. Eyebrows—scaliness, crusting, bushiness, joining, absence, lice
    2. Eyelashes—scaliness, crusting, absence, lice
    3. Eyelids—erythema, edema, discoloration, epicanthal folds, styes, upward slant, excessive blinking or squinting, ptosis, mases
    4. Orbit—edema, discoloration, alignment, Dennie's sign or allergic shiner in orbitopalpebral grooves
    5. Bulbar conjunctiva—redness, increased vascularity, jaundice, dryness, chemosis, pterygium, hemorrhage
    6. Palpebral conjunctiva—redness, pallor, dryness, cobblestone apperaance, exudate, chalazion
    7. Extraocular muscles (see Chap. 20—cranial nerves III, IV, and VI)
    8. Lacrimal apparatus—exudate, excess tearing
    9. Sclera—jaundice, erythema
    10. Cornea—scarring, ulcerations, opacities
    11. Iris—dullness, each of a different color
    12. Lens—cat's-eye sign, opacity
    13. Fundus—presence or absenceof red reflex
    14. Optic nerve (see Chap. 20—cranial nerve II)
    15. Pupil—symmetry of size, reaction to light (See Chap. 20—cranial nerve III)
    16. Globe—exophthalmos, sunken appearance, blank look
    17. Vision screening (see text, Visual Acuity)

Source: G. M. Scipien et al. (eds.), *Comprehensive Pediatric Nursing,* 3d ed., McGraw-Hill, New York, 1986, p. 1373.

Allergic Responses of the Eye

These responses of the eye may occur at any age, depending on the specific allergy, and include edema of the lids, chemosis, hyperemia (redness), conjunctivitis, Dennie's sign, and allergic shiners. *Chemosis* is defined as edema of the bulbar conjunctiva. In *allergic conjunctivitis,* the palpebral conjunctiva is milky, pale, and edematous. *Vernal conjunctivitis* involves both upper and lower palpebral conjunctivae, the upper containing hard, flattened papillae. The child complains of lacrimation, itching, and photophobia. Exudate is stringy and mucoid and contains eosinophils. *Edema of the eyelids* is due to local irritants such as hair spray, powder, and nail polish. Both Dennie's sign and allergic shiners involve the lower orbitopalpebral grooves. In *Dennie's sign,* lines radiate from the inner corner of the eye, slant downward, and end in a slight upward swing. *Allergic shiners* ("black eyes") are noted because of edema and discoloration of these grooves.

Hearing

Hearing and the development of language are closely associated. Babies with normal hearing and hearing-impaired infants progress through the same stages until about 7 months of age, when babbling diminishes in both.

In the first day or two of life, gelatinous tissue is present in the neonate's middle ear. This debris hinders the movement of the ossicles and eardrums. Thus, the newborn responds only to high-intensity sounds. After absorption, sound frequency and intensity can be discriminated.

At birth, accumulated vernix caseosa is present in the external auditory canal. This material is absorbed during the first week. Until absorption takes place, it is difficult to visualize the tympanic membrane. Thus otoscopic examination is not a routine part of neonatal assessment in the newborn nursery.

Unusual ear configuration and abnormal placement may be indicative of other auditory anomalies or other body system abnormalities. For example, deformity and near absence of the auricle are associated with anomalies of the external canal and middle ear; failure of formation of the external canal and ossicular anomalies result in conductive hearing loss; and low-set ears may be indicative of renal abnormalities or mental retardation. An infant who has a cleft palate or submucosal cleft is prone to ear infections and may have a conductive hearing loss.

Newborn vocalizations, when not crying, are described as chirps. By 4 weeks of age, infants begin to have speech discrimination. At this time their vocalizations consist of cooing (and crying). Sensitivity to sound increases with age (Table 21-3). By 3 months of age, infants babble. They attempt to imitate sounds at 7 months of age, when babbling diminishes. At this time hearing-impaired infants begin to develop gestures rather than imitate sounds in an effort to communicate. By the end of the first year an infant with normal hearing utters his first meaningful word. At 2 years of age toddlers have an expressive vocabulary of about 50 words. Children progress to approximately 2000 words and four- to five-word sentences by 5 years of age.

The basis for learning, language acquisition, and communication is established during the preschool years. Late-onset or previously undetected hearing loss may be recognized in preschoolers because of delays in progress

TABLE 21-3 Normal Values for Auditory Threshold and Sound Localization

Age, Mo	Threshold, dB	Localization Ability
3-4	50-60	Begins to turn head to the side at which the sound is heard
4-7	40-50	Turns head directly toward the side of a signal but cannot locate a sound above or below
7-9	30-40	Directly locates a sound source to the side and indirectly below
9-13	25-35	Directly locates a sound source to the side and below

Source: M. Tudor (ed.), *Child Development,* McGraw-Hill, New York, 1981, p. 376.

TABLE 21-4 Risk Factors Arranged by Age Groups

History	Maternal infections with rubella or viral infection
	Family history of childhood hearing impairment
Neonates	Birth weight less than 1500 g
	Apgar score of 5 or less at 5 min
	Unconjugated bilirubin over 20 mg 100 ml
	Asphyxia with acidosis
	Congenital defects of ear, nose, or throat
Infants and toddlers	Meningitis
	Middle ear effusions
	Major infections treated with aminoglycosides
Preschool	Speech delays
	Balance problems
	Infections; meningitis and viremia
	High fevers
	Recurring otitis media
	Behavior problems
School-age children and adolescents	Academic delays
	Inattentive behavior
	Speech disorders
	Allergic syndromes
	Noise-induced hearing loss
	Acoustic trauma
	Accidents

Source: G. M. Scipien et al. (eds.), *Comprehensive Pediatric Nursing,* 3d ed., McGraw-Hill, New York, 1986, p. 618.

as described above and in school-age children and adolescents because of academic delays. Risk factors for hearing impairments by age groups are listed in Table 21-4.

There are two types of hearing loss; conductive and sensorineural. In *conductive hearing loss,* there is a reduction of sound without distortion of clarity. In *sensorineural hearing loss,* sounds are distorted; hence, discrimination is difficult. High frequencies are affected more than low frequencies are unless there is severe involvement, in which case both are impaired.

Conductive hearing losses, the more common type in children, are associated with impacted cerumen or a foreign body in the external canal, otitis media, congenital malformations (e.g., external atresia and otosclerosis), trauma, and tympanic membrane perforation. Sensorineural hearing losses, the more serious but less common type, may be hereditary, congenital, or secondary to ototoxic drugs, trauma, or infection (e.g., *Haemophilus influenzae* meningitis, mumps, rubella, and rubeola).

When assessing hearing, the nurse must keep sequential development in mind. As with vision, appraisal involves the collection of subjective and objective data (Table 21-5).

Common Screening and Diagnostic Tests
Taste

The four primary modalities used in taste testing are sweet, sour, salt, and bitter substances. Receptors for sweet and salty tastes are greatest in the tip of the tongue,

TABLE 21-5 Assessment of the Ear

I. Subjective data
  A. Presenting problem (alone or in combination)
    1. Malformed auricle ("My baby has a funny-looking ear.")
    2. Decrease in or absence of babbling ("He doesn't babble like he used to.")
    3. Sleep disturbances ("She was crying all night, and she has a fever.")
    4. Repeated otitis media ("I think she has another ear infection, the third one this year.")
    5. Delay in language acquisition ("He's 2 years old, and he's not talking.")
    6. Impacted cerumen ("I can see wax when I look in his ear.")
    7. Foreign body ("She stuck a bean in her ear.")
    8. Noise pollution ("He has that hi-fi so loud all the time that I think he can't hear as well as he used to.")
  B. History of presenting problem
    1. Onset—sudden or gradual
    2. Duration—length of time present
    3. Frequency—constant, intermittent, completely absent for a time and then present
    4. Type (some examples)
      (a) Exudate in external canal—color, consistency, odor, amount
      (b) Language acquisition—misarticulation errors; stuttering; voice problems; organic speech problems; inability to recall words, phrases, and other parts of speech; omission of connecting words and phrases; use of gestures and pantomime to be understood; making persistent noises
      (c) Foreign body—bean, pea, insect
    5. Progression—better or worse than when first noted
    6. Circumstances—better or worse with activity, at night, during day, in classroom, during one-to-one interactions
    7. Current treatment—medicines, over-the-counter drugs, home remedies; type, frequency, duration, and effect of medicines and remedies; speech therapy
    8. Associated symptoms
  C. Past history
    1. Prenatal history—trauma, anorexia, maternal systemic disease (e.g., rubella, cytomegalovirus)
    2. Perinatal history—birth weight below 1500 mg, serum bilirubin levels greater than 20 mg/100, significant asphyxia associated with acidosis, cleft palate or submucosal cleft
    3. Ototoxic drugs
    4. Meningitis
    5. Repeated ear infections and/or frequent colds
    6. Trauma
    7. Any of the presenting problems noted above
  D. Family history
    1. Hereditary childhood hearing impairment
    2. Allergies
II. Objective data
  A. Temperature, pulse, respirations, blood pressure (3 years and above)
  B. Growth measures
    1. Length or stature
    2. Weight
    3. Head circumference
  C. Ears
    1. Pinna—shape, size, malformations, nodules, lesions, placement, skin tags, swelling, tenderness, asymmetry
    2. External canal (using otoscope)—patency, discharge, narrowing, redness, pain, foreign bodies, cerumen
    3. Tympanic membrane (using otoscope)—short process of malleus, umbo, long process of malleus, light reflex, color, mobility, bullae, bulging, perforation, retraction
    4. Hearing screening (see text below for common screening and diagnostic procedures)
  D. Eyes—vision screening (see text below for common screening and diagnostic procedures)
  E. Nose—see Table 21-2
  F. Mouth—cleft palate or submucosal cleft
  G. Language and speech—part of developmental assessment by listening to child talk and screening with R-PDQ and/or DDST

sour is at the sides, and bitter sensations are experienced in the most posterior region. Since more complex flavors result in stimulation of both gustatory and olfactory sensations, they are not used. Because dry solids are ineffective, the substances tested need to be in solution.

The tongue is withdrawn and grasped with a gauze square. A moist applicator is used to place crystals of salt, sugar, and other substances on different areas of the tongue. Saliva converts the crystal to a liquid form. The tongue is then wiped clean, and the child is asked to describe what is being sensed.

Several variable affect taste. For example, irradiation of the head and neck can impair this sense, and excessive dryness can also alter it. There are some medications which can cause misinterpretations and distortions of the sense of taste. Examples include penicillamine, procarbazine, vincristine, and vinblastine. In addition, children di-

agnosed with Bell's palsy lose taste in about one-half of the tongue.

While the precise nature of how taste buds are stimulated is unknown, testing for taste can be difficult in infants and young children who are unable to report what they are experiencing. In those situations, it is important for a nurse to observe facial and bodily responses to substances. For example, an infant who is given a sweet substance begins to suck for more, whereas a toddler is likely to pucker when tasting a sour substance or object vehemently to a bitter substance by spitting or attempting to remove it from his mouth. An older child who knows these different tastes is able to describe them.

Smell

For a substance to be perceived as an odor, it must be volatile or have the capability to spread in the air in very small particles. It must be soluble in water or lipids. Smell, the least understood of all the senses, is determined by cranial (olfactory) nerve I.

A number of nonirritating substances can act as olfactory stimuli in identifying the intactness of cranial nerve I. Swabs of cotton are saturated with liquids of familiar substances, such as lemon, vanilla, and oil of peppermint. With the patient's eyes closed and one nostril occluded, the saturated cotton swab is placed under the child's patent nostril. After inhaling the substance, he is asked to identify the odor. After testing of one nostril, the procedure is repeated for the other nostril. Cooperation of the child may be a problem in ascertaining the ability to smell. It may be difficult to determine whether the child cannot identify the odor itself or if there is a problem in smelling the substance. The olfactory nerve is considered intact if the smell is detected in the nostrils, even though the patient cannot specifically identify the odor.

Anosmia, or the loss of smell, is not rare. Although it is more common in adults (e.g., among heavy smokers), it is often found in children who have allergic rhinitis and chronic rhinitis.

Visual Acuity

Many of the problems which result in decreased visual acuity are preventable if they are detected early. Eye examinations should be part of a well-child examination (see Chap. 6 and the assessment section above); however, a visual history also should be taken to identify those behaviors which indicate the presence of visual difficulty. They include parental observations of roving eye movements, nystagmus, photophobia, items held up close to the eyes, sitting close to the television, grimacing, facial contortions, rhythmic body movements, and pressing or rubbing the eyes. Since the critical period for developing acute vision occurs between 1 and 6 years of age, testing should begin early in life and should continue at regular intervals. In infancy, visual acuity can be estimated by performance, such as following a light or bright object. During the third or fourth year, it can be measured fairly accurately using Snellen E cards or the Snellen E chart. When the letter E is presented, a child of normal intelligence can be asked to point his fingers in the direction toward which the E is pointed. Preschoolers need to be instructed immediately before the procedure. A brief training period can facilitate a better understanding of what is desired by the tester. When the child understands what is expected, the chart or card is placed 20 ft from him for the actual test. The tester asks the child to read the 20/30 or 20/40 line, working up or down the chart, depending on the child's progress. Typically, preschoolers are more interested in close objects, showing little interest in activities across the room. If such is the case, vision can be tested at 10 ft and the findings can be transposed to obtain an accurate acuity reading. Using E cards in testing a very young child is less confusing; however, one disadvantage may be the child's inability to indicate the direction toward which the legs of the letter point. If a set of E pic-

TABLE 21-6 Passing Scores for the Snellen E or Alphabet Chart

20/20 line	Fourth grade and up
20/30 line	4 years through third grade
20/40 line	Below 4 years

Source: M. U. Barnard et al., *Handbook of Comprehensive Pediatric Nursing,* McGraw-Hill, New York, 1981.

tures is given to the child, he can then choose the symbol being held by the tester, thus eliminating the problem.

While picture cards are sometimes used in testing very young children, a major problem may be the child's inability to recall the word which identifies the picture. Also, the picture may be unfamiliar. The Allen cards are probably best because they consist of items most children know, such as a birthday cake, a telephone, and a Christmas tree.

These examinations should be done on *all* children before the start of school, midway through elementary education, and just before beginning high school as well as at 2-year intervals thereafter. The Snellen alphabet chart (obtainable from the National Society for the Prevention of Blindness) is the most accurate method for screening visual acuity in older children. As the child stands 20 ft from the chart, the examiner tests each eye separately, beginning at the 20/30 or 20/40 line and working up or down depending on the child's ability. Visual acuity is noted as a fraction; the top number is the distance from the chart, and the bottom number is the last line read correctly. With all letters on one line exposed, a passing score is one in which the child is able to read a majority of letters on that line (Table 21-6). The vision of both eyes together will not be worse than that of each eye separately. Any child with a two-line difference between eyes or one who is unable to read the age-appropriate lines must be evaluated further.

Vision screening kits are available to parents whose children do not have access to formal screening programs in their communities. They can be obtained free of charge from the National Society for the Prevention of Blindness (Fig. 21-4).

When poor vision or blindness is suspected on the basis of screening tests, the infant or child should be referred to an ophthalmologist for further evaluation. For the blind child, several electrophysiological tests are available. Each records the eye's response to light at a different level, as follows:

1. The electroretinogram (ERG) at the sensory retinal level
2. The electrooculogram (EOG) at the retinal pigment epithelial level
3. Visual evoked potentials (VEPs) at the cortical level (Apt and Gaffney, 1987)

Increasing numbers of nurses are becoming involved in day care centers and preschool nurseries. In improving the health services offered, many have initiated vision

SYMBOL CHART FOR 10 FEET
Snellen Scale

FIGURE 21-4   The Snellen E chart for screening preschoolers. *(From G.M. Scipien et al. [eds.], Comprehensive Pediatric Nursing, 3d ed., McGraw-Hill, New York, 1986, p. 1375.)*

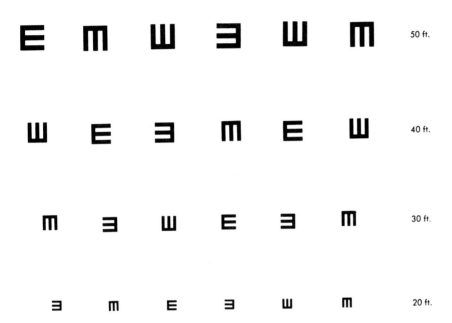

20 ft.
Equivalent

50 ft.

40 ft.

30 ft.

20 ft.

testing as an integral component of assessment or have done screenings after teachers have identified problems in their young students. While those efforts are laudable, greater efforts must be directed toward educating parents and the general public.

Color Blindness
Color blindness, or the inability to distinguish between certain colors, is common in males and rare in females. Sometimes parents note that the child is slow in learning colors and ask to have a test done. The test is a simple one and should be performed early, especially in boys. In addition, the results obtained are not reversible, and so individuals are tested only once.

This eye problem is an inherited disorder and consists of three different classifications. The protanopic type involves red, blue, and green sensitivity, while the dueuteranopic type affects green, brown, purple, and gray colors. A third extremely rare form, tritanopia, involves yellow and blue colors.

A child is shown a series of Ishihara plates, which consists of figures made up of dots on a background of other colorful dots. When asked to name or trace the figure present within a plate, a child who is color-blind is unable

to do so because he cannot identify the figure's presence. The only clue available is its color, which he cannot "see."

While most kindergarten students can be tested easily, the Guy color vision test may need to be used with younger children. The Ishihara plates are utilized in conjunction with matching figures. When asked to identify the symbol present, a child merely selects the appropriate matching figure.

Children who are color-blind must be identified early, especially in view of the increasing use of colored educational materials, such as color-coded reading tests, in elementary schools. While color blindness may result in wearing mismatched colors of clothing, there are other serious safety issues. These boys may not be able to distinguish the red, amber, or green traffic lights from street lamps or the red brake lights of cars. Adolescents may need occupational counseling, particularly if color coding is a component of their vocational choice.

Auditory Evaluation
Many of the problems associated with decreased hearing are preventable if they are detected early. Auditory screening, including a hearing history, should be a part of every well-child examination to identify behaviors which

may indicate a hearing loss (as discussed in the section on assessment and noted in Table 21-5). The revised Denver Developmental Screening Test (DDST) and the Revised Denver Prescreening Developmental Questionaire (R-PDQ) are appropriate screening tools from birth to 6 years of age. Developmental milestones have to be obtained in the history and observed by the examiner. For example, any delays in head control, sitting, standing, and walking can signify vestibular damage.

In pediatric ambulatory settings, nurses who have received special training administer auditory screening tests. For example, 3- and 4-year-old children may be tested by the VASC auditory screening method. The child is first given a practice period to ensure that he understands what is expected of him. Once the nurse believes that the child understands, the earphones are put in place. A recorded voice names different objects, and the child is asked to point to a picture of the object. Each ear is tested separately. Older children are tested for intensity and freqnency using an audiometer. The sound stimuli consist of various tones. If hearing loss is suspected at any age, the child is referred to an audiologist for further testing. Audiologists have several methods by which to test infants and children. These techniques include electrophysiological testing, sound field testing, impedance audiometry, play audiometry, and conventional audiometry.

Electrophysiological Testing (Evoked Response Audiometry)

The brainstem evoked auditory response (BEAR) is the most accurate test for a child of any age. It is particularly useful for assessing newborns who have been in a neonatal intensive care unit and children who have developmental disabilities. Brain waves that respond to sound are measured through scalp electrodes. Both conductive and sensorineural hearing losses can be determined.

Sound Field Testing

This method usually is not used until 6 months of age because the normal infant does not begin to localize on the lateral plane until that time. Testing takes place in a soundproof booth. The baby is seated on the parent's lap, facing the examiner's window. Speech stimuli, noise, and warble tone are fed into loudspeakers located to the infant's right and left. For speech stimuli, the speech awareness level only is tested until 2 years of age. (Speech reception cannot be determined until 2 or 3 years of age, and speech discrimination is possible in the testing situation by 3 or 4 years of age.) The infant's localization to sound stimuli is observed and recorded. Specific information about each ear may not be obtained since responses are given by the better ear if a hearing deficit is present.

Impedance Audiometry

Impedance audiometry (tympanometry and acoustic reflex testing) is an objective means of assessing eustachian tube function, middle ear pressure, tympanic membrane mobility, and mobility and continuity of the middle ear ossicles. Stapedial reflex testing may supply information regarding the presence of conductive, cochlear, or retrocochlear pathological conditions. The reliability of impedance testing results prior to 7 months of age is questionable.

In this procedure, an earplug attached to the machine seals the external canal. Pressure to the external canal and eardrum is varied automatically. Reflected sound is recorded on a graph. When the middle ear is filled with fluid, sound is reflected. Thus this test confirms the presence of fluid behind the tympanic membrane. The results are interpreted by a physician, a nurse who has had special training, or an audiologist.

Play Audiometry

This method is used with children from 2 to 5 or 6 years of age. The child may be tested with or without earphones; the advantage of earphones is that they supply specific information about each ear. In either event, the child is first conditioned through praise to respond to sound stimuli. Reactions, e.g., dropping a block in a box in response to the tester's voice or to a tone, are observed and recorded. The procedure is done in a soundproof room. A speech discrimination score may not be determined until 3 or 4 years of age.

Conventional Audiometry

For children 5 to 6 years of age and older, conventional audiometry is used. The sound stimuli consist of various pure tones presented through earphones in a soundproof booth. The child indicates that the sound is heard by raising his hand. To test sensorineural hearing levels, a bone vibrator is placed on the child's mastoid. The child raises his hand upon hearing the sound produced. With these techniques, both conductive and sensorineural deficits can be determined.

Common Nursing Measures

A child who is undergoing treatment for a health problem involving the nose, eyes, or ears often faces the prospect of a surgical correction. Depending on his age, the child may or may not understand the reason or be prepared for what will happen to him.

Surgical intervention usually results in a change in breathing, seeing, or hearing which may be permanent or temporary. After surgery, there may be a temporary diminution of function due to edema and/or the packing or dressing. It is important for a nurse to know the physician's plans in order to interpret those plans for the child and parents and prepare them for the postoperative course. Since procedures are changing rapidly and health care facilities have specific policies regarding care, only basic nursing principles are included in the following section.

Nursing Diagnoses

An alteration in sight, hearing, taste, or smell can occur in the presence of a deviation from normal. Many nursing diagnoses can be developed for a child who experiences such an impairment. While the list is not all-inclusive, some nursing diagnoses that can apply to these children and their families include the following:

Sensory/perceptual alteration (visual, auditory, kinesthetic, gustatory, tactile, olfactory)

Pain

Altered oral mucous membranes

Impaired verbal communication

Potential for infection

Self-care deficit (bathing/hygiene, feeding, dressing/ grooming, toileting)

Knowledge deficit related to the alteration

Social isolation

Ineffective individual coping

Ineffective family coping

Nursing Management of Children with Impairments

Children with visual or auditory deficits are admitted to hospitals for a wide variety of problems which may or may not be related to their sensory impairments. The nursing interventions suggested here are the most common, successful methods of delivering care to these children. Most of them are independent nursing actions determined by the child's needs and developmental stage as well as the nurse's knowledge base (Chap. 9).

The Visually Impaired Child

In obtaining a nursing history (Chap. 5), it is essential to identify how long the child has been blind, what self-help skills he has mastered, and his daily routine. If parents elect to remain with the child during the hospitalization, they may interpret the many new and different sounds and smells which prevail. If not, the primary nurse needs to be available for an extended time in order to enhance his orientation. It also is essential for a nurse to know the degree of visual impairment because this information is helpful in determining the amount of supervision needed and the types of activities in which the child may participate. These data are recorded in the chart and Kardex and shared with the associate nurse and playroom personnel so that all providers know the child's capabilities as well as his limitations.

Each visually impaired child should be walked around the pediatric unit by a nurse who provides an additional commentary on the noises within the vicinity, answers the questions which arise, and allows the child to identify specific landmarks. In the room, the child needs the freedom to familiarize himself with the placement of furniture and all the objects present to develop his concept of spatial relationships. Once the child has oriented himself spatially, it is very important for the furniture to remain in its proper place.

When a procedure is done, an explanation should always be provided; however, a visually impaired child also should be allowed to handle the equipment beforehand whenever possible. Safety is a real concern, and the beds of these children must be at the lowest possible height from the floor. Siderails should be up unless someone is in the room. Again, safety and possible disorientation in waking necessitate such action. Restraints are not used on these children unless there is absolutely no alternative because the use of their hands is critical to tactile stimulation.

Whenever a nurse enters or leaves the room, the child is verbally informed of her presence before she departs. It also is important for each provider to identify himself or herself on entering the room.

These children should always have sighted roommates, preferably of the same chronological age, especially if the parents do not plan to room-in. In addition to providing company, roommates furnish invaluable verbal input and decrease the likelihood of withdrawal by a visually impaired child.

Nursing interventions must focus on encouraging the independence of these children and maintaining the self-care skills they have mastered. The adjustment of visually impaired children to hospitals can be facilitated by nurses who recognize their special needs.

The Hearing Impaired Child

A child with a hearing impairment may have to be hospitalized for an unrelated health problem. A nurse needs to know the degree of impairment and how long the deafness has been present. This information should be incorporated into the nursing history. In addition to assessing the child's abilities and determining his developmental level, it is critical for a nurse to know the comunication pattern used by the child and his family members. Is it signing, finger spelling, or lipreading? Many times a combination of methods is used, depending on the age of the child and the time when the impairment was diagnosed. For example, lipreading may be the primary method of comuniating with a child who has had normal hearing. If a hearing aid is used, the nurse needs to become familiar with the particular model. Parents often are pleased to demonstrate its use and maintenance.

The child and parents are oriented to the unit, as described in Chap. 9. Although parents should be encouraged to room-in, they may elect not to do so. In that instance, the primary nurse should allow extra time for the admission in order to provide the explanations which are essential. One important aspect of the child's orientation involves the use of a call bell. With the child's hearing affected, the intercommunication system in the nurses' station must be labeled appropriately so that all personnel answering it know that a hearing-impaired child is in the room. In addition, it is most important for the nurse who responds to the call bell *to go into the room to do so.* These children need to be involved in any play programs in the pediatric unit or in a playroom. However, playroom personnel must be informed about the child's hearing deficit and about an effective method of comunicating with him. It is hoped that his roommate also can be helpful where diversional activities are concerned.

When a procedure is to be done, efforts should be made to communicate an understandable explanation to the child. If it is a procedure in which the nurse is not in the child's vision, it is wise to obtain the assistance of another nurse who maintains visual contact and continues the explanation. It is important to touch the child *before* speaking so that he knows the nurse is present and can concentrate on what is being communicated. If the child is asleep, he should be awakened slowly and very gently. A child with a hearing aid often turns the device off for a nap or sleep. Sometimes a parent or nurse turns on the hearing aid while the child is being aroused. If this practice is part of the child's routine, it should be done carefully, especially in regard to volume control.

It is not unusual, unfortunately, for children who are severely affected to be considered developmentally delayed because of speech patterns which are not clear or because they may not understand what is being verbally said to them. An initial developmental assessment rules out such an erroneous and invalid conclusion. The nurse who provides care to a hearing-impaired child also must be extremely conscious of facial expressions, which convey a great deal to a child who relies almost exclusively on visual input.

Nursing interventions focus on encouraging the independence of children with hearing impairments. To do so, however, it is essential for a primary nurse to communicate the presence of a hearing impaired child to the associate nurse and to place this information on the chart and Kardex. Communicating with a hearing-impaired child is not a problem provided that the method for doing so has been shared with everyone involved.

Nasal Surgery

Preoperatively, these children and adolescents need to be prepared for what they can expect before and after surgery. Usually they are NPO (nothing by mouth) for 6 to 8 hours, and young children who are given general anesthesia are medicated with atropine to decrease secretions. Adolescents frequently are awake during these procedures, which are done under local anesthesia. This type of surgery necessitates a nasal packing at the conclusion of a procedure, and the child needs to be informed beforehand. Waking up in the recovery room and not being able to breathe nasally can be anxiety-provoking and frightening if it is unexpected.

The packing consists of $\frac{1}{2}$-in gauze which can be petrolatum-impregnated, plain, unfilled gauze, or another type desired by the physician. It is held in place by strips of adhesive tape under the nose which may need changing as they are soiled by drainage. If the packing is accidentally dislodged, the physician must be notified immediately. Hemorrhage is a potential problem which can be identified by the presence of blood on the packing, in vomitus, or in sputum. The back of the throat should always be examined for blood when a child appears to be swallowing frequently. Tarry stools are seen in some children for 1 to 2 days postoperatively.

With the packing in place, a child breathes through the mouth, making oral hygiene an important nursing function. Although fluids can be given soon after recovery from anesthesia, once solid foods are started, most of these children have a poor appetite. The diminished intake is related to two basic causes: the loss of smell and the presence of nasal packing. Most children and adolescents prefer an extensive list of liquids, at least until the packing has been removed. Although there is a degree of discomfort, especially immediately after surgery, it is primarily related to the presence of nasal packing.

The head of the bed is in semi-Fowler's position after surgery to decrease the amount of local edema which can develop. These children also should be asked not to cough if possible, because they may start bleeding. If the surgery is performed on the external portion of the nose, there may be some periorbital discoloration and edema, which is relieved by the application of ice packs.

When the packing is removed 48 hours or more after insertion, the child or adolescent needs to be told to refrain from blowing the nose for at least 48 hours because some bleeding can occur. Usually no medications are prescribed at discharge; however, instructions need to be given regarding follow-up visits to the clinic or physician's office.

Eye Surgery

Any child who is about to experience eye surgery needs thorough preparation; however, it is *imperative* when one or both eyes are to be bandaged after a procedure. Not being able to see what is going on can precipitate incredible fantasies and fears in the mind of a creative, imaginative child. It is important for the child to know that although the dressings are in place after surgery, when they are removed he will be able to see again. Using a blindfold to simulate eye patches and practicing how to use the call bell with the blindfold in place enhance a child's understanding of what "it will be like afterward."

If both eyes are to be dressed after the procedure, it is important for a child to become familiar with the immediate environment and to meet those providers who will care for him postoperatively. With eye dressings in place, sounds which were not heard previously take on unusual and anxiety-provoking meaning. While he is interacting with various professionals involved in providing care, the unusual meaning of sounds is yet another stressor with which the child must contend.

Preoperatively, the instillation of eye medications is necessary to dilate the pupils. It is most important for a nurse to administer them properly and at the times *scheduled* in order to prepare the eyes correctly for a procedure.

Children usually receive general anesthesia for eye surgery; therefore, foods and fluids are withheld for about 6 hours beforehand. In addition, atropine is administered with a drug of the physician's choice to facilitate induction.

After surgery, children are frequently restless after recovery and attempt to remove their dressings. Parents, grandparents, or significant others should be asked to saty with the child. This arrangement is one which needs to be planned before admission. Having a parent or an uncle or aunt at the bedside can be comforting and reassuring for a child. More importantly, however, that adult may eliminate the need for using restraints which a child resists. When parents elect to remain with the child, it is important for a nurse to stay with them until they are comfortable with what is expected of them. If it is impossible for a family member to be present, a nurse may be assigned to care for the young patient; however, when she is absent from the bedside, restaints need to be in place. Concern centers on the child removing the dressing and damaging the operative site. The less restriction imposed, the less the anxiety and the greater the cooperation; however, protecting the eyes is critical, and so restraints may be necessary. Elbow restraints, which are far less inhibiting than wrist restraints, prevent the child from removing the dressings.

Postoperatively, nursing care focuses on preventing any increased intraocular pressure or stress on the suture line. The serious complications of hemorrhage or infection may be present in a child who complains of sharp pain in the operative site.

If the surgery is unilateral, the child is positioned on the unaffected side. He is asked to lie reasonably quiet and to try not to cough, sneeze, or move his head suddenly. However, these requests can make compliance difficult. When fully awake and sufficiently distracted by appropriate quiet activities, these children are cooperative.

Clear fluids are resumed after recovery, and they should be given slowly. Vomiting increases intraocular pressure, and vomitus can contaminate the dressing, making a change essential.

When the dressing is removed, the eye may be red, edematous, and encrusted, and so both parents and child should be prepared for its appearance. The eye can be rinsed gently with warm saline to alleviate the discomfort.

If the child is to be discharged on ophthalmic medications, his parents should be shown how to instill them and administer them before leaving. Reviewing signs of infection enables them to identify its presence early. Parents need to be encouraged to call if they have any questions about the child's progress. While the physician may impose few restrictions on the activities of a young child, older children and adolescents may not be able to participate in contact sports for several weeks after eye surgery.

Ear Surgery

Usually ear surgery is necessary when there is a prolonged infection which is not responding to treatment; however, it also may be considered for cosmetic reasons. A child who has had a unilateral mastoidectomy returns to his room with a pressure dressing in place, as does a child who experiences an otoplasty. In the former, hearing is reduced slightly, but in the latter, it is reduced substantially because the pressure dressing is wrapped around the entire head, with only the face exposed. Preparation for that eventuality is an important nursing action.

Since general anesthesia is given to most of these children, food and fluids are withheld after midnight and the child is premedicated to decrease secretions and facilitate induction. A myringotomy and the insertion of ventilating tubes which facilitate drainage and allow for an air exchange between the middle and outer ear do not necessitate a dressing. However, any exudate must be cleaned from the outer ear with hydrogen peroxide. Fluids and foods are gradually introduced. Pain is not a common complaint, and recovery is rapid. When tubes have been inserted, discharge teaching should include measures parents must take to protect the ear, especially during shampooing or bathing. An effective method of preventing water from entering the ear canal is to cover the affected ear with sterile cotton coated with petroleum jelly. In addition, children should be instructed not to do any swimming as long as the tubes are in place.

Elbow restraints may be used on a child who has a dressing in place. While drainage from an otoplasty is almost nil, serosanguineous drainage is expected after a mastoidectomy. If bright red blood is evident, a physician should be notified immediately. The child should be positioned on the unoperated side; he will have pain and will develop edema. Since nose blowing increases air pressure in the eustachian tube and thus causes additional discomfort, it should not be done. When the child is allowed out of bed, he may complain of being dizzy as a result of middle or inner ear stimulation during surgery. Ambulating the child slowly is helpful.

When mastoid dressings are changed, sterile technique and proper disposal of materials are important. The drain and packing are usually removed 3 to 4 days after surgery. However, swimming, showers, and shampoos are not permitted until the incision is completely healed, which takes about 10 to 14 days.

Methods of Enhancing Adaptation

Contact Lenses

Although eyeglasses are worn to correct refractive errors or to normalize vision, there are situations in which contact lenses are preferable. Contact lenses can be used in children 8 to 10 years of age; however, their use frequently is deferred until adolescence, when their cosmetic effects are highly desired. In addition, contact lenses may be used successfully in infants who have had congenital cataract surgery. A complete ophthalmic examination prior to fitting is important to rule out any existing pathological problem. If contact lenses are not used properly or if they fit poorly, they can impair visual acuity. Wearing contact lenses eliminates common problems such as broken eyeglasses, loosened frames, and dirty lenses. Some disadvantages of wearing contact lenses include the time-consuming process of teaching a child how to insert and remove them and the initial discomfort experienced in adjusting to them. There are three types.

Hard contact lenses are made of a hard plastic material. They are less expensive and longer lasting than other types; however, adjustment periods may be difficult. They cannot be worn during sleep and should not be worn while swimming. Hard lenses require daily cleaning, which takes time. While they are used by adolescents who play football, basketball, or soccer, participating in sports such as racquetball or tennis necessitates the use of protective eye guards in order to prevent injury from a ball traveling at a high velocity.

Soft contact lenses are made of a flexible, hydrophilic plastic and are much easier to become accustomed to wearing; however, they are more expensive and have a shorter life span. Although they also require daily cleaning, the solutions used are more expensive and the process itself is complicated. These lenses tend to absorb aerosols, such as hair sprays, or colognes which can irritate the cornea, which decreases the likelihood of the lens popping out or being dislodged. However, when a soft lens is lost or damaged, it is extremely difficult to reproduce, and the duplicate may not be as comfortable as the initial lens.

Recently, contact lenses which can be worn for *extended* periods of time have been developed. They are quite expensive; however, the prospect of having good vision 24 hours a day is especially appealing. These lenses can be worn for weeks at a time, with a visit to the ophthamologist at specific intervals for cleaning. There is no need to remove them for either sleep or daily cleaning. Since these contact lenses are not removed every day, there is a greater risk of infection and ocular irritation.

Nursing Management

A nurse needs to know the initial instructions given so that they can be reiterated in patient teaching. The school-age child or adolescent should be responsible, motivated, and sufficiently mature to follow the instructions regarding cleaning solutions and lens care. It is important for these children and adolescents to adhere to the initial schedule developed for adapting to the wearing of contact lenses.

Because both hard and soft contact lenses require the use of a variety of solutions, care must be taken not to contaminate these liquids or eye kits. Serious eye infections can occur if proper precautions are not taken. Some of the solutions used can cause the eyes to become red or sensitive to light. It is important for these children and adolescents to know that redness, pain, photophobia, irritation, and any changes in vision are serious symptoms which need to be communicated to their physicians.

A nurse should know how to remove hard or soft contact lenses from the eyes of a patient who is unable to perform the task. Once the presence of contact lenses has been ascertained and the type worn has been identified, one can proceed to remove them. When hard contacts are present, placing both thumbs at the corners of the eyelashes with the lids open traps the lens, causing both dislodgement and ejection. Soft lenses can be removed by pulling the upper lid upward with the thumb, dislodging the lens and enabling the nurse to lift it off the cornea. The rubber bulb of a glass eye dropper also may be used. After the bulb is wet and compressed, it may be lowered onto the lens, which can be lifted up and off the cornea with gentle manual suction.

Artificial Eye

With a penetrating wound to the eye or in the presence of a malignancy, it may be necessary to remove the globe from its socket. All the extraocular muscles are cut as close as possible to the globe and then approximated with sutures to a plastic implant which permits coordinated movement with the real eye. The prosthetic conformer remains in place until the edema subsides an there is no evidence of infection in the socket.

A permanent prosthesis may be inserted as early as 3 or 4 weeks after the enucleation. The artificial eye may be made of glass or plastic. Although a glass eye lasts much longer if it is not broken, it is heavier.

Once it is in place, it is not necessary to remove the plastic prothesis for cleaning because the child's tears lubricate and cleanse the eye. If any mucus appears, the prosthesis should be cleaned thoroughly. It can be removed by pressing down on the lower lid while applying gentle pressure to the upper lid. Once it is out, the eye needs to be cleaned immediately and cautiously handled to prevent scratching its surface area. No special solutions are necessary for this procedure. The eye can soak in hot (not boiling) water for several minutes.

Wetting the artificial eye before reinserting it facilitates replacement. With the narrow portion of the shell held toward the nose, the lids are separated, the lower lid is everted while the upper lid is raised, and the prosthetic eye is slipped gently into place.

Teaching a child and the parents how to care for the artificial eye and socket is critical. If the child is young, the parents must become skillful in removing and reinserting the prosthesis. School-age children and adolescents can learn these procedures and assume the associated responsibilities. It is essential to stress thorough hand washing prior to handling the prosthesis. While some tearing can be expected, any increase in the amount, duration, or appearance needs to be reported to the ophthalmologist promptly.

Since children are active and prone to injury, safety glasses are often prescribed despite the fact that vision in the remaining eye is normal. Some anxiety may be generated, and so it is important for a nurse to explain the rationale for such a prescription. Once an enucleation is performed, it is imperative to protect the remaining eye to ensure a degree of vision for the child and successful adaptation to a minimal handicap.

Hearing Aids

Hearing is essential for language development. When a moderate or profound hearing loss is identified, the use of a hearing aid enables the infant or child to receive some sound stimuli. However, these devices are helpful only in the presence of conductive hearing loss. Sound waves are unable to reach the inner ear.

A hearing aid is used to amplify sound through the use

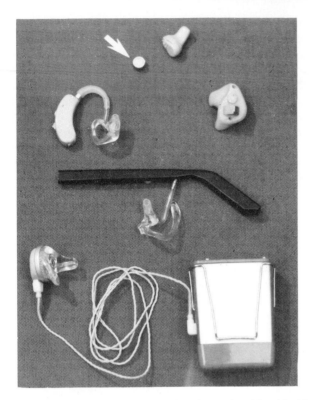

and determine whether it is in working order. The ear mold can usually be washed in warm water with mild soap. It must be dried thoroughly before being reinserted. A critical nursing function is evaluating the child's response to the hearing aid. If it has been present since infancy, the child views it as a part of himself. However, if its use is more recent, there may be some resistance to its utilization; for example, an 11-year-old girl may not use her hearing aid because of its presence behind her ear or because she does not want her friends to see her with it. The nurse may suggest that she wear her hair long to cover its placement behind her ear.

In working with hearing-impaired children who use such devices, a nurse constantly needs to be alert to situations in which the hearing aid can be damaged. For example, if x-rays are to be taken, the hearing aid should be removed because radiation can affect its function. If a child's hair is to be washed or if he wants to take a shower, the hearing aid must be removed so that it is not damaged by the water.

If the child is admitted for unrelated surgery, the hearing aid should be left in place until anesthesia has been administered. At that time, personnel in the operating room remove the aid, label it, and take it to the recovery room, where it will be kept until the child arrives. It is usually reinserted before the child is fully recovered.

The early identification of infants and children, especially those at risk, improved testing methods, and the use of hearing aids have been instrumental in decreasing the numbers of hearing-impaired children who receive no sound stimuli whatsoever. Although some causes of conductive hearing loss are preventable, educating the public continues to be a major need.

Sensory Problems in the Newborn and Infant

Ophthalmia Neonatorum

The term *ophthalmia neonatorum* refers to any acute conjunctivitis in the newborn. The most common origins are chemical, bacterial, and chlamydial. In acute conjunctivitis, the usual manifestations are tearing, discharge, conjuctival hyperemia, chemosis, papillae, pseudomembrane, and preauricular and submaxillary lymphadenopathy.

Chemical conjunctivitis is secondary to the prophylactic instillation of silver nitrate into a newborn's eyes. Hyperemia, chemosis, and discharge occur within 24 hours and last 24 to 48 hours. Treatment consists of keeping the eyes clean with sterile water irrigations.

Bacterial conjunctivitis occurs 3 or more days after birth; however, gonococcal conjunctivitis may appear as early as 2 days of age (or as late as 21 days if silver nitrate was instilled prophylactically). Gonococcal conjunctivitis is considered the most serious form of conjunctivitis because of the associated potential for blindness.

Gonorrheal conjunctivitis is usually contracted from an infected mother during the birth process. Both eyes are affected. Clinical manifestations include a profuse pu-

FIGURE 21-5 Types of hearing aids. Below is the older aid with a battery pack worn on the body and a wire connected to the ear mold. Next is the earpiece containing a battery and mold worn in the ear. Above to the left is the behind-the-ear battery with ear mold. To the right is a small ear canal mold with battery. Above is the newer smaller mold worn in the ear. The arrow identifies the smaller battery used for the newer hearing aids. *(From S.M. Lewis and I.C. Collier [eds.], Medical-Surgical Nursing, 2d ed., McGraw-Hill, New York, 1987, p. 369.)*

of a microphone. The sound waves are converted into electrical impulses and then amplified, which allows them to cross the tympanic membrane. There are four kinds of hearing aids. The most common type is placed behind the ear. Another type is designed for fitting into the frames of eyeglasses. The body type contains the power source in a case which is suspended from around the neck or kept in a pocket. The fourth type is a very small device which fits into the ear itself (Fig. 21-5). All models have batteries, volume controls, and off and on switches.

Generally, infants and children are admitted to the hospital for a variety of problems with hearing aids in place. However, it is important for a nurse to assess the child or parent's knowledge regarding the hearing aid, its maintenance, and its function as well as to examine the ear to determine the presence of irritation. Parents usually are extremely conscientious about keeping the hearing aid clean and in good working order. However, the parents of young infants may need additional anticipatory guidance, especially in regard to experimentation by the infant, who may take the hearing aid apart or mouth it.

A nurse needs to know how to care for a hearing aid, especially how to clean it, change the battery, reinsert it, rulent discharge, redness and chemosis of the conjunctiva, and edematous eyelids. If it is contracted in utero from premature rupture of the membranes, corneal ulcers may result. Diagnosis is confirmed with a positive smear and culture. Treatment consists of aqueous crystalline penicillin G, intramuscular (IM) or intravenous (IV), 100,000 U/kg/d for at least 7 days. If the gonococcal strain is penicillin-resistant, cefotaxime or gentamicin is substituted in appropriate doses. The neonate's eyes are irrigated immediately with saline, which is continued every hour to eliminate discharge. These newborns require contact isolation for at least 24 hours after appropriate therapy has been instituted. Resolution occurs within 3 to 4 days.

Occasionally gonococcal conjunctivitis has occurred in newborns given only silver nitrate prophylaxis. If the mother is known to have gonorrhea at the time of birth, the baby is given a single dose of penicillin G, IV or IM — 50,000 U for full-term and 20,000 U for low-birth-weight neonates.

Chlamydial conjunctivitis occurs 5 to 23 days after birth. It is usually unilateral and presents with a watery discharge which becomes progressively purulent. Papillae are present, and occasionally there is a pseudomembrane. It is caused by the *Chlamydia trachomatis* organism, subtypes A through K. This obligate intracellular organism which is descended from bacteria is the most common infectious cause of ophthalmia noenatorum. Diagnosis is made from a positive tissue culture and smear for inclusion bodies and for direct immunofluorescence. Treatment consists of oral erythromycin 50 mg/kg/d in four divided doses for 14 days. To avoid reinfection of the newborn, both parents must be treated. In children and adolescents, this eye infection may be acquired through inadequately chlorinated swimming pools or secondarily through sexual transmission from contaminated hands to the eyes.

Dacryostenosis, a congenital obstruction of the vasolacrimal drainage system, must be differentiated from chlamydial conjunctivitis. Neonates with dacryostenosis have constant tearing and discharge from birth, usually in one eye only. This condition generally resolves by 6 to 8 months. If resolution does not occur, the infant is referred to an ophthalmologist. Once dacryostenosis is diagnosed, parents are taught to express material from the lacrimal sac by means of massage several times a day until resolution occurs or a referral is made.

Nursing Management

In this age of early discharge from the newborn nursery, there may be problems in identifying ophthalmia neonatorum of any cause. Newborns may leave the hospital with their parents as early as 5 hours of age. The constant tearing in and discharge from the eye of a newborn with dacryostenosis may be equated with the chemical conjunctivitis resulting from silver nitrate or may not be noted. Gonorrheal conjunctivitis does not appear until 2 to 3 days of age, and chlamydial conjunctivitis occurs between 5 and 23 days of age. Thus, parents must be instructed to contact the pediatrician immediately if exudate persists beyond 2 to 3 days of age or appears after 3 days of age.

Control measures for ophthalmia neonatorum include the instillation of one of the following in each eye:
1. 1% silver nitrate solution
2. 1% tetracycline ophthalmic ointment
3. 0.5% erythromycin ointment

Prophylaxis may be delayed up to 1 hour after birth to allow for parent-newborn bonding. Silver nitrate is not effective for chlamydia. In areas where this infection is prominent, erythromycin or tetracycline ophthalmic ointment is recommended. In areas where this infection is rare, silver nitrate is the preferred prophylactic agent, particularly if *Neisseria gonorrhoeae* infections are prevalent.

To instill prophylactic agents, each eyelid is wiped gently, using sterile cotton. Then two drops of silver nitrate solution or one or two ribbons of ophthalmic ointment are put in the lower conjunctival sac of each eye. To spread the ointment, the eyelids are massaged gently. After 1 minute, excess solution or ointment is wiped away with sterile cotton.

Newborns who subsequently develop gonorrheal conjunctivitis are hospitalized and treated as described above. Contact isolation consists of the following:
1. Placing the baby in a private room or sharing a room with others who have the same infection
2. Having personnel wear masks if they will be in close contact with the newborn
3. Using gowns if soiling is likely
4. Washing the hands after touching the neonate or after touching potentially contaminated articles and before giving care to another baby
5. Discarding contaminated articles or preparing reusable articles for decontamination according to hospital policy
6. Teaching parents contact isolation

Parents should be reassured that prompt and adequate treatment results in a complete cure.

Infections of the Ear

The most common ear problem in infants and children is *otitis media,* a middle ear infection and effusion. Several factors must be considered in order to understand this condition. It involves a system which includes several components: nares, nasopharynx, eustachian tube, middle ear, and mastoid air cells. The eustachian tube connects the middle ear with the posterior nasopharynx. Its lining is continuous from the nares to the middle ear cleft. Infants have a shorter, wider tube which forms a relatively straight line, while in older children the angle is more acute. The three physiological functions of the eustachian tube were enumerated above under Physiology of the Ear. If any one of the three is compromised, the usual result is effusion and infection of the middle ear. Ventilation of the middle ear is accomplished through swallowing and yawning. Reflux of nasopharyngeal secretions into the middle ear is apt to occur with swallowing when supine. A little-understood eustachian tube dysfunction is present in children who have otitis media. Whether reflux or dysfunction is the precipitating factor, otitis media may result as fluid persists in the middle ear. The following precipitating factors are also considered:

1. Age—more common in the first 2 years of life
2. Sex—more common in males
3. Familial predisposition—more common in children with a family history in parents and siblings
4. Socioeconomic status—more prevalent among the poor
5. Season of the year—higher incidence during cold months

In addition, infants who have cleft palate and those who have Down's syndrome are more apt to have otitis media than are those in the general population. Respiratory infection with respiratory syncytial virus, influenza virus A or B, and adenovirus may be associated with acute otitis media. Generally, the younger the child is at the time of the first attack, the greater the number of episodes of otitis media that are expected.

The most common causative agents of otitis media in all age groups are *Streptococcus pneumoniae* and *H. influenzae.* Other organisms less commonly recovered from middle ear exudate include group A beta-hemolytic streptococcus, *Staphylococcus aureus, N. catarrhalis,* and various gram-negative bacilli (*Escherichia coli, Klebsiella pneumoniae, Pseudomonas aeruginosa,* and various *Proteus* species).

Otitis media is generally subdivided into two types: *acute suppurative* and *nonsuppurative.* Synonyms for nonsuppurative otitis media in common usage are secretory otitis media, serous otits media, otitis media with effusion, glue ear, and catarrhal otitis media. Nonsuppurative otitis media may precede or follow the suppurative form. The clinical manifestations of both may be similar, subtle, or absent. A definite diagnosis of suppurative versus nonsuppurative can be established only after culture of the middle ear effusion (as accomplished through a myringotomy).

Clinical findings are variable and nonspecific. Infants may present with all or several combinations of the following: irritability, crying spells, sleeping difficulties, diarrhea, feeding problems, tugging or rubbing the ear, high fever, rhinitis, and cough. Older children may have rhinitis and cough, irritability, loss of hearing, or ear pain. Otoscopic examination of the tympanic membrane (TM) reveals abnormalities, but there is no agreement by physicians on what is diagnostic. Findings include hyperemia (but the TM may be gray or orange); bulging, as denoted by partial or complete obscuration of the bony landmarks; absence of the light reflex; and impaired mobility of the drum. The constant, most critical features are fluid behind the eardrum and diminished mobility as determined by pneumatic otoscopy.

Paradise (1980) delineated the difficulties in distinguishing suppurative from nonsuppurative otitis media. In suppurative otitis media, the contour of the eardrum ranges from normal to bulging; its color may be red, pale yellow, or white; its luster is variable; its light reflex may be present or absent; it may be translucent early in the disease process but is generally opaque (or at times an air-fluid level is noted); and mobility is generally decreased. In nonsuppurative otitis media, the contour ranges from retracted to normal to slightly bulging; the color may be pink, grayish white, amber, or bluish; the luster is variable; the light reflex may be present or absent; the eardrum is usually opaque but may demonstrate an air-fluid level; and its mobility is impaired. Impedence testing after 6 months of age is used by some physicians to confirm the presence of middle ear effusion (see Common Screening and Diagnostic Tests above).

Occasionally, an infant or child will present with exudate in the external canal. A typical history for an infant is that he was irritable and having sleep disturbances but suddenly was quiet and slept well, and drainage was discovered on the crib sheet. The history for an older child is that he complained of severe ear pain and subsequently fell asleep; drainage was discovered on the pillowcase in the morning. Both are indicative of a ruptured TM.

Rupture of the tympanic membrane must be distinguished from *otitis externa,* which is an infection of the skin of the external canal. Differences include age, time of year, and causative organism. Otitis externa is seen frequently in children from 5 years of age through young adulthood. It is especially common in the summertime, affecting many children who spend a great deal of time swimming. Generally, the ear canal is swollen and discharges a purulent exudate. Common organisms include *staphylococcus, Pseudomonas,* and other gram-negative bacteria.

Treatment consists of instillation of an acidic solution containing polymyxin or neomycin. In severe cases corticosteroids are used to reduce the inflammatory process. When the child is swimming, earplugs are recommended after an initial episode. A simple prophylactic measure is the instillation of 2 or 3 drops of white vinegar (5% acetic acid) before and after swimming.

In the absence of myringotomy or before its results are known, antibiotic therapy is instituted (Table 21-7). If a culture of the middle ear effusion has been done, specific antibiotics sensitive to the offending organism are used. Decongestants are of questionable value, although some physicians believe that they improve tubal drainage and ventilation. Acetaminophen 10 mg/kg every 4 hours may be given for pyrexia. Criteria for myringotomy (incising the TM) vary with physicians. A constant criterion is lack of response to antibiotic therapy in 48 to 72 hours. Other criteria include evidence of severe earache which requires immediate relief, a critically ill child, and a child with compromised defenses.

Infants and children with spontaneously ruptured TMs must be treated with antibiotics. In nonsuppurative otitis media, children who have not recently been treated are usually given a 10-day to 2-week course of antimicrobial therapy. Children who are prone to several ear infections per year may be placed on sulfisoxazole or ampicillin twice a day prophylactically, particularly during the cold months of the year.

If effusion persists, tympanometry should be done.

NURSING CARE PLAN

21-1 *The Child with Otitis Media*

Clinical Problem/Nursing Diagnosis	Expected Outcome	Nursing Interventions
Ear pain<hr>Pain related to infected tympanic membrane	Child's pain will be alleviated, and he will be able to interact with environment in comfort	Assess degree and location of pain Observe for ear tugging Administer antibiotics, ear drops, and analgesics as ordered Teach parents proper medication, administration techniques, side effects, and time schedule Assess effectiveness of analgesics and antibiotics; note ability of child to sleep and play regularly
Fever and/or irritability<hr>Hyperthermia (temperature 38.5°C)	Child's temperature will return to normal (37.5°C)	Monitor temperature for elevation Report temperature >38.5°C Properly administer antibiotics and/or antipyretics as ordered Gradually decrease body temperature Administer tepid sponge; with fever, avoid shivering Assess for clinical signs and symptoms of febrile seizure activity (maintain adequate airway; ensure child's safety; enforce seizure precautions; administer anticonvulsants if ordered) Comfort and support child through interventions; involve parents to increase sense of security
Hearing impairment Vertigo<hr>Sensory/perceptual alteration (auditory)	Child's normal hearing sensation and vestibular function will be preserved	Assess signs and symptoms of hearing loss (changes in behavior, responsiveness to voice and noise from toys) Support child through auditory testing during hospitalization Teach parents to detect early signs of otitis media (ear tugging) to ensure prompt treatment Encourage parents to avoid putting child to sleep with bottle to decrease likelihood of further infections
Suppurative complications (mastoiditis, meningitis, brain abscess)<hr>Potential for infection	Child will be protected from life-threatening sequelae through control of infection	Closely monitor vital signs for subtle changes Monitor for signs of sepsis (fever, lethargy, increased irritability, hypotention, neck stiffness, etc.) Assess for signs of mastoiditis (persistent purulent drainage and enlarged lymph nodes) Assess for signs of brain abscess (formation (fever, abnormal facial neurological exam, seizure activity)

Children whose TMs have reduced compliance, as recorded on the tympanogram, are further evaluated for the use of tympanostomy tubes. Although the tubes allow immediate drainage of fluid in the middle ear and improved hearing, there are possible drawbacks. Since the middle ear and mastoid air cells no longer form a closed chamber, the eustachian tube's protective function may be compromised in that nasopharyngeal secretions can enter the middle ear. Use of tympanostomy tubes has become widely accepted in nonsuppurative otitis media, but indications for their use, long-term benefits, and possible hazards have not been established. The tubes generally stay in place for 6 to 7 months.

Middle ear effusion is accompanied and/or followed by mild to moderate hearing loss for variable periods. Regardless of whether the hearing deficit is transient or permanent, language skills suffer when the child's ability to hear is compromised. Indeed, Teele et al (1984) found a strong association between time spent with middle ear effusions in the first 6 months of life and speech and language delay at 3 years of age. Whether it will persist through later years is not known. Hence, the detection and treatment of middle ear effusion is imperative to the child's development. Any child who has had even one episode should have periodic audiometric follow-up.

Although mastoiditis, an inflammation of the mastoid air cells, was a common complication in the preantibiotic era, it is now relatively rare. It can occur when a perforated eardrum is not recognized (and thus the child is not treated for otitis media), when there is inadequate treatment of a child with otitis media, and when follow-up appointments for evaulation of progress are not kept. Mastoiditis may be acute or chronic in nature.

In *acute mastoiditis,* the child has a history of draining ears, redness, severe pain, fever, and retroauricular swelling. In the *chronic stage*, the child has a history of perforated eardrum with draining over a period of time and mastoid infections. Conductive hearing loss is common, and surgery usually is necessary (mastoidectomy and tympanoplasty with reconstruction of the eardrum and the hearing apparatus of the middle ear). Early recognition of tympanic perforation, adequate treatment of otitis media, and diligent follow-up of these children by the clinic nurse or community health nurse can further decrease the incidence of this complication.

Nursing Management

Generally, children with ear infections are treated in ambulatory settings. Nurses in these settings need to help parents understand the mechanisms by which otitis media can occur. Knowing that the lining of the eustachian tube is continuous from the nares to the middle ear cleft, the nurse should explain that for some children, an episode of nasopharyngitis will be accompanied by otitis media. It probably occurs more frequently in infants and young children because the angle of the eustachian tube is less acute at that age. The nurse should ask in what position the infant is fed and should explain that reflux of nasopharyngeal secretions or of formula into the middle ear can occur when the infant swallows while supine. The nurse should also emphasize the importance of giving antibiotics as prescribed in order to maintain adequate blood levels and to ensure an adequate treatment course. She should explain the side effects of the chosen antibiotics (Table 21-7). Parents should be instructed not to discontinue medications if side effects occur but to call the primary provider, who will assess the situation. Parents also need to know the relationship between the child's ability to hear and language development. They should be instructed to call the primary provider if the child does not show improvement in 2 to 3 days. The importance of keeping the follow-up appointment in 10 days to 2 weeks in order to evaluate progress is stressed. If tympanocentesis, tympanometry, audiometry, or tympanostomy tubes are prescribed, reasons for their need and a description of the procedure should be offered.

Nasopharyngitis

Acute nasopharyngitis (the common cold) involves the nasopharynx, the accessory paranasal sinuses, and frequently the middle ear. Although the causative agent includes a large number of viruses, the principal ones are rhinoviruses. The incubation period is 12 to 72 hours, and the infectious period lasts from a few hours before to 24 to 48 hours after symptoms have appeared. It is transmitted by droplet infection. Predisposing factors are suspected to be teething, poor nutrition, chilling, exposure to dampness and cold, degree of susceptibility and resistance, and allergy.

Clinical manifestations in infants and young children differ from those in older children. Before 3 months of age, infants are usually afebrile. Children above 3 years of age usually have low-grade fever and are more prone to persistent sinusitis. Infants over 3 months of age are febrile, often as high as 38.9 to 40°C (102 to 104°F). Sneezing, irritability, and restlessness are common. Within a few hours, nasal discharge appears. Nasal obstruction interferes with sucking during feedings. The eardrums may be

TABLE 21-7 Antibiotics for Children Who Have Acute Otitis Media

Drug	Indications	Action	Method	Dosage	Side Effects
Amoxicillin	Acute otitis media (AOM) caused by susceptible strains of gram-positive and gram-negative organisms	Bacterial	Orally	50 mg/kg/d q 8 h Maximum dose <40 kg: 375 mg tid Maximum dose >40 kg: 500 mg tid	Anemia, eosinophilia, leukopenia, thrombocytopenia, thrombocytopenic purpura, nausea, vomiting, diarrhea, erythematous maculopapular rash, urticaria, overgrowth of nonsusceptible organisms Anaphylaxis: fever and chills Interactions: bacteriostatic antibiotics (amoxicillin given at least 1 h before chloramphenicol, erythromycin, and tetracycline)
Cefaclor	AOM due to *Haemophilus influenzae, Sreptococcus pneumoniae, Escherichia coli, Pseudomonas mirabilis, Klebsiella,* and staphylococci	Bactericidal	Orally	40 mg to 50 mg/kg/d q 8 h (not to exceed 1 g/d)	Anemia, eosinophilia, transient leukopenia, lymphocytosis, dizziness, headache, nausea, vomiting, diarrhea, anorexia, overgrowth of *Monilia,* maculopapular rash, hypersensitivity, fever

Source: G. M. Scipien et al. (eds.), *Comprehensive Pediatric Nursing,* 3d ed., McGraw-Hill, New York, 1986, p. 1384.　　　　*Continued.*

TABLE 21-7 Antibiotics for Children Who Have Acute Otitis Media—cont'd

Drug	Indications	Action	Method	Dosage	Side Effects
Erythromycin in combination with sulfisox-azole	AOM due to suscep-tible strains of *H. influenzae*	Bacteriostatic	Orally	Erythromycin: 50 mg/kg/d q 6 h Sulfisoxazole: 150 mg/kg/d q 6 h	Erythromycin: (see Chap. 23) Sulfisoxazole: agranulocytosis, aplastic anemia, purpura, erythema multiforme, gener-alized skin eruptions, epider-mal necrolysis, exfoliative dermatitis, urticaria, pruritis, photosensitivity, abdominal pain, nausea, vomiting, diar-rhea, anorexia, headache, convulsions, toxicnephrosis, serum sickness, drug fever
Sulfamethoxazole-trimethoprim	AOM due to suscep-tible strains of *H. influenzae* and *S. pneumoniae*	Bacteriostatic	Orally	40 mg sulfa per kg/d (8 mg trimethoprim) q 12 h or <10 kg: ½ tsp q 12 h 10-15 kg: 1 tsp q 12 h 15-20 kg: 1½ tsp q 12 h >20 kg: 2 tsp q 12 h	Agranulocytosis, aplastic ane-mia, hemolytic anemia, mega-loblastic anemia, leukopenia, thrombocytopenia, nausea, vomiting, diarrhea, anorexia, abdominal pain, stomatitis, headache, convulsions, toxic nephrosis, skin manifestations as with sulfisoxazole, hyper-sensitivity, serum sickness, drug fever, jaundice

congested for 2 or 3 days. Since infants react systemically to infection, vomiting and diarrhea may be present.

Treatment consists of antipyretics for fever, malaise, and irritability; tepid-water sponge baths for fever over 39.4°C (103°F); fluids at frequent intervals; and saline nose drops. Use of Neo-Synephrine nose drops has de-creased, particularly for children in the first 8 months of life. They supply short-term relief but cause a rebound vasoconstriction, thus increasing congestion. The result is a chemical rhinitis. If prescribed, they should be used sparingly. Oil-base drops are never given, since they may be aspirated and cause lipid pneumonia. Nose drops are never given for more than 4 or 5 days. Overuse of nose drops can irritate the nasal mucosa.

Nursing Management

Unless complications such as febrile convulsions and su-perimposed infection ensue, infants are treated on an am-bulatory basis. Therefore, the nurse's role is mainly one of teaching and counseling the parents. Parents must under-stand how to give the exact amount of antipyretic and nose drops and at what times. They need to know how and when to give a tepid-water sponge bath. The nurse should discuss the importance of fluids, prevention of ex-coriation of the skin due to exudate, and prevention of secondary infection. Parents should also be alerted to the signs and symptoms of complications and urged to call if any appear.

Sensory Problems in the Toddler
Strabismus (Squint, "Crossed Eyes")

Eye movement is controlled by the muscles of the eye, and any imbalance in extraocular muscles results in one or both eyes deviating rather than functioning as a unit; this condition is known as *strabismus*. In early infancy movements of the eye bear little relationship to one an-other; however, by the sixth month convergence should be established.

There are several types of strabismus. *Internal strabis-mus* (convergent, also called *esotropia*) results in the eye turning inward. It may be congenital (established by 4 to 6 months of age) or acquired (noted between 18 months and 4 years of age). In order for the child to see more clearly, he must accommodate, and in doing so conver-gence results. Most children are farsighted (hyperopic), requiring greater accommodation, hence the frequency of this type of strabismus. *External strabismus* (divergent, also called *exotropia*) occurs when the eye turns "out" and may be intermittent (onset in infancy) or constant (later onset). Exotropia is associated with little or no re-fractive error. *Vertical strabismus* may be hypertropic, when the eye is above the visual axis, or hypotropic, when the eye is below the visual axis. These children have ocular deviations as a result of overactive or under-active oblique and vertical rectus bulbi muscles.

Amblyopia, or the loss of vision without any apparent organic cause, can occur in the deviating eye when one eye is preferred. If it is not corrected by age 6 years, the visual deficit is permanent.

Refractive errors are a major cause of strabismus. The high degree of hyperopia in children gives rise to the overconvergence which results in convergent strabismus. Conversely, myopia is responsible for an underconvergence and divergent strabismus. Corneal scarring, cataracts, and optic atrophy all interfere with vision, interrupt fusion, and result in strabismus.

Treatment may entail any one or all four of the of the following. After an eye examination, glasses may be prescribed to correct the refractive error and control the excessive accommodation. The eye will then be in a better position to develop binocular vision. In addition, strong miotics may be prescribed to produce peripheral rather than central accommodation, thereby lessening convergence. The second step in treatment may include an occlusion of the straight eye with elastic tape, forcing the squinting eye into activity. The third step may involve orthoptic training, with exercises especially devised for these children to perform. This ocular physical therapy is concerned with restoring binocular function or assisting in its development. The last option is surgery. One of two types of procedures may be employed. When a *resection* is done, the extraocular muscles are shortened, while a *recession* refers to a lengthening of these muscles.

Nursing Management

Successful treatment of a child with strabismus is related to the teaching of parents and children. The care is long term and necessitates office or clinic visits every 6 to 12 months for several years.

If glasses are prescribed, children should be taught how to care for them and how to clean them. If they break, replacement is imperative. Some children may need encouragement to wear these prescription lenses. Patients with occlusive patches should wear them constantly during the 6- or 8-week period in which they will be utilized. If they become loose or are removed, they too should be replaced immediately. Since the parents and children may not understand the rationale, a nurse should spend time explaining why the "straight," good eye is patched, and her comments should focus on improving the amblyopia. The teacher should be contacted so that he or she knows why the child's schoolwork may be substandard initially.

When all conservative efforts to correct the strabismus have not been as successful as desired by the ophthalmologist, surgery may be performed. Surgery usually is done in a day surgery facility. Preoperative teaching includes preparing the child for eye patches (if they are used by the surgeon) and restraints in the recovery room. The child may engage in normal activities upon his return home. Children who attend day care, preschool, or elementary school may resume attendance in 1 week.

Parents are taught to instill eye drops or ointments as prescribed. The importance of follow-up appointments is stressed, since the aim is to prevent recurrence of amblyopia and to determine the need for further surgery.

Foreign Bodies in the Eye

A child knows when particles of wood, sand, plastic, or paper enter the eye because the discomfort is immediate. Most *conjunctival foreign bodies* can be removed easily after everting the upper lid and locating the object. A moist cotton-tipped applicator may be used to snatch the particle from the conjunctiva. The eye also can be flushed with a saline solution. Foreign bodies can be removed without any damage to vision.

Corneal foreign bodies are more difficult to remove. They are painful, they cause lacrimation, and children persistently complain of a scratchy sensation whenever the eye is moved. They are potentially more serious than foreign bodies which are confined to the conjunctiva. If relief is not achieved by irrigating the eye or using a moistened applicator, the child should be seen immediately by an ophthalmologist.

Nursing Management

A young child who has "something in his eye" needs reassurance that the foreign body will be removed; however, a degree of cooperation is necessary. As a last resort, the child is restrained with the help of parents. Most of these particles of dust or eyelashes can be retrieved with a moistened applicator or gentle flushing with saline.

If the pain and discomfort continue, the child should be seen promptly by an ophthalmologist, who can confirm the presence of a corneal foreign body using fluorescein stain. A wide-spectrum ophthalmic antibiotic is prescribed, and parents need instruction in its administration. An eye patch may be necessary if the child is young and does not refrain from rubbing the eye. With the surface area of corneal epithelium abraded, there is a potential for infection; therefore, parents should be instructed to return the child to the clnic or doctor's office 24 hours after the incident so that the eye can be reexamined.

Foreign Bodies in the Ear

Young children may place a variety of objects within the external auditory canal, including beads, erasers, pebbles, and food. A playmate may also be the culprit. Whether it is accidental or purposeful is irrelevant, for it is a foreign body and may result in certain clinical manifestations.

The object may be identified readily, or weeks may go by before its presence is known. Insects within the ear cause a great deal of noise and discomfort, and as a result they are easily and frequently found. While a rough-edged plastic object may damage the ear, substances of a vegetal source (pea, bean) tend to swell and set up a local inflammatory response which results in deafness. An obstruction may also be caused by an overaccumulation of cerumen.

A complaint of deafness may be the first indication of the presence of a foreign body. Pain and cellulitis are other clinical manifestations, especially if the object is vegetal in nature.

Foreign bodies should not be removed by anyone other than a physician. If a person is not skilled in performing this procedure, additional damage to the ear may occur. Unless it is clearly visible and within easy reach and unless the patient is cooperative, the object is removed under anesthesia with forceps. It is essential the object be identified before treatment is begun. Cerumen is most easily removed after a solution of hydrogen peroxide or sodium bicarbonate is instilled to soften the wax and then the auditory canal is irrigated with warm water. Instilling oil or water drowns the insect, and irrigations remove it from the canal. Other objects such as rubber or beads may be removed by instilling oil or soap and then irrigating the auditory canal. Irrigating vegetabal objects such as a bean or pea should be avoided because the irrigating solution may be absorbed, increasing the object's size.

Nursing Management

A nurse may become involved in irrigating the auditory canal, and it is important that the patient's cooperation be obtained through a simple explanation. Restraints may be necessary for the child's safety. Syringing is done with a 20-ml syringe. A soft No. 5 or No. 8 rubber catheter is an effective device to use, because it decreases the possibility of injury. A commercially manufactured ear irrigation machine may also be used. Ear drops are usually prescribed and should be instilled properly. An important aspect of caring for these children is teaching the patient to refrain from placing objects in his ear. He in turn may be responsible for teaching his playmate to refrain from performing the identical act.

Foreign Bodies in the Nose

Through exploration, toddlers discover that small objects can be placed in the nostrils. Such *foreign bodies* include erasers, pebbles, cherry stones, beads, nuts, and paper wads. Rarely is any small object pushed deeply into the nostril by the child. Initially it is anterior and not forced farther unless parents, the child, or other unskilled people push it deeper in their efforts to remove it.

If the mother is unaware that her toddler has placed a foreign body in his nose, her first clue may be his complaint of soreness when his nose is touched. He may also have local obstruction and sneezing due to irritation. *Hygroscopic bodies,* such as peas and peanuts, increase in size

as they absorb fluid. These objects cause discomfort soon after placement in a nostril. Smooth, hard objects which are hygroscopic may not produce symptoms for weeks or months or may cause swelling and obstruction through mucosal irritation. If infection ensues, a purulent, malodorous, or even bloody discharge is noted. Whenever a child complains of or presents with unilateral nasal obstruction and discharge, a foreign body should be suspected as the causative agent. Examination with a nasal speculum or nasoscope confirms the diagnosis.

Removal is accomplished promptly to prevent aspiration and local tissue necrosis. After the instillation of a local anesthetic, the object is removed with either forceps or a nasal suction apparatus. Infection disappears shortly, and usually no other treatment is needed. Some pediatricians have found that a foreign object may be moved into the anterior nasal chamber for easy removal by occluding the unobstructed nostril with the finger and blowing into the mouth, as in cardiopulmonary resuscitation.

Nursing Management

Nurses providing routine well-child care should alert mothers to the toddler's bent for placing small objects in his nose as he explores his body in relation to his environment and discuss methods of prevention. Mothers should be aware of the signs and symptoms produced by these foreign bodies and realize the importance of having a physician remove them before necrosis occurs or the object is aspirated into the lower respiratory tract. Nurses should be aware of signs and symptoms so that appropriate and immediate referral is made for removal of the foreign object.

Periorbital Cellulitis

Periorbital cellulitis is a serious inflammatory problem because the infectious process can affect the eye or the central nervous system. Frequently, the eyelids and adjacent structures are involved. There is pain, tenderness, and edema (especially of the eyelids), and sometimes there is conjunctivitis as well as drainage from a wound in the area. While the swelling is not clearly demarcated, it has a very distinctive magenta discoloration. The child may also have a concurrent upper respiratory infection or otitis media.

The most common causative organism in children under 5 years of age is *H. influenzae* type B. With a history of trauma and a break in the skin, *S. aureus* and group A beta-hemolytic streptococcus are suspected causes. A variety of cultures (nose, eye, blood) are done in order to identify the specific microorganism; however, vigorous intravenous antibiotic therapy is instituted until the results of these cultures are obtained. Antibiotic sensitivity test also are done to facilitiate the solution of the most effective drug. Other diagnostic tests which may be used are x-ray of the chest, orbit, and sinuses and ultrasound and computerized axial tomography (CAT) scan of the orbit.

Nursing Management

These infants and toddlers are admitted as emergencies, without any preparation for hospitalization. In addition, the affected eye is so edematous that it is closed and very painful to the child. A parent can be very helpful in assisting providers in obtaining various cultures and starting intravenous therapy. Since most of these children are very young, four-point restraints may be necessary to ensure the maintenance of the intravenous line, especially when the parents are not present.

The major thrust of treating a child with periobital cellulitis focuses on the administration of prescribed antibiotics. They must be prepared properly and administered at the times ordered so that drug blood levels can be maintained, thereby maximizing their therapeutic effect. The results of antibiotic treatment are dramatic, with the

NURSING CARE PLAN

21-2 The Child with Periorbital Cellulitis

Clinical Problem/Nursing Diagnosis	Expected Outcome	Nursing Interventions
Congestion of eyelids, edema, erythema, discomfort, and irritability Pain related to bacterial infection	Child's pain will be alleviated Child will be able to rest and sleep in comfort	Document location and severity of edema: note degree of eye opening Assess child for signs of proptosis Apply local warm packs to affected site q 2 h Discourage child from rubbing eye Properly administer antibiotics and/or analgesics as prescribed
Fever Hyperthermia (temperature 38.5°C) related to bacterial infection	Child's temperature will return to 37.5°C	Assess eye for drainage; note amount, color, and consistency of drainage Obtain culture for C + S Monitor temperature q 2 h; notify physician of temperature of 38.5°C Administer antipyretics as ordered Document effectiveness of antipyretic measures Properly administer antibiotics (accurate dose and time schedule) Institute other cooling methods (tepid baths, loose clothing, fluids, cool room)
Risk for complications: systemic infection (headaches, stiff neck, nasal drainage, tachycardia, and hypotension) Potential for infection (secondary) related to localized infectious process	Child's vital signs will be stable, indicative of absence of secondary infection	Monitor vital signs and neurological status q 4 h Assess for clinical signs of systemic infection (lethargy, irritability, fever, change in vital signs, increased heart rate hypo/hypertention, increased respiratory rate); report above findings promptly to physician
Visual impairment Sensory/perceptual alteration (visual) related to infection	Child's visual acuity will remain intact	Assess child for changes in behavior (ability to track toys and objects; abiity to maintain appropriate eye contact) Assess pupillary reflexes; EOM's with vital signs Support child through ophthalmologic examinations
Anxiety and withdrawal Anxiety related to unfamiliar environment and experiences of hospitalization	Child will receive support and comfort from parents and providers Child will express his feelings through medical play	Encourage parents to participate in child's care Comfort child after painful procedures, e.g., IV heplock placement Provide child with security object (favorite toy or blanket) Encourage child to work through traumatic experiences in medical play (place IV in doll, draw blood from doll, etc.)

edema subsiding and the child able to open the eye in 24 to 36 hours. The magenta discoloration persists for several days. The eyelid and surrounding facial area become very dry and start to peel. A nurse can apply a very thin layer of petrolatum jelly to the upper lid and to the affected cheek and forehead.

Some hospital policies require isolation until culture results are obtained. In these cases, parents and other visitors need to be told why these measures are being instituted and what protocol they should follow during a visit. When they understand, compliance is not an issue.

Sensory Problems in the Preschooler
Refractive Errors

The extent of visual impairment can be diagnosed by an ophthalmologist, regardless of the infant or young child's age or occupation, with a retinoscopic examination in which the refractive state of an eye can be determined (Fig. 21-6). The examination is facilitated with the use of cycloplegic drugs (atropine, scopolamine, homatropine, or cyclopentolate), which eliminate the ability of the eye to accommodate.

FIGURE 21-6 An ophthalmologist examines a preschooler's eyes. *(Courtesy of Media Center, Eunice K. Shriver Center for Mental Retardation, Inc., Waltham, Mass. From G.M. Scipien et al. [eds.], Comprehensive Pediatric Nursing, 3d ed., McGraw-Hill, New York, 1986, p. 1392.)*

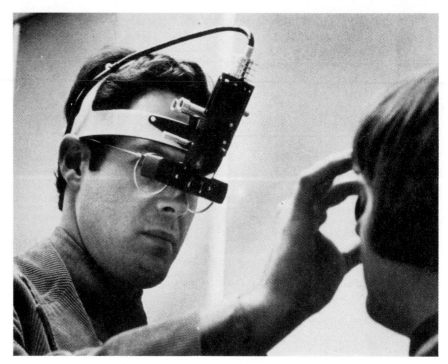

FIGURE 21-7 Hyperopia and myopia. *(From G.M. Scipien et al. [eds.], Comprehensive Pediatric Nursing, 3d ed., McGraw-Hill, New York, 1986, p. 1392.)*

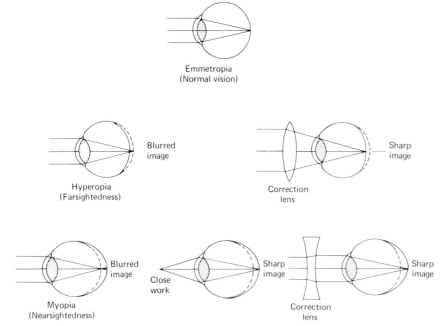

Hyperopia (Farsightedness)

Hyperopia is a refractive error in which parallel rays of light focus behind the retina (Fig. 21-7). In these situations distance vision is usually better than close vision. Hyperopia is common in all infants and normal for most children. As a child grows, the eye also grows slightly, and the hyperopia diminishes; however, in some instances farsightedness persists into adulthood.

The child may be symptom-free or complain of frontal headaches with pain which localizes over one eye. Frequently there is squinting to "see better" or a toy or book is held up close to the eyes while the child is being examined.

Glasses are usually prescribed to correct the refractive error. If distance vision is impaired, glasses should be worn at all times. In some instances the child's symptoms are those of insufficient accommodation for close work, and glasses may be prescribed for reading only.

Myopia (Nearsightedness)

Myopia is a refractive error in which parallel rays of light focus in front of the retina (Fig. 21-7). Myopic children usually see well when doing close work and have difficulty viewing objects in the distance. The cause is an increased anterioposterior diameter of the eye. It is frequently diagnosed at the start of school when the teacher notices that the child cannot see the blackboard from the back of the room.

Prescription eyeglasses are corrective, and children should be encouraged to use them to learn what good vision is. Since there is some resistance to wearing glasses, they should be used in the classroom; however, whether they are worn during play activities is a decision the child should make.

Astigmatism

When there is an irregular curvature of the anterior surface of the cornea which results in an aspheric surface, the entering rays of light are not regularly refracted and astigmatism is present. When an astigmatic child looks at the symbol + and focuses on the vertical bar, the horizontal bar will not be in focus. Conversely, when he focuses on the horizontal bar, the vertical bar will not be clear. Uncorrected astigmatism causes squinting, burning, and fatigue. These children have an intense dislike for prolonged close work. Eyeglasses are usually prescribed. In some instances visual improvement is not obtained with the use of glasses, and contact lenses, which act by neutralizing the irregularity of the corneal surface, may be indicated.

Nursing Management

Many children with refractive errors are diagnosed early, but the nurse who observes children may identify a previously unrecognized visual problem. In the course of meeting other health needs, parents may ask about the use of medications, exercises, or vitamins which may improve the visual acuity of their children. None of these measures are effective in hyperopia, myopia, and astigmatism, and parents should be advised accordingly. These conditions necessitate prescription lenses, and parents as well as children must understand that they are to be worn appropriately. In general, contact lenses are not recommended until adolescence because of economic and maturity factors. Since these problems are long-term, regular clinic or office visits—every 6 to 12 months—should be encouraged.

Trauma to the Eye

Blows to the eyeball by blunt objects such as stones, baseballs, and fists may cause damage which ranges from pain to severe intraocular destruction. Corneal abrasions may occur from paper, tree branches, or fingernails. In addition, defective aluminum twist-off caps on soft drink bottles can inflict serious injuries (Editorial Staff, 1984).

A common result of such a blow is hemorrhage into the anterior chamber, a condition known as *hyphema.*

Most hyphemas occupy less than one-third of the anterior chamber. Absorption occurs in 1 week, and the child suffers no serious consequences. Children who have a small hyphema, i.e., one that fills less than 25 percent of the anterior chamber, can be treated at home. The injured eye is patched, and the child is placed on bed rest with limited ambulation. A child who has a larger hyphema is hospitalized and placed on complete bed rest for 5 to 7 days. The affected eye is patched, and the child cannot engage in any activity which requires near accommodation, e.g., reading (Apt and Gaffney, 1987). Three to 5 days after the injury, a second hemorrhage which tends to be more severe than the initial episode may occur. Thus these children require careful, ongoing evaluation. If rebleeding is not evident after 5 days, limited ambulation is begun. Ongoing long-term follow-up is important, since glaucoma or cataracts can develop years after such accidents.

Nursing Management

A child who has received a blunt injury which results in hyphema is placed on bed rest, with a unilateral eye patch in place. Ophthalmic topical steroids and dilating medications are given as frequently as every 2 hours. It is important to adhere to the eye medication schedules to maximize their effectiveness. The injury is very painful, the eyelid is very edematous, and the child may be uncooperative when the prescribed medications have to be instilled. The assistance of another nurse may be necessary. When the eye patch is removed, the eye must be evaluated, especially in regard to any edema or drainage (color, amount, consistency) which is present as well as overall responses to treatment. These children are afraid of losing their sight; therefore, support, reassurance, and presence are critical nursing functions. They usually are sedated, and whenever possible they should be in a quiet environment, away from the activity of a nurses' station, in a room with dimmed lighting. An important consideration is the type of diversional activity in which to involve the child. Those types which do not require near accommodation, such as word games, story telling, visiting with peers, and listening to a radio, are appropriate. These children also need a primary nurse who allows them to vent their feelings and express their fears and who explains all aspects of the treatments they receive. The need for follow-up visits is an important issue in discussions with the child or parents because of complications (glaucoma, cataract) which may develop at a later date. Their early identification is essential to effective treatment.

Trauma to the Nose

Trauma to the nose may occur as a result of a fall, an auto accident, being hit by a baseball, or colliding with another person. While the fractures are severe, they are easily reduced. The cosmetic damage done tends to become more apparent in adolescence if it is not reduced at the time of the accident.

Almost all external fractures of the nose have an associated subluxation, a fracture of the nasal septum, or both.

Since fractures may occlude one side of the nares, breathing is difficult; rhinitis and chronic sinusitis may develop. If the bone is displaced, a physician reduces the fracture by applying pressure to the convex surface of the nose with one or both thumbs.

Common symptoms of trauma to the nose are epistaxis, edema, and ecchymosis. While bleeding is associated with hemophilia, rheumatic fever, or purpura, it is also present when an injury has been severe enough to fracture the nose. If a nosebleed occurs, the child is placed in an upright, forward position and instructed to stop talking and to breathe through his mouth. The nose is compressed between the nurse's fingers for 15 to 20 minutes. It is important that the pressure applied be adequate and constant in order to be effective. After the blood flow has stopped, ice packs can be applied over the bridge of the nose. Cotton plugs with petrolatum may be inserted into the nares to remain there for about 4 hours if a small amount of bleeding persists.

If bleeding continues, a physician may insert cotton pledgets saturated with vasoconstrictors such as phenylephrine and epinephrine (1:1000) into the nares in an effort to control the bleeding. If bleeding persists, nasal packing may be necessary. Generally, prophylactic antibiotics are given.

Nursing Management

When the child is brought to the emergency room, it is important for the nurse to obtain an accurate history regarding the circumstances of the injury and the symptoms that the child is experiencing. An x-ray may be needed, particularly if edema is present. If the child has a septal hematoma, drainage and packing may be done to prevent the formation of an abscess and damage to the septal cartilage. If reduction is needed, edema must have subsided sufficiently (about 3 to 5 days) for the physician to evaluate the extent of deviation. During nosebleeds, children may swallow blood, producing nausea and precipitating the vomiting of "coffee-ground" material. The nurse needs to reassure the child and parents and explain what is happening.

In addition to trauma causing nosebleeds, young children may initiate hemorrhage by picking their noses and rupturing distended vessels in the anterior, inferior section of the nasal septum. Applying liberal amounts of petrolatum to the encrusted areas and teaching the child to refrain from picking his nose should be initiated to decrease the likelihood of such occurrences.

The nurse needs to emphasize prevention of accidents whenever she is involved in discussing health with parents and children. Such education is important in reducing the incidence of traumatic events.

Allergic Rhinitis

Both seasonal and perennial allergic rhinitis are seen in children, usually not before 4 or 5 years of age. Foods are often the allergens in the first year or two of life. Later, inhalants are more important.

Seasonal allergic rhinitis (hay fever, rose fever) is caused by sensitivity to molds, pollens, and house dust. Allergy to molds may depend on the weather. Reactions to pollens (rose fever) coincide with the pollinating season of several grasses and also occur in the early spring with tree pollens. Sensitivity to ragweed pollen is manifest from mid-August to early October. House dust is the most common allergen during the winter months, particularly with central heating. Clinical manifestations include sneezing, itching of the nasal mucosa, profuse lacrimation and rhinorrhea, and often allergic conjunctivitis. Olfaction and gustation are decreased. The nasal mucosa is edematous, pale, and wet.

Perennial allergic rhinitis has no seasonal pattern and is caused by sensitivity to house dust, wool, feathers, and molds. It is manifested by mild congestion and sniffling, mouth breathing, postnasal drip, and complaints of an itchy nose. Several facial mannerisms may be indicative of perennial allergic rhinitis: the allergic salute, nose wrinkling, and mouth wrinkling. All are utilized to relieve nasal itching. In the *allergic salute,* the child uses one hand to push the nose upward and backward not only to relieve itching but also to move the swollen turbinates away from the septum, thereby allowing freer air passage. After 2 years of pronounced saluting, a transverse nasal crease occurs just above the bulbous portion of the nose. Nasal mucosa may be pale, edematous, and wet; with purulent discharge, it may be inflamed as in acute nasopharyngitis. Differential diagnosis may then be made via nasal smear. Eosinophilia is present in allergic conditions, whereas polymorphonuclear cells are seen with infection. Recurrent epistaxis due to persistent nose picking and mouth breathing is common in perennial allergic rhinitis, and allergic shiners may be present.

Diagnosis is made through a detailed present, past, and family history; eosinophilia on nasal smears; and scratch test. By x-ray, the mucosa of the maxillary sinuses may appear thickened, and polyps may be seen. Treatment includes a comprehensive program aimed toward removal of causative allergens, desensitization to incitants which cannot be avoided, and control of infection. Immediate treatment for symptomatic relief is provided by antihistamines, oral decongestants, and nasal sprays.

Nursing Management

Nurses providing routine well-child care who observe that a child has allergic shiners, conjunctivitis, allergic facial mannerisms, and/or a transverse nasal crease should refer that child for an allergic evaluation. Other clues include reddened nasal mucosa, sneezing, an itchy nasal lining, and rhinorrhea. A thorough history will add to the data base. Once an allergic basis has been determined, the parents will need to know how to allergy-proof the house. The nurse should also provide health teaching in relation to medications and prevention of infection.

Since medications are used to treat this disorder, it is important to teach parents the side effects of all drugs used. Parents should be instructed to observe the child's response to a particular medication. Some children may respond to a drug initially; however, after several weeks the antihistamine may appear to lose its effectiveness. Therefore, parents should be told to notify a nurse or physician of the recurring symptoms. Often, switching to another class of antihistamine provides significant relief for the child.

Sensory Problems in School-Age Children and Adolescents

Sinusitis

Sinusitis is an inflammatory process involving the frontal (ethmoid) or sphenoid sinuses. Bacterial infections of the sinuses can occur in infancy as well as throughout childhood, but they are most common in the school-age period. Sinusitis may be acute or chronic, involving the maxillary, ethmoid, and/or frontal sinuses. The most frequently involved microorganisms include the filtrable viruses of acute rhinitis, *S. pneumoniae*, staphylococci, and streptococci. While sinusitis itself may be symptomatically severe, the real danger lies in the infectious process invading adjacent structures.

The signs of *acute sinusitis* accompanying an upper respiratory infection include a fever, purulent nasal discharge with nasal congestion, headache, and periorbital or facial swelling which is tender to touch. The periorbital edema and redness of the skin involved indicate a bone and periosteal infiltration. When the purulent material is trapped within a sinus, there may be subsequent necrosis of the bone, venous thrombosis, and finally bone sequestra. The passing of pus from the sinus into the orbit of the eye, especially in ethmoid sinusitis, may cause permanent blindness as a result of a thrombosed orbital vein. Other complications of sinus infections include otitis media, meningitis, orbital cellulitis, and optic neuritis. A severe frontal sinus infection which has ocular involvement may produce an epidural abscess secondary to an erosion of the frontal sinus. Treatment involves nasal and nasopharyngeal cultures and smears, which are examined immediately for identification of the microorganisms involved. Systemic antibiotics and vasoconstrictors are employed. Drainage of the frontal sinus followed by antibiotic irrigations of this cavity may be necessary.

Chronic sinusitis may be caused by hypertrophied adenoids. Allergic irritants may also be responsible for a chronic condition. In warm climates, diving into swimming pools may cause an irritation and dental caries may cause maxillary sinusitis. Clinical manifestations include a chronic cough from a persistent postnasal drip, a constant, purulent discharge, a recurrent headache, frequent sneezing, and mouth breathing. Chronic sinusitis tends to aggravate the respiratory problems of asthmatic children. Treatment depends on the cause, which may be difficult for the physician to identify. If systemic antibiotics and nasal decongestants do not relieve the symptoms, adenoidectomy and sinus irrigation may be necessary.

Nursing Management

The aim of therapy is to provide a tract whereby the purulent material is drained from the affected sinus. If hospitalization is necessary, these patients are frequently febrile, and so their temperatures are monitored often. Antipyretics and cool sponges should be utilized as frequently as ordered or necessary. Fluids are encouraged, and humidifiers which are effective in liquefying secretions may facilitate the draining process. Nose drops are frequently ordered and should be administered after a thorough, gentle cleansing of the nasal passages. In assessing a patient's response to therapy, the nurse should focus on the temperature returning to normal and the type of drainage being produced. It is especially important to note the color and the tenaciousness of the material, for as there is a response to treatment, the drainage becomes clear and more liquid.

Warm compresses applied to the periorbital edema may be soothing for a young patient. Accompanying eye drainage may be purulent, and its presence should be noted. It is important to assess frequently the extent of the tissue involved, its color, and the patient's ability to open his eye. Identifying a change in the child's behavior or neurological status may determine the existence of a complication. For example, if he covers his ear with his hand or complains that his ear hurts, it may indicate otitis media. Other changes in his neurological status may demonstrate the presence of an epidural abscess. A physician should be notified immediately.

Sinusitis may partially obstruct the airway, impairing the senses of smell and taste. The nurse should explain this change to the child and his parents. Health teaching about proper diet, care of the teeth, and/or allergies should be provided, along with instruction about prescribed treatments.

Trauma to the Eye

The eye can sustain a variety of injuries which may result in a number of long-term problems. A *blunt injury* occurs after one is hit by a closed fist, a hockey puck, a baseball, or a stone. When the eye is struck, it dimples inward, raising the intraocular pressure. If there is a very sudden increase, the impact may fracture the orbital floor, which is a very serious complication.

The consequences of these types of traumatic insults extend from ecchymosis and edema to corneal abrasion, dislocated lens, anterior chamber hemorrhage (discussed in the section on preschoolers above), and retinal detachment. Exploding firecrackers also have a particularly dangerous concussive effect.

A *penetrating* injury may scratch or perforate the cornea or extend to a collapse of the vitreous humor, in which case the eye will be lost. Flying pieces of objects, such as metal, glass, and wood, and darts have caused this type of trauma. Constant pain and tearing are some of the complaints of children with corneal abrasions, while excruciating pain and instant blindness will be verbalized by an adolescent who has sustained an extensive penetrating eye injury. Cataracts can develop as a result of very minor penetrations (Tumulty and Resler, 1984). Infection is a major complication because these objects are contaminated.

NURSING CARE PLAN

21-3 The Child with a Blow-Out Fracture

Clinical Problem/Nursing Diagnosis	Expected Outcome	Nursing Interventions
Pain	Child's eye pain will be alleviated	Administer analgesics as ordered; (assess side effects and adverse reaction)
Pain related to orbital fracture		Apply ice in first 24 h
		Position child comfortably
Disturbed vision Entrapment of eye/ repositioning of eye	Child will report any decreased visual acuity, swelling, double vision, exudate, feelings of pressure in eye	Assess neurological status with vital signs: note eyelid swelling, edema, pupillary reflexes, EOMs, visual acuity, ability to track objects, scleral hemorrhagic eye injections, and presence of foreign material
Sensory/perceptual alteration (visual)		Keep eye clean and surrounding area dry
		Teach child to avoid rubbing, irritating eye
		Explain all aspects of care and procedures
		Evaluate child's understanding of what is happening to him
Fear and anxiety	Child will be comforted and supported through painful procedures	Encourage parents if appropriate to support and comfort child after treatment and medical interventions
Anxiety related to emergent medical treatment		Provide opportunities for the child to share his feelings
		Explain all procedures in depth and evaluate results of teaching done
At risk for infection of surrounding sinuses	Child will be free of sinus infection	Monitor temperature
		Notify physician of temperature >38.5°C
		Obtain cultures as ordered
		Administer antipyretics as ordered
Potential for infection related to trauma		Assess for presence of sinus pain and headaches
		Note presence of purulent nasal drainage and nasal congestion
		Properly administer antibiotics as ordered
Nasal stuffiness	Child's nasal decongestion will decrease, and his nares will remain patent with decreased postnasal drainage	Properly administer nasal decongestants and/or nasal antihistamines as ordered
Ineffective airway clearance related to nasal congestion		Facilitate expectoration of nasal secretions

A sudden blow to the back of the head can precipitate the accumulation of fluid between the choroid and retina, resulting in a *retinal detachment*. These clients complain of floating spots, flashes of light, smoky vision, or blacked-out areas of their visual fields. They may be admitted for surgical intervention.

A serious complication of sudden increased intraorbital pressure is a *blow-out fracture* of the orbital floor. The force of the blunt injury is transmitted to the walls of the orbit. The floor of the orbit fractures or blows outward because its structure is the weakest. Crepitus in the lid, edema, ecchymosis, and sometimes a zygomatic fracture are found on x-ray. It may be necessary to admit these adolescents in order to wire their jaws, a procedure which enhances healing.

Chemical trauma is due to the corrosive nature of acids of alkalis which reach the eyes. Household cleaning materials, aerosol sprays, plumbing supplies, and a variety of agents used in chemical experiments can cause these types of injuries. Acid burns usually are self-limiting if infection does not develop. However, alkalis are more serious because they continue to dissolve eye tissue by forming toxic alkaline products which penetrate deeper and deeper into the affected tissue.

Nursing Management

When children or adolescents are brought to the hospital for eye injuries, it is imperative for the nurse to notify an ophthalmologist immediately. The nursing history should include the nature of the injury (blunt, penetrating, chemical), the treatment given at the scene, and the problems which have developed as a result. Patients with more severe injuries are admitted for observation and treatment.

The danger of infection is significant in a child who has received a penetrating injury because the foreign object is contaminated when it enters the eye. While the child may be sedated and requires pain medications, the administration of prescribed antibiotics is most important. They must be given on time, in the proper dose, and by the correct route.

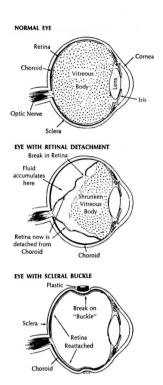

NORMAL EYE

Retina
Cornea
Choroid
Vitreous Body
Lens
Optic Nerve
Iris
Sclera

EYE WITH RETINAL DETACHMENT

Break in Retina
Fluid accumulates here
Shrunken Vitreous Body
Retina now is detached from Choroid
Choroid

EYE WITH SCLERAL BUCKLE

Plastic
Break on "Buckle"
Sclera
Retina Reattached
Choroid

FIGURE 21-8 Eye with detached retina; eye with scleral buckle (bottom). *(From D.A. Jones et al. [eds.], Medical-Surgical Nursing, 2d ed., McGraw-Hill, New York, 1982, p. 1416.)*

When an adolescent has experienced a detached retina, he is placed on bed rest, in a quiet room, with bilateral eye patches in place. Eye medications are administered as ordered to keep the pupils dilated. Surgical intervention involves the application of a scleral buckle, a silicone implant which results in an indentation of the affected eye (Fig. 21-8). After surgery, specific orders include raising the head of the bed and positioning the head itself. A pressure dressing is in place. The greatest challenge for a nurse is related to preventing increased intraocular pressure which results from vomiting, straining, or coughing. With contact sports forbidden because of possible recurrence, a nurse needs to spend time with an athletic adolescent who faces this lifetime restriction. Discharge planning should emphasize the restriction of weight lifting for about 3 months because this activity also raises intraocular pressure. It is beneficial for a nurse to involve peers in selecting activities in which the adolescent may participate and to explain his limitations to his peers so that these relationships can be maintained.

When a blow-out fracture complicates an eye injury, it is painful and requires the administration of analgesics. Ice packs and cold compresses also relieve the pain and edema. Any eye drainage which develops should be reported to a physician promptly. When the zygomatic fracture must be immoblized, the jaw is fixed, using wires or rubber bands. Postoperatively, the head of the bed is elevated and the patient is kept on his side. The wired jaw necessitates a fluid diet, and a plastic straw or asepto syringe can be used for feedings. When they are started, it is

important to have suction on standby. The patient should be on his side or in a sitting position when he is being fed. Whenever fluids are taken, the oral cavity needs to be rinsed with water afterward. Diligent mouth care is an essential nursing activity which should be done every 2 hours. With the mouth wired shut, *wire cutters must be taped conspicuously to the head of the bed.* If the airway becomes obstructed from choking, vomiting, or cyanosis, the wires or rubber bands *must* be cut immediately. The jaw remains wired for several weeks; and so oral hygiene is a major teaching focus for the nurse.

A young patient with a severe chemical burn is hospitalized. Topical steroids and antibiotics are administered, and on occasion it may be necessary to debride dead tissue in order to identify the extent of the injury and enhance healing. It is important to be honest in reassuring these children about the restrictions they are experiencing, especially in regard to the temporary loss of vision, *if* such is the case. The healing process is lengthy (5 or 6 weeks), and so teaching with an emphasis on the need to comply with the treatment plan is critical to recovery.

The types of eye injuries described above are in many instances avoidable. The prevention of such accidents should be emphasized whenever a nurse is involved in teaching health to children or parents. Relevant safety issues should be incorporated in the anticipatory guidance provided to the parents of very young children. For example, toddlers should not be allowed to run with sticks or pencils, and forks should never be used as weapons at the table. Children should not be allowed to handle firecrackers because of the associated dangers. Whenever chemicals are used, safety glasses should be worn. Advocation of the use of safety belts in cars and helmets in contact sports or on recreational vehicles needs to be intensified. The improper care of contact lenses, the harmful effects of aerosol sprays, and the danger inherent in sharing eye makeup are all topics for discussion with children and adolescents. In addition, everyone should know what to do in the event of a chemical burn to the eye. It *must* be irrigated with clean tap water for 20 to 30 minutes, longer if the substance is an alkali, and the child should be taken to the nearest health care facility for evaluation. It is important for nurses to become much more involved in teaching good eye care, emphasizing safety factors which have a direct effect on vision.

Trauma to the Ear

The ear can be damaged by a hard blow to the head (punch, bat, ball), a sharp or foreign object being placed in the ear, swimming and diving accidents, certain ototoxic drugs, and sound pollution. Repeated middle ear infections (otitis media) and their inadequate treatment can result in perforations of the tympanic membranes which decrease their mobility. Some prenatal infections and congenital malformations can continue and result in some type of hearing loss.

The symptoms which a child demonstrates vary and depend on the source as well as the type of injury sustained. If he has received a severe blow to the head or in-

TABLE 21-8 Extent of Hearing Loss

Degree	Range, dB	Effect of Loss	Child Needs
Mild	26-40	Has difficulty hearing soft voices, distant voices, or sounds; misses some information	Seat selection in front of classroom; training in speech reading
Moderate	41-55	Hears conversation at 3-5 ft; has defective speech; is delayed in language development	Testing and fitting for hearing aid
Moderately severe	56-70	Hears only very loud speech; experiences almost no auditory input during group activities or from distant voices	Early use of hearing aid; special language programs as early as 1 yr of age
Severe	71-95	Hears shouted voices at very close range	Amplification aid as soon as possible after birth; enrollment in infant stimulation programs for hearing-impaired
Profound loss (deaf)	Above 95	Has residual hearing in some frequencies	Amplification aids very early; carefully selected academic settings

serted an object which penetrates the tympanic membrane, the pain is sharp and there is loss of hearing in the affected ear. If a foreign object has been introduced into the external canal and allowed to remain undetected, it may go unnoticed until drainage develops. A fracture of the temporal bone results in a hearing loss with an accumulation of blood behind the eardrum. If it involves the lower portion of the bone, there is paralysis of the facial nerve; however, if there is a longitudinal fracture through the inner ear, there is permanent hearing loss (Table 21-8).

Conductive Hearing Loss

In a conductive hearing loss the obstruction, which can be impacted wax or a foreign object (eraser, pea), results in an interruption in the transmission of sound waves from the external ear to the inner ear. Although a temporary hearing loss develops with an effusion, it is the permanent scarring of the tympanic membrane which reduces its mobility and hence its sensitivity to sound waves. The inner ear is not affected in any way.

Congenital malformations affecting any part of the hearing apparatus also can cause conductive hearing loss. There may be a partially developed auricle or pina, an atresia of the external canal, or an anomaly which affects the inner ear and results in a fixation of the ossicles. Some of these malformations are identified at birth; however, others which are not visible on a physical examination may go undetected until problems of language development become evident. Hearing aids are helpful to some infants and children who are experiencing a conductive hearing loss. In children who were born with congenital anomalies, some of the malformations are surgically correctable.

Sensorineural Hearing Loss

This type of hearing loss is the most serious, because it is not treatable and is permanent. Some hereditary causes are associated with certain disorders such as Alpert's, Treacher Collins, and Usher's syndromes. Prenatal infections such as rubella and cytomegalovirus also contribute to a sensorineural hearing loss.

Drug-induced damage to the ears can occur on occasion with the use of certain medications. Aminoglycosides, which are capable of destroying sensory cells, causing the loss of inner ear function, include amikacin, tobramycin, and gentamicin. Streptomycin also is considered an ototoxic drug. This devastating side effect reinforces the need for nurses to know the recommended doses of medications and to compute the precise amounts. In addition, the destructive effect of certain drugs may not be evident during aggressive treatment, which makes follow-up for screening and testing crucial.

In the work setting, regulations developed by the Occupational Safety and Health Administration (OSHA) require the use of special muffs or plastic inserts when noise levels are above 85 dB. However, there are no such controls during recreational activities, in which noise levels far exceed 85 dB. Sound pollution has contributed to significant numbers of people developing a sensorineural hearing loss through acute exposure to recreational sounds of rock 'n' roll music, model airplanes, and snowmobiles. The increased use of Walkman-type tape players and radios has many audiologists concerned because of the levels at which they are set (*U.S. News and World Report*, 1987). Sound energy is transmitted directly to the inner ear with plugs or earphones that cover the ear, and at full volume these items generate 115 dB. If a person walks by an individual wearing a headset and hears what that person is listening to, the level is dangerously high. Sets with volume controls labeled 1 to 10 should *never* be set above 4. If school-age children and adolescents do not use these sets properly, as their loss increases, they will turn up the volume controls and create even more damage to the inner ear.

Nursing Management

When a child is brought to the emergency room, a nurse needs to obtain accurate information regarding the accident and the symptoms the child has demonstrated (pain, loss of hearing, drainage). If x-rays reveal a fractured temporal bone, a nurse monitors the teenager for signs of neurological involvement, especially complaints of a persistent earache; the degree of facial paralysis; or an increase in a hearing impairment. Any changes should be recorded carefully and reported promptly to a physician. If surgery is required, the reader is referred to the section on common nursing measures at the beginning of this chapter.

While a nurse computes and administers ototoxic drugs properly, follow-up is extremely important when the client is a pregnant teenager or is a child who is being treated for a severe infection, such as meningitis. A nurse also needs to know drug interactions because the ototoxicity of a medication may be potentiated in the presence of another drug. In addition, a nurse needs to monitor blood levels of these ototoxic drugs whenever such medications are given.

When a nurse is working with patients, anticipatory guidance should include proper ear washing (washcloths, not cotton-tipped applicators), removal of cerumen (instill mineral oil; irrigate with a Water Pik to remove wax), and safety issues, especially the need to supervise toddlers who are playing with sharp objects. Adolescents need to be urged to use helmets when they participate in contact sports to decrease the likelihood of trauma to the ears.

Nursing interventions for a child or adolescent with a perforated tympanic membrane focus on teaching and stressing the need to keep water out of the ear canal. Such patients should not take showers or go swimming until the perforation heals. When hair needs to be washed, petroleum jelly applied on a cotton ball and inserted in the outer ear and a mold created from Silly Putty are effective methods of keeping water out of the ear.

A nurse has to become involved in preventing injuries which result in hearing impairments, especially those which are permanent. A hearing loss occurs slowly and progressively. The increased use of headsets with subsequent permanent hearing loss should be a major health care concern.

Learning Activities

1. Assign clinical students to care for children and adolescents admitted for eye surgery or periorbital cellulitis or to care for a hearing-impaired child hospitalized for a nonrelated health problem.
2. Invite the mother of a deaf infant to class so that she may share her feelings and describe to the class the impact that the hearing impairment has had on the family.
3. Design and supervise a sensory deprivation experience for students over a 24-hour period. Place eye patches over both eyes of a student and assign another student to lead the visually deprived student through all the activities of daily living. Obtain pairs of protective earmuffs, place them in the proper position on another student to obliterate all sound, and then proceed to carry out normal activities for the prescribed period. Have the students describe their experiences in class.

Independent Study Activities

1. Volunteer to participate in vision and hearing screening programs at a local nursery school.
2. Develop a teaching plan for a child with otitis media which includes an explanation of the problem and the importance of parental compliance in the treatment of the problem.

Study Questions

1. Color perceived by the eye depends on:
   A. The aqueous humor.
   B. The wavelength absorbed by photosensitive pigments of the retina.
   C. The lens.
   D. The vitreous humor.
2. The sense of touch is well developed in the neonate, particularly in the:
   A. Chest, tongue, lips, and ears.
   B. Arms, chest, tongue, and lips.
   C. Legs, tongue, lips, and forehead.
   D. Tongue, lips, forehead, and ears.
3. In Dennie's sign:
   A. There is edema and discoloration of the lower orbitopalpebral grooves.
   B. There is edema of the lower eyelids.
   C. Lines radiate from the inner corner of the eye, slant downward, and end in a slight upward swing in the lower orbitopalpebral grooves.
   D. There is edema of the bulbar conjunctiva.
4. Newborns who develop gonorrheal conjunctivitis are hospitalized and require:
   A. Reverse isolation. C. Contact isolation.
   B. Enteric isolation D. Strict isolation.
5. In children who have nasal surgery, a nurse needs to realize that their diminished oral intake is related not only to the nasal packing but also to:
   A. The loss of smell. C. A feeling of nausea.
   B. A feeling of fullness. D. The edema present.
6. If a child has stuck a bean or pea in his ear, the nurse:
   A. Remove the foreign object using ear irrigation.
   B. Can remove the foreign object using an ear spoon.
   C. Needs to refer the child to a physician.
   D. Needs to instill ear drops.
7. The mother of a 7-year-old girl who has allergic rhinitis tells the nurse that her daughter has a crease above the tip of her nose. She asks what the crease means. The nurse explains:
   A. Nose wrinkling as a means of relieving itching.
   B. The allergic salute, its purpose, and its result.
   C. Mouth wrinkling in allergic rhinitis.
   D. Dennie's sign.

8. A common result of nonperforating injury to the eye by blunt object is:
   A. Corneal break.
   B. Prolapsed iris.
   C. Sympathetic ophthalmia.
   D. Hyphema.

9. Sinusitis may be secondary to:
   A. Optic neuritis.   C. Dental caries.
   B. Otitis media.   D. Respiratory infection.

10. When an adolescent who has sustained a blow-out fracture secondary to blunt eye trauma complains of limited jaw movement, a nurse should notify the physician because of the possibility of :
    A. A zygomatic fracture.
    B. Nasal sinus perforation.
    C. Dental fractures.
    D. Mandibular fracture.

11. When responding to the call light of a visually impaired child, it is important for a nurse to:
    A. Answer the call light promptly.
    B. Go into the room.
    C. Touch the child before speaking to him.
    D. Address the child upon entering the room.

Organizations Providing Additional Information

Alexander Graham Bell Association for the Deaf
3417 Volta Place, N.W.
Washington, DC 20007
202-337-5220

Better Hearing Institute
P.O. Box 1840
Washington, DC 20013
1-800-424-8576

American Council of the Blind
1010 Vermont Avenue, N.W., Suite 1100
Washington, DC 20005
1-800-424-8666

American Foundation for the Blind
15 W. 16th Street
New York, NY 10011
1-800-232-5463

References

Apt, L., and W.L. Gaffney: "The Eyes," in A.M. Rudolph and J.I.E. Hoffman (eds.), *Pediatrics*, 18th ed., Appleton & Lange, Norwalk, CT, 1987.

Editorial Staff: "Blinding Missiles: Soft Drink Twist-off Bottle Caps," *Sightsaving*, 53(1):2-7, 1984.

Kamenir, S.: "Hands-on Skills for Dealing with Hearing Aids," *Canadian Nurse*, 78:44-45, 1982.

Paradise, J.L.: "Review Article: Otitis Media in Infants and Children," *Pediatrics*, 61(5):917-943, 1980.

Teele, D.W., et al.: "Otitis Media with Effusion during the First Three Years of Life and the Development of Speech and Language," *Pediatrics*, 74(2):282-287, 1984.

Tumulty, G., and M. Resler: "Eye Trauma," *American Journal of Nursing*, 84:740-743, 1984.

U.S. News and World Report, "Loud Noise from Little Headphones," Oct. 12, 1987, p. 77.

Bibliography

Goldberg, R.: "Identifying Speech and Language Delays in Children," *Pediatric Nursing*, 10:252-259, 1984.

22

The Musculoskeletal System

Objectives

After reading this chapter, the student will be able to:
1. Describe the functions of the musculoskeletal system.
2. Identify appropriate subjective and objective data to be elicited during assessment of the child and family.
3. Understand the purpose of diagnostic tests and medical treatment.
4. Explain general nursing measures appropriate for pediatric clients who have musculoskeletal problems.
5. Delineate specific nursing measures appropriate to the care of pediatric clients who have various musculoskeletal problems.

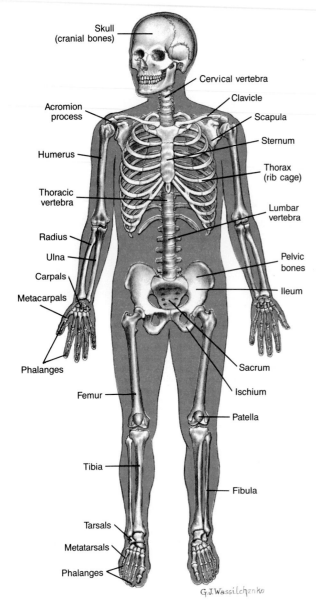

Skull
(cranial bones)

Cervical vertebra

Clavicle

Acromion process

Scapula

Sternum

Humerus

Thorax
(rib cage)

Thoracic vertebra

Lumbar vertebra

Radius

Ulna

Pelvic bones

Carpals

Ileum

Metacarpals

Phalanges

Sacrum

Femur

Ischium

Patella

Tibia

Fibula

Tarsals

Metatarsals

Phalanges

G.J.Wassilchenko

FIGURE 22-1   Anterior view of the human skeleton. *(From L.L. Langley et al., Dynamic Anatomy and Physiology, McGraw-Hill, New York, 1958, p. 53.)*

The adult skeleton is composed of 206 bones. Many more bony pieces can be identified at birth, but by the twenty-fifth year union and ossification of most bones have been completed, reducing the initial number. An anterior view of the skeleton is presented in Fig. 22-1.

Bone

Bone functions both as a structure and an organ. As a structure, it provides a framework for the body, acts as a lever for skeletal muscles, and protects vital organs such as the brain, spinal cord, heart, and lungs. As an organ, it contains tissue for the production of erythrocytes and stores calcium, phosphorus, and other minerals.

Bone reacts to injury or disease in three basic ways: (1) local death *(necrosis)*, (2) alterations in the way new bone cells are deposited, and (3) alterations in bone resorption.

When the blood supply to an area of bone is completely stopped, *avascular necrosis* (local death due to inadequate blood supply) occurs. The resultant dead bone encourages further bone destruction in the area.

Alterations in bone *deposition* and bone *resorption* take place in bone which is alive. Bone is deposited in sites that are subjected to stress and is resorbed from sites that receive little stress; normally a balance of these two processes exists. Reactions to abnormal conditions may occur in an entire bone, in part of a bone, or in all the bones of the body.

Fractures

Several different kinds of fractures occur. Fractures are classified according to the way in which the bone fragments relate to one another and to the surrounding tissue.

Compound fractures are those in which a bone fragment pierces the skin. Infection of bone from dirt or other environmental contaminants may occur. *Simple* fractures, on the other hand, are those in which the skin over the fracture site is not broken. A *depressed* fracture is one in which the broken segment is displaced inward toward the center of the bony cavity. For example, a blow to the head can drive a segment of the skull into the cerebral cavity. A *pathological* fracture is one that results from a disease that weakens the bone. Bones that have been eroded by cancer, for example, may break spontaneously or under slight pressure (Fig. 22-2).

After a fracture, local bone deposition increases in order to form *callus,* a substance that develops temporarily at the site of the fracture. Composed of bone cells, cartilage, and the bone minerals calcium and phosphorus, callus stabilizes the bone fragments to some degree. Fig. 22-3b shows how callus looks on x-ray film.

The healing and reforming processes that repair a fracture are divided into three stages: (1) Callus forms around the broken edges and becomes progressively firmer and less mobile. (2) When callus is firm enough so that no movement occurs at the fracture site, *clinical union* has taken place. (3) Consolidation of the fracture has oc-

TYPE OF FRACTURE	DEFINITION
1. Transverse	1. Usually produced by angulating force; once the fragments are aligned and immobilized, stability is assured
2. Oblique	2. Fragments tend to slip by one another unless traction is maintained
3. Spiral	3. Produced by twisting or rotary force; reduction difficult to maintain
4. Greenstick	4. Caused by compression force in long axis of the bone; often seen in children under age of ten
5. Compression	5. Usually produced by severe violence applied to cancellous bone, such as the spine
6. Comminuted	6. Always more than two fragments
7. Impacted	7. Produced by severe violence, driving bone fragments firmly together
8. Avulsion	8. Produced by forcible contraction of a muscle which pulls off a fragment of bone
9. Fracture dislocation	9. In addition to fracture there is a subluxation or dislocation of the joint

FIGURE 22-2   Types of fractures. *(From J. Barry, Emergency Nursing, McGraw-Hill, New York, 1978, p. 319).*

FIGURE 22-3   Healing and remodeling of a fractured humerus in a newborn. *(A)* At birth, *(B)* 3½ weeks (the ball-shaped shadow is callus), and *(C)* 5½ months. *(Courtesy of Indiana University School of Medicine.)*

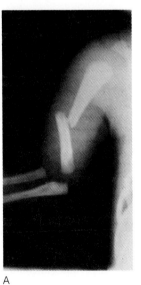
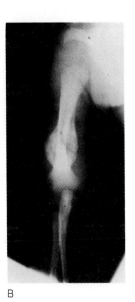
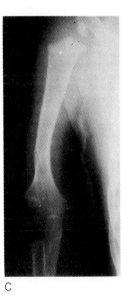

A   B   C

curred when all callus is replaced by mature bone. Sharp edges are smoothed off by bone resorption and deposition. The remodeling process is illustrated in Fig. 22-3.

Healing of a fracture varies a great deal with age. More time is required for healing as a person gets older. For example, a fracture of the femoral shaft at birth is united in 3 weeks. At age 8 years, the same fracture requires 8 weeks for union; at 12 years, 12 weeks is re-

FIGURE 22-4 Clinical terms used to describe movement. (*Adapted from L. L. Langley et al., Dynamic Anatomy and Physiology, 4th ed., McGraw-Hill, New York, 1974, p. 124.*)

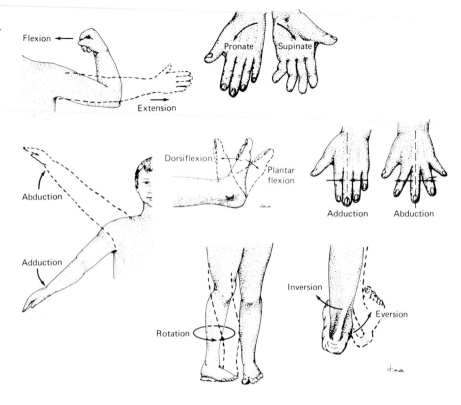

quired; at 20 years through adulthood, 20 weeks is needed for healing.

Epiphyseal Plate

The epiphyseal plate is the anatomic structure near the ends of the long bones which produces new bone cells to cause growth during childhood. Normal growth requires an intact epiphyseal plate, normal blood supply, and intermittent pressure from weight bearing and activity. Like bone, each epiphyseal plate reacts in limited ways to abnormal conditions. Reactions include (1) increased growth, (2) decreased growth, and (3) torsional (twisted or spiral) growth. A prolonged increase in blood supply to the epiphyseal plate stimulates growth; hypoxia retards it. A complete lack of blood supply results in necrosis and completely stops growth in the affected bone. Torsional growth, producing a spiral deformity, occurs when growth is abnormal in one part of an epiphyseal plate and normal in the rest.

Joints

A joint is a junction between two or more bones. Joints have several functions: They segment the skeleton, permit motion between segments, and allow for varying amounts of growth between the segments. Its construction varies. Joints are classified as fibrous, cartilaginous, and synovial. Motion is very limited in *fibrous* joints, found between the bones of the skull in childhood. Slightly movable *cartilaginous* joints include the epiphyseal plates and the symphysis pubis. *Synovial* joints, the most movable, appear at the elbow, shoulder, and fingers. Movements

and the terms used to describe them are illustrated in Fig. 22-4.

Skeletal Muscle

Skeletal muscles provide active movement and maintain the posture of the skeleton. They are called *voluntary* muscles because they can be controlled at will. Microscopic cross striations account for their other name, *striated* muscles.

Each muscle fiber is innervated by an axon and activated by biochemical changes that result from axon activity and cause the fiber to contract. The energy for muscle action is thought to be derived from the breakdown of adenosine triphosphate (ATP). Actual contraction seems to result from movement of special myofilaments in the myofibril, a subunit of the muscle fiber. As these myofilaments move closer together, the entire fiber contracts and shortens.

Each muscle fiber obeys the *all-or-none law:* It contracts maximally or not at all. Therefore, the number of individual fibers that contract determines whether a contraction is weak or powerful. The total number of muscle cells is established at birth; however, dead muscle cells do not regenerate but are replaced by fibrous tissue. Enlargement of a muscle after sustained physical exercise is a result of hypertrophy of existing muscle cells, not an increase in their number.

Dysfunction or injury of any part of the single motor unit (an individual muscle fiber and its connections in the nervous system) can cause a reaction in skeletal muscle. *Disuse atrophy,* which is manifested by weakness and a decrease in the size of a muscle, results from lack of normal use. A persistent shortening of a muscle is a muscle *contracture* and occurs when the muscle is maintained in a shortened position over a prolonged period. While a muscle becomes stronger and larger when it is repeatedly exercised against resistance, the resulting *hypertrohy* of muscle fibers will be temporary unless it is kept up by persistent exercising. *Ischemic necrosis* of a muscle occurs within 6 hours after arterial occlusion, which can be caused by spasm, thrombosis, or embolism.

Movement

Movement depends on the nervous system, muscles, bones, joints, ligaments, and tendons. *Ligaments* bind the bones together, while *tendons* connect muscle to bone at a joint. Both are composed of tough, relatively inelastic collagen fibers and cells. When skeletal muscles contract, tendons exert force on the joints, and movement of the skeleton results.

Movement may be involuntary (reflex) or voluntary. *Involuntary,* or reflex, movement may be elicited by receptors for temperature, pressure, touch, pain, proprioception, or stretch. The lower motor neuron is involved in this type of movement. Sensory impulses are sent by way of the sensory neuron to the spinal cord, the motor neuron originating in the spinal cord is excited, and motor impulses are sent back down to the muscle fiber, causing it to contract. Voluntary movement is under the control of the motor cortex. The upper motor neuron carries impulses from the motor cortex to the spinal cord. The lower motor neuron is then stimulated and causes the muscle fiber to contract.

Assessment of the Musculoskeletal System

Assessment of the musculoskeletal system requires interviewing skills for history taking as well as keen observational skills in conducting the physical examination. Although separated from the neurological assessment, both systems are closely related and interdependent. This section will focus on the particular functions of the musculoskeletal system.

History

The health history is elicited by questioning both parents and child. If the *present illness* involves the musculoskeletal system, several questions are presented: (1) date of onset of symptoms and/or date when the alteration was recognized; (2) any trauma prior to onset of signs and symptoms; (3) kind, duration, and degree of symptoms; (4) time of injury, type of first aid; and method of transportation to a health care facility; (5) chronological course of the disease, including any therapy.

The *past health history, patient profile,* and *review of systems* vary somewhat with the different age groups. Specific items for questioning are presented in Table 22-1. For *family history,* information is gathered about past and present illnesses or defects involving the musculoskeletal system in family members, including spinal curvature, muscle weakness, hip dysplasia, joint stiffness or swelling, and deformities of extremities. Several musculoskeletal problems have a genetic basis.

Physical Examination

Examination of the musculoskeletal system involves mainly inspection and palpation. A measuring tape is helpful to assess symmetry and length of opposite parts. The examination begins with general observations of the body and its parts as a whole and proceeds to very specific observations and palpation of each joint and digit. Clothing should not obscure observations; the diaper is removed from the infant, and only underpants are worn by the older child. The gown of the adolescent must be parted at the back for examination of the spine. The legs, feet, and gait are evaluated without any socks, shoes, or leg coverings.

Several other points are helpful. The newborn period is critical. Some abnormalities begin as minor ones in the newborn but progress to major problems if not treated early (e.g., foot and hip deformities). When assessing temperature, color, and size of a part or muscle strength, it is best to compare one side of the body or one extremity with the other. In this way, individual variations are considered. Epiphyseal fractures may result in limb length discrepancies. To measure true limb length, the ends of the measuring tape are placed on the anterior superior spine of the pelvis and on the medial malleolus of the ankle. This measurement from bone to bone is more accurate than is measurement from soft tissue landmarks. Measurements may be required over several years as follow-up after an epiphyseal fracture. In exploring range of motion, both active and passive, the number of degrees of flexion and extension at the angle of the joint provides an objective description of limits. Range of motion is frequently decreased in conditions affecting the musculoskeletal system. Assessment of circulation in an extremity is especially important after surgery or casting.

Recording of vital statistics gives helpful clues regarding musculoskeletal status. Height or length (stature) directly reflects bone growth. Weight measurements reflect organ growth. The length (or stature)/weight ratio can depict obesity, which frequently complicates immobilizing disorders, as well as metabolic or hormonal alterations which predispose to certain diseases (e.g., a slipped upper femoral epiphysis often occurs in tall, thin teenagers or those who are obese). Elevated vital signs may indicate an inflammatory process, as in juvenile rheumatoid arthritis.

Other major sections of the musculoskeletal examination include assessment of the extremities, joints, back and spine, general body contour and alignment, and movement. The examination varies according to the developmental needs of the child and the problems which typically occur in each age group. Suggested sequences for conducting the exam in different age groups are presented in Table 22-2.

TABLE 22-1 Health History of the Musculoskeletal System in Different Age Groups

I. Newborn and infant
  A. Prenatal
    1. Medications taken
    2. Infections
    3. Surgery or procedures
    4. X-rays
  B. Labor and delivery
    1. Breech or unusual presentation
    2. Forceps
  C. Postnatal (type of problem, treatment, response)
    1. Congenital musculoskeletal deformities
    2. Fractures or other birth injuries
  D. Developmental milestones
    1. Gross motor: controls heads, sits, rolls over, stands, walks
    2. Fine motor: grasps (pincer), reaches, passes hand to hand
  E. Dietary habits
    1. Vitamin D—fortified milk
    2. Vitamin and iron supplements
  F. Review of systems
    1. Joints: congenital deformity or signs of injury or disease (swelling, pain, refusal to move, stiffness, heat, redness)
    2. Muscles: swelling, weakness, soreness
    3. Bones: fractures (deformity, heat, redness, pain, swelling) or deformities (e.g., tibial torsion, dysmelia)
    4. Movement: decrease in movement or activity level (refusal to move the involved limb may indicate pain)
II. Toddler and preschooler
  A. History of musculoskeletal congenital deformities, injuries, or disease requiring hospitalization or surgery
  B. Developmental milestones
    1. Gross motor: walks forward and backward, balances on one foot, kicks, jumps, pedals tricycle, hops on one foot, walks heel-to-toe
    2. Fine motor: scribbles, stacks blocks, copies shapes, draws freehand
    3. History of milestones during infancy
  A. Dietary habits
  B. Play and activity level
  C. Self-help skills: independence/dependence
  D. Perceptions of illness and body image
  E. Review of systems (refer to newborn and infant above)
III. School-age and adolescent
  A. History of musculoskeletal deformities, injuries, or disease requiring hospitalization or surgery
  B. Development
    1. Achievement of early milestones
    2. Participation in sports activities, either organized or informal
  C. Dietary habits: balanced diet, regular mealtimes, adequate intake for growth and sports activity needs
  D. Independence in self-help skills if child is disabled
  E. Perceptions of illness and body image
  F. Review of systems (refer to newborn and infant above)
  G. Sports evaluation: to elicit from both child and parents the above information, the following questions are suggested by the American Orthopaedic Society for Sports Medicine (1981)
    1. Have you ever had an illness, condition, or injury for which you had to go to the hospital overnight or for an emergency room visit or an x-ray? Have you ever had a problem that caused you to miss a game or practice, see a doctor, or require an operation?
    2. Are you now under the care of a physician for any reason? Have you been in the past?
    3. Do you currently have any medical problems or injuries?
    4. Have you ever had an injury to your bones or muscles, such as a broken bone, joint sprain, ligament tear, muscle pull, head injury, neck injury or nerve pinch, dislocated joint, back trouble?

TABLE 22-2 Physical Examination of the Musculoskeletal System in Different Age Groups

I. Newborn and infant
  A. General assessment
    1. Position: on parent's lap or examination table with clothing on
    2. Observations: general body configuration and spontaneous movements
  B. Examination of the hips
    1. Position: supine position on the examining table; diaper should be removed
    2. Assessment: Ortolani test is performed by the physician or nurse-practitioner. The position of the examiner's hands is illustrated in Fig. 22-5. With the newborn infant supine, the examiner moves the flexed hip into adduction while pressing the femur downward. In this position an abnormal hip becomes dislocated. The examiner then moves the thigh into abduction while lifting the femur upward. As the femoral head slides into the socket, a click is elicited, the sign of a positive test for dislocated hip. After 1 mo of age, this is less useful and limitation of hip abduction is the most reliable sign. Asymmetrical gluteal creases are an unreliable sign in the newborn, as these creases are a normal variation
  C. Observation and palpation of the neck and upper extremities
    1. Position: supine position on the examining table with clothing removed
    2. Assessment: neck is observed and palpated. In torticollis, a lump is felt on one side of the neck and range of motion is decreased. The clavicles are palpated, and full range of motion of the shoulders is done to make sure no clavicular fracture exists. The hands are examined for extra digits and webbing between fingers. A simian crease in the palm is suggestive of Down's syndrome
  D. Observation and palpation of the lower extremities
    1. Position: supine position on the examining table
    2. Assessment: muscle tone and strength in the legs are evaluated, as well as symmetry in shape
    3. Position: prone on the examining table
    4. Observation: child's gross motor skills, including abiity to raise his head and shoulders from the table, to crawl, roll over, and reach or grasp an object, are observed
    5. Position: standing position with support from the examiner as needed

Continued.

6. Evaluation: general body tone, head control, and the ability to bear weight on the legs are evaluated. Slight bowleggedness is a normal variation in infancy. The position of the feet is observed; the feet should point straight ahead. In *metatarsus adductus* the heel is straight and in line with the leg, but the front half of the foot turns inward. A more severe clubfoot deformity, *talipes equinovarus,* involves abnormal turning of the ankle as well. Both conditions need referral for treatment

E. Evaluation of the spine and sitting ability
   1. Position: if over 4 mo of age, sitting position, with support from the examiner
   2. Observation and palpation: normal spinal curvature of the infant is a C shape, which will progress to the S curve of the adult; skin on the lower back should be assessed for dimples, cysts, or tufts of hair, all indicative of spina bifida

II. Toddler
   A. General observations
      1. Position: on parent's lap or nearby, with clothing on
      2. Assessment: general appearance, growth, and body proportion are observed, as well as child's behavior
   B. Palpation of hands and feet
      1. Position: on parent's lap or nearby, with socks and shoes removed
      2. Assessment: palpation of hands and feet provides a playful, nonthreatening way to initiate contact during the examination
   C. Evaluation of the upper and lower extremities
      1. Position: supine position on the examining table or the parent's lap, with diaper or underpants removed
      2. Evaluation: symmetry and anatomy of the lower extremities. Range of motion of the hips. *Tibial torsion* can be tested for with the child supine and the knees facing upward. The forefoot and hindfoot should be in line with knees. The same test may be done with child prone and the knee bent; foot should be in a neutral position. In tibial torsion tibia is in a twisted position, either internally or externally, causing feet to turn inward or outward
      3. Position: sitting position on examining table or parent's lap, wearing only diaper or underpants
      4. Observation and palpation: of upper and lower extremities. Range of motion is assessed. Subluxation of the radius, most common in 2- to 4-year-olds, is indicated when passive range of motion is possible in all directions except supination
      5. Position: young toddler stands on examining table with whatever support is needed. If learning or able to walk, child is placed on the floor and supported by parent or examiner
      6. Observation: of back, symmetry of lower extremities, configuration of lower legs and feet, and gait. *Pes valgus* (toeing out) and *pes varus* (toeing in) may be causing or caused by tibial torsion. If these conditions persist, referral is needed. Observation is made for *genu varum* (bowleggedness) and *genu valgum* (knockknees). In genu valgum, the medial malleoli are more than 1 in apart when the knees are touching. This latter condition may be normal in children between 2 and 3½ years of age. In assessing the toddler's gait, the examiner expects it to be broadbased with very little balance

III. Preschool
   A. General assesment
      1. Position: depending on comfort level, seated on examining table, in a nearby chair, or on parent's lap
      2. Observations: of general appearance, growth, and body proportion as well as behavior
   B. Assessment of upper extremities
      1. Position: sitting, wearing only underpants
      2. Observation and palpation: of upper extremities, including range of motion
   C. Assessment of lower extremities
      1. Position: supine on examining table, wearing underpants only
      2. Observation and palpation: of lower extremities, including range of motion; tibial torsion is noted
      3. Position: standing on the floor wearing only underpants
      4. Observation: configuration of the lower legs (genu varum or valgum) and feet (pes varus or valgus)
   D. Assessment of the spine
      1. Position: standing on the floor with the back to the examiner; observations are made in the upright and forward bending positions
      2. Observation and palpation: of the back, for scoliosis or other spinal deformity; complete screening exam is included in that section (see Table 22-8)
   E. Observation of gait
      1. Position: standing on floor
      2. Assessment: child is instructed to walk away from and then return to examiner. The shy preschooler may need to be accompanied by parents. The examiner notes smoothness of movement and position of arms, legs, and toes. Toes should point straight ahead, and the opposite arm and leg should move forward at the same time. Abnormalities should be described in relation to the specific phase and stage. The two phases are the stance phase and the swing phase. The *stance phase* begins when the heel strikes the ground. Heel strike is the first of three stages: the heel strike, midstance, and push-off. The *swing phase* also consists of three stages: acceleration, swing-through, and deceleration
   F. Observation of gross motor skills
      1. Position: standing on the floor
      2. Assessment: preschooler is learning such skills as jumping, hopping, and skipping; examiner observes the symmetry, smoothness, and ease with which these skills are performed

IV. School-age and adolescent
   The following examination protocol has been developed by the American Orthopaedic Society for Sports Medicine (1981) as an orthopedic screening examination for participation in sports.
   A. General assessment
      1. Instructions: stand straight with arms at sides
      2. Observation: symmetry of upper and lower extremities and trunk. Common abnormalities include swollen or enlarged joints and asymmetrical waist (indicative of leg length discrepancy or scoliosis)
   B. Examination of neck
      1. Instruction: look at ceiling; look at floor; touch right (left) ear to shoulder; look over right (left) shoulder
      2. Observations: ability to touch chin to chest, ears to shoulders and look equally over shoulders; previous neck injury may be indicated by loss of range of motion

Continued.

TABLE 22-2 Physical Examination of the Musculoskeletal System in Different Age Groups—cont'd

C. Examination of upper extremities
  1. Instructions: shrug shoulders while examiner holds them down
  2. Observations: trapezius muscles appear equal with equal strength on both sides; neck or shoulder problems may be indicated by loss of strength or muscle bulk
  3. Instructions: hold arms out from sides horizontally and lift while examiner holds them down
  4. Observations: deltoid muscles should be equal in size with equal strength
  5. Instructions: hold arms out from sides with elbows bent (90°); raise hands back vertically as far as they will go
  6. Observations: hands go back equally and achieve an upright vertical position; loss of external rotation may indicate a shoulder problem such as an old dislocation
  7. Instructions: hold arms out from sides with palms up; straighten elbows completely and then bend them completely
  8. Observations: movement should be equal in left and right arms; loss of flexion or extension may indicate an old elbow injury
D. Examination of the forearms and hands
  1. Instructions: hold arms down at sides with elbows bent (90°); supinate palms, then pronate palms

  2. Observations: palms should go from facing the ceiling to facing the floor; failure to achieve these positions may indicate old forearm, wrist, or elbow injury
  3. Instructions: make a fist; open hand and spread fingers
  4. Observations: fist should be tight and fingers straight when spread; protruding knuckles or swollen, crooked fingers may indicate old finger fractures or sprains
E. Examination of the spine
  1. Instructions: with back to examiner, stand up straight; then bend forward slowly to touch toes
  2. Observations: screening for scoliosis; this exam is coverd in detail in the section on scoliosis and is outlined in Table 22-8
F. Examination of lower extremities
  1. Instructions: stand on heels; raise up to stand on toes; child is facing away from examiner
  2. Observations: symmetry of calf muscles, with equal raising of both heels; wasting of calf muscles may indicate an Achilles tendon injury or old ankle injury
  3. Instructions: stand facing the examiner; squat on heels; duck walk four steps and stand up
  4. Observations: distance between the heel and buttock should be equal both left and right. Knee flexion is equal when walking. At completion, child rises straight up. The maneuver should be painless.

Common Diagnostic Tests

X-Ray Examinations

X-ray films are widely used in orthopedics for diagnosing or ruling out fractures, tumors, some foreign bodies, and various other disturbances of the bones and joints. X-ray films are useful not only for diagnosing fractures and other problems but also for monitoring treatment effectiveness and healing.

The child's role in x-ray film studies of the skeletal system is only to refrain from moving for the fraction of a second. The nurse's role is to inform and prepare the youngster so that he can cooperate without undue fear or anxiety. X-ray equipment is huge and can have an alien quality that small children and school-age children find alarming. The novice pediatric nurse can best prepare herself to help children in the x-ray department by going along with clients and soliciting their descriptions and "explanations" of what takes place there.

Muscle Enzyme Studies

Several enzymes are released from damaged or dying muscle cells and are then found in abnormally high concentrations in blood specimens of persons with muscle trauma and muscle disease. These enzymes include lactic acid dehydrogenase (LDH), aldolase, the transaminases (SGOT and SGPT), and creatine phosphokinase (CPK). These enzymes are also normally present in liver cells and cardiac muscle, and serum levels rise in diseases of those organs as well as in skeletal muscle disorders. Surgery and exercise also produce elevated serum enzymes.

Serum enzymes are nonspecific indicators of damage to the heart, liver, brain, or muscle. When liver disease, brain injury, and heart damage can be ruled out, serum enzymes are indicative of skeletal muscle disorder. CPK is most concentrated in the voluntary muscles and hence is the best muscle enzyme for diagnosing muscle disease. Serum CPK is measured in children suspected of having muscular dystrophy. Retesting is done to assess the progress of the disease.

Common Nursing Measures

Nursing Diagnoses

Table 22-3 lists nursing diagnoses that are particularly relevant in the care of children with musculoskeletal disorders. Some apply to virtually every client (for example, impaired physical mobility), while others, such as altered tissue perfusion, are rare and generally occur only when complications arise. The relatively rare nursing diagnoses are included to give students a comprehensive overview of the client's situation and to alert them to watch for complications.

Anxiety is a special problem for children whose mobility is restricted, since physical activity plays a major role during childhood and adolescence in (1) coping, (2) social activities and peer status, (3) learning, and (4) self-concept.

Constipation readily develops in association with immobility. Moreover, constipation may arise whenever self-

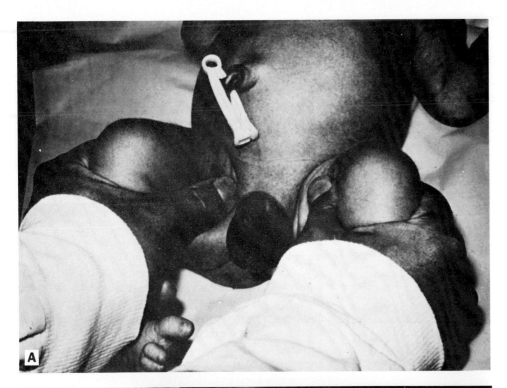

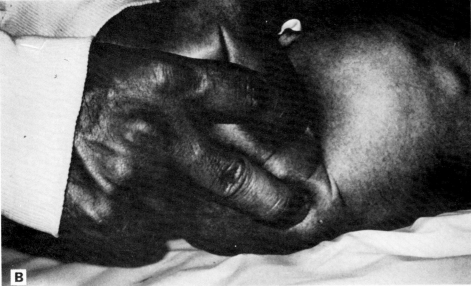

FIGURE 22-5   The Ortolani test is the most reliable method to detect a dislocated hip before 1 month of age. *(Photos courtesy of Richard Lindseth.)*

concious children or teenagers are expected to use bed-pans, as may be required if the child is in traction or a body cast.

Pain may be caused by trauma, muscle spasm, anxiety, pressure points under casts, and surgery. Pain following fracture is of special concern until the nurse can rule out the possibility that nerves or blood vessels are being compressed by bone fragments or by the cast. Compressed nerves or vessels can cause irreversible loss of function or even of a limb; early recognition and intervention are critical, as will be explained in a later section.

Coping can fail when a client experiences birth defects, trauma, or other conditions (such as cancer) that can lead to orthopedic disorders in childhood or adolescence. These circumstances are often accompanied by guilt on the part of the parents and child, anxiety, fear, immobility, deformity, pain, separation of family members, and the difficulties children and families experience when hospitalization is necessary. Permanent impairment in either function (e.g., limping) or appearance (e.g., amputation) obviously strains coping resources.

Diversional activities including play during childhood

TABLE 22-3 Nursing Diagnoses That May Often Apply in the Care of Children and Adolescents with Musculoskeletal Disorders

Anxiety
Body image disturbance
Comfort, alteration in: pain
Constipation
Coping, ineffective family: compromised
Coping, ineffective individual
Diversional activity deficit
Fear
Grieving, dysfunctional
Growth and development, altered
Infection, potential for
Injury, potential for
Knowledge deficit
Mobility, impaired physical
Nutrition, altered: potential for more than body requirements
Pain
Parenting, altered: potential
Role performance, altered
Self-care deficit
Self-esteem disturbance
Skin integrity, impaired: potential
Social interaction, impaired
Tissue integrity, impaired
Tissue perfusion, altered (peripheral)

Source: North American Nursing Diagnosis Association, 3525 Caroline Street, St. Louis, MO 63104.

and many of the social activities that are so important to development in childhood and adolescence. Any disorder of mobility, physical skill, or coordination calls for resourceful substituting of activities that promote mental health and human development.

Fears of children may or may not be verbalized and are likely to include fear of procedures (venipuncture, cast removal), fear of equipment (traction apparatus, x-ray machine), fear of pain or further injury from being touched and moved, fear of permanent disfigurement or disability, and the fears that accompany hospitalization (loss of peer status, failure in school).

Grieving is a prominent nursing diagnosis when loss of limb or life is threatened, as in serious trauma and malignant disease. Loss of social role, such as athlete or student, and loss of even seemingly small hopes, such as being able to participate in a particular event, can also induce grieving.

Alteration in growth and development is potentially applicable to all pediatric clients with birth defects, traumatic injuries, limited mobility, and the like. The promotion of normal growth and development is of course always a prominent goal in pediatric nursing whether or not the client's musculoskeletal system is affected.

Clients with musculoskeletal problems are at risk for *infection* if the skin has been broken in an accident or as an unavoidable part of their therapy (e.g., for surgical repair of a fracture or for the insertion of traction devices that attach to the bones). Casts and skin traction also create the potential for skin irritation that can progress to infection unless good nursing care is provided. Immobility creates the risk of respiratory infection such as stasis pneumonia.

Children and adolescents with musculoskeletal disorders may have to make special efforts to prevent *injury* if their strength or balance is impeded. As an obvious example, a client with a leg cast or a degenerative disease of the lower extremities will have trouble with balance and is at risk for injurious falls.

Knowledge deficit is a universally applicable nursing diagnosis that reminds nurses of their responsibility to teach. In pediatric nursing particularly, knowledge deficit consists not only of not knowing but also, in the words of the folk philosopher, "knowing so many things that just ain't true." Broken bones and casts generate many mistaken ideas and alarming fantasies in children's minds, perhaps because the word *broken* when applied to toys and household items often means broken into separate pieces that may not be amenable to reassembly. Preschoolers and school-age children have expressed the misconception that a plaster cast is a substitute for a limb rather than a protective cylinder around it. The nurse must assess clients' mistaken ideas as well as their lack of knowledge. Parent teaching is always part of pediatric nursing when the client has a musculoskeletal disorder.

Impaired physical mobility is obviously common and is a major focus of orthopedic nursing. The special challenge with children and adolescents is to keep to an absolute minimum the detrimental effect reduced mobility has on the attainment of developmental tasks.

Alterations in nutrition occur when immobility and other aspects of illness or hospitalization interfere with appetite. In this regard children with muscle and bone disorders are not different from children with other kinds of health problems. The potential for intake that exceeds caloric needs, however, is particularly common among inactive clients, and obesity is a frequent complication of disorders, such as muscular dystrophy, that produce long-term underactivity.

The potential for *alteration in parenting* is enormous in orthopedic disorders that induce permanent disability. If a child has been injured in circumstances that can be interpreted as parental neglect or failure to supervise, parents' guilt can be a heavy burden. Parents frequently blame themselves for all their children's injuries and illnesses: "If only I . . ."; "I should have. . . ." Congenital defects and familial diseases are also likely to cause guilt feelings. The diagnosis of altered parenting may pertain to the client's siblings in situations in which parents are so fully occupied with caring for the ill child that they have difficulty realizing and meeting the requirements of their other children.

Self-concept disturbances are not rare among pediatric clients with musculoskeletal problems. *Body image* may be severely interfered with by disability or deformity and is also hampered by traction equipment, casts, prostheses, crutches, and the like. *Self-esteem* in childhood and adolescence depends to a great degree on peer status and on the ability to perform games and other physical activities. A "normal" appearance is also of central importance to self-esteem. *Role performance,* from participating in play groups to sex roles, is inseparably tied in with self-concept.

Loss of *skin integrity* can occur because of traction and casting, as will be discussed later, and appliances such as braces can also lead to skin breakdown. Failure to preserve skin integrity can result in serious and usually needless complications. An ulcer caused by a toy or other foreign object placed inside a cast can easily become infected. A child who wears leg braces and has poor circulation because of paralysis can be sidelined for days or weeks if blisters or abrasions develop as a result of inattention to a small wrinkle in a stocking.

Social interaction has been alluded to already. Family relations, peer interactions, and social mobility can be impeded by orthopedic disorders.

Tissue integrity and *tissue perfusion* are at risk in numerous musculoskeletal disorders, especially those which can cause compression of nerves or blood vessels. These topics will be discussed at length later in this chapter. Nerves or arteries can be caught between fragments of a broken bone. Neurovascular occlusion from edema that develops inside a cast can cause permanent paralysis or gangrene. A similar edema phenomenon called *compartment syndrome* can also lead to tissue death from swelling inside a fascia sheath; the inflexible fascia binds the edematous tissue inside it, and as the swelling increases, perfusion of the muscle fails and necrosis and nerve damage follow. Skilled observation and early recognition of neurovascular occlusion, followed promptly by intervention to relieve the compression (by splitting the offending cast or by surgical incision to release tissue encased in a fascia compartment), prevent deformity.

Nursing Management
Care of the Child with Multiple Trauma
Motorcycle and automobile accidents, lawn mower injuries, and falls are just a few of the causes of multiple trauma in children. Injuries to the musculoskeletal system often include fractures, dislocations, and associated soft tissue injuries. Although other body systems may take priority in regard to immediate treatment, disabilities from musculoskeletal injuries are longer lasting and are often of more concern to the child and his family.

Assessment of the *skeletal* system after trauma begins with observation for obvious deformity, swelling, and pain. Fractures and dislocations should be splinted before moving the extremity to prevent further injury, minimize pain and immobilize the limb. The splint is applied above and a joint below the fracture with the limb in a position of maximum comfort and relaxation. For upper extremity fractures, a padded arm board or right-angle splint can be used and a right angle or a Thomas splint (Fig. 22-12) is appropriate. When the patient has arrived wearing a plastic air splint, the physician should be present during removal since improper removal can cause further injury to

the limb. Splinting should not be done when an extremity is so deformed that it does not conform to the splint; instead, the extremity should be left in its position and immobilized with sandbags.

The possibility of a coexisting neck injury should always be considered in trauma. The patient should not be moved until an x-ray has confirmed that the cervical vertebrae are intact. When an injury to any part of the spine is suspected, the child should be moved only as an immobilized unit with a board or flat object as a splint. When turning is necessary, it should be done by *logrolling,* a method of turning the body as a rigid unit. A drawsheet often facilitates logrolling, and an adequate number of staff members should help with this procedure.

Whenever possible, the nurse should seek information from a witness to the accident concerning the time and events leading to the injury. The type of accident often indicates the type of injury to be suspected; for example, a diving accident makes one suspect trauma to the cervical spine. If parents or relatives are available, they should be questioned about the time of the child's last meal, allergies, and his past medical history. Some type of progress report at intervals can help relieve the anxiety of family members waiting outside the emergency area.

Preoperative and Postoperative Care
The aims of musculoskeletal surgical procedures are to improve function and ability, prevent or correct deformity, and relieve pain. Surgical manipulations (Table 22-4) are usually done to reduce fractures or dislocations by passive movements of the parts. Surgical operations involve incisions and repair or reconstruction of tissues; soft tissues (muscles, tendons, and ligaments), nerves, joints, or bones may be involved.

Preoperative preparation centers on the child's and family's understanding of the surgery and the child's readiness to cooperate with postoperative care. The nurse reinforces information given by the physician concerning an-

TABLE 22-4 Terms Used to Describe Common Surgical Procedures

Term	Definition
Arthrodesis	Stabilization or fusion of a joint
Arthroplasty	Reconstruction of a joint
Arthrotomy	Surgical opening and exploration of a joint
Epiphyseodesis	Fusion of an epiphysis to its diaphysis
Laminectomy	Removal of the vertebral lamina for decompression of spinal nerves
Myotomy	Cutting into a muscle
Osteotomy	Division of a bone
Tendon lengthening	Division of a tendon followed by resuturing in an elongated position
Tendon or muscle transfer	Transfer of the origin or insertion of a tendon or muscle into the place of a paralyzed or damaged one
Tenotomy	Division of a tendon

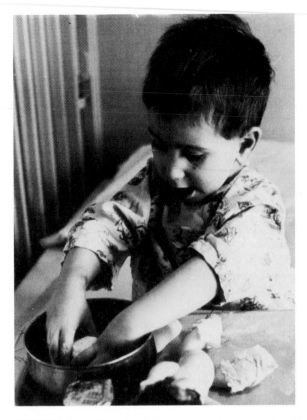

FIGURE 22-6 Child casting doll as preoperative preparation. *(Courtesy of James Whitcomb Riley Hospital for Children, Indianapolis; photo by G. Dreyer.)*

esthesia, the time of surgery, the surgery itself, and the child's postoperative appearance. The child may enjoy manipulating rolls of plaster and applying a cast on a doll similar to the cast he will wear after surgery, as illustrated in Fig. 22-6. Special functions which will be required postoperatively may be practiced before the child goes to surgery. If he is to be immobilized, he should try voiding into a bedpan in bed. Other routines which can be rehearsed are turning or logrolling, coughing, and deep breathing.

Postoperatively the nurse assesses circulation and function in peripheral parts of the extremity. At 1- to 2-hour intervals, observations are made of color, warmth, swelling, pulses, sensation, and movement in the limb. The fingers or toes are pressed to see if they blanch and show rapid return of color. Drainage on the cast or bandage should be recorded. Stains on the cast are outlined with a pen and labeled as to the time observed. The nurse must be aware of early warning signs that the cast is too tight or circulation is insufficient (Table 22-5). If any of these signs are observed, they should be reported to the physician at once. Their presence usually means that the cast must be *bivalved* (split apart) to restore circulation and function to the extremity.

Positioning during the immediate postoperative period is intended to maintain the original shape of the cast and to support the child in anatomic postures. Pillows and blanket rolls are used for padding and support. The cast is

TABLE 22-5 Neurovascular Checks*

Severe pain or pain that is not relieved by analgesics
Persistent swelling that is not relieved by elevating the limb
Pulselessness
Coldness to touch
Discoloration: pallor or cyanosis
Distorted sensation: numbness, tingling, or burning
Inability of client to move a previously functional part

*Neurovascular checks are made at the part of the extremity distal to the injury or surgical site and distal to a cast. Danger signs may indicate compression of nerves or blood vessels and require immediate notification of the physician.

elevated to prevent swelling. A footboard, special shoes, or splints prevent foot drop in the paralyzed patient. The child should be turned every 2 hours to promote circulation and facilitate drying of the cast, which should also be left uncovered. In the supine position, the child's head should be slightly elevated during drinking and eating in order to prevent choking.

Casts

Casts are used for immobilization of body parts, maintenance of position, or correction of deformity. The most common cast material is plaster of paris. However, fiberglass casts also are being used on children. Approximately 24 to 48 hours is required for the plaster cast to dry completely. The cast dries from the outside to the inside; therefore, it may feel dry on the outside but still be wet on the inside. It should remain uncovered during drying, and the patient should be turned every 2 hours so that moisture can evaporate from its surface. Heat lamps or heated fan dryers should never be used for drying.

During cast application, the child is positioned as directed by the physician. To minimize movement at a fracture site, manual traction on the extremity or a strong steady pull on each side of the fracture site is exerted while the cast is being applied. A special orthopedic cast table is usually required when body or hip spica casts are applied. Various types of casts are shown in Fig. 22-7.

Casts which are made of fiberglass are useful in special circumstances. The advantages of this material are that it is stronger and lighter than plaster and can be immersed in water if the physician permits. Soaking should not be prolonged, and soap should be used sparingly around the cast. Drying is accomplished by blotting with towels or blowing with a hair dryer set at a low temperature. Rough edges can be finished off with an emery board or a nail file.

Cast Care

After cast application, circulation and function in the limb should be assessed for all patients every 1 or 2 hours and then less frequently. Parents of children who are sent home from the hospital immediately after cast application must be informed about the signs of a tight cast (Table 22-5). They are instructed to return to the physician with-

FIGURE 22-7 Types of casts. *(From H. Moidel et al., Nursing Care of the Patient with Medical-Surgical Disorders, McGraw-Hill, New York, 1971, p. 881.)*

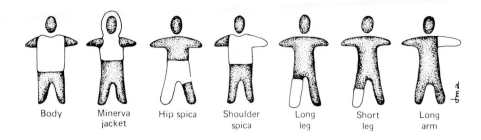

Body   Minerva jacket   Hip spica   Shoulder spica   Long leg   Short leg   Long arm

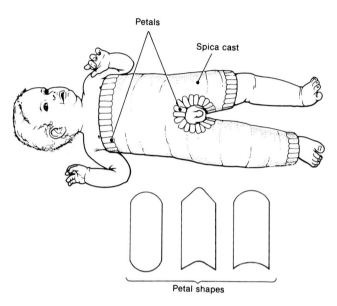

FIGURE 22-8 Spica cast finished off with adhesive tape petals; samples of petals.

out delay if any of these signs appear. To prevent unnatural molding of the cast, the wet cast is supported on pillows on a firm base or mattress, and the child is turned at 1- or 2-hour intervals. The nurse handles the cast with the palms instead of the fingers to prevent indentations in the soft plaster. Abduction bars built into the cast to keep the legs apart should never be used as handles to move the cast.

When the cast is dry, rough edges are finished off by petaling. Strips of adhesive tape are cut and secured over rough or unfinished edges as illustrated in Fig. 22-8. Each petal overlaps the previous one until the entire edge is covered. The skin at cast edges is checked for signs of soreness, and tight edges causing irritation are stretched or cut away. Complaints of pain or burning or an offensive odor from the inside of the cast should be investigated since these symptoms may indicate that a sore is forming or has become infected. Powders and lotions should not be used inside the cast; skin underneath cast edges can be massaged with alcohol. Itching under the cast is eliminated by blowing cool air through the cast with an Asepto syringe or hair dryer. Some physicians insert a strip of gauze through the cast which can be used to massage the skin gently and eliminate itching. Sharp objects such as

knitting needles may injure the skin and are not suitable as scratchers. Skin care is particularly important for a neurologically damaged child who lacks sensation under the cast.

Keeping the cast clean and dry is a challenge with infants or children who are incontinent. The child may be placed on a frame which allows urine and feces to drain into a bedpan below, or he may be returned to his crib with plastic-covered pillows used for support. With the head of the frame or bed elevated, urine and feces drain away from the cast by gravity. Plastic wrap is tucked around cast edges, although it cannot be taped onto the cast until it dries. When the cast is dry, inner edges around the diaper areas may need to be cut away to allow for care after defecation and voiding. Edges of the dry cast are covered with adhesive tape petals, after which plastic wrap is tucked under the inside edge and secured to the outside of the cast with tape. A child who is in bed can be kept dry by the use of a folded diaper or sanitary pad which is tucked under the cast edges and changed frequently. The diaper (or pad) is held in place by another diaper which is fastened around the cast. Plastic 24-hour urine collecting bags may also be used, but they often cause skin irritation. When a cast becomes soiled, it can be cleaned by removing soiled tape petals and wiping with a damp cloth.

For all children in casts, bowel and bladder function should be assessed regularly. Constipation and poor urinary drainage may result from immobilization. A fracture bedpan can be used to facilitate toileting. The child's head and shoulders should be elevated, and a folded pad should be placed over the back edge of the bedpan. Administration of suppositories or mild laxatives may be necessary for a child who is constipated. The urine should be checked for signs of infection, especially in a child who has a neurogenic bladder. An adequate fluid intake should be maintained. A low-calcium diet may be prescribed in an effort to prevent urinary calculi.

Home Care

To prepare the parents for home care of the child, the nurse should demonstrate turning, positioning, and handling of the child in the cast and also clarify the child's mobility limits with parents. Bathing, skin care, diaper care, bowel evacuation, and treatment of problems in these areas are discussed, and activities of care are practiced. Parents should be aware of warning signs that the cast is too tight (Table 22-5) or the child is outgrowing the cast, and they should know what to do if problems ensue. Other safety measures should be discussed, such as elevating the child's head during eating and drinking to prevent choking; preventing the small child from dropping crumbs, coins, or other small objects down into the cast which could cause skin breakdown; and using body mechanics when lifting and transporting the child.

Normal daily activities at home may need to be altered for the child in a cast, although the child should be treated as normally as possible within activity limits. Clothing has to be purchased in larger sizes or constructed differently. A wagon, wheelchair, or stretcher is needed to transport a child in a heavy cast, while crutches may be required for an older child in a long leg cast. A creeper or padded board on wheels provides mobility for a young child in a body or spica cast. Simple tasks such as washing hair or bathing may need to be modified. A sponge bath may have to be substituted for a tub bath. Spray hoses aid hair washing over the sink, but an older child in a body cast may have to wash his hair by leaning over the edge of the bed with a pan placed on a low stool below. Flexible drinking straws made from plastic tubing used in aquariums facilitate drinking for the child who cannot sit. Teachers for the home-bound may be required for the child to continue schoolwork.

Cast Removal
When the cast is to be removed, the cast cutter, an electric saw with a vibrating (*not* rotating) circular blade, is frightening to children. The child may believe that the saw will cut off his limb. The cutting noise is also upsetting. Children can be helped to deal with anxiety by wearing a special set of soundproof earmuffs or by observing the saw lightly touched to the operator's palm. During the actual procedure, the child should be held very still and the procedure should be carried out as quickly and safely as possible. Short casts, such as clubfoot casts, can be soaked off with the physician's permission in order to avoid use of the saw. Parents can be instructed to immerse the cast in a vinegar-water solution (about 1 part vinegar to 4 parts water) and unwind the softened bandages. When a cast is removed, support is provided for all joints which were immobilized. Dead skin and sebaceous material are removed gently by rubbing with alcohol, repeated washing, or applying oil for a few hours, followed by washing.

Traction
Traction is the application of a pulling force to a part of the body. Force is exerted either manually or mechanically. Traction is used in the treatment of fractures, joint dislocations, contractures of muscles causing deformity, and muscle spasm. The specific aims of traction in the treatment of a fracture are to correct displacement of fragments in the fractured bone, immobilize the fracture during healing, and reduce muscle spasm around the fracture site, thereby reducing pain. Traction may also be used to decrease spinal curvature or joint dislocations, stretch the shortened fibers of contracted muscle, and treat muscle spasm unassociated with a fracture.

The type of traction is selected in accordance with the age of the patient and the goals of treatment. Skin traction is used for younger children when mild forces of traction are sufficient. Skeletal traction is used in children when greater traction force is required. Traction may be continuous or intermittent. When used for reduction and immobilization of a fracture, it is continuous and should not be interrupted for dressing or any other activity. When traction is intermitttent, it may be disconnected temporarily as specified by the physician. Traction may be applied by a traction device fastened to the end of the bed (*fixed traction*) or balanced by cords with pulleys and weights (*balanced traction*).

Skin Traction
In *skin traction* the pulling force is applied directly to the skin and indirectly to muscles and bones. Skin traction may be applied by a sponge rubber boot or adhesive straps. When the latter method is used, the adhesive straps are applied by the physician because of the risk of circulatory compromise. Weights are attached to the boot or straps by cords which pass over one or more pulleys. If the physician specifies, the foot of the bed may have to be raised so that the child's own weight provides countertraction. Skin traction is contraindicated if skin rash or hypersensitivity, soft tissue damage in the area, vascular insufficiency, swelling, or neurovascular compromise is present.

One type of skin traction is *Bryant's traction,* which is used to reduce hip dislocation in children under 3 years of age. Both lower extremities are suspended from an overhead rod with the hips at right angles, as shown in Fig. 22-9. This type of traction should be used only in a child weighing less than 35 lb because of the risk of circulatory complications. With the legs in an overhead position, blood has to be pumped against gravity to reach the feet. Circulation is further compromised in a child weighing over 35 lb because the amount of weight needed for traction causes stretching of the popliteal muscle and therefore compression of the blood vessels to the lower extremity. Bryant's traction should be used *only* to treat hip dislocation in the young child. Pediatric orthopedic surgeons have taken the position that Bryant's traction is not to be used to treat fractures of the femur in children because circulatory complications happen frequently in the noninjured leg.

In Bryant's traction, the amount of weight applied is the amount needed to keep the buttocks just barely off the bed. The nurse should be able to pass one hand under the child's buttocks as they clear the bed. The nurse also checks that the traction bandages are continued to a point well above the knee and up to the hips. Bandages should be rewrapped daily, not just checked, in order to prevent circulatory compromise. The knee should be in a slightly flexed position to prevent stretching of the popliteal mus-

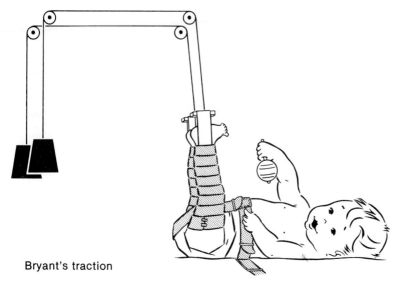

Bryant's traction

FIGURE 22-9   Bryant's traction, used to reduce hip dislocation. *(From G. Carini and J. Birmingham, Traction Made Manageable, McGraw-Hill, New York, 1980, p. 129.)*

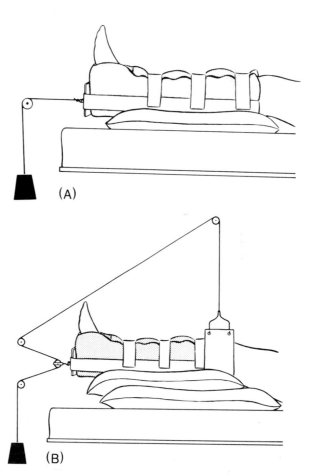

FIGURE 22-10   Skin traction to the lower extremity. *(A)* Buck's extension traction. *(B)* Russell's traction. *(From G. Carini and J. Birmingham, Traction Made Manageable, McGraw-Hill, New York, 1980, pp. 87-88.)*

cle. A small notch cut in the tapes at the ankle allows the child to move the foot without causing constriction at the ankle. A jacket restraint or T strap is necessary to keep the child in the desired position. Caution must be taken if sandbags are used as restraints along the side of the trunk, as sandbags tend to slip down and adduct the hips. Shock blocks are often used to allow countertraction.

Buck's extension traction (Fig. 22-10A) is another method of applying traction to the lower extremity. One or both legs rest on the bed, and the traction force is applied by weights directly at the end of the bed. Often a boot device is worn on the foot. A pillow is placed under the leg to keep pressure off the heel. Countertraction is provided by elevating the foot of the bed approximately 6 in. This type of traction is used in immobilizing a fractured hip or an injured knee or proximal tibia.

Skin traction to the lower extremity is also applied by *Russell's traction,* as illustrated in Fig. 22-10B. In this traction, two pulling forces are applied to the knee. A sling under the distal thigh applies force to the back of the thigh. A sponge rubber boot or adhesive straps are applied to the leg, and weights are attached which exert force on the long axis of the leg. The resultant pulling force is along the axis of the femur. Therefore, this traction is used to reduce and immobilize fractures of the femoral shaft. When the child is positioned in traction, both the hip and knee remain slightly flexed. The lower leg is elevated on pillows so that it is parallel to the bed. The amount of weight is less than that required in Buck's extension traction. Because of the double-pulley system at the foot, the amount of traction force is double the amount of weight. In Russell's skin traction, countertraction is provided by elevating the foot of the bed approximately 6 in.

Skin traction to the upper extremity is achieved by *sidearm traction, overhead 90-90 traction, or Dunlop's traction* (Fig. 22-11). Fractures of the humerus, elbow, or shoulder are treated by these methods. If the skin ap-

proach is not indicated in one of these injuries, the skeletal approach can be used. In *sidearm traction,* adhesive straps are applied to the upper arm and forearm by the use of woven cotton elastic (Ace) bandage wraps. Longi-

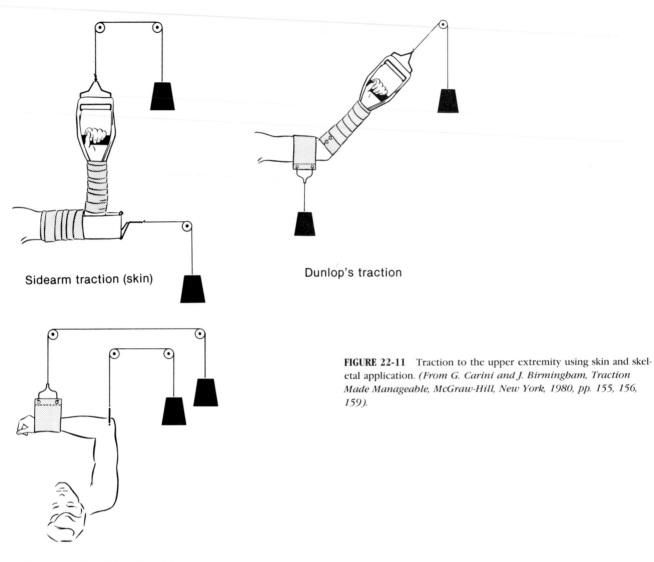

Sidearm traction (skin)

Dunlop's traction

Overhead 90–90 traction (skeletal)

FIGURE 22-11   Traction to the upper extremity using skin and skeletal application. *(From G. Carini and J. Birmingham, Traction Made Manageable, McGraw-Hill, New York, 1980, pp. 155, 156, 159).*

FIGURE 22-12   Leg in Thomas splint and Pearson attachment. *(From G. Carini and J. Birmingham, Traction Made Manageable, McGraw-Hill, New York, 1980, p. 109.)*

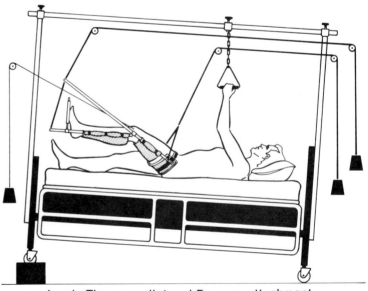

Leg in Thomas splint and Pearson attachment

tudinal traction is applied to the upper arm to exert force on the humerus. The forearm is pulled upward to hold the upper extremity in the lateral position. Countertraction is accomplished by elevating the bed with shock blocks on the same side as the traction force or by placing a folded blanket under the mattress on the affected side. A special frame can be clamped to the bed which allows the head of the bed to be elevated without disrupting the traction. *Dunlop's traction* is used specifically to reduce supracondylar fractures of the humerus. The shoulder is held in abduction, and the elbow is held in a 45-degree extended position. Skin traction is applied to the forearm and attached to the weights. A second force is applied by a sling with weights hanging from the distal portion of the upper arm. As in Russell's traction, the line of pull is in a third direction. A molding force results which brings the bone fragments into correct position. Countertraction is achieved by elevating the side of the bed toward the traction. In both of the above traction methods, the arm is abducted and held in a lateral position. This position is in contrast to *overhead 90-90 traction,* in which the arm is suspended over the upper chest. Although skin traction can be used, skeletal application is more common. The upper arm is held in a position perpendicular to the body by means of a weight pulling on the elbow. The forearm is suspended in a sling to provide support. This method allows more freedom of movement and also has the advantage of lessened edema.

A special skin traction setup which exerts pressure around the spinal column is *Cotrel traction.* A head halter and pelvic girdle are used to exert traction indirectly on the spinal column and paraspinous muscles in preparation for surgery. Scoliosis patients may use this type of traction continuously or intermittently. Pressure areas at the chin and iliac crest need special preventive care. It is imperative that the traction be adjusted to fit the patient correctly. The main pull should be off the occipital area, with minimal pull off the chin. When the patient is in full extension, the nurse should be able to place one hand under the lumbar region.

Skeletal Traction

In *skeletal traction* a direct hold on the bone is obtained by means of metallic devices. Certain children's fractures are best reduced and immobilized by skeletal traction. For example, a compound fracture of the long bones and an unstable fracture of the long bones that has multiple fragments both require skeletal traction. Metallic devices most often used are Kirschner's wires and Steinmann pins. A *Kirschner,* or *K,* wire is a small-gauge stainless steel wire. Because of its small diameter it has several advantages: A smaller opening can be made in the skin, there is less destruction of bone cells, and infection is less likely. A disadvantage of the K wire's small gauge is that it can cut through bone if very heavy traction is applied. The Steinmann pin is larger in diameter and stronger than the K wire. Both pins and wires are inserted completely through the bone, and traction forces are applied to them. Crutch-

field tongs and halo pins utilized to apply traction of the cervical spine are imbedded in the skull. All sites of entry for pins, wires, or tongs should be treated as surgical wounds. These areas may be kept very clean by wiping with Betadine solution or applying Neosporin or Bacitracin ointment daily. Some physicians prefer to let these areas crust over or cover them with plaster signs of pintract infection noted around the sites of entry or exit of metallic devices, include redness, swelling, heat, pain or purulent exudate. The child should be cautioned not to touch the area around the pin site and not to move around excessively in traction, since these activities can contribute to development of an infection.

The nurse should be aware of various types of skeletal traction. Traction to the cervical spine is accomplished by Crutchfield tongs or a metal halo fastened to the skull by pins. It is important to maintain the proper position of the patient in cervical spine traction. A turning frame such as a Stryker frame is often used. Another important nursing function is assessment of the child's neurological status. Movement of the extremities, strength of hand grips, and sensory complaints such as numbness, tingling, and loss of sensation are evaluated. Traction to the upper extremities may be by skeletal means. Sidearm skeletal traction is applied by the use of a Kirschner's wire through the olecranon. Other parts of the traction setup are the same as in sidearm skin traction. Overhead 90-90 traction is most often used with a skeletal application and may include a Kirschner's wire through the olecranon. When skeletal traction is required for the lower extremities, three sites commonly are used for pin insertion: (1) the distal femur and (2) proximal tibia, both used for fractures of the femur, pelvis, and acetabulum, and (3) the calcaneus or heel site, for compound or unstable fractures of the tibia. Fractures of the hip and femur are managed by the use of a Thomas splint with a Pearson attachment (Fig. 22-12).

Nursing Care for Children in Traction

When caring for a patient in traction, the nurse checks for neurovascular disturbance in the extremities. The vascular (circulatory) status is assessed by checking the quality of pulses distal to the injury, capillary filling (blanching sign), amount of swelling color, warmth, and increase in pain upon motion. The neurological status is evaluated by testing for normal sensation distal to the injury as well as pain, numbness, and tingling. Motor function is also assessed distal to the injury. The most serious complication of vascular occlusion is *compartment syndrome,* which occurs because of the compression of structures within a confined area as a result of secondary edema. Normally, there is an increase in edema secondary to the injury. Should edema formation continue, the increased pressure within the closed spaces of the tissue compartment obstructs venous circulation and causes arterial occlusion, which results in inadequate circulation and ischemia. In the forearm this syndrome is better known as *Volkmann's ischemic contracture.* A vicious cycle of edema and ischemia is established and, if allowed to go unchecked, will result in nerve and muscle damage. A contracted, paralyzed, and nonfunctioning extremity is the outcome. Signs of compartment syndrome are severe pain, absence of peripheral pulses, pallor and coolness of the skin, puffy swelling, paresthesia, and paralysis. The nurse must avoid giving analgesics for severe and persistent pain. Instead, when this syndrome is suspected, constricting bandages should be loosened, traction weights should be decreased, and the physician should be notified immediately.

The nurse should know the type of traction being used and its purpose. A diagram of the traction setup can be taped to the bed to assist the nurse in checking that traction is maintained correctly. The prescribed amount of weight must be attached at all times. Weights should hang free; ropes must be in the center track of the pulleys; and the footplate should not rest against the foot of the bed. Pressure from tapes on the following points should be avoided: dorsalis pedis artery (inside of top of foot), peroneal nerve (outer aspect of the calf just below the knee), and Achilles tendon (back of heel). The child's body alignment must be such that the purpose of traction is accomplished. Restraints and sandbags may be necessary to maintain body alignment. When indicated, countertraction is provided by the use of shock blocks under the legs of the bed on the same side as the traction apparatus. A firm mattress over bed boards helps eliminate sagging and maintain proper body alignment. Siderails should be on all traction beds to provide safety, security, and support.

The types of movement, exercise, and position changes allowed for the child are clarified with the physician. *Traction is not interrupted for any nursing activity* without specific orders. Clothing and diversional activities must be adapted to the traction apparatus. The child's bed can be pulled into the hall or playroom for group activities. Mobiles and toys can be suspended from the overhead bar. Measures are taken to prevent foot drop, especially in a neurologically damaged patient, by putting a box or special boot next to or on the unaffected foot. Flexion contractures of the hip are prevented by lowering the backrest of the bed several times a day unless contraindicated. Unaffected body parts are exercised actively or passively several times a day to maintain range of motion and muscle tone. Deep-breathing exercises are done to assist with ventilation.

Skin care for the child in traction is important. The child should lie on smooth, clean, and dry bedsheets. When the bed of a larger child is changed, two folded sheets are often more convenient than a single sheet. One sheet is applied from the head of the bed to the level of the splint, while the other covers the lower half of the bed under the splint. A trapeze bar assists the older child in lifting his shoulders off the bed for his bath and back care. The sacral area is another body part which is likely to become sore and irritated. Both the back and sacral area should be lifted off the bed and massaged two or three times a day. Devices which help to prevent skin breakdown include an "egg crate" mattress, a water mattress, and sheepskin pads. Skin over the heels, ankles, and elbows is inspected daily for signs of pressure from the bed or bandages. Heel and elbow protectors as well as pillow supports help prevent pressure problems. Frequent diaper changes prevent skin breakdown in the perineal area of the incontinent child. Daily assessments of bowel and bladder function should accompany skin care. A fracture bedpan assists the older child in toileting. Constipation and urinary infections are complications which can often be prevented by early nursing interventions. Proper nutrition is an important consideration to meet the body's demands for healing and to prevent skin, bowel, and bladder complications.

Bed Rest and Immobilization

Bed rest provides total body rest for acute conditions such as osteomyelitis. The patient in traction or in a spica or body cast is also forced to maintain bed rest to some degree. Remaining in bed for prolonged periods has several potential hazards, however, to both the physical and psychological well-being of the child. The effects of immobility may be greater than the effects of the illness or injury itself.

Physical Effects of Decreased Mobility

Physiological effects of immobility involve all major body systems. The *musculoskeletal* system suffers because normal movement and stresses from weight bearing are diminished. In muscle, disuse atrophy occurs as a result of tissue breakdown and loss of muscle mass. Wasting of the muscle is accompanied by weakness. The contraction of some muscles and the stretching of others may cause such disabilities as flexion contractures or foot drop. In the absence of normal joint movement, collagen fibers generating within the joint become fibrotic and create joint contractures. Demineralization of the bone (osteoporosis) weakens it and leaves it prone to pathological fractures. The *integumentary* system is particularly at risk in areas where the bone surface is near the skin. Pressure points include the sacrum, occiput, trochanter of the femur, and ankle. Circulation is impeded in these areas, manifested as redness. If pressure is not relieved, a large blister forms. The discolored area gradually becomes black and hard. Over several days, the necrotic tissue sloughs off, leaving a deep decubitus ulcer. *Circulatory* disturbances include orthostatic hypotension, increased workload of the heart, and thrombus formation. Without muscular contractions, blood tends to pool in dependent areas. Edematous tissue is especially prone to infection and trauma. The *respiratory* system reacts to a lessened demand for oxygen by altering the respiratory rate. Respirations become slower and more shallow. Chest expansion may be limited by a body cast, by the prone position, or by abdominal distention. More effort may be required to expand the lungs. The maintenance of one position allows the collection of bronchial secretions, which may result in development of hypostatic pneumonia, atelectasis, or respiratory acidosis. The *gastrointestinal* system's functions of intake and elimination are affected by immobility. Reduced energy requirements contribute to a diminished appetite and decreased intake of nutrients. A child who must lie supine is at greater risk for aspiration of food and fluids. Bowel elimination is altered by decreased muscle activity, changes in diet, loss of efficiency in defecation, and psychological difficulties during defecation. Constipation is a common problem and has been found to occur more often in children who have been toilet trained and have achieved bowel control. The *urinary* system is affected by changes in position during urination, alterations in gravitational force, and increased excretion of calcium from the bones. Stasis of urine in the kidney pelvis is complicated by large amounts of calcium which must be excreted; formation of calculi may be the result. Because the patient has difficulty voiding in the supine position, the bladder may become distended. Overflow incontinence and urinary infections are potential complications.

Nursing interventions need to prevent complications. A regular active exercise program is prescribed, using all unaffected joints and extremities. Passive exercises are prescribed for patients whose unaffected limbs are paralyzed. Frequent change of position is essential, preferably every half hour to hour. Special beds, such as the Stryker frame, may be indicated. Other devices used to prevent skin breakdown are an egg crate mattress, sheepskin pads, and sheepskin ankle and elbow protectors. A diet consisting of adequate fluids and bulk foods helps prevent constipation and urinary infection. A regular bowel elimination schedule can be established. Suppositories may aid in bowel evacuation. A child who is paralyzed should continue regular bowel-training programs in the hospital. After prolonged immobility, the child should be allowed to return to normal function gradually. Stiff joints can usually be worked out through play by a young child, while an older child may need physical therapy for rehabilitation. The child should build up his activity tolerance slowly to allow the heart to regain its optimal capabilities.

Psychological Effects of Decreased Mobility

Immobility has many psychological effects. The child views the inability to move as a threat to self-preservation. Immobilization implies surrender and passivity to the child and reactivates the struggle between dependence and independence. No longer can the child rely on freedom of movement to discharge tension, express dissatisfaction and aggression, or explore and master the environment. He may feel he is being "held captive" as he becomes a victim of his fears and fantasies. Distortions in body image often result from immobilization. The initial experience in being immobilized constitutes a crisis, since the child is confronted with new tasks that he cannot master quickly with existing coping mechanisms. New tasks include (1) learning new ways to cope constructively with frustration, (2) doing the grief work necessary to cope with changes in self-image and body image as well as the loss of pleasure from activity, self-care, and independence, and (3) establishing new patterns of interaction with his environment which provide gratification and restore self-esteem.

Immobilization has particular psychological effects on children in each age group. The *infant* copes with stress primarily through movement. Through touch, vision, and movement the infant develops a conception of his body image. Immobilization poses a threat to coping and to his development of body image. It also deprives him of much-needed physical contact through holding and cuddling. The *toddler* has an overwhelming need for movement. Any limitation on his newly gained motor skills results in an immediate threat to security. His typical reaction is to resist by climbing over siderails, tearing off restraints, or trying to walk in a cast. Screaming and crying also register protest. The *preschooler* has the same need for autonomy as does the toddler. His heightened feelings of vulnerability when immobilized predispose him to increased fears and fantasies of bodily injury and of being out of control. The *School-age* child is deprived of many sources of pleasure and learning and many normal coping patterns such as controlling behaviors and motor activity. His reaction, may be a combination of depression, hostility, and frustration. The *adolescent* is extremely stressed by mobility restrictions because they decrease his long-sought freedom and independence. He may be embarassed by the lack of privacy imposed or feel deprived of normal peer contact. The fantasies that arise from immobilization worry the adolescent who fears being "different" from his peers. *Parents* have their own reactions when a child is immobilized. The process of bonding may be interrupted if the newborn has restrictions as to positioning. Fears about unknown equipment, lack of knowledge about how to handle and care for the child, and feelings of loss of control are common among parents. The interpersonal relationship between the parent and child may be stressed. The parent receives less contact comfort from the child. Parents may not understand the immobilized child's acting-out behaviors, and this misunderstanding can lead to feelings of anger and frustration in the parent.

Nursing interventions can assist the child in dealing with immobilization. Problems with boredom are minimized by providing regular activities in a structured daily schedule. Schoolwork can be continued in the hospital. The child often enjoys having a television, radio, record player, tape recorder, or telephone available. All these measures increase sensory stimulation for the child. The nurse also tries to extend the physical space of the child. The chlid's bed is pulled into the hall or playroom for group activities. For the child who cannot sit up, special glasses with prismatic lenses allow him to see people and activities in front of him. The prone position may be facilitated by having the child lie on a stretcher or Stryker frame with his arms free. Peers are encouraged to visit the child in his room. Parents need help in adjusting to the unfamiliar environment so that they can be supportive to the child. Providing opportunities for play is another aim of the nurse. Games provide the child with important tactile and kinesthetic feedback. Mirrors give visual feedback to the child. The pleasure associated with play is an important distraction from feelings of restriction. It is also important for the nurse to promote independence in the immobilized child. The child can help to plan his activities, and he gains a sense of control when he is allowed to make choices about daily activities. Self-care activities can be adapted so that he is able to perform them despite physical restrictions.

Exercise

Therapeutic exercise is intended to increase muscle strength or to maintain or regain joint movement. Exercises are classified as active, passive, and resistive. Only *active exercises* strengthen muscles, and they are executed by the child himself as a natural part of his daily activities. Active exercise is dynamic when it produces motion and is static when no motion is produced *(isometric exercise). Passive exercise* is performed by external forces and is most valuable for patients with paralyzed or contracted muscles. Range of motion exercises prevent deformity by maintaining movements in joints. Contractures may be treated by passive stretching of muscles. *Resistive exercise* is active exercise performed by the patient against an external resistive force, such as iron weights, sandbags, or elastic bands. This type of exercise allows the patient to improve muscle strength and coordination and to build muscle hypertrophy.

Rehabilitation

As long as physical and social barriers exist, the ability of the physically handicapped child to develop to his potential remains limited. Nurses can participate in eliminating barriers through community action and individual assistance to children and families. Local community resources can be made available to the handicapped child in conjunction with an overall treatment program which helps the child maximize his individual resources.

The most simple and concrete suggestions are the most helpful to a child and family. For example, the little girl on crutches who would like to carry her doll with her can do so when a sling-type carrier is devised. Aprons or clothes with big pockets are useful for both boys and girls. Lightweight bicycle baskets can be attached to walking frames and pushers for use as carryalls. During play outdoors in cold weather, children who are paralyzed should be checked every 15 to 20 minutes to ensure that their legs and feet are warm. Electric blankets and heating pads should not be placed on the paralyzed child's bed since they can cause burns. For the child who is incontinent, absorbent garments can be cut from colorfully designed flannel material and constructed to look more like underpants than diapers. Plastic wastebaskets can be cut out and converted into bathing chairs to help a child with poor trunk control sit in the bathtub. Parents are often exceptionally creative in adapting equipment and devising activities for the child. The nurse works closely with other interdisciplinary team members and with parents to provide a wide range of experiences which lead to maximum independence and self-esteem in the child.

The management role of the nurse cannot be overemphasized in the rehabilitation of children with long-term disabling conditions. On the hospital unit, the nurse not only manages the care of the immediate problem but also investigates the need for follow-up in other areas, such as urology and neurosurgery. The nurse considers the long-term implications of short-term problems. For example, a child admitted for surgery and casting and his parents need information not only about the cast but also about the ways the cast may affect school attendance or urinary drainage. In the outpatient department, the nurse functions as a liaison between the family and the hospital. This role often involves orienting the family to the hospital system, clarifying medical treatment, adapting plans for use at home, and exploring hospital or community resources. The outpatient nurse is particularly concerned about continuity with colleagues: staff nurses on hospital units, community health nurses, and school nurses.

Musculoskeletal Diseases and Dysfunctions in the Newborn

Fractured Clavicle

The clavicles are the bones most often fractured during delivery and also the bones most commonly fractured during childhood. A clavicular fracture may be incomplete or complete. If the fracture is incomplete at birth, no pain or disability may be noticed at first, but in the second or third week of life a large callus will be discovered at the fracture site. The complete fracture is disclosed immediately after birth by the infant's refusal to move the affected arm, crying with pain when his arm is moved, and tenderness at the fracture site. The Moro reflex is reduced on the affected side. Diagnosis is confirmed by x-ray. The usual treatment for fracture in the newborn consists of a triangular sling and/or a figure-of-eight bandage worn underneath the clothes for 2 weeks.

The tumbling preschooler is also especially prone to a fracture of the clavicle during childhood. Treatment in the toddler consists of immobilization in a figure-of-eight bandage. In a child over 10 years of age, the figure-of-eight bandage is applied to reduce the fracture, and if the child is very active, a plaster cast is added over the bandage.

Nursing Management

In the nursery, the nursing staff must know how to apply appropriate slings. The figure-of-eight bandage passes around the anterior side of the shoulder and then crosses and ties posteriorly between the shoulder blades. Cotton or gauze pads should be placed in each axilla to protect the infant's skin from rubbing by the bandage. It needs to be tightened daily so that it fits snugly around the shoulders; however, it should not be applied so tightly as to exert pressure on vessels or nerves. Maximum pressure should be exerted over the distal part of the shoulders, and lifting of the affected arm should be avoided. A triangular sling may be used to support the elbow, thereby holding the arm up against the chest so that the shoulder does not sag.

The nurse's teaching prepares parents to care for the child in the bandage or sling. Parents should be asked to demonstrate positioning and handling of the infant in the sling during activities such as bathing, dressing, and feeding. Parents need to know how to tighten the bandage each day as it stretches and how to reapply it if it comes off.

Brachial Plexus Injuries

Paralysis of the upper limb may be caused by traction to one or more components of the brachial plexus. These injuries occur in large babies when delivery is difficult.

Signs of the injury vary according to the part of the brachial plexus which is injured. The *upper arm* type of injury (Erb-Duchenne) involves damage to the fifth and sixth cervical nerve roots in the upper trunk of the plexus. The upper arm lies by the side of the body, with the forearm pronated and the elbow slightly flexed. Swelling and tenderness may appear in the supraclavicular region in the first few days of life. The *whole arm* type involves all the cords of the plexus, resulting in complete paralysis of the limb. This injury is less common than the upper arm type. The *lower arm* type is the rarest and involves paralysis of the hand. There is an abnormal posture of a limb and movement is absent.

The course of paralysis depends on the degree of damage to the nerves, which may range from slight stretching to complete rupture. If the injury is mild, recovery is spontaneous in the first month. In moderate injuries, recovery is slow and incomplete. In severe injuries with complete rupture of the nerves, no recovery is to be expected, and with increasing age there may be severe wasting of the paralyzed muscles.

Without treatment, fixed adduction and medial rotation of the shoulder usually develop in a few days. The treatment of choice is early motion, in which passive range of motion exercises are instituted as soon as the diagnosis is made. On rare occasions, the "Statue of Liberty" splint is indicated. The arm is held in abduction and external rotation in this splint.

Spontaneous recovery occurs to some degree in more than half of infants with the upper arm type of injury. For an infant with any type of injury in whom no recovery has taken place by the end of 2 years, reconstructive surgery has to be considered. In severe cases which cannot benefit from such surgery, amputation above the elbow may be desired during adolescence, followed by fitting with a prosthetic limb.

Nursing Management

Nurses play a major role in detecting brachial plexus injuries as they care for the infant in the nursery, and it is their responsibility to teach parents how to care for the baby after discharge. When passive range of motion exercises are prescribed, the nurse carries out the exercises and demonstrates them to parents. These exercises include shoulder movements of abduction (the arm is moved out to the side and straight up), flexion (the arm is moved forward and straight up), and external rotation (the arm is rotated outward). Other movements are flexion-extension of the elbow, pronation-supination of the forearm, and flexion-extension of the wrist and fingers.

Parents should practice doing exercises before the child is discharged so that they can continue to perform them correctly at home. The purpose of these exercises should also be explained to parents. Use of the "Statue of Liberty" splint requires much care by the nursing staff to prevent posterior dislocation of the shoulder; therefore, the child's arm and shoulder should be supported carefully and moved cautiously.

The parents of a child with a brachial plexus injury should be given an estimate of the severity of damage and expectations for future growth by the physician. When the child is older, he should be helped to understand his disability and the reasons for reconstructive surgery. If amputation is considered, the adolescent should make this decision, utilizing information and support from his family and medical personnel.

Clubfoot (Talipes Equinovarus)

Involved in talipes equinovarus are equinus, adduction, and inversion of the hindfoot and adduction and inversion of the forefoot (Fig. 22-13a). The incidence of this common congenital abnormality of the foot varies from 1 to 4.4 per 1000 births and is twice as common in males as in females. An equinovarus deformity may be present at birth in association with other defects, such as myelomeningocele; however, management of clubfoot due to paralysis differs from treatment of talipes equinovarus as an isolated deformity.

The cause is not known. The most widely accepted theory is that of arrested development during the ninth and tenth weeks, when the embryonic foot goes through a stage of equinus and inversion. Because the insult occurs early, it more often leads to the *rigid* type of clubfoot. Later in development, malposition and abnormal intrauterine pressures are thought to be at fault. The type of deformity caused later in development is more *flexible* and involves joint tissues instead of bone.

In the rigid type of clubfoot, the only bony deformity at birth is in the talus, a major bone of the foot; there are no primary abnormalities of muscles, tendons, nerves, or vessels. The foot can be only partially corrected by man-

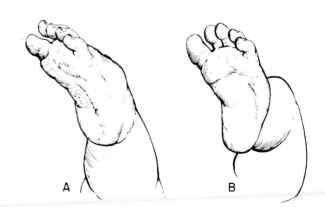

FIGURE 22-13   Congenital foot deformities. *(a)* Clubfoot. *(b)* Metatarsus adductus. *(Courtesy of Indiana University School of Medicine.)*

ual pressure. In the flexible type of clubfoot, abnormal bony relationships are present, but they are not severe. Soft tissues do not show severe shortening initially, and it is possible to correct the foot by manual pressure. Without treatment, however, all deformities progress as they did in utero. Contractures worsen, and the clubfoot becomes more rigid.

Treatment for both rigid and flexible deformities should begin within the first week of life if possible. Gentle manipulation is followed by immobilization with plaster casts, elastic splints, or adhesive strapping. Weekly manipulations and cast changes are needed owing to rapid growth. For an additional 3 months, correction is held at night by bivalved casts and during the day with corrective shoes and passive exercises. If the foot is not corrected after 3 to 4 months, surgery probably will be needed to correct bony deformity, release tight ligaments, or elongate or transplant tendons.

Metatarsus Adductus

Also called metatarsus varus, metatarsus is an adduction or varus deformity of the forefoot. The anterior portion of the foot, including all metatarsals, is adducted as well as supinated (Fig. 22-13b). There is usually an associated internal tibial torsion deformity. The incidence is 2 per 1000 live births, and it is often bilateral. Metatarsus adductus is one of the causes of pigeon-toed gait.

If the deformity is minimal, treatment consists of stretching exercises five or six times daily by parents and attention to sleeping posture. Habitually sleeping with the feet turned in aggravates the deformity. Initially, treatment involves plaster casting to achieve a gradual reduction of the deformity. After 6 to 12 weeks, a Denis Browne boot splint is worn nightly. This splint is worn for a few months to maintain the correction and to treat the accompanying internal tibial torsion. Corrective shoes are worn during the daytime for the first year.

The deformity becomes more rigid with each month it is undetected. If it remains untreated after walking begins, the child may toe in, walk clumsily, and trip over his feet. In untreated severe metatarsus adductus, a soft-tissue-releasing operation or osteotomy may be required.

Nursing Management

Nurses play a role in early detection and referral of an affected child to an appropriate physician or clinic. Parents need an overall view of the treatment program to understand the importance of regular cast or splint changes. They can be taught to soak off old casts before a clinic appointment by immersing the cast in a vinegar-water solution of about 1 part vinegar to 4 parts water and then unwrapping the plaster. When a new cast is applied, parents should be instructed about ways to support the cast until it dries and to observe for signs of circulatory impairment.

If the child is fitted with a Denis Browne splint, the nurse should discuss its use with parents. The child's feet may be slipped into special boots or shoes attached to the splint, or the feet may be strapped to the splint by adhesive tape. The nurse can demonstrate these care measures: application of the removable splint, use of socks to protect the feet, checking the skin for reddened areas, and use of the splint key to tighten shoes against the bar if they become loose. The nurse should clarify for parents the times the splint is to be worn. The child who requires surgery receives preoperative and postoperative care as described earlier in this chapter.

Congenital Hip Dysplasia

Congenital hip dysplasia denotes an abnormality of the hip joint at birth. The unstable hip can become subluxed or dislocated upon manipulation. In subluxation of the hip, the femoral head rides on the edge of the acetabulum. In dislocation of the hip, the femoral head is completely outside the acetabulum. When the hip is subluxed or dislocated, the bony development of the acetabulum becomes progressively abnormal. Hip dysplasia may be unilateral or bilateral (Fig. 22-14).

Several theories of the cause of hip dysplasia have been suggested. Laxity of the ligaments around the capsule of the hip joint is the most widely accepted cause, and it is thought to result from action of maternal sex hormones which relax maternal ligaments in preparation for labor. Other important causative factors include malposition in utero and environmental factors after birth. The former is often associated with a breech presentation, dislocation being 10 times more common after a breech delivery than after a vertex presentation. Factors in the environment include the position in which an infant is carried during its early months.

Physical findings depend on the age of the child and the type of dysplasia (unstable, subluxed, or dislocated). The most reliable test to detect the dislocated hip at birth is the *Ortolani test*. After 1 month of age, the Ortolani test is less useful, and limited abduction of the hip becomes the most reliable sign. The femur appears shortened when the infant lies on a table with his knees and hips flexed at right angles. Asymmetry of skin folds of the thigh and popliteal and gluteal creases result in deeper creases on the affected side (Fig. 22-15). These creases may be present at any age, but they are unreliable for diagnosis in the newborn. After 1 year of age, when the infant has begun to walk, he has a typical limp to his gait—a ducklike waddle or "sailor's gait." The child shifts the weight of his

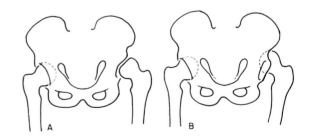

FIGURE 22-14 Unilateral hip dysplasia in the newborn. *(A)* Left subluxed hip and *(B)* left dislocated hip, with normal hips on both right sides. *(Courtesy of Indiana University School of Medicine.)*

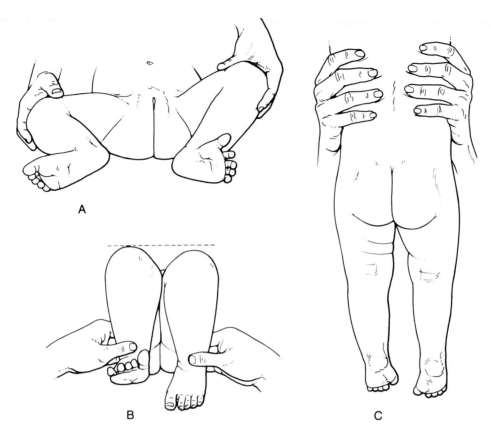

FIGURE 22-15 *(A)* Full hip abduction on the right and limited hip abduction on the left. *(B)* Right knee is higher than left knee. *(C)* Asymmetry of gluteal folds.

trunk over the dislocated hip when he stands on it. Another sign is a positive Trendelenburg's test: When the child stands on the side of the dislocated hip, the pelvis drops on the opposite normal side; when he stands on the normal side, the pelvis on that side stays up in the horizontal position.

Treatment which begins under 2 months of age is most successful. The hip is reduced by gentle manipulation and maintained by splinting the hips in abduction with a Frejka pillow or other abduction splint. The splint is used continuously for approximately 2 to 3 months, followed by night splinting for another month. Normal development of the hip can then be expected.

By the second to the eighteenth month, a contracture of the hip adductors has developed. The child who is diagnosed at this time is first placed in Bryant's traction, to pull the femoral head down to the acetabulum. An older child who has been standing or walking may need to be placed in skeletal traction on the affected side, with skin traction on the normal side. The hips are gradually moved into wide abduction after the femoral head has been brought into the socket. After a period of approximately 21 days, gentle closed reduction is done. If a reduction is evident on x-ray, the hips are immobilized in a hip spica

cast or metal splint for 4 to 6 months. Open reduction may be needed if closed methods are unsuccessful.

The older the child when treatment is begun, the less potential for normal hip development. With increasing age and progressive weight bearing, soft tissue contractures become more rigid and the contour of the acetabular socket and femoral neck becomes more abnormal. Skeletal traction followed by closed or open reduction and a hip spica cast are accepted treatments between the ages of 1½ and 3 years. In the child of 4 to 7 years, skeletal traction and open reduction are usually necessary. Osteotomy may also be necessary. By 8 years and older it is best to postpone treatment for bilateral dislocation, although when dislocation is unilateral, attempts may be made to improve the stability of the hip by surgery.

Nursing Management

Every nurse concerned with the care of newborn infants should be aware of the clinical signs and tests used to diagnose congenital dislocation of the hip. Although the nurse does not generally perform the Ortolani test, she can be aware of suspicious signs such as asymmetric creases and limitation of abduction. In the infant, these signs are much more significant. Additional observations should be made of the child who is walking, including watching for the ducklike waddle and positive Trendelenburg's sign. The routine practice of picking up an infant by both feet to place the diaper underneath should be discouraged in the care of all infants and must be avoided in the infant with congenital hip disease.

When dysplasia is found early, the newborn or infant is fitted with a Frejka pillow splint or another abduction device such as the Illfeld splint. The nurse should explain the splint's purpose and demonstrate its application to parents. As the nurse observes parents applying the splint, instructions should be given about handling the child in such a way as to keep hips abducted. Clothing worn under the splint should protect the child's skin from any irritation caused by the appliance. Two pillow covers are provided with the Frejka pillow splint so that one can be worn while the other is being laundered. It is important that the nurse clarify with parents the times the splint is to be worn and how long it can be removed for bathing, dressing, and diaper changes.

A child who is hospitalized for treatment faces several months of immobilization in traction and spica casts. Parents need information and anticipatory guidance about the care of the child. If they feel comfortable with equipment used in treatment and are informed adequately, they will be better able to enjoy and play with the child during the course of his immobility.

Musculoskeletal Diseases and Dysfunctions in the Infant and Toddler

Osteomyelitis

Osteomyelitis is primarily a disease of children. Long bones that are rapidly growing, such as the femur, tibia, humerus, and radius, are most often involved. In 80 to 90 percent of the cases, *Staphylococcus aureus* is the responsible organism. *Streptococcus, Proteus,* and *Pseudomonas* are other causative agents. Bacteria enter through infections on the skin, such as scratches, pimples, and boils, or through the mucous membranes after nose or throat infections. An open fracture or other wound may also serve as a portal of entry. When bacteria have been introduced, a traumatized area in a bone seems to attract bacteria and provide a locus for osteomyelitis.

Because a bone is a rigid closed space, the edema and hyperemia at the beginning of infection cause a sharp rise in pressure within the bone. Severe and constant pain is felt in the area. With formation of pus, pressure on local blood vessels may be so great that necrosis of bone results. Pus also strips the periosteum from bone, interfering with its blood supply. When infection spreads through the cortex to the periosteum, pain becomes even more severe.

Without treatment the area of infection continues to enlarge, and septicemia may develop. The infection penetrates the periosteum into the soft tissues, where it produces cellulitis and then an abscess. If the joint capsule is penetrated, septic arthritis results. Metastatic focuses of infection are carried to other bones by the septicemia. Without treatment, the child acquires a chronic form of osteomyelitis.

The first symptom experienced with this disease is pain in the involved area. The child is unwilling to move the limb. Septicemia results in just 24 hours, as evidence by weakness, lack of appetite, and fever. A few days are required for soft tissue swelling, redness, and heat to be produced as the infection spreads beyond bone. In infants, signs of osteomyelitis are more diffuse. Little or no fever may be present, but irritability, loss of function in the involved limb, tenderness, and swelling may be noted. Early diagnosis is based on clinical signs alone. X-ray is valuable only after several days, when destruction of bone has taken place.

Treatment begins immediately in the hospital. After blood cultures have been taken, intravenous antibacterial therapy is instituted. Bed rest and analgesics make the child more comfortable. The affected extremity is rested by removable splints or traction to reduce pain, prevent movement which spreads infection, and prevent contractures in soft tissues. If clinical signs have not improved within 24 hours, decompression of the infected bony area must be done in surgery. At that time, pus is removed for culture and pressure in the bone is relieved.

Inadequate treatment usually leads to chronic osteomyelitis. The presence of infected dead bone prevents healing. Because this bone separates from live bone, resorption and deposition of new bone do not take place, and antibiotics cannot reach it. The child is no longer acutely ill, but local signs of inflammation are present. Treatment is more radical in the chronic form of disease. Removal of the dead bone usually must be accomplished by surgery, followed by drainage of the area. The nursing management of children with osteomyelitis is similar to care provided to clients with septic arthritis and is described in the following section.

Septic Arthritis

Acute septic or suppurative arthritis is an inflammation of the joint caused by pus-forming organisms. Infants and children of 1 or 2 years of age are most often affected, although this disease appears in all age groups. The hip joint is the site of highest frequency, with the knee and elbow second. More than one joint may be involved.

Infection, most commonly caused by a staphylococcus or streptococcus organism; is spread to the joint through the bloodstream from a distant infection such as otitis media. Extension of infection may travel from a neighboring bone focus, especially at the hip. At the knee, penetrating wounds are a primary cause. Inflammation begins in the synovial membrane. Synovial fluid thickens as pus is formed. The pus rapidly destroys articular cartilage. Disintegration of cartilage may be followed by osteomyelitis in the underlying bone.

There are signs and symptoms in the toddler who may be able to point out the painful joint, and he guards it from movement. Other signs include spasms of the muscles around the joint, swelling of tissues, fever, and an elevated white blood cell count.

In the infant, septic arthritis is found most frequently in the hip. Pathological dislocation and necrosis of the femoral head complicate the disease. Because the entire femoral head, including the epiphyseal plate, is composed of cartilage, it may be destroyed completely.

Treatment must be immediate. Fluid for culture is obtained by needle aspiration. Antibiotic treatment is started locally by joint instillation. Surgical exploration of the joint (arthrotomy) is more effective to remove pus and irrigate the joint. Postoperatively, closed infusion and drainage are used commonly and are continued until drainage is sterile. Immobilization of the joint by casting is necessary to prevent dislocation. If damage to the joint is permanent, reconstructive procedures may be needed. Although treatment is similar in osteomyelitis and septic arthritis, failure of treatment in septic arthritis can lead to more permanent disability.

Nursing Management

The nurse's role in early detection and in support during hospitalization is similar in osteomyelitis and septic arthritis. When a child is seen with chief complaints of fever and a swollen, tender extremity, the nurse should think primarily of acute osteomyelitis. A history of puncture wounds, tonsillitis, or upper respiratory infection increases the likelihood of thie diagnosis. Signs of septic arthritis which can be recognized early by the nurse include a painful and swollen joint, guarding the joint against movement, fever, and irritability. Assessment of the site is more difficult in an infant or toddler who cannot describe where he hurts. A child who is suspected of having either of these disorders should be referred to a physician for immediate diagnosis and treatment.

When the child is admitted to the hospital, he should be placed in bed and helped to rest as much as possible. The nurse assists the physician in securing blood and wound cultures and instituting intravenous therapy. Drugs which are often given intravenously include penicillin and nafcillin. Analgesics are administered to make the child more comfortable. Skin traction, splints, or casts are applied to immobilize the involved limb or joint. The nurse should check the peripheral circulation of the limb for signs of circulation impairment in a cast or traction. Vital signs are monitored every 4 hours or more frequently in the presence of fever or postoperatively. If closed infusion and drainage are used, the nurse is responsible for monitoring the fluids and keeping accurate intake and output records. A well-balanced diet should be consumed by the child. High-protein snacks, such as milk shakes, can be supplied between meals. Small, frequent feedings may be necessary when anorexia is a frequent complaint.

When early treatment has been effective and the child does not feel particularly ill, appropriate stimulation becomes a part of nursing care. Play activities can be brought to the child, or he can be taken to them in bed or in a wheelchair. The child's parents need to be involved in his care. They should be helped to understand his mobility limitations as well as his needs for socialization.

Care is evaluated on the basis of whether (1) infection is eradicated by early and complete treatment, (2) the child's comfort is maintained, (3) complications of therapy are prevented, (4) parents and child cope adequately with long-term illness, and (5) follow-up is maintained to detect chronic disease or growth disturbance.

Osteogenesis Imperfecta

Also known as "brittle bones," osteogenesis imperfecta is a connective tissue disorder that primarily affects bone. It is manifested by a fragile skeleton, thin skin and sclera, poor teeth, macular bleeding, and hypermobility of the joints. The tendency of the fragile bones to fracture on slight trauma is an outstanding characteristic of the disease. The pathology is in bone formation. Collagen remains in an immature form. Instead of normal compact bone, a coarse, immature type of bone is produced.

A *congenital* type of osteogenesis imperfecta in which multiple fractures occur during delivery or in utero is rare. Osteogenesis imperfecta *tarda* is less severe and becomes evident at some time in childhood.

In the tarda type, the child is often seen by a physician for the first time following a fracture. The number of fractures which continue to occur during childhood varies greatly. Lower limbs are more frequently affected. Refracturing is common because of limb deformity and disuse atrophy resulting from immobilization.

The pain, deformity, and swelling which result from a complete fracture are the same as those in a normal child. With an incomplete fracture, however, pain may not be a complaint because soft tissue injury is minimal. A deformity often develops in the injured limb with continued activity. Fractures heal at a normal rate. Callus formation may be minimal or occasionally so excessive that it may be misdiagnosed as osteogenic sarcoma. Bone formed following a fracture is of the same poor quality as that which it replaces.

Growth may be retarded from curvature of the limbs and spine and by multiple injuries at the epiphyseal ends. Extremities tend to be thin and long. Kyphosis and scoliosis are common as a result of compression fractures of the vertebral bodies. The skull is misshapen, with protrusion of the frontal and parietal regions.

Skeletal muscles are poorly developed, and the child is generally weak. Hypermobility of joints results from excessive laxity of the ligaments and capsule. The skin is thin, and subcutaneous hemorrhages may occur. Teeth, often discolored, are affected because of deficiency of dentin. They break easily and are prone to caries, and fillings are not retained. The scleras may appear blue, although vision is unaffected. Deafness due to osteosclerosis or pressure on the auditory nerve may be a problem later.

The prognosis varies in the tarda type. If the condition is severe in early childhood, disabling deformities are likely to develop unless constant care is taken to minimize them. The severity is likely to decrease at puberty. With maturity, the patient also learns how to prevent falls and fractures.

There is no specific treatment. The child should be taught to avoid unnecessary risks. Active sports and gymnastics activities should be prohibited. With fractures, immobilization should be reduced to a minimum since disuse atrophy increases the likelihood of more fractures. Bowing or torsional deformities may require multiple osteotomies of long bones and intramedullary metal rods. These rods serve the dual purpose of correcting deformity and providing support to prevent further fractures and deformity. Braces, crutches, or wheelchairs are sometimes prescribed as added protection against fractures.

Nursing Management

Early recognition of fractures is important in treatment; therefore, both parents and the child need to be taught the signs of fractures. They need instruction on how to splint the fracture site or wrap the extremity in an elastic bandage before the trip to the hospital. Treatment of fractures and correction of deformities often involve traction and/or immobilization in casts. A hip spica cast is used for lower extremity fractures in severely affected children. Circulation checks and cast care are important. In the hospital, the nurse must handle the child gently to avoid further fractures. The child himself as well as his parents can give the nurse the best guidance about safe handling techniques. Modifications may need to be made in clothing, diapering or toileting, bathing, and feeding activities for a child who is severely affected.

Limitation of activity and frequent hospitalizations place stress on both the child and his family. As the child assumes independence, close monitoring by parents is impossible. It is essential that the child be helped to understand his disability so that he gradually can assume responsibility for the precautions required. Interest in activities other than the gross motor type should be encouraged by parents and nurses. School should be continued during the older child's admissions to the hospital. Parents need information concerning recurrence risks and may want to be referred to a genetic counseling service.

Tibial Torsion

Both external and internal tibial torsion are rotational deformities of the tibia. When the knee is facing forward, the foot is rotated inward (internal torsion) or outward (external rotation). It is usually secondary to myelomeningocele or cerebral palsy.

Internal tibial torsion is a common cause of intoeing in young children. Some degree of torsion is common in all infants and corrects itself with growth. If the child continually assumes postures which aggravate the torsion, it may increase. Two positions which have this effect are sleeping on the knees with the feet turned inward and sitting on top of inturned feet.

Treatment consists of training the child to avoid harmful postures during sleeping and sitting. If the deformity is so severe that the child over 2 yeras of age trips over his feet when walking, a night splint may be utilized to hold the feet in external rotation, which influences the growth of the epiphyseal plate to achieve correction. The Denis Browne splint is commonly used as a night splint for this purpose. If conservative measures are unsuccessful, surgical correction may be necessary.

Nursing Management

The nurse's attention initially is directed toward detection of torsional deformities. Children with suspected deformities should be referred for diagnosis and treatment. As part of treatment the nurse clarifies for parents the postures which the child is directed to assume. Instructions are given concerning use of the Denis Browne splint.

Fracture of the Femur

Displaced fractures of the femur are common in childhood and usually involve the middle third of the femoral shaft. The strong periosteum of the femur remains intact even with much displacement of fragments, but because the fracture is very unstable, it should be splinted as soon as it is discovered.

Reduction of a simple closed fracture may be achieved by mechanical or manual traction. If mechanical, the child is placed in balanced skin traction (Russell's traction). When the femur is relatively stable and painless, traction is discontinued, and a hip spica cast is used for immobilization until clinical union of the fracture. Another approach for a simple closed fracture is manual reduction followed by immediate casting, usually under anesthesia (Fig. 22-12).

Healing always takes place by temporary overgrowth of bone. The ideal position for uniting bone fragments is one of intentional shortening; fragments are placed side to side with overriding of about 1 cm. The shortening is compensated by overgrowth within 1 year.

Nursing Management

A displaced fracture of the femoral shaft appears to the nurse as an angulation, external rotation, and shortening deformity of the thigh which is swollen and very painful. Splinting should be done immediately. The child should be moved as little as possible for x-rays and other examinations to prevent further displacement of the fracture and pain.

A serious complication that can occur after reduction is compartment syndrome. Ischemic damage to muscles and nerves can also result from femoral artery spasm, which is aggravated by excessive traction.

Nursing Care Plan 22-1 describes the treatment for a child with a fractured femur.

Musculoskeletal Diseases and Dysfunctions in the Preschooler

Juvenile Rheumatoid Arthritis

The cause of juvenile rheumatoid arthritis (JRA) is unknown, but the evidence suggests that the primary prob-

NURSING CARE PLAN

22-1 The Child with a Fracture of the Femur

Clinical Problem/Nursing Diagnosis	Expected Outcome	Nursing Interventions
Pain, edema, irritability Pain related to fractured femur	With the administration of analgesics, child will be comfortable	Assess type of pain, location, severity and character; document assessment Properly administer analgesics with the knowledge of side effects, appropriate dose/kg Promote immobilization of femur Institute splinting of femur immediately Elevate splinted extremity as ordered by physician Apply ice bags to injured extremity during first 24 h after trauma

Imposed restrictions on movement secondary to cast or traction
Increased risk for atelectasis, skin breakdown, constipation
 	
Impaired physical mobility (level III) related to therapeutic and mechanical restrictions
	Child will tolerate traction; remain in body alignment; be free of complications
	Child will maintain muscle strength in uninvolved extremities with active/ passive ROM
	Child will actively participate in isometric exercises indicated in plan of care
		Clarify with physician appropriate exercises, positions, and movements client can safely tolerate
		Child in traction:
		  Note type, purpose, and weight of traction
		  Maintain proper body alignment
		  Provide client with firm orthopedic mattress
		  Ensure safety and proper functioning of siderails, overbed triangle lift, mechanical equipment
		  Closely monitor proper functioning of traction apparatus (weight/ pulley strings in straight alignment without obstruction)
		  Encourage lung expansion breathing exercises 4-5x q 1 h
		  Provide meticulous skin care (see interventions for potential impairment of skin integrity)
		  Prevent constipation: encourage high-fiber diet with adequate fluid intake
		  Assess circulation and neurovascular status of extremities q 1 h, document assessment
		Child with cast immobilization:
		  The circulatory and neurovascular status of the affected extremity will be maintained free of complications
		  Assess circulatory and neurovascular status of extremities q 1 h, note color, capillary refill, quality of pulses, warmth, sensory/motor function; document findings
		  Assess for presence of localized pain, tight points
		  Support contour of cast and body alignment with pillows
		  Assess cast for presence of drainage (circle site, write the date and time circle was made) and foul-smelling odor
		  Promote social interaction, age-appropriate activities; involve play therapist, OT to provide therapeutic play
		  Promote active/passive ROM of unaffected extremities; encourage recommended isometric exercises
		  Ensure safety in child's position during and after meals to prevent aspiration

Risk of compartment syndrome
Mechanical pressure from cast, traction, soft tissue trauma
 	
Potential impaired tissue integrity related to risk from alteration in circulation secondary to cast, traction, trauma
	With frequent assessments and the early detection of alterations, tissue in the child's involved extremity will be perfused adequately	Monitor vital signs with BP q 4 h
		Assess and document neurovascular integrity of extremities q 1-2 h
		  Note bilaterally
		    Color/pallor
		    Peripheral pulses
		    Capillary refill
		    Swelling
		    Motor/sensory function
		    Pain/tight points from immobilization apparatus
		Immediately notify physician of presence of circulatory compromise

Continued.

NURSING CARE PLAN 22-1 The Child with a Fracture of the Femur — cont'd

Clinical Problem/Nursing Diagnosis	Expected Outcome	Nursing Interventions

Pink areas on skin over bony prominences
 	
Potential impaired skin integrity related to immobility and/or mechanical pressure
	Given frequent skin care, and taking steps to prevent tissue breakdown, child's skin integrity will be maintained	Frequently assess exposed skin (especially pressure points) for
		  Pink/reddened areas
		  Excoriated skin
		  Presence of blisters on skin
		  Breakdown
		  Skin rash
		Document findings, note exact size in centimeters
		Apply circular massage to exposed skin areas; concentrate treatment over sacrum, back, elbows, heels
		Provide child with a sheepskin, egg crate, or H_2O mattress to decrease contact irritation over pressure points
		Wash skin with mild, nonirritating soap; dry skin thoroughly
		Provide smooth, clean, dry bed linens
		Change child's positioning q 2 h to promote ROM
		Assess skin areas at cast edges for irritation, breakdown
		Petal cast edges with mohair/tape
		Alcohol on skin areas near cast edges q 2-4 h
		Prohibit use of foreign objects to scratch skin under cast or use of powders or lotions under cast
		Tuck plastic wrap around edges of buttocks window and around cast edges near perineum
		Support contour of cast with pillows
		Promptly report complaints of burning, pain, foul odor from cast

Constipation Constipation related to immobility and/or pain medication	With an adequate intake of liquids and a diet high in fiber, child will maintain normal bowel habits	Promote diet high in fiber bulk, fruits Encourage adequate fluid intake Offer fruit juices at frequent intervals Assess need for mild stool softener (e.g., Colace)

Atelectasis
 	
Potential ineffective breathing pattern related to immobility and/or pain medications
	Through the use of breathing exercises and incentive spirometry, child will demonstrate maximum lung exertion, with breath sounds clear in all lobes	Teach and assist child with breathing exercises
		  Coughing and deep breathing
		  Incentive spirometer
		Encourage breathing exercises 4-5 x q 1 h
		Change child's position q 2 h
		Maintain HOB elevated to 30-45° angle if appropriate
		Assess quality of breath sounds in all lung fields; note adventitious sounds; compare bilaterally
		Assess for respiratory compromise

Elevated temperature, 37.5°C
 	
Potential for infection related to trauma, complications of immobility
	Child will remain free of secondary infections	Assess client for early signs of infection
		Closely monitor vital signs q 2-4 h
		Monitor temp q 2 h if febrile
		Report temperature elevation 37.5°C promptly to MD
		Note presence of tachycardia, changes in BP
		Obtain cultures properly as ordered
		Promptly administer antipyretic measures as indicated
		Child with cast:
		  Note presence of foul odors from cast
		  Note color, amount, odor of drainage from cast
		  Assess for warm spots over cast surface
		  Assess for presence of localized diffuse pain

Anorexia Altered nutrition related to pain, immobility	By encouraging a high protein intake, child's nutritional intake will be adequate in promoting wound healing	Promote diet high in protein, vitamin D to support wound healing Calculate appropriate Kcal for age Encourage small and frequent high-caloric, high-protein snacks (shakes, peanut butter)

Clinical Problem/Nursing Diagnosis	Expected Outcome	Nursing Interventions
Loss of control ——— Impaired social interaction related to potential for body-image disturbance	Child will demonstrate independence with ADL within limitations Child will maintain developmental milestones and demonstrate increasing levels of self-esteem	Promote regular structured age-appropriate activities in daily plan of care Maintain school activities; facilitate tutoring Promote social interaction with family, siblings, peers Encourage cards from classmates, tape recordings from siblings, friends Provide consistent nursing care Provide choices in plan of care, i.e., time of cast care; request child's assistance in cutting out cast petals Involve play therapist, OT to provide age-appropriate games, crafts, medical play (i.e., casted/or immobilized doll)

lem is either a hypersensitivity response in which normal immune mechanisms are exaggerated or a reaction to unknown infectious agents. The peak age is during the preschool years. There are three subgroups of JRA. *Pauciarticular* disease is limited to only a few joints and affects about 45 percent of children with JRA. Large joints are characteristically involved. The distribution of affected joints is often asymmetrical. *Polyarticular* JRA affects about 35 percent of children with chronic arthritis. Any synovial joints of the body may be affected, although those of the lumbodorsal spine are generally spared. A symmetrical polyarthritis of the small joints of the hands and feet is characteristic. Larger joints (knees, ankles, and elbows) are affected in most patients. Fever, anemia, and growth retardation may also occur. *Systemic-onset* JRA, characterized by extraarticular manifestations, affects about 20 percent of these patients. Chronic arthritis, generally polyarticular in distribution, usually begins during the first few months of disease.

The pathology begins in the synovial membrane, with inflammation, edema, and proliferation of cells. Granulation tissue causes the swelling. As the disease progresses, scar tissue replaces granulation tissue, and the joint may become contracted. The muscles are affected by inflammation in muscle tissue as well as by joint immobility, aggravating contractures.

Symptoms at the onset vary. Some children become ill suddenly, while in others symptoms appear very gradually. The clinical manifestations may be limited to the peripheral joints, or they may appear as a generalized systemic illness. When the onset involves *peripheral* joints, swelling is usually the first sign noticed by the parent. There is some limitation of motion, a limp, and mild warmth over the joint which accompanies the swelling. Tenderness and pain are present when swelling has occurred suddenly. The onset of *systemic* involvement is usually more sudden and includes high and intermittent fever, rash, malaise, pallor, subcutaneous nodules, lym-

phadenopathy, liver and spleen enlargement, and pericarditis as well as arthritis in one or more joints.

The clinical course is variable, involving exacerbations and remissions. Pain on motion is the major complaint of a child, but instead of voicing his discomfort, he may walk with a limp or refuse to move the extremity. Morning stiffness is manifested by the child's inability to get out of bed in the morning or difficulty arising from a nap. A *rheumatoid rash* is a salmon-pink macular rash which appears intermittently on the chest, thighs, axilla, and upper arms. The rash is seen most often in systemic disease. Subcutaneous nodules are found in some affected children, usually on the fingers, toes, wrist, or elbows. For about three-fourths of children, fever occurs intermittently, and it is often accompanied by other systemic symptoms. *Iridocyclitis,* or inflammation of the iris and ciliary body develops several years after the onset of the disease. Joint deformities, including subluxation, dislocation, and contracture, are seen in more severe cases. *Synovectomy* (resection of the diseased synovial membrane) or releases of the joint capsule and contractures about the joint may be helpful. Growth disturbances sometimes result from abnormal influences on the epiphyseal plate.

Diagnosis of juvenile rheumatoid arthritis depends mainly on the history and clinical symptomatology. According to the official criteria, arthritis must be present for 6 consecutive weeks before a diagnosis of JRA can be made. There are no specific diagnostic laboratory tests for this disease. Tests such as sedimentation rate, rheumatoid factors, antinuclear antibodies, and histocompatibility types are positive in some patients.

Nursing Management

In JRA, the child and his parents face a disease with many unknowns. The parents may feel guilty, and the child often attributes the illness to his "bad" behavior. A nurse can help family members understand that the course of the disease is unpredictable and may continue for several

TABLE 22-6 Drugs Used in Treatment of Juvenile Rheumatoid Arthritis

Drug	Action	Route	Side Effects or Toxicity
Aspirin	Anti-inflammatory, analgesic, antipyretic	PO*	Hyperventilation, CNS* depression or excitation, GI* irritation, tinnitis
Indomethacin	Anti-inflammatory, analgesic, antipyretic	PO	Nausea, other GI distress, headache, dizziness, drowsiness, tinnitis, weight gain from edema, rash
Naproxen	Anti-inflammatory, analgesic, antipyretic	PO	Nausea, other GI distress, dizziness, headache, rash, weight gain from edema, tinnitis
Tolmetin sodium	Anti-inflammatory, analgesic, antipyretic	PO	Nausea, other GI distress, headache, weight gain from edema, tinnitis, rash
Gold	Unknown	IM*	Rash, nephritis, thrombocytopenia, neurotoxicity
Steroids	Anti-inflammatory	PO, IM, IV*, intraarticular	Masking of infection, GI distress, vascular disorders, hypertension, blurry or dim vision, osteoporosis, euphoria or other mental disturbance, glycosuria, weight gain from edema, appetite stimulation

*PO = oral; CNS = central nervous system; GI = gastrointestinal; IM = intramuscular; IV = intravenous.

years. Long-term encouragement becomes necessary as the parents and child experience the inertia of a daily therapy program as well as recurring episodes of acute illness.

The child is hospitalized during acute episodes of joint inflammation and systemic illness. The nurse checks to see that the child's bed has a firm mattress which resists sagging. Pillows should be kept from under painful joints to prevent stiffness and contractures. The child may be allowed up if he can tolerate the activity, but if the inflamed joints are too painful to move actively, they should be moved passively at least twice a day by the physical therapist or nurse. Both of these disciplines should work together to reinforce the treatment program. The child is encouraged to do his exercises actively as soon as he is able. Warm compresses to joints, hydrotherapy, and paraffin oil baths often facilitate joint movement. Warm baths or showers in the morning help the child overcome morning stiffness. Diversional activities also encourage movement. When splints are used to rest warm, swollen joints, the child may have difficulty adjusting to them, especially during sleep. Nurses must know how to apply splints properly in addition to helping the child adjust to the splint.

Drug therapy is an important part of treatment. Drugs are not curative, but they can satisfactorily suppress synovitis in most affected children. An important point for teaching is that drugs should be taken regularly, even when the child feels well. Aspirin is still the initial drug of choice. Drugs used in treatment of JRA are described in Table 22-6.

The community nurse, who may have played a role in the detection of the disease, is also responsible for follow-up care. This nurse may administer gold intramuscularly, and it is essential that the patient be monitored closely for side effects. Encouragement and supervision are given for the prescribed exercise or play program and for warm baths to overcome morning stiffness. For a child who attends school, provisions may need to be made to allow him to move around every hour. The nurse should ensure that every child with this disease receives a slit-lamp ophthalmologic examination four times a year for detection of iridocyclitis. These examinations are important even when the disease is in remission. Regular follow-up should be made for symptoms such as visual disturbance, chest pain, and skin rashes, and any new or unusual symptoms should be reported to the physician promptly.

The prognosis is improving for this disease as medical care progresses. On the whole, 75 to 80 percent of children survive the disease without serious disability. Follow-up is essential since there may be unexpected recurrences of disease after years of remission. The serious type, systemic-onset JRA, is rarely fatal as a result of modern drug therapy. Children at greatest risk for joint destruction are those with systemic-onset disease and those with polyarthritis. Iridocyclitis, seen most often in children with pauciarticular JRA, can lead to permanent loss of vision and even blindness if it is not detected early. Despite the risk of complications, most children recover completely and without continuance into adulthood.

Nursing Care Plan 22-2 describes the treatment for a child with rheumatoid arthritis.

Legg-Perthes Disease

Legg-Perthes disease is one of a group of diseases called the *osteochondroses.* Vascular disruption to the femoral head causes necrosis and variable deformity of the upper femoral epiphysis. The age of onset is usually between 3 and 11 years, and the disease may be present for 2 to 8 years, after which time it spontaneously resolves itself. The condition is unilateral in about 85 percent of cases, and it tends to recur in families.

The pathophysiology of the disease can be divided into four phases. The first phase, *avascularity,* begins with spontaneous interruption of the blood supply to the upper femoral epiphysis. Bone-forming cells in the epiphysis die, and bone ceases to grow, although its density does not change. The second phase is the period of *revascularization.* New blood vessels are sent into the dead bone, and both bone resorption and deposition take place. How-

22-2 *The Child with Juvenile Rheumatoid Arthritis*

Clinical Problem/Nursing Diagnosis	Expected Outcome	Nursing Interventions
Fever Hyperthermia	Given antipyretics and sponge baths, the child's temperature will return to and remain normal (37 to 37.5°C)	Monitor temperature q 2 h while febrile Notify MD for temp 38.5°C or as specified Properly administer antipyretics or salicylates as ordered Provide tepid bath for high spiking fever Document effectiveness of antipyretic measures Assess for alterations in vital signs
Joint pain Irritability Pain	Child will experience less discomfort and greater joint mobility Child will interact with environment in comfort	Properly administer anti-inflammatory medications as ordered (be knowledgeable about side effects and indications of toxicity of all meds) Children on gold treatment: check urine for protein q 4 h Apply warm compresses and moist heat to affected joints Elevate affected extremities Encourage early morning warm bath or shower Consult physical therapy about indications for hydrotherapy, paraffin oil baths, or splints to rest swollen joints
Musculoskeletal impairment Immobility Impaired physical mobility	Child will have improved joint mobility and ROM	Interventions for joint pain as above Participate and aid in daily PT/OT regimen Provide reinforcement of teaching exercises suggested by therapist Provide active/passive ROM bid Provide diversional activities to increase movement Provide firm mattress Avoid use of pillows under painful joints to prevent increased stiffness and contractures Promptly administer analgesics and anti-inflammatory medications appropriately prior to exercises
Iridocyclitis Visual impairment Sensory/perceptual alteration (visual)	After the child's pain resolves, visual acuity will improve	Encourage and support through periodic ophthalmologic exams Note signs of early iridocyclitis: redness, eye pain, photophobia
Anemia Alteration in normal hemodynamic parameters: pallor	The intake of a diet high in iron, vitamins, and protein will result in improved color and hematologic values	Assess color, capillary refill Assess changes in vital sign parameters (tachycardia, hypo/hypertension, tachypnea) Guaiac stool q 4 h and prn Encourage adequate nutritional intake rich in iron, vitamins, and protein
Lowered self-esteem (secondary to growth retardation) Self-esteem disturbance related to growth retardation	Child will maximize his or her ability to adjust to psychological stress Child will participate in a therapy regimen with good compliance	Promote activities which enhance strengths Provide interaction with peers who share similar concerns and experiences with JRA Encourage intervention by ancillary supports: OT, PT, child psychologist, social worker, play therapist Inform school nurse about medication and exercise regimen and need to move q 1 h during school day
Complications from therapy: salicylates, gold, and other nonsteroidal anti-inflammatory drugs Potential for injury related to pharmacologic treatment	By encouraging small frequent feedings, maintaining alkalinity of the stomach and taking medications properly, the child will be free of GI bleeding, gastritis, and alterations in hematologic values or impaired renal function	Administer correct dosage of medications at proper intervals and know side effects of all medications Encourage small, frequent meals Administer ASA with meals/antacids Check stool guaiac q 4 h Educate client and family about proper medication administration and precautions for medical therapy

ever, the new bone is not strong, and pathological fractures occur. Pain and limited motion develop in the hip joint. The third phase involves *healing*. Dead bone is removed and replaced by new bone. The fourth phase of *residual* deformity takes place when healing is complete and the contour of the hip joint is fixed. Subluxation of the hip, flattening of the epiphysis resulting in the incongruity of joint surfaces, and limitation of motion may lead to degenerative joint disease in later life.

Clinical symptoms begin in phase 2. Pain may be felt in the hip during the initial period. The child walks with a protective limp and has limited movement in the hip joint. Disuse atrophy develops in muscles of the upper thigh.

In general, the earlier the age of onset, the better the results of treatment. Success is diminished by the fact that symptoms do not occur until phase 2, when damage has already been done to the femoral head. Treatment is aimed at preventing abnormal forces on the femoral head during revascularization (usually lasting 2 to 4 years) and the third phase of healing. Most physicians begin treatment with bed rest and traction to the limb during the painful initial period. An attempt is made to locate the femoral head deep in the acetabulum, protecting it while revascularization and growth occur. This process is accomplished by weight bearing in abduction plaster casts or abduction braces to allow deeper seating of the femoral head or by use of a hip sling to rest the affected leg. A surgical osteotomy of the femur may prevent or correct subluxation. Treatment is considered to be successful if the hip joint allows normal function after resolution of the disease.

Nursing Management

When the child is admitted to the hospital with Legg-Perthes disease, he is uncomfortable and may need analgesics for relief of pain. If bed rest and traction are instituted and abduction casts are applied. Immobilization is often difficult for the child to accept. After the initial period of discomfort, he feels well and wants to be up and out of bed. The preschool child has difficulty understanding why he must stay in bed or wear special appliances. All children can benefit from explanations and visual aids about the disease and its treatment. During immobilization, the child should participate in activities which keep him occupied and stimulate his development. Play should include exercise for uninvolved extremities. A teacher may be required for the school-age child, and special activities with peers should be arranged. During hospitalization, the nursing staff can demonstrate such management to parents and help them plan for care at home.

Duchenne's Muscular Dystrophy

Duchenne's muscular dystrophy is a progressive muscle disorder which is genetically determined. The more common form is found only in boys because it is transferred as a sex-linked recessive trait. Muscular dystrophy usually starts in the preschool years. The pathogenesis is unknown, although a biochemical defect in muscle tissue is suspected.

The child appears normal during infancy, and no abnormality appears until he begins to walk. At age 3 to 5 years, the child typically has flat feet, develops weakness in his legs, and begins to stumble and fall. Weakness in the pelvic muscles causes difficulty in climbing stairs and getting up off the floor to a standing position. The child must "climb up his legs" with his hands to arise from the floor, a characteristic sign of the disease known as *Gowers' sign*. Although wasting of the muscles is progressive, muscles appear to grow larger or hypertrophy, especially in the calves. Histological changes show a variation in size of muscle fibers, degeneration of the fibers, and fatty infiltration between muscle bundles.

The course of this disease is relentless, without remissions. Lordosis develops as the pelvis rotates forward because of muscle weakness. To compensate, the child assumes a waddling gait and begins to walk on his toes. As walking becomes more precarious, the child fears falling and spends more time in a wheelchair. Confinement to the wheelchair usually begins between 7 and 10 years of age. Scoliosis develops and progresses to the extent that vital organs are displaced. Contractures of the elbows, feet, knees, and hips may develop during immobilization. Few boys survive beyond 20 years of age. The most frequent causes of death are respiratory infection, respiratory acidosis, and cardiac complications.

Diagnosis is made from the history and various tests. The enzyme CPK is elevated early in the course of the disease. An electromyogram (EMG) may be done to establish whether muscle weakness is caused by abnormal nerves or muscles. A muscle biopsy is performed surgically to confirm the diagnosis.

Without a cure for this disease, children face progressive disability and death. Normal amounts of exercise, dietary supervision, light braces, special aids and equipment, and supportive relationships with staff are all part of the treatment program to help make the disease more bearable for children and their families.

Nursing Management

The diagnostic period in muscular dystrophy involves frightening and uncomfortable tests for the child. One of these tests is the EMG, in which thin, wirelike needles are stuck into the child's muscles while a recording of muscle contractions is made on a screen. After explaining the test to parents, the nurse can plan with them for preparation of the child. Reassurance that the test is not a punishment is important for the preschooler. Whenever possible, the nurse who is working with the child should accompany him.

Preparation for muscle biopsy is also required. The child and his parents need to understand that the child will be asleep during the procedure, that only a tiny part of the muscle will be removed, and that there will be a small incision after surgery. Postoperatively, the child's vital signs are monitored frequently until stable and then every 4 hours. Drainage from the incision is recorded as well as observations about pain and the effect of analgesics. Before discharge, parents need instructions on keeping the incision clean and dry and allowing return to normal activity. When a positive diagnosis is made on biopsy, parents need additional explanations about the disease from the physician, followed by clarification and emotional support by the nurse.

During the course of the disease the goal is to keep the child as independent as possible and provide supportive interaction for the family and child. An interdisciplinary team supervises continued care. The child is encouraged to continue normal activities to prevent atrophy of uninvolved muscles. Attention is given to diet in an efort to prevent or reduce obesity, which makes walking more difficult. Light braces may be fitted to delay progression of abnormal postures or to support weakened muscles. For the child to benefit from bracing, his parents must reinforce the treatment program and supervise proper wearing of the brace. Ramps may have to be installed in the home and architectural barriers which hinder independent mobility may have to be reduced. An electric wheelchair allows mobility for the older child with upper extremity weakness. Correct positioning of the feet and adjustment of footrests on the wheelchair is important to prevent foot drop and other ankle deformities. Portable lifts are useful when a child is unable to transfer himself or is too heavy to lift. Prolonged bed rest and inactivity should be avoided because of their weakening effects.

Other measures for independence in daily activities are planned to compensate for the child's weakness. Clothing may need to be modified so that the child can dress himself. Large rings on zipper tabs in the front of clothing allow easier manipulation. Toileting is difficult, requiring special planning or the use of a bedside commode or bedpan. Bathing, washing hair, and self-feeding may also need to be modified in accordance with the child's abilities and the home situation. Operation of special equipment should be demonstrated by staff to parents and by parents to staff. Parents also need information about the genetic transmission of Duchenne's muscular dystrophy, for which genetic counseling can be helpful.

Fractures of the Forearm

When a child falls and catches himself with his hands, forces are transmitted to the wrist and forearm, causing fractures in those parts. Fractures of the forearm usually involve injury to both the radius and the ulna. They may be incomplete (greenstick) or complete.

A *buckle* fracture in the distal third of the forearm is common in young children. This is a compression fracture resulting in "buckling" of the thin cortex which surrounds bone. It heals completely after several weeks in a cast. A *greenstick* fracture in the distal or middle third of the forearm must first be reduced by closed manipulation (manipulation to realign the bone without a surgical incision). *Complete* fractures are reduced by closed manipulation and immobilized in plaster casts.

Nursing Management

The nurse may assist with the reduction and immobilization of fractures as well as supervision of the child in a cast. Closed reductions of fractures are usually done by applying manual traction to the forearm with the elbow flexed, while wrapping the arm in a circular plaster cast from the axilla to the midpalm. After casting, the arm should be elevated for 24 to 48 hours with ice bags applied to the forearm; and frequent checks of circulation are made. A triangular sling, which ties at the back of the neck, can be used to support the hand, forearm, and elbow. If the child is cared for at home during this time, instructions should be given to parents about care of the cast, circulation checks and use of the sling. X-rays are taken at intervals to visualize alignment of bone fragments. After several weeks, the cast is removed and the child is allowed free use of his arm.

Supracondylar Fracture of the Humerus

The most common and most serious type of fracture around the elbow is a supracondylar fracture of the humerus. The incidence of complications is high. The usual injury is falling on the hand with the elbow flexed. The forces of injury are transmitted through the elbow joint to the humerus.

Treatment varies according to the extent of damage. The undisplaced fracture requires only immobilization of the arm with the elbow flexed for 3 weeks. Most displaced fractures are treated by closed reduction. If reduction is confirmed by x-ray, the arm is immobilized in a plaster cast held by a sling around the neck. After reduction, the child is admitted to the hospital for observation. The peripheral circulation should be checked for signs of compartment syndrome. Although the cast is worn for only 3 weeks, elbow stiffness is always present after removal. Stiffness should be alleviated by the child's own active movements; passive exercises should be avoided. In a few dislocated fractures, reduction is very unstable and excessive swelling or circulatory impairment is present. These fractures are treated by skeletal traction through a pin in the olecranon. The extremity is placed in either overhead arm traction (Smith's) or sidearm traction (Dunlop's) (see Fig. 22-11).

Complications which may occur in addition to compartment syndrome are peripheral nerve injury and malunion. The prognosis for recovery is good. If residual deformity is severe, a supracondylar osteotomy is required to restore the appearance and function of the elbow.

Nursing Management

Observations are made in the hospital to ensure that the fracture is held in a reduced position and to check for signs of complications. The position of the cast or alignment of traction is observed at regular intervals. Peripheral circulation and neurological function in the forearm and hand are checked every hour for the first 24 to 48 hours and then less frequently to detect signs of compartment syndrome and peripheral nerve injury. Persistent pain may be a sign of compartment syndrome and should not be masked by careless use of analgesics. Before discharge, the nurse demonstrates to parents the application of the collar and cuff neck sling or triangular sling and its proper fit to hold the arm in alignment. If the child is wearing a long arm or shoulder spica cast, this care is also discussed with parents.

Crush Injury

Crushing injuries caused by household machinery account for thousands of accidents every year in children. Today modern machines, such as lawn mowers, cause extensive damage to soft tissues. A variety of forces produce injury: compression, contusion (bruising), heat from friction, laceration, and avulsion. The extent of damage is determined by the force of the machinery, the amount of the extremity contacted, the duration of exposure, and the forces used to extricate the extremity.

After the injury, edema and hemorrhage develop. Extensive hematomas may accumulate in spaces created by separation of the skin and subcutaneous tissue from the underlying fascia. Subfascial hematoma and severe muscle damage are manifested by pain on passive extension of the body part. Fractures may be present in cases of severe injury.

In the emergency room, the extremity is cleaned, hematomas are drained, lacerations are sutured, and wounds are dressed. A bulky pressure dressing is applied, and the extremity is elevated. Tetanus antitoxin and antibiotics are given. Damage is difficult to assess initially, and progressive damage can result from edema and the swelling caused by hematomas; therefore, many children are hospitalized for observation. When dressings are changed 24 hours after injury, the extremity is reevaluated. Areas of skin with full-thickness loss are prepared for grafting. Hematomas are drained. If significant swelling, skin loss, or paralysis is present, the child remains in the hospital for further observation and treatment. The child who is able to be discharged at that time is instructed to elevate the extremity for 48 hours and to continue wearing the pressure dressing. Return appointments are made for periodic changes of the dressing.

Nursing Management

When a child with a crush injury arrives in the emergency room, the nurse or physician should collect information from relatives about the injury. Important facts to know are the age and type of the machine, the area of the extremity crushed, the time of exposure, and the actions required to extricate the extremity.

Aseptic technique is used for treatment of wounds. The extremity is cleansed with a mild detergent solution, after which hematomas are drained and wounds are dressed. A bulky pressure dressing is applied to immobilize the extremity. Antibiotic therapy is instituted after the administration of tetanus toxoid.

On the pediatric unit, the extremity is elevated. An affected upper extremity is suspended from an intravenous

(IV) drip pole or similar apparatus. These patients may be allowed out of bed pushing their IV poles. An affected lower extremity is elevated on pillows, and the child must remain in bed or on a stretcher. Circulation in the fingertips or toes is assessed every 1 to 2 hours. Analgesics can be given before dressings are changed to make the child more comfortable.

When the child is discharged, parents should receive instructions from the nurse on how to elevate the extremity and rewrap the dressings which come off. If medications are prescribed, instructions about the drug and its administration are given to parents. The importance of keeping follow-up outpatient visits which require dressing changes is stressed. Mobility limits and the amount of activity allowed also need to be elaborated at this time.

Musculoskeletal Diseases and Dysfunctions in the School-Age Child and Adolescent

Athletic Injuries

Americans have seen an enormous expansion in scholastic and community-based sports programs for youth in recent years. These programs provide the exercise that vitally contributes to health and fitness. Important needs of the child and adolescent can be met through sports participation. The normal evolution of independence can be fostered by the relationship with a team, the responsibilities of team membership, and the process of winning and losing. The young person's need for acceptance can be met by teammates, peers, coaches, and parents as long as the primary goals of the program are having fun and developing skills.

Growth is the single quality that is unique to the young athlete. It produces change in body size, proportion, and composition. Increase in strength, change in body functions, and maturation of behavior are also part of the growth process. Unfortunately, the growing musculoskeletal system is susceptible to injury. Because the epiphyseal plates have not closed in the young growing athlete, he is prone to types of injuries different from those of his adult counterpart. The preadolescent athlete, even when engaged in contact sports, runs less risk of injury than does his counterpart at the high school or college level. The significantly lower rate of injury among preadolescents in contact sports can be attributed to lower impact velocity produced by smaller children.

Injury to young athletes can be attributed to two mechanisms: the recurrent microtrauma of training and exposure of growing bones and joints to excessive impact trauma in heavy contact sports. Children are susceptible to many of the same injuries as adults, including sprains, strains, and contusions, as well as long-bone fractures of their extremities. Four special types of injuries can be sustained by children as a result of musculoskeletal trauma: (1) growth plate injuries, (2) injuries to the epiphysis or end of the bone, (3) avulsions (pulling away) of tendons at the site of insertion on the bone, and (4) stress frac-

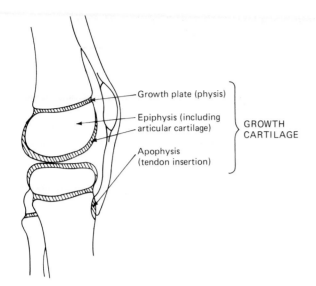

FIGURE 22-16 Sites of growth cartilage in the knee. These areas are particularly susceptible to injury in the growing athlete. *(From R.H. Strauss [ed.] Sports MEdicine and Physiology, Saunders, Philadelphia, 1979; reprinted by permission of Holt, Rinehart and Winston.)*

tures due to excessive or rapid training techniques. (Fig. 22-16).

The growth plate is more susceptible to deforming forces than either the ligaments of nearby joints or the outer shafts of the long bones. Therefore, a heavy blow or twist to the extremity of a child can result in disruption or fracture through the growth plate (Fig. 22-17). Loss of limb length, angular deformity, or joint incongruity can result from this type of injury. Both the knee and the ankle are particularly prone to develop subsequent problems after growth plate injury. Any injury around these joints should not be dismissed until damage to the growth plate is ruled out. Treatment of growth plate injuries consists of immobilization, often requiring casting.

The epiphysis is covered by the articular cartilage and forms part of the joint. During childhood, the articular (joint) surface and the articular cartilage appear to have a special susceptibility to injury. An impact of sufficient intensity can injure the articular cartilage, cause pieces to be knocked free into the joint, and grow to such size that they inhibit joint function. *Osteochrondritis dissecans* is the term for this disorder. Early arthritis can also result. The elbow, knee, hip, and ankle are most susceptible to this type of injury. Complaints of persistent pain in the joint are indicative of the problem. If such an injury is detected early, treatment consists of rest or immobilization by casting the extremity. Surgery is sometimes required to remove fragments that are already free in the joint.

Avulsion is an injury which has a unique incidence in children. Avulsions can occur in both the upper and lower extremities in the young athlete. Hockey players are prone to develop avulsion of the adductor muscles in the groin. Track and soccer players may suffer avulsions of the hamstring muscle and hip flexors at their insertions on the hip and lower pelvis. *Little League elbow*, seen in school-age baseball pitchers, involves overstretching of the elbow muscles and tendons which results in an avulsion fracture of the medial and lateral epicondyles of the humerus. Sudden injury can result in such excruciating pain that it may be mistaken for serious fracture. Surgery may be required to reattach the tendon to the site of avulsion from the bone. Less severe injuries can heal satisfactorily with rest and immobilization alone.

Stress fractures result from slow but progressive loss of bony substance at one particular site. If the process continues long enough, a complete fracture can occur. In young athletes, stress fractures are usually caused by the rapid increase of a specific training activity over a short period of time. The athlete involved in running activities is particularly likely to develop a stress fracture of the tibia below the knee. The runner experiences moderately severe pain while running, before changes in the bone can be seen on x-ray. Early treatment, including rest and immobilization, can prevent the bone from completely fracturing, which would require prolonged cast treatment or operation. Another location susceptible to stress fracture is the spine. As the gymnast repeatedly bends and puts pressure on the spine, a stress fracture can occur between the anterior and posterior parts of lower spinal vertebrae. This singular condition is known as *spondylolysis*. When the upper spine has slipped forward, the condition is called *spondylolisthesis*. Early detection is necessary to prevent a potentially serious problem. Early treatment consists of rest and immobilization of the spine. Surgical spinal fusion is required for more serious disorders that do not respond to conservative treatment or when further slipping occurs.

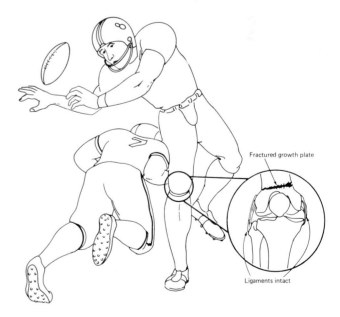

FIGURE 22-17 The growth plate is more susceptible to injury in the growing athlete than are the surrounding ligaments. *(From R.H. Strauss [ed.], Sports Medicine and Physiology, Saunders, Philadelphia, 1979; reprinted by permission of Holt, Rinehart and Winston.)*

Injury Prevention

Early attention to complaints of pain and dysfunction and suspicion of growth cartilage or stress injuries are important ways of preventing serious injury to the young athlete. The injured athlete should not reenter competitive sports until adequate healing has taken place. The overall athletic program should be evaluated by the health professional to assure that some essential requirements are met. Intelligent coaching, capable officiating, and use of the best facilities and equipment possible are important aspects of any program. The potential athlete should be counseled as to his or her suitability for a particular sport. The child's size, maturity, and level of conditioning can be assessed in regard to the requirements of the desired sport. Maturational age rather than chronological age should be the main criterion for placement in a sport. Alterations should be made in certain rules or tactics to decrease the risk of injury to the young athlete. An example of this measure is the Little League's limit on pitching among school-age baseball pitchers. Use of protective equipment such as padding and helmets helps prevent injuries, as does the enforcement of safety rules and regulations in sports activities. Proper conditioning is another factor in the prevention of unnecessary injury. Precautions should be taken in weight training for conditioning. The use of heavy-weight or low-repetition techniques must be avoided in training. Growth plate injuries and rupture of tendons have been reported in children lifting excessive weights. Children should lift weights under proper supervision using the low-weight, high-repetition technique.

Epiphyseal Plate Fractures

Fracture injuries of the epiphyseal plate account for 15 percent of all fractures in children. Trauma causes separation through the weakest area of the plate, the area of calcifying cartilage. Since the plate gets its blood supply from the epiphysis, disruption of the vessels to the epiphysis causes both the epiphysis and the plate to become necrotic, and growth ceases. With trauma, separation of the plate is more likely than tearing of the ligaments or dislocation of the joint.

Treatment for these injuries is different from that for typical fractures. Some types of epiphyseal fractures require open reduction and internal fixation. Immobilization may be shorter than for a fracture of the metaphysis in the same bone; however, longer follow-up is essential to detect any disturbance in growth. Such disabilities are progressive, with retardation of growth occurring for several months, followed by an arrest in further development. If the entire epiphyseal plate stops growing, the affected limb will be shorter than the other, normal limb. If the damaged bone is one of a pair, as with the radius and ulna, an angulatory deformity becomes evident and progresses with growth.

In the leg-length discrepancy, surgical procedures are sometimes done to correct the differences in length. In *epiphyseal plate arrest,* the epiphyseal plate in the longer leg is prevented from further growth by bone grafts or metal staples. *Epiphyseal plate stimulation* increases the circulation to the epiphyseal plate of the shorter leg so that it is stimulated to grow faster.

Nursing Management

It is imperative that parents keep follow-up appointments for the child after epiphyseal plate fractures and that they be aware of the risk of growth disturbances. The community or outpatient nurse encourages parents to keep regular appointments and checks the length of the affected limb. True length of the leg is assessed by measuring from the anterior superior iliac spine to the medial malleolus of the ankle. This measurement should be compared with the length of the normal leg, and any discrepancies must be reported to the physician. The length of time necessary for follow-up is at least 1 year, possibly longer.

Slipped Upper Femoral Epiphysis

In slipped upper femoral epiphysis, the head of the femur becomes displaced both downward and backward off the neck of the femur. Weakness of the epiphyseal plate allows the epiphysis to slip off the femoral neck in reaction to force. If the gradual slipping continues and separation of the epiphysis and the femoral neck is complete, the blood supply is likely to be interrupted, resulting in avascular necrosis of the femoral head.

Early symptoms include fatigue after walking or standing, mild pain in the hip which may be referred to the knee, and a slight limp. A progressive external rotation deformity develops in the lower limb. Movements of internal rotation, flexion, and abduction become restricted, and x-ray confirms the diagnosis.

This problem is found most frequently in boys between 10 and 16 years of age. The disorder is most common in very tall, thin, rapidly growing children and in obese, inactive children with underdeveloped sexual characteristics.

The slip or separation is reduced by gentle manipulation, and threaded pins are inserted surgically across the epiphyseal plate for stabilization. The aim of treatment is to prevent further slipping. Weight bearing is not allowed until the epiphysis is joined to the femoral neck.

Nursing Management

When slipped upper femoral epiphysis is suspected, the young person should be referred to a physician as soon as possible and instructed to avoid unnecessary weight bearing. After admission to the hospital, bed rest is instituted with the affected leg in an internally rotated position. The rationale for traction and surgical procedures must be clarified for the child and his family. In consultation with the dietitian, a weight-reduction diet for the obese child should begin in the hospital. Both the child and his parents should be involved in planning for the diet in the hospital and at home. Rest and prevention of abnormal forces on the affected hip are prescribed when the child is at home. Normal daily activities and school activities must be revised if weight bearing is not allowed. Mobility limits must be understood clearly by child and parents.

NURSING CARE PLAN

22-3 *The Child with Slipped Upper Femoral Epiphysis*

Clinical Problem/Nursing Diagnosis	Expected Outcome	Nursing Interventions

Pain (leg, hip, knee)
 	
Pain related to femoral head displacement
	With analgesics and reduced weight-bearing, child's leg pain will be alleviated and permanent physical disability will be prevented	*Preoperative:*
		  Reduce weight bearing
		  Properly institute splinting and traction
		  Administer analgesics as ordered
		Postoperative:
		  Continue bed rest, splinting, traction, analgesics as ordered

Limp Impaired physical mobility	Through appropriate nursing intervention, child will be free of permanent physical disability	Immediately reduce weight bearing and promote bed rest preoperatively Maintain muscle strength of unaffected extremities with ROM, isometric exercises as ordered Consult physical therapy for therapeutic exercise program
Obesity Altered nutrition: more than body requirements	With nutritional counseling, child's dietary habits will improve and a weight loss will occur	Consult dietician to plan an appropriate weight-reduction program for age Reinforce teaching of improved dietary habits to child and family Provide written information, i.e., dietary charts to promote compliance Encourage child to participate in plan of diet program
Potential for destruction of skin surfaces Impaired skin integrity	Child's skin will remain intact	Provide sheepskin, H$_2$O mattress, egg crate under pressure points Reposition child q 2 h Observe skin for pink reddened areas; presence of excoriation Thoroughly wash and dry skin (especially between skinfolds) Apply circular massage to promote skin circulation
Sensory deprivation Sensory/perceptual alteration (sensory deprivation)	Child will be provided with diverse environmental and age-appropriate stimuli	Promote age-appropriate activities (medical play, art therapy, music, relaxation techniques) Involve OT, play therapists in plan of care to provide arts, crafts, structured daily intervention
Constipation Constipation	A diet high in fiber, fruits, and vegetables will enable the child to maintain normal bowel patterns Child will have regular bowel movements	Encourage diet high in fiber, fruits, vegetables Encourage fluid intake Assess need for mild stool softener or laxative

Follow-up care emphasizes monitoring of the opposite hip for bilateral involvement. The nurse's teaching can help both child and family understand the disease process and the importance of early recognition of symptoms in the opposite leg.

Nursing Care Plan 22-3 describes the treatment for a client with slipped epiphysis of the femoral head.

Osteogenic Sarcoma

Children, adolescents, and young adults are victims in three-fourths of all cases of osteogenic sarcoma (osteosarcoma). This malignancy affects males twice as frequently as females. The tumor arises from osteoblasts, or bone-forming cells, with the most common site being the metaphysis of a long bone. More than half these lesions found at the lower end of the femur, the upper end of the tibia, or the upper end of the humerus are sites of active epiphyseal growth.

Pain is the only consistent symptom; it begins intermittently but becomes more intense and continuous. Joint function is limited as the tumor grows. Because this neoplasm is very vascular, swelling over the tumor site feels warm and overlying veins are dilated. Pathological fractures may take place. X-ray shows a characteristic formation, but a positive diagnosis requires surgical biopsy.

Other diagnostic tests are carried out when the patient is first admitted to the hospital. Blood tests include a complete blood count, platelet count, and liver function studies such as alkaline phosphatase, transaminase, and protein electrophoresis. Urinalysis is routinely done, as are bone studies, including x-rays of the lesion, bone survey, and bone scan. Computerized axial tomography of the lungs and the tumor site is performed. These tests are done for evaluation of the lesions as well as screening for other lesions.

Because pulmonary metastases are seen early, osteogenic sarcoma is a tumor that has had a poor prognosis. At present, the 5-year survival rate is 55 percent. No consistent response has been shown to any single treatment. The tumor is not particularly radiosensitive; therefore, amputation is the treatment of choice if no evidence of metastases is shown on x-ray. Chemotherapy is inititiated either before or after surgery and involves treatment with high-dose methotrexate in combination with such drugs as doxorubicin (Adriamycin), cyclophosphamide, actinomycin D, vincristine, and cisplatin (Greene, 1982). Radiation therapy is rarely used.

When metastases are present or the tumor is nonresectable, treatment is by chemotherapy. Drugs are administered for pain. In cases of severe pain or deformity, amputation may be done for palliative instead of curative reasons.

Nursing management is discussed with Ewing sarcoma.

Ewing Sarcoma

This neoplasm develops from primitive bone marrow cells. It usually occurs between the ages of 5 and 15 years. The incidence for males is twice that for females. Shafts of the long bones, including the femur, tibia, and humerus, are common sites.

The lesion tends to extend longitudinally in the involved bone and develop early metastases to the lungs, other bones, and lymph nodes. Tumor cells grow so rapidly that they soon perforate the cortex of the bone to form a large soft tissue mass. This mass is palpable and tender. Pain at the site of the bony lesion becomes increasingly severe. As the lesions outgrow their blood supply and degenerate, toxic products enter the bloodstream and cause fever and leukocytosis.

Hematologic studies done before diagnosis include hemoglobin, hematocrit, white blood cell count, and platelet count; blood chemistry includes determinations of serum glutamic oxaloacetic transaminase (SGOT), alkaline phosphatase, and uric acid. A 24-hour urine test for vanillylmandelic acid (VMA) or total urinary catecholamines is done to rule out neuroblastoma, a tumor in which these substances are elevated. Other diagnostic measures include urinalysis, bone marrow aspiration, chest x-ray and tomograms, bone survey, bone scan, and x-ray of the involved area. A surgical biopsy confirms, the diagnosis.

The 5-year survival rate with Ewing sarcoma is approximately 60 percent. The primary treatment is high-dose radiotherapy (Greene, 1982). Chemotherapy is used to prevent metastases. Vincristine, cyclophosphamide, dactinomycin, and doxorubicin are the drugs of choice.

Surgical removal of the tumor or involved limb may be done in selected cases.

Chemotherapy

Chemotherapy is used to inhibit growth of tumor cells in major lesions as well as to prevent or inhibit microscopic metastases. Drugs which are commonly used for treatment of osteogenic sarcoma and Ewing sarcoma are listed in Table 22-7. If these drugs prove ineffective, investigational drugs may be tried. All side effects of chemotherapeutic drugs should be reported to the physician so that measures can be taken to counteract them or the drugs can be discontinued. Nurses are in the best position to observe side effects and help relieve them if the drug must be continued. Baseline studies can serve as comparisons to later symptoms.

In response to either radiation or chemotherapy, mouth ulcers may appear. Good oral hygiene should include regular cleansing of gums and teeth and the use of mouthwashes. Nausea and vomiting should not be ignored; instead, every effort should be made to find a schedule of administration and an antiemetic drug which will give relief. Constipation may require the use of a stool softener. Before the child loses his hair *(alopecia)*, he should be prepared for this possibility and encouraged to purchase a wig if he wishes.

Special considerations are required for some drugs. Hemorrhagic cystitis caused by cyclophosphamide (Cytoxan) can be detected by routine testing for blood in urine. High fluid intake or hydration with intravenous fluids is necessary when this drug is administered. Oral doses of the drug should be given in the morning so that the child has all day to drink extra fluids. High-dose methotrexate is combined with citrovorum factor (folinic acid-SF, Leucovorin) rescue in the treatment of osteogenic sarcoma. Because cancer cells absorb methotrexate much more rapidly than normal cells do, normal cells can be "rescued" from much of the toxicty of methotrexate by the citrovorum factor. The citrovorum is usually given orally 1 to 2 hours after methotrexate infusion and continued at 6-hour intervals until acceptable serum methotrexate levels are reached. Normal cells pick up the citrovorum factor, which acts as an antidote, and the cells are not destroyed. Renal damage is a serious complication of high-dose methotrexate. Excretion is through the kidneys, and in an acid environment the methotrexate tends to precipitate in the renal tubules. Therefore, electrolyte solutions containing sodium bicarbonate are administered to keep the urine alkaline, and adequate hydration is essential. A major side effect of cisplatin is renal toxicity. This complication is minimized by the presence of normal renal function prior to drug administration. It is essential to maintain aggressive hydration and diuresis during and after cisplatin infusion.

Amputation

Amputation is *therapeutic* in the case of a neoplasm and is therefore done to prolong life, decrease pain, or increase

TABLE 22-7 Drugs of Choice for Treatment of Osteogenic Sarcoma and Ewing Sarcoma

Drug	Specific Action	Route of Administration*	Toxic and Side Effects
Doxorubicin (Adriamycin)	Unknown; believed to retard DNA synthesis	IV	Oral ulceration, anorexia, nausea and vomiting, alopecia, cardiac toxicity; extravasation causes induration
Cisplatin (Cis-Diamminedichloroplatinium LL; CPDC)	Unknown; believed to promote inhibition of DNA synthesis and bind with cell membranes	IV	Renal toxicity, nausea and vomiting, electrolyte disturbance, mild myelosupression, auditory disturbance
Cyclophosphamide (Cytoxan)	Prevention of cell division	IV or PO	Leukopenia, hemorrhagic cystitis, alopecia, nausea and vomiting
Dactinomycin (actinomycin D, Cosmegen)	Inhibition of protein synthesis	IV	Bone marrow depression, nausea and vomiting, alopecia; injection site extravasation causes induration
Methotrexate	Folic acid antagonist; inhibition of DNA synthesis	IV	Bone marrow depression, kidney and liver toxicity, oral and gastrointestinal ulcerations, nausea and vomiting, diarrhea, rash, fever, pneumothorax
Vincristine sulfate (Oncovin)	Arrest of cells in metaphase	IV	Neurotoxicity (jaw pain, paresthesia, foot drop, constipation) alopecia; extravasation causes induration

*IV = intravenous; PO = by mouth.

Source: Adapted from P. Flummerfelt and M. Morse, "Injectable Chemotherapeutic Agents," drug sheet utilized at James Whitcomb Riley Hospital for Children, Division of Pediatric Hematology-Oncology, 1980.

function. Amputation is physically and psychologically distressing for the child and his family. On admission to the hospital, an assessment should be made of the child's behavior and relationships with his parents. When amputation is therapeutic, the nurse has time to help the patient and family prepare for surgery through explanations and interviews. Feelings need to be expressed. Preoperatively the child may act out his overwhelming fears of disfigurement and death by hostile reactions and refusal to cooperate with the hospital staff. Postoperatively all children should be provided with some means for expressive play or expression of their feelings. Since loss of a body part can be compared with death of a loved one, the child feels extreme sadness and grief. Parents often have guilt feelings about the disease. Both child and parents need support in working through the grief process.

During surgery every attempt is made to cover the stump with a flap of healthy skin so that scars or nerve endings are not over the weight-bearing portion of the bone. Nursing care postoperatively aims to prevent bleeding, minimize swelling, maintain body alignment, and decrease pain. A plaster cast or compression bandage is usually applied. The stump may be elevated on pillows, although elevation must be done judiciously to avoid contractures which would interfere with the use of a prosthesis. If an immediate postoperative lower limb prosthesis is used, a plaster cast is applied around the stump after surgery. When the cast is dry, a temporary prosthesis is secured to the plaster and the patient begins walking or using the prosthesis.

Phantom limb sensations may be very disturbing and confusing to the child. Feelings such as burning, itching, throbbing, or sharp pain may be perceived in the phantom limb. Over a period of 1 or 2 years, the phantom sensations decrease until the distal portion merges with the stump. The child needs to be supported in understanding that these sensations are normal and will gradually decrease.

Adjustment to the loss of a limb is a difficult, long-term process. Nurses can help the child accept the stump by treating it in a matter-of-fact way, without negative projections or undue concern. When the child looks at the stump or touches it, he can begin to accept its reality; therefore, these activities should be encouraged when the child is ready for them. He should also be encouraged to discuss future activities and relationships such as modifications in clothing, use of the prosthesis, returning to school, and meeting old friends.

The child and family should begin caring for the stump in the hospital. Daily washing with soap and water should be accompanied by checks for skin irritation or breakdown. Exercises for muscle strengthening are taught by the physical therapist. The permanent prosthesis is usually fitted a few months after the stump is healed. The prosthesis is removed at night, and stump and socket hygiene follows. The stump is cleansed with an antiseptic soap and then dried thoroughly. The socket of the prosthesis is washed with mild soap, rinsed, and dried. The stump sock or bandage should be changed daily and washed with a mild soap. Skin disorders should be reported to the physician promptly so that necessary adjustments can be made in the prosthesis. The prosthesis will

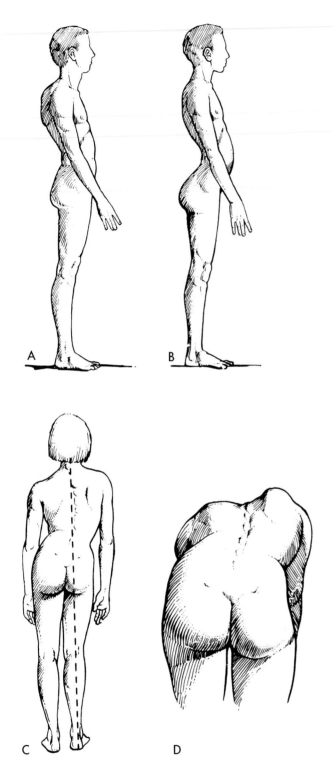

FIGURE 22-18 Spinal deformities: *(a)* kyphosis, *(b)* lordosis, *(c)* scoliosis (standing), and *(d)* scoliosis (bending forward). *(Courtesy of Indiana University School of Medicine.)*

need frequent replacement as the child grows. Regular follow-up in an amputee clinic is important to ensure that the child wears and benefits from his prosthesis.

Nursing Management

Diagnosis of a neoplasm has a tremendous impact on the child and his family. If the diagnosis is given too early and then reversed, the family members may be so frightened that they cannot believe the more favorable diagnosis. If the diagnosis of a neoplasm is given too late, the family members may have such false hope that the decision for lifesaving amputation will be postponed. The nursing staff must be honest with the child and family from the beginning. The child will not accept amputation or long-term chemotherapy without a good understanding of the problem. The physician usually talks with parents first and gives parents the choice of whether they or the physician or both together will talk with the child. It is important to use a term the child can understand yet at the same time educate the child about the meaning of terms which will inevitably be heard, such as "cancer" or "tumor." Older children need specific information, and they resent not being told about the diagnosis or treatment.

Nurses need to find out from the physician and the parents what the child has been told and what terms were used. It is important that nurses do not avoid the child or his family, for they can offer support and should be available to listen. Often a child or family members will confide in the nurse instead of the physician, thereby partially relieving themselves of fears and misconceptions.

In evaluating nursing interventions, the nurse notes the achievement of these outcomes: The child, siblings, and parents understand and cope adequately with diagnostic measures and diagnosis; the child and family progress through the grieving process appropriately; the child's comfort is maximized; illness and its complications are eradicated or controlled by therapy as long as possible; complications of chemotherapy, radiation therapy, or amputation are prevented or minimized; the child and family understand and cope adequately with the therapy program and long-term illness.

Curvature of the Spine
Types of Curvature

Spinal deformities include kyphosis (humpback), lordosis (swayback), and scoliosis (lateral curvature) as shown in Fig. 22-18. These deformities may occur alone or in association with other conditions.

Kyphosis is a fixed flexion deformity of the spine which most often appears in the thoracic spine. The vertebral deformities in the infant with myelomeningocele may assume the form of a kyphosis. It is also produced by a decrease in weight bearing and muscular control, as seen in muscular dystrophy and poliomyelitis. *Adolescent kyphosis* is a disorder affecting both girls and boys which begins at puberty and progresses until vertebral growth has stopped in the late teens. The child with adolescent kyphosis has "poor posture" or "rounded shoulders," but as the curvature progresses, moderate back pain may be a complaint. Treatment is conservative, including spinal exercises, sleeping without a pillow and with boards under the mattress, body casts, and the Milwaukee brace modified to treat kyphosis.

Lordosis is an increase in the normal inward curvature in the lumbar area of the back, causing a hollow back deformity. It rarely occurs in isolation but most often forms to compensate for other abnormalities. Whenever kyphosis is present in the spine, lordosis may form above or below it.

Scoliosis involves a lateral curvature of the spine. *Nonstructural* scoliosis is caused by changes outside the spine, such as poor posture, pain, or leg length discrepancy. Because the curve is flexible, it corrects by bending to the opposite side. *Structural* scoliosis is a curvature in which the vertebral bodies are rotated in the area of the greatest or major curve. Structural scoliosis may be idiopathic or due to another abnormality such as neurofibromatosis or paralysis. Treatment is by bracing, casting, and often spinal fusion. Untreated scoliosis leads to degenerative joint disease. Respiration may be affected, and pain may be progressive.

Idiopathic Scoliosis

In 70 percent of cases of scoliosis, the cause is idiopathic. Types of idiopathic scoliosis are differentiated by age group: infantile (birth to 3 years), juvenile (4 to 9 years), and adolescent (age 10 until growth ceases). More severe curves are several times more common in girls. Boys and girls are equally affected by idiopathic scoliosis, but some other factor, such as hormones, influences the progression of the curve so that more girls are seen for treatment. In both boys and girls with the adolescent type of scoliosis, a right thoracic curve is the most common.

The lateral curvature progresses with growth, making secondary changes in the vertebrae and ribs. Vertebrae are wedge-shaped in the middle of the curve from pressure on one side of the epiphyseal plate of the vertebral bodies. Typically, the curve begins slowly and is concealed by clothing. An uneven hemline may be the first clue that a problem exists. When it is noticed that one shoulder blade is higher than the other or one hip is more prominent, a significant curve exists.

The prognosis is better when curvature is mild, begins at an older age, and less growth remains. Treatment is instituted to prevent progression of mild scoliosis and stabilization as well as correction of more severe scoliosis. Treatment may be conservative, operative, or a combination of the two.

Many types of conservative treatments have been tried. Exercises alone and plastic body jackets have been unsuccessful. The Milwaukee brace is the most successful type of spinal brace and is widely used in the treatment of scoliosis (Fig. 22-19). In the older child the brace may prevent the need for surgery; in the younger child it may keep the curvature from becoming worse. In the last few years several types of new braces have appeared. One

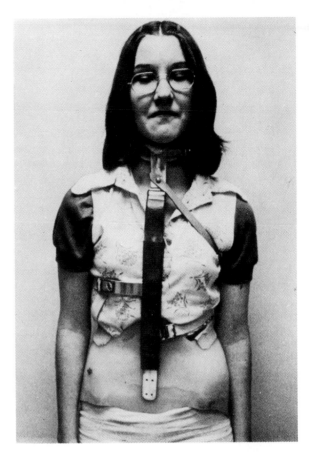

FIGURE 22-19   Milwaukee brace (blouse is worn under brace for purpose of photograph only). (*Courtesy of James Whitcomb Riley Hospital for Children, Indianapolis; photo by G. Dreyer.*)

such brace is the Boston brace, used to correct lumbar curves.

The Milwaukee brace is fitted individually to combine forces of longitudinal traction and lateral pressure. Exercise programs should be prescribed in conjunction with its use. Supervised by the physical therapist, exercises are designed for two purposes: (1) to increase muscle strength of the torso to counteract the effects of splinting and (2) to assist actively in correcting the abnormal curves and rib deformities. The increased strength gained from exercises helps the patient maintain an improved position after he has begun to remove the brace parttime. In school a full program of physical education usually can be maintained, with the exception of contact sports, trampoline, and gymnastics.

Operative treatment is usually done after 10 years of age. Preoperatively, curvatures may be corrected by plaster casts, Cotrel traction, or halofemoral traction. In surgery, the curvature is corrected, and the involved area of the spine is stabilized. Moderate curvatures may be treated by spinal fusion and immobilization in a body cast. In severe curvature, mechanical correction of the curve is accomplished by means of a Harrington rod or other instrumentation, followed by spinal fusion and the wearing of a body cast for several months. Postoperatively, when the patient is out of the cast, activities should be limited and strenuous exercise or sports which are likely to end in falls (i.e., horseback riding) should be avoided.

Nursing Management

The nursing role in idiopathic scoliosis begins with detection. With early case finding, conservative treatment is more likely to be effective. School nurses and community health nurses are conducting successful screening programs which refer schoolchildren to physicians for early diagnosis and treatment. All children in grades 5 through 8 (ages 10 through 13) should be screened yearly for scoliosis. Boys strip to the waist; girls may wear a brassiere or halter top and shorts or a bathing suit. The nurse conducts a simple, systematic examination of the back on each child (Table 22-8 and Fig. 22-20).

When surgery is required, various casts may be used preoperatively for correction of the curvature. The *localizer* cast is a body cast which utilizes cephalopelvic traction as well as pressure directly over the major curves to give correction. Cotrel's *E-D-F cast* (elongation, derotation, and flexion) is most effective in correcting the rib hump of severe thoracic curves. The *surcingle cast,* which extends up over the occiput, also provides correction of the rib hump. Patients are usually hospitalized overnight after cast application so that necessary adjustments can be made in the cast before discharge. The nurse should check the cast for uncomfortable or tight

---

TABLE 22-8 Examination of the Back Used in Routine Scoliosis Screening

Position of Student and Examiner	Observations by the Examiner*
Student standing erect, feet together, arms hanging straight down, back to examiner	Head not balanced over body? Shoulder level unequal? One shoulder blade more prominent than other?
Examiner seated, observing student's back	Waistline uneven? Distances between arms and body unequal? Hip level unequal? Spine curved?
Student bending forward at the waist, back parallel with floor, feet together, knees unbent, arms hanging freely, palms together, with back and then front to examiner. Examiner seated, observing rear and front of student	Difference in level between two sides of the back? Hump on one side of the upper back? Compensating hump on opposite side of lower back?
Student standing erect and then forward bending (positions above), with side to examiner. Examiner seated, observing side view of student	Thoracic gibbus (hump)? Lumbar lordosis (sway back)? Thoracic gibbus persisting on forward bending?

*If findings are positive, there is a possibility of scoliosis.

Source: Adapted from *Scoliosis Screening for Early Detection,* Multi Video International, Inc., Minneapolis, Minn. 55435, 1975.

---

points and help the patient adjust to wearing it. Movements in the cast are restricted; ambulation is often difficult at first; and sleep is uncomfortable until the child adjusts to the cast.

Normal activities such as bathing, dressing, and washing hair must often be modified. Skin care in the cast includes keeping the skin clean and dry and preventing sore areas at pressure points. Clothing must be loose or purchasd in larger sizes to be worn outside the cast. Washing the hair can be made easier by the use of spray hoses on faucets or by lying with the head extended over the side of the bed above a washpan. Stretchers or reclining wheelchairs may be necessary for mobility, and trips to and from the hospital require the use of an ambulance, station wagon, or van for the nonsitting or nonambulating patient. The nurse can help the child and parents plan for these activities during hospitalizations and outpatient visits.

The patient who is just beginning to wear the Milwaukee brace gradually increases his time in the brace until he is wearing the brace 23 hours a day. To protect the skin, he should bathe daily out of the brace, apply alcohol to pink skin areas or areas where the brace presses, and avoid the use of creams, lotions, or powders under the brace since these products can irritate the skin. A smooth-fitting undershirt or stockinet should be worn under the brace to protect the skin. Other clothing is worn outside the brace. If there is skin breakdown, the physician should be consulted, and the brace must not be worn until the skin heals. Adjustment may need to be made in the brace to reduce pressure points. Low-heeled shoes increase comfort and safety in ambulation.

The nurse can be a very real help to the child and parents in adjusting to or coping with the cast or brace. The mental preparation for cast or brace wearing can be much more important than the physical preparation in terms of the difficulties experienced by the adolescent and his parents. Withdrawal, self-consciousness, denial, and fear of peers' reactions are commonly experienced by the adolescent, while his parents often feel guilt or discomfort in their role of enforcing therapy. As the nurse gets to know a particular patient and family, she can become an emphathetic listener and facilitate their attempts at problem solving. The school or community health nurse can help ease an adolescent's return to the classroom by interpreting his needs to teachers and administrators.

Traction may be used before surgery to stretch out soft tissue structures or correct spinal curvature. *Cotrel dynamic traction,* used for preoperative stretching, consists of a leather head halter, pelvic apparatus, and foot stirrups. The patient is usually in traction for only 10 to 15 minutes each hour, with exercise periods during the daytime hours. Intermittent traction allows him to carry on many normal activities out of traction. The nurse checks equipment and instructs and supervises the patient during the exercise sessions. Sheepskin padding is needed at potential pressure points at the chin and pelvis, and the skin should be checked for signs of breakdown. *Halofemoral traction* corrects severe and resistant curves. Pins

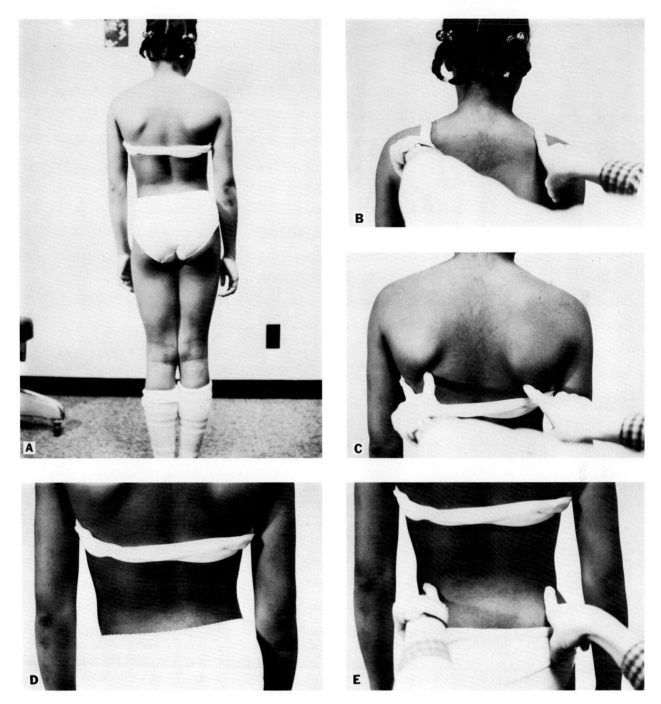

FIGURE 22-20   Observations indicative of scoliosis, taken from a routine screening exam. *(A)* Head is not balanced over body, *(B)* shoulders are not level, *(C)* scapulae are not symmetrical, *(D)* space between arms and waist is not symmetrical, *(E)* pelvis is not level.

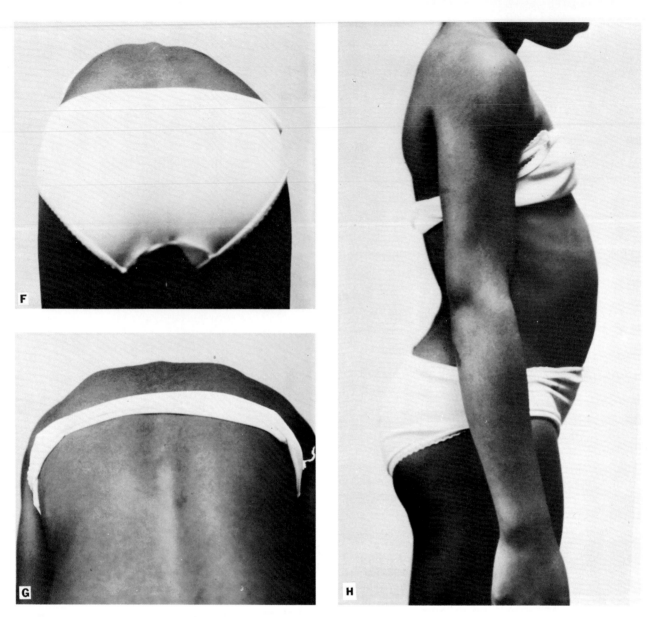

FIGURE 22-20, cont'd. *(F)* hump is present in lumbar region, *(G)* hump is present in thoracic region, and *(H)* thoracic kyphosis and lumbar lordosis are present. *(Photos by Chuck Isaacson.)*

which attach the halo to the skull and insert into the distal femur for femoral traction should be kept clean by daily nursing care. In addition to checking the traction setup, the nurse monitors the patient for signs of complications such as pain, skin trauma, joint contractures, neurological deficits, and organ displacement. Organ displacement is manifested by respiratory distress and internal bleeding or compression. Other complications of halofemoral traction are anorexia, thrombophlebitis, hypertension, respiratory compromise, and sensory or social deprivation. By gradual addition of heavier weights, dramatic correction is achieved. Surgery is performed after adequate correction, and the patient may be returned to traction postoperatively.

Preoperative preparation includes explanations about the surgery. Explanations about care immediately before surgery, anesthesia, postoperative care, and postoperative appearance are given to the child and his parents. The child practices deep breathing, logrolling, lying on a Stryker frame or special mattress, leg exercises, eating, and use of the fracture bedpan while laying flat in bed. If the child is to be transferred to the intensive care unit postoperatively, a preoperative visit for both child and parents is helpful. Visiting with other postoperative scoliosis patients also helps the child and his parents know what to expect.

Postoperative nursing care must be gentle but at the same time aggressive enough to prevent complications.

The patient is usually returned without a cast but with a dressing over the back incision. A hospital bed is most comfortable postoperatively, although it should have a firm mattress and be placed so that it is not easily jogged. If a Stryker frame or Circo-Electric bed is used, special care should be taken to increase the patient's feelings of comfort and security. Postoperative nursing functions include logrolling at 2-hour intervals, caring for the urethral catheter, monitoring intravenous and central venous pres sure lines, monitoring blood transfusions, administering analgesics or antibiotics, supervising coughing and deep breathing, and assisting with comfort and safety.

Nursing observations are made for signs of complications and include vital signs to assess for hypovolemia, shock, respiratory difficulties, or infection; intake and output for signs of urinary retention or fluid imbalance; neurological checks in the lower extremities to detect deficits in sensory or motor function; drainage from the incision and wound healing for signs of bleeding, hematoma, dehiscence, or infection; skin over bony prominences to note red or sore areas; unusual pain which might indicate displacement of the rod; circulation in the lower extremities to screen for thrombophlebitis; and gastrointestinal symptoms for signs of superior mesenteric artery syndrome with paralytic ileus, abdominal distention, and pain.

The adolescent's psychosocial status and his parents' teaching needs are also considered by the nurse postoperatively. To prevent boredom in the hospital or home, a schedule can be devised to make each part of the day meaningful. Schooling should be initiated and plans made for tutoring or returning to school at home. On the basis of interest, games, crafts, and other activities are planned which can be adapted to his mobility limitations. To assist with schoolwork and recreational activities, prism glasses, bedboards, and easels are recommended. Peer interaction is arranged by bringing other patients or friends into the adolescent's hospital room or planning for friends to visit at home. Ideally, parents spend several days caring for the child in the hospital before discharge so that they can become familiar with cast care, turning and positioning, supervision of activities, and other care needs. The child is discharged in a body cast, and the community health nurse receives a referral for follow-up supervision at home.

Adolescents treated for scoliosis have many concerns about their bodies and body images. In the cast, the adolescent may feel unreal or unlike his real self. Girls often are concerned about breast development and the effect of treatment on other bodily functions. They may be worried that the cast will prevent growth or change the shape of their breasts or that menstruation will temporarily cease in the cast. Feelings of vulnerability are common, aggravated by disrobing during cast application or the restrictions imposed by casts or traction. Most teenage girls adjust well, however, because of their desire to look better and to please their parents and the medical staff. The acceptance of the treatment program by parents is a crucial factor in the child's acceptance.

Nursing Care Plan 22-4 describes the treatment for a child with scoliosis.

 NURSING CARE PLAN

22-4 The Child with Scoliosis

Clinical Problem/Nursing Diagnosis	Expected Outcome	Nursing Interventions

Child and family requesting information concerning scoliosis and individual therapy program	Child and family will verbalize and demonstrate knowledge of scoliosis, therapy program, and discharge instructions individualized to child's needs	Educate child and family about scoliosis and indicated therapy regimen
		Utilize visual aids, i.e., model of spinal column, cast, brace, in presentation of information
		Teach exercises specifically ordered by MD or PT to strengthen muscles
		Provide teaching for child with Milwaukee brace:
		Instruct child and family to:
		  Observe skin integrity
		  Remove brace immediately when skin irritation noted, gradually increase tolerance
		  Bathe out of brace bid
		  Apply alcohol to pink areas
		  Avoid use of lotions or creams that soften or irritate skin
		  Wear a thin cotton shirt under the brace
		  Wear low-heeled shoes to assist ambulation
		Nurse and occupational therapist will assist with adjustment to bathing, walking, sleeping, and dressing and will support compliance

Knowledge deficit related to lack of prior experience with scoliosis and treatment		

Continued.

Clinical Problem/Nursing Diagnosis	Expected Outcome	Nursing Interventions
		Provide teaching for child with cast immobilization:
		Teach child and family cast care:
		Instruct to check color, temperature, capillary refill of extremities bilaterally
		Teach them to report above changes in extremities and presence of pain, or foul-smelling odor from cast
		Assist child and family with adjustments to hygiene, positions for sleeping, use of pillows for support
		Provide preoperative teaching for child requiring surgery (rod placement):
		Instruct and have child demonstrate understanding of the following:
		Coughing and deep breathing exercises
		Use of incentive spirometer
		Logrolling
		Use of fracture bedpan
		Lying on orthopedic bed/Stryker frame
		Prepare child and family for:
		O_2 mask/nasal cannula
		Cardiac monitor leads
		Postop catheters, i.e., intravenous therapy, Foley catheter, CVP, arterial line
		Familiarize with equipment; teach purpose of monitoring
		Arrange preop visit to the ICU to prepare for postop recovery
		Facilitate meeting with child who can share experiences with scoliosis, therapy, surgery, to strengthen compliance incentives
		Assist child and family with understanding of alterations in activity, i.e., avoid vigorous gymnastics and horseback riding
		Encourage promotion of independence with ADL
		Contact school nurse to support compliance with treatment
		Facilitate follow-up care for home therapy program with MD, PT, OT
		Facilitate screening for other family members
Nausea and vomiting Anorexia Urinary retention ——————— Potential fluid volume deficit related to surgical losses, vomiting	Given the appropriate observations and interventions, the child will maintain fluid, electrolyte, and acid-base balance	Monitor vital signs with BP q 2 h
		Monitor CVP for fluid balance (clarify acceptable v.s. parameters with MD), report alterations in v.s. promptly
		Monitor ABGs for acid-base balance
		Assess client for fluid depletion: tachycardia, hypotension
		Monitor strict I&O
		Measure urine output via Foley catheter q 2 h
		Check urine: specific gravity, blood, protein, glucose
		Assess hydration status: note skin turgor, presence of moist mucous membrances, tears
		Monitor serum electrolytes (Na, K, Cl) and CBC (Hbg, hct)
		Properly and promptly administer replacement of colloid and crystalloid fluids as indicated by clinical status, lab values, and MD order
		Accurately assess and measure surgical wound dressings for the volume, color, and consistency of drainage (weigh dry dressing pads before reapplication)
Pink areas on skin over bony prominences ——————— Potential impaired skin integrity related to immobility	Given the appropriate interventions, the child will maintain skin integrity and skin circulation will be promoted	Log roll q 2 h
		Place sheepskin directly under pressure points
		Wash skin folds with mild nonirritating soap
		Wash Betadine (from surgery), urine, stool, wound drainage thoroughly from skin
		Thoroughly pat areas dry; avoid vigorous rubbing
		Protect skin from tape burns and sheet burns
		Provide clean dry gown, bed linens; avoid wrinkles in sheets under client
		Maintain clean and dry dressings
		Perform circular massage on exposed bony prominences and skin areas after turning

Clinical Problem/Nursing Diagnosis	Expected Outcome	Nursing Interventions
		Closely observe skin condition for presence of pink or red areas, openings in skin, rashes, edema, blisters; document presence, location, exact size of findings in cm
		Encourage diet high in protein, vitamins A and C to promote wound healing
		Casted child:
		Petal cast edges
		Apply alcohol on skin areas at cast edges
		Child with brace:
		Bathe out of brace bid.
		Apply alcohol on pink areas
		Gradually increase tolerance to brace
		Avoid use of lotions that soften or irritate skin
Pain Tachycardia Diaphoretic Pain related to surgery	Child will be able to rest and sleep with comfort Child will tolerate logrolling, breathing exercises with comfort Child will verbalize relief from pain	Properly administer ordered analgesics (preferably IV route) immediately postoperatively
		Observe s/s of respiratory depression; decreased respiratory rate; shallow respirations
		Coordinate logrolling, breathing exercises with pain medication (allow 30 min for effectiveness of meds)
		Encourage use of calming music with favorite tunes and use of Walkman to promote relaxation
		Document description of pain, type, location, effectiveness of analgesia
		Encourage visits from parents and significant others to comfort child, hold hand, rub forehead
Imposed restrictions of movement Impaired physical mobility related to brace, cast, surgery (rod placement)	Given the appropriate interventions, the child will maintain skin integrity, be free of pulmonary complications, have soft and regular bowel movements, and achieve optimal level of ROM and muscle strength	Logroll q 2 h (roll child as one unit with minimum of two nurses)
		Ensure proper use of Stryker frame or Circo-Electric bed
		Position pillows behind back and between legs to increase comfort and maintain body alignment
		Massage exposed skin areas to increase circulation to skin
		Assess skin condition at pressure points
		Encourage child to cough and deep breathe/use incentive spirometer 4-5 × q 1 h
		Promote diet high in fiber; encourage adequate fluid intake
		Assess presence of abdominal distention, pain, bowel sounds
Surgical incision susceptible to infection Potential for infection related to surgical wound	Child will experience wound healing without infection	Monitor child for alterations in vital signs: tachycardia, hypotension, elevated temperature
		Report elevated temperature (>38.5°C); notify MD of culture results, administer ordered antipyretics
		Properly administer prescribed IV antibiotics
		Assess surgical wound for amount, color, consistency, odor of drainage
		Note quality of wound healing, color of wound edges
		Protect integrity of wound; splint and support incision during coughing and deep breathing and logrolling
		Assess would for bleeding, hematoma formation, dehiscence
Restricted lung expansion Structural deformity Pain Shallow respirations Ineffective cough Potential ineffective breathing pattern related to musculoskeletal impairment	Child will maintain a patent airway and will receive adequate oxygenation as evidenced by O_2 saturation of 95 mmHg	Preoperatively assess pulmonary function results (note degree of impairment from structural deformity)
		Note preop O_2 saturation
		Monitor respirations for depth, rate, regularity
		Assess quality of breath sounds throughout lung fields
		Postoperative:
		Assess child for s/s of respiratory compromise; note color, teachypnea, PaO_2, quality of breath sounds
		Monitor ABG, pulse, oximetry for adequate O_2 saturation values
		Provide O_2 therapy via mask/nasal cannula as indicated
		Promote maximal lung expansion with coughing and deep breathing exercises; incentive spirometry 4-6× q 1-2 h

Continued.

NURSING CARE PLAN 22-4 The Child with Scoliosis —cont'd

Clinical Problem/Nursing Diagnosis	Expected Outcome	Nursing Interventions

Altered sensorimotor function
 	
Potential for injury: risk of neurological impairment related to surgical implantation of vertebral rod
	Child's neurologic status will be stable, with intact sensorimotor function	Assess neurological status with vital signs:
		  Note pupil size and reactivity to light
		  Check soft/sharp distinction with pin on extremities bilaterally
		Note abiity to move toes, plantar flexion
		Check strength of upper and lower extremities bilaterally
		Assess neurovascular status and peripheral perfusion of extremities:
		  Note pulses (strength/quality), color, warmth of exremities bilaterally
		  Prevent rod displacement injury by careful logrolling (turn body as one unit and use minimum of two nurses)
		Report change in affect, level of consciousness, sensorimotor function immediately to physician

Sensory deprivation Diversional activity deficit	Child will be provided with environmental and social stimuli appropriate for his developmental level	Encourage activities to decrease boredom: Use of Walkman with favorite music Drawing and painting Participation in appropriate games Peer interaction/visits on unit and with friends Use of VCR Provide with favorite books Schoolwork Encourage participation in ADL (practice modifications in activity) Encourage and support creative ideas for dealing with limitations in movement
Lack of participation in social activities Verbalizes self-conscious feelings and concerns Avoids peer contact Body-image disturbance	Child will enjoy interaction with peers and participate in social and school activities with self-confidence	Explore child's feelings about self, family, friends, body changes and characteristics Explore and address concerns related to sexuality and breast development Utilize art therapy to gather more information about child's perception of body image Encourage child to participate in plan of care (contribution of creative suggestions in coping with altered ADL) Provide opportunity for choice and control in plan of care, i.e., time of cast care, cutting out cast petals Ensure privacy during care and examinations Facilitate contact with a peer with scoliosis who can share experiences in coping with conservative treatment or surgery to further encourage verbalization of fears and concerns about being different Encourage cards from friends Encourage peer interaction Promote activities that enhance strength, self-esteem (art, crafts, talking to peer on unit about experiences) Assist family to support independence of the child

Study Questions

1. Clinical union of a fracture is considered to have taken place when:
   A. Callus formation can be demonstrated on x-ray film.
   B. The fracture has been reduced and a cast has been applied.
   C. Callus is firm enough that no movement occurs.
   D. All callus has been replaced by bone.

2. When the knees of a preschooler are held together by the examiner, if the feet remain apart, the child has:
   A. Genu valgum.   C. Coxa valgum.
   B. Genu varum.   D. Coxa varum.

3. The Ortolani test is indicative of skeletal abnormality if:
   A. The knees are not level.
   B. The baby does not have pain.
   C. A click is felt or heard in the joint.
   D. Normal range of motion is impossible.

4. In instruction the parents of a child with osteogenesis imperfecta, it is essential to teach them:
    A. How to recognize and splint a fracture.
    B. How to administer vitamin D.
    C. How to check radial and pedal pulses.
    D. How to prepare high-protein meals.

5. When a cast is to be applied on a preschooler after orthopedic surgery, a most appropriate nursing intervention is:
    A. Showing the child rolls of plaster of paris.
    B. Allowing the child to apply a cast to a doll.
    C. Taking the child to the cast room.
    D. Explaining the procedure days beforehand.

6. When a metallic device is used to apply traction directly to bone, it is called:
    A. Bryant's traction.
    B. Russell's traction.
    C. 90-90 traction.
    D. Skeletal traction.

7. With a diagnosis of Legg-Perthes disease, the teaching and counseling done by a nurse must include its:
    A. Lengthy course.
    B. Rapid resolution.
    C. Extensive rehabilitation.
    D. Debilitating sequelae.

8. A test in which thin, wirelike needles are stuck into a child's muscle while a recording of muscle contractions is made is called an:
    A. Electrokymogram.
    B. Electromyogram.
    C. Electronystogram.
    D. Electroretinogram.

9. When working with a child who has muscular dystrophy, the primary goal of care is to:
    A. Provide a high-protein, high-calcium diet.
    B. Increase the child's participation in physical activities.
    C. Promote bowel regularity.
    D. Keep the child as independent as possible.

10. A child who has sustained a supracondylar fracture of the humerus is usually placed in sidearm traction known as:
    A. Dunlop's traction.
    B. Smith's traction.
    C. 90-90 traction.
    D. Bryant's traction.

11. The phantom pain which follows an amputation for a neoplasm is disturbing and confusing to a school-age patient; therefore, it is important for a nurse to:
    A. Diversify the activities in which the client is involved.
    B. Tell the client to report any such experiences immediately.
    C. Counsel the child about the prosthetic devices available.
    D. Explain that the sensations are normal and expected.

12. In screening for scoliosis, the nurse asks the child to:
    A. Jog around the room to assess symmetry of movement.
    B. Bend forward at waist to inspect symmetry of shoulders, hips, and scapulae.
    C. Bend sideways to determine any limitations.
    D. Sit and then bend forward to identify any evidence of an uneven waist.

13. When an older infant diagnosed with congenital hip dysplasia is placed in Bryant's traction, a nurse monitors proper position by:
    A. Checking to see whether all weights are hanging freely.
    B. Keeping the infant in a jacket restraint.
    C. Passing one hand under the infant's buttocks.
    D. Rewrapping both sets of elastic bandages daily.

14. When skin traction is instituted, the pulling force is applied directly to the:
    A. Muscle.
    B. Skin.
    C. Bone.
    D. Weights.

15. A child in a body spica needs to be assessed daily for:
    A. Hyperreflexia.
    B. Hydration.
    C. Constipation.
    D. Anorexia.

16. A nursing intervention which facilitates joint movement in the child with juvenile rheumatoid arthritis is:
    A. Placing pillows under affected areas.
    B. Massaging painful joints gently.
    C. Applying warm compresses.
    D. Raising the foot and head of the bed.

17. Stress fractures result from the slow loss of bony substance at a particular site and are commonly caused by:
    A. Jogging over very irregular terrain.
    B. A rapid increase in a training activity over a short period.
    C. Excessive training activities over a long period of time.
    D. Sudden change in weight distribution on impact with the ground.

References

American Orthopaedic Society for Sports Medicine: "For the Practitioner: Orthopaedic Screening Examination for Participation in Sports," *Pediatrics in Review*, 2:229-239, 1981.

Bonsett, C., and J. Glancy: "Prophylactic Bracing in Pseudohypertrophic Muscular Dystrophy," *Journal of the Indiana State Medical Association*, 68(3):181-187, 1975.

Drummond, D., et al.: "Spinal Deformity: Natural History and the Role of School Screening," *Orthopedic Clinics of North America*, 10(4):751-759, 1979.

Greene, P.E.: "Malignant Bone Tumors," in *Nursing Care of the Child with Cancer*, D. Fochtman and G.V. Foley, (eds.), Little, Brown, Boston, 1982.

Bibliography

Carini, G., and J. Birmingham: *Traction Made Manageable*, McGraw-Hill, New York, 1980.

Ferholt, J.D.: *Clinical Assessment of Children: A Comprehensive Approach to Primary Pediatric Care*, Lippincott, Philadelphia, 1980.

Hilt, N., and S. Cogburn: *Manual of Orthopedics*, Mosby, St. Louis, 1980.

Jaffe, N.: "Advances in the Management of Malignant Bone Tumors in Children and Adolescents," *Pediatric Clinics of North America*, 32(3):801-810, 1985.

Rennebohm, R., and J.K. Correll: "Comprehensive Management of Juvenile Rheumatoid Arthritis," *Nursing Clinics of North America*, 19(4):647-662, 1984.

Smith, N.J. (ed.): "Symposium on Sports Medicine," *Pediatric Clinics of North America*, 29(6):1305-1440, 1982.

Strauss, R. (ed.): *Sports Medicine and Physiology*, Saunders, Philadelphia, 1984.

23

The Respiratory System

Objectives

After reading this chapter, the student will be able to:
1. Describe the functions of the respiratory system.
2. Identify the basic subjective and objective data to be obtained in assessing a child.
3. Understand the purpose of diagnostic tests and medical treatment.
4. Describe general nursing measures appropriate for pediatric clients who have problems involving the respiratory system.
5. Delineate specific nursing interventions appropriate for pediatric clients who have problems involving the respiratory system.

Anatomy and Physiology

The main function of the respiratory system is to maintain adequate oxygen and carbon dioxide exchange between the body and the environment. The anatomic structures of the respiratory system are shown in Fig. 23-1. Respiration consists of two phases, external and internal. *External respiration* occurs in the alveoli, where inspired oxygen is exchanged for carbon dioxide, which is expired. *Internal respiration* occurs as oxygen from the alveoli is carried by the arterial circulatory system to the capillaries, through the capillary wall into the tissue fluid surrounding the cells, and across the plasma membrane. Carbon dioxide passes in the opposite direction by the same route until it reaches the capillaries, where it enters the venous blood to be transported to the lungs for exhalation.

External Respiration

Several muscles are involved in respiration. Normally, only the inspiratory muscles (those which elevate the chest cage) are used. Expiration is the result of elastic recoil of the lungs when the inspiratory muscles relax. The diaphragm is the most important inspiratory muscle. Diaphragmatic movements account for 80 percent of inspired air volume, while rib movements are responsible for the other 20 percent. If inspiratory effort is great, the scalene and pectoralis minor muscles assist in raising the rib cage.

Two pleural membrane layers are found in the thoracic cavity, one covering the lungs and one lining the thoracic cavity. Since the pleural layers are in intimate contact, the pleural space is potential rather than actual. Both layers are moist, causing surface tension, which in turn causes the lung wall to follow the thoracic wall. Surface tension is present in the alveoli and respiratory passages because of the fluids lining them. The alveoli secrete a lipoprotein called *surfactant* which tends to decrease surface tension. If surfactant were absent, lung expansion would be difficult. As the lung decreased in size during expiration, surface tension would increase, causing atelectasis.

Surface tension is not the only reason why the pleural space remains potential. Intrapleural pressure is below atmosperic pressure. Thus, the lungs maintain their elasticity. Intrapulmonary pressure (pressure within the lungs) is exactly atmospheric at the conclusion of expiration, no air is flowing, and there is free communication between the atmosphere and the alveoli via the airways. During inspiration, intrapulmonary pressure decreases as the lungs and chest expand, and air enters the lungs. If the chest wall were pierced, the lungs would collapse.

During expiration both intrapleural and intrapulmonary pressures increase. However, intrapleural pressure never reaches atmospheric pressure. Intrapulmonary pressure becomes greater than atmospheric pressure, and air moves out of the lungs. Normal expiration is due to relaxation of the muscles of inspiration. During a forced expiration intercostal and abdominal muscles are utilized.

Internal Respiration

Most of the oxygen transported to tissues is in the form of oxyhemoglobin. The extent to which oxygen combines with hemoglobin depends on the partial pressure of oxygen in blood, the pH of blood, and tissue temperature. Alveolar oxygen partial pressure is greater than blood oxygen partial pressure. Therefore, oxygen from the alveoli diffuses into arterial blood. Most of this oxygen combines with hemoglobin, while the remaining 3 percent is carried in physical solution. A blood oxygen partial pressure (PO_2) of 100 mmHg ensures 90 percent saturation. With partial pressures from 10 to 60 mmHg, the degree to which oxygen combines with hemoglobin rapidly in-

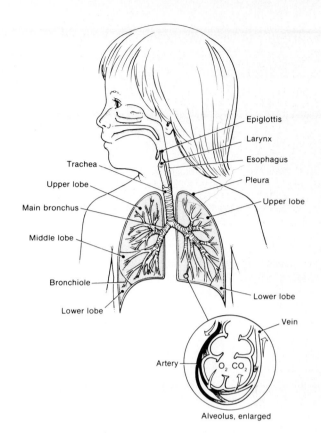

FIGURE 23-1 The respiratory system.

creases. Since pulmonary disease moderately reduces the PO_2 in the alveoli and the arteries, this plateau from 60 to 100 is important in regard to oxygen supply to the tissues.

The PO_2 of blood depends on the amount of oxygen molecules which are free in solution (only gas molecules which are free in solution can create gas pressure). The oxyhemoglobin does not contribute to this pressure. As blood enters the capillaries, tissue PO_2 is lower than blood PO_2. Therefore, the free plasma oxygen diffuses into the tissues. Since plasma PO_2 is now lower than that of the erythrocytes, oxygen is released from oxyhemoglobin and diffuses into the plasma (Table 23-1).

The pH of the blood is determined by hydrogen ion concentration. An increase in hydrogen ion causes a decrease in pH. The more acidic the blood is (decrease in pH), the less affinity hemoglobin has for oxygen. Tissue temperature affects the formation of oxyhemoglobin in a manner similar to that of pH. Tissue temperature is elevated when tissue is engaged in active metabolism. The release of oxygen from hemoglobin is facilitated as blood flows through these tissue capillaries during active metabolism and by an increase in the chemical 2,3-diphosphoglycerate (2,3-DPG) in the red blood cell.

Once arterial blood has supplied oxygen to the tissues via diffusion through the capillary walls, carbon dioxide diffuses out of the tissue into the venous blood, where 8% remains in physical solution and 25% combines with hemoglobin. The remaining 67% is converted into bicarbon-

TABLE 23-1 Normal Arterial Blood Gas Values

Measurement	Normal	Definition
pH	7.35-7.45	Acidity or alkalinity of blood in terms of hydrogen ion concentration
$PaCO_2$	35-45 mmHg	Partial pressure of carbon dioxide in arterial blood
PaO_2	80-100 mmHg; 40-60 mmHg in newborns	Partial pressure of oxygen in arterial blood
SaO_2	95-100%	Saturation of oxygen—plotted on an oxyhemoglobin dissociation curve—affected by pH, PCO_2 and temperature
HCO_3	22-26 meq/liter	Bicarbonate ion, the basis of the buffer system
H_2CO_3	1.05-1.35 meq/liter	Carbonic acid, formed by carbon dioxide and water, is 3% of PO_2 the ratio of hydrogen ion to carbonic acid is usually 20 to 1)

Source: M. J. Smith et al. (eds.), *Child and Family: Concepts of Nursing Practice,* 2d ed., McGraw-Hill, New York, 1987, p. 663.

ate and hydrogen ions primarily in the red blood cells. The hydrogen ions in excess of the amount needed to maintain normal pH of the blood are eliminated by the kidneys (assuming normal renal function). As venous blood flows through the lung capillaries, hydrogen and bicarbonate combine to produce carbonic acid which breaks down to carbon dioxide and water. Now that blood PCO_2 is greater than alveolar PCO_2, carbon dioxide diffuses through the capillary walls into the alveoli, from which it is expired into the atmosphere. Carbon dioxide moves much more easily across the alveoli than oxygen does. Hence, with disease, the PO_2 changes first.

Ventilation

Ventilation, or the process of acquiring oxygen and removing carbon dioxide, is regulated in several ways. Within the medulla oblongata and pons in the brainstem is a group of neurons known as the *respiratory center.* There are inspiratory and expiratory neurons which fire alternately back and forth indefinitely, causing the act of respiration.

Increased carbon dioxide in inspired air and an increase of the hydrogen ions in the blood which diffuses into the cerebrospinal fluid increase ventilation. Chemoreceptors, located in the carotid and aortic bodies which transmit signals to the respiratory center, are stimulated by hypoxia, and ventilation increases. When hypoxia and hypercapnia (increased CO_2) are prolonged and severe, the respiratory center is depressed.

The Hering-Breuer reflex limits lung inflation and deflation, thereby preventing overdistention and overcompression. The Hering-Breuer receptors in the bronchioles and, possibly, in the walls of the alveoli stimulate the respiratory center by way of the vagus nerve to inhibit inspiration as the lungs fill and allow expiration to occur. As the lungs deflate, the receptors work to stimulate inhibition of expiration. If these reflexes are not intact, respiratory arrest can occur much more quickly than it will if they are intact.

Assessment

The infant and child's respiratory system (see Fig. 23-1) differs from the adult's in several ways. The neonatal lung has immature ductlike structures rather than true alveoli. After birth, rapid alveolorization of these structures occurs. The alveoli enlarge and triple in number by 3 months of age. Growth continues during childhood, but there is disagreement in the literature as to when alveoli complete their growth. At maturity, the alveolar diameter has quintupled and the number of alveoli has increased fifteenfold. The weight of the lungs doubles by 6 months of age, triples by 1 year, and is 10 times greater at maturity than in the neonatal period. With age, then, there is an increase in lung volume and a decrease in respiratory rate.

Neonates are obligatory nasal breathers until 3 to 4 weeks of age, at which time they can learn to breathe through the mouth. Respirations are mainly diaphragmatic with a gradual transition to mainly costal by 7 years of age. Average respiratory rates are given in Chap. 6. Since infants and children have smaller airway lumens from the trachea to the terminal bronchioles, obstruction with small amounts of mucus more readily occurs. The loosely attached mucosa lining the bronchioles and the larger proportion of soft tissue in the lungs increase the potential for edema. Respiratory and coughing efforts are less effective or sustained, because the accessory muscles of respiration are not completely developed. Since the upper airway is narrow, enlarged tonsils and adenoids can interfere with breathing. When assessing the pediatric patient, the nurse should keep these differences in mind.

Assessment of the infant or child's respiratory system involves the collection of subjective and objective data. Subjective information is gleaned from the parents and/or child (if age, vocabulary, and status permit). Objective information is obtained through physical examination and laboratory and diagnostic procedures. The techniques of and approach to eliciting a history and performing a physical examination are discussed in Chaps. 5 and 6. Assessment is ongoing; that is, initial assessments are made on the basis of subjective and objective data, care is planned and implemented, intervention is evaluated, further assessments are made, the care plan is updated, and so forth (Chap. 5).

Subjective data include the child's presenting problem, the history of the presenting problem, past history, and family history (Table 23-2). *Objective data* include

TABLE 23-2 Assessment of a Pediatric Patient with Respiratory Problems

I. Subjective data
  A. Presenting problem (singly or in combinaiton)
    1. Cough ("He has a bad cough.")
    2. Respiratory difficulty ("She's not breathing right.")
    3. Congestion and/or rhinorrhea ("He has a runny nose" or "He's stuffed up.")
    4. Sore throat ("She says her throat hurts.")
  B. History of presenting problems
    1. Onset—sudden or gradual
    2. Duration—length of time present
    3. Frequency—constant, intermittent, completely absent for a time and then present
    4. Type
      (a) Cough—dry, hacking, moist, barking, productive (color of sputum)
      (b) Respiratory difficulty—rapid, slow, shallow, or deep respirations; retractions; wheezing
      (c) Rhinorrhea—color, consistency, odor, amount
    5. Progression—better or worse than when first noted
    6. Circumstances—better or worse with activity, at night, during day; present at night only; better or worse with change of position (e.g., sitting, lying); anxious
    7. Current treatment—medications, over-the-counter drugs, home remedies, vaporizer; type of treatment, frequency, duration, and effect
    8. Associated symptoms (onset, duration, and so on)—pain (location), flaring of the nares, cyanosis, pallor, anorexia, vomiting, decreased fluid intake, decreased urination, diarrhea, large bulky stools, constipation, depressed or bulging fontanel (infants), dry mucous membranes and lips, hoarseness, dysphagia, disturbed sleeping patterns, change in behavior (e.g., fatigue, restlessness, irritability)
  C. Past history
    1. Prenatal, birth, and perinatal (Chap. 5)
    2. Respiratory problems (e.g., frequent colds, respiratory distress syndrome, bronchopulmonary dysplasia, pneumonia; hospitalizations; treatment)
    3. Exposure to others who are ill (family, friends, schoolmates)
    4. Allergies (e.g., asthma, hay fever)
    5. Immunization status
  D. Family history
    1. Respiratory problems (e.g., tuberculosis, cystic fibrosis)
    2. Allergies (e.g., asthma, hay fever)

II. Objective data
  A. Growth measuremens and vital signs
    1. Length or stature (length up to 36 mo; stature thereafter)
    2. Weight
    3. Head circumference
    4. Temperature, pulse, respirations
  B. General appearance—alert, irritable, lethargic, and so on; growth percentiles
  C. Skin—color, turgor, dryness, rash, irritation (Chap. 19)
  D. Head (infants)—anterior fontanel depressed, soft and flat, bulging (Chap. 20)
  E. Eyes—sunken, dry, glazed, bright, moist (Chap. 21)
  F. Ears—tympanic membrane (mobility, landmarks, light, reflex, color)
  G. Nose—flaring of the nares, rhinorrhea
  H. Mouth—mucosa dry, lips dry and cracked
  I. Throat—color, exudate, enlarged tonsils, hoarseness, cough, dysphagia
  J. Lymph nodes—enlarged, tender
  K. Chest
    1. Inspection
      (a) Respiratory pattern (rate, depth, rhythm: Table 23-3)
      (b) Restractions (intercostal, subcostal, supraclavicular, suprasternal; Chap. 17)
    2. Palpation—stability of ribs, vocal fremitus (during crying or speaking), equality of expansion
    3. Percussion—resonance, dullness
    4. Auscultation—decreased breath sounds, abnormal breath sounds (rales, rhonchi, wheezing), prolonged inspiration or expiration
  L. Heart—rate, rhythm, murmurs (Chap. 24)
  M. Gastrointestinal system (Chap. 26)
    1. Observation—anorexia, vomiting, constipation, diarrhea, large and bulky stools
    2. Auscultation—bowel sounds (paralytic ileus)
    3. Palpation—descended liver (flattened diaphragm)
  N. Urinary system—decreased urinary output (Chap. 27)
  O. Neurological system—muscle tone, response to pain, level of consciousness (Chap. 20)

Source: G. M. Scipien et al. (eds.), *Comprehensive Pediatric Nursing,* 3d ed., McGraw-Hill, New York, 1986, p. 844.

length or stature, weight, and head circumference measurements; temperature; blood pressure; a complete physical examination; and diagnostic tests as ordered by the physician. Serial growth measurements, if available, are helpful in determining whether lack of adequate oxygenation over a period of time has affected growth (e.g., in cystic fibrosis). Weight and length or stature measurements are necessary to determine medication dosages and amounts of fluid intake needed. Respiratory problems may stem from the upper or lower airways; occur in conjunction with middle ear, gastrointestinal, neurological, and cardiac problems; and herald the onset of some communicable diseases. Fluid and electrolyte disturbances may develop. Thus, particular attention must be paid not only to the child's respiratory system but also to other body parts (Tables 23-2 and 23-3).

Impending respiratory failure may be evidenced by combinations of the following signs: severe inspiratory retractions, use of accessory muscles of respiration, decreased respirations, cyanosis, poor skeletal muscle tone, decreased response to pain, and depressed level of consciousness. Laboratory tests in support of assessment are a $PaCO_2 \geq 75$ mmHg and $PaO_2 < 100$ mmHg in 100% oxygen.

TABLE 23-3 Classification of Respiratory Patterns

Type	Rate	Rhythm	Depth	Respiratory Cycle
Eupnea (normal)	Infant: 30 to 60; Child: 15 to 25	Smooth and even	Variable	Active inspiration; passive expiration
Tachypnea	Increased	Regular or irregular	Within normal range or decreased	Active inspiration; passive expiration
Bradypnea	Decreased	Regular or irregular	Normal to increased	Active inspiration; passive expiration
Apnea	Variable	Irregular	Variable	Active inspiration; temporary cessation in the resting expiratory phase
Hyperpnea	Normal or inceased	Regular	Increased	Active inspiration; usually prolonged and deep; passive expiration
Hypopnea	Normal or increased	Regular	Shallow	Shallow, active inspiration; passive expiration
Apneusis	Decreased	Regular or irregular	Variable	Active inspiration; cessation during inspiration; passive expiration
Cheyne-Stokes respiration	Variable	Regular increases and decreases in rate	Sequential changes from increased to decreased	Active inspiration; passive expiration with recurring periods of apnea lasting 10 to 15 s
Kussmaul's respiration	Variable	Regular or irregular	Increased	Active inspiration; passive inspiration
Biot's respiration	Variable	Irregular	Shallow	Shallow breathing followed by apnea

Source: M. J. Smith et al. (eds.), *Child and Family: Concepts of Nursing Practice,* 2d ed., McGraw-Hill, New York, 1987, p. 660.

Common Diagnostic Tests

It is most important for a nurse to know the many procedures used to identify a pathogen, visualize anatomic parts, and assess a child's pulmonary function. Such information is essential if explanations are to be accurate, the child is to be cooperative, and the teaching done is to be effective.

A *throat culture* is done to identify the presence of group A beta-hemolytic streptococcus (GABHS) in the pharynx. There are now tests for rapid detection of group A streptococci. One of these antigen detection tests can be read in 15 minutes. However, if the results are negative, a throat culture is sent to the laboratory to ensure that the test was not falsely negative. Under sterile conditions, the cotton plug is removed from the mouth of a sterile test tube. One or two sterile swabs are removed from the test tube or from a sterile package (for rapid detection tests). The child is asked to open his mouth. The nurse depresses his tongue with a tongue depressor and swabs the entire pharyngeal area in a circular motion. The swabs are replaced in the sterile test tube and the cotton plug is reinserted. The tube is labeled and sent to the laboratory. To gain the child's cooperation during this procedure, the nurse explains that the back of the throat will be "tickled" with the swab. The child also is asked to breathe through his mouth to prevent gagging. Preliminary results are available in 24 hours and final results in 48 hours.

A procedure in which the nurse plays a vital role is a *laryngoscopy,* usually performed to determine the cause of an obstruction, such as a foreign body. Proper positioning is extremely important. The child is placed on a flat surface, with the neck in slight extension and the jaw forward. After the child is suctioned and slightly hyperventi-

lated with a mask or bag, the physician inserts a laryngoscope blade into the mouth. Generally, a straight blade is used for infants and small children and a straight or curved blade is utilized for older children.

Although a laryngoscopy is often an emergency procedure, both procedure and purpose need to be explained to the child and/or parents. The infant or toddler must be mummy-wrapped (Chap. 10) so that the nurse can hold the head at a proper angle to ensure slight hyperextension only. Exaggerated hyperextension inhibits good visualization. While the nurse can offer support during the procedure by talking softly or stroking the child, it is important afterward to allow the young client an opportunity to express his true feelings about the event (e.g, drawing his perception of the procedure, pounding blocks to vent anger, or restraining a doll).

There are usually two reasons for performing a *bronchoscopy:* (1) to visualize the trachea, bronchi, and orifices of the bronchi directly to determine the cause of an obstruction (foreign body, congenital anomaly, stenosis), bleeding sites, or the origin of purulent secretions and (2) to aspirate secretions for laboratory examination. The procedure, always done in the operating room, is highly specialized, with rigorous monitoring of the child's vital signs and supplemental oxygen provided to minimize the possibility of complications. The postprocedure nursing responsibilities are substantial. It is necessary to observe for upper airway obstruction, and aerosol therapy or intermittent positive pressure breathing (IPPB) may be instituted to reduce the laryngeal edema. Signs of upper airway obstruction include hoarseness; croupy (barking) cough; stridor, particularly on inspiration; prolonged expiratory phase; increased respiratory rate (60 or more); and retractions, especially supraclavicular, suprasternal, and sternal. In addition, mediastinal or subcutaneous emphysema and pneumothorax are possible consequences; hence, total assessments and diligent monitoring of vital signs are essential for early diagnosis.

Gastric washings are done to determine the presence of tubercle bacilli in gastric juices, especially in children who are too young to cough up their secretions. Since the procedure is uncomfortable and must be carried out on 3 successive days, the child objects more vehemently with each day's proceedings. After the child is kept NPO and the specimen is collected before breakfast. Infant feeding tubes (Nos. 5 through 10) are used for the infant while Levine or stomach tubes (Nos. 10 through 16) are more efficient in older children. Placing the tube in a bowl of ice cubes prior to the procedure facilitates its insertion. The depth of insertion, determined by measuring the length of tubing from the bridge of the nose to the xyphoid process, is marked on the distal end of the tubing. It is inserted orally in infants and intranasally in older children. A 20- to 30-ml syringe (regular tip for feeding tubes and catheter tip for Levine tubes) is attached to the tube, and aspiration is done to confirm placement. If no gastric contents are obtained, the tube may be in the trachea, which is further confirmed by the child's coughing. Once it is in the stomach, the gastric juices are aspirated and placed in a sterile container. Then the stomach is lavaged with sterile water, and the washings are aspirated, added to material in the container, labeled, and sent to the laboratory for culture.

The *iontophoretic sweat test,* which identifies the amount of sweat sodium (Na) or chloride (Cl), is a test for cystic fibrosis. After washing the volar surface of a child's forearm with distilled water and drying the area, a 3- by 3-in gauze square with 6.4% pilocarpine hydrochloride is placed under a positive electrode. The process is repeated using a wet 0.04 N H_2SO_4 gauze square, under a negative electrode. The current is slowly raised to 150 µA and maintained for 12 minutes; then it is slowly decreased to zero. The gauze and electrodes are removed. Then the stimulated forearm is washed again with distilled water and dried. Using sterile gloves and forceps, previously weighed gauze is removed from a sterile, preweighed flask and applied to the volar surface. A piece of plastic, previously washed and dried to ensure that it is free of Na and Cl, is placed over the gauze and sealed tightly with adhesive. After 1 hour the gauze is removed with forceps and returned to the flask. It is important to wear gloves or use paper towels when handling the flask because it has been preweighed and sweat from the tester's hands can change its weight. When this procedure is completed, the flask is labeled and sent to the laboratory.

While this diagnostic test is not as traumatic as those mentioned previously, the potential for altering its results is great. It is essential to explain the procedure to the child and parents, emphasizing the fact that sweat from one's hand can easily affect the final values. The task of protecting the prescribed body area is especially difficult

if the patient is an infant or a toddler, and the use of restraints may be necessary.

Pulmonary Function Tests

There are many pulmonary function tests which can be ordered to help in identifying the severity of a respiratory problem, evaluating changes in the lungs, or determining the effectiveness of treatment protocols. While they are done frequently on adults, they are not ordered as often in pediatrics because they require the participation and hence the cooperation of the child. While 3- and 4-year-olds may be "conditioned" to learn what is necessary to complete a particular test, for the most part, these tests are not performed on children less than 6 or 7 years of age. However, there are health problems, such as cystic fibrosis or asthma, which require pulmonary function tests at certain intervals.

The more commonly done tests provide information about airway resistance regarding trapped air, airway obstruction, and ventilation. Most of them require the use of spirometry or flowmeters. The test for *functional residual capacity* (FRC) measures the total amount of gas in the lungs at the end of the respiration, while a child is at rest. *Tidal volume* (TV) identifies the amount of gas inhaled or exhaled with each respiration. *Total lung capacity* (TLC) measures the total amount of gas in the lungs at the end of a full respiration, while the child is at rest. The greatest amount of gas a child can exhale after a full inspiration is called *vital capacity* (VC), while the amount of gas which remains in the lungs after a full expiration is called *residual volume* (RV).

The nurse is in a position to work with the tester and parents in preparing the child to cooperate when undergoing these various pulmonary function tests. A nurse may be the one who "conditions" the preschooler to the use of a mouthpiece, or parents may be asked to perform this task. Whether or not parents display any inclinations to become involved in the care of their child, the nurse should invite their participation. Then the nurse is provided with an opportunity to share information with and listen to parents. Another possible outcome is that parents may be invited to accompany the child when he is scheduled for testing.

A major responsibility for the nurse is to prepare the child. In order to ensure their cooperation, children need to become familiar with the methods used for mouth breathing with the nostrils closed during spirometry. Closing nostrils is accomplished with a nose clip or by an adult closing the child's nostrils between two fingers. If they are to be tested with a spirometer or flowmeter, children are usually more cooperative if they are allowed to familiarize themselves with the mouthpiece.

In addition, demonstrations of mouth breathing with nostrils closed and the use of a mouthpiece by the tester, nurse, or parents may be well-accepted by the child who then returns the demonstration. Cooperation and collaboration among tester, child, nurse, and parents ensures the successful completion of these procedures.

General Nursing Measures

Nursing Diagnoses

The respiratory problems of children are diverse. Some are acute, others may be chronic with acute exacerbations, and still others may be life-threatening. It is essential for a nurse to develop a nursing diagnosis on the basis of the data available. Some examples of nursing diagnoses the nurse should consider include the following:

Impaired gas exchange
Ineffective airway clearance
Ineffective breathing pattern
Potential fluid volume deficit
Altered tissue perfusion
Pain
Potential activity intolerance
Anxiety related to the emergency situation
Knowledge deficit related to the health problem
Sleep pattern disturbance
Hopelessness
Impaired home maintenance management (mild, moderate, severe, potential, chronic)

Methods of Improving Oxygenation

It may be necessary for a nurse to use oxygen therapy for a wide variety of respiratory problems. However, it also may be critical for improving the oxygenation of children with other health conditions, such as cardiac disorders and neurological problems.

When the nurse is administering oxygen to a child, certain facts need to be remembered, for this commonly used gas may have harmful effects on some structures in the body, particularly in the case of a newborn. The amount of oxygen given should be determined by monitoring the PO_2 level, and it should be commensurate with the cellular needs of the body at that time.

It is most important to prevent oxygen toxicity in the neonate. Increasing amounts of oxygen may create an inability on the part of a newborn to assimilate the gas, consequently increasing his oxygen needs. The direct toxic effects are related to alveolar oxygen concentrations which eventually cause ciliary damage in the form of paralysis, interstitial thickening, bronchopulmonary dysplasia, and other pathophysiological changes. It is not clear how much oxygen for what period of time results in these changes; however, concentrations below 40% are considered to be safe. It is probably a combination of a high *inspired oxygen* (FIO_2) and positive pressure which produces the most damage. Therefore, physicians in some medical facilities have begun using negative pressure respirators on newborns, while others are using pressures as low as possible.

Although the physiological effects of hypoxia may occur at an arterial PO_2 level of 50 mmHg, cyanosis usually does not become evident until the arterial PO_2 level falls below 32 to 40 mmHg. (Since cyanosis is related to the amount of unsaturated hemoglobin, a child with anemia may not appear to be cyanotic as early as a patient with a high hematocrit.) In many medical centers the PO_2 and PCO_2 levels are monitored simultaneously. It is important to remember the danger associated with PO_2 levels above 100 mmHG—retrolental fibroplasia. The American Academy of Pediatrics has recommended that arterial PO_2 determinations be available in every hospital where continuous oxygen is administered to very young patients over a period of time.

Certain safety principles are vigorously adhered to when oxygen therapy is in effect, since oxygen supports combustion. Electrical equipment must not be used while oxygen is being administered. The clothing or linen used should not be made of wool or synthetic fibers which may produce static electricity. Alcohol or oil should not be used on an infant or child receiving oxygen within a confined environment.

As the patient's condition improves, termination of therapy should be gradual in order to allow him to adjust to normal atmospheric oxygen concentrations. In an incubator, the rate of oxygen flow can be decreased or the air vents may be opened. In a mist tent, zippers may be opened or a section of the plastic canopy may be flipped over the top of the tent. In either instance, it is important to observe the patient and to note his responses to decreased oxygen concentrations. Any distress, increase in respiratory rate, retractions, or cyanosis should be reported to a physician immediately, and methods of increasing oxygen intake should be considered.

Incubator or Hood

In closed incubators 40 to 100% levels of oxygen can be administered to newborns or infants. It is imperative that oxygen analyzers be used every 2 hours to identify appropriate concentrations in addition to monitoring blood gases. Oxygen levels greater than 40% should not be administered unless there is cyanosis or unless they have been ordered specifically by a physician.

Oxygen should always be moisturized before it is delivered to an incubator, and this process is facilitated by the passage of the gas through a type of water vessel or nebulizer (Fig. 23-2). Sterile water should always be used unless medications or other agents which liquefy secretions are to be utilized.

Since inhalation equipment is a source of contamination, daily cleaning is imperative. All equipment should be changed every 7 days. Cultures of oxygen tubing, water, nebulizers, and the interior of incubators should be taken at least every 3 days.

Closed incubators have a significant loss of heat and oxygen because of imperfectly fitted plastic lids, uncovered vents, and the frequent opening of portholes, thereby contributing to a depletion of the desired heat and oxygen concentrations. If the patient's condition necessitates oxygen levels above 40%, plastic circular hoods should be used to maintain that concentration. Maintenance of heat will then be the problem with which the nurse must contend, for while 34°C (93.2°F) may be necessary for small infants, others may need only a supplemental temperature of 30°C (86°F). Fluctuations in a young patient's environment result in a lowering of body temperature and the immediate, rapid metabolism of still

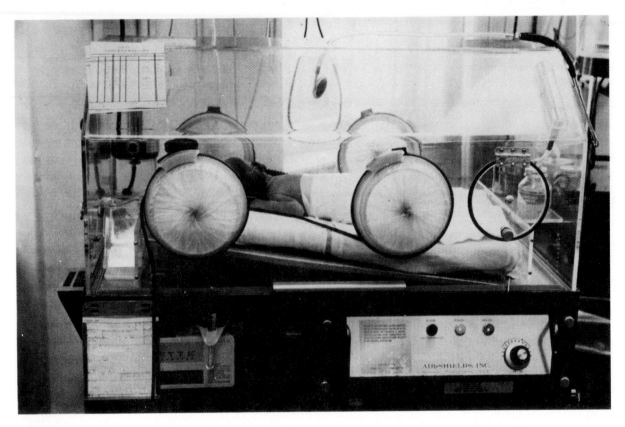

FIGURE 23-2   A neonate in a closed incubator receiving oxygen and humidity. *(Courtesy Children's Hospital Medical Center, Boston.)*

larger amounts of oxygen. Simultaneous recordings of the infant's body temperature and the temperature of his environment are essential notations for a nurse to make when working with preterm or newborn babies. Members of the health team should coordinate their individual activities to prevent fluctuations of heat and oxygen which may contribute further to the debilitating status of a young patient. Open incubators deliver radiant heat while procedures are being done or nursing care is being given, and with the utilization of a circular hood the desired humidified oxygen concentration can be maintained without exposing the patient to stressful variations.

Whenever oxygen is being administered, it should be warmed to 31 to 34°C, depending on the baby, and should always be humidified. Thermal sensors are present in a baby's face, and a blast of cold oxygen produces a typical neonatal response to cold stress, including oxygen deprivation, metabolic acidosis, rapid depletion of glycogen stores, and a reduction of blood glucose levels.

Using a Mist Tent
Mist tents are usually utilized to increase oxygen levels in young children. Obviously, the size of the patient determines the most appropriate equipment. The mist tent is frequently used with older infants, toddlers, and preschoolers.

The mist tent is portable and easy to assemble and facilitates observation of a young patient. Another distinct

advantage is that all working parts of a tent are outside the canopy, away from a curious young child's reach. One disadvantage for nursing personnel is that the tent needs to be opened frequently for treatments, procedures, or the monitoring of vital signs, and entry results in the lowering of both oxygen and humidity concentrations. Thought should be given to organizing nursing functions and coordinating procedures which will be done by other health team members, too. Consideration should be given to maintaining the desired humidity and oxygen concentrations as well as providing the patient with substantial periods of rest.

Occasionally a face mask is used simultaneously to supplement oxygen intake. The young child may resist it initially, and a nurse should offer support to the patient by staying with him until he becomes accustomed to it. Since it is placed over his nose and mouth, caution should be exercised whenever its use is contemplated. In objecting to its utilization, a toddler can cause it to slip above the nose and possibly cause injury to the eyes. Frequent adjustments are imperative. It is essential for the nurse to evaluate the youngster's response to this additional therapeutic measure.

When oxygen therapy is instituted, a nurse should check the tent for tears or malfunctioning zippers, which make it difficult to achieve the desired humid, oxygenated environment. It is important to smell the mist being released to be positive that the tubing is not carrying a noxious chemical or the remains of a solution which was not adequately rinsed out after use by a previous patient. The mist tent should be flooded with condensation before the patient is placed inside and covered with a cotton blanket. While a supersaturated aerated mist provides the desired relief, the condensation necessitates frequent changes of clothing and linen to prevent chilling of the patient.

As the child improves, he takes a more active interest in his surroundings and demonstrates a desire to play with toys. While he is in the supersaturated environment, it is important to select carefully the kind of toys he will play with and the material of which they are made. For example, stuffed animals and other cloth toys tend to absorb the moisture (becoming excellent media for the growth of microorganisms), and they should not be used within this humidified canopy. A very favorite teddy bear may not be able to tolerate the mist tent as well as his young friend can. Toys which retard absorption, are washable, or are easily cleaned appear to be the most suitable.

Whenever oxygen therapy is begun, a nurse must know how to use the equipment involved in its delivery to a patient. This health care provider must know the models available, the various regulatory devices that are utilized in conjunction with this treatment, and the methods used in determining oxygen and humidity levels. It is the nurse who must maintain the desired concentrations, evaluate the functioning of the equipment, and determine the effectiveness of the treatment in relation to the young patient's respiratory status.

Endotracheal Intubation

There are situations in which an infant or child is unable to maintain a satisfactory respiratory status and an artificial method must be instituted. The modality of treatment depends on the child's health problem, with the ultimate decision being made by the physician. An *endotracheal (ET) tube* is used to maintain an adequate upper airway and to stabilize the trachea during a tracheostomy. It may be placed in the oral cavity or through the nares. While orotracheal tubes are selected during emergencies or when the child needs upper airway assistance for less than 12 to 18 hours, nasotracheal tubes are preferred in situations which demand upper airway support for longer periods of time (up to 1 week; 3 weeks for neonates). If, in the opinion of a physician, such support is necessary for a more extensive period of time, a tracheostomy is performed.

The advantages of a nasotracheal tube over an oral route include ease in oral/pharyngeal suctioning and hygiene (reducing the buildup of secretions and lessening the likelihood of infection) and better stabilization of the tube (reducing the possibility of tracheal erosion and accidental extubation).

The equipment utilized for inserting an ET tube includes a laryngoscope and blades, endotracheal tubes, a ventilator bag with a 15-mm adaptor, several sizes of face masks and suction catheters, adhesive tape, and tincture of benzoin. The sources of oxygen and suction need to be checked to ensure that they are working properly. When all is in readiness, the child is placed on a firm surface with the neck in slight extension and the jaw pulled slightly forward. After gentle suctioning of the mouth and nose, the child is hyperventilated by Ambu bag and mask for no more than 1 minute.

If the physician elects to use the orotracheal route, the laryngoscope blade is inserted into the mouth and advanced along the right side. When it is in place, the ET tube is then passed along the side of the blade until it is located midway between the vocal cords and carina. It is necessary to auscultate the child's lungs immediately after placement to be sure that the tube has not slipped into the right primary bronchus. Confirmation of placement is also done by x-ray.

The placement of a nasotracheal tube is more complicated. After the ET tube is inserted into a naris and guided into the posterior oropharynx, the laryngoscope blade is put into the mouth and advanced until it is in the proper position. Then the laryngoscope blade is removed, and ET tube placement is confirmed by auscultation and x-ray.

Stabilizing the ET tube is critical to its effectiveness. After the child's cheeks have been painted with tincture of benzoin, both ends of 1-in tape (about 4 in long) are split lengthwise. The upper left strip is wound around the ET tube several times and taped to a cheek. The left lower strip is also placed around the tube and taped to a cheek. The identical maneuver is repeated with the remaining strip of tape.

If artificial ventilation is to be used, a 15-mm connecting tube must be attached to the ET tube. It is also necessary to utilize a sleeve cut from an ET tube one size larger than the tube in place. All joints are taped separately. Finally, an appropriate ventilator is selected and connected to the child (Chap. 17).

Cuffs are not used for children under 10 years of age. For those over 10 years, the cuff is inflated to a minimum volume which provides a tracheal seal. However, it must be deflated hourly for 2 to 5 minutes to reduce the possibility of tracheal necrosis.

The ET tube is kept free of secretions by suctioning, usually hourly. During this procedure, the ventilator is disconnected from the ET tube and 0.25 to 0.50 ml of normal saline is placed into the tube and followed by ventilation for 1 minute. The child's head is turned to one side. With a gloved hand, the premeasured catheter is passed 1 cm beyond the end of the ET tube. After it has been pulled back 1 cm, suction is applied as the catheter is withdrawn over a 5-second period. Then the child's ET tube is connected to the ventilator at pressures 25 percent greater than usual for 2 minutes and returned to its previous reading. Since the opposite side must be suctioned too, the ventilator is again disconnected, normal saline is instilled, and the child's head is turned in preparation for repeating the procedure.

Tracheostomy

A tracheostomy may be performed on infants or children who have upper airway obstruction, cardiopulmonary failure, or neurological problems which interfere with an adequate O_2–CO_2 exchange. Tracheostomy tubes most often are made of lightweight plastic or silastic rather than metal. Since they are soft and pliable, they conform easily to the shape of the trachea, which is an important consideration in neonates and young infants with short, flexible necks. Most of these disposable tracheostomy tubes are radiopaque, which allows their positions to be confirmed by x-ray.

Equipment needed for the procedure includes a surgical tracheostomy set, ET tube, bronchoscope, disposable suction equipment, twill tape, various sizes of tracheostomy tubes (Nos. 00, 0, 1, and 2), and suction catheters. Other supplies are sterile gloves and drapes, normal saline, an Ambu bag and adaptor, suction and oxygen (in working order), and adequate lighting. When the surgical procedure has been completed, the tracheostomy tube is held in place by attaching twill tape to each hole on this winged tube and tying the ends at the back of the neck. The tie always needs to be assessed at the conclusion of the procedure. It is done by placing one's finger between the tape and the infant's neck. If it fits snugly, the knot is satisfactory. These tubes are changed weekly.

With inspired air bypassing the normal filtering, humidifying, and warming functions of the upper airway, it is necessary to do so artificially. The child can be placed in a mist tent or connected to a special "collar," nebulizer, or "T" tube for the delivery of warm, humidified air to the tracheostomy (Fig. 23-3). Such an attachment prevents the formation of a mucous plug and loosens secretions. The tube must be patent at all times.

As long as the tracheostomy tube is in place, the following equipment should be available at the bedside: a sterile tracheostomy tube (same size), a sterile hemostat, an endotracheal intubation set, and an Ambu bag with an adaptor that fits the tracheostomy tube. The hemostat can be used to open the stoma if extubation occurs.

After a tracheostomy, frequent suctioning (every 30 minutes) is necessary to maintain patency by keeping the airway clear of secretions and preventing any oxygen deficit. Attention is given to the color, amount, and consistency of these secretions. The amount of normal saline

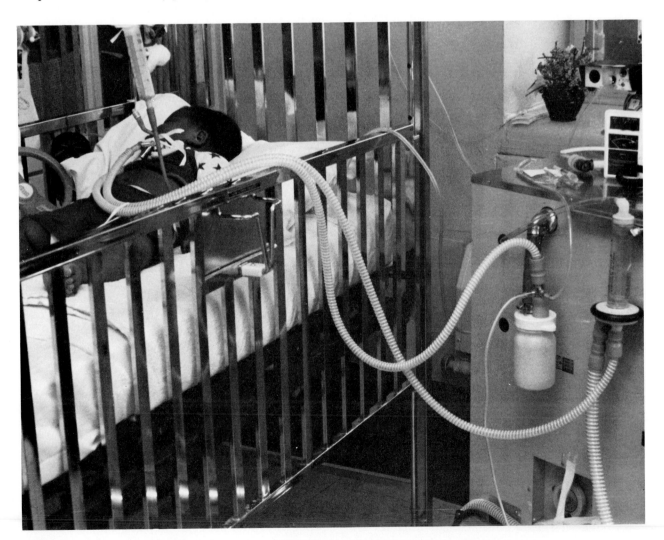

FIGURE 23-3 The bedside of a child with a permanent tracheostomy and ventilatory assistance. Humidified oxygen is being administered. Note the suspended gastrostomy tube. *(Courtesy Pediatric Nursing Department, Boston City Hospital, Boston, Mass.)*

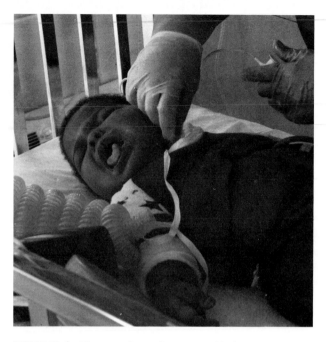

FIGURE 23-4 The gag reflex is demonstrated before suctioning is started. The nurse's thumb controls the suction pressure, which is not applied during insertion of the catheter. *(Courtesy Pediatric Nursing Department, Boston City Hospital, Boston, Mass.)*

(0.5 to 2 ml) instilled prior to sunctioning depends on the size of the child. Suctioning is done whenever a young patient demonstrates signs of mucus accumulation, such as noisy breathing, coughing, or bubbling of secretions from the tracheostomy.

After the child's head has been turned toward one side to suction the opposite bronchus, the sterile catheter is moistened with saline and inserted into the tracheostomy without applying any suction. When gagging is demonstrated (Fig. 23-4), the suction tip is withdrawn while it is rotated in a circular manner. The intermittent suctioning takes approximately 10 to 20 seconds. Both catheter and glove are discarded after a single use because sterile technique must be carried out at all times. After the nurse has evaluated the child's air exchange, the procedure is repeated on the opposite side.

A child who has a tracheostomy must be observed constantly, and so placement within close proximity to a nurses' station is ideal if intensive care is not required. While the patient's vital signs are being monitored, it is also important to maintain good hydration and nutrition. The stoma site must be observed for bleeding, crust formation, or irritation. It should be cleaned frequently, especially if the client is a neonate or young infant with a short neck. Slight hyperextension can correct the problem. Nurses need to be alert to the signs of increasing respiratory distress and the development of complications which may be evident by changes in color (pallor or cyanosis), restlessness, nasal flaring, changes in pulses and blood pressure, retractions, dyspnea, and noisy respira-

tions. Complications other than accidental extubation or blockage of the tube as a result of tenacious secretion include tracheal edema, subglottic stenosis, pneumothorax, pneumomediastinum, tracheitis, aspiration pneumonia, and emotional dependency on the tracheal tube.

The most frightening aspect of a tracheostomy for a young child is the inability to cry out or speak with the tube patent. The pleading, frightened eyes of an infant who is crying silently or a toddler who is vigorously objecting to the suctioning without uttering a sound also are stressful scenes for anxious parents to witness. Young patients who can understand need to be reassured that the loss of speech is temporary. Explanations to parents and patients should be simple, in language they can understand. While the nurse provides an opportunity for the child to express his feelings about this treatment through play therapy, parents need conferences away from the bedside so that their apprehensions can be lessened. Parents should become involved in the child's care if they wish to do so.

When a tracheostomy tube is to be removed, a progressively smaller tube is inserted each morning after suctioning, until the child can tolerate a No. 0 or 00 tube. At that point the tube is plugged for 48 hours. If the child does not experience any respiratory difficulty and appears to be tolerating the plug, the tracheostomy tube is totally removed. Air leaks from the site usually close off in less than 72 hours.

In cases where the tracheostomy is permanent, nurses need to do a great deal of parent teaching, so that the parents will be comfortable in caring for the child after discharge. Parental anxieties must be lessened if learning is to take place. A nurse needs to assess their level of stress and devise a plan for diminishing it. Once teaching begins, it must include suctioning, cleaning, and changing the tube. Constant feedback is possible if the nurse takes time to demonstrate the care and observe parents as they perform these tasks. Parents can increase their levels of comfort and confidence by means of such endeavors. Printed detailed instructions, a hospital phone number, and a list of available community resources should be reviewed with and given to them prior to discharge. Ideally, some contact with a community health nurse who will follow the family is a great reassurance to parents in making this transition. One important point for a nurse to remember is that parents return to a home which does not have an abundance of sterile supplies readily available to them. Specifically, they will need to purchase or rent a suction machine and to obtain suction catheters, gloves, ½-in twill tape, a medicine dropper, bandage scissors, and a humidifier prior to leaving the hospital. They should be instructed to make normal saline by adding 2 tsp of uniodized salt to 1 qt of water. Also, it is wise to recommend the purchase of a bulb syringe for use when the child and parents are away from home. Adequately preparing parents for these new responsibilities is a critically important nursing function.

Respiratory Problems in the Infant

Sudden Infant Death Syndrome

The most common cause of death during the first year of life (exluding the first week of life) is the sudden infant death syndrome (SIDS) or "crib death." SIDS was defined in 1969 as "the sudden, unexpected and unexplained death of an apparently healthy infant" (Friedman et al., 1981, p. 543). Increasingly, the terms "near miss for SIDS" and "aborted SIDS" are appearing in the literature. Members of the National SIDS Foundation suggest that *infantile apnea* be substituted for these two terms, since apnea has many causes, both known and unknown. The relationship of apnea to SIDS is under investigation but has not been fully clarified.

It strikes 1 out of every 350 live-born infants each year. SIDS is seen more frequently in low-birth-weight infants and those who live in overcrowded settings, is more common in males (3 out of 5), is more prevalent during the winter months, and occurs almost exclusively while the infant is asleep. Its peak incidence is at 2 to 4 months of age, but it is rarely seen before 3 weeks or after 8 months of age.

When an apparently healthy, symptomless infant is put to bed and found lifeless sometime later, SIDS should be considered. A positive diagnosis is made on autopsy. The common findings include a minor inflammation of the middle ear and/or respiratory tract, petechiae over the pleura, and pulmonary edema, often hemorrhagic. Many theories have been postulated to account for these sudden, unexplained deaths with minimal postmortem findings. Physiological variations in heart and respiratory rates during sleep are normally kept under control by the carotid body network and brainstem reflexes in response to blood gas changes. For unknown reasons, whether poor autonomic development and instability or delayed chemical or autonomic development of the brainstem, these mechanisms probably fail to work. The infant most likely suffers progressive hypoxia and hypercapnia and finally cessation of respiration. Current research is focused on ventilatory control of parents of SIDS victims, the relationship between apnea (> 20 seconds) and SIDS, methods of decreasing apneic periods and excessive periodic breathing, the relationship between BPD and SIDS, and hormonal imbalance.

No known way of preventing SIDS exists. The treatment lies in supporting parents and siblings who not only grieve over the death of the infant but also wonder if they could have prevented the death. People who may come in contact with the family after the infant's death—police officers, fire fighters, coroners, doctors, nurses—need to understand the nature of SIDS so that they can guard against thoughtless remarks. Someone who is knowledgeable about SIDS and skilled in helping families deal with grief (whether nurse, doctor, or other health professional) should provide information and counseling as early as possible.

Nursing Management

The three most common *parental concepts* of the cause of sudden infant death are suffocation, choking, and unsuspected illness. If the infant was seen by a physician (a routine visit) before death, both parents and physician wonder what signs and symptoms were missed. When SIDS occurs, the victim is often rushed to a hospital emergency room by emergency medical personnel, police officers, or family members. Hospital emergency room personnel who are aware of their own feelings about death and grief and knowledgeable about SIDS and parental reactions to it are better equipped to help parents who are overwhelmed by a previously healthy infant's death. Parental acting-out behavior will then be accepted. Some parents may need time alone while others may need continual support from emergency room personnel. Some parents may need to touch, hold, and rock the dead infant before saying a final good-bye. During the acute phase of grief, which may last several weeks, parents at first express disbelief that the infant is dead. They speak of the infant in both past and present tenses. They may also express anger, helplessness, loss of meaning of life, fear of going insane, and guilt regarding the death. Physical symptoms may include "whirling around," "pressure in the head," "heartache," and "stomach pain." A sad expression, sighing, insomnia, and restlessness are associated with these strange visceral sensations.

After the acute phase of grieving, parents often have mood fluctuations. Their hostility may be directed toward friends and relatives, and they have difficulty concentrating. Denial of the infant's death may be expressed in behavior, such as preparing the infant's food and bath. Many parents dream about the infant and are afraid of being left at home alone. Parents who have no close ties are apt to move from the area after the infant's death. The preceding description of the grief reaction is normal and follows Lindemann's classic description.

If nurses are to help families with their grieving, they must be able to discuss the symptoms of grief with the parents and assure them that they are not going insane. Some physicians make referrals to a skilled public health nurse who realizes that parents will be upset and may be unable to utilize factual information immediately. Therefore, the nurse may have to make several home visits in order to repeat the factual information and assist the parents with the grieving process. Many parents decide to have another child and may need support, factual information, and counseling during the decision-making process, pregnancy, and the first year of the subsequent child's life.

Members of the National Foundation for Sudden Infant Death have proposed a compassionate and medically sound procedure for handling SIDS. The procedure includes mandatory autopsies in all cases of sudden infant death. Results of the autopsy would be relayed promptly to parents by a physician, nurse, or other health professional who is knowledgeable about SIDS and skilled in helping parents deal with their grief. Coroners and medical examiners would be informed of criteria for diagnosing SIDS on autopsy, and the term *sudden infant death syndrome* would be utuilized on the death certificate.

The strategy to accomplish these proposals would include provision for dissemination of information to instruct the public, including those most likely to come in contact with the family; alliance with professional medical and health organizations; and involvement with the government on local, state, and national levels to ensure the necessary legislation for compassionate and medically sound handling of all cases of sudden infant death. Nurses can be prime movers of appropriate legislation by contacting their legislators, disseminating information to them, and helping to instruct the public, who in turn can contact legislators.

Bronchiolitis

In *acute bronchiolitis* a blockage of the egress of air from the alveoli results in overdistention of the lungs, dyspnea, cyanosis, and exhaustion. It occurs during the first 2 years of life, with the peak incidence at 6 months of age. It is most often seen in the winter and early spring. Viral invasion causes widespread inflammation of the bronchial mucosa, and tenacious exudate within the lumens of the bronchioles acts like a ball valve. Respiratory syncytial virus (RSV), the most common offender, is discussed below. Air may be permitted to enter the alveoli during inspiration, but the orifice closes and traps air during expiration. The lungs become progressively distended, and many alveoli lose their normal function of aerating blood (atelectasis). If a critical portion of alveoli is affected, adjacent alveoli cannot compensate for the inadequate ventilation. As a result, hypoxia occurs, carbon dioxide is elevated, pH decreases, and the infant is in respiratory acidosis. Small areas of pneumonia may be present in the lungs.

Symptoms of acute bronchiolitis include flaring of alae nasi and an overdistended chest which collapses poorly on expiration and retracts intercostally and subcostally on inspiration. Respirations range from 60 to 80 per minute and are labored but shallow because of lung distention. Varying degrees of cyanosis may be present. The infant is restless, has a hacking cough, eats and sleeps poorly. Activity, crying, and feeding exaggerate the symptoms. Fever may be absent, intermediate, or high, or the infant may be hypothermic. The acute phase lasts 2 to 3 days after the onset of cough and dyspnea. When this critical period is over, recovery is dramatic and rapid. A very small percentage of affected infants may require assisted ventilation when they become exhausted.

If bronchiolitis is mild, the infant may be treated at home. Criteria for hospitalization include one or more of the following signs: cyanosis, a respiratory rate greater than 60, retractions, or nasal flaring while at rest; $PaO_2 <$ 60 mmHg and $PaCO_2 > 45$ mmHg; and 2 months of age or younger (Simkins, 1981a). Supportive treatment at home includes the use of a vaporizer, semi-Fowler's position (e.g., placing in an infant seat), increased fluid intake,

and antipyretics for fever. Parents are instructed to call the physician if the infant becomes cyanotic, if the respiratory rate increases beyond 60 breaths per minute, or if retractions or nasal flaring occur.

Since the causative agent is viral, there are no antimicrobial agents which are therapeutic. Tracheostomy is not indicated because the obstruction is at the bronchial level. The value of corticosteroids is questionable. One dose of epinephrine may be given to see if there is any response. Otherwise, since bronchodilating drugs increase restlessness and oxygen requirements, they are usually contraindicated. However, if RSV is the causative organism, theophylline may be given to prevent apnea. Otherwise, treatment is symptomatic. High humidity to liquefy secretions and decrease edema and oxygen for dyspnea are readily supplied through the utilization of a mist tent, oxygen tent (Fig. 23-5), hood, or nasal cannula. Since anxiety and restlessness accompany dyspnea, they will be allayed through an adequate supply of oxygen.

Positioning is important. Putting the infant in semi-Fowler's position with slight extension of his neck allows for fuller chest expansion and a clearer airway. Extreme neck extension or flexion must be avoided.

If the infant tires easily when sucking and because of tachypnea, he is placed on "nothing by mouth," and intravenous fluids are started. Tachypnea in itself may have a dehydrating effect, and supplemental intravenous fluids may be given along with oral fluids. Respiratory acidosis is helped through the administration of appropriate parenteral fluids, with better perfusion of the lungs and ventilation and blood flow (V/Q) ratio.

Nursing Management

Observation of the infant's vital signs, skin color, skin turgor, and anterior fontanel and accurate recording and reporting of these observations are extremely important nursing activities during the critical 48 to 72 hours following the onset of cough and dyspnea. These data, in conjunction with findings on auscultation and palpation and laboratory findings, provide important clues to the infant's status. They also alert the nurse to impending respiratory acidosis and secondary dehydration.

The nurse checks the oxygen tent frequently to ensure its proper functioning in providing high humidity and oxygen at a comfortable temperature. The higher oxygen content aids in breathing, and the mist helps to liquefy secretions, thus making coughing less distressing to the infant. In the presence of moist rales, postural drainage is initiated if the infant can tolerate it. Suctioning is done as needed. The infant's response to oxygen therapy is evaluated through observation of his color, the nature of his respirations, the degree of restlessness, and determination of arterial blood gases. If the infant's nares are blocked, he will breathe through his mouth. Nasal secretions should be removed with cotton-tipped applicators or cotton cones. Positions as described above should be maintained to aid in oxygenation.

If fluids are tolerated, the infant is offered water be-

FIGURE 23-5 An infant in a mist tent receiving oxygen and humidity to relieve his respiratory distress. *(Courtesy Children's Hospital Medical Center, Boston, Mass.)*

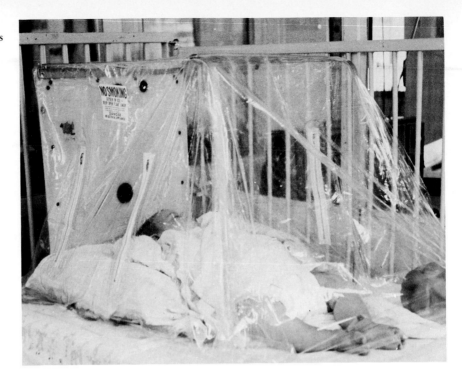

 NURSING CARE PLAN

23-1 *The Child with Bronchiolitis*

Clinical Problem/Nursing Diagnosis	Expected Outcome	Nursing Interventions
Labored shallow respirations, tachypnea, retracting, flaring nares, cough, and expiratory wheeze	Child's respiratory distress will decrease (respiratory rate 60 breaths/min) Child's oxygenation needs will be met: $PaO_2 > 60$ mmHg $PaO_2 < 35\text{-}45$ mmHg Child's airway will remain patent	Monitor vital signs q 1-2 h while in acute respiratory distress Assess heart rate for regularity, rate, and rhythm: report findings of tachycardia or bradycardia, hypotension or hypertension, and/or ectopy or irregular rhythm promptly Assess perfusion: note strength of peripheral pulses, color and warmth of extremities, and quality of capillary refill Assess respiratory status for signs of adequate gas exchange: note respirations for rate, quality, and depth; observe color of nailbeds and mucous membranes; assess quality and symmetry of chest expansion on inspiration and expiration
Ineffective breathing pattern related to lower airway obstruction		Assess breath sounds for equality and quality of aeration in all lung fields: assess for diminished breath sounds; note presence of crackles and expiratory wheezing Assess degree of respiratory distress: observe for tachypnea, dyspnea, nasal flaring, retracting, grunting, difficulty eating, color changes, cyanosis, changes in behavior, increased irritability, restlessness, and fatigue Note presence of hacking cough (productive and/or nonproductive) Monitor child for acute increase in severity of respiratory distress; assess for signs of atelectasis and pneumothorax Evaluate need for cardiorespiratory monitoring in a child with moderate to severe distress Monitor oxygen saturation values via external pulse oximeter probe; titrate oxygen as orderd to maintain O_2 saturation > 95 mmHg; monitor arterial blood gas values as indicated Properly administer cool humidified oxygen via mist tent or hood (maintain child's temperature under cool mist) Maintain patency of airway (bulb suction)

Continued.

NURSING CARE PLAN 23-1 The Child with Bronchiolitis —cont'd

Clinical Problem/Nursing Diagnosis	Expected Outcome	Nursing Interventions
		Properly obtain respiratory secretions for culture to detect the presence of respiratory syncytial virus (RSV), bacterial pneumonia, and parainfluenza
		Institute appropriate respiratory isolation precautions for RSV bacterial pneumonia; enforce strict hand washing practices
		Observe respiratory status and signs of increased distress during feeding; out of oxygen source (hood or tent)
		Maintain nothing by mouth (NPO) for respiratory rate > 60 breaths/min; avoid nasogastric tube placement in nonintubated child; place oral gastric tube in infants with respiratory distress if indicated
		Properly administer prescribed medications: antibiotics, bronchodilators, and/or corticosteroids
		Monitor for side effects of all medications; monitor theophylline levels closely
		Position child in semi-Fowler's position with slight neck extension; position with head of bed elevated to 30-40°; present hyperextension and hyperflexion of neck
		Perform chest physical therapy as indicated by chest x-ray; auscultate breath sounds; closely monitor tolerance of procedure; conserve energy and promote rest between treatments
		Reposition child to mobilize secretions: promote adequate ventilation to all lobes
		Assure adequate hydration to liquefy secretions for effective airway clearance
NPO secondary to respiratory distress Increased insensible water losses secondary to respiratory distress	Given the appropriate nursing care, child's fluid and electrolyte balance will be maintained	Monitor intake and output volumes; monitor electrolyte values; report and correct imbalances as ordered
		Assess for signs of dehydration; observe for sunken fontanel, sunken eyes, dry mucous membranes, absence of tears, poor skin turgor, decreased urine output, and urine specific gravity > 1.025
		Administer intravenous fluids as ordered: note patency and placement of IV while NPO for respiratory distress
Potential fluid volume deficit related to altered PO intake; respiratory distress		During recovery phase, encourage PO feeding with a respiratory rate < 60 breaths/min: feed slowly with frequent rest periods
Rectal temperature > 38.5°C	Child's temperature will return to normal range (37-37.5°C)	Monitor temperature every h while febrile; report temperature > 38.5°C to physician
		Administer antibiotics as ordered
Hyperthermia related to respiratory infection		Administer antipyretics as ordered and evaluate their effectiveness in controlling fever
		Obtain blood, urine, and respiratory secretions for cultures
Rectal temperature < 36.5°C	Child will maintain normothermic rectal temperature (37°C)	Monitor temperature q 2 h
Hypothermia related to therapeutic use of cool, humidified oxygen mist		Prevent unstable temperature in mist tent; maintain dry bed linens; change clothing when damp; keep child dry and well covered; protect head from evaporative heat loss (make hat from stockinette material); collect moisture deposits around tent itself

tween feedings. If he cannot be removed from the mist tent because of his respiratory status, the nurse supports his head and back with one hand while holding the bottle with the other. If the infant's breathing is labored, medications and feedings are given very slowly. The nurse notes the infant's behavior during a feeding to ascertain the need for stopping oral feedings. The rate and flow of any intravenous fluids are observed frequently to prevent over- or under-hydration and/or electrolyte imbalance. The presence of either can be determined through urine specific gravity determinations (< 1.008 = overhydration; > 1.025 = dehydration). Parents need support, particu-

Clinical Problem/Nursing Diagnosis	Expected Outcome	Nursing Interventions
Increased respiratory distress: labored breathing, irritability, restlessness, difficulty feeding, respiratory rate > 60, O_2 saturation < 95 mmHg	Child will conserve energy and oxygen reserves	Monitor child for signs of increasing distress, especially in relation to activity and exertion of energy Reduce physiological stressors: maintain patent airway, adequate oxygenation, normothermia; provide adequate hyration; maintain NPO when respiratory rate < 60 breaths/min; maintain constant oxygen levels in mist tent Reduce psychosocial stressors: encourage parental participation in care (comforting, holding, and cuddling); provide security object (favorite blanket or toy); provide pacifier for sucking needs; promote calm, quiet, restful environment; organize care to limit disturbances and increase length of rest periods in mist tent
Activity intolerance and Fatigue related to insufficient oxygenation secondary to lower airway obstruction		

larly during the acute phase. Approximately 50 percent of these infants subsequently develop asthma.

Respiratory Syncytial Virus (RSV)

A virus which has its greatest effect on very young infants is respiratory syncytial virus. It is the most common cause of bronchiolitis, and because treatment is supportive, caring for these infants is both frustrating and anxiety-provoking.

The prevalence and frequency of RSV mandate its inclusion here. RSV occurs in annual outbreaks during January, February, and March. It usually involves the lower respiratory tract, commonly infects males more than females, and is seen frequently in lower socioeconomic groups living in crowded conditions.

The incubation period is about 4 days. Some symptoms include coryza, pharyngitis, fever, and otitis media, and on auscultation there are diffuse rhonchi, fine rales, and wheezing. Infants who are severely ill have retractions, respiratory rates in excess of 70 breaths per minute, hyperexpanded chests, cyanosis, apneic spells, and poor air exchanges. In some young infants the cough can be severe and paroxysmal so that it resembles pertussis.

Diagnosis is made on the basis of mucus sent to the virology laboratory. Treatment is symptomatic, and antibiotics are not ordered; however, humidified oxygen and fluids (intravenous or PO) are ordered. Physicians at some medical centers also utilize ribavirin in conjunction with aerosol therapy, but this treatment plan has not been totally accepted (Ray, 1988). Despite its stormy course, the prognosis is good except for young infants who have other health problems affecting the cardiovascular, pulmonary, neuromuscular, or immunologic systems.

Nursing Management

The diagnosis depends on the nurse aspirating nasopharyngeal mucus and sending the specimen to the virology laboratory promptly. On hospitalization, these infants are isolated because RSV is considered contagious and cross-infection is a major problem during its annual outbreak.

It is imperative for a nurse to assess the respiratory status and hydration of an infant who is infected with RSV. Because medical treatment is based on symptoms, a nurse needs to monitor these infants closely. Oxygen and humidity usually are provided by mist tent or hood, depending on the age and size of the infant. He should be kept in an elevated position to maximize chest expansion. Oxygen concentrations must be taken and recorded approximately every 2 hours. If ribavirin is used, the nurse needs to know when it is started and when it is to finish, because this aerosol treatment usually is given continuously for 20 out of 24 hours. Although the respiratory therapy department may be responsible for its administration, the nurse who cares for the young client *must* know the correct time parameters. Ribavirin therapy is reasonably new, and the long-term adverse side effects are unknown; hence, in some institutions pregnant women are advised not participate in caring for infants who are receiving such treatment.

Arterial blood gases are done at frequent intervals. While it is essential for the nurse to know the latest results, it is also important for her to identify the amount of blood being withdrawn, especially in the case of small infants.

A major nursing problem relates to the hydration status of the young client. If his respiratory rate is very rapid, he may be struggling for air and becoming more and more exhausted. Many infants become mildly to moderately dehydrated. Some may be able to take fluids by mouth, while others may need intravenous fluids. If they are difficult feeders because of their high respiratory rates, physicians may order than to be NPO. Their intravenous rates must be monitored at least every hour because of the danger of fluid overload. A urine specific gravity should be done with every void and recorded. It is essential to maintain an accurate intake and output record for these infants.

The experience is frightening for parents who are observing the labored respirations of their infant. They may not understand why antibiotics are not ordered, why the intravenous line is necessary, and why improvement is so slow. They need a significant amount of information, support, and understanding. They also should be told that the infant may be excreting the virus for 3 or more weeks. Since transmission occurs by the respiratory route, it is essential for parents to understand that after discharge neonates or young infants should not have contact with the baby until after that period of time has passed.

Croup

Croup is a term applied to several conditions characterized by cough, inspiratory stridor, hoarseness, and signs of respiratory distress. Bacterial croup is seen more commonly in the 3- to 7-year age group, while viral croup is seen more frequently from 3 months to 3 years of age. Males, for no known reason, have a higher incidence of croup. The disease seems to occur more often in cold weather. Parainfluenza viruses account for the majority of infectious croup cases. Epiglottitis, a bacterial form, is discussed later in this chapter. Clinical varieties of viral croup include laryngitis, laryngotracheobronchitis (the most common form), and acute spasmodic croup.

Laryngitis is usually mild except in the young infant. The high obstruction causing respiratory distress in the infant is due to edema of the vocal cords and subglottic area. With laryngotracheobronchitis (LTB), as the name suggests, the infection extends downward from the larynx to the bronchi. Children who have acute spasmodic croup for little or no apparent reason develop episodes of severe laryngospasm at night.

Laryngitis begins with an upper respiratory infection followed by sore throat, cough, and croup. When the clinical course is severe, obstruction occurs in the subglottic area. Marked hoarseness, deep suprasternal and substernal retractions, severe inspiratory stridor, dyspnea, and restlessness occur. As the course progresses, air hunger and fatigue appear, at which time the infant alternates between periods of agitation and exhaustion secondary to decreased PO_2 and increased PCO_2.

The onset of LTB is characterized by an upper respiratory infection which lasts for several days before cough and inspiratory stridor indicate the advent of respiratory distress. As the bronchi and bronchioles become involved, expirations become labored and prolonged and the infant appears restless and frightened. Fever may be slight, or the temperature may reach 39.4 to 40°C (103 to 104°F).

The illness lasts for several days, a week, or longer. It is initially distinguished from epiglottitis by its slower onset as opposed to the explosive onset and more rapid course of epiglottitis.

If croup is mild, the infant may be treated at home. Criteria for hospitalization include stridor and retractions at rest, tachypnea ($>$ 60 breaths per minute at rest), increased heart rate, cyanosis (particularly circumoral), and restlessness (hypoxia) (Simkins, 1981b). Supportive home treatment is the same as that described for bronchiolitis. Parents are instructed to call the physician if symptoms increase (e.g., retractions, tachypnea, cyanosis).

Acute spasmodic laryngitis occurs most commonly between 1 and 3 years of age. Since anxious and excitable children seen more prone to this condition and a familial predisposition may be present, allergy and psychological factors may be implicated along with viruses. After mild to moderate coryza and hoarseness, the child awakens at night because of respiratory distress. He exhibits a barking, metallic cough, noisy inspiration, anxiety, and fright. The child is afebrile. His respirations are slow and labored with supraclavicular, suprasternal, substernal, and intercostal retractions. His pulse is rapid, and his skin is cool and moist. If the child becomes excited, dyspnea increases and intermittent cyanosis may occur. Severe symptoms usually last several hours and then decrease. Increasingly milder attacks may occur on one or two subsequent nights. Eventual recovery is complete.

The aim of treatment is to ensure adequate exchange of oxygen and carbon dioxide at the alveolar level. High humidity with cold mist aids in preventing the drying of secretions and in reducing mucosal edema. If an infant is in severe respiratory distress, oral feedings may be discontinued and parenteral fluids may be given. Thus, physical exertion is lessened, and the probability of aspiration of vomitus is decreased. Serial determinations of urine specific gravity are done to monitor over- or underhydration. Cyanosis may be an indicator for intubation or tracheotomy. When oxygen is administered to alleviate anoxia and apprehension, the infant must be observed carefully for other clinical signs of an impending need for more aggressive treatment. Although increased restlessness may mean increased hypoxia, blood gases must be drawn for confirmation. While indications for a tracheotomy include advancing cyanosis, tachycardia, and restlessness, some physicians elect to intubate young patients for 24 hours. The inhalation of racemic epinephrine is also beneficial.

Sedatives are *contraindicated*, since restlessness is one of the criteria for ascertaining the need for tracheotomy. In those rare instances where sedation may be essential because of extreme agitation and fright, chloral hydrate or paraldehyde (never intravenously) may be given, since neither dries secretions or depresses the respiratory center. No medications are of value in treating viral croup, with the exception of subemetic doses of syrup of ipecac to relieve laryngeal spasm in spasmodic croup. Emetic doses of ipecac result in vomiting due to probable vagal stimulation.

Nursing Management

Frequent reassurance by the nurse will help keep the infant calm and quiet and may be accomplished through the nurse's tone of voice, touch, and physical presence. The nurse must observe the infant frequently. Careful noting, recording and reporting of the degree of hoarseness; type of cough; type and severity of retractions; degree of stridor, cyanosis, and restlessness; presence of labored and prolonged expirations; pyrexia; and tachycardia are essential in determining the infant's progress. The pattern of increased heart rate, decreased respiratory rate, and decreased stidor indicates an emergency. Stridor decreases as the infant moves less air. Heart rate increases in response, and respiratory rate decreases as PCO_2 rises above 60 or 70 mmHg.

The nurse should note the infant's behavior during feedings. If he becomes tired, oral feedings may be discontinued and parenteral fluids started. Rate of flow, amount, and type of intravenous fluid must be recorded at least every hour. Signs of infiltration of parenteral fluids should be reported immediately and recorded.

If an infant suffers an attack of croup at home, instant steam may be provided by fully turning on all hot water taps in a closed bathroom. The infant may then be placed in an atmosphere of high humidity. This procedure may be done in lieu of cold mist, but cold mist vaporizers for home use are commercially available. If a hot mist vaporizer is used, parents are cautioned to place the vaporizer out of the child's reach to prevent burns. Whether a hot or cool mist machine is used, parents are instructed to disassemble and clean the machine daily to prevent the formation of molds. In the hospital, the infant is placed in tent with oxygen and mist and is positioned in an infant seat to enhance chest expansion.

If a high fever is present, sponge baths with tepid water may be given. These sponge baths last approximately 15 minutes. If at any moment during that time cyanosis, weak irregular pulse, slow shallow respirations, or chills occur, the sponge bath should be discontinued because of impending circulatory collapse.

Increased restlessness, pulse rate, and fever and the presence of dyspnea and retractions *before cyanosis occurs* are indications for a tracheotomy. At some centers, nasotracheal tubes may be used in place of a tracheotomy tube. The infant may have an anxious expression on his face because of his inability to aerate his lungs adequately. An alert nurse will report the advent of these manifestations to the physician.

After a tracheotomy has been performed, the nurse observes the infant for and reports restlessness, extreme fatigue, dyspnea, cyanosis or pallor, fever, rapid pulse, retractions, noisy respirations, bleeding, crepitance, and infection around the incision. Symptoms of obstruction in the tracheotomy tube include blue or ashy color, especially of the infant's ears, face, and lips; noisy, moist respirations; substernal retractions; restlessness or apprehension; and increased pulse rate. Adequate suctioning and changing should prevent obstruction in the tracheotomy tube. The infant's arms are restrained to prevent his removing the tube with random arm movements. The nurse may assure the infant through tone of voice, touch, and physical presence. The infant is provided with oxygen and mist, usually by means of a mist tent. Immediately following a tracheotomy, the infant is suctioned frequently and then every hour. As he improves, his need for suctioning decreases.

Since the infant cannot cry, he needs a sense of trust in himself and others. Trust is provided through the love of his mother and the nurse caring for him. Vital signs are taken as ordered or more frequently, according to the nurse's assessment. Changing the infant's position frequently prevents pooling of secretions. The infant is offered small amounts of water at frequent intervals unless oral feedings are contraindicated. Arm restraints may be removed under the nurse's supervision to provide range of motion exercises.

Parents need factual information and constant reassurance during the acute phse of the illness. After an explanation of the child's condition and reasons for treatment and nursing measures, parents can determine, with the nurse's help, the degree of their involvement in the care of the child. This involvement can pave the way for the infant's return home.

Sometimes an infant with LTB is discharged with the tracheotomy tube in situ. Parents who have been involved in the care of the infant know how to carry out procedures and are aware of danger signals. They are also cautioned to be careful when bathing the infant to prevent water from entering the tube. If parents need help in caring for the infant at home, a referral is made to a community health nurse.

Pertussis

The infant has no temporary immunity to pertussis (whooping cough) in the first few months of life and is highly susceptible to this communicable disease. The highest mortality from pertussis occurs in the first year of life.

Pertussis, an acute infection, is caused by a bacterium known as *Bordatella pertussis* or *Haemophilus pertussis* and is spread by droplet infection or direct contact. It is characterized by a paroxysmal cough which ends in a prolonged inspiration or "whoop" and, frequently, vomiting. The structures most affected are bronchi and bronchioles. Some inflammation may be seen in the trachea, larynx, and nasopharyngeal mucosa. Lymphocytes and some neutrophils infiltrate the respiratory passages, causing an interstitial pneumonitis. Small mucous plugs in the bronchioles cause obstructive emphysema and atelectasis.

Symptoms may occur from 7 to 14 days after exposure. The disease proceeds in three stages: catarrhal, spasmodic or paroxysmal, and convalescent. The entire course lasts about 6 weeks.

The *catarrhal stage* has an insidious onset with a mild cough, usually at night. For the following 10 days to 2 weeks the cough becomes progressively more severe and occurs during the day. Coryza, sneezing, and sometimes hoarseness occur. The infant may be anoxic. Recovery of the causative organism from nasopharyngeal swab culture during this phase is helpful in making the diagnosis.

At the end of 10 days or 2 weeks of the catarrhal stage, the infant enters the *spasmodic,* or *paroxysmal,* stage. During a severe paroxysm, a series of explosive efforts occurs. The infant's face becomes red from this exertion and may even turn cyanotic. As the paroxysm ends, a sudden inspiratory whoop occurs. This episode may be followed by vomiting or by coughing up or swallowing large amounts of thick, tenacious, mucoid sputum. In small infants, choking spells may occur in place of the characteristic whoop. After the coughing spasm, sweating, congestion of neck and scalp veins, mental confusion, convulsions (especially in infants), and exhaustion may occur. Paroxysms are aggravated by excitement, sudden changes in temperature, activity, and inhalation of irritating fumes such as smoke.

The *convalescent stage* begins about the fourth week of the clinical course. The number and severity of paroxysms decrease, vomiting subsides, and appetite returns. An intercurrent respiratory infection may cause a recurrence of all major symptoms of the disease process.

Pertussis is readily recognized during the paroxysmal stage. Sequelae include hemorrhages (epistaxis, hemoptysis, conjunctival extravasations, and intracranial hemorrhage), respiratory tract infections (otitis media, bronchopneumonia, atelectasis), nervous system complications (encephalitis), and digestive tract complications (emaciation due to prolonged vomiting and hernias due to straining on coughing and vomiting). Residual conditions include bronchiectasis and pulmonary fibrosis due to severe respiratory complications and epilepsy, mental retardation, and personality changes due to cerebral edema and intracranial hemorrhage.

The infant with suspected pertussis is isolated to prevent spread of the disease. Oxygen and humidity are ordered to ensure the liquefying of secretions and adequate oxygenation. Although antibiotics do not alter the course of this disease once the infant has become infected, they are ordered to eradicate *B. pertussis* from secretions, thereby putting others at lower risk. Erythromycin or ampicillin may be prescribed for this purpose.

Nursing Management

Since pertussis is highly contagious, the infant is placed in isolation. Spread of the disease must be prevented, and the affected infant must be protected against secondary infection. Though paroxysms of coughing are inevitable, they can be decreased if the nurse enters the room quietly and talks to the infant before touching him or lowering the cribside. All sudden noises and sudden changes in temperature should be avoided. By maintaining a quiet environment, the nurse minimizes excitement (laughter, fright, crying) in the infant.

During paroxysmal coughing spells, the nurse reassures the infant by talking to him in a quiet voice. She supports the infant's muscles to prevent any weakening of abdominal musculature during these severe paroxysms. The

infant is kept in a humidified environment to liquefy secretions. Oxygen is given if he becomes cyanotic, and chilling is avoided. Sometimes an infant's respirations cease after a paroxysm, and the nurse provides artificial respiration. If he vomits or has excessive mucus, he is suctioned in order to maintain a patent airway. Meticulous nose and mouth care is given to prevent excoriation of the skin around the nose and lips due to nasal secretions. If the infant convulses after a coughing spasm, he is protected from hurting himself and from occluding his airway.

It is important to offer the infant small, frequent feedings to maintain his nutritional status. If he vomits a feeding during a coughing episode, the infant should be refed in 20 to 30 minutes. Since exhaustion is common, it is important for a nurse to observe the infant's overall status and take the time needed to ensure an adequate oral intake.

In order to assess the infant's progress, the nurse must observe, report, and record the severity and frequency of paroxysms; the amount, type, and frequency of vomiting; the infant's color before, during, and after coughing episodes; the type and amount of mucus; and the condition of the infant after a paroxysm. The nurse should also observe, report, and record any signs and symptoms of complications and/or sequelae.

Whooping cough is frightening to parents. They need constant reassurance and factual information during the course of the disease. They are taught isolation technique in order to spend time with the hospitalized infant and, if they desire, become involved in his care. Parents may also need information about immunization schedules and booster "shots" for any eligible sibling.

Pneumonia

Pneumonia may be caused by several organisms. Clinically, they may be difficult to distinguish. Pneumococcal pneumonia that is caused by *Streptococcus pneumoniae* is presented here. Other types are described briefly in Table 23-4.

The highest incidence of pneumococcal pneumonia is during late winter and early spring. It occurs most frequently in the first 4 years of life. In infants, bronchopneumonia is more common, whereas in older children one or more lobes are involved in the disease process without affecting the remainder of the bronchopulmonary system. The clinical course in older children is similar to that in adults. In bronchopneumonia, there is a consolidation of scattered lobules and the mucosa is inflamed.

The infant usually has a mild upper respiratory tract infection of several days' duration characterized by a stuffy nose, fretfulness, and decrease in appetite. This initial phase is followed by an abrupt onset of fever from 39.4 to 40.6°C (103 to 105°F), restlessness, apprehension, and respiratory distress. The infant may have a generalized convulsion due to high fever. Observation of the infant may reveal flushed cheeks; circumoral cyanosis; flaring of the alae nasi; supraclavicular, suprasternal, intercostal, and

TABLE 23-4 Types of Pneumonia

Organism (Age)	Signs and Symptoms	Laboratory Reports	Treatment
Chlamydia trachomatis 2-14 weeks	Possible history of maternal cervicitis or *C. trachomatis* vaginitis Possible history of purulent conjunctivitis beginning at 3-21 days of age (average 7-10 days) Nasal discharge, tachypnea, cough Possible snorting respirations without discharge Possible concomitant otitis media Gradually increasing tachypnea and cough (at times paroxysmal and stacatto) Crepitant inspiratory rales on auscultation, but prominent wheezing unusual Possible severe respiratory distress and periods of apnea	Possible findings: Eosinophils $> 300/mm^3$ Elevated IgA, IgM, and/or IgG Decreased PaO_2 and $PaCO_2$ Positive culture of nasopharyngeal aspirates X-ray: symmetrical interstitial infiltrates and hyperexpansion bilaterally	Symptomatic and supportive Erythromycin for 14-21 days
Staphylococcus (under 1 yr)	History of furunculosis, recent hospitalization, or maternal breast abscess; respiratory infection, upper or lower, for several days up to 1 week followed by abrupt change—fever, cough, respiratory distress, tachypnea, grunting respirations, sternal and subcostal retractions, cyanosis, anxiety Lethargy if undisturbed, irritability if roused Pyopneumothorax, pneumatoceles, and empyema as clinical course progresses	White blood cell count (WBC): normal range in young infant, $20,000/mm^3$ with predominant polymorphonuclear leukocytes in older infants Positive tracheal aspiration and/or pleural tap culture X-ray: patchy infiltration or dense (bronchopneumonia or lobar)	Symptomatic and supportive Oxygen Semi-Fowler's position Parenteral fluids during acute phase Methicillin or penicillin G for 3 weeks IV or IM Thoracentesis Closed chest drainage with extensive involvement for 5-7 days Hospitalization 6-10 weeks
Streptococcus group A (3-5 yr)	Mild prodromal symptoms followed by sudden onset of high fever, chills, respiratory distress Clinical course similar to staphylococcal; complications: empyema and bacterial foci in bones and joints	Elevated WBC with polymorphonuclear leukocytes predominating Elevated antistreptolysin O titer Positive culture X-ray: disseminated infiltration	Symptomatic and supportive Penicillin G Thoracentesis Closed drainage
Haemophilus influenzae (infants and young children)	Mild or severe. Insidious onset Clinical course subacute and prolonged, of several weeks' duration; signs and symptoms similar to pneumococcal; signs and symptoms in young infants associated with bacteremia and emphysema Complications: bacteremia, pericarditis, cellulitis, empyema, meningitis, pyarthrosis	Bacteremia Positive cultures Moderate leukocytosis with lymphopenia X-ray: lobar consolidation	Symptomatic and supportive Ampicillin
Mycoplasma pneumoniae (school-age and adolescence [see section on adolescent])	History of fever, malaise, *headache,* muscle pain, and anorexia followed by rhinitis, dry hacking cough, and sore throat Progression of cough from nonproductive to productive (seromucoid to mucopurulent) Occasional fine crepitant rales and wheezing on auscultation Less ill than with bacterial pneumonias	Normal white blood cell count (WBC) usually Increased cold agglutination titer or complement fixation titer X-ray: diffuse or patchy infiltrates	Symptomatic and supportive Erythromycin or tetracycline (if over 8 yr of age) Possible treatment at home, if not toxic
Virus (see Table 23-7 for types) (any age)	History of upper respiratory infection for several days; conjunctivitis with Coxsackie virus Mild to high fever Slight to severe cough Possible progression from malaise to prostration	Normal WBC usually X-ray: diffuse or patchy densities	Symptomatic and supportive Possible treatment at home, if not toxic

subcostal retractions; tachypnea; and tachycardia. On auscultation, decreased breath sounds, crackling rales, and pleural friction rub may be heard. Breath sounds on the opposite side may be exaggerated. A cough appears as the clinical course progresses. Abdominal distention may be due to swallowed air or paralytic ileus. Meningism may be present. On x-ray, a patchy infiltration of one or several lobes is found, and the causative organism is recovered in secretions. The prognosis is favorable.

Penicillin G is the most effective antimicrobial agent in the treatment of pneumococcal pneumonia (Table 23-5). If the infant is allergic to penicillin, erythromycin or cephalothin is an effective agent. Treatment is symptomatic and supportive: bed rest, an abundance of oral fluids, and antipyretics for fever. Oxygen and mist are administered to alleviate respiratory distress and anxiety. Intravenous fluids are given to combat dehydration and electrolyte imbalance.

Nursing Management

An infant who has pneumonia needs rest and should be disturbed as little as possible. His respiratory status is assessed frequently, and appropriate measures are instituted. Fluids are necessary to maintain electrolytes and a normal specific gravity, but the infant should not be forced to eat since he is anorexic. Intravenous therapy may be necessary. The infant may tend to lie on the affected side to relieve pain. Frequent position change will prevent the pooling of secretions and maintain adequate circulation. Postural drainage and clapping may be necessary to assist the infant in relieving congestion. Both parents and infants need reassurance, particularly during the acute phase.

Taking an accurate temperature is important in preventing febrile convulsions. If the infant's temperature is 38.9°C (102°F), the nurse administers the prescribed antipyretic. A fever of 39.4°C (103°F) or above necessitates a sponge bath with tepid water. A distended abdomen may be indicative of constipation, paralytic ileus, or swallowed air due to mouth breathing. A rectal tube may provide some relief for constipation and swallowed air. Excoriation due to copious nasal discharge may be prevented through effective skin care.

The spread of a staphylococcal infection is a night-

TABLE 23-5 Antibiotics Used in Treating Pneumonia

Drug	Indications	Method	Dosage	Side Effects
Bactericidal agents				
Penicillin G	Moderate to severe systemic infections	Orally Intramuscularly Intravenously	25,000-100,000 U/kg/d PO q 6 h 25,000-300,000 U/kg/d IM or IV q 4 h	Polyarthritis, hemolytic anemia, thrombocytopenia, leukopenia; neuropathy and convulsions with high doses; rash, urticaria, maculopapular eruptions, edema Thrombophlebitis if given IV Overgrowth of nonsusceptible organisms Anaphylaxis: fever and chills Interaction: bacteriostatic antibiotics (penicillin given 1 h before bacteriostatic antibiotics): if PO, given 1-2 h before or 2-3 h after meals
Ampicillin	Systemic infections with susceptible strains of gram-positive and gram-negative organisms	Orally Intramuscularly Intravenously	50-100 mg/kg/d PO q 6 h 100-200 mg/kg/d IM or IV q 6	Anemia, thrombocytopenic purpura, eosinophilia, leukopenia Nausea, vomiting, diarrhea, glossitis, stomatitis: thrombophlebitis as with penicillin Overgrowth as with penicillin Hypersensitivity: chills, fever, rash, pruritis, urticaria, anaphylaxis Interaction: as with penicillin: if PO, given 1-2 h before or 2-3 h after meals
Cephalothin sodium	Severe respiratory (and other) infections	Intramuscularly Intravenously	20-40 mg/kg IM q 6 h 14-27 mg/kg IV q 4 h	Transient neutropenia, eosinophilia, hemolytic anemia Malaise, dizziness, headache, paresthesia Nausea, vomiting, diarrhea, anorexia, glossitis, abdominal cramps, pruritis ani. oral candidiasis Nephrotoxicity: genital moniliasis Maculopapular; erythematous rash Urticaria Hypersensitivity; dyspnea Thrombophlebitis as with penicillin At injection site: pain, induration, sterile abscess, warmth, sloughing

TABLE 23-5 Antibiotics Used in Treating Pneumonia—cont'd

Drug	Indications	Method	Dosage	Side Effects
Methicillin sodium	Systemic infections with staphylococci	Intramuscularly Intravenously	100-200 mg/kg/d q 4-6 h	Eosinophilia, hemolytic anemia, transient neutropenia Neuropathy (convulsions with high doses) Glossitis and stomatitis Overgrowth as with penicillin Hypersensitivity as with ampicillin Thrombophlebitis and interaction as with penicillin
Nafcillin sodium	Systemic infections with staphylococci	Orally Intramuscularly Intravenously	50-100 mg/kg/d PO q 4-6 h 100-200 mg/kg/d IM or IV q 4-6 h	With high doses, transient leukopenia, granulocytopenia, and thrombocytopenia Nausea, vomiting, diarrhea Overgrowth as with penicillin Hypersensitivity as with ampicillin Thrombophlebitis and interaction as with penicillin (if PO, given 1-2 h before or 2-3 h after meals)
Oxacillin sodium	Systemic infections with staphylococci	Orally Intramuscularly Intravenously	Same as nafcillin	Granulocytopenia, thrombocytopenia, eosinophilia, hemolytic anemia, transient neutropenia Neuropathy, oral lesions, nephritis, hepatitis Hypersensitivity as with ampicillin Thrombophlebitis and interaction as with penicillin (if PO, given 1-2 h before or 2-3 h after meals)
Bacteriostatic agents Erythromycin	Severe respiratory (and other) infections caused by group A beta-streptococci, *Streptococcus pneumoniae, Mycoplasma pneumoniae, Bordatella pertussis, Corynebacterium diphtheriae,* and *Chlamydia trachomatis*	Orally Intravenously	30-50 mg/kg/d PO, q 6 h 15-20 mg/kg/d IV q 4-6 h	With high doses intravenously, hearing loss Abdominal pain, cramping, nausea, vomiting, diarrhea, hepatitis; urticaria and rashes Anaphylaxis: fever Overgrowth of nonsusceptible bacteria or fungi Interactions: possible antagonism with clindamycin and lincomycin (not given with erythromycin); antagonism with penicillin (given 1 h after penicillin: if PO and not enteric coated, given 1 h before or 2 h after meals
Tetracycline	Infection caused by sensitive gram-positive and gram-negative organisms and *M. pneumoniae*	Orally Intramuscularly Intravenously	Children over 8 yr: 50 mg/kg/d PO q 6 h 15-25 mg/kg/d IM (maximum 250 mg) single dose or divided q 8-12 h 10-20 mg/kg/d IV q 12 h	Neutropenia, eosinophilia, hepatotoxicity with IV doses: dizziness, headache Pericarditis Sore throat, glossitis, dysphagia, anorexia, nausea, vomiting, diarrhea, epigastric pain, stomatitis, enterocolitis Rash, urticaria, photosensitivity, increased pigmentation Interactions: decreased absorption with food; milk and other dairy products; antacids; laxatives which contain calcium, aluminum, or magnesium; iron products (thus, tetracyclines given 1 h before or 2 h after food, dairy products, antacids, and laxatives and 2 h before or 3 h after iron products)

mare in a pediatric unit. The infant is placed on strict isolation, and meticulous precautions are observed by all who care for him. The nurse may have to intervene with allied hospital personnel by teaching them the importance of carrying out strict isolation technique. The infant needs oxygen therapy and blood determinations for electrolytes, hemoglobin, hematocrit, white blood cell count and differential, and so forth. Therefore, the nurse aids in the prevention of spread of a staphylococcal infection by ensuring the observance of strict isolation technique by hospital personnel.

Cystic Fibrosis

Cystic fibrosis is a hereditary disease of the exocrine glands. Although the basic genetic defect is unknown, investigators agree that it is transmitted as an autosomal recessive trait. Cystic fibrosis occurs most often in Caucasians and is one of the most common serious and chronic childhood diseases in this country. Thick, tenacious excretions of some mucus-producing glands cause obstructions mainly in the pancreatic ducts and bronchi. The secretory acini and ducts are dilated, and the exocrine parenchyma suffers secondary degeneration. The pancreas, and often the salivary glands, are firmer, smaller, and thicker than normal. With pulmonary involvement, the bronchioles are the structures first occluded, followed by the main bronchi. Eventually, chronic lung disease results, followed by emphysema due to obstructive overinflation. In trying to adapt to bronchial obstruction and pulmonary hypertension, the heart develops a right-sided ventricular hypertrophy. Secretions from sweat and parotid glands demonstrate an abnormal chemical composition. (The mother may state that the infant's skin tastes salty.) Children with cystic fibrosis are extremely susceptible to respiratory infections, although the immune response is normal. Approximately 50 percent of these children live to the age of 18 years or older.

Clinical manifestations include meconium ileus, chronic pulmonary disease, pancreatic insufficiency, and cirrhosis of the liver. Meconium ileus occurs in only 10 to 20 percent of these children. Most affected children have chronic pulmonary disease. Its onset may occur weeks, months, or years after birth. It begins with a dry, nonproductive cough followed by signs of generalized bronchiolar obstruction with secondary infection. Some degree of respiratory distress is evident and may be severe. With subsequent respiratory infections the manifestations are repeated and eventually may result in death. As thick, tenacious secretions accumulate in one or more bronchi, obstructions and dilatation result. The disease state progresses through irreversible bronchial damage to pulmonary insufficiency followed by death. Without bronchial damage, antibiotics may hold the disease process in check. As the pulmonary disease progresses, the functioning alveoli are overaerated, causing chest distention. The child displays a barrel-shaped chest. Clubbing of fingers and toes may also be noted. *Pseudomonas* and *Aspergillus* are the most common pathogens recovered from the child's nasopharynx, sputum, and lungs. Complications include lobar atelectasis, lung abscesses, asphyxia, hemoptysis, spontaneous pneumothorax, emphysema, and cor pulmonale. Sinusitis may be demonstrable via x-ray, and the child may have a nasal voice, postnasal drip, and polyps.

Over 80 percent of children with cystic fibrosis have pancreatic involvement. Pancreatic insufficiency manifests itself through symptoms of intestinal malabsorption. Although the child has a voracious appetite, he may appear strikingly undernourished. His abdomen is distended, and stools are frequent, bulky, fatty, and foul. Since most children are given prepared vitamins orally, vitamin deficiencies, with the exception of vitamin E, are usually absent. Diagnosis is made through family history, increase in sweat electrolyte concentration, absence of pancreatic enzymes, and chronic pulmonary disease. Although all four diagnostic criteria may not be present, (1) a combination of increased sweat electrolytes and either pulmonary disease or pancreatic insufficiency or (2) a combination of pulmonary and pancreatic manifestations suggests cystic fibrosis.

The pilocarpine iontophoresis sweat test is simple and reliable in diagnosing this condition. A sweat chloride above 60 meq/liter is diagnostic and levels from 50 to 60 meq/liter are suggestive. Sweat sodium values are approximately 10 meq/liter higher than values for chloride. Chronic lung disease with emphysema is demonstrable by x-ray. Pulmonary function tests reveal increased residual lung volume, decreased ventilatory flow rates, increased airway resistance, and uneven gas distribution throughout the lungs. Pancreatic deficiency may be determined through examination of duodenal contents for pancreatic enzyme activity and a stool for trypsin content. Trypsin is absent in over 80 percent of affected children. Stools are also examined for fat content, and various other fat absorption tests may be ordered. Steatorrhea is present if the amount of fat in the feces is excessive. Serum electrolytes are normal unless the child has severe pulmonary disease.

Approximately 97 percent of affected males are sterile as a result of abnormal development of the vas deferens, epididymis, and seminal vesicles. In affected females, increased viscosity and dehydration of mucous secretions in the vagina lead to reduced fertility.

Treatment of these children requires an interdisciplinary approach by the physician, nurse, physical therapist, and medical social worker. The child is allowed as nearly normal a life as possible, and care is taken to prevent his dominating the family. Children with severe pulmonary involvement need repeated intensive antibiotic therapy in the hospital, as do those with moderate pulmonary involvement when they have acute pulmonary exacerbations. The choice of drug is based on the results of culture and sensitivity of the offending pathogens. Physicians are not in agreement on continuous antibiotic therapy. Physical therapy is provided to promote bronchial drainage. The use of a mist tent is controversial, because some physicians believe it is a source of pathogens. If oxygen therapy is needed, blood gas levels are monitored frequently to prevent carbon dioxide narcosis.

23-2 *The Child with Cystic Fibrosis*

Clinical Problem/Nursing Diagnosis	Expected Outcome	Nursing Interventions
Tachypnea Dyspnea Cough Pulmonary congestion Crackles Atelectasis Decreased activity intolerance Chronic respiratory infections Ineffective airway clearance related to excessive mucus secretions; viscous airway secretions Ineffective breathing pattern related to respiratory infections	Child will be able to remove viscous secretions from airway and maintain clear passages as demonstrated by O_2 saturations > 95 mmHg Child will experience optimum pulmonary function, after pulmonary infections are detected and treated Child and family will demonstrate meticulous compliance with daily pulmonary infection measures; individual therapeutic regimen	Monitor vital signs q 2-4 h Auscultate breath sounds throughout all lung fields: note quality and equality of aeration and presence of crackles, wheezes, and diminished breath sounds; observe symmetry of chest expansion (inspiration/expiration) and length of inspiratory/expiratory phase of respiration Note rate, quality, and regularity of respirations and observe color of nailbeds and mucous membranes Assess for signs of respiratory distress: tachypnea, dyspnea, labored respirations with activity and/or stress, nasal flaring, retractions, grunting, restlessness, fatigue, and irritability Monitor for pulsus paradoxus, edema, increased abdominal girth, and abdominal pain Assess child for signs of advanced disease: marked increase in anterior-posterior diameter of chest; dyspnea and/or tachypnea on exertion; decreased excursion of thoracic cage; audible crackles, wheezing, difficulty eating, weight loss, clubbing, and cyanosis Auscultate breath sounds before and after pulmonary treatments to evaluate effectiveness Administer aerosol treatments properly with mucolytics, bronchodilators, and expectorants Perform vigorous chest percussion, vibrations, and postural drainage q 2 h during acute respiratory infection, concentrating on specifically affected areas, and q 4 h during recovery phase Determine maintenance of pulmonary therapy (aerosol/chest physical therapy routine; frequency and duration) based on individual child's respiratory assessment and clinical response to treatment Assist child in expectorating secretions; observe color, amount, consistency; culture samples as necessary; suction nasopharyngeal passages if necessary Promote maximum lung expansion with deep breathing exercises and incentive spirometry; position upright with head of bed elevated Monitor oxygenation: observe color of nailbeds; mucous membranes; use external pulse oximeter for O_2 saturation; examine ABGs Observe for increased respiratory distress during chest therapy, activity, feeding, interruption of oxygen therapy Administer O_2 properly to maintain oxygen saturation > 95 mmHg Provide humidified O_2 by mask, oxyhood, or mist tent Administer antibiotics as ordered and monitor placement and patency of IV line Prevent dehydration by encouraging generous PO fluid intake to liquefy bronchial secretions; administer IV fluids as ordered Conserve child's oxygen and energy reserves; organize care to ensure periods of uninterrupted sleep and rest Explain all aspects of aerosol therapy and chest physical therapy to parents Teach parents to perform chest physical therapy and postural drainage Teach parents basic skills required to use a nebulizer, properly administer medications by nebulizer, and give antibiotics as ordered Provide ample opportunities for parents to demonstrate pulmonary care measures until they are comfortable doing them Advise parents not to purchase cough suppressant preparations Explain importance of coughing to remove mucus Teach parents importance of adequate hydration in liquefying secretions, offering liquids and juices often Teach parents signs of respiratory infections and respiratory distress and when to contact pulmonary clinic for guidance, direction, and evaluation of child Assist family in identifying and obtaining equipment for home care (oxygen and supplies for aerosol therapy) Evaluate need for community health nurse referral to support parents and child at home

Continued.

Clinical Problem/Nursing Diagnosis	Expected Outcome	Nursing Interventions
Fatigue Weakness Dyspnea with increased play activity	Child will enjoy play and sports activities to promote growth and development without increased respiratory distress	Monitor child for increased respiratory distress: note increased distress in relation to activities and expenditure of energy
		Conserve energy reserves during periods of pulmonary infection; promote rest periods between nebulizer treatments, chest physical therapy, and other procedures
Activity intolerance related to pulmonary congestion; decreased air exchange		Provide quiet diversional activities during recovery (art, crafts, building toys) and increase activity level gradually
		Encourage participation in school activities and sports events and ensure the replacement of Na and H_2O losses by drinking lots of fluids
		Reassure parents that exercise and sports activities are effective methods of loosening secretions for expectoration and promoting child's level of self-confidence and self-esteem
Failure to gain weight and/or grow Weight loss	Child's increased caloric intake will promote weight gain	Obtain serial growth measurements of length, height, weight, and head circumference and plot on growth chart
		Document caloric intake for caloric count and instruct parents to monitor type and amount of food ingested
Altered nutrition: less than body requirements due to inadequate caloric intake; pancreatic enzyme deficiency; poor digestion and absorption of fat and fat-soluble vitamins; increased caloric needs secondary to stress of chronic illness	With addition of vitamins, minerals, and extracts, child's digestive ability will improve and fats as well as proteins will be absorbed	Incorporate child's favorite foods into therapeutic diet plan
		Replace pancreatic enzymes with extracts such as pancrelipase (Cotazym), pancrease, and viokase; they are titrated to individual child's clinical response with goal of increasing weight, decresing number of stools, and increasing form of stools
	Child's stools will decrease in number and bulk	Administer enzymes with meals and snacks (doses of certain enzymes are proportional to food ingested)
		Administer vitamins and mineral supplements: A, D, and E; children with liver disease and those receiving large amounts of antibiotics require evaluation for additional sources of B complex, K, C, and folic acid; children who have diarrhea and those who fail to thrive may need additional sources of zinc
		Administer supplemental fat-soluble vitamins (A, D, E, and K) in water-soluble preparations; administer multiple vitamin preparations as ordered
		Give sodium chloride preparations as ordered, especially during bouts of high fever, diarrhea, and diaphoresis and in hot weather
	All members of family will comply with therapeutic nutritional regimen to optimize their health	Collaborate with nutritionist; refer family to counseling for meal planning assistance
		Promote diet high in protein, carbohydrates, and calories (approximately 130% RDA) to support growth and weight gain; administer dietary supplements (medium-chain triglycerides) as ordered; stress well-balanced meals and frequent high-caloric, high-protein snacks (peanut butter, cheese)
		Provide written instructions for meal plans and encourage ongoing nutritional evaluations
Lethargy Weakness Muscle cramps Alkalosis Hyponatremia Hypochloremia	Child will remain in fluid and electrolyte balance	Monitor child for elevated temperature and increased sweating
		Institute measures to decrease sweating: avoid excessive room temperatures; overdressing, and excessive exercise in hot weather
	Child will experience minimized acute sodium and chloride losses	Promote frequent rest periods and intake of large amounts of fluids in hot weather
		Administer NaCl supplements with excessive sweating in hot weather or during exercise
Fluid volume deficit (and electrolyte imbalance) related to impaired sweat gland function; high Na, Cl, and K content in sweat	Child and family will be able to prevent and/or recognize signs of electrolyte depletion and intervene appropriately	Report muscle cramping, lethargy, fatigue, and changes in behavior or levels of consciousness promptly
		Monitor electrolyte values and promptly report signs of imbalance
		Assess child's hydration: measure specific gravity; calculate output; examine mucous membranes and skin turgor as well as anterior fontanel in infant

Clinical Problem/Nursing Diagnosis	Expected Outcome	Nursing Interventions
		Explain to parents excessive NaCl losses in children with cystic fibrosis; stress losses in hot weather and during excessive exercise; review signs of dehydration and NaCl losses and urge them to consult physician for prompt treatment
Signs and symptoms of congestive heart failure	Child will experience increased cardiac output following prompt treatment	Encourage child and parents to comply with vigorous chest physical therapy and postural drainage to decrease frequency of respiratory infections
Decreased cardiac output related to progressive or advanced pulmonary disease	Child and family will demonstrate meticulous compliance with pulmonary care to prevent infections and progression of pulmonary disease	Monitor vital signs; observe changes from baseline; look for presence of dyspnea, tachypnea, and tachycardia

Assess child for signs of congestive heart failure: difficulty feeding, edema, weight gain, hepatomegaly, fatigue, restlessness, rales, pneumonia, diminished peripheral pulses, cool extremities, and decreased urine output

Provide supportive therapy during congestive heart failure: conserve oxygen and energy reserves; promote frequent rest periods; provide small, frequent feedings; administer cool, humidified oxygen; and administer digoxin and diuretics as ordered |
| Fear
Anxiety
Denial
Poor compliance with daily treatments | Child and family will develop constructive coping mechanisms for optimal family functioning

Child and family will receive support and comfort from health team members | Assess child and family's experiences with prior illnesses and hospitalizations

Identify psychosocial impact of disease on child and family

Identify stressors within family unit; provide assistance; approach in warm, caring, supportive manner

Evaluate knowledge of cystic fibrosis, required treatments, and long-term management; identify presence of cystic fibrosis in family history; clarify existing myths about cystic fibrosis |
| Altered family processes related to stressors of chronic illness | | |
| | Child and family will comply with therapeutic treatment regimens to optimize child's health | Explain to parents critical importance of complying with treatment program, especially pulmonary care, giving dietary supplements, and meal planning as well as administering all medications properly

Provide written instructions for all aspects of home care

Discuss and make arrangements for genetic counseling; include all family members |
| | Child and parents will benefit from community support systems | Review with child and family all available support systems: community resources—Cystic Fibrosis Foundation, American Lung Association, Crippled Children's Programs, Sick Children's Services (state); these organizations provide information, financial support, and home care equipment

Discuss need for follow-up with cystic fibrosis center, pediatrician, pulmonary specialist, and nutritionist

Refer child and family to psychologist or family counselor if necessary for ongoing support

Provide ample opportunities for child and parents to verbalize their fears and concerns; clarify questions

Assess child for signs of disturbances in body image resulting from progressive illness and repeated hospitalizations; monitor for decreased interest in play and/or school activities and peer interactions

Provide emotional support to child and family through all aspects of care

Encourage child and family to incorporate all therapeutic measures into routine daily activities with as much normality as possible to optimize normal growth and development of child

Facilitate and encourage child and family members to seek out and participate in support groups for parents and siblings of children with cystic fibrosis; they offer support and information and promote helpful strategies for coping with cystic fibrosis |

When the child returns home, physical therapy and aerosol by nebulizer at night are continued indefinitely. Some physicians believe there is too great a risk of increasing the resistance of bacteria to antibiotics, but others believe that severely ill patients cannot be controlled adequately without this therapy. They recommend that antibiotic therapy be instituted by parents whenever the child has an elevated temperature and difficulty breathing. Drugs include tetracycline (over 8 years of age), erythromycin, and oxacillin 25 to 60 mg/kg/day, depending on the child's clinical response. At times, aerosol antibiotic therapy may be recommended (neomycin solution 50 mg/ml or colistin 5 to 10 mg/ml plus isoproterenol) two or three times per day. At times expectorants and bronchodilators may be helpful. During the winter months especially, a dry atmosphere may be combatted with nebulization of aerosol via tent. In summer, temperatures within the tent may be uncomfortable. A room air conditioner will help decrease the heat.

Pancreatic deficiency is treated through a high-calorie, high-protein, moderate-fat diet in addition to pancreatic enzymes. A double dose of liposoluble vitamins prepared in a water-miscible liquid is given daily. Pancreatic extract is given with each meal.

Excessive perspiration in hot weather results in a great loss of sodium and chloride. An intravenous saline infusion to prevent cardiovascular collapse may be necessary. Thus, during hot weather supplemental sodium chloride is given orally.

Nursing Management

Observation, recording, and reporting of the character of feces aid in assessment of pancreatic activity, while observation, recording, and reporting of the child's respiratory status aid in assessment of pulmonary problems. Adequate preparation of the child, if he is old enough to understand, for sweat iontophoresis, chest x-ray, pulmonary function tests, nasopharyngeal cultures, duodenal aspiration, and stool collection ensures cooperation.

Nursing care for children receiving oxygen therapy is the same as that previously described. Although a physical therapist may be providing chest therapy to promote bronchial drainage, it behooves the nurse to know these techniques in the event that the therapist cannot always come at specified times.

Unfortunately, infections are common. While it is critical for a nurse to obtain cultures correctly, administering systemic antibiotics properly and noting the child's responses to these treatments also are very important nursing activities. Generally, these children are treated with aminoglucosides such as gentamycin, amikacin, and tobramycin, while the more common antipseudomonal penicillins prescribed are carbenicillin and ticarcillin.

As the child nears discharge, the nurse should stress the importance of treating him as nearly normally as possible. For example, the child should be allowed to exercise and play according to his individual tolerance. The school-age child should attend regular classes when phys-

ically able. Parents should be included in the child's care whenever possible. Before he returns home, they must learn how to perform physical therapy to the chest (percussion and drainage), administer aerosol bronchodilators, evaluate breathing exercises, administer other medications properly, and know methods of giving pancreatic enzymes with meals. Parents are also instructed in ways of trying to prevent respiratory infection and are encouraged to ask questions and discuss fears.

Complying with follow-up visits is imperative if pulmonary changes are to be identified early; therefore, nursing efforts must be directed toward explanations which emphasize the need to do so. These visits allow providers to identify children who may require hospitalization for a thorough pulmonary clean-out or indicate the need for changes in maintenance protocols.

Cystic fibrosis is a progressive, devastating disease which has death as its inevitable outcome. Once its presence is identified, the nurse is involved in teaching the child and family basic principles which encompass care so that the child's health status can be maintained at a maximum level of wellness. The repeated hospitalizations, the worsening pulmonary symptoms, and the deterioration that occurs over time also require a nurse to be honest, patient, supportive, and understanding.

Respiratory Problems in the Toddler

Aspiration of Foreign Objects

Toddlers who are up and about, investigating the environment, are particularly prone to the aspiration of a variety of objects and foods. Aspiration occurs most frequently in children from 6 months to 3 years of age. The severity of the problem depends on what has been aspirated and the degree of obstruction. Although there is choking, gagging, wheezing, or coughing initially, there may be a symptom-free period for days or weeks when the original precipitating episode is forgotten. The time interval produces little pathological change or a total respiratory response.

Laryngeal-Tracheal Aspiration

A foreign body located in the larynx or trachea causes severe respiratory distress, hoarseness, a croupy cough, aphonia with hemoptysis, and dyspnea with wheezing; cyanosis may also occur. If the object is opaque, it can be detected on roentgenographic examination; however, if it is nonopaque, it can be identified by the physiological effects produced. A direct laryngoscopy confirms the diagnosis and provides access to the foreign body.

Bronchial Aspiration

Symptoms related to aspirated objects which lodge in the bronchi are affected by the degree of obstruction and the local pathological changes which have occurred. A nonobstructive foreign body may produce few symptoms even after a prolonged period, while an obstructive object may produce signs and symptoms and pathological changes quickly. If there is a slight obstruction, wheezing will be present, but in a more severe form, emphysema or atelectasis may be produced with subsequent chronic pulmonary disease. Metallic or plastic aspirants may produce obstructions because of their size and injury to tissue because of their shape. If the foreign body is of a vegetal source, such as a peanut, bean, pea, or watermelon seed, it has a tendency to swell to many times its size and is serious because bronchitis may develop with a resultant cough, fever, and dyspnea. Most of these objects are radiolucent, and so they are not seen on x-ray. An asymmetrical auscultation is most significant.

If signs, symptoms, and history suggest aspiration of a foreign object, treatment depends on its location. When the object is in the primary bronchus, or in a more distal position, it is usually removed by bronchoscopy.

Nursing Management

These toddlers are usually frightened, coughing, wheezing, and cyanotic. Relieving the child's distress, gaining his confidence, and establishing a meaningful relationship with his parents will promote trust between the child and the nurse. Although he may not fully comprehend them, procedures should be explained to him. Since these admissions are usually of an emergency nature, initial preparation of the patient is limited to bare essentials.

An important nursing observation after a bronchoscopy or laryngoscopy is the patient's ability to reestablish his swallowing reflex. The clear fluids initially offered should be given slowly and cautiously. When the child has reacted fully and has no difficulty swallowing, fluids should be urged because they tend to decrease the amount of soreness experienced. The patient should also be observed for laryngeal edema which causes an airway block and increases respiratory distress. Monitoring respirations and identifying any breathing difficulty (increased respiratory rate or retractions) are important.

After the object has been removed, vigorous CPT is done every 4 hours, preceded by nebulized bronchodilators. These children may be placed in mist tents to provide them with additional amounts of oxygen and humidity.

Since he has been hurt, the toddler usually rebels by crying and screaming, which tend to increase the irritation of the respiratory tract. An effort should be made to calm him. His parents may be of tremendous assistance.

Total prevention is impossible. However, the numbers of aspirations seen annually can be decreased if efforts are made to educate parents and the public. Ideally, all parents of young children should be taught how to manage airway obstruction (Chap. 12). Hot dogs, round candies, nuts, sunflower seeds, popcorn, and other similar edibles should not be offered to infants or toddlers. Parents also need to check toys for small, removable parts, such as the wheels of a car or the eyes on stuffed animals. Toddlers should be discouraged from force-feeding younger siblings in play and also should be taught not to run with food or other objects in their mouths. Aspiration of foreign objects is a health problem over which adults can exert some control.

Chemical Pneumonia

The severity or intensity of the manifestations of chemical pneumonia depends on three factors which should be considered in every case of aspiration or ingestion: the material ingested, the individual child's response to that substance, and the amount involved. Most chemical pneumonias seen in clinical pediatrics fall into one of two categories: hydrocarbon and lipoid pneumonias. Some authorities believe the aspiration of lipoids and hydrocarbons during swallowing, vomiting, or gastric lavage is the cause of lung involvement.

Hydrocarbon Pneumonia

Several thousand children under 6 years of age accidentally ingest hydrocarbons each year. These substances are classified as either aliphatics or aromatics. The *aliphatic* hydrocarbons are kerosene, gasoline, furniture and floor polishes, pesticides, and Stoddard solvent in paint thinners. The *aromatic* hydrocarbons include benzene, xylene, and toluene compounds found in paint removers, airplane glue, and other plastic-binding products. There are combinations of both types in some products, and all of them can affect the lungs as well as the central nervous system. The usual amount aspirated into the lung by children is estimated to be 2.5 to 4.0 ml. At least 12 ml/kg is needed to produce toxic effects (Einhorn, 1987). Thus, most children are asymptomatic or have mild respiratory discomfort at the time of ingestion.

Symptomatic children may complain of a burning feeling in the mouth and throat. They choke and gag, become cyanotic, cough, complain of nausea, and vomit. More serious manifestations include tachycardia, nasal flaring, tachypnea, retractions, and grunting. In association with this chemical pneumonitis, children become febrile with temperatures ranging from 38 to 40°C (100 to 104°F). Pleural effusion may develop, as manifested by rales, rhonchi, and wheezes. Blood gases may be abnormal. Central nervous system manifestations are variable and include dizziness, hypotonia, lethargy, irritability, convulsions, and unconsciousness.

Changes in the lungs may not be evident for 2 to 6 hours and may progress for as long as 72 hours. Follow-up x-rays demonstrate a return to normal in 5 to 15 days. Respiratory symptoms may not appear for several hours, even though x-ray results are abnormal. Conversely, they may be evident before changes are noted on x-ray. Given these inconsistencies, all asymptomatic children are observed for 8 hours. If they remain symptom-free, they are not hospitalized.

Symptomatic children are admitted to an intensive care unit for observation. The first aim of treatment is to prevent further aspiration if possible. The second aim is to provide cardiorespiratory support. To prevent further aspiration, the child is placed in an upright or semirecumbent position and is disturbed as little as possible. Cardiocirculatory support, if needed, consists of airway maintenance, oxygenation, ventilation, and maintenance of acid-base balance and renal function.

Gastric lavage is indicated if the child has ingested

1. A camphorated hydrocarbon, an insecticide, or turpentine
2. A chlorinated hydrocarbon (e.g., carbon tetrachloride, DDT, or chlordane)
3. An alkylaromatic substance (e.g., xylene, toluene), benzene, or gasoline
4. A hydrocarbon containing an organophosphate or metal

Children who are comatose or have a depressed gag reflex are intubated before lavage is begun. The child is placed on his right side, and his head is lowered. It is imperative that suction be immediately available. In fully conscious children, some physicians may use syrup of ipecac for gastric evacuation.

Nursing Management

These young children need very careful respiratory monitoring, since deterioration of their status can be determined by an increase in respiratory rate, increasingly labored respirations, or dyspnea. Frequently these patients are febrile, and antipyretic administration as well as other cooling measures should be carried out as ordered by the physician. Observations of vital signs, which is done hourly initially, can be decreased appropriately as the patient's condition stabilizes or improves.

Gastroenteritis may be a problem; therefore, the patient's output should be recorded at the bedside after each stool. His skin turgor should be assessed carefully, as should his state of hydration. Parenteral fluids may be started, and they must be monitored closely. The institution of oxygen therapy with humidity is common, and all the equipment should be checked frequently, including a measurement of oxygen levels at 3-hour intervals with a Beckman analyzer or another device.

Observing the patient and evaluating his comfort are essential components of nursing care. Cyanosis and dyspnea may occur, and observation is thus imperative. The child's position should be changed every 3 hours to prevent additional pulmonary complications. Postural drainage, if needed, should be done conscientiously. Since drowsiness may be a clinical manifestation, the patient's level of consciousness should be monitored. Although twitching, convulsions, and coma are rare, the nurse may be involved in preventing these sequelae through the use of observational skills.

Parents of children who have accidentally ingested a harmful substance are usually overwhelmed by the sudden onset of symptoms, the emergency measures, and the equipment used. They may verbalize feelings of negligence or guilt, and it is important to listen to them and understand the emotions they are experiencing.

It is important to review basic safety with parents. They should be advised not to transfer solutions from the original containers to other bottles. Toddlers associate contents with the shape of familiar bottles, inadvertently

consuming a hydrocarbon instead of the juice or tonic usually found in those bottles. All toxic substances and drugs should be kept in locked containers away from toddler accessibility. Also, "Mr. Yuk" labels should be placed on all household products. The parents of toddlers should have a 1-oz bottle of syrup of ipecac on hand at all times. In addition, the telephone numbers of the local poison control center and family physician shold be prominently posted.

Nurses need to urge legislation which mandates safe packaging and the use of warnings on labels. They can also speak to parents' groups and visit nursery schools. In performing these types of services nurses can increase the awareness of adults and also teach young children prevention.

Lipoid Pneumonia

Lipoid pneumonia, caused by the aspiration or accumulation of oil in the alveoli, is a chronic condition which may occur in children with cleft palates, in debilitated infants with improper swallowing or depressed cough reflexes, and in children who are force-fed or maintained in a horizontal position. Aspiration of milk is a common cause of lipoid bronchopneumonia in the first year of life. Administering substances with oily bases such as mineral oil, castor oil, and cod liver oil to crying toddlers may result in lipoid pneumonia.

Vegetable oils such as olive oil, cottonseed oil, and sesame oil are the least toxic and least irritating lipoids. They are not hydrolyzed by lung lipases, cause little damage, and are removed mainly by expectoration. Animal oils, such as cod liver oil, are very dangerous because they have a very high fatty acid content; when hydrolyzed by lung lipases, the liberated fatty acids combine with those present in the originally aspirated substance and produce severe inflammatory responses.

After aspiration an initial interstitial, proliferative inflammatory response occurs. The second phase involves the development of diffuse, proliferative fibrosis, which is followed by the formation of multiple, localized nodules. A cough is present, and dyspnea may be evident in severe cases; however, there may be no other manifestations unless there is a superimposed infection. Secondary bronchopneumonic infections are common. Roentgenographic chest films reveal patchy to nodular infiltrations or densities, especially in the right lung.

The prognosis is dependent on the extent of involvement, whether administered oil preparations are continued, and the overall physical status of the young child. Treatment is symptomatic, and the prevention of secondary infections is essential. Surgical resection may be considered later if pulmonic involvement is localized to one segment or lobe.

Nursing Management

It is imperative for nurses to remember the causes of lipoid pneumonia. Although feeding a child slowly is time-consuming, particularly if he objects to eating or is debilitated, the nurse must do so if the likelihood of aspiration is to be decreased. Cradling the child or holding him upright while he is being fed may enhance his oral intake. If the child is bottle-fed, the hole in the nipple must not be too large or the flow of fluid may be too much for the child. If the hole is too small, his oral intake will not be adequate. There should be an ongoing evaluation of his sucking and swallowing reflexes. It is also important that such information be placed on the young patient's Kardex or in his nursing care plan to assist personnel in identifying nursing problems and successful interventions.

Realistically, toddlers may resist certain oily base medications which the nurse is attempting to administer. Where possible, water-miscible vitamins should be given to these children. Castor or mineral oil should be administered very carefully. Several methods of gaining the child's cooperation are explored and evaluated. When parents are expected to continue the medication at home, sharing what has been learned by the staff is most helpful for them.

Proper positioning of the young patient is another nursing function, for if changes are not considered, hypostatic pneumonia may be an additional complication. Placing a child on his side or abdomen lessens the possibility of aspiration and is essential if he has a tendency to regurgitate or vomit after feedings. Parents may need some instruction about administering feedings, vitamins, and other medications. Including them in the care of the child, where feasible, decreases their anxiety and apprehension.

Asthma

Asthma is the most common cause of chronic disease in children under 17 years of age, and its prevalence is increasing. There are many factors which precipitate this largely reversible obstructive process.

The most common allergens which cause asthma in children are inhalants such as house dust, mold spores, airborne pollens (trees, grasses), and feathers as well as the saliva and dander of dogs, cats, and other animals. Certain foods such as egg whites, cow's milk, chocolate, wheat, and other cereal grains can result in asthma, especially in infants. In addition, certain factors aggravate asthma, such as respiratory infections, rapid changes in temperature and barometric pressure, the pollutants found in large cities, strong odors, tobacco smoke, and stress within the family. Vigorous, sustained exercise for 6 to 8 minutes, which results in an apical rate exceeding 170 beats per minute, can also cause bronchospasm. It may also be induced by aspirin. In some children, a specific cause can be identified; however, in many instances, a combination of factors provokes the onset or aggravation of asthma.

An acute attack, which may have a gradual or abrupt onset, consists of bronchospasm, mucosal edema, and the hypersecretion of tenacious material from the bronchi. As the spasm and edema increase, there is tightness in the chest, accessory respiratory muscles are utilized, and wheezing becomes audible. There may be paroxysmal coughing. In a severe attack, these children are diaphoretic, anxious, and cyanotic. Characteristically, rales are heard throughout the lung fields and there is a prolonged expiration accompanied by wheezing.

Older children and adolescents frequently sit upright with their shoulders hunched forward as they utilize accessory respiratory muscles. Infants who appear to be comfortable in a supine position may have wheezing on inspiration and expiration.

With frequent asthmatic episodes over a long period of time, chronic emphysema may develop because of the thickening of the bronchiolar walls and the child's persistent effort to aerate his lungs. Physical characteristics of this chronic condition include prominent sternum, rounded back, and increased anteroposterior chest circumference which produces the "barrel chest" so typically found in asthmatic children.

A diagnosis of asthma is more likely in the presence of the following data: a family history of asthma, repeated attacks of bronchiolitis in the infant, eosinophilia, immediate positive response to epinephrine, sudden onset without preceding respiratory infection, or extremely prolonged expiration. Eczema in infancy may be a precursor of asthma in childhood.

The diagnosis is based mainly on clinical findings. When a febrile incident precedes an attack, wheezing may occur for a day or two after the appearance of rhinorrhea. Resolution may take place in a few hours or a few days. An abrupt onset may be accompanied by a coughing paroxysm. As the attack progresses, increasing dyspnea, prolonged expiration, and expiratory rales occur. If the attack is severe, pulmonary ventilation is decreased. Flaring of the alae nasi, retractions, cyanosis, and hypercapnia indicate the air hunger which results. The child becomes restless and tired, his heart and respiratory rates increase, his sputum becomes tenacious, and he may perspire.

Early in an acute attack, the PCO_2 will be lowered because the child is hyperventilating. A normal PCO_2 in asthma is a sign of CO_2 retention and early respiratory failure. When it exceeds 50 to 60 mmHg, the pH is apt to fall rapidly, and respiratory acidosis increases. At this time, assisted ventilation is necessary.

Confirmation of the diagnosis of asthma is made through chest x-ray, examinations of the sputum and peripheral blood, tests for hypersensitivity, and pulmonary function tests. Chest x-ray *may* indicate hyperventilation during an asthmatic attack through elevation of the rib cage, depression of the diaphragm, and increased translucency of the lung fields. Bronchial obstruction and infection may result in pneumonic consolidation, revealed in segmental or lobar collapse or patchy shadows.

In asthma, sputum is mucoid or mucopurulent. Bronchial casts and eosinophilia are present. With superimposed infection, bacteria and pus cells may be found.

Although the best evidence of an allergic causation for asthma is obtained through careful history taking, skin testing for allergens may support an allergic basis for the disease process. Skin testing is accomplished through pricking or scratching especially prepared antigens into the skin of the forearm or through intradermal injection.

NURSING CARE PLAN

23-3 The Child with Asthma

Clinical Problem/Nursing Diagnosis	Expected Outcome	Nursing Interventions
Decreased breath sounds Expiratory and/or inspiratory wheezing Dyspnea and retractions Prolonged expiratory phase of breathing Cyanosis Anxiety and/or restlessness Ineffective airway clearance related to bronchospasm	Child's airway will remain patent with blood gas values reflective of adequate oxygenation (PaO$_2$ > 60 mmHg, PaCO$_2$ < 45 mmHg, pH 7.35-7.45) Child will demonstrate improved aeration and quality of breath sounds in all lung lobes	Assess severity and progression of respiratory distress q 30 min during acute phase of asthmatic attack Monitor vital signs q 30-60 min Observe for decreased breath sounds, wheezing, retracting, grunting, cyanosis, or use of accessory muscles Note respiratory rate, depth, regularity, and symmetry of chest expansion Identify duration of inspiratory and expiratory phases of breathing and observe for prolonged expiratory phase Assess nailbeds and mucous membranes for cyanosis Observe child for increased anxiety, restlessness, and changes in behavior and levels of consciousness Assess apical rate for rhythm, regularity, and presence of pulsus paradoxus Monitor arterial blood gas values for signs of respiratory failure decreased PaO$_2$ < 60 mmHg; elevated PaCO$_2$ > 45 mmHg, and lowered pH < 7.35) Administer humidified oxygen by face mask to maintain PaO$_2$ > 60 mmHg, PaCo$_2$ < 45 mmHg, and pH 7.35-7.45 Administer sodium bicarbonate properly as ordered to treat acidosis Titrate oxygen therapy properly as indicated by clinical status and ABG values Clarify with physician acceptable vital sign parameters and expectations for notifying physician Obtain accurate body weight on admission for drug dosage calculations Administer bronchodilators IV or by nebulizer; monitor vital signs during administration and note changes in rhythm, regularly, rate of apical pulse, and blood pressure; monitor theophylline levels closely and assess for signs of toxicity (nausea, vomiting, restlessness) Determine need for cardiorespiratory monitor for child requiring frequent (q 1-2 h) isoproterenol (Isuprel) nebulizer treatments or continuous IV bronchodilator therapy with beta$_2$-adrenergic agents Auscultate breath sounds before and after treatment; assess and document effectiveness of therapy in reducing respiratory distress Administer steroids and prescribed medications; assess and document effectiveness of all treatments Avoid administration of sedatives in nonintubated child to prevent masking signs of respiratory depression Hydrate child adequately Elevate head of bed 40 to 45° to promote maximum lung expansion: assist child in leaning forward with arms extended over pillow or bed table to optimize lung expansion

Clinical Problem/Nursing Diagnosis	Expected Outcome	Nursing Interventions
Unable to rest or sleep Restlessness Fearful facial expression Difficulty cooperating with oxygen therapy Anxiety related to respiratory distress; stressors of hospitalization and required therapy	Child will experience an alleviation of anxiety-induced symptoms of increased respiratory distress Child will be able to rest comfortably Child will feel safe and secure during hospitalization	Encourage age-appropriate and parental support and participation in care such as child holding face mask and holding child on lap for nebulizer treatments Provide child and parents with reassurance and support; address their fears, concerns, and questions Assess level of understanding by child and parents of required treatments and procedures and appropriate interventions Promote adequate rest periods for child: encourage parents to take time out for diversion Provide quiet, restful environment Provide young child with security blanket or toy and allow school-age child or adolescent to express fears, experiences, and concerns about illness Determine need for psychological intervention for parent and/or child to enhance family's coping with chronic illness
Dyspnea Vomiting NPO Potential fluid volume deficit related to respiratory distress; altered intake	Child will remain in fluid and electrolyte as well as an acid-base balance	Assess child for signs of dehydration: dry mucous membranes, depressed anterior fontanel, absence of tears, poor skin turgor, decreased urine output, and urine specific gravity > 1.025 Monitor intake and output hourly Monitor urine specific gravity; dipstick for ketones, protein, glucose, and blood on every voiding until stable; document results Test emesis for blood; note amount and color; document results Administer intravenous fluids correctly Monitor child for signs of electrolyte imbalance; note alterations in vital signs; note muscle cramping; monitor electrolytes as they are obtained Promote calm, quiet, supportive environment to reduce anxiety Support parents so they can comfort and support child through treatments, procedures, and therapy Reassure, calm, and support child, especially during acute respiratory distress
Dyspnea with activity Fatigue Restlessness Activity intolerance and Fatigue related to respiratory distress	Child will conserve energy and oxygen reserves Child will have adequate periods of rest and sleep	Institute measures to reduce respiratory distress as cited previously Organize care and treatments to minimize disturbances and optimize length and frequency of rest periods; conserve energy and oxygen reserves; keep child off oral feeding (NPO); encourage bed rest Promote calm, quiet environment, free of allergens and known irritants (minimize cold stress and noise) Monitor child's physiological and psychological tolerance of invasive procedures (IV placement, arterial blood gases); support child through them Encourage parental participation in calming measures which enhance child's sense of security Institute measures which have a calming effect and promote rest and/or sleep (back massage, being read to, listening to music) Encourage PO liquids once child's respiratory status stabilizes; avoid intake of excessively cold fluids Advance child's dietary intake slowly (both liquids and solids) as respiratory status improves Provide age-appropriate instruction related to anatomy and physiology

Continued.

NURSING CARE PLAN 23-3 The Child with Asthma—cont'd

Clinical Problem/Nursing Diagnosis	Expected Outcome	Nursing Interventions
Newly diagnosed asthmatic child requesting information Noncompliance with medications, treatments, and/or prior teaching Knowledge deficit related to: diagnosis of asthma; medications and treatments	Child and parents will verbalize and redemonstrate understanding of medications (dose, route, times, actions, side-effects, toxic signs), chest physical therapy, and pathophysiology and signs of asthma as well as methods of preventing asthmatic attacks	Provide age-appropriate instruction related to anatomy and physiology of the respiratory system (use charts and coloring books from American Lung Association), pathophysiology of asthma, medications (dose, times, route, side effects, and toxic symptoms), stressing need to take *exact* prescribed dosage; proper administration and strict use of nebulizer/aerosol therapy Evaluate child and family's understanding and knowledge of what has been taught Review environmental factors which precipitate attacks such as smoke, dust, animals, known allergens, and irritants; avoid vigorous exercise and excessive cold Provide written instructions regarding medication schedule, treatment protocol, etc. Teach child and parents signs of respiratory distress and impending asthmatic attack and explain what they need to do promptly Consult with respiratory therapist and teach parents how to perform physical therapy; teach child breathing exercises and relaxation exercises Instruct child and parents about importance of consuming large amounts of liquids Arrange follow-up visits to allergy clinic Refer family to community resources, e.g., American Lung Association, for variety of children's workshops which focus on coping, prevention, and exercise Assess need for psychological counseling in coping with chronic illness Known asthmatic child Assess understanding of previous teaching and reinforce weak areas and/or deficiencies Explore child's feelings about illness and required care as well as feelings about self Encourage verbalization of issues which affect compliance with care to optimize child's health Document home medication regimen in nursing history; note theophylline level on admission to assess compliance Encourage participation in planning care; facilitate peer support system with other children who have asthma so they may share frustrations, methods of coping, and feelings

Intradermal injection causes a more severe wheal and erythematous flare than does pricking or scratching the skin.

Increased airway resistance may be discovered through an increase in total lung capacity (TLC), functional residual capacity (FRC), and residual volume (RV) and a decrease in force vital capacity (FVC), forced expiratory volume in 1 second (FEV_1) and maximum midexpiratory flow rate (MMEFR) (particularly MMEFR 25-75), and peak flow rate (PFR). Vital capacity (VC) may be normal or decreased (Buckley, 1987). Serial recordings of FEV_1 and MMEFR 25-75 using simple spirometry are valuable in determining progress and evaluating the effect of various therapeutic agents in the long-term management of children with asthma. Inexpensive flowmeters for de-

termining PFR are available for home use. In the majority of children, asthma may be brought under control with appropriate treatment.

Treatment consists of preventive measures, managing the acute attack, and long-term management. Preventive measures include hyposensitization, removal of incitants, and the use of bronchodilators. Treatment by hyposensitization seems to be most effective in seasonal asthma. A child who has gross pollen sensitivity is given a preseasonal course of pollen antigen injections. Although hyposensitization of children who are allergic to house dust, animal danders, molds, and various insects has been less effective in treatment than has hyposensitization to pollens, it is utilized in children who cannot avoid contact with such antigens. Removal of offending antigens is a more effective step in the general management of an asthmatic child, and the child may have to forgo having certain household pets.

The severity of the attack and the degree of obstruction determine the type of treatment protocol instituted. The drugs described in Table 23-6 are some of the medications used in treating moderately severe episodes of asthma. They are administered orally, subcutaneously, or intravenously; by nebulizer; or by specially designed inhalers.

Increasing a child's oral fluid intake is mandatory; however, if the child is demonstrating substantial distress, it may not be possible. Furthermore, fluid losses from vomiting, diaphoresis, and hyperventilation can threaten electrolyte balance, necessitating parenteral therapy. To prevent fluid accumulation around the small bronchioles, fluid replacement is generally 1 to 1½ maintenance requirements. If acidosis develops as a result of a continuously inadequate gaseous exchange, sodium bicarbonate is given intravenously. Correcting the acidosis may reestablish responsiveness in an epinephrine-fast child. Humidified oxygen delivered by mask is usually indicated, and vigorous chest physical therapy may be done. Mist tents offer no advantage and interfere with observation.

When a child fails to respond to the aggressive therapy described above, he is in *status asthmaticus.* Administration of bronchodilators is continued, and serum theophylline levels are monitored. Metaproterenol or isoetharine may be given by mask or nebulizer, and methylprednisolone may be administered intravenously. During a prolonged or unusually severe attack, the child may be unable to move tenacious secretions from the bronchioles. In addition, air is trapped within the alveoli. Fatigue and diminishing pulmonary function result, breath sounds become diminished or absent, and cyanosis appears. With the resultant rise of the arterial PCO_2 a mixed acidosis occurs: respiratory acidosis due to retention of carbon dioxide and metabolic acidosis due to anoxia. If the PCO_2 rises above 60 mmHg, assisted ventilation is usually prescribed. Positive pressure breathing by mask may be intermittent or continuous (Fig. 23-6). If the child is unable to help in this method for any reason, assisted ventilation is provided via an endotracheal or nasotracheal tube. When an endotracheal tube is in place, aspiration of secretions from the bronchial tree is facilitated and bronchial lavage with warm physiologic saline solution may be accomplished. Sometimes a tracheostomy is necessary to provide adequate assisted ventilation and bronchial lavage. Cupped-hand percussion to the chest and postural drainage may facilitate bronchial aspiration.

A child who is receiving such care requires the cooperation of the physician, anesthesiologist, nurse, inhalation therapist, and physical therapist. Also, continuous monitoring of body temperature, electrocardiograms, central venous pressure, and peripheral arterial pressure require an intensive care setting. Arterial blood must be examined frequently for pH, PCO_2, and PO_2 in order to provide adequate control of ventilation. The child's electrolyte balance is identified through determination of serum sodium,

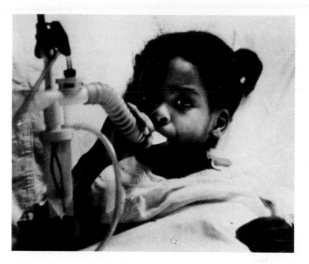

FIGURE 23-6 A preschooler administering her own intermittent positive pressure breathing. *(Courtesy Boston City Hospital.)*

potassium, and chloride values. The heroic measures taken to save the child in status asthmaticus may result in complications such as pneumomediastinum, pneumothorax, subcutaneous emphysema, cardiac arrest, and tracheal or glottic stenosis.

Long-term management of an asthmatic child consists of adequate drug therapy, avoidance of precipitating factors, and humidified indoor air at 40 to 50 percent during the cold months of the year. Precipitating factors include known allergens, respiratory infections, and respiratory obstruction due to enlarged tonsils and adenoids. Known allergens are avoided if possible. Respiratory infections caused by bacteria are treated with specific antibiotics. Emotional factors rarely serve as a primary trigger. Since tonsillar and adenoid tissues diminish after adequate allergic management, their removal is not undertaken unless the child fails to respond to an adequate program of allergic management, including hyposensitization. The physical therapist can teach the child how to improve ventilation by controlling his breathing pattern.

Children with asthma are at risk for complications of influenza infections. The Committee on Infectious Diseases of the American Academy of Pediatrics has recommended that they receive yearly immunizations of killed influenza vaccine (Committee on Infectious Diseases, 1986).

Children with mild asthma do not need daily medication. If symptoms occur, they are advised to use albuterol, metaproterenol, or terbutaline, two actuations every 6 hours, by metered dose inhaler. The specific drug is prescribed by the physician.

Several alternative daily antiasthma drug treatments are prescribed for children who have moderate asthma, that is, children who wheeze one or two times per week and cough intermittently. Some physicians prefer to use a sustained-release theophylline preparation by mouth every 8 to 12 hours while others advocate cromolyn sodium inhalations three to four times a day by Spinhaler or home nebulizer. Either treatment is supplemented with an adrenergic drug by mouth or by inhalation as needed (Table 23-6). Children who do not respond to this therapy are said to have severe asthma. For these children, steroid therapy is added (Table 23-6).

Metered dose inhalers (MDIs) may be difficult for some children to use, particularly if they cannot coordinate actuation with inspiration. Many physicians recommend the use of a spacer device attached to the MDI. With spacers, the drug is more likely to be delivered to the small airways (the target site). Hand et al. (1988) have suggested that spacers be used for inhalation of steroids to reduce the incidence of oral candidiasis and dysphonia and adrenergics in children who have coordination difficulties.

There is no uniform agreement regarding the technique of MDI usage. At this time, it seems appropriate to follow the manufacturer's instructions for use. According to Hand et al. (1988), the most important steps are the slow, steady inhalation coordinated with actuation and then holding the breath for at least 10 seconds. The recommended time between actuations cited in the literature varies from 1 minute to 15 minutes.

Exercise and sports are not prohibited for children who have asthma. A child whose asthma is under control must be evaluated individually for tolerance of duration and intensity of effort. For many children, use of an adrenergic by MDI 15 minutes before exercising or engaging in a sport will prevent wheezing and coughing.

Nursing Management

Advances in clinical pharmacology have improved the management of children with asthma and have increased the responsibilities of pediatric nurses. In addition to precisely computing and properly administering medication, nurses play a major role in observing the patients, noting their responses to the drugs used, monitoring infusions, and analyzing blood gas results.

While aminophylline, the drug of choice, is being in-

TABLE 23-6 Bronchodilators for Asthmatic Children

Drug	Action	Dosage*	Side Effects	Nursing Implications
Albuteral sulfate (Proventil, Ventolin) (90 µg per actuation)	Adrenergic: relaxes smooth muscle of bronchi; is more effective by inhalation	Oral: 6 mo to 9 yr, 2 mg q 6 h; > 9 yr, 4 mg q 6 h Metered dose inhaler: ≥ 7 yr, 1-2 inhalations q 4-6 h	Tremors, tachycardia, palpitations, increased blood pressure, dizziness, nausea, heartburn	Improvement in pulmonary functions begins within 15 min; maximum effect occurs within 60-90 min; effects continue 4 to 6 h; children must be taught proper use of inhaler (and spacer, if indicated) For exercise-induced asthma, inhaler should be used 15 min before exercise or sporting events
Aminophylline, theophylline, ethylenediamine (IV: 25 mg/ml; PO: 100 and 200 mg)	Relaxes smooth muscle of respiratory tract	*Not currently receiving theophylline:*† *Children 6 mo to 9 yr* IV loading dose: 6 mg/kg; maintenance for next 12 h: 1.2 mg/kg/h; maintenance beyond 12 h: 1.0 mg/kg/h. *Children 9-16 yr* IV loading dose: 6 mg/kg/maintenance for next 12 h: 1.0 mg/kg/h; maintenance beyond 12 h: 0.8 mg/kg/h; orally: 7.5 mg/kg for an acute asthmatic attack; 5 mg/kg q 6 h for maintenance	Nausea, vomiting, epigastric pain and diarrhea; cardiovascular effects include hypotension, ventricular tachycardia, and other irregularities; central nervous system hyperirritability, seizures, circulatory collapse	When this drug is being given IV, patient *must* be attached to a cardiac monitor to identify arrhythmias which can develop; it should be infused *slowly* to prevent circulatory collapse or cardiac arrest; seizures may occur; a nurse must be in attendance to monitor rate of flow; therapeutic theophylline level is 10-20 µg/ml, while toxic signs may develop with concentration > 20 µg/ml

*IV = intravenous; IM = intramuscular; SC = subcutaneous.
†For children currently receiving theophylline products, the loading dose is 0.5 mg/kg—deferred until a theophylline level is obtained.
Adapted from G. M. Scipien et al. (eds.), *Comprehensive Pediatric Nursing*, 3d ed., McGraw-Hill, New York, 1986, pp. 886-889.

TABLE 23-6 Bronchodilators for Asthmatic Children—cont'd

Drug	Action	Dosage*	Side Effects	Nursing Implications
Beclomethasone dipropionate (Beclovent, Vanceril) (inhaler: 10 mg)	Steroid: is a topical anti-inflammatory adrenocorticosteroid which acts on bronchi and bronchioles; is used by those who require long-term glucocorticosteroids and those who do not respond to conventional treatment	Metered dose inhaler: 6-12 yr: 1-2 inhalations (50 μg each) four times per day, with 60 s between inhalations; should not exceed 10 inhalations per day	Dysphonia and mild oral candidiasis. Spacer devices reduce these problems (Hand et al., 1988) *Caution:* When some patients on systemic corticosteroids are switched to aerosol therapy, they develop adrenal insufficiency and death can ensue	Patients who are receiving bronchodilators by inhalation concurrently are encouraged to use them 15-20 min before inhaling beclomethasone; delay maximizes respiratory penetration; these patients need to be taught good oral hygiene to decrease likelihood of fungal infections; child is cautioned against use of inhaler for acute asthmatic attack
Cromolyn sodium (Aarane, Intal) inhalation capsules: 20 mg each for use with Spinhaler turboinhaler)	Prophylactic: has a local effect on mucosa of lungs and prevents release of histamine as well as other substances which trigger allergic responses	1 capsule (20 mg) inhaled q 6 h *only* in children over 5 yr of age	Bronchospasm, nasal congestion, coughing, and pharyngeal irritation; other effects: urticaria, exfoliative dermatitis, dizziness, dysuria, nausea, and headache	When administered, capsule must be used with Spinhaler so that powder can be inhaled Parents and child need to understand the drug is ineffective if capsule is taken orally; it should not be taken to prevent an acute asthmatic attack Corticosteroid doses may need to be decreased when it is evident that cromolyn is effective
Epinephrine adrenalin chloride [ampules: 1:1000 (aqueous) with 1 mg/ml]	Adrenergic: dilates bronchioles to relieve bronchospasm in asthma	0.01 ml/kg SC; can be repeated twice at 20- to 30-min intervals; maximum dose is 0.3 ml; it is rapid-acting (3-10 min); Sus-Phrine is a long-acting epinephrine suspension which can be effective for up to 6 h; it may be ordered following a response to *first* dose of epinephrine; dosage: 0.005 ml/kg	Arrhythmias, nausea, headache, palpitations, vomiting, hypertension, pallor	A nurse should be in attendance monitoring child's response to drug; tissue necrosis can occur at local injection site; using a tuberculin syringe to administer epinephrine decreases likelihood of medication error
Isoetharine (Bronkosol-2, Dey-Lute)	Adrenergic: relaxes smooth muscle of bronchi	Nebulizer (1:1000 solution): 0.5 ml in 1.5 ml saline q 4-6 h Metered dose inhaler: 2 inhalatioins q 4-6 h	Nervousness, palpitations, agitation, hand tremors, loss of sleep	Children must be taught proper use of inhaler (and spacer if indicated) Parents are taught use with nebulizer (.e.g., PulmoAide) for infants and young children
Isoproterenol (Isuprel, Proternol) (tablets: 10 and 15 mg; nebulizer: 1:100, 1:200; inhalant mistometer; 1:500; ampule: 1.0 mg per 5 ml)	Adrenergic: relaxes smooth bronchial muscle in bronchospasm	Nebulizer (1:200 solution): 0.1-0.5 ml in 2 ml H_2O q 4-6 h; IV: 0.05-4.0 μg/min Metered dose inhaler: 1-2 inhalations q 4-6 h	Arrhythmias, nervousness, headache, palpitations, hypertension (excessive inhalation can aggravate the asthma)	It should *not* be administered *with* epinephrine because serious arrhythmias can develop; sublingual and oral absorption is unreliable

Continued.

TABLE 23-6 Bronchodilators for Asthmatic Children—cont'd

Drug	Action	Dosage*	Side Effects	Nursing Implications
				The drug is rapid-acting A nurse must be present, especially during inhalation When given IV, infusion rate is monitored closely Child's response to this medication must be evaluated
Metaproterenol sulfate (Alupent, Metaprel) [tablets: 10 and 20 mg; syrup: 10 mg per 5 ml; metered dose inhaler: 15 ml (225 mg)]	Adrenergic: relaxes smooth muscle of bronchi in bronchospasm; is more effective by inhalation	Oral: *6-9 yr or < 60 lb*—10 mg three or four times per day; *over 9 yr or > 60 lb*—20 mg three or four times per day. *Not recommended for children under 6 y of age* Metered dose inhaler: 1-2 inhalations q 4-6 h with 1 min elapsing between inhalations; *not* to exceed 12 inhalations per day Nebulizer: 5 drops in 2 ml saline	Nausea, vomiting, headache, tachycardia, hypertension, dizziness	This drug has an extremely rapid onset: 1 min after inhalation, 15 min after tablet is swallowed Patients must be instructed regarding inhalation therapy If syrup is used, container needs to be agitated before pouring off a dose
Prednisone	Steroid: promotes bronchodilation; induces smooth muscle contraction	Oral: 2 mg/kg initial dose in divided doses for 2-3 days; then single dose (before 9 A.M.) for 2-3 days; then progressively decreased doses on alternate days down to 1 mg/kg; introduction of beclomethasone during tapering; tapering continued until, if possible, only beclomethasone therapy	Increased weight; edema, disturbance of linear growth and pituitary adrenal axis, cushingoid features, hirsutism, striae, easy bruising, increased susceptibility to infection, increased blood pressure	Importance of minimal exposure to infection and of adherence to prescribed schedule are stressed
Theophylline (Slo-Phyllin, Elixophyllin) [tablets: 100 and 200 mg; syrup: 80 mg per 5 ml; gyrocaps (time-release): 60, 125, and 250 mg]	Relaxes smooth muscle of bronchi in bronchospasm	Oral: initial dose of 16 mg/kg/24 h in 3 divided doses for 2-3 days; then maintenance dose q 12 h: 1-8 yr—24 mg/kg/24 h; 9-11 yr—20 mg/kg/24 h; 12-15 yr—18 mg/kg/24 h (these dosages represent averages and may be lower if serum theophylline level remains in 10-20 μg/ml range after 2-3 days of 16 mg/kg/24 h schedule)	Nausea, vomiting, palpitations, headache, insomnia	Taking drugs with meals lessens gastric discomfort When started, vital signs should be monitored Patients need to be instructed on keeping appointments because theophylline levels must be monitored Increased theophylline levels can result from concurrent use with erythromycin, clindamycin, lincomycin
Terbutaline sulfate (Brethine, Bricanyl) (tablets: 2.5 and 5 mg; ampule: 1 mg/ml)	Adrenergic: relaxes smooth muscle of bronchi; is more effective by inhalation	*Children 12-15 yr* 0.075 mg/kg or 1.5 mg three times per day; *SC:* 0.01 mg/kg to maximum of 0.25 mg/kg *Not recommended for use in children less than 12 y of age*	Headache, tremors, tachycardia, nausea	Patients should be advised to take only prescribed dose; exceeding that dose can be extremely harmful Patient should be advised to notify clinic or physician if medication does not improve breathing

fused, the child is observed for an indication of its effectiveness. These children are usually attached to cardiac monitors to facilitate identifying arrhythmias, which may develop while the drug is being given. Dangers associated with a rapid intravenous administration (severe and/or fatal circulatory failure) mandate diligent regulation of flow. Explanations need to be provided to children who become upset about blood work. Serum theophylline levels are evaluated frequently to ensure that optimum therapeutic levels of 10 to 20 μg/ml are achieved. It is important for the nurse to know that aminophylline suppositories are contraindicated because of erratic absorption and increased risk of toxicity. These children need to be evaluated constantly for drug side effects and signs of toxicity.

On admission to a unit or while in status asthmaticus, these children should be assessed every half hour. Their lung fields need to be auscultated to evaluate wheezing, the presence of rales, and the quality of aeration. There may be subtle changes in the degree of distress, respiratory rate, and retractions, and so vital signs, including blood pressure, are done at least hourly. In addition, a child's level of consciousness should be checked frequently, especially in a severe attack.

When humidified oxygen is ordered, it should be given by face mask, ensuring an adequate oxygen supply. A nurse cannot rely on the child's color as an indication of distress because a significant amount of hemoglobin must be desaturated before cyanosis becomes evident. A comfortable position for an older child to assume is accomplished by placing a pillow on the overbed table directly in front of the patient, allowing him to extend his arms over the table and rest on the pillow. It also allows for greater lung expansion.

Oxygen, which is given by face mask or nasal prongs, must always be humidified to decrease the likelihood of drying secretions. While face masks are the most efficient, they are also the most problematic for toddlers and preschoolers. The correct size is always selected; however, young children must be observed constantly to ensure that the proper position is maintained. It is essential for the nurse to monitor the amount of oxygen being administered and to assess the quality of the mist being produced if this therapy is to be effective.

Chest physical therapy (CPT) may be an integral component of any treatment protocol. It is usually done following the administration of an inhaled bronchodilator to facilitate the removal of copious, tenacious secretions. Through percussion, vibration, and postural drainage as well as coughing, these secretions can be removed. However, a nurse should auscultate the lung fields before *and* after the procedure to evaluate its effectiveness.

Since parenteral fluids are given to these patients, it is important to maintain patency and a constant rate of flow ordered by the physician. With dehydration contributing to inspissation of mucus, adequate hydration is critical. It can be measured by performing a specific gravity test.

Because these patients are exhausted and have an increased respiratory rate, eating is difficult; it is not unusul

for them to refuse solids. An effective strategy is to provide smaller, more frequent meals in an unhurried atmosphere.

In those rare situations where infused fluids and medications, other drugs, or humidified oxygen do not reverse a bronchospasm, the child may be in status asthmaticus. During this life-threatening crisis, respiratory failure can occur. In addition to the previously described treatment, arterial lines are established to monitor blood gases closely, and a loading dose (5 mg/kg) of aminophylline is given intravenously over 20 minutes. A maintenance dose is run for 1 hour and then altered according to serum theophylline levels until a level of 10 to 15 μg/ml is achieved. Serum levels are then monitored every 12 hours. Corticosteroids are prescribed. If the child's PCO_2 rises above 55 mmHg, assisted ventilation is usually considered. These children are critically ill and should be in intensive care settings or admitted to a unit where one-to-one care can be provided.

Although these children are in substantial distress and the nurse is involved in performing a variety of essential functions, it is imperative to supply them with explanations of all that is happening. Comforting, reassuring, and consoling him through touch as well as speech can allay the child's fears and anxieties. Being unable to breathe is a frightening experience. If parents are present, they too must be given explanations, which can be brief initially and elaborated on later. As the child improves, the nursing focus moves from action-oriented responsibilities to patient teaching. Considering the long-term management of children with asthma, efforts need to be directed toward preventing frequent recurrences and maintaining normal pulmonary function.

A survey of the home environment is essential to remove causative allergens which provoke asthmatic symptoms. Feather pillows need to be exchanged for those made of foam rubber. Curtains, wool rugs, or wool blankets should be removed and replaced by synthetic fibers or plastic materials.

It may be necessary to displace the family pet, which is an especially difficult experience for everyone involved. The child's room needs to be dusted daily when he is not present, and all dust-collecting items must be removed. Room air conditioners may be recommended to decrease the presence of airborne allergens.

Both parents and child also need to understand why the child should not be exposed to respiratory infections or strong odors such as paint and tobacco smoke. They can trigger an acute episode. If a food is suspected, it is removed for several months and sensitivity will be determined at a later date.

A physical therapist usually teaches the adults how to percuss and vibrate while the positions assumed for postural drainage are demonstrated. In long-term care, CPT is generally reserved for children who also have cystic fibrosis. For children with asthma only, the newer bronchodilators and increased fluid intake appear to control the viscosity of bronchial secretions. Since abdominal breathing exercises have shown that a child can exert some control over the symptoms of asthma, they should be taught to these children.

Any teaching plan developed for an asthmatic child or family should include the anatomy and physiology of the respiratory system as well as the pathophysiology of asthma. Since symptom control is determined by drug compliance, administering the correct dose at the appropriate time is a critical self-help skill. Actions of each of the medications, their side effects, and symptoms of toxicity must be explained in detail, with time for questions. Demonstrations and return demonstrations should be included. Both child and parents are taught how to use and care for a nebulizer or other type of aerosol therapy. In each instance, the nurse *must* emphasize the precise method of administration. For example, when metaproterenol is inhaled, it is important for the school-age child or adolescent to comply with the time allotment between doses in order to maximize its effectiveness. While abuse decreases its beneficial results, overabuse can be fatal. If these children are to live with this chronic health problem and manage themselves effectively, they must learn to recognize the symptoms of asthma and begin appropriate drug use early. Greater compliance can result in fewer hospitalizations and fewer visits to an emergency room and can decrease the amount of time lost from school.

A nurse involved in patient teaching must realize it is not done once, prior to discharge. Teaching begins when the client and parents are ready to learn. It is done as thoroughly as possible to ensure understanding of this disease. These basic principles will be repeated many times at the clinic or in the physician's office. If the child is unable to understand, parents are the learners; however, as the child grows and develops, he assumes more responsibility for initiating the treatment protocol.

If the patient attends school, a conference with the mother, school nurse, homeroom teacher, principal, and gym teacher can facilitate everyone's understanding of this health problem as it may affect performance. When drug schedules are devised, efforts should be made to avoid the need for taking medications during school hours. It is a critical issue for adolescents who may be perceived as different by peers who do not understand asthma.

Children who suffer from exercise-induced asthma will need additional counseling. Certainly, they can participate in some sports (baseball, football) which demand running for short periods of time. Playing basketball or soccer and jogging may be ruled out because of the nature of these sports. Some of these children excel in swimming, bowling, and ice skating. If the child is interested in music, he should be encouraged to play one of the wind instruments, which is physically beneficial because of the breathing exercises which can be done while using the instrument.

It is important to treat children with asthma as individuals who are able to identify their capabilities and interests as they assume more responsibility for their own health. Certainly, with time, self-management skills need to be refined in order to decrease the number of acute attacks. Most importantly, these children must be allowed to grow and develop in order to experience childhood and adolescence as normally as possible.

Respiratory Problems in the Preschooler and School-Age Child

Epiglottitis

Epiglottitis, an infectious form of croup, is seen more commonly in children from 3 to 7 years of age, whereas croup of viral origin is seen more in infants and younger children. The onset, often abrupt, is preceded by a minor upper respiratory infection in approximately one-fourth of affected children. Epiglottitis is a severe, rapidly progressive infection of the epiglottis and surrounding area and is most commonly caused by *Haemophilus influenzae* type B. Children may progress from an asymptomatic state to one of complete airway obstruction in *2 to 5 hours.*

In younger children the presenting symptom is sudden onset of high fever, while in older children the initial complaints are severe sore throat and dysphagia. The rapid progression of the disease is exhibited within minutes or hours of onset when the child displays severe respiratory distress with inspiratory stridor, cough, dysphagia, hoarseness, irritability, and restlessness. The child's temperature can range from 37.8 to 40.6°C (100 to 105°F) with an average of 39.4°C (103°F). With dysphagia, drooling may occur.

A younger child may assume a position of neck extension, but other meningeal signs are absent. The older child seems to prefer leaning forward in a sitting position, mouth open with tongue protruding. The severity of disease in some children is displayed in a rapid progression to a shocklike state characterized by pallor, cyanosis, and seeming loss of consciousness.

Observation of the child reveals severe respiratory distress and inspiratory stridor with flaring of the alae nasi and suprasternal, supraclavicular, intercostal, and subcostal inspiratory retractions. On examination of the child's oral cavity, pharyngitis and excessive mucus in the faucial regions are usually visualized. When the child's tongue is depressed with a blade, a large, edematous cherry-red epiglottis is seen. This finding is pathognomonic of epiglottitis. The use of a tongue depressor (which is discouraged if epiglottitis is suspected) to visualize the epiglottis may lead to sudden and complete obstruction in a child who is seriously ill. Therefore, the following equipment must be immediately available when this procedure is performed on a seriously ill child with the suspected diagnosis of epiglottitis: suction, oxygen, self-inflating bag, laryngoscope, and nasotracheal tubes of appropriate sizes. A throat culture is deferred until a later time, since sudden obstruction may occur. On palpation of the neck, a mild to moderate cervical adenitis may be found. Use of auscultation may reveal diminished bilateral breath sounds indicative of poor air exchange. If mucus is present in the upper respiratory tract, rhonchi will be heard.

Endotracheal intubation is imperative for a child who displays increasing fatigue, heart rate, and respiratory rate. If intubation is difficult, a tracheostomy may be necessary. Prior to intubation the child is kept in an upright position and is oxygenated for 3 to 5 minutes. The child is placed in the intensive care unit. Once a blood culture has been obtained, antimicrobial therapy is instituted. Many physicians prefer intravenous cefuroxime 75 mg/kg/d. When intravenous antibiotics are discontinued, systemic antibiotics are given for 10 days.

Supportive measures include high humidity with cold mist, parenteral fluids, and reduction of fever. The child is usually extubated in 48 to 72 hours, without complications. Most children can be discharged in less than 1 week.

Nursing Management

The place in a hospital—emergency room, operating room, or elsewhere—where the child undergoes intubation depends on his condition and the protocol of the particular hospital. The nurse's first contact with the child and his parents may be in a hectic emergency room. The physician will most likely be the one who first talks with parents and explains procedures. The nurse can later reinforce what the physician has said. If an intensive care unit is not available, a nurse should be in constant attendance. The nursing care for a child with epiglottis is essentially the same as that described for an infant with laryngotracheobronchitis following tracheotomy, taking into consideration the age of the child. If the child has a nasotracheal tube in place rather than a tracheostomy, accidental extubation must be avoided. Since the preschooler's great fear is bodily harm, the child needs much reassurance once a patent airway has been restored. A patent airway is maintained. The child is observed frequently for signs of obstruction. Intravenous fluids are monitored closely, and medications are administered as ordered by the physician.

Epiglottitis generally occurs only once. Since the experience is frightening to the child and his parents, they appreciate knowing that it is unlikely to happen again.

Acute Pharyngitis

In most upper respiratory infections, pharyngeal involvement is present. In its strictest sense, acute pharyngitis refers to all infectious conditions in which the principal site of involvement is the throat. Since the presence or absence of the tonsils does not affect the frequency, course, or complications of or susceptibility to the illness, the term *pharyngitis* includes tonsillitis and pharyngotonsillitis. The peak incidence of the disease occurs between the fourth and seventh years of life. Though pharyngitis is generally caused by viruses, group A beta-hemolytic streptococci are found in approximately 15 percent of affected children.

Clinically, it is difficult to distinguish viral from streptococcal pharyngitis because of overlapping signs and symptoms. In *viral* pharyngitis, the onset is gradual with early signs of fever, malaise, and anorexia. Within a day or so the child complains of a sore throat, which reaches its peak in a day or two. Rhinitis, hoarseness, and cough are commonly noted. Usually, pharyngeal inflammation is slight. Moderately enlarged and firm lymph nodes are generally discovered.

In *streptococcal* pharyngitis, the child's initial complaints may consist of headache, abdominal pain, and vomiting. Although fever occasionally does not occur for several hours, initial symptoms may be accompanied by a fever of 40°C (104°F). In several hours, the child may complain of a sore throat, which may be mild or severe enough to make swallowing difficult. Some children have tonsillar enlargement, exudation, and pharyngeal erythema. Others have only mild erythema, with slight tonsillar enlargement, and no exudate. Tender anterior cervical lymphadenopathy occurs early, and fever may last from 1 to 4 days. If the child is severely ill, he may be incapacitated for as long as 2 weeks.

Since 10 to 15 percent of normal children carry group A streptococci in their throats, a positive throat culture does not necessarily provide conclusive evidence of streptococcal pharyngitis. Physicians differ in their approach to diagnosis. Some will not institute antibiotic therapy unless the throat culture is positive. Others will not order a throat culture but will give an antibiotic to the child. If a clinical response is not noted within 24 hours, streptococcal infection is ruled out unless complications are present. Complications which follow streptococcal pharyngitis include sinusitis, otitis media, and, rarely, meningitis.

No known specific therapy is available for viral pharyngitis. Streptococcal infections respond well to penicillin. A one-time-per-episode long-acting penicillin is recommended to eliminate the compliance problem. The dosage is benzathine penicillin G 600,000 U intramuscularly (IM) for children less than 60 lb (27.3 kg) and 1,200,000 U IM for children over 60 lb (27.3 kg). In children less than 12 years of age and greater than 60 lb in weight, some physicians may use a mixture of 900,000 U of benzathine and 300,000 U of procaine penicillin. Oral penicillin therapy (500 to 675 mg daily in three to four divided doses), if prescribed, is continued for 10 days. If the child is allergic to penicillin, either erythromycin estolate (20 to 40 mg/kg/d in two to four divided doses) or erythromycin ethyl succinate (40 to 50 mg/kg/d in three to four divided doses) is a satisfactory substitute.

Late sequelae of streptococcal pharyngitis include rheumatic fever (onset in 2 to 4 weeks) and glomerulonephritis (onset in 1 to 2 weeks). Thus, prompt treatment is essential.

Many parents ask about tonsillectomy. The efficacy of this surgery remains controversial. However, most experts agree that indications include

1. Recurrent documented pharyngitis (viral or bacterial)
2. Severe upper airway obstruction due to hyperplasia (adenoidectomy may also be necessary)
3. Suspicion of malignancy of the tonsils

Tonsillectomies most often are done in day surgery centers. It is imperative that parents be apprised of how to monitor the child's pulse and determine the presence of the signs and symptoms which indicate hemorrhage and/or obstruction to the airway.

Nursing Management

Most children with acute pharyngitis are treated at home. Care is symptomatic. The child needs rest, and quiet play activities are provided. When a child's fever is 38.9°C (102°F), the prescribed antipyretic is given. If his temperature is 39.5°C (103°F), a sponge bath with tepid water is given. Excoriation around the nostrils due to rhinitis can be prevented by gently swabbing with cotton-tipped applicators and using a soothing skin ointment. The child should be observed for allergic reactions to penicillin.

If the child has a sore throat, either hot or cold compresses to the neck provide relief; the child can decide which method he prefers. If the child knows how to gargle, warm saline gargles are effective in relieving the pain of a severely sore throat. Acetaminophen may also be prescribed. If the child experiences pain on swallowing, cool bland liquids are tolerated well. No attempt should be made to force the child to eat. The nurse explains to the child and parents that the incubation period is generally 2 to 4 days (range, 1 to 7 days). Approximately 5 percent of close contacts (family, friends, schoolmates) develop the infection. The child is usually not contagious after a 24-hour period of appropriate antibiotic therapy and may return to school or the day care center once he is well clinically.

Respiratory Problems in the Adolescent

Viral Respiratory Infections

About one-half of all respiratory infections in children and adolescents are caused by viruses which can be identified in the laboratory. A majority of these infections are not influenced by antibiotics, and the treatment is symptomatic. It is important to understand the great variation in the frequency of viral infection, which changes from season to season and area to area.

To compound the problem further, one virus may result in the presentation of multiple symptoms, and several viruses may also be involved in one clinical syndrome. While the respiratory tract is limited in its responses to an infection, the clinical manifestations presented by a patient depend on the resistance of that person.

Many viruses change their antigen properties over a period of years; therefore, vaccines and natural infections fail to provide protection to the host. Although some vaccines are available for immunization against respiratory diseases due to influenza, parainfluenza, adenovirus, and rhinovirus, they are of limited value. In the case of the influenza virus, the vaccine is usually prepared from the most recent, current antigenic variant, and good immunity can be induced for a short period of time.

Influenza pneumonia can be very serious in some children and adolescents. This viral infection leads to a decrease in lung compliance, an increase in alveolar fluid, and an increase in pulmonary venous pressure; therefore, patients with heart disease, cystic fibrosis, and asthma are prone to pulmonary decompensation.

Three large categories of viral agents are responsible for many respiratory infections seen in pediatrics: the myxovirus, the adenovirus, and the picornavirus groups. The most common viruses within each category are included in Table 23-7.

Nursing Management

Viral upper respiratory infections are common in children and adolescents. Often hospitalization is not necessary. A proper diet and an adequate amount of sleep strengthen a person's resistance to these infections. The nurse should teach the concepts of good health whenever the opportunity arises.

In almost all instances treatment is symptomatic. If a child is febrile, fluids should be encouraged and antipyretics should be given as ordered. Complaints of "aches and pains" may require confinement to bed. Isolation decreases exposure and hence communicability. Adenoviruses may cause a conjunctivitis which a youngster finds bothersome, and compresses may be helpful. Ulcerations, found in herpangina and located in the oropharynx, are uncomfortable. Mouthwashes will bring relief.

Patients with asthma, cystic fibrosis, and heart disease may become more seriously ill as a result of pulmonary complications. In those instances, assessing their respiratory status and administering humidified oxygen may be necessary. Viral infections render any patient more susceptible to secondary bacterial infections such as *S. pneumoniae,* staphylococcus, and streptococcus.

Primary Atypical Pneumonia
(Mycoplasma pneumoniae)

Pleuropneumonia-like organisms (PPLO) are the smallest known microorganisms of the genus *Mycoplasma.* Within this group, *M. pneumoniae* is the cause of a respiratory problem identified as primary atypical pneumonia. It is recognized as a major cause of respiratory infections in late school-age children and adolescents and as being responsible for the development of bronchitis and upper respiratory disease. While the prevalence varies from year to year, the lowest incidence is usually found during the summer months. The disease spreads readily among high school and college students.

Adenoviruses, influenza viruses A and B, and parainfluenza viruses have also been the cause of atypical pneumonia. After an incubation period of 10 to 20 days, there is a rapid onset of fever, malaise, and persistent cough. Chills, headache, and conjunctivitis occasionally develop. Rhinitis will be evident, enlarged cervical nodes are present, and decreased breath sounds are heard.

The microorganism is usually isolated from the nasopharynx, and x-ray findings show an infiltration from the hilum to the periphery. Usually this disease lasts 1 to 2 weeks with otitis media occasionally developing. Tetracycline and erythromycin are the drugs of choice.

TABLE 23-7 Common Viral Infections

Virology/ Epidemiology	Clinical Manifestations	Laboratory Results	Treatment
Myxoviruses			
INFLUENZA VIRUS			
Influenza virus type A has a tendency to develop many variant strains; this type is encountered in epidemic form, rising abruptly and spreading rapidly, especially from early autumn to late spring; types B and C provide immunity which is type-specific and strain-specific; its duration is short; although it has a low mortality rate, morbidity rate can be 10-30% of the population; entry is through mucus-producing respiratory epithelial cells	Incubation period of 1-2 days followed by chills, aches, pains, and temperatures of 38.3-40°C (101-104°F); some diseases such as croup, bronchitis, bronchiolitis, and upper respiratory infections (URIs) can occur in presence of virus because of damage to epithelium	Blood counts are usually within normal limits, but leukocytosis may be present; nasal and throat washings are used to identify causative agent	Primarily symptomatic; secondary infections by staphylococci are common in children, and antibiotics may be ordered until bacterial cultures are obtained
PARAINFLUENZA VIRUS			
These infections are endemic, and they are more commonly found in colder months	Mild rhinitis, pharyngitis, and fever which lasts 1-2 days; type 1 is commonly associated with croup; type 3 is responsible for some bronchitis and bronchiolitis found in children; all four types are found in adolescents and adults suffering from URIs	Nasopharyngeal cultures are used to identify the virus	Supportive in all instances
Adenoviruses			
About 28 different types of adenovirus are known to humans; they are more common in summer months, but there are peaks in winter and spring; types 3, 4, and 7 have been involved in epidemics; types 1, 2, 3, and 5 are prevalent in infants and children; entry through conjunctiva as well as respiratory tract	Temperatures up to 39.4-40°C (103-104°F) lasting 1-10 days, sore throat, conjunctivitis, headache, and listlessness; adult respiratory distress (ARD) is associated with this virus; its onset is gradual; temperature is 37.8-40°C (100-104°F); chills, headache, and malaise are characteristic; coryza, cough, and sore throat appear less commonly	Pharyngeal, ocular, and lower respiratory tract secretions are used in identification; antibody titer rises during convalescence, which aids in diagnosing cause; it is used to identify an adenoviral infection but gives no clue regarding specific type	Symptomatic: secondary bacterial infections are rare
Picornaviruses			
RHINOVIRUS (FORMERLY CALLED "COMMON COLD VIRUSES" OR CORYZAVIRUSES)			
There are two large subgroups, H and M; M strains occur in winter and spring months, while H strains are common in summer and fall; rhinoviral infections are transferred from one person to another; viruses are recovered from nasal secretions and throats prior to onset of illness and 1-6 days after; incubation period is 2 days	Symptoms of cold including a slight sore throat, nasal stuffiness, sneezing, mild headache, and fever	Identification of virus is from nasopharyngeal secretions	Symptomatic; complications include otitis media, sinusitis, and a bacterial superimposed infection: antibiotics are contraindicated unless a secondary bacterial infection occurs

Continued.

TABLE 23-7 Common Viral Infections—cont'd

Virology/ Epidemiology	Clinical Manifestations	Laboratory Results	Treatment
ENTEROVIRUSES			
Coxsackie viruses A and B			
There are 23 types of Coxsackie group A and 6 types of Coxsackie group B; it is transferred from person to person by direct contact, flies, and dogs; communicability highest in home environment; it has been recovered from nasopharyngeal secretions and feces. Incubation period ranges from 1-14 days with a mean of 3-5 days; Coxsackie B viruses are found in outbreaks of febrile respiratory illnesses in families, camps, and institutions, especially in summer and fall	All signs indicate acute respiratory illness; A9 is sometimes found in patients with pneumonia; A21 is frequently cultured out in adolescents with respiratory problems, while B3 and 5 have been found in patients with croup, bronchiolitis, and pneumonia	Isolation of virus in laboratory confirms diagnosis; there is an increase in antibodies	Complete recovery after symptomatic treatment, except in newborn infants who may have cardiovascular anomalies as a result of a group B maternal infection in first trimester
Coxsackie A, types 1-6, 8, 10 and 22 have been associated with herpangina, a febrile, acute, self-limiting disease; it is seen in summer months; onset is rapid; incubation period is 2-4 days	Temperature to 40.6°C (105°F) for 1-4 days with anorexia, dysphagia, sore throat, headaches, abdominal pain, red pharynx, ulcers of soft palate, uvula, and other areas of oropharynx	White blood cell count is normal or just slightly elevated	Symptomatic; recovery is usually uncomplicated after symptomatic treatment
ECHOVIRUSES			
About 30 types of echovirus are known; infection is much more common in warm seasons, in lower socioeconomic conditions, and among children; it is more frequently found in feces than in oropharynx; occasionally an exanthum has been associated with echo infections	Echovirus type 11 is found in children with acute respiratory infections; pharyngitis and conjunctivitis are also seen in these patients; symptoms of aseptic meningitis may occur; certain types produce muscular weakness similar to poliomyelitis	Causative agent is identified after culturing oropharyngeal secretions; antibody titer rise is significant	Symptomatic

Nursing Management

Symptomatic treatment is important. Humid aerosol therapy is effective in loosening tenacious mucus. Postural drainage also should facilitate its removal. These adolescents must have extended rest periods and more than an adequate amount of fluids. They should be encouraged to assume this responsibility for themselves. Intravenous therapy may be instituted in a young child who is hospitalized and dyspneic. Since adolescents and college students may develop this disease more than any other age group, health teaching should be done routinely. The need for a balanced diet and adequate sleep should be emphasized.

Tuberculosis

Tuberculosis (TB) is caused by the tubercle bacillus *Mycobacterium tuberculosis*. It is usually inhaled by droplets from someone with active pulmonary disease. Although the most common primary site is the lung, the tubercle bacillus is capable of migrating to various other organs of the body through the blood and lymphatic systems. When TB is present in parts of the body other than the pulmonary system, it is called miliary tuberculosis. This bacillus ultimately may affect the genitourinary system, bones, joints, and subarachnoid space as well as the meninges.

There is no evidence of a genetic predisposition to tuberculous infection, but the following factors should be considered: the resistance of the person, the defenses of the host, the virulence of the invading organisms, the size of the infecting dose, and the number of bacilli present.

Although TB deaths have decreased with effective antimicrobial treatment, the numbers of new active cases have not kept pace. There are certain groups of people who continue to be especially prone to the disease. For example, in recent years a greater incidence of TB among younger age groups of Hispanics than among patients of other ethnic groups has been noted. Also, nonwhites in the United States have a mortality rate two to five times greater than that of whites. Living conditions and socioeconomic factors affect its incidence, since there are many opportunities for reinfection. Children, especially those under 3 years of age, have a diminished resistance to the bacilli and develop miliary TB and TB meningitis. In puberty and adolescence there is an increased susceptibility because of reinfection and the metabolic changes which occur during that period of growth. Some investigators believe that the influx of immigrants from southeast Asia and the Philippines ultimately may have an effect on the epidemiology of this disease in America (Stead and Dutt, 1981). Their concern stems from the fact that in those regions of the world there is a high incidence of drug resistance encountered in treating TB. Chronic fatigue, chronic illness, and malnutrition may also reduce resistance to TB.

Once the invasion into the parenchyma of the lung has occurred, the bacilli create a small inflammatory area, the primary focus. Simultaneously, bacilli begin to migrate through the lymphatics to the nearest lymph nodes which drain the area. The combination of the primary focus and the regional lymph node involvement is known as the *primary complex.*

In the affected area of the lung polymorphonuclear leukocytes accumulate, followed by the formation of epithelioid cells. In the process of proliferating, they surround the bacilli and create the typical walled-off tubercle formation. Eventually the lesion becomes calcified in children.

The incubation period for TB varies, with 2 weeks the minimum and 10 weeks the maximum; however, the average range appears to be 3 to 5 weeks. At the end of that time hypersensitivity is evident in the positive tuberculin reaction which occurs if the causative organisms are present in the body of the host. There may be no other symptoms present in the child except the positive skin test. Although an early diagnosis is imperative, no obvious clinical manifestations can be identified.

Tuberculin skin testing appears to be the most effective method of determining the infectious process in chil-

dren. A positive skin test signifies only that the child has been infected with the tubercle bacilli at one time or another. It does not signify an active or inactive infection, nor does it define acuteness or chronicity. The size or intensity of the reaction is not related to the severity of the disease. If the procedure were done routinely on all children in addition to those identified as coming in contact with an active adult TB patient, chemotherapy could be instituted more quickly, thereby decreasing the possibility of its innumerable complications.

The preparation used in tuberculin skin testing is purified protein derivative (PPD). It can be given into the volar surface of the forearm by intradermal injection or through the use of various mutiple puncture tests (Tine, Heaf) (Table 23-8). The latter are usually considered for screening purposes, and their positive results need to be verified by a Mantoux test. The standard dose of PPD is 5 TU (tuberculin units) in 0.1 ml Tween-stabilized solution. It is important to remember that the results of tuberculin tests are affected by recent live virus vaccinations, some infectious diseases, and corticosteroids or immunosuppressive agents.

In addition to a positive tuberculin reaction, the bacillus itself must be found in order to confirm the diagnosis, and a gastric washing is performed for this purpose. Children tend to swallow organisms which reach the pharynx from the lungs. A gastric lavage done on three successive mornings after an overnight fasting period aids in identification.

There are no known antimicrobial agents which eradicate the causative organism, and the aim of treatment is to arrest the existing condition and prevent complications. Drugs of greatest efficacy in treating TB in children are listed in Table 23-9. They have largely been responsible for the drastic reduction in deaths from TB. This disease is seldom treated with only one drug because that practice may lead to the emergence of a resistant strain. With *para*-aminosalicylic acid (PAS) poorly tolerated by young children, rifampin and isoniazid are the most frequent medications prescribed. Triple-drug therapy is utilized only in the presence of the most serious forms of tuberculosis such as TB meningitis and miliary TB.

Several attempts have been made to introduce artificial immunity against TB, the most successful of which is

TABLE 23-8 Common Methods of Tuberculin Skin Testing

Test	Method of Administration	Reading Time Interval	Results
Mantoux	0.2 ml of purified protein derivative (PPD) is injected intradermally under skin; a wheal *must* be produced	48-72 h	Area of induration is measured at greatest transverse diameter: <5 mm, negative; 5-9 mm, questionable; 10 mm, positive
Heaf gun	Heaf gun injects concentrated PPD with six punctures simultaneously 1 mm in depth	3-7 days	Presence of four or more papules is positive
Tine test	Four tines predipped in PPD are pressed into skin	48-72 h	One or more papules 2 mm or larger is positive

TABLE 23-9 Drugs Used in Treating Tuberculosis

Drug/Action	Dosage	Side Effects	Nursing Implications
Ethambutal dihydrochloride (Myambutal)—antitubercular	15 mg/kg/d in two divided doses orally; NB: *not* used in children under 13 yr	Retrobulbar neuritis with loss of visual acuity; defects in visual fields; inability to distinguish between red and green colors (all effects are reversible); gastrointestinal tract disturbances such as anorexia, nausea, vomiting, and abdominal pain	A visual acuity examination is done before this drug is started; patient needs to be advised this type of examination will be done monthly; since blurred or impaired vision can develop using this drug, patient must be instructed to call physician or clinic promptly; these symptoms disappear
Isoniazid (INH)—penetrates cell membrane; moves freely into cerebrospinal fluid and caseous tissue; prevents complications	10-20 mg/kg/d; maximum daily dose 300 mg given orally, intramuscularly, or intrathecally	Allergic reactions; gastrointestinal disturbances such as nausea, vomiting; jaundice; neurotoxic signs such as peripheral neuritis, seizures	Liver function tests done before beginning treatment; patient teaching focus is on need to take drug as ordered and notify physician or clinic should nausea and vomiting, tingling or numbness of extremities, or jaundice develop
Kanamycin—inhibits growth of tubercule bacillus; *used when patient is streptomycin-resistant*	15 mg/kg/d in 2-4 divided doses intramuscularly	Auditory impairment and vestibular damage with symptoms such as dizziness, vertigo, tinnitus, and hearing loss; nephrotoxic signs: an increase in blood urea nitrogen, serum creatinine, and proteinuria	It should be given slowly, with sites rotated; forcing fluids reduces toxicity; patients must be advised to notify physician or clinic when balance and hearing are affected: urine is monitored for volume, casts, blood cells; audiometric testings should be done
Para-aminosalicylic acid (PAS)—has bacteriostatic effect on bacilli; also acts to delay resistance to streptomycin	200-300 mg/kg/d in three or four divided doses orally	Gastrointestinal disturbances such as nausea, vomiting, abdominal pain; hypokalemia; severe allergic reactions	Patient instructed to drink large amounts of fluids because hydration decreases likelihood of side effects; drug should not be stored in bathroom medicine cupboard where moisture will decompose PAS; patients advised that taking drug with meals decreases gastric upset
Rifampin—antimicrobial	10-20 mg/kg/d; maximum daily dose 600 mg orally	Gastrointestinal disturbances; urticaria; rashes; leukopenia; thrombocytopenia; headache; drowsiness and other general symptoms	Patient should be told to take drug on empty stomach with large glass of water; this drug can change color of urine, feces, saliva to an orange-red, patient should be advised: should any adverse effects become evident, patient should call physician or clinic
Streptomycin—inhibits growth of tubercle bacillus	20-40 mg/kg/d up to maximum dose of 1 g intramuscularly	Auditory impairment and vestibular damage with symptoms such as vertigo, tinnitus, and hearing loss (hypersensitivity may include exfoliative dermatitis)	Sites must be rotated: adverse effects reviewed with patient; any evidence of hearing loss or equilibrium imbalance must be reported immediately; audiometric tests should be done

bacillus Calmette-Guèrin (BCG) vaccine. The practice of protecting vulnerable children with BCG has declined, since equal or greater protection is provided through administering isoniazid daily.

Complications of TB may appear within 1 month after the onset of the primary infection; however, most complications are evident within 6 months to a year. The most serious, meningeal and miliary TB, may be evident within

3 months. As bacilli are disseminated and migrate to other parts of the body (before hypersensitivity), some of the infecting organisms may die or their subsequent development may be arrested by the host. In the latter case, these tubercle bacilli lie dormant, and when the host's resistance is lowered by injury, disease, or malnutrition, they may become active again.

Nursing Management

Nurses in schools, public health agencies, outpatient departments, and inpatient settings have a role to play in identifying tuberculous children. Follow-up of a known contact is imperative, since an early diagnosis decreases the likelihood of some of the aforementioned complications.

Skin testing and long-term chemotherapy are essential preventive measures. Now, only children with draining lesions, renal disease, or chronic pulmonary TB are isolated. The daily use of isoniazid, particularly where contacts have been established, produces the protection desired. In view of the severity of the disease in adolescents, special attention should be devoted to case finding. Systematic testing of these persons in schools and camps may facilitate the process.

Since TB is difficult to diagnose in its early stages, when a diagnosis is important, routine skin testing should be incorporated in all existing pediatric admitting policies unless testing has been done within the previous year. A positive tuberculin reading should precipitate a most conscientious search for the contact because it is extremely rare for a single person in a household to acquire this disease. The community health nurse may be the initiator of the investigation, which could involve roentgenograms on all adults who have had contact with the child.

The adolescent is the most difficult person to involve in diversional activities, for he is missing peer group interactions essential to his developmental age. Fortunately, bed rest and isolation are being kept to a minimum with current chemotherapeutic programs. However, concerted efforts should be made to maintain group contact. A phone by his bed or active correspondence with friends may decrease the possibility of boredom or despair. Active participation in the health team's planning for his care and rehabilitation permit him to have some control over his environment.

Arrangements for a tutor or "home to classroom" intercommunication device permit adolescents with TB to participate in classroom activities. Fortunately, teenagers on chemotherapy who are afebrile are allowed to resume normal activity, including attendance at school. The only exception is participation in vigorous contact sports.

Long-term antimicrobial therapy is imperative for arresting the tuberculous infection and preventing complications. Administering medications to small children may be a nursing problem. Flavored syrups such as isoniazid may be used to disguise the taste of the medication. Tablets may be pulverized and mixed in applesauce, jam, or jelly. If the patient is hospitalized, recording successful interventions to nursing problems on the chart is helpful to all members of the staff.

A poor appetite initially is a typical problem; thus, selecting proper foods and those which he will eat is not an easy task. In the acute, early phase of the disease the diet should be high in calories and protein. Allowing the child to select his menu will usually increase the likelihood of his consuming it.

Since many adolescents with TB are from low-income families, parents may need some guidance in budgeting their food money so as to be able to purchase essential foods. In collecting data during history taking, the nurse may identify a potential problem and need to approach members of other disciplines and appropriate agencies for additional financial allowances. Arranging a consultation between the family and a nutritionist may result in improved nutritional intake for all family members.

The amount of teaching to be done by a nurse caring for a patient with TB is great. Parents have many questions about this infectious disease, particularly the mode of transmission and its communicability to adults and other children in the family. In their fears and anxieties are to be relieved, discussions should focus on the needs which they verbalize. The importance of maintaining chemotherapy in spite of the absence of symptoms; the need for a diet rich in protein, calcium, and phosphorus; and the need for adequate rest should be integrated in discussions with parents or the teaching plan developed by the nurse. Long-term follow-up should be stressed. Although this disease is under control, it is far from eradication.

Learning Activities

1. Assign clinical students to care for children who have diverse acute and chronic respiratory problems.
2. Invite the parent of a child with cystic fibrosis to class and ask that adult to share his or her thoughts about the impact of this chronic disease on the family.

Independent Study Activities

1. Develop a nursing care plan for a 3-year-old who has been admitted repeatedly for acute asthmatic attacks, with a focus on teaching and developmental needs.
2. Visit a local branch of the American Lung Association in order to have a better understanding of the extent of their involvement in educating the public about a variety of common respiratory health problems.

Study Questions

1. The PO_2 of blood depends on:
   A. The amount of oxyhemoglobin.
   B. The amount of oxygen molecules free in solution.
   C. A decreased hydrogen ion concentration.
   D. A decreased tissue temperature.

2. To prevent a typical neonatal response to cold stress during the administration of oxygen, it is important for the nurse to:
   A. Keep the neonate wrapped in warm blankets.
   B. Place the newborn in a closed incubator.
   C. Warm the oxygen to 31 to 34°C and humidify the oxygen.
   D. Use a circular hood.

3. When caring for a child with a tracheostomy who is accidently extubated, the first action of a nurse should be to:
   A. Call a physician.
   B. Open the stoma with a hemostat.
   C. Use an Ambu bag.
   D. Perform deep endotracheal suctioning.

4. The neonate does not learn to breathe through his mouth until about age:
   A. 3 to 4 weeks.   C. 7 to 8 weeks.
   B. 5 to 6 weeks.   D. 9 to 10 weeks.

5. The iontophoretic sweat test is used in diagnosing:
   A. Asthma.   C. Cystic fibrosis.
   B. Pneumonia.   D. Apnea.

6. After a young infant treated for RSV is discharged, parents need to be advised to keep the child away from other small infants because:
   A. The baby continues to shed RSV virus.
   B. The baby is susceptible to a variety of other childhood diseases.
   C. He is more likely to become reinfected with respiratory syncytial virus.
   D. He is more likely to acquire pertussis.

7. A toddler is seen in the emergency room because of wheezing. The parents tell the nurse that a week ago the child had an episode of choking, gagging, wheezing, and coughing. This information prompts the nurse to attempt to determine through further questioning whether the child has:
   A. Allergies.
   B. Asthma.
   C. Aspirated a foreign object.
   D. Been hyperventilating.

8. Children who have ingested hydrocarbons are placed in an upright or semirecumbent position to:
   A. Provide cardiocirculatory support.
   B. Prevent further aspiration.
   C. Prepare them for gastric lavage.
   D. Enhance observation.

9. The mother of an asthmatic child asks the nurse if he should have his tonsils and adenoids out. The nurse explains that:
   A. These tissues are enlarged during an attack, and so they should be removed.
   B. These tissues are not affected.
   C. These tissues usually diminish in size in response to adequate allergic management.
   D. While adenoids may be removed, tonsils never are.

10. A therapeutic serum theophylline level is:
   A. 10 to 20 μg/ml.   C. 6 to 10 μg/ml.
   B. 5 to 15 μg/ml.   D. 20 to 30 μg/ml.

11. Spacer devices are used as an adjunct to metered dose inhalers for children who:
   A. Wheeze one or two times a week.
   B. Are preparing to exercise.
   C. Cannot take theophylline.
   D. Cannot coordinate actuation with inhalation.

12. A mother tells the nurse that her child has "strep throat" and is on antibiotics. She wonders how long the child will be contagious. The nurse says that the period of contagion generally lasts:
   A. 2 to 4 days.
   B. 1 to 7 days.
   C. The first 24 hours of antibiotic therapy.
   D. Until he has finished the antibiotic therapy.

13. A positive tuberculin skin test in children signifies:
   A. An active infection.
   B. An inactive infection.
   C. The severity of the disease.
   D. An infection with the tubercle bacilli at one time or another.

14. A teenager with tuberculosis who is receiving rifampin and isoniazid states that his urine, feces, and saliva are an orange-red color. The nurse explains that:
   A. The change in color is due to the interaction of the two drugs.
   B. It is not unusual to see these changes when taking isoniazid.
   C. It is not unusual to see these changes when taking rifampin.
   D. It is essential for him to see a physician immediately.

Organizations Providing Additional Information on Asthma and Cystic Fibrosis

Allergy Rehabilitation Foundation
810 Atlas Building
New York, NY 10019

American Lung Association
1740 Broadway
New York, NY 10019

Asthma and Allergy Foundation of America
1302 18th Street, NW, Suite 303
Washington, DC 20032

Cystic Fibrosis Foundation
6000 Executive Boulevard, Suite 307
Rockville, MD 20852

Health Education Associates
14 North Lake Road
Columbia, SC 29223

References

Buckley, R.H.: "Allergy," in A.M. Rudolph and J.I.E. Hoffman (eds.), *Pediatrics,* Appleton & Lange, Norwalk, Conn., 1987.

Committee on Infectious Diseases: *Report of the Committee on Infectious Diseases,* American Academy of Pediatrics, Elk Grove, Ill., 1986.

Einhorn, A.H.: "Petroleum Hydrocarbon Poisoning," in A.M. Rudolph and J.I.E. Hoffman (eds.), *Pediatrics,* Appleton & Lange, Norwalk, Conn., 1987.

Friedman, S.B., et al.: "Statement on Terminology from the National SIDS Foundation," *Pediatrics,* **68**(4):543, 1981.

Frost, L., G.M. Kieckhefer, and C. Rubino: "Incorporating Research into a Community Asthma Program," *Pediatric Nursing,* **14**(3):197-200, 1988.

Hand, S.H., B. Thorarinsson, and W.A. Speir: "The Uses and Types of Spacer Devices," *Consultant,* **28**(5):142-145, 1988.

Mack, J.E.: "Ribavarin: An Antiviral Agent with Promise," *Pediatric Nursing,* **14**(3):220-221, 1988.

Ramsey, A.M., and A.S. Sirokey: "The Use of Puppets to Teach School-Age Children with Asthma," *Pediatric Nursing,* **14**(3):187-190, 1988.

Ray, C.G.: "Ribavirin," *American Journal of Diseases of Children,* **142**(5):488-489, 1988.

Simkins, R.: "The Crisis of Bronchiolitis," *American Journal of Nursing,* **81**(3):514-516, 1981a.

———: "Croup and Epiglottitis," *American Journal of Nursing,* **81**(3):519-520, 1981b.

Stead, W.W., and A.K. Dutt: "What's New in Tuberculosis," *American Journal of Medicine,* **71**:1-4, 1981.

Wells, P.W., and S. Meghdadpour: "Research Yields New Clues to Cystic Fibrosis," *MCN: The American Journal of Maternal-Child Nursing,* **13**(3):187-190, 1988.

24

The Cardiovascular System

Objectives

After reading this chapter, the student will be able to:
1. Identify the basic subjective and objective data to be obtained in assessing the cardiovascular status of a child.
2. Understand the purpose of diagnostic tests.
3. Explain general nursing measures appropriate for pediatric clients who have cardiovascular problems.
4. Identify common congenital heart defects.
5. Delineate specific nursing measures appropriate to the care of children with various cardiovascular problems.
6. Identify risk factors in chidlren which relate to cardiovascular disease in adults.

Although the heart is not the first organ to make its appearance in the embryo, it reaches a functional state long before any of the other organs do and is functional while still in a relatively primitive stage of development. By the end of the third week the heart is beating, and by the fourth week principal divisions of the heart are recognizable. The majority of fetal cardiac development occurs between the fourth and tenth weeks of fetal life. Most forms of congenital heart defects occur as a result of aberrations in this stage of development.

Cardiovascular Anatomy and Physiology
Fetal Cardiovascular Anatomy and Physiology

The fetal circulation is anatomically and physiologically different from the adult circulation in several important ways. Fetal blood is oxygenated in the placenta, which is a low-resistance circulatory pathway. Fetal arterial oxygen tension (PaO_2) is lower than adult levels (at approximately 25 mmHg), and fetal hemoglobin binds more readily to oxygen than adult hemoglobin does.

The major factor influencing the pattern and distribution of fetal blood flow is the relative vascular resistance in the pulmonary and systemic circuits. In the fetus, pulmonary vascular resistance is very high and systemic vascular resistance is low.

Two major structural differences in the fetal circulation are the *foramen ovale* and the *ductus arteriosus*. The foramen ovale is a flapped opening in the atrial septum that allows shunting of blood from the right to the left atrium. The ductus arteriosus allows blood flow between the pulmonary artery and the aorta. Oxygenated blood returning to the fetal heart from the placenta enters the right atrium through the superior and inferior venae cavae. Most of this blood flowing from the right to the left atrium through the foramen ovale passes to the left ventricle and to the aorta and is distributed primarily to the head and upper extremities. Blood returning to the right atrium via the superior vena cava enters the right ventricle and the pulmonary artery where most of this blood is

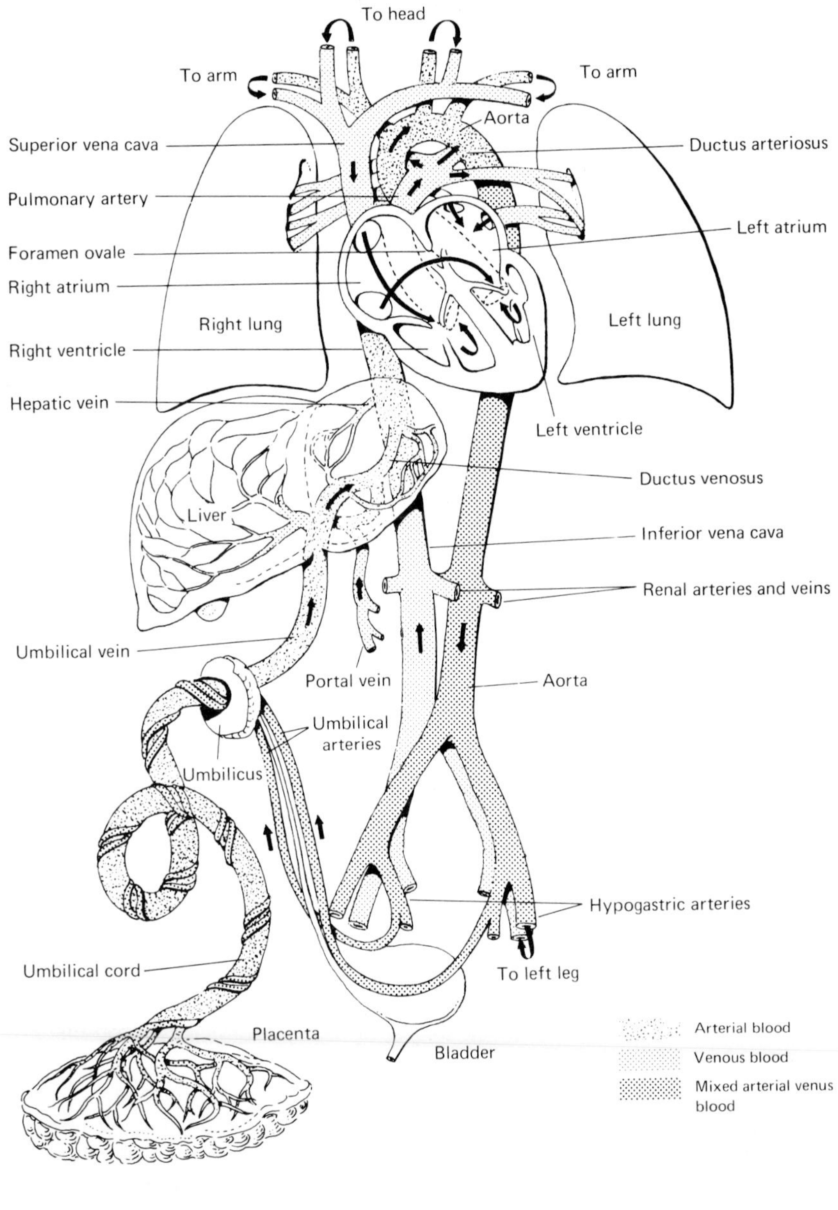

FIGURE 24-1   Fetal circulation. (*Reprinted with permission of Ross Laboratories, Columbus, OH 43216 from Ross Clinical Education Aid No. 1, © 1957 Ross Laboratories.*)

diverted through the patent ductus arteriosus into the aorta. Only a small amount of blood enters the distal pulmonary arteries to nourish lung tissue (Fig. 24-1).

At birth, the child takes a first breath and begins pulmonary oxygenation of the blood, which causes a rise in the arterial oxygen tension (PaO_2), a potent stimulus for constricting the ductus arteriosus. The rise in PaO_2 produces pulmonary vasodilatation, resulting in a fall in pulmonary vascular resistance. Pressures on the right side of the heart begin to fall, and the foramen ovale flaps shut. Clamping the umbilical arteries causes systemic vascular resistance to rise. All these changes begin at birth but may take hours or months to complete (Fyler, 1980). The ductus arteriosus usually begins fibrous infiltration within 72 hours and eventually is converted into a ligament. Pulmonary vascular resistance drops sharply at birth and continues to fall to final levels the first 4 to 8 weeks of life. At this time, pulmonary pressure and pressures on the right side of the heart equal the pressures seen in normal adults. The foramen ovale closes within 2 months of life in most normal children. Systemic vascular resistance and systemic arterial pressures in the full-term neonate rise from a mean of 50 mmHg in the first 12 hours, to a mean of 90 mmHg in the 1-year-old infant.

Adult Cardiovascular Anatomy and Physiology

The basic function of the heart is to pump oxygenated blood and essential metabolites to the tissues of the body and remove metabolic waste products from the peripheral

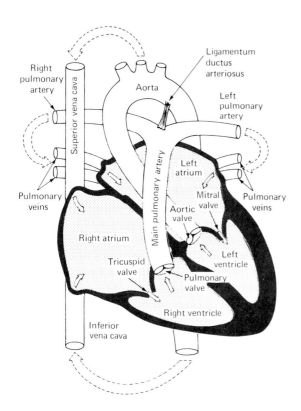

FIGURE 24-2 Bloodflow through the normal heart. (*Reprinted with permission of Ross Laboratories, Columbus, OH 43216 from Ross Clinical Education Aid No. 7, © 1961 Ross Laboratories.*)

tissues. It is a muscular pump that propels blood into the arterial (delivery) system and collects blood from the venous (return) system (Fig. 24-2). Blood moves through the heart by passive filling and muscular contraction of the atria and ventricles. Valves within the heart open and allow blood flow because of differences in pressure within its chambers. Venous blood returns from general systemic circulation through the inferior and superior venae cavae to the right atrium. The inferior vena cava drains blood from the lower half of the body; the superior vena cava drains blood from the upper half of the body. Blood supplying the myocardium returns to the right atrium via the coronary sinus. The blood returning in the venous system after releasing oxygen to peripheral tissues is dark red in color with an oxygen saturation of approximately 75%. This venous blood flows from the right atrium through the tricuspid valve to the right ventricle. The tricuspid valve separates the right atrium and the right ventricle and prevents regurgitation of blood during ventricular contraction (systole). This oxygen-poor venous blood is ejected by the right ventricle through the semilunar pulmonary valve into the pulmonary artery and to the lungs. As blood passes through the pulmonary capillaries, its red blood cells lose carbon dioxide and bind oxygen from the alveolar air in preparation for reentry into the systemic circulation. Oxygenated blood is bright red in color, with an oxygen saturation of approximately 97%. This blood returns to the left atrium via the pulmonary veins. After passing through the mitral (bicuspid) valve to the left ventricle, the blood is pumped through the semilunar aortic valve into the systemic circulation. As the blood passes through the systemic capillary bed, its red blood cells surrender the oxygen to metabolizing tissues and accumulate carbon dioxide and other metabolic waste products.

Assessment of Cardiopulmonary Function in Children

Although cardiovascular diseases still constitute the leading causes of illness and death among combined age groups in the United States, recent statistics indicate a decline in mortality due to heart diseases. Prevention and sophisticated treatment methods are largely responsible for this trend. A careful health history and physical assessment by the nurse are of primary importance in the evaluation and management of a child with confirmed or suspected cardiac disease.

The Health History Interview

The *symptoms* of cardiac problems and the *degree of severity* of the symptoms are equally significant, and pertinent information should be elicited from the parents or child early in the history. It is important to determine the length of time the child has experienced symptoms, precipitating or alleviating factors, and the effect of the symptoms on the child's activities of daily living. Some children with cardiac disease may be asymptomatic because the condition has not yet created hemodynamic complications or because the heart has compensated for the problem with slight hemodynamic changes. Therefore, it is important for the nurse to question parents carefully about the child's prenatal, perinatal, and family histories during the interview.

Since the heart is one of the earliest organs to develop in the embryo, it is vulnerable to the effects of teratogens and alterations in maternal physiology during pregnancy. The detrimental effects of rubella virus on the developing heart have been known for some time. There is a growing incidence of congenital heart defects related to maternal exposure to Coxsackie virus. While some drugs and chemicals have the *potential* to affect the developing heart, *very few drugs* have been linked firmly to congenital heart defects in offspring. Those drugs include thalidomide and trimethadione. Congenital heart defects have been found in approximately one-half of infants born with fetal alcohol syndrome and in approximately 5 percent of infants born to insulin-dependent diabetic mothers.

Patent ductus arteriosus is present in nearly 80 percent of preterm infants with birth weight less than 1200 g or gestational age less than 30 weeks and is also seen with increased frequency in neonates who experience perinatal hypoxemia (Hazinski, 1984a). Neonates who are small for gestational age also have a higher incidence of congenital heart defects (patent ductus arteriosus, atrial septal defect, tetralogy of Fallot) than do normal infants.

A family history of premature coronary artery disease (myocardial infarction before age 50), hypertension, and hypercholesterolemia among parents, grandparents, or siblings should be noted. A child with familial hypercholesterolemia and/or documented hypertension requires long-range follow-up as well as dietary counseling. The nurse should plan to counsel the chid to avoid smoking and obesity, since both can increase the child's risk of hypertension and/or coronary artery disease.

If the child is old enough, a profile of his lifestyle and daiy activities should be included in the history-taking interview. He/she can relate information about symptoms, the effect they have on play, school performance, and relationships with peers. The existence of behavioral, family, and environmental stressors may be difficult to identify. Family behavior patterns, the child's diet, usual forms of exercise, and use of tobacco, acohol, and drugs (e.g., oral contraceptives) can suggest factors which may place the child at risk for cardiovascular disease later in life.

General Assessment and Skin Color

Effective oxygenation of the blood and tissues requires adequate respiratory and cardiovascular function. Often cardiovascular disorders produce respiratory symptoms, and so a nurse requires skills in assessing both systems. The degree of the child's distress dictates the sequence of the nurse's assessment. If the child is extremely unstable, the nurse should focus on evaluating vital organ functions; if the child is ambulatory and in no distress, a more complete, more organized assessment may be undertaken.

Before disturbing the child, the nurse should note the position a child assumes for comfort. A child in congestive heart failure prefers the semi-Fowler's position, and a child with severe tetralogy of Fallot interrupts play to squat or assumes the knee-chest position in bed. The child's color, heart rate, respiratory rate and effort should be noted during sleep and during activity. Large discrepancies between sleep and wake states, should be discussed with a physician. Excessive irritability and extreme lethargy may indicate cardiorespiratory compromise.

Mucous membranes are assessed when the nurse evaluates skin color and capillary oxygenation, since these tissues are least affected by variations in skin pigment. *Central cyanosis,* a blue color of the mucous membranes and nailbeds, indicates arterial oxygen desaturation. Usually, central cyanosis is not visible until there is 5 g of reduced hemoglobin present per 100 ml of capillary blood and is usually detected at arterial oxygen saturations of 75 to 85%. The degree of cyanosis visible depends on the total amount of hemoglobin present and its saturation. It is not a reliable indicator of the degree of hypoxemia present. An anemic patient may be profoundly hypoxemic before cyanosis is observed, while a polycythemic patient may appear extremely cyanotic at modest levels of arterial oxygen desaturation.

Acrocyanosis, or peripheral cyanosis, is normal in the newborn and thought to be due to vasomotor instability. It is observed in extremities or around the mouth of the newborn, but does not involve mucous membranes or nailbeds and it disappears with increased warmth or activity.

Since arterial oxygen desaturation may be caused by either cardiac or respiratory disease, a nurse needs to document the distribution and degree of cyanosis and precipitating or alleviating factors. Cyanosis which *decreases* with cry is *respiratory* in origin and is relieved by increased tidal volume during vigorous cry. Cyanosis that *increases* with cry is *cardiac* in origin, since the expiratory phase of crying decreases pulmonary blood flow and increases right-to-left intracardiac shunting in cyanotic heart disease. Cyanosis that is respiratory in origin improves with oxygen administration, but cardiac cyanosis does not.

Decreased cardiac output in children causes mottling or pallor of the skin rather than cyanosis. Decreased capillary filling time and decreased skin temperature are also noted when low cardiac output is present.

Chronic arterial oxygen desaturation eventually leads to clubbing of fingernails (Fig. 24-3). Normally, the nail makes an angle of 20 degrees or more with a projected line of the digit; clubbing causes diminution in this 20-degree angle. This angle may be obliterated so that the digit and plate lie in a strainght line, or the nail may turn downward with severe involvement.

Respiration

The newborn breathes with shallow, irregular respirations. The normal newborn respiratory rate is approximately 40 to 60 breaths per minute during sleep and 60 to 80 breaths per minute while awake. Since the newborn's respiratory rhythm is so irregular, it should be observed and counted during a full minute, and the alertness

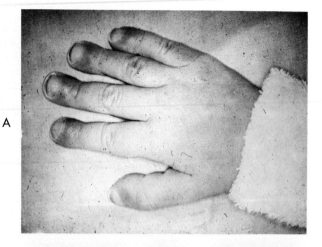

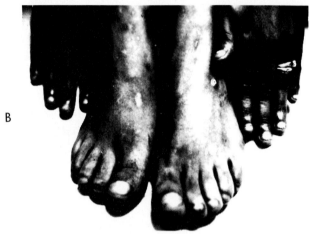

FIGURE 24-3 *(A)* Clubbing in an infant. *(B)* Clubbing and cyanoses in an adolescent. *(Courtesy James F. Shira.)*

TABLE 24-1 Normal Respiratory Rates in Children*

Age	Breaths per Minute
Infants	30-60
Toddlers	24-40
Preschoolers	22-34
School-age children	18-30
Adolescents	12-16

*Always consider the patient's normal range and note that respiratory rate will increase in the presence of fever or stress.

Source: M. Hazinski, "The Cardiovascular System," in J. Howe (ed.), *The Handbook of Nursing,* Wiley, New York, 1984.

TABLE 24-2 Normal Heart Rate Ranges for Children*

Age	Beats per Minute
Infants	120-160
Toddlers	90-140
Preschoolers	80-110
School-age children	75-100
Adolescents	60-90

*Always consider the patient's normal range and note that heart rate will increase in the presence of fever or stress and will decrease during sleep and vagal stimulation.

Source: M. Hazinski, "The Cardiovascular System," in J. Howe (ed.), *The Handbook of Nursing,* Wiley, New York, 1984.

(asleep, awake, or crying) of the neonate should be noted with the rate (Table 24-1).

The abdomen of an infant usually moves with respiration. Retraction of the chest, grunting, and rapid or labored respiration indicate distress. An infant with respiratory difficulty may take a long time to feed, may stop frequently because of shortness of breath, and may vomit after feedings.

With the older child, respirations tend to slow to about 20 to 30 breaths per minute (Table 24-1). A respiratory rate persistently above 40 breaths per minute is abnormal. The rate, depth of inspiration, and shortness of breath should be recorded. A child with respiratory distress may: need to take a breath before completing a sentence; stop to catch his breath while other children his age continue with their activity; sit up at night or prop up his head on a pillow to facilitate breathing.

Heart Rate and Pulse

Cardiac output is a product of stroke volume and heart rate. Since the child's heart rate and rhythm may vary with breathing patterns and level of activity, the rate should be counted for a full minute. Normal heart rates are more rapid for infants and slower for older children (Table 24-2). The heart rate always should be evaluated with the child's general appearance, level of activity, and indirect evidence of cardiac output. A more rapid heart rate is expected in a frightened, active, or critically ill child, because tachycardia is the fastest method of increasing cardiac output in the presence of a normal or slightly reduced stroke volume. A slower heart rate is normal when the child sleeps. When recording the child's heart rate, the nurse also should note the quality of peripheral pulses, warmth and color of extremities, color of mucous membranes, and capillary filling times.

Peripheral pulses should be described as decreased, normal, or bounding. Decreased or thready pulses are present with decreased cardiac output. Lower extremity pulses may be decreased or absent in the presence of thoracic coarctation of the aorta. Peripheral pulses may be bounding *(waterhammer pulse)* in the presence of patent ductus arteriosus, or other disorders. The nurse also should note any variability in the strength of pulses.

Blood Pressure

The Second Task Force on Blood Pressure Control in Children-1987 recommends that annual blood pressure measurements be incorporated into the continuing health care of all children 3 years of age and older. Because age and size are important variables to consider in obtaining blood pressure readings, selection of a proper size cuff is essential. The length and width of the inner inflatable bladder rather than the outer (and larger) cloth covering are used to determine the appropriate size cuff. The inner bladder should be long enough to encircle the extremity completely with or without overlapping, and the cuff width should be sufficient to cover approximately 75 percent of the upper arm length.

Since apprehension and fear can influence blood pressure, it is important to give the child a short age-appropriate explanation before attempting blood pressure measurement. If possible, the pressure should be taken in a relaxed environment which contains a minimum of external stimuli. With the child comfortably seated, the cuff is applied snugly and the extremity is positioned at heart level. Blood pressures of infants are obtained while they are in the supine position. The cuff is inflated rapidly to approximately 20 to 30 mmHg above the point where the radial pulse disappears. The cuff pressure is released *slowly* whie the examiner asucultates over the brachial artery. Deflation at a rate greater than 2 to 3 mmHg/s may contribute to an inaccurate reading. The onset of a clear tapping sound that is produced when the cuff pressure on the vessel is released is known as the *first Korotkov sound,* which is recorded as the systolic pressure. The point at which the tapping sounds become muffled and low-pitched is known as the *fourth Korotkov sound.* The fourth Korotkov sound is used as the measure of diastolic blood pressure in infants and children up to 12 years of age. The *fifth Korotkov sound* is the point at which all

sound disappears and is the diastolic reading for adolescents (U.S. National Heart, Lung, Blood Institute, 1987). Use of a Doppler electronic device facilitates a more accurate measurement of blood pressure in neonates and critically ill infants than the standard mercury sphygmomanometer. When a Doppler device is not available and an infant's blood pressure is not audible by the standard method, the *flush* method may be used (Chap. 6). It is important for the nurse to remember that the flush blood pressure can provide an indication of only the child's *mean* arterial pressure.

The use of blood pressure percentile charts is advocated to plot a child's blood pressures over time in much the same manner as length/stature and weight are plotted on a growth chart (Figs. 24-4, 24-5, 24-6). The blood pressure percentile chart is a tool for observing a child's blood pressure pattern during the period of growth and maturation. It is important that these percentile charts *not* be used to evaluate an isolated blood pressure measurement of a given indivudual. Rather, multiple measurements over several visits are averaged. If this reading is between the 90th and 95th percentile for the child's age, the result is compared with the 90th percentile readings and growth parameters at the bottom of Figs. 24-4, 24-5, or 24-6. Children who are tall for age and/or have excess lean body mass for age have a normal BP. Conversely, for children who are judged to be obese, dietary treatment and periodic BP measurements are advocated. Those children who are neither tall for age nor heavy for age are moni-

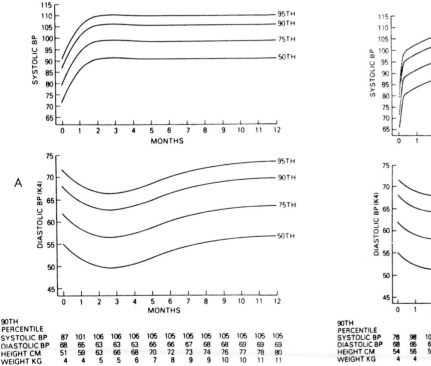

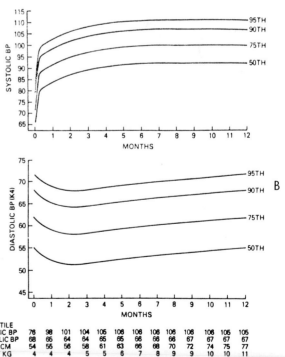

FIGURE 24-4 Age specific percentiles of BP measurements in (a) boys and (b) girls—birth to 12 months of age; Korotkoff phase IV (K4) used for diastolic BP. *(Reproduced by permission of Pediatrics, 79[1]:5-6, 1987.)*

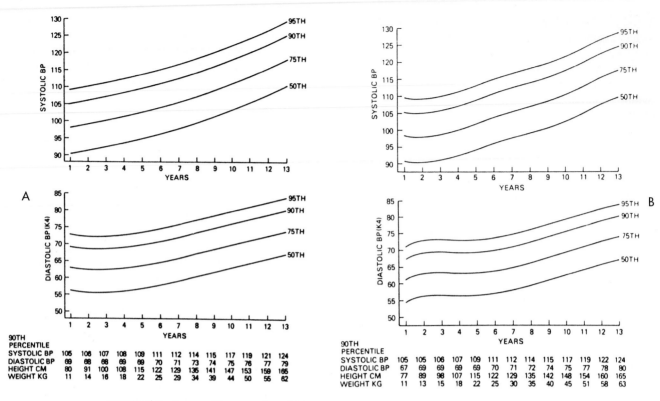

90TH PERCENTILE													
SYSTOLIC BP	105	106	107	108	109	111	112	114	115	117	119	121	124
DIASTOLIC BP	69	68	68	69	69	70	71	73	74	75	76	77	79
HEIGHT CM	80	91	100	108	115	122	129	135	141	147	153	159	165
WEIGHT KG	11	14	16	18	22	25	29	34	39	44	50	55	62

90TH PERCENTILE													
SYSTOLIC BP	105	105	106	107	109	111	112	114	115	117	119	122	124
DIASTOLIC BP	67	69	69	69	69	70	71	72	74	75	77	78	80
HEIGHT CM	77	89	98	107	115	122	129	135	142	148	154	160	165
WEIGHT KG	11	13	15	18	22	25	30	35	40	45	51	58	63

FIGURE 24-5 Age specific percentiles of BP measurements in *(a)* boys and *(b)* girls—1 to 13 years of age; Korotkoff phase IV (K4) used for diastolic BP. *(Reproduced by permission of Pediatrics, 79[1]:6, 1987.)*

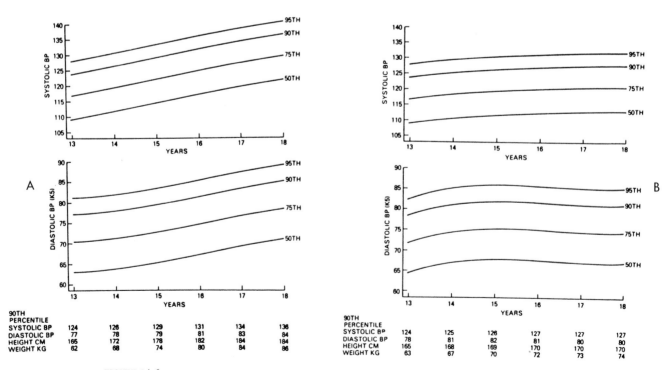

90TH PERCENTILE						
SYSTOLIC BP	124	126	129	131	134	136
DIASTOLIC BP	77	78	79	81	83	84
HEIGHT CM	165	172	178	182	184	184
WEIGHT KG	62	68	74	80	84	86

90TH PERCENTILE						
SYSTOLIC BP	124	125	126	127	127	127
DIASTOLIC BP	78	81	82	81	80	80
HEIGHT CM	165	168	169	170	170	170
WEIGHT KG	63	67	70	72	73	74

FIGURE 24-6 Age-specific percentiles of BP measurements in (a) boys and (b) girls—13-18 years of age; Korotkoff phase V (K5) used for diastolic BP. *(Reproduced by permission of Pediatrics, 79[1]:6-7, 1987.)*

tored at least every 6 months. Children who have readings above the 95th percentile are evaluated further through diagnostic procedures (National Heart, Lung, Blood Institute, 1987).

Blood pressure in the lower extremities also can be measured. Normally, arm and leg systolic pressures are equal in children under 1 year of age. Beyond that age the systolic readings in the upper extremities should be up to 40 mmHg higher. If lower extremity blood pressures are lower than expected, coarctation of the aorta should be suspected.

An additional determination that is made is the *pulse pressure,* which is the difference between the systolic and diastolic values in millimeters of mercury. Generally there is a difference of 20 to 50 mmHg. A widened pulse pressure results from any disorder causing increased stroke volume and/or a decreased peripheral resistance, including hypertension, aortic regurgitation, thyrotoxicosis, patent ductus arteriosus, arteriovenous fistulas, and coarctation of the aorta. A narrowed pulse pressure results from disorders causing increased peripheral resistance, decreased stroke volume, or decreased intravascular volume, including tachycardia, severe aortic stenosis, constrictive pericarditis, and pericardial effusions. Atrial fibrillation may cause a decrease in pulse pressure as a result of the absence of the atria's synchronous contractions. A weak pulse is felt when there is a narrowed pulse pressure due to the decrease in stroke volume.

Normally the pulse pressure decreases slighty with inspiration. This phenomenon results from a decrease in intrathoracic pressure which allows blood to return more freely to the right side of the heart. Blood freely enters the pulmonary circulation: therefore, less blood returns to the left side of the heart. During respirations of normal depth, no *palpable* variation in pulse volume is demonstrated, although an inspiratory diminution of 2 to 3 mmHg may be noted and can be accentuated in abnormal states.

A *paradoxical pulse,* or *pulsus paradoxus,* is defined as a significant drop in arterial pressure during normal end-inspiration, with a rise or little fall in the venous pressure. Diminution of the pulse volume may be palpated or demonstrated with the manometer. If a manometer is used, disappearance of the first Korotkov sound or of pulses during inspiration is noted while deflating the cuff 10 mmHg or more. This phenomenon may be observed after cardiac surgery, when pericardial tamponade or paramediastinal effusion is present, or with constrictive pericarditis or tension pneumothorax.

Another change in pulse pressure that is evaluated is *pulsus alternans.* There is a normal interval between beats, but the pulse waves alternate between those of greater and those of lesser amplitude, indicating myocardial weakness. In less severe situations the difference may not be palpable, but it can be detected by measuring the blood pressure by the auscultatory method. As the cuff is deflated from high pressure, the sounds from the alternate beats are first audible; as the pressure declines, the number of sounds is suddenly double. This phenomenon may be distinguished from pulses accompanying *bigeminal rhythm* in which the intervals between pulses are inconsistent. Pulsi bigemini are the result of premature ventricular contractions rather than myocardial failure.

Arrhythmias

In doing an apical pulse, particular attention should be given to the rate and rhythm of the beats heard because an abnormality in either rate or rhythm should be investigated further. An electrocardiogram helps determine whether the disturbance is normal or abnormal. If a child demonstrates low cardiac output from the arrhythmia, action may be taken immediately to treat the arrhythmia and its cause.

A *sinus arrhythmia* is a normal irregularity in the child's heart rhythm. With this rhythm, the heart rate speeds up at the end of inspiration and slows down at the end of expiration. It requires no treatment.

Sinus tachycardia is present when the heart rate exceeds the normal range. It is present with fear, fever, exercise, or anemia. It also may be a sign of cardiovascular distress, such as congestive heart failure, since tachycardia is the first response to a decrease in stroke volume. It requires no treatment unless the heart rate is so rapid that ventricular diastolic filling time and stroke volume are compromised significantly.

Paroxysmal atrial tachycardia (PAT) is a tachyarrhythmia characterized by the sudden onset of a heart rate between 130 and 300 beats per minute. PAT is most commonly observed in male infants less than 6 months of age. Mothers usually report a history of feeding problems, irritability, and vomiting. With such a rapid heart rate, ventricular diastolic filling time, stroke volume, and coronary artery perfusion are drastically reduced. If the episode of PAT persists beyond 24 hours, symptoms of congestive heart failure usually develop and tachypnea, dyspnea, heptaomegaly, and pallor may be noted.

These paroxysmal episodes may subside spontaneously with a reutrn to the normal rate. They may be terminated by unilateral carotid sinus massage, deep breathing (if the patient is old enough to comply), the Valsalva maneuver, gagging (physically induced), or vomiting. If congestive heart failure is present, the child requires urgent medical treatment. A digitalis derivative is required to slow the heart rate, and diuretics may be given to relieve systemic and pulmonary venous engorgement. Treatment with a digitalis preparation also will be required if the episodes of PAT are repeated (Fink and Mandel, 1983).

Sinus bradycardia is a heart rate below 90 beats per minute in infants and below 60 in children. Brief periods of sinus bradycardia may be observed in the neonate, particularly during sleep, or in the physically fit adolescent. This rhythm is rarely normal in other children. It can occur with forms of heart block, which may be congenital or surgical in origin. If the heart rate is so slow that cardiac output is compromised, treatment with chronotropic drugs, such as isoproterenol, or a pacemaker may be required.

Ventricular tachycardia is a rapid rhythm that produces ventricular depolarization at a rate of 100 to 250 times per minute. It is associated with a dramatic fall in stroke volume and cardiac output, since ventricular diastolic filling time and coronary artery perfusion are reduced. It indicates myocardial irritability and may be caused by electrolyte imbalance, hypoxia, acidosis, myocardiopathy, anesthesia, drug overdose, or neurological disease. Pulses and blood pressure usually are reduced with the onset of ventricular tachycardia, and ventricular fibrillation may ensue. *Resuscitation is necessary if blood pressure and systemic perfusion are compromised drastically.*

Ventricular fibrillation is characterized by chaotic electrical activity which prevents uniform cardiac depolarization and contraction. External cardiac massage must be begun immediately to maintain circulation, or death results. It is rare in children unless severe acid-base or electrolyte imbalance is present or death is imminent.

Heart Sounds and Murmurs

Variations in normal heart sounds and/or the presence of heart murmurs often are noted in children with cardiac problems (Fig. 24-7). The first sound heard on auscultation (S_1) indicates the systolic part of the cardiac cycle. It is synchronous with the apical or carotid pulse and represents the closing of the mitral and tricuspid valves. The second sound (S_2) corresponds to the closing of the aortic and pulmonary semilunar valves during the diastolic phase of the cycle. The second heart sound is split during inspiration, because decreased intrathoracic pressure causes the pulmonary valve to close later than the aortic valve. This normal splitting of the second heart sound during inspiration is called *physiological splitting* of the second sound. The third heart sound (S_3) is heard best at the apex of the heart while the child is supine or lying on the left side. It is caused by a rapid diastolic filling which follows opening of the mitral and tricuspid valves. While accentuated with conditions resulting in ventricular dilatation, it frequently is noted in children with normal hearts. The fourth heart sound (S_4) results from forceful atrial contraction and blood ejection into a noncompliant ventricle. It is heard just before the first heart sound and is very similar to the third heart sound. This sound is almost never a normal finding and is indicative of congestive heart failure (CHF), anemia, or another disease.

Gallop Rhythm

A gallop rhythm consists of the first and second sounds acompanied by either a third or a fourth sound. Children with fevers or other systemic illnesses may develop a gallop rhythm with tachycardia in the absence of cardiac decompensation. If the child has the signs and symptoms of CHF, however, and tachycardia with a gallop rhythm is heard, the implication may be that myocardial function is severely depressed.

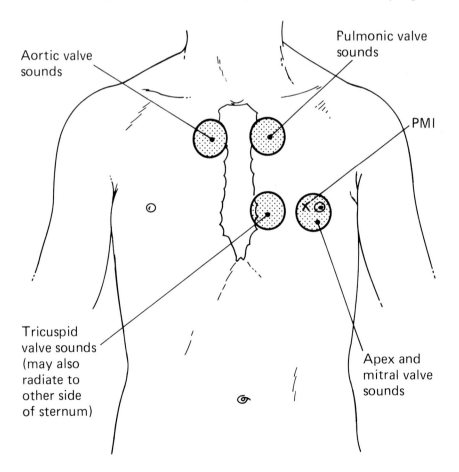

FIGURE 24-7 Major auscultatory areas of the chest. (*M. Hazinski: "The Cardiovascular System," in J. Howe [ed.], The Handbook of Nursing, Wiley, New York, 1984.*)

Aortic valve sounds

Pulmonic valve sounds

PMI

Tricuspid valve sounds (may also radiate to other side of sternum)

Apex and mitral valve sounds

Functional (Innocent) Murmurs

A functional murmur is the sound made by the turbulence of blood flowing through a normal heart and may be present in up to 70 percent of normal children. This type of murmur is caused by the normal function of the heart and great vessels. It is not significant and disappears as the child reaches adulthood. They may be loud in anxious or febrile patients and generally are widely transmitted in thin-chested children. A murmur is classified as "innocent" when the chest x-ray and electrocardiogram are normal and there is no evidence of organic heart disease. Three types of murmurs account for most functional murmurs.

Vibratory or "Twanging String" Murmur

This murmur is the most characteristic innocent murmur, described as a grade 1 to 3 musical murmur heard in early systole in the third or fourth left intercostal spaces along the left sternal border. Commonly heard in young children between the ages of 2 and 7 years, these murmurs may persist into adolescence and young adulthood and change in quality with a change in position.

Venous Hum

A *venous hum* is a continuous murmur heard in both systole and diastole under the right and/or left clavicles in young children. It is usually heard with the bell of the stethoscope during auscultation of neck vessels and is due to altered venous flow patterns. Obliteration or change in these sounds can be accomplished by applying pressure at the point of maximum intensity or by lifting or turning the child's head. It may increase with exercise or anemia and is more evident when a child is in an upright position.

Pulmonary Ejection Murmur

This *pulmonary ejection murmur* does not transmit widely. It is heard best in the second and third intercostal spaces at the sternal border. Short in duration, its intensity is increased by exercise, fever, and the supine position. It is thought to be caused by the rapid flow of blood across normal pulmonary valves and has no significance.

Bruits

A *bruit* is a localized murmur or other sound related to blood flow through a vessel. A bruit in the neck may originate in the carotid artery (carotid bruit) at its point of origin from the innominate artery. Bruits may be heard in the neck vessels if aortic stenosis or pulmonary stenosis is present. Bruits heard in the carotid vessels of young children are rarely significant.

A significant cranial bruit is continuous, usually very loud, and seen in the presence of an emerging problem. For example, a significant cranial bruit usually is accompanied by an increase in the head size of an infant. Almost all neonates have audible bruits in their heads, but they are not significant in the absence of other symptoms.

Rheumatic Murmurs

Systolic murmurs arise primarily at the apex of the heart of the young adult and are considered rheumatic in origin until proved otherwise. They are caused by mitral valve insufficiency. The diastolic murmur associated with aortic regurgitation is heard most frequently along the left sternal border, usually in the third or fourth interspace.

Murmurs Associated with Congenital Heart Defects

Patent Ductus Arteriosus

The most common murmur heard in neonates and infants is the murmur of a patent ductus arteriosus (PDA). Initially it appears as a systolic murmur in the newborn; however, if the ductus remains open, this murmur becomes continuous as blood begins to flow through the ductus during diastole as well as systole. When the blood flow becomes turbulent, the machinerylike murmur of a patent ductus is noted. While heard best under the left clavicle, this murmur may transmit to the second and third intercostal spaces along the left sternal border.

Ventricular Septal Defect

Another common congenital heart murmur heard in newborns and infants is associated with a ventricular septal defect (VSD). Caused by blood flow from the left ventricle through the VSD and directly into the pulmonary artery, it is loud, harsh, and holosystolic (or pansystolic). It is most audible in the third or fourth intercostal spaces along the left sternal border. At times a palpable thrill may be felt at the site of the murmur.

Atrial Septal Defect

The murmur heard in the presence of a secundum atrial septal defect (ASD) is caused by the large blood flow across the pulmonary valve. Fully oxygenated blood returning to the left atrium moves through the ASD, into the right atrium, across the tricuspid valve to the right ventricle during diastole, then across the pulmonic valve during systole. It is most audible in the second and third intercostal spaces along the left sternal border. *Fixed* splitting of the second heart sound, the pathognomonic auscultatory finding associated with this defect, results from prolonged right ventricular ejection time and consistently later closure of the pulmonary valve.

Stenotic Murmurs

Murmurs associated with aortic or pulmonary valve stenosis may be heard at any age. The murmur ocurs when blood is ejected across a valve which does not open fully. They begin after the first heart sound, increase in intensity during systole, and then decrescendo before the second sound is heard.

The systolic murmur of aortic stenosis is heard loudest in the second right intercostal space and is transmitted into the neck vessels. In infants and small children, it may be noted along the left sternal border. In the presence of valvular pulmonary stenosis, an ejection murmur caused by blood flow across the narrow pulmonary valve has the characteristics of an aortic stenosis murmur.

The murmur heard in an infant or child with coarctation of the aorta results from turbulent blood flow across the narrowed aortic segment, usually located in the thoracic aorta. It is heard best under the left clavicle and usually is heard posteriorly at the tip of the scapula on the left side.

Other Murmurs

The murmurs heard in other types of congenital heart lesions frequently are caused by a combination of murmurs. For example, a child with tetralogy of Fallot demonstrates the murmurs of pulmonary stenosis and a VSD. In a child with pulmonary atresia, there is no outlet from the right ventricle to the pulmonary artery; with no blood crossing the pulmonary valve, there may be no murmur. If an infant has transposition of the great vessels without a VSD, there will be no characteristic associated murmur; however, if a VSD is present, the VSD murmur described above is heard.

A murmur is insignificant unless congenital heart disease or another cardiovascular pathological condition is present. When the diagnosis of a functional murmur is made, parents have many questions which need to be answered with honest reassurance. Appropriate explanations can avoid needless worry and concern on the part of the family.

Additional Physical Assessments

The nurse must carefully evaluate exercise tolerance in the pediatric patient to separate activity limitations enforced by the family from actual intolerance of physical activity due to illness or cardiovascular disease. With most congenital heart defects, exercise to the limits of the child's tolerance usually is allowed. In general, children with CHF tire and cease activity before myocardial damage occurs. Children with cyanotic heart disease due to pulmonary outflow tract obstruction may squat instinctively to increase pulmonary blood flow during physical activity. If a cyanotic child has a history of hypoxic episodes—profound cyanosis with hypoxemia and loss of consciousness—physicians usually limit activity and plan immediate surgery to increase the child's pulmonary blood flow. Those with critical aortic stenosis who have angina or syncopal episodes or who have evidence of left ventricular strain on ECG should be placed on very *strict* activity limitation, since they are at risk for developing arrhythmias and sudden death.

Children with cardiac conditions that cause increased pulmonary blood flow seem to have more difficulty than normal in managing pulmonary infections. Parents complain that the child takes a long time to recover from upper respiratory infections. Pneumonia complicates the management of children with a large pulmonary blood flow (as in left-to-right shunts) or those with greatly enlarged hearts. Poor weight gain and small body size may be found in children with cardiac failure or cyanotic forms of congenital heart disease.

CHF leads to the most frequently described symptom complex occurring in children with cardiac disease. Because of its significance in the nursing care and medical

treatment of these children, CHF is covered in a separate section in this chapter.

Diagnostic Tests

In addition to a thorough history and physical examination, the diagnosis of abnormal heart conditions in children is confirmed using electrocardiographic, echocardiographic, radiological, and certain hematologic tests.

A nurse who is familiar with these procedures is in a unique position to teach. Through information sharing, audiovisual aids, and visits to different departments, the fear, anxiety, and apprehension generated by thoughts of these diagnostic studies can be lessened appreciably.

Electrocardiographic Tests

Electrocardiographic methods utilize the body surface to measure the sequence, rate, and magnitude of electric currents generated by the heart. The *electrocardiogram* (ECG) is a recording of cardiac depolarization and repolarization in response to the electrical impulses which originate in the heart. It *is not* used to evaluate adequacy of the cardiac contraction following the depolarization. In the normal heart, depolarization of the atria results in a first wave, the P wave. The Q, R, S, and T waves are related to the depolarization and repolarization of the ventricles. The shape of the normal Q, R, S, and T waves is shown in Fig. 24-8.

The *vectorcardiogram* is a form of ECG which records three leads simultaneously and is used to identify more precisely the true time and spatial relationship between electrical impulses and myocardial responses. The image frequently is deformed when various cardiac lesions are present.

A *phonocardiogram* is a graphic representation of sounds which originate in the heart and great vessels. This measurement accurately times intracardiac sounds which are too rapid or too subtle to be detected by auscultation.

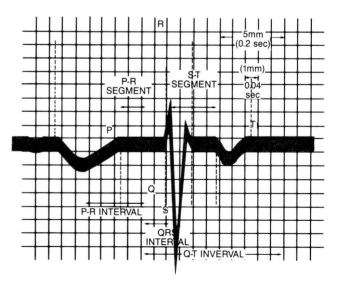

FIGURE 24-8 Normal ECG pattern.

Echocardiography

This cardiac diagnostic technique is a painless, noninvasive procedure which employs ultrasound. A small transducer sends sound beams through the chest wall and into the heart and then receives the sound bouncing off valves, cardiac chambers, and great vessels. These echoes are transformed into images on an oscilloscope, photosensitive paper, or a photograph. The image allows determination of anatomic relationships, measurement of intracardiac chamber or structure size, and indirect evaluation of function.

Radiologic Tests

Certain roentgenographic and fluoroscopic tests are performed to aid in the diagnosis of heart defects. Alone, x-ray and fluoroscopy do not provide conclusive diagnoses. The radiologist examines pulmonary vascular markings, cardiac size and contour, and great vessel and visceral position for indications of abnormalities.

Cardiac Catheterization and Angiocardiography

Cardiac catheterization involves passage of a small, soft radiopaque catheter into the cardiac chambers and vessels under fluoroscopy to diagnose cardiovascular defects, identify their severity, and evaluate their effects on overall cardiovascular function. It also is performed approximately 1 year after cardiac surgery to evaluate the repair and assess cardiovascular function.

The objective is to enter as many of the chambers of the heart and the great vessels as possible to (1) determine intracardiac and intravascular pressure, (2) measure oxygen saturations, (3) measure cardiac output, (4) evaluate the function of the aortic, mitral, pulmonary, and tricuspid valves, (5) visualize major intracardiac structures and shunts, (6) evaluate hemodynamics, and (7) perform diagnostic or palliative procedures such as His bundle mapping and balloon atrial septostomy.

Catheterization can be done through either the right or the left side of the heart. In infants and young children, the catheter is inserted most often through a femoral artery or vein; percutaneous puncture or cutdown is used. Umbilical artery catheterization may be preferred in the neonate. A cutdown in the antecubital vein or a brachial arteriotomy may provide access for older children.

Angiocardiography, the injection of a radiopaque contrast medium, frequently is performed with cardiac catheterization. X-ray films done provide valuable information concerning intracardiac hemodynamics, shunts, obstruction, and valve function. Although the injection of radiopaque media introduces the risk of an adverse reaction, its diagnostic potential is valuable and may be required for infants with cyanotic congenital heart disease regardless of the immaturity of the child or the severity of the symptoms. It is also indicated when a neonate does not respond to treatment for CHF within 12 hours or when a child with symptoms of cardiovascular disease does not have a definitive diagnosis.

Nursing Mangement of the Child Undergoing Cardiac Catheterization

Preparing the child and parents prior to these tests is a nursing responsibility. Information regarding the preparatory measures, the procedures, what the child can expect to see and do during the tests, and what the child may expect after the procedures should be presented in logical sequence and in language appropriate to the child's age and cognitive development.

Preparation of the child usually is done 1 day before the procedure. An older child or adolescent who is hospitalized more than 1 day before the tests may be ready earlier for information about the procedures planned. Questions should be answered succinctly and honestly. Visual aids, such as photographs or drawings of the cardiac catheterization lab or a miniature facsimile of the lab and equipment, are effective in helping the child understand. The nurse should accompany the child to the laboratory and/or remain with him during the procedure.

The parents should be present during the nurse's initial explanation to the child. Afterward, parents should have an opportunity to meet privately with the nurse. Often they will not verbalize their concerns about the child's diagnosis until the nurse directs attention to their needs.

The goals in the nursing management of a child undergoing cardiac catheterization and angiocardiography are to (1) promote the child's optimal condition before, during, and after the test, (2) detect adverse reactions to the procedures, and (3) prevent complications after the procedures. Frequently, the nurse accompanies the child to the cardiac lab. If a familiar nurse remains with him during the procedure, additional comfort and support for the child may be provided. Since the procedure usually lasts from 1 to 3 hours (but may be as long as 5 hours), the nurse should be sure the child is positioned carefully to avoid muscle strain and pressure on blood vessels and peripheral nerves. All extremities are cushioned carefully before the procedure and restrained to prevent movement which could cause damage to or contamination of the catheterization site.

Vital signs are monitored carefully during the first 48 hours following the procedures. Blood pressure, pulse, and respirations are recorded every 15 minutes for several hours after the catheterization. Because cardiovascular compromise may result in multisystem body changes, the nurse needs to observe the infant for indications of cardiopulmonary arrest. *Bradycardia* may occur as a result of hypoxia, acidosis, or the effects of sedation or anesthesia during the procedure. If it is accompanied by hypotension, cardiac arrest is imminent. Episodes of alternating tachycardia and bradycardia also may precede cardiac arrest.

The nurse must assess the circulation of the catheterized extremity frequently. If an arterial site was used, the pulses and perfusion of the extremity must be monitored closely. Evidence of mottling, coolness, pallor, and decreased pulse intensity should be reported immediately to a physician. Arterial spasms or thrombus require immediate intervention to prevent irreversible tissue damage; thrombectomy or a heparin drip may be ordered. If a *venous* catheterization was performed, the nurse monitors the child for cyanosis or edema of the extremity, an indication of venous obstruction. If they are observed, the extremity should be elevated to facilitate venous return. Since edema may compromise arterial circulation to that extremity, any decrease in pulses is reported to a physician immediately (Hazinski, 1984b).

Hypotension is a potential problem after cardiac catheterization. Inadvertent cardiac perforation with resultant tamponade is manifested by hypotension during or immediately after the procedure. The nurse needs to check the dressing for evidence of bleeding at the site every 15 minutes. Hemorrhage causes tachycardia, weak thready pulses, and cool extremities before a decrease in blood pressure is observed. Bradycardia is a very late sign of deterioration due to hemorrhagic hypovolemia.

If a percutaneous approach to the femoral artery is used a pressure dressing should be placed over the site for at least 30 minutes at the end of the procedure and the child remains in bed with the involved leg extended for 6 to 8 hours after catheterization. These children should be examined for evidence of bleeding, since blood may pool under the hip and thigh, under the thigh muscles or fascia lata, or in the retroperitoneal space.

These children are monitored for rhythm disturbances which result from catheter manipulation during the procedure or from hypoxemia, acidosis, myocardial irritability, and electrolyte imbalance. If arrhythmias are observed after the catheterization, the nurse should notify a physician and prepare to provide emergency resuscitation if the arrhythmia becomes life-threatening. When recovered, the child can begin taking clear liquids and advance to his usual diet.

The catheterization wound is kept covered and dry, and strict asepsis is maintained when changing dressings. Since endocarditis may develop from infection, any evidence of fever or inflammation should be investigated immediately. The physician needs to be notified of any heat, erythema, or discharge observed at the entry site. Wound cultures are usually ordered.

Adverse effects of cardiac catheterization and angiocardiography decrease significantly when they are done after 2 or 3 years of age. However, older children and adolescents remain vulnerable to the problems discussed above.

Hematologic Tests

Congenital heart defects may produce hematologic abnormalities. The development of these abnormalities depends on the type and severity of the defect, the child's age, the physiological effects of the condition, and the existence of other abnormal conditions. No blood test is diagnostic of congenital heart disease. Abnormal results of blood tests are usually a sign of the consequences of the child's heart disease.

Infants and children with cyanotic congenital heart disease, are likely to have increased hemoglobin and hematocrit values, which result from chronic arterial oxygen desaturation. Because oxygen tension in the circulating blood is low, erythocyte production is increased (to increase oxygen-carrying capacity). In some children, *secondary polycythemia* develops. It is characterized by an increased number of red blood cells. Polycythemia secondary to cyanotic cardiac defects is accompanied by an increase in the blood volume and blood viscosity.

In newborns, polycythemia secondary to congenital heart defects results in a hemoglobin level exceeding 23 g/100 ml of blood and a hematocrit above 70 percent. In older infants and in children, hemoglobin levels above 16 g/100 ml of blood and hematocrits above 55 percent suggest secondary polycythemia.

However, a child with a cyanotic heart condition may have anemia. If it is present, the hemoglobin may be near or within normal limits, and the cyanosis is deceptively less severe, although arterial oxygen content may be reduced significantly. The hemoglobin concentration of a child in heart failure must be monitored closely, because a mild anemia (10 g/100 ml blood) may place additional work on an already failing heart.

A platelet count and platelet function studies are done. Children with cyanotic congenital heart diseases and secondary polycythemia may have *thrombocytopenia*, which is associated with a defect in platelet function. It has been observed that platelet function returns to normal after corrective surgery and elimination of the polycythemia.

The chief indicator of tissue oxygenation is the *oxygen content* of arterial blood. It can be determined from the hemoglobin concentration, the *oxygen saturation* of the hemoglobin, and the arterial *oxygen tension* (PaO_2). Normal arterial oxygen saturation is 97%, and normal oxygen tension is 80 to 100 mmHg. Hypoxemia (reduced arterial oxygen tension) may be respiratory or cardiac in origin. If the child's oxygen tension fails to increase significantly while he breathes 100% oxygen, the hypoxemia is probably cardiac in origin.

General Nursing Measures

Nursing Diagnoses

Although there are many congenital heart defects and cardiovascular problems, there are common nursing diagnoses and general nursing measures related to the care of these children. Some examples of nursing diagnoses related to cardiovascular problems in children include the following:

Activity intolerance (actual or potential)
Altered nutrition: less than body requirements related to difficulty in eating and decreased intake
Decreased cardiac output related to decreased myocardial contractility and/or increased systemtic resistance
Fluid volume excess related to edema and fluid retention
Impaired gas exchange related to pulmonary congestion and tissue hypoxia
Anxiety related to tests and procedures
Altered family processes related to a critically ill child

Activity intolerance requires planning for care activities and collaboration among caregivers. Nursing care activities such as feeding, physical care, vital signs, and medication administration should be grouped to allow for maximum periods of rest. Members of other disciplines must carry out their activities within the planned times.

Careful monitoring and recording of intake and output are necessary to assure adequate caloric intake, maintain fluid restriction if indicated, and document the effect of diuretics or other medications. Daily weights or weights before and after the administration of diuretics are also necessary in monitoring nutritional status and fluid retention or loss. In the infant, diapers must be weighed dry and after urination. One gram of weight converts to 1 ml of urine volume.

Promotion of oxygenation is a major concern in providing nursing care. Humidified oxygen, positioning, and suctioning may all be necessary. Oxygen should be humidified and provided as ordered using a head hood, croupette, face mask, or nasal cannula as appropriate for and tolerated by the infant or child. In Chap. 23, there is a discussion of the methods used to meet a child's oxygenation needs.

Positioning the infant or child in a semi-Fowler's position eases respiratory effort by decreasing pressure on the diaphragm from an enlarged liver and by reducing pulmonary vascular congestion as blood pools in the dependent areas. An infant seat or cardiac chair facilitates this position in young infants. This position also decreases the possibility of aspiration of feedings or secretions.

Suctioning can be done with a bulb syringe or nasotracheal catheter. The use of a nasotracheal catheter requires a catheter size appropriate for age, sterile technique, and skill in doing the procedure. The suctioning must be done quickly to minimize interference with oxygenation and patient distress.

Since infants are vulnerable to hypothermia, care must be taken to maintain body temperature. Radiant-heat warmers maintain warmth and allow for easy observation of a young infant.

The nurse must have an excellent knowledge of the medications used in managing cardiac problems. Cardiac output is increased through the use of digoxin. The amount ordered and the volume should be double-checked by another nurse before administration. Careful observation of the infant or child for signs of toxicity is needed to identify problems early. Signs and symptoms of digitalis toxicity include bradycardia, arrhythmias, anorexia, nausesa, vomiting, dizziness, and visual symptoms. However, in young children, clinical signs may be absent and arrhythmias may be the only manifestation (Behrman and Vaughan, 1983).

Special Nursing Problems in Cardiac Care of Children

Cardiopulmonary Emergencies

The nurse must be thoroughly familiar with the signs of cardiac and respiratory arrest and must always be pre-

pared to administer resuscitative measures whenever they are indicated. *Cardiopulmonary arrest* may be defined as cessation of effective ventilation and/or circulation of blood. Cardiopulmonary arrest can occur without prior warning in any individual, regardless of age.

The *signs of cardiac arrest* are an absence of the heartbeat and an absence of carotid and femoral pulses. Arrest of the heart and circulation may be due to asystole, ventricular fibrillation, or cardiovascular collapse related to arterial hypotension. *Respiratory arrest,* identified by apnea and cyanosis, may be caused by an obstructed airway, depression of the central nervous system, or neuromuscular paralysis. Cardiopulmonary resuscitation, foreign body aspiration, and the Heimlich maneuver are discussed in Chap. 12.

Congestive Heart Failure

Congestive heart failure includes clinical signs and symptoms which indicate myocardial dysfunction or cardiac output insufficient to meet the metabolic demands of the body. In children, it may be caused by defects producing an increase in cardiac preload or afterload, impaired cardiac contractility, or alterations in sequence or rate of cardiac contraction (Hazinski, 1984a). In pediatrics, it is caused primarily by a wide variety of congenital heart lesions; however, it may occur secondary to systemic disease affecting the renal or pulmonary systems.

As the heart attempts to compensate, its rate increases and cardiomegaly develops. When the cardiac dysfunction is severe, the stroke volume decreases. Tachycardia occurs in an effort to maintain an adequate cardiac output despite a decrease in stroke volume. The urinary output diminishes. Diaphoresis occurs. If all these compensatory measures fail, cardiac output decreases.

With increased systemic vascular resistance and renal vasoconstriction, renal blood flow and glomerular filtration are reduced. Sodium and water are retained.

Diaphoresis is a common sign of heart failure in children, especially in neonates and infants. A mother often complains that the child's head is "sweaty" or that the sheets at the head of the bed are damp after the infant has taken a nap.

In children, biventricular failure usually is seen. Increased cardiac end-diastolic ("filling") pressures result in *systemic and pulmonary venous engorgement.* Pulmonary venous engorgement and interstitial edema produce a decrease in lung compliance and an increase in breathing. Signs and symptoms of pulmonary venous engorgement include tachypnea (one of the earliest signs), dyspnea, retractions, nasal flaring, and gruting. If the child has a respiratory infection or heart failure from severe obstruction in the left side of the heart or in the aorta, rales may be present, but they may not occur as a result of defects producing high pulmonary blood flow (such as a VSD). Dyspnea and respiratory distress may be reduced by placing the child in a semi-Fowler's position, which allows maximal diaphragmatic excursion during spontaneous inspiration.

Signs and symptoms of systemic venous engorgement

include hepatomegaly (one of the first signs) and periorbital edema. Jugular venous distention may be difficult to see in the short neck of an infant, and dependent edema is seen rarely unless CHF is severe.

A young patient with CHF may be pale and easily fatigued. The newborn or infant, although hungry, has a great deal of difficulty feeding, for as he sucks, he becomes tired and falls asleep exhausted. After a short nap he wakes up screaming, hungry, and anxious to eat, only to have the vicious cycle repeated. This situation is particularly challenging to the pediatric nurse faced with supplying an adequate nutritional and fluid intake to the infant. The parents may be very anxious. They need a great deal of reassurance and information which explains what is happening to the baby and why the monitoring of nutritional and fluid intake is critical to the infant's well-being.

Nursing Management

In caring for a child in CHF, the goals are to (1) improve myocardial contractility, (2) reduce energy requirements, and (3) remove accumulated fluid and sodium. Treatment includes digitalization, bed rest, diuretics, and fluid restriction. A low-sodium diet and the administration of oxygen may also be ordered.

Digitalis improves the force of the ventricular contraction, and it is helpful in most cases of CHF. Digoxin is the most frequently used digitalis preparation in pediatrics because it is well tolerated, rapidly absorbed, and quickly excreted. It always should be administered cautiously. The nurse must check and recheck the calculation, the dose, and the route when administering digitalis. If any arrhythmias are noted, the digitalis should be stopped and a physician should be notified.

When a digitalis preparation initially is prescribed for the child, a digitalization dose is administered in three or four divided amounts over a 12- to 24-hour period to establish therapeutic levels of the drug. The *oral* digitalizing doses are listed in Table 24-3. Preterm infants and chil-

dren with myocardiopathies generally receive lower digitalizing doses than those listed. Intravenous doses are calculated at two-thirds of the oral dose. The child initially receives 50 percent of the digitalizing dose and then receives another 25 percent of the dose 6 to 8 hours later. The final 25 percent of the digitalizing dose is administered 6 to 8 hours after the second dose, but only after a rhythm strip is obtained. If the rhythm strip reveals toxic effects of the digitalis, including bradycardia, heart block, or premature atrial or ventricular contractions, the third dose is held and a physician is notified. Once the child has received the full digitalization dose without complications, he is placed on maintenance digoxin; the maintenance dose is one-eighth of the digitalizing dose, given every 12 hours.

The dosage of digoxin is calculated to provide a therapeutic range which relieves the congestive failure without toxic symptoms. However, patients and tolerance levels vary. These children need to be observed closely while they are being digitalized. Vital signs are monitored hourly, and a nurse can evaluate the progress of therapy by a careful assessment of the patient and his behavior. Digoxin toxicity is a serious complication; therefore, observing the patient for decreased appetite, bradycardia, nausea, vomiting, diarrhea, and the appearance of arrhythmias is essential. Preterm infants are particularly vulnerable to toxicity as their immature renal system delays excretion of the drug.

Electrocardiograms usually are obtained before and during digitalization in order to complete baseline data. Tracings are obtained on a regular basis and whenever toxicity is suspected. While heart block is the most common arrhythmia which occurs with digitalis toxicity, nearly every kind of arrhythmia has been associated with the administration of this drug. Therefore, the nurse should notify the physician of *any* irregularity in the child's heart rate or rhythm and obtain an order to hold the digoxin until toxicity has been ruled out or reversed.

To reduce energy requirements, the patient is placed on bed rest and handled minimally. Small frequent feedings (at least every 3 hours) assure that the infant's nutritional and fluid needs will be met without exhausting the infant with prolonged feedings.

It is desirable to place an infant in an infant seat or cardiac chair. In this orthopneic position the liver impinges minimally on the diaphragm, venous return to the heart and lungs is diminished, and pulmonary congestion may be relieved. An older child is propped up in bed with his head elevated to produce similar results. Skin care is very important, as is regular, frequent positional change.

Diuretics and oral fluid restrictions are employed to facilitate the removal of accumulated fluid and sodium when there is pulmonary or systemic edema. Total fluid intake may be restricted and gradually increased as the child responds to therapy. The parenteral route is used for diuretic therapy when rapid diuresis is indicated. Furosemide is the drug of choice for rapid diuresis. It may be administered parenterally (1 to 2 mg/kg per dose) when

---

TABLE 24-3 Total Digitalizing Doses for Children (Digoxin)

Child's Age	Dosage of Digoxin*
Neonate	0.044-0.066 mg/kg (0.02-0.03 mg/lb)
2 weeks-2 yr	0.066-0.088 mg/kg (0.03-0.04 mg/lb)
2-10 yr	0.044-0.066 mg/kg (0.02-0.03 mg/lb)
10 yr to adult	2-3 mg (average)

*Intravenous dosage should be two-thirds of given dosages.
Note: Above doses should be given in divided doses approximately as follows (may be slight variation in various institutions). For digitalization: one-half of digitalizing dose given intially, one-quarter of digitalizing dose given 6-8 h later, last one-quarter of digitalizing dose given after 6-8 h more. For maintenance: one-eighth of digitalizing dose given 12 h later and every 12 h thereafter.

Source: M. Hazinski, "The Cardiovascular System," in J. Howe (ed.), *The Handbook of Nursing,* Wiley, New York, 1984.

heart failure is severe, and orally (1 to 4 mg/kg per dose) for less acute diuresis. Since furosemide is ototoxic in infants, it should be used cautiously when the patient is receiving other ototoxic agents. The thiazide diuretics (chlorothiazide and hydrochlorothiazide) are the most frequently used agents for long-term maintenance therapy in children. Spironolactone, which can be used for long-term diuretic therapy in children, results in potassium sparing, and so it is particularly useful for a child who develops hypokalemia from chronic furosemide or thiazide therapy (Hazinski, 1984a).

Whenever the child receives diuretics, the nurse must be careful to note the exact time of administration as well as the child's urine output. If the child fails to respond to the diuretic, it may indicate worsening heart failure or renal damage.

Diuretic agents can produce electrolyte imbalance, so the child's serum electrolytes are monitored carefully during therapy. The most frequent and most serious electrolyte disturbance encountered during diuretic therapy is potassium depletion. Hypokalemia potentiates digoxin toxicity, which increases the likelihood of arrhythmias. Therefore, oral preparations of potassium chloride usually are ordered when the patient is receiving digoxin and a potassium-wasting diuretic. In some instances the physician may elect to offset potassium loss by adding a potassium-sparing diuretic, such as spironolactone, to therapy with a thiazide or furosemide.

Once the therapy has begun, the patient's weight is monitored every 8 hours to document fluid loss and evaluate the effectiveness of the diuretic. Weight sheets should be located at the bedside, readily accessible. The child should be weighed at the same time of day, with the same amount of clothing, on the same scale. Daily weight changes of 50 g or more in an infant, 200 g or more in a child, and 500 g or more in an adolescent should be rechecked and then reported to a physician.

Since CHF produces sodium and fluid retention, restricted sodium intake may be indicated. Low-sodium formula is available for infants. In an older child, if sodium intake is limited to less than 1 g a day, the diet is low in protein and generally unpalatable. These children may become problem eaters. An astute nurse who identifies the problem and contacts a nutritionist skilled in and knowledgeable about appropriate substitutions may alleviate a potentially serious problem. Whether or not a *salt-restricted* diet is ordered, excessively salty foods such as bacon, ham, and potato chips should be avoided while heart failure is severe and diuretic therapy is being regulated.

Oxygen therapy may be utilized when caring for a patient with heart failure, especially if a concurrent respiratory infection is present. A croupette, a head hood, a nasal cannula, or a face mask may be used.

Systemic vasodilation has been found to be useful in the treatment of severe or chronic CHF in children. It is thought that the systemic vasodilatation reduces left ventricular afterload and improves cardiac output. Nitroprus-

side, dobutamine, isoproterenol, or nitroglycerine may be administered. The nurse must monitor systemic perfusion and be alert for the development of hypotension.

Congenital Cardiac Malformations*

There are 35 recognized types of congenital heart malformations; nine common lesions represent 90 percent of these anomalies. Congenital cardiac malformations may be categorized in various ways. A useful classification is based on two clinical features: the presence or absence of cyanosis and the amount of pulmonary blood flow (increased, normal, or decreased). *Cyanosis* refers to visible blue coloring of the skin and mucous membranes which occurs when there is hypoxemia or reduced arterial oxygen saturation. It is important to know that the signs and symptoms seen in a patient depend on the degree of severity and/or the presence of coexisting defects.

Children with acyanotic congenital heart defects demonstrate a wide variety of symptoms. Acyanotic defects which cause CHF in the first weeks of life include severe obstruction of the left side of the heart or of the aorta, and combined shunt lesions (e.g., a VSD with coarctation). Uncomplicated defects that produce high pulmonary blood flow under high pressure result in demonstrating CHF at 4 to 8 weeks of age, when pulmonary vascular resistance falls. Cyanotic defects usually produce symptoms at birth or within the first months of life. Some anomalies, such as secundum ASD and small VSDs, may not produce significant symptoms and go undetected until the child is older.

Acyanotic Heart Defects with Increased Pulmonary Vascularity

The combination of increased pulmonary vascular markings and acyanosis indicates the presence of a cardiac defect that permits the passage of blood from a high-resistance pathway on the left side of the heart to a low-resistance pathway on the right side of the heart or the shunting of oxygenated blood into the pulmonary circulation. Since the physical and laboratory findings depend on the volume of blood shunted, a nurse can anticipate a wide variety of symptoms. Many of these patients are asymptomatic. However, the larger the volume of blood shunted, the more commonly symptoms appear. In general, the clinical manifestations include CHF, tachypnea, and poor growth.

Ventricular Septal Defect
A *ventricular septal defect* (VSD) is an abnormal opening in the ventricular septum; which is most commonly lo-

---

*Because the problem of congenital heart lesions in the nursing care of children with cardiovascular defects is so extensive and serious, the format of the following section of this chapter differs from that of other chapters. Rather than grouping cardiac diseases and defects according to the age groups in which they occur most frequently, they are divided here into congenital and acquired problems. Congenital defects present serious problems for neonates, infants, and toddlers, while acquired heart diseases are more commonly seen in older children.

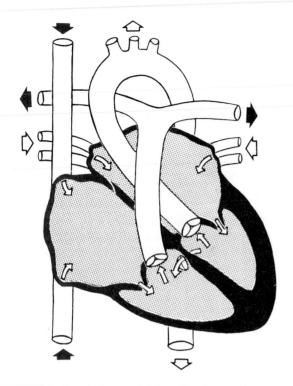

FIGURE 24-9 Ventricular septal defect. *(Reprinted with permission of Ross Laboratories, Columbus, OH 43216 from Ross Clinical Education Aid No. 7, © 1961 Ross Laboratories.)*

cated in the upper portion of the septum (Fig. 24-9). The magnitude and direction of the shunt are determined by the size of the opening and the relative resistances to flow into the pulmonary and systemic vascular circuits. Once pulmonary vascular resistance falls, the shunt is usually left-to-right. Any condition that increases resistance to left ventricular outflow (aortic stenosis and coarctation of the aorta) increases the magnitude of the left-to-right shunt. Small septal defects produce no symptoms and may require no treatment. Such defects do not become larger as the child grows older, and about 50 percent close spontaneously. However, if the defect is large and the shunt correspondingly great, pressure between the right and left ventricles becomes equal, producing increased pulmonary blood flow under *high pressure.* This type of shunt can produce pulmonary hypertension, with an increase in pulmonary vascular resistance. If this large defect is not repaired within a few months or years, irreversible pulmonary hypertension may develop.

Since there is little flow through the defect until pulmonary vascular resistance falls, it may not be detected at birth. In many patients the murmur is not heard until 6 weeks of age, when sufficient blood flows through the defect to cause a murmur. Many children are asymptomatic throughout childhood. Their main risk is the development of bacterial endocarditis. Children with larger defects may develop CHF, which does not develop until after the first month of life.

A harsh pansystolic murmur, heard best in the third and fourth left intercostal spaces, is the classic finding in

patients with a VSD. The heart size may be normal in patients with small left-to-right shunts and normal pulmonary resistance, while cardiomegaly may be present if a moderate or large VSD is present.

A cardiac catheterization demonstrates an increased oxygen saturation of blood in the right ventricle and the pulmonary artery, which is proportional to the volume of oxygenated blood shunted from the left ventricle. In small defects, a small increase is found.

The prognosis for these children is good in most instances. There is a low lifetime incidence of bacterial endocarditis, which can be prevented by administering antibiotics prophylactically. Prophylactic antibiotics should be taken during episodes of bacteremia or when dental work and other forms of surgery are performed. A small VSD which produces insignificant hemodynamic changes is not closed for the purpose of preventing endocarditis.

Patients who develop CHF or significant left-to-right shunts often need surgical treatment, which requires open-heart surgery. Smaller defects may be sutured closed, while larger defects are closed with the insertion of a prosthetic patch. Surgical mortality is approximately 1 to 4 percent. Operative risk is higher and postoperative complications are more likely when significant pulmonary hypertension or CHF is present preoperatively. Mortality and morbidity increase when the VSD is not an isolated cardiac defect but part of a more complex intracardiac problem. If a large VSD is present and surgical repair is impossible (due to the child's illness or the complexity of additional intracardiac defects), a closed-heart palliative procedure called a *pulmonary artery banding* may be performed in order to reduce blood flow and pressure within the pulmonary circulation. If very high pulmonary vascular resistance is present, the sudden surgical closure of the septal defect can cause acute right ventricular failure, because the right side of the heart is unable to generate sufficient pressure to maintain normal flow into the high-resistance pulmonary circulation. A promising approach that gives the right ventricle and pulmonary circulation time to adjust gradually to the new circulatory conditions imposed by surgery is the use of perforated patches to correct these septal defects. The patches contain one or more small openings that eventually close completely, but closure is gradual enough to allow the heart to adjust. These patches provide a means of closing defects which were previously considered inoperable due to severe pulmonary hypertension.

Atrial Septal Defect
At birth the foramen ovale is open and gradually closes during the first few months of life. A true ASD is located most commonly near the foramen ovale and is called a secundum ASD (Fig. 24-10). The size and direction of the shunt through an ASD are determined by the relative resistances of the right and left ventricular outflow tracts. Since the right ventricle is more compliant and pulmonary vascular resistance is low, blood flow is left to right through an uncomplicated ASD.

This shunt causes a right ventricular volume overload

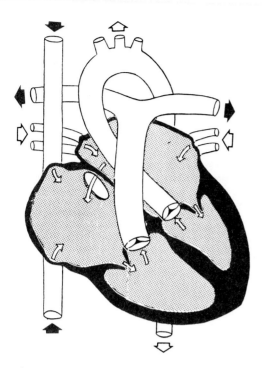

FIGURE 24-10 Atrial septal defect. *(Reprinted with permission of Ross Laboratories, Columbus, OH 43216 from Ross Clinical Education Aid No. 7, © 1961 Ross Laboratories.)*

and increased pulmonary blood flow; however, it is under low pressure. Most children do not develop CHF and are asymptomatic.

A systolic pulmonary ejection murmur, is heard best at the left upper sternal border because of the increased flow across the normal pulmonary valve. The pathognomonic auscultatory finding due to an ASD is fixed splitting of the second heart sound.

In a cardiac catheterization increased oxygen content in the right atrium is demonstrated. Pulmonary artery pressures are normal.

The prognosis for these children is good. A child with an ASD is asymptomatic and has only the auscultatory findings described above. Normally, cyanosis is not present, but it may be noted if CHF or pulmonary hypertension develops. The child may experience decreased exercise tolerance or severe respiratory infections. The risk of bacterial endocarditis is low (Hazinski, 1984a).

When an ASD results in cardiac enlargement or pulmonary blood flow which is twice as great as the systemic blood flow, surgical repair is indicated. Open-heart surgery is done. The defect may be sutured directly or a patch may be placed over the defect. The operative risk in either procedure is low. The optimal age for surgical treatment is between 1 and 4 years. Postoperative complications include arrythmias and heart block. Heart failure occurs postoperatively if the left ventricle is small.

Patent Ductus Arteriosus

Patent ductus arteriosus (PDA) (Fig. 24-11), the most common congenital cardiac anomaly found in neonates with congenital rubella syndrome, is often present in con-

junction with coarctation of the aorta. Nearly 80 percent of preterm infants with a birthweight less than 1200 g have a PDA.

The ductus arteriosus is a fetal structure that allows blood flow from the pulmonary artery to the aorta in utero. It normally constricts within 72 hours of birth; the most potent stimulus for constriction is thought to be the rise in the neonate's arterial oxygen tension (PaO_2) following the first breath. Preterm infants have an increased incidence of PDA because many of them have respiratory disease which causes hypoxemia so that their arterial oxygen tension does not rise normally after birth.

If the ductus arteriosus remains patent beyond the first weeks of life, shunting of blood from the aorta to pulmonary artery (left to right) occurs once pulmonary vascular resistance drops. The size and effect of the shunt are determined by the length and width of the ductus as well as the relative pulmonary and systemic vascular resistances. When pulmonary vascular resistance is high (e.g., in the neonate or preterm infant with pulmonary vasoconstriction secondary to lung disease), there may be negligible left-to-right shunting through the ductus. If the PDA is long and narrow, it may not permit much blood flow, and the child may remain asymptomatic with only a slight increase in pulmonary blood flow. Most patients with a PDA beyond the neonatal period demonstrate few symptoms.

If pulmonary vascular resistance is low and the ductus is short and wide, there will be a large shunt from the aorta to the pulmonary artery (left to right), producing increased pulmonary blood flow under high pressure. Clini-

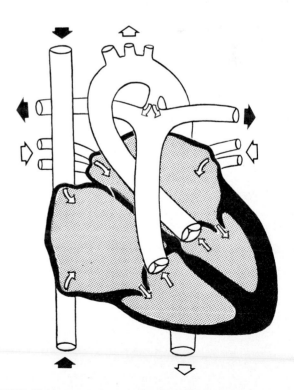

FIGURE 24-11 Patent ductus arteriosus. *(Reprinted with permission of Ross Laboratories, Columbus, OH 43216 from Ross Clinical Education Aid No. 7, © 1961 Ross Laboratories.)*

NURSING CARE PLAN

24-1 The Child with Patent Ductus Arteriosus

Clinical Problem/Nursing Diagnosis	Expected Outcome	Nursing Interventions
Anxiety and stress associated with unknown experiences of cardiac disease, hospitalization, and surgery	Child and family will be provided with emotional support adequate to promote optimal coping with illness, hospitalization, and surgery	Assess child and family's previous experiences with illness, hospitalization, and surgery Assess child and family's understanding of cardiac defect and required treatment Identify learning needs for child and family preoperatively, precatheterization, and after hospitalization
Knowledge deficit related to preparation for cardiac catheterization and surgery and home care		
Altered family processes related to ill child and stressors of hospitalization and illness		Develop teaching plan based on child's cognitive and developmental level: individual fears and coping strategies need to be identified and included in plan to provide maximal psychological support to child
	Parents will become actively involved in preparing child for cardiac catheterization and surgical intervention	Involve parents in preparing child; ask them how they believe child can best be prepared and separated; ask them to identify particular fears child may have and succesful comforting measures; this information must be communicated to all members of health care team
	Child and parents will be given tour of relevant hospital areas, meeting other nurses who will provide care to child	Familiarize child and family with sights, sounds, surroundings, equipment, procedures, sensations, and routines of postcatheterization/postoperative unit Explain to parents need to be present to support child as he is prepared for catheterization, surgery, another line, and/or new intervention; provide child with favorite toy or security object Introduce child and family to nurses who will be caring for child postoperatively and after catheterization
	Child and family will participate in development of teaching plan that meets their individual needs	Develop teaching plan for family, taking into consideration timing, pace, cultural and educational factors, and language barriers; timing and pace of preoperative teaching must be identified and considered in developing teaching plan; do not overwhelm family with details that may increase anxiety and fear Observe child and family for signs of discomfort indicating need for rest from teaching and evaluate their ability to process information provided
	Play activities will be integrated in plan of care to enable child to express feelings about what he is experiencing	Support child to master stressors of hospitalization, surgery, and postoperative care through use of play (provide child with doll, bandages, ECG leads, miniature IV bottles, syringes, etc.; role-play experiences child will have or has had to assess child's response and fears and to prepare child for certain sights (demonstrate use of surgical masks and gowns and prepare older child for diverse sounds in intensive care unit to allay his fears) Promote use of therapeutic play or art therapy to help child work through fears, express feelings about experiences, and master stressors Assessment of gathered data from observing child play, making comments, and expressing feelings must be documented and communicated to all health care team members Involve child in diversional play activities on pediatric unit or in playroom

Clinical Problem/Nursing Diagnosis	Expected Outcome	Nursing Interventions
	Parents will actively care for child during hospitalization	Encourage parental participation in child's care: identify with parents what aspects of care they are comfortable performing; encourage their comforting role as parents; they may need increased support in immediate postoperative period in terms of how to comfort child because they may be intimidated by the equipment; facilitate contact and bonding between parents and child
		Encourage parents to address child's concerns honestly with explanations appropriate for child's age
		Provide adequate time for child and family to express their fears and concerns and to ask questions and clarify misconceptions
		Facilitate communication between family and health care team
		Carefully assess child and family for individual sources of fear and anxiety and ensure prompt intervention to maximize coping mechanisms
		Facilitate appropriate referral for financial support
		Ensure adequate periods of rest for both child and family
	Both parents and child will be taught how to perform any procedures that may be necessary after discharge, especially recognizing signs of infection	*Discharge Teaching*
		Teach parents and child proper wound care, importance of keeping site clean and dry, and assessing wound for signs of infection (erythema, tenderness, inflammation, drainage, and elevated temperature); tell parents to report signs of infection immediately to pediatrician and/or cardiology clinic
		Advise parents to seek prompt medical attention for signs of respiratory infection (rapid breathing, difficulty feeding, elevated temperature)
	When taught about all prescribed medications and need for prophylactic antibiotics and given written instructions regarding home care, parents and child will understand management protocol to be followed	Provide teaching for all prescribed medications, including proper dose, route, administration, time schedule, side effects, and clinical indications for use
		Teach parents and child importance of antibiotic prophylaxis for dental work and surgical procedures; advise them to consult with pediatrician prior to scheduled dental work or surgery
		Teach parents several feeding techniques if they experienced problems previously
		Explore possibility of family members learning cardiopulmonary resuscitation (CPR) prior to discharge
		Clarify for parents when child can return to school and discuss limitations on physical activity (e.g., strenuous sports activity); reassure parents that children limit their own activity
		Encourage activities that promote child's growth and development; stress importance of consistent school attendance
		Communicate with school nurse to identify child's health care needs
		Provide family with written instructions for all aspects of home care
		Encourage school-age children and adolescents to participate actively in their care and plan for discharge; elicit their help in writing out specific instructions and developing their own schedules for specific teaching (e.g., medication schedule)
		Provide parents and child adequate opportunity to verbalize and/or redemonstrate understanding of teaching to enhance their confidence
		Provide family with written list of phone numbers to facilitate contact with health care team (primary nurse, clinical nurse specialist, cardiologist, cardiac clinic, pediatrician, etc.)
		Evaluate need for community health nurse referral to support family with health care issues which arise at home
		Provide family with opportunity to contact support groups for parents of children with cardiac defects
		Provide family with instructions for follow-up visits with cardiology clinic, cardiac surgeon, and pediatrician

Continued.

Clinical Problem/Nursing Diagnosis	Expected Outcome	Nursing Interventions
Fatigue Restlessness Irritability ——— Activity intolerance related to insufficient oxygenation secondary to decreased cardiac output	Child will maintain optimum circulatory and pulmonary function	Preoperative and precardiac catheterization Monitor apical pulse for rate and regularity; auscultate chest at second intercostal space of midclavicular line for continuous machinelike murmur Note presence of bounding peripheral pulses, widened pulse pressure, and low diastolic pressure
Congestive heart failure as evidenced by tachycardia, tachypnea/dyspnea, hepatomegaly, decreased urine output, cool extremities, and weak pulses	Through appropriate observations and interventions, child will conserve energy stores.	Monitor child for signs of CHF Assess child for signs of decreased cardiac output (tachycardia, poor peripheral perfusion, peripheral vasoconstriction, cool pale extremities, decreased peripheral pulses, delayed capillary refill, diaphoresis, decreased urine output (< 1 ml/kg/h) Assess child for signs of systemic venous enlargement (hepatomegaly, jugular neck vein distention, periorbital edema) Assess child for signs of pulmonary venous enlargement (tachypnea, dyspnea, and frequent or current respiratory infections) Assess respirations for rate, depth, and regularity and observe equality of chest expansion Auscultate breath sounds for equality and quality of aeration in all lung fields Assess child for signs of respiratory distress (tachypnea, retractions, nasal flaring, use of accessory muscles, and grunting) Monitor precatheterization and preoperative arterial blood gas values, hemoglobin and hematocrit values, complete blood count (CBC), blood urea nitrogen (BUN), electrolytes, and urinalysis Properly administer prophylactic antibiotic therapy as ordered preoperatively Provide supportive measures for CHF Administer oxygen therapy properly as indicated and prevent oxygen toxicity Assess child's ability to feed by mouth; note presence of increased distress with feedings; provide frequent rest periods In presence of respiratory infection, promote pulmonary hygiene measures; provide chest physical therapy, encourage deep breathing exercises, administer humidified oxygen, and encourage child to participate actively in breathing exercises Monitor intake and output volumes (strict) Measure daily weights at same time and on same scale every morning (note presence of IV boards, etc., with weight) Identify and document child's medication history on admission
	Child's cardiac status will improve as result of medications administered	Administer digoxin and diuretic therapy properly as ordered (provide adequate potassium replacement; ensure fluid and electrolyte balance Monitor child for signs of digoxin toxicity (dysrhythmia, nausea, vomiting); monitor digoxin levels closely Document child's baseline heart rate prior to digoxin therapy; consult with physician when rate is lowered significantly for age Properly administer prostaglandin inhibitors such as indomethacin as ordered; carefully monitor for any side effects (impaired renal function) and know the contraindications
	Given appropriate nursing care, child's systemic perfusion, vital signs, electrolytes, and respiratory status will be maintained at optimal levels	*Postcardiac catheterization care* Assess child for signs of cardiovascular compromise; monitor pulse, blood pressure, and respirations q 15 min Observe child for evidence of dysrhythmia and note effect on systemic perfusion, tachycardia, bradycardia, and hypotension or hypertension Assess for signs of cardiac tamponade (decreased systemic perfusion, pulsus paradoxus, and decreased systemic arterial pressure)

Clinical Problem/Nursing Diagnosis	Expected Outcome	Nursing Interventions
		Assess circulation of catheterized extremity: note quality of arterial perfusion: palpable pulses; immediately after catheterization, note color and temperature of catheterized extremity
		Monitor for increased coolness, blanching, or mottling of the extremity; report signs of altered arterial perfusion immediately
		Catheterized extremity should progressively increase in warmth, pink color, and capillary refill time
		Observe extremity for signs of venous obstruction; note presence of edema, decrease in pulse intensity, and cyanosis: elevate extremity to promote venous return; notify physician immediately of vascular compromise to prevent tissue damage
		Assess systemic perfusion; note warmth of extremities; color of nailbeds and mucous membranes; presence, strength, and quality of peripheral pulses; and capillary refill time
		Auscultate breath sounds for quality and equality of aeration in all lung fields; assess rate, depth, and regularity of respirations; observe child for equality of chest expansion and evidence of apnea, dyspnea, or restlessness; monitor oxygen saturation values hourly; monitor hemoglobin/hematocrit (Hgb/Hct) values; properly administer oxygen therapy as indicated: report oxygen saturations < 95 mmHg
		Maintain normothermia (rectal temperature 37°C); use overbed warmers or lights safely to warm child; avoid rapid warming or wide fluctuations in body temperature
		Enforce bed rest 6-8 h after catheterization
	Child's catheterization site will be free of hematomas or infection	Assess catheterization site q 15 min for signs of bleeding or hematoma formation; apply direct pressure and ice to site in presence of bleeding and promptly notify physician of persistent bleeding
		Protect catheterization site from infection; keep site clean and dry and provide dry sterile dressing; observe the site for drainage, erythema, and tenderness and obtain wound culture as indicated
		Monitor serum electrolytes and Hgb/Hct values and promptly report imbalances to physician
		Carefully document intake of fluids, contrast media, medications, and output volumes such as blood loss as well as blood samples taken for laboratory analysis during catheterization
		Monitor volume of urine output; note color and concentration of urine; test RBCs, Hgb, and protein
	Child's vital signs, systemic perfusion, respiratory status, and blood and elecrolyte values will demonstrate maximum function of all body systems	*Postoperative nursing care*
		Monitor vital signs q 5-15 min for first several hours postoperatively
		Consider child's defect, preoperative clinical condition, and individual response to cardiac physiology, quality and complexity of surgical repair, and intraoperative complications; assess heart rate; observe child for tachycardia, bradycardia, and dysrhythmia (note effect on systemic perfusion); assess blood pressure for hypotension or hypertension and monitor closely until stable
		Observe for signs of decreased systemic perfusion and low cardiac output; observe for signs of hypovolemia (hemorrhage, cardiac tamponade, decreased systemic perfusion, pulsus paradoxus, and decreased arterial systemic pressures)
		Assess warmth of extremities, color of mucous membranes and nailbeds, presence and quality of peripheral pulses, and capillary refill time
		Maintain patent airway
		Monitor arterial blood gas values; report results indicating hypoxemia, hypercapnia, and acidosis
		Auscultate breath sounds for equality and quality of aeration in all lung fields
		Assess breath sounds for changes in pitch and intensity
		Observe symmetry and equality of chest expansion; observe respirations for rate, depth, and regularity
		Observe child for signs of increased respiratory effort (tachypnea, retractions, nasal flaring, and grunting); report signs of respiratory distress immediately for prompt restoration of adequate ventilation

Continued.

Clinical Problem/Nursing Diagnosis	Expected Outcome	Nursing Interventions
		Observe child for shallow breathing and splinting of incision secondary to pain of thoracotomy incision; assess closely for decreased lung aeration and signs of respiratory infection
		Ensure adequate pain control to optimize respiratory management, (morphine sulfate 0.1 mg/kg as ordered)
		Provide pulmonary hygiene measures as clinically indicated; encourage deep breathing, chest physical therapy, and use of incentive spirometry and elevate head of bed; ensure adequate pain control prior to pulmonary hygiene measures
		Maintain normothermia (rectal temperature 37°C, skin temperature 36-36.5°C)
		Monitor temperature q 30 min-1 hr postoperatively; properly use overbed warmer or overbed warming lights to establish normothermia; prevent wide fluctuations in child's body temperature; prevent exposure to extremes in environmental temperature; notify physician if rectal temperature > 37°C in presence of poor systemic perfusion
		Maintain patent effective chest tube drainage system at 20 ml negative pressure as ordered; closely monitor amount, color, and type of drainage; notify physician immedately of excessive blood loss (blood loss usually decreases 3-4 h postoperatively)
		Monitor strict intake and output; monitor hourly urine volumes and report output < 0.5 ml/kg h; measure urine specific gravities q 4 h postoperatively; note presence of RBCs, HgB, and protein in urine sample; document volumes of blood used for laboratory tests and ABGs to help identify sources of blood loss and cause of decreased HgB/Hct values
		Carefully assess child's fluid balance; confer with physician if intake significantly exceeds output; obtain accurate daily weights; regulate amount and type of fluid needs to minimize salt and water loads as ordered
		Maintain NPO and ensure patency of nasogastric tube during immediate postoperative period
		Monitor CBC, HgB, Hct, and platelet count results; administer fresh whole blood, packed red cells, platelets, and fresh-frozen plasma (FFP) as ordered; ensure adequate supply of typed and cross-matched blood on standby for immediate use as needed
		Monitor serum electrolytes; observe for signs of hypo/hyperkalemia, hypocalcemia, hypoglycemia, and acidosis and promptly report and correct electrolyte and acid-base imbalances
		Identify pharmacologic agents that may be needed, such as protamine, vasoactive drugs, emergency drugs, and calcium gluconate; prepare medications, calculating dose for child's weight in kg and keep them available at the bedside for immediate use if needed postoperatively
		Assess child postoperatively for signs of congestive heart failure; compare findings with preoperative clinical assessment
		Assess for signs of systemic venous engorgement (hepatomegaly, periorbital edema, and jugular neck vein distention)
		Assess for signs of pulmonary venous engorgement (tachypnea, increased respiratory effort, weight gain, and altered arterial blood gas values)
		Properly administer digitalis and diuretics postoperatively as ordered; consult medical history to confirm child's preoperative maintenance dose
		Assess neurological status; observe pupil size and response to light bilaterally
		Note quality of movement and strength in all extremities; observe response to tactile and auditory stimuli; observe for signs of seizure activity (maintain patent airway and monitor ABG and serum electrolyte values); notify physician promptly
		Maintain clean, dry, intact environment for surgical incision and all catheter sites; observe incision for signs of inflammation (erythema, drainage, tenderness, and warmth)
		Provide meticulous care to all invasive sites with strict asepsis and strict hand washing techiques

Clinical Problem/Nursing Diagnosis	Expected Outcome	Nursing Interventions
		Monitor temperature for elevations and report temperature > 38°C
		Properly obtain wound, blood, urine, and tracheal aspirate cultures as needed
		Administer antipyretics as ordered
		Properly administer prophylactic antibiotics as ordered
		Minimize cardiovascular and oxygen requirements; comfort and calm child during all aspects of care and contact
		Devise adequate rest periods and sufficient uninterrupted periods of sleep free of treatments
		Provide child with optimal pain relief with prescribed analgesics
		Maintain normothermia; prevent exposure to extremes in environmental temperature
		Maximize caloric and protein value of all PO intake; provide small frequent feedings to increase tolerance of diet and minimize energy expenditure
Congenital heart defects Invasive procedures Invasive lines Poor nutritional status	Child will remain free of infection	Evaluate child's medical history, especially immunization record and exposure to communicable disease
		Note child's experience with frequent respiratory infections; promote pulmonary hygiene measures (deep breathing exercises, chest physical therapy as tolerated, and humidified oxygen)
		Protect child's skin integrity
		Optimize child's nutritional status
Potential for infection related to cardiac disease and invasive procedures		Promote good oral hygiene
		Provide meticulous care to all invasive catheter sites and IV sites according to unit policy with strict asepsis and strict hand washing techniques
		Maintain clean, dry, intact environment for incision and all catheter sites; observe child for signs of infection; monitor for temperature elevations > 38°C rectally and provide antipyretics as ordered; assess for increased respiratory secretions; properly obtain wound, blood, urine, and tracheal aspirate cultures as needed; observe wound and invasive sites for signs of infection (drainage, tenderness, erythema, and inflammation)
		Ensure prompt removal of invasive catheters when child has stabilized
		Properly administer prescribed antimicrobial therapy preoperatively and postoperatively; teach parents importance of antibiotic prophylaxis for future dental or surgical procedures; teach parents proper wound care and how to assess for presence of infection (wound or respiratory); encourage parents to seek prompt medical intervention
Poor weight gain Poor appetite Vomiting and/or diarrhea Fatigue Tachypnea and/or labored respirations	Child will demonstrate adequate progressive weight gain for age Child will maintain optimal fluid and electrolyte balance	Assess and document trends in weight loss or gain
		Weigh child daily (twice a day as needed), at same time and on same scale; plot weight on graph to monitor trends
		Obtain child's length, weight, head circumference, and abdominal girth on admission; follow serial measurements during hospitalization and in outpatient follow-up visits
		Obtain detailed nutritional history, including child's diet, daily caloric consumption, appetite, ability to tolerate feeding (degree of dyspnea and/or fatigue), number of ounces taken at one feeding, and length of time required to feed
Altered nutrition; less than body requirements related to fatigue, increased energy expenditure, and increased caloric needs		Identify child's unique feeding preferences: specific type of nipple, warmth of formula, favorite foods, etc.
	Child will tolerate a diet rich in protein, carbohydrates, calories, and vitamins to promote wound healing and growth	Optimize child's caloric intake (children with cardiac defects require approximately 150-200 kcal/kg/d); provide formulas high in caloric density; enrich caloric value of formula with cereal, microlipids, polycose, and other preparations of sugar, protein, carbohydrate, and fat supplements
		Offer older children high-calorie, high-protein, vitamin-enriched snacks between meals frequently
		Collaborate with nutrition specialist to calculate increased caloric needs for child with cardiac disease, provide suggestions for special high-caloric formulas, and provide counseling for meal planning

Continued.

NURSING CARE PLAN 24-1 The Child with Patent Ductus Arteriosus—cont'd

Clinical Problem/Nursing Diagnosis	Expected Outcome	Nursing Interventions
	Infant will be given small, frequent feedings, using nipples which decrease energy expenditure	Encourage small frequent feedings q 2-3 h and time limit feedings to 30-45 min per feeding to prevent fatigue
		Use soft easy-flow nipples (premie nipples) to decrease sucking effort
		Provide frequent adequate rest periods between feedings
		Feed child immediately after sleep and rest periods
		Minimize energy expenditure after feeding; promote calm, quiet environment
		Assess child's ability to tolerate feedings; if child is vomiting and markedly distressed and fatigued, assess need for enteral feedings; monitor child's ability to absorb feedings, check residuals, and monitor for diarrhea; support infant's need to suck, provide with pacifier, hold, cuddle, during feedings PO or nasogastrically; assist in evaluating need for total parenteral nutrition to meet the caloric and nutritional needs of severely compromised child
	Parents will become actively involved in providing care to child, especially in regard to maintaining nutritional needs	Encourage parents to feed child as much as possible during hospitalization to familarize them with feeding techniques prior to discharge
		Teach parents to avoid administering medications such as digitalis and diuretics in bottle to prevent altering taste of formula and to ensure precise administration of prescribed medications
		Assess effectiveness of the nutritional support interventions in promoting wound healing and growth

cal symptoms, such as CHF, similar to those seen with a large VSD may ensue.

The classic auscultatory finding is a continuous machinerylike murmur at the left intraclavicular area. When the shunt is small, a systolic murmur may be the only finding. Large shunts produce a continuous murmur. Most patients with a PDA are asymptomatic and a murmur is the only evidence of disease.

CHF caused by a large left-to-right shunt occurs in approximately one-fourth of affected individuals during early infancy. If it does, other lesions such as VSD, ASD, and coarctation of the aorta are suspected. CHF also may develop in preterm infants who have a patent ductus but no other associated cardiac defects.

Cardiac catheterization is usually not necessary to document a PDA when the clinical picture and echocardiogram are typical. Catheterization is done on infants with CHF to exclude other lesions.

The PDA may be eliminated through closed-heart surgery. Surgical mortality is very low and postoperative complications are minimal in the asymptomatic patient. Surgical mortality and postoperative complications are considerably higher, however, in the symptomatic preterm infant. In these patients, therefore, efforts may be made to induce ductus closure with the oral administration of indomethacin, a prostaglandin inhibitor.

The success reported with indomethacin closure of the ductus varies from 50 to 90 percent in preterm neonates. Permanent closure of the ductus seems more likely when treatment is initiated during the first 14 days of life. The recommended maximum total dose of indomethacin is 0.6 mg/kg. Initially an oral, rectal, or intravenous dose range of 0.1 to 0.2 mg/kg is given. This dose may be repeated twice at 12- to 24-hour intervals. In addition to administering the drug, nursing responsibilities include careful monitoring of urinary output because indomethacin has been observed to cause reduced renal blood flow. Use of indomethacin is contraindicated in the presence of bleeding, necrotizing enterocolitis, thrombocytopenia, and overt infection.

Spontaneous closure of a PDA after infancy is extremely rare. Without surgical intervention, the life expectancy is shortened and the patient is at increased risk for the development of pulmonary hypertension. Bacterial endocarditis, a complication of late childhood, may result in the development of pulmonary and systemic emboli. Surgical intervention is necessary if the ductus has not closed during infancy.

Acyanotic Heart Defects with Normal Pulmonary Vascularity

Whenever there is an obstruction causing increased resistance to blood flow, the chamber proximal to the obstruction must generate higher than normal pressures to maintain normal blood flow through the area of resistance (pressure = flow × resistance). The greater the obstruc-

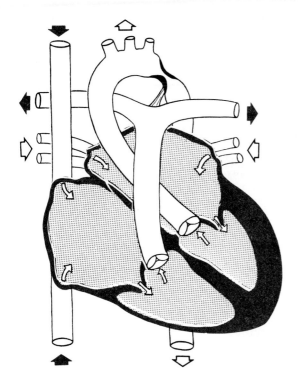

FIGURE 24-12 Coarctation of the aorta. *(Reprinted with permission of Ross Laboratories, Columbus, OH 43216 from Ross Clinical Education Aid No. 7, © 1961 Ross Laboratories.)*

tion (resistance), the higher the pressure that must be generated by the proximal chamber to maintain flow. Increased resistance results in proximal chamber hypertrophy in a degree proportional to the amount of obstruction. Mild obstruction results in minimal changes. Severe aortic or pulmonary obstruction results in significant ventricular hypertrophy and critical obstruction may cause CHF.

Coarctation of the Aorta

Coarctation of the aorta is a narrowing of the aortic lumen which most commonly occurs in the thoracic aorta, near the junction of the ductus arteriosus (Fig. 24-12). It is the adult or *postductal* type of coarctation. With postductal coarctation, collateral circulation develops to carry blood around the narrow area into the descending aorta. While collateral vessels succeed in maintaining descending aortic *flow*, the *pressure* in the descending aorta still is reduced. The patient demonstrates hypertension in both upper extremities and hypotension in both lower extremities. Unless the coarctation is severe or is accompanied by an additional defect such as a VSD or PDA, upper extremity hypertension is often the only sign of the defect.

With *preductal* coarctation, the ductus arteriosus usually supplies blood flow to the descending aorta; therefore, there is little stimulus for the development of collateral circulation during fetal life. As a result, the infant develops acute distress when the ductus arteriosus begins to constrict after birth. CHF and a severe decrease in sys-

temic circulation also occurs. If the coarctation is located in the aortic arch, between the innominate and left subclavian arteries, there is a discrepancy between right and left arm blood pressures; there is hypertension in the right arm and hypotension in the left arm and lower extremities. Preductal coarctation is often tubular rather than discrete. The result is narrowing of a significant portion of the aortic arch, causing severe symptoms in the neonate.

Severe coarctation in any form causes CHF in infancy. Approximately 15 percent of all patients with uncomplicated coarctation develop symptoms in infancy. If the coarctation is accompanied by another lesion, particularly one causing increased pulmonary blood flow (PDA or VSD), development of CHF in the first weeks of life is more likely. Most patients with coarctation who develop symptoms in the first 6 months of life have severe coarctation or an associated congenital heart lesion and require early surgical intervention. Approximately 35 percent of patients with coarctation of the aorta have a significant additional congenital heart lesion, and many have a bicuspid aortic valve.

The most obvious signs of coarctation are upper extremity hypertension (above the 95th percentile for age) with lower extremity hypotension. Lower extremity blood pressure normally exceeds upper extremity blood pressure by up to 40 mmHg beyond the first year of life; therefore, if leg blood pressures are equal to or lower than arm blood pressures or if a significant discrepancy between upper extremity blood pressure exists, coarctation should be suspected. With significant coarctation, lower extremity pulses are often absent. With severe coarctation and development of CHF, all peripheral pulses are usually diminished and decreased systemic perfusion and metabolic acidosis are present.

A systolic murmur associated with flow through the postductal coarctation may be heard over the child's back, between the scapulae. Bruits may also be heard over the intercostal arteries if the arteries have enlarged to provide collateral flow. A murmur may be absent with preductal coarctation.

Cardiac catheterization reveals the location and severity of the coarctation. Affected individuals have an increased risk of developing bacterial endocarditis.

Preoperative and postoperative mortality is highest for infants with severe CHF in the first 6 months of life. These children require aggressive management of heart failure before surgical repair is attempted. Surgical repair of coarctation generally entails closed-heart surgery. The narrowed aortic segment is removed, and the remaining segments of the aorta are reanastomosed. During infancy, a portion of the subclavian artery or prosthetic material may be utilized in the aortic reanastomosis to enlarge the aorta and reduce the possibility of later restenosis. The incidence of restenosis is highest in children who are repaired under 1 year of age. Restenosis usually produces significant residual hypertension. There is also an increased incidence of persistent hypertension if the coarctation is not repaired during early childhood.

24-2 *The Child with Coarctation of the Aorta*

Clinical Problem/Nursing Diagnosis	Expected Outcome	Nursing Interventions
Anxiety and stress associated with unknown experiences of cardiac disease, hospitalization, and surgery	Given individualized teaching and emotional support, child and family will be able to cope with stresses of illness, hospitalization, and surgery	Prepare child and family for hospitalization experiences, cardiac catheterization, surgery, and home care Individualize teaching and psychosocial supportive interventions according to child's cognitive and developmental level
Knowledge deficit related to preparation for cardiac catheterization, surgery, and home care		
Altered family processes related to an ill child and stressors of hospitalization and illness		See Nursing Interventions for Knowledge Deficit in the Nursing Care Plan of a Child with Patent Ductus Arteriosus
Hypertension Headache and/or dizziness	Through appropriate interventions, child's energy needs will be conserved and child will have improved circulatory and respiratory function.	Monitor apical pulse for rate, rhythm, and regularity of beats; auscultate chest posteriorly between the scapulae for systolic aortic murmur over coarctation
Fatigue and decreased exercise tolerance		Measure and record blood pressure values in upper and lower extremities bilaterally; note presence of hypertension in upper extremities and hypotension in lower extremities (lower extremity blood pressures may be ≤ upper extremity blood pressures
Congestive heart failure, pallor, and cool lower extremities		Compare blood pressure values in both right and left extremities (blood pressure measurements may be greater in right extremity compared with left secondary to increased blood flow to innominate artery)
		Compare strength and quality of brachial pulses
Actvity intolerance related to insufficient oxygenation secondary to decreased cardiac output		Assess presence, quality, and strength of lower extremity pulses; they may be absent or weak
		Assess for presence of bounding pulses proximal to defect and weak or absent pulses distal to defect; consult cardiac catheterization data for child's individual cardiac physiology
		Assess perfusion to lower extremities; note presence of cool, pale lower extremities; note evidence of leg pain or cramping with exercise caused by decreased lower extremity blood flow; observe child for fatigue with activity, decreased activity tolerance, and altered level of consciousness (dizziness, fainting, headache, and change in behavior)
		Assess child for signs of congestive heart failure (tachycardia, tachypnea, dyspnea, decreased urine output, hepatomegaly, cool extremities, and weak pulses); provide supportive measures (oxygen, digoxin, and diuretics) as ordered; see Nursing Interventions for Activity Intolerance (assessment and management of congestive heart failure) in Nursing Care Plan 24-1
		Provide postcardiac catheterization care; see Nursing Interventions for Activity Intolerance in Nursing Care Plan 24-1
		Provide postoperative care; see Nursing Interventions for Activity Intolerance, providing postoperative care, in Nursing Care Plan 24-1
		Monitor blood pressure constantly via arterial line and cuff pressure for evidence of hypertension; compare with blood pressure values preoperatively; administer antihypertension medications as prescribed; administer vasodilators as ordered to control hypertension; evaluate hypertension and effectiveness of management in outpatient follow-up care
		Assess child's tolerance of pain; administer analgesics as ordered (morphine sulfate 0.1 mg/kg IV); ensure adequate control of pain to optimize control of hypertension

Clinical Problem/Nursing Diagnosis	Expected Outcome	Nursing Interventions
		Assess for signs of congestive heart failure; implement appropriate nursing measures
		Assess systemic perfusion: observe for cool, pale, mottled extremities and weak pulses; constantly monitor temperature, color, pulses, and perfusion of lower extremities; evaluate signs of improvement or deterioration in perfusion postoperatively
		Monitor child for evidence of respiratory distress (alterations in arterial blood gas values, metabolic acidosis, hypoxemia, labored respirations, retracting, flaring, and grunting); maintain patent airway, optimize oxygenation, and monitor chest x-ray reports; ensure adequate control of postoperative pain to optimize respiratory management
		Monitor for signs of excessive bleeding; monitor chest tube drainage for excessive blood loss; monitor complete blood count, hemoglobin, and hematocrit values; monitor for signs of chylothorax (increased respiratory distress, decreased aeration of lung on involved side, and milky chest tube drainage); monitor amount, color, and consistency of chest tube drainage; report signs of excessive bleeding and/or respiratory distress immediately to physician
		Assess child for abdominal pain and tenderness; follow white blood cell count, note evidence of fever, measure abdominal girth, assess for abdominal distention and vomiting, ausculate for presence of bowel sounds, and monitor for gastrointestinal bleeding; report above signs to physician
		Monitor child's neurological status: assess lower extremity movement and sensation as well as motor and sensory function; compare strength and quality of reflexes bilaterally
Congenital heart defect Invasive procedures Invasive lines Poor nutritional status	Given individualized teaching, child and/or parents will be able to verbalize early signs of infection and know whom to contact	Prevent infection: closely monitor child for signs of infection and intervene promptly; see Nursing Interventions for Potential for Infection in Nursing Care Plan 24-1
Potential for infection related to increased susceptibility secondary to cardiac disease and invasive procedures		
Poor weight gain Poor appetite Vomiting Diarrhea Fatigue Tachypnea Labored respirations	Given appropriate antibiotics prior to invasive procedures, child will remain free of infection	Optimize child's nutritional status and maximize caloric intake; see Nursing Interventions for Alteration in Nursing Care Plan 24-1
Altered nutrition: less than body requirements related to fatigue, increased energy expenditure, and increased caloric needs	Through necessary interventions, child will gain weight appropriate for age and will reach fluid and electrolyte balance To promote wound healing and growth, child will progressively tolerate a diet rich in protein, carbohydrates, calories, and vitamins	

Pulmonary Stenosis

Pulmonary stenosis refers to any lesion that obstructs the flow of blood from the right ventricle. There are various types of obstructions, but generally the pulmonary valve cusps are altered or distorted in their development so that they fuse and form a membrane with a small opening in the center. The stenotic pulmonary valve is dome-shaped with a narrowed central orifice. Because of the restricted pulmonary valve orifice, the level of right ventricular pressure must increase to maintain normal blood flow into the pulmonary artery. With an increased right ventricular pressure, right ventricular hypertrophy and occasionally right atrial enlargement occur. Pulmonary stenosis can be present with other congenital heart defects. In about one-third of affected patients there is an associated ASD.

Patients with pulmonary stenosis are asymptomatic, although decreased exercise tolerance may be present. In severe valvular obstruction, right ventricular end-diastolic pressure increases, elevating the right atrial pressure and fostering a right-to-left atrial shunt through a patent foramen ovale; it causes central cyanosis. CHF occurs also. Occasionally, some patients complain of precordial pain.

Patients with valvular pulmonary stenosis have an ejection murmur over the pulmonary area. This systolic murmur is maximal at the upper left sternal border with radiation to the suprasternal notch.

Cardiac catheterization and angiocardiography document the degree and location of stenosis. Catheterization shows right ventricular hypertension with normal pulmonary artery pressures. Pulmonary blood flow is decreased in severe stenosis. Right atrial pressure may be elevated in moderate or severe stenosis.

Patients with *mild* stenosis are asymptomatic and do not have reduced life expectancy. Their stenosis is not progressive, surgery is not required, and the incidence of subacute bacterial endocarditis is extremely low (though antibiotic prophylaxis is recommended). Patients with *severe* stenosis often are symptomatic and require surgical relief of the stenosis. Indications for surgery include dyspnea, angina, syncope, CHF, evidence of decreased right ventricular function, and development of cyanosis. Infants who demonstrate critical pulmonary stenosis require emergency surgery.

Aortic Stenosis

Obstruction to flow from the left ventricle to the aorta may be located below the aortic valve, at the aortic valve, or just above the valve. Regardless of the site of obstruction, left ventricular pressure must be increased to maintain normal aortic flow. Left ventricular hypertrophy occurs. Dilation and cardiac failure may develop with severe forms of aortic stenosis. Many children with this lesion have other forms of cardiovascular disease.

Valvular aortic stenosis, the most common form of obstruction to left ventricular outflow, is caused by fusion of valve commissures, so the size of the valve orifice is reduced. Subvalvular stenosis, the second most common form of obstruction, is usually caused by formation of a

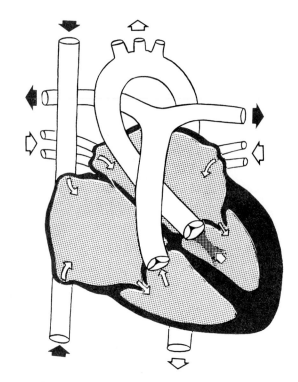

FIGURE 24-13 Subaortic stenosis. *(Reprinted with permission of Ross Laboratories, Columbus, OH 43216 from Ross Clinical Education Aid No. 7, © 1961 Ross Laboratories.)*

membrane below the aortic valve (Fig. 24-13). *Supravalvular* aortic stenosis is rare and is caused by constriction of the aorta just above the aortic valve and the coronary arteries.

Most children with the lesion have mild aortic stenosis and are asymptomatic. During the school years an initial referral is made because of the presence of a systolic aortic murmur at the right upper sternal border.

With moderate aortic stenosis, left ventricular hypertrophy develops. An ejection click and an aortic murmur may be heard. Peripheral pulses may be decreased in intensity and there may be a narrow pulse pressure. These patients are checked carefully for any evidence of severe aortic stenosis. Syncope, CHF, angina, and decreased exercise tolerance are all indicators for restricted activity and immediate surgical relief of the aortic stenosis.

Critical aortic stenosis in the neonate results in CHF and ultimately can cause low cardiac output, metabolic acidosis, and death unless medical and surgical intervention are skilled and aggressive. The development of critical aortic stenosis in an older child also produces the same symptoms; however, the stenosis develops more gradually so that the onset is less precipitous.

A cardiac catheterization demonstrates left ventricular hypertension unless cardiac output is reduced as a result of severe stenosis. Data collected reveal the specific location as well as the severity of the obstruction.

With severe forms of subvalvular and valvular aortic stenosis, coronary blood flow to the thickened myocardium may be inadequate, particularly during times of exercise. These patients are at risk for sudden arrhythmias and sudden death. Activity restriction is necessary once the child demonstrates severe obstruction. The reason for such restriction must be explained carefully to the child and parents, and surgery should be scheduled immediately. The incidence of bacterial endocarditis is significant in patients with aortic stenosis and so antibiotic prophylaxis is required even after surgical intervention.

Aortic stenosis is often a progressive disease. Open-heart surgical intervention is necessary when there is evidence of significant obstruction. An aortic valvulotomy relieves valvular stenosis temporarily, though aortic insufficiency and restenosis often result. Ultimately, a repeat valvulotomy or aortic valve replacement may be necessary. If the subvalvular stenosis is due to a membrane, it can be removed successfully. If muscular subvalvular aortic stenosis is present, resection is more difficult, mortality is higher, and residual stenosis is more likely. Supravalvular aortic stenosis also may be relieved surgically.

Surgical mortality is extremely high in critically ill neonates (approximately 50 percent or higher) and in children of any age with symptoms of critical stenosis and left ventricular strain. Postoperative complications include CHF, heart block, hemorrhage, arrhythmias, and low cardiac output.

If the aortic stenosis is relieved successfully without creating aortic insufficiency, the child tolerates normal activity. However, he needs to be monitored for recurrence, progression of the stenosis, or development of bacterial endocarditis. If significant aortic insufficiency is created, future valve replacement will be necessary and activity tolerance will not be normal.

Cyanotic Heart Disease (Right-to-Left Shunts)

In children with cyanotic congenital heart disease, an abnormality is present that permits some of the systemic venous return to bypass the lungs and enter the systemic arterial circulation directly. Right-to-left cardiac shunts result from two types of cardiac alterations: conditions that permit mixture of the systemic and pulmonary venous return and conditions that result in severe obstruction to pulmonary blood flow. *Whenever the patient has cyanotic congenital heart disease, it is imperative that no air be allowed to enter intravenous lines, since this air may be shunted into the systemic arterial circulation, producing a cerebral air embolus* (stroke) (Hazinski, 1984a).

Common congenital defects resulting in cyanosis may be divided into those with increased pulmonary vascularity (transposition of the great vessels, total anomalous pulmonary venous connection, and truncus arteriosus) and those with decreased pulmonary vascularity (tetralogy of Fallot, tricuspid atresia, and Ebstein's malformation). Cyanosis in the newborn and young infant presents a problem different from that of cyanosis in the older child. An older child may have symptoms and not be in acute distress, but a cyanotic newborn presents an emergency situation. Tetralogy of Fallot is the most common lesion

causing cyanosis in the infant. Transposition of the great vessels is the most comon cause of cyanosis in the newborn. A cyanotic newborn also may suffer from lung disease, and should be considered the cause of cyanosis.

With chronic arterial oxygen desaturation, red blood cell formation is stimulated, which results in polycythemia. Clubbing of the nailbeds is observed.

Cyanotic Heart Defects with Increased Pulmonary Vascularity

With most of these defects, a septal defect is one of several anomalies present. Oxgenated and venous blood mix within the heart or great vessels. Since pulmonary vascular resistance is lower than systemic vascular resistance, more blood enters the pulmonary circulation. The higher the pulmonary blood flow, the greater the amount of oxygenated blood returning to the heart. These children are at risk for the systemic consequences of polycythemia.

Transposition of the Great Vessels

In this condition the aorta arises from the right ventricle, and the pulmonary artery from the left (Fig. 24-14). However, the great veins are not similarly transposed, so the pulmonary veins deliver oxygenated blood into the left side of the heart, which pumps it back to the lungs. Unoxygenated blood from the body returns to the right side of the heart, which pumps this blood back into the systemic circulation. There must be another congenital heart defect, such as a PDA, an ASD, or a VSD, which allows mix-

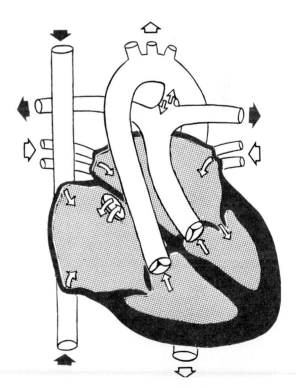

FIGURE 24-14 Complete transposition of the great vessels. *(Reprinted with permission of Ross Laboratories, Columbus, OH 43216 from Ross Clinical Education Aid No. 7, © 1961 Ross Laboratories.)*

ing of the oxygenated and venous blood, or the child will not survive.

Most neonates demonstrate cyanosis within the first hours or days of life. Occasionally, a PDA temporarily increases pulmonary blood flow so that cyanosis is minimal. If the infant has no other septal defect, cyanosis, hypoxemia, and metabolic acidosis develop rapidly as the ductus constricts, and the infant dies without treatment.

A large ASD is the best lesion for the child with transposition, because it allows the best mixing of oxygenated and venous blood. Once pulmonary vascular resistance falls, an ASD causes increased pulmonary blood flow, but it is well tolerated because the increased flow is under low pressure. A VSD allows some mixing of oxygenated venous blood but it often causes the development of CHF. If a VSD *and* pulmonary stenosis are both present, mixing of oxygenated and venous blood is facilitated, yet the pulmonary stenosis prevents excessive pulmonary blood flow and the development of CHF. There is no characteristic murmur associated with transposition of the great vessels.

A cardiac catheterization reveals systemic arterial oxygen desaturation and systemic pressures in the right ventricle. The angiocardiography demonstrates the abnormal great vessel position. Usually once the diagnosis of transposition is confirmed, a balloon-tipped catheter is inserted, passed through the patent foramen ovale (or the existing ASD), and inflated. As it is pulled back from the left to the right atrium, the balloon tears the atrial septum. This septostomy (Rashkind) allows better mixing of oxygenated and venous blood in the atria and improves arterial oxygen saturation. This procedure reduces hypoexmia sufficiently so that acidosis is eliminated, and the child is able to grow larger to undergo complete surgical correction of the transposition within the first months of life. If the Rashkind septostomy is inadequate, a surgical procedure called a Blalock-Hanlon septectomy may be performed to remove more of the atrial septum. This procedure, however, has become less popular recently, since complete surgical correction may be performed safely during the neonatal period (Hazinski, 1984a).

The neonate requires aggressive management of hypoxemia and acidosis in the first days of life. While the VSD improves arterial oxygen saturation, it may predispose the child to the development of CHF.

If the Rashkind septostomy or a Blalock-Hanlon septectomy can increase the child's arterial oxygen saturation (and content) sufficiently to prevent severe hypoxemia and acidosis, corrective surgery may be performed electively in the first year of life (or the first several months of life). However, if the neonate demonstrates profound hypoxemia and metabolic acidosis and is unresponsive to prostaglandin administration, surgical intervention will be necessary in the neonatal period.

There are several types of corrective open-heart operations for patients with transposition. The selection depends on the presence and types of associated defects and on the preference of the cardiovascular surgeon.

Two procedures, the Senning and the Mustard procedures, provide redirection of systemic and pulmonary venous return using an intraatrial baffle created from atrial septum (Senning) or pericardium (Mustard). After repair, systemic venous return from the venae cavae is diverted to the mitral valve and then into the left ventricle and pulmonary artery. Pulmonary venous blood is diverted to the tricuspid valve and then to the right ventricle and the aorta.

Recently, renewed attempts have been made to relocate the great vessels to their appropriate ventricles surgically. While the great vessels can be moved, the coronary arteries are more difficult to relocate; they must be reimplanted into the "new" aorta. Recently, this procedure, the Jatene operation, has been performed during the first days or weeks of life with a relatively low mortality. It is hoped that infants who survive the early surgical repair will have improved long-term survival, with fewer sequelae.

Children with transposition of the great vessels have a significant incidence of pulmonary vascular disease, particularly if the defect is not repaired until after 1 year of age. These children still should receive antibiotic prophylaxis at times of increased risk of bacteremia, since they are at risk for the development of bacterial endocarditis even after surgical repair.

Total Anomalous Pulmonary Venous Connection

In total anomalous pulmonary venous connection (TAPVC), the pulmonary veins fail to join the left atrium.

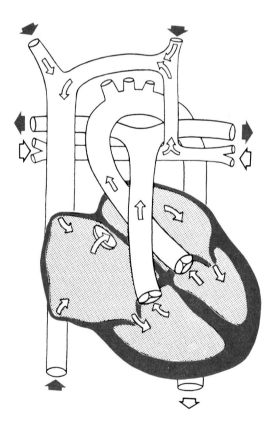

FIGURE 24-15 Total anomalous pulmonary venous return. *(Reprinted with permission of Ross Laboratories, Columbus, OH 43216 from Ross Clinical Education Aid No. 7, © 1961 Ross Laboratories.)*

As a result, pulmonary venous blood ultimately enters the right atrium through the superior vena cava, inferior vena cava, or coronary sinus (Fig. 24-15). Since the right atrium receives both pulmonary and systemic venous return, pulmonary blood flow is increased. If stenosis is present at the junction of the pulmonary veins and the systemic circulation, severe pulmonary vascular obstruction, pulmonary edema, and CHF can result.

Since pulmonary and systemic venous blood both enter the right atrium, an ASD must be present to allow flow to the left side of the heart. The amount of blood flow through an unrestrictive ASD is dependent on relative pulmonary and systemic vascular resistances.

Most patients with TAPVC develop cyanosis and/or CHF in the first year of life; many develop these symptoms in the first month of life. The degree of cyanosis is usually inversely related to the amount of pulmonary blood flow.

Surgical repair usually is performed during infancy, utilizing cardiopulmonary bypass, hypothermia, and circulatory arrest. Operative mortality may be high if the patient is extremely ill preoperatively. Postoperative complications include bleeding, arrhythmias, CHF, low cardiac output, and respiratory insufficiency.

The prognosis for these children is guarded, since operative mortality is significant and obstruction may develop later at the junction of the left atrium and the pulmonary veins. Pulmonary vascular disease develops early in all of these patients and contributes to later mortality. Following surgical repair, the child requires close medical follow-up and antibiotic prophylaxis at times of increased risk of bacteremia.

Truncus Arteriosus

The *truncus arteriosus,* a single large vessel, arises from both ventricles astride a large VSD (Fig. 24-16). A single, malformed semilunar valve is also present. The output of both ventricles is ejected into the common truncus. Systemic and pulmonary arterial blood mix incompletely in this trunk.

Pulmonary blood flow usually is increased, causing the development of CHF in the first weeks of life. Cyanosis is usually present and varies inversely with the amount of pulmonary blood flow.

If pulmonary blood flow is increased, aggressive management of CHF is required within the first weeks of life. If severe CHF persists, pulmonary artery banding may be performed to reduce the volume and pressure of pulmonary blood flow until the child grows and is in more stable condition to undergo surgical repair.

Recently, correction has been performed successfully in infants less than 6 months of age with the use of cardiopulmonary bypass and hypothermia.

A child who requires repair in infancy will need several other operations as he grows. These children always require antibiotic prophylaxis at times of increased risk of bacteremia to prevent the development of bacterial endocarditis.

Cyanotic Heart Defects with Decreased Pulmonary Vascularity

Tetralogy of Fallot

This anomaly is the most common cause of cyanotic congenital heart disease. The malformation called tetralogy of Fallot includes a VSD, dextroposition of the aorta (so that it overrides the VSD), hypertrophy of the right ventricle, and pulmonary infundibular stenosis (Fig. 24-17). The right ventricle must generate higher pressures to maintain flow through the area of obstruction. If pulmonary infundibular stenosis is severe, the aorta and systemic circulation (through the VSD) provide less resistance to flow, and a right-to-left shunt develops. Since the aorta is located directly over the VSD, the venous blood shunted from the right ventricle enters almost directly into the aorta, producing systemic arterial oxygen desaturation. The degree of cyanosis is related to the degree of pulmonary obstruction. Right ventricular hypertrophy is present and pulmonary blood flow is reduced once cyanosis is apparent. The left atrium and ventricle may be reduced in size because of the small amount of pulmonary venous return.

Cyanosis is often not apparent at birth. Since the pulmonary infundibular stenosis usually increases as the child grows, cyanosis generally develops during the first year of life. The cyanosis characteristically increases with cry or exertion. Exercise tolerance usually is reduced. The child may interrupt play to squat, since the knee-chest position seems to help increase pulmonary blood flow. CHF does not develop once pulmonary blood flow is reduced.

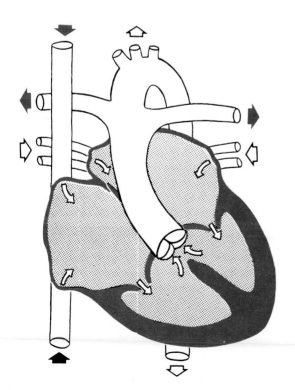

FIGURE 24-16 Truncus arteriosus. *(Reprinted with permission of Ross Laboratories, Columbus, OH 43216 from Ross Clinical Education Aid No. 7, © 1961 Ross Laboratories.)*

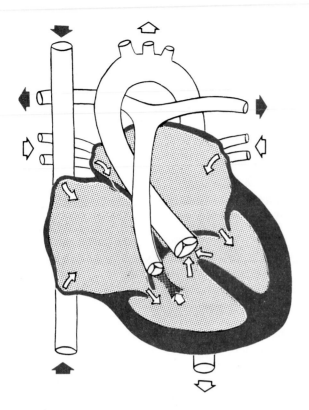

FIGURE 24-17 Tetralogy of Fallot. *(Reprinted with permission of Ross Laboratories, Columbus, OH 43216 from Ross Clinical Education Aid No. 7, © 1961 Ross Laboratories.)*

In severe forms of tetralogy, the pulmonary infundibulum may go into spasm, causing a severe and sudden decrease in pulmonary blood flow, increased right-to-left shunt, and hypoxemia. The infant becomes profoundly cyanotic and often loses consciousness. These spells may be relieved by placing the child in a knee-chest position. Administration of oxygen and morphine or a beta-adrenergic blocker such as propanolol may be required to increase pulmonary blood flow. If the child has a history of these "tet" spells, surgical palliation or correction is required on an urgent basis.

On physical examination, a harsh systolic murmur is heard along the left sternal border, and the second heart sound appears single. With severe forms of tetralogy, bronchial collateral vessels contribute to pulmonary blood flow, causing continuous murmurs heard over the child's back. Polycythemia and other systemic consequences of chronic arterial oxygen desaturation will be present.

Cardiac catheterization demonstrates arterial oxygen desaturation and the presence of the VSD. Angiocardiography delineates the size and anatomy of the pulmonary outflow tract and pulmonary artery.

Indications for surgery include severe hypoxemia and cyanosis, the presence of acidosis, and a history of "tet" spells. If the distal pulmonary arteries are small, a surgical shunt may be created to increase pulmonary blood flow and allow the arteries to grow before surgical correction is attempted. All these shunts should produce increased

NURSING CARE PLAN

24-3 The Child with Tetralogy of Fallot

Clinical Problem/Nursing Diagnosis	Expected Outcome	Nursing Interventions
Anxiety and stress associated with unknown experiences of cardiac disease, hospitalization, and surgery	Given individualized teaching and emotional support, child and family will be able to cope with stress of illness, hospitalization, and surgery	Prepare child and family for hospitalization experiences, cardiac catheterization, surgery, and home care Individualize teaching and psychosocial supportive interventions according to child's cognitive and developmental level; see Nursing Interventions for Knowledge Deficit in Nursing Care Plan
Knowledge deficit related to preparation for cardiac catheterization, surgery, and home care		
Altered family processes related to ill child and stressors of hospitalization and illness		

Clinical Problem/Nursing Diagnosis	Expected Outcome	Nursing Interventions
Increased irritability Acute arterial oxygen desaturation episodes Cyanosis Syncope Distress with play Fatigue Activity intolerance related to insufficient oxygenation secondary to decrease in pulmonary blood flow ("tet spells") and arterial oxygen desaturation	Given nursing care directed toward energy conservation and increasing pulmonary blood flow, child will have improved circulation and respiratory function	Monitor apical pulse for rate, rhythm, and regularity of beats: auscultate the chest at the 2d to 3d intercostal space, left sternal border, for a harsh systolic ejection murmur radiating over anterior and posterior lung fields Observe child's color; note presence of cyanosis at rest and evidence of clubbing of toes and fingers; assess degree and severity of cyanosis with crying and increased activity; assess degree of respiratory distress and fatigue with activity. Assess child for signs of decreased cardiac output: tachycardia, decreased peripheral perfusion, peripheral vasoconstriction, cool pale extremities, decreased peripheral pulses, sluggish capillary refill, and decreased urine output ($< 1cc/kg/h$). Monitor child for signs and symptoms of congestive heart failure; provide supportive measures as previously outlined; see Nursing Interventions for Activity Intolerance in Nursing Care Plan 24-1 Assess respirations for rate, depth, and regularity; observe quality and equality of chest expansion; auscultate breath sounds for equality and quality of aeration in all lung fields Monitor child for signs of respiratory distress: tachypnea, labored respirations, retractions, nasal flaring, grunting, and cyanosis Monitor child for frequency and severity of hypercyanotic episodes or tet spells as evidenced by squatting at play, irritability, diaphoresis, cyanosis, acute arterial oxygen desaturation, altered level of consciousness, and syncope; assist child to knee-chest position. Monitor child's arterial blood gas values or oxygen saturation via pulse oximetry; notify physician promptly Administer prostaglandin E_1 to maintain ductal dependency to increase pulmonary blood flow as ordered Administer beta-adrenergic blocking agents: keep morphine sulfate, propranolol, phenylephrine, and sodium bicarbonate available for immediate use to relieve infundibular spasm Teach parents how to recognize and intervene during hypercyanotic episodes; teach them to place child in a knee-chest position and to notify physician Monitor arterial blood gas values, complete blood count, hemoglobin, hematocrit (Hct), platelet count, blood urea nitrogen, creatinine, and urinalysis results, along with precardiac catheterization and postoperative record for a baseline comparison Provide postcardiac catheterization care; see Nursing Interventions for Activity Intolerance in the Nursing Care Plan for a Child with Patent Ductus Arteriosus Provide postoperative care; monitor child for postoperative complications: excessive bleeding, arrhythmias, increased cyanosis, hypoxemia, acidosis, decreased cardiac output, congestive heart failure, and altered neurological status; see Nursing Interventions for Activity Intolerance in the Nursing Care Plan for a Child with Patent Ductus Arteriosus
Focal neurological deficits: hemiparesis and seizures Irritability Fever Potential for injury (neurological insult, cerebral embolus/brain abscess) related to polycythemia (Hct 60%) and chronic oxygen desaturation	Given appropriate nursing observation to detect complications from polycythemia and chronic oxygen desaturation, child will receive prompt treatment and potential for neurological injury wil be reduced	Monitor child's neurological status for signs of cerebral embolus; observe child for evidence of focal seizure activity, focal neurological deficits (hemiparesis), and transient loss of consciousness; notify physician promptly with above findings Maintain patent airway; administer medications as prescribed; protect child from injury; monitor vital signs closely and perform ongoing neurological assessments Observe child for changes in sensation, level of consciousness, and pupillary response (equality and reaction to light); assess motor and sensory function and response to environment and stimuli Monitor child for signs of brain abscess; observe child for evidence of fever, headache, anorexia, and signs of meningitis; see Nursing Care Plan for the Child with Meningitis (Chap. 20)

Continued.

NURSING CARE PLAN 24-3 The Child with Tetralogy of Fallot—cont'd

Clinical Problem/Nursing Diagnosis	Expected Outcome	Nursing Interventions
		Monitor child for signs of increased intracranial pressure: increased irritability, headache, vomiting, drowsiness, change in behavior and feeding patterns, increased head circumference and bulging fontanels in infants, and alterations in vital signs (hypertension, bradycardia, and widened pulse pressure)
		Administer antibiotic therapy as prescribed
		Prepare child and family for surgery as indicated; monitor vital signs and neurological status closely; administer medications and antipyretic measures as ordered; maintain patent airway
		Maintain and optimize child's hydration status to prevent hemoconcentration
		Prevent dehydration; recognize and treat fever, vomiting, and diarrhea promptly
		Monitor lab values for evidence of coagulopathies: presence of microcytic anemia and decreased platelet count or function; report alterations in hematologic lab results and correct coagulopathies as ordered
		Monitor hemoglobin and Hct laboratory values; maintain optimal hemoglobin levels
		Teach parents to notify physician of changes in child's ability to walk, behavior, activity level, and evidence of fever, vomiting, and diarrhea to ensure prompt treatment; explain importance of preventing dehydration to decrease risk of polycythemia
Fever Irritability<hr>Potential for infection (brain abscess and endocarditis) related to bypass of blood through the lung's filtering system; turbulent intracardiac blood flow	Child will respond positively to treatment of infection as evidenced by return of fever to normal and disappearance of irritability Given appropriate antibiotic prophylaxis prior to dental work or surgical procedures, child will remain free of infection	Monitor child for elevated temperature > 38.5°C rectally; notify physician; administer antipyretic measures as ordered; obtain blood and body fluid cultures as needed; administer antibiotic therapy for brain abscess or bacterial endocarditis as prescribed; instruct parents to administer antibiotic prophylaxis prior to dental work or surgical procedures Inform parents of need to consult physician prior to invasive procedures to ensure antibiotic prophylaxis; teach parents to report evidence of fever and malaise; prevent infection and detect signs of infection early; see Nursing Interventions for Potential for Infection in Nursing Care Plan 24-1
Poor weight gain Poor appetite Vomiting Diarrhea Fatigue Tachypnea and labored respirations<hr>Altered nutrition: less than body requirements related to fatigue, increased energy expenditure, and increased caloric needs	Through necessary interventions, child will gain weight appropriate for age and will reach fluid and electrolyte balance To promote wound healing and growth, child will progressively tolerate a diet rich in protein, carbohydrate, calories, and vitamins	Optimize child's nutritional status; maximize child's caloric intake; see Nursing Interventions for Alteration in Nutrition in Nursing Care Plan 24-1

pulmonary blood flow and result in increased arterial oxygen saturation and decreased cyanosis. The Blalock-Taussig shunt, or subclavian-to-pulmonary arery shunt, is the shunt of choice for even small infants. In this procedure the child's own subclavian artery is used; it is separated from the arm circulation and sewn to the pulmonary artery so that it provides flow from the aorta through the subclavian artery to the pulmonary artery. More recently, prosthetic material has been utilized to create a shunt between the child's subclavian artery and the epilateral pulmonary artery. These shunts are created from polytetrafluoroephylene (Gor-tex or Impra RTM), and they can be constructed to allow increased shunt flow as the child grows. Complications are few and include those of a thoracotomy. Once a subclavian artery-pulmonary artery shunt has been performed, the nurse will not be able to obtain a conventional indirect blood pressure reading from the brachial artery of the involved arm; the other arm always should be used for indirect blood pressure measurement and any arterial blood sampling. This need should be noted on the child's chart.

A Waterston-Cooley shunt also may be created between the ascending aorta and the pulmonary artery. This shunt is more difficult to eliminate when later surgical correction of the tetralogy is performed. In addition, CHF and later pulmonary hypertension may result if the shunt is too large.

The prognosis is best for a child with minimal infundibular stenosis and cyanosis. If the neonate has severe tetralogy and has severe cyanosis and hypoxemia in the first days of life, the pulmonary arteries may be small, making surgical repair difficult. This infant usually requires a shunt, followed by complete repair when the pulmonary arteries have grown (usually in several months or years). If effective pulmonary blood flow can be achieved and no CHF or arrhythmias are present, the child does very well. These children require antibiotic prophylaxis at times of increased risk of bacteremia to prevent bacterial endocarditis.

Other Cardiac Conditions that Occur in Children

Acute Rheumatic Fever

Rheumatic fever, a collagen disease, is an important cause of acquired heart disease in children. It is difficult to determine its incidence accurately since the diagnostic criteria vary and the disease is not a reportable one in the United States. Even with the increased treatment available for streptococcal infection, rheumatic fever still occurs, though its incidence is declining.

Acute rheumatic fever is a systemic inflammatory disease that develops 10 or 14 days to 6 weeks (if reinfection occurs) after a group A, beta-hemolytic streptococcus infection, and it is found most often in children between the ages of 5 and 14 years. The diagnosis is based on the application of the modified Jones criteria for acute

rheumatic fever. The presence of two major criteria or one major and two minor criteria strongly suggests that the child has acute rheumatic fever. Major criteria include arthritis, carditis, chorea, erythema marginatum, and subcutaneous nodules. The minor criteria consist of a fever, a previous streptococcal infection, arthralgia, leukocytosis, an elevated erythrocyte sedimentation rate, a positive C-reactive protein, a prolonged PR interval on ECG, prior history of rheumatic fever, and the presence of rheumatic heart disease.

There appears to be an inherited tendency or familial predisposition to rheumatic fever since children of parents who had rheumatic fever contract acute rheumatic fever more readily than do children of parents with no history of the disease. It also seems to occur more frequently in lower socioeconomic groups, where overcrowding, poor nutrition, and poor hygienic conditions contribute to a higher incidence of this acquired disease. Rheumatic fever is more common in the spring on the east coast and in the winter on the west coast of the United States.

Since acute rheumatic fever occurs in school-age children, this disease is often diagnosed during a routine school physical examination. Early diagnosis is difficult because symptoms may be vague. General symptoms such as malaise, pallor, loss of weight, and loss of appetite frequently are associated with rheumatic fever; however, the course of illness varies and may not include all these symptoms.

In about 50 percent of children with rheumatic fever the parents describe a cold or sore throat 10 days to 6 weeks before the onset of illness. This illness might have been treated with an antimicrobial agent either transiently or in an inadequate dosage. The severity of the upper respiratory infection might have been average, and its duration usually no more than 2 to 4 days. Other children may experience a low-grade fever, complain of abdominal pain, or have spontaneous nosebleeds or dyspnea on exertion for a period of time.

The acute attack of rheumatic fever may follow the infection and consist of (1) a fever of 38 to 39°C (100.4 to 102.2°F), (2) leukocytosis, (3) elevation of the erythrocyte sedimentation rate, (4) mild or occasionally severe anemia, and (5) lassitude, irritability, and moderate weight loss. After the acute phase, the child may experience some of the specific manifestations of rheumatic fever—arthritis, carditis, and chorea. Other symptoms may include epistaxis, abdominal pain, and skin manifestations. The typical lesions of rheumatic fever occur in the connective tissue of the arteries, subcutaneous tissue, and the heart.

Rheumatic changes in the heart are of great concern. Carditis may cause permanent cardiovascular changes and may be fatal. It is seen in approximately 50 percent of patients with rheumatic fever and is usually evident within 2 weeks of the acute rheumatic fever.

While inflammation of the pericardium, myocardium, and valves occurs, the mitral and aortic valves are the most susceptible to damage. Rheumatic carditis is responsible for the majority of organic mitral valve lesions and eventually causes mitral stenosis or insufficiency.

Mitral insufficiency is the most common rheumatic heart lesion seen in children. Most forms are mild and produce no symptoms. The heart sounds are normal, except for a systolic apical murmur and left atrial enlargement. If severe mitral regurgitation occurs, symptoms of pulmonary venous engorgement, dyspnea, CHF, and exercise intolerance usually develop early in life. Atrial fibrillation and pulmonary hypertension develop if chronic mitral regurgitation is present. Some degree of mitral stenosis usually is associated with mitral insufficiency.

With mild *mitral stenosis,* the patient may be asymptomatic. With severe mitral stenosis, increased left atrial size is present. In addition, left atrial and pulmonary venous pressures are elevated, and pulmonary edema, dyspnea, orthopnea, and exercise intolerance may result. With chronic mitral stenosis, pulmonary hypertension develops and may produce right ventricular failure.

Aortic regurgitation usually develops during or soon after the episode of acute rheumatic fever, and it occurs more often than does aortic stenosis. Mild aortic insufficiency causes no symptoms.

The myocardial lesion primarily involved in rheumatic fever is the formation of Aschoff's bodies. With inflammation, there is a cellular response to the altered collagen common to perivascular connective tissue, and the result is the formation of nodules known as *Aschoff's bodies.*

Pericarditis can be detected by means of a friction rub. The heart sounds become distant, dull, and muffled with the development of a large effusion. Poor cardiac pulsations and feeble heart sounds should be noted by the nurse. A ventricular diastolic gallop is commonly present in acute rheumatic carditis. CHF may develop during the acute phase of rheumatic fever, producing symptoms of systemic and pulmonary venous engorgement.

ECG tracings reveal transient changes. Prolongation of the PR interval (first-degree block) is the most frequent abnormality.

Arthritis, the most common complaint of children with rheumatic fever, involves several joints simultaneously or in succession. They are tender, swollen, and painful to move and remain in this condition as the disease runs its course in 3 weeks or less. Usually large joints such as the knees, ankles, wrists, and elbows are involved.

Sydenham's chorea involves the nervous system and is manifested by muscular twitchings, weakness, and purposeless movement. At first the child may show evidence of not concentrating in school, exhibiting mood swings, being hyperirritable, and demonstrating other signs of inappropriate behavior. Jerky, involuntary movements become evident. This involvement may begin 2 to 6 months after the initial infection. The muscular weakness can be so extreme the child cannot sit up or even talk. The symptoms gradually subside after a period of time.

The skin manifestations of rheumatic fever are erythematous areas with irregular borders, sharply demarcated and often of a transient nature. Erythema marginatum is often seen with carditis.

Rheumatic nodules are a major and specific manifestation of rheumatic fever. These subcutaneous nodules attached to tendon sheaths have a symmetrical distribution over the scapulae, elbows, edge of the patella, the vertebrae, and the occiput. They are painless and freely movable under the skin. Although they may be found in other conditions, they occur in severe or chronic forms of the rheumatic activity. They may last a few days or a few weeks.

The major aim of therapy is to prevent permanent cardiac damage through rapid treatment of rheumatic fever, minimization of cardiac inflammatory process, and maximization of cardiac function. Bed rest during the acute febrile part of the illness is not necessary unless heart failure is present. Careful observation for recurrence of signs and symptoms, especially those of CHF, is important. CHF must be treated aggressively (see Congestive Heart Failure, above). Management can prevent valvular damage or minimize the progression of existing valvular damage. Improvement of cardiac function and general symptomatic relief during the acute phase is an important goal.

The first priority in antibiotic treatment is eradication of the streptococcal infection and prevention of further episodes of rheumatic fever. Penicillin is the drug of choice except for children who are sensitive to the drug. In such cases, erythromycin is selected. It is given in oral form unless the child has had previous episodes of carditis or rheumatic fever; then parenteral antibiotics are given. For long-term prophylaxis in a child who is allergic to penicillin, sulfonamides, particularly sulfadiazine, and erythromycin are considered most effective. The length of therapy varies, but patients with severe cardiac involvement usually are maintained on lifelong prophylaxis.

Corticosteroids are considered when patients have symptoms of severe CHF or arthritis. If steroids are prescribed, the nurse must monitor the patient's fluid and electrolyte balance even more carefully. The combination of steroid therapy and stress may lead to the development of gastric ulcers.

Aspirin does not alter the duration of an acute rheumatic attack. It does contribute to the child's comfort, especially when he is febrile or when joint pain is present. In addition, it may reduce the inflammatory process associated with carditis or arthritis. The medications selected, their dosage, and the duration of use vary. They are highly individualized to meet the needs of patients who have a wide variety of symptoms.

Nursing Management

Optimum cardiac function and relief of pain are prime nursing concerns. Antibiotics are started after the diagnosis is confirmed. Vital signs are evaluated at routine intervals. In the presence of carditis and CHF, steroids, diuretics, and digoxin may be ordered. Explanations of these drugs and their effects should be provided to the child and parents. The mood swings often demonstrated by a child receiving steroid therapy are frightening and preparation for such behavior is important.

Since the child frequently receives salicylates, it is important for a nurse to evaluate his response to the aspirin (i.e., lowering temperature, relieving pain). The signs of toxicity and the effects of salicylates on clotting time (bleeding tendencies) are critical nursing assessments.

The arthritis is so painful that the weight of a blanket may be unbearable, especially in an older child who appears to have more severe joint pain than does a younger client. Initially, positioning is a major problem, and the nursing interventions instituted need to be evaluated and revised constantly in order to decrease the child's discomfort most expeditiously.

Assessing hydration is another important nursing function, particularly since excessive fluids augment CHF. It is essential to monitor the intake and output closely, determine urine specific gravity, and evaluate hydration through assessment of mucous membranes as well as skin turgor.

If choreic activity develops, a child may experience extreme frustration in regard to the lack of control over these movements. Most children do not understand their outbursts of anger and need patience and understanding in addition to safety measures (siderails up, staying with a child who is in a wheelchair) which prevent injury. On occasion their frustration levels become so high that children who already are anxious become more apprehensive, thereby increasing choreiform movement and causing exhaustion.

Some children in the acute phase do not feel acutely ill. Others withdraw, while still others, especially adolescents, become belligerent and require a great deal of patience on the part of the nurses and/or family members caring for them. It is important for a nurse to understand and anticipate the needs of these children and to encourage them in the making of decisions such as menu selection and bath time. The restlessness and boredom these children experience can challenge even the most creative and innovative nurse. A telephone, quiet games with ambulatory clients, and visits from friends are helpful until that time when there are no specific limits on physical activity.

Hospital confinement often results in missing an appreciable amount of schooltime, which can be a significant event for the late school-age child or adolescent. Parents can be requested to bring in books so that the patient can make an effort to keep up with schoolwork. After the acute phase is over, large blocks of time are available for performing this normal task.

There is a possibility that the patient can develop rheumatic fever again following another group A beta-hemolytic streptococcal infection. Therefore, the nurse plays a vital role in follow-up care. Teaching the child and family about the disease, its course, and the drugs being used should be done routinely. In addition, it is critical to stress why the medications should be continued, the clinic or doctor visits kept, and the affected child protected from family members with respiratory infections.

The American Heart Association recommends that all patients who currently have or have had acute rheumatic fever should be placed indefinitely on a program of prophylaxis. Such a recommendation markedly reduces the frequency of recurrences. This long-term treatment and hospitalization is an emotional and financial burden on the child and family. Health team members must be cognizant of individual family needs, including those which can be met best by the community health nurse, social worker, teacher, or nutritionist.

The prognosis varies; however, marked cardiomegaly and/or the presence of significant CHF at the time of acute rheumatic fever are the most consistent precursors of later rheumatic heart disease. When treatment is instituted promptly and there is a good response, the prognosis is favorable.

Hypertension

Hypertension is a condition in which either systolic or diastolic blood pressure consistently exceeds the 95th percentile for any given year of life (Table 24-4). There is growing evidence to suggest that cardiovascular diseases which become evident during adulthood may have their origin during the first or second decade of life. The identification and control of high blood pressure in children currently is being given high priority because hypertension is known to predispose an individual to severe degenerative cardiovascular problems, most specifically cerebrovascular accident and myocardial infarction. It is therefore important that measures be instituted as early in life as possible which eliminate or minimize the detrimental effects of hypertension on the future health of affected individuals and others who may be at risk.

TABLE 24-4 Classification of Hypertension by Age Group

Age Group	Significant Hypertension (mm Hg)	Severe Hypertension (mm Hg)
Newborn 7 d	Systolic BP ≥96	Systolic BP ≥106
8-30 d	Systolic BP ≥104	Systolic BP ≥110
Infant (<2 yr)	Systolic BP ≥112 Diastolic BP ≥74	Systolic BP ≥118 Diastolic BP ≥82
Children (3-5 yr)	Systolic BP ≥116 Diastolic BP ≥76	Systolic BP ≥124 Diastolic BP ≥84
Children (6-9 yr)	Systolic BP ≥122 Diastolic BP ≥78	Systolic BP ≥130 Diastolic BP ≥86
Children (10-12 yr)	Systolic BP ≥126 Diastolic BP ≥82	Systolic BP ≥134 Diastolic BP ≥90
Adolescents (13-15 yr)	Systolic BP ≥136 Diastolic BP ≥86	Systolic BP ≥144 Diastolic BP ≥92
Adolescents (16-18 yr)	Systolic BP ≥142 Diastolic BP ≥92	Systolic BP ≥150 Diastolic BP ≥98

Source: Reprinted by permission of *Pediatrics*, 79(1):7, 1987.

It has been difficult for experts to determine the actual incidence of hypertension among children and adolescents. It is estimated that approximately 1 to 2 percent of children and up to 11 or 12 percent of adolescents in the general population are hypertensive. Both *primary* and *secondary* forms of hypertension have been observed in children and adolescents. *Primary hypertension* (formerly called essential hypertension) is a form of high blood pressure which cannot be attributed to an identifiable cause, whereas *secondary hypertension* results from a structural abnormality or an underlying pathophysiological process. Generally, the more severe the hypertension and the younger the child, the more likely that the hypertension is secondary in nature. A well-documented history, a thorough physical examination, and radiological and laboratory tests usually identify the etiology of secondary hypertension in a child. In Table 24-5, the most common causes underlying secondary hypertension in children and adolescents are listed.

Primary hypertension is associated with many interacting factors. Although the precise manner in which these variables interact to produce hypertension is not understood, heredity, environment, and life-style seem to exert a significant influence on the blood pressures of individuals at all ages. An individual's baseline blood pressure has the strongest relationship to the risk of hypertension later in life. There is evidence to suggest that an individual's blood pressure remains at the same general place in the blood pressure distribution curve throughout life. Therefore, if an individual's blood pressure is in the 50th percentile at age 10, he is likely to have a blood pressure around the 50th percentile at age 18 and at age 45, pro-

TABLE 24-5 Common Causes of Secondary Hypertension in Children and Adolescents

Renal system
Chronic glomerulonephritis
Acute or chronic pyelonephritis
Renovascular alterations or defects
Cardiovascular system
Coarctation of the aorta
Large patent ductus arteriosus
Arrhythmias
Endocrine system
  Adrenal disease (excess catecholamines, mineralocorticoids, or glucocorticoids)
Central nervous system
  Increased intracranial pressure
  Encephalitis
  Tumors
Collagen diseases
Drugs, toxins, and chemicals
  Sympathomimetics
  Amphetamines
  Methylphenidate
  Long-term high-dose therapy with corticosteroids
  Oral contraceptives
  Testosterone therapy
  Lead poisoning
  Foods high in tyramine

vided that he does not develop an illness which affects blood pressure regulation. This relationship between blood pressure measurements obtained on the same person at different points in time is known as *blood pressure tracking*. Examples of percentile charts suitable for use in tracking children's blood pressures over a period of time are provided in Figs. 24-4, 24-5, and 24-6. If the child demonstrates blood pressures that are near or above the 95th percentile for age and sex on at least three occasions, the child's three BP readings are averaged. If the average reading is equal to or greater than the 95th percentile, diagnostic evaluation is warranted, and the child may be a candidate for pharmacotherapy. Readings between the 90th and the 95th percentiles are considered high normal. In those children who are tall for age and/or have excess lean body mass for age, such averaged blood pressure readings may be assessed as normal rather than high normal [National Heart, Lung, Blood Institute (NHLBI), 1987].

In addition to the individual's baseline blood pressure average, the presence of hypertension in one or both parents, and possibly in siblings, seems to be a strong predictor of primary hypertension in adult life. The incidence of primary hypertension is significantly higher in adult blacks, especially males, than in whites, but the influence of race on children's blood pressures is unclear at this time.

The danger of hypertension lies in its "silent" nature. When there are symptoms to suggest the presence of hypertension, the disease may already be quite severe. In children, the symptoms include blurred vision, severe headaches, marked irritability, focal or generalized seizures, and occasionally severe back or abdominal pain. Physical examination may reveal papilledema, retinal hemorrhages or exudates, constriction of the retinal arteries, and abdominal masses. Radiological and laboratory studies may demonstrate left ventricular hypertrophy and altered renal function.

When a child is found to have a suspiciously high blood pressure, caution should be utilized because labeling a child as hypertensive, even when his blood pressure is high, is likely to produce unnecessary emotional stress for the child and his family. Many children and adolescents with borderline high blood pressure require only periodic blood pressure measurement. Adolescents may manifest transient elevations in blood pressure related to their suden growth spurt and hormonal changes.

The decision to initiate specific treatment measures is made only after complete evaluation of the child. Severity and duration of hypertension, age, race, sex, and the presence of risk factors are considered carefully in determining whether treatment is indicated. Pharmacologic treatment is reserved for children with severe hypertension (Table 24-4). It is recommended for children with significant hypertension *only* if they fail to respond to nonpharmacologic therapy over a period of time. The latter intervention mode is used with both groups (NHLBI, 1987).

Nonpharmacologic treatment is tailored to the individual child. Counseling topics include family history, over-

TABLE 24-6 Drugs Used for Treatment of Hypertension in Children and Adolescents

Diuretic agents	*Agents acting on the adrenergic system*
Hydrochlorothiazide	
Chlorthalidone	Propranolol
Spironolactone	Methyldopa
Furosemide	Guanabenz
	Atenolol
Vasodilators	Clonidine
Hydralazine	
Minoxidil	*Angiotensin conversion inhibitor*
Diazoxide	
Nitroprusside	Captopril

weight, lack of exercise, stress, and tobacco use—all cardiovascular risk factors. A weight reduction program is begun for the overweight child. For all children who have significant or severe primary hypertension, a regular aerobic exercise program is developed, and a decrease in salt intake with a concomitant increase in potassium-rich foods is recommended. Children experiencing stress associated with family life or school are offered support to help them cope (NHLBI, 1987).

The Second Task Force on Blood Pressure Control in Children has advocated a specific protocol for use in treating children with antihypertensive agents. Several pharmacological agents used to treat hypertension in children and adolescents are listed in Table 24-6.

Nursing Management

Nurses have a particularly significant role in the identification and management of this pediatric health problem. Often, it is the nurse who first identifies the existence of elevated blood pressure in a child. The nurse may be responsible for conducting additional measures to confirm or rule out abnormal blood pressure in a child or adolescent.

The nurse also assumes important responsibilities in relation to health maintenance, teaching, and counseling for the families of children with borderline or true hypertension. Lack of compliance with the prescribed treatment and the required follow-up visits have been cited repeatedly as the major obstacle to successful treatment of hypertension in children and adolescents. Noncompliance among pediatric patients may be 50 percent or more. Adherence to treatment appears to be better in young children who are dependent on their parents for administration of medications, but success is highly dependent on the quality of teaching and support the parents receive from health care providers. Often an older child will feel and look well, and so he inadvertently or deliberately skips the medication. If the child has also been placed on sodium or caloric restriction, it will be even more difficult for him to adhere to the treatment plan.

While the nurse should avoid creating undue fear or preoccupation with illness in the child and family, both the parents and child (if he is old enough) should clearly understand the reason for treatment and the importance of adhering to the prescribed treatment. Compliance is highly dependent on the parents' and patient's ability to recognize the seriousness of the illness and the importance of treatment.

Teaching includes an explanation of hypertension; the administration, action, and side effects of medications (if they are prescribed); dietary modifications; an exercise program; and the importance of return visits to the clinic or health provider. For some patients, teaching about avoidance of associated risk factors, such as smoking, is also indicated. Adolescent girls who have been taking oral contraceptives may need teaching about alternative forms of birth control. Success is highly dependent on the learner's motivation. The nature of the prescribed treatment influences patient compliance. Generally, the greater the number of drugs prescribed and the greater the frequency of administration, the less likely it is that the treatment will be successful. Moreover, when the therapy requires a change in habits or life-style (e.g., dietary restriction), compliance is less likely to occur. It may be necessary for the nurse to assess the patient's and family's motivation and consider approaches that promote motivation before attempting to give instruction. A small peer support group, for example, effectively enhances motivation and compliance in older children and adolescents.

Atherosclerosis

Although *atherosclerosis*, a condition characterized by fatty deposits on the walls of arteries, has been associated with middle-aged and older adults, the atherosclerotic process is beginning to receive attention from those concerned with the prevention of cardiovascular conditons in children. Major risk factors associated with the development of atherosclerosis and coronary heart disease include hypercholesterolemia, hypertension, and smoking. Obesity, hyperglycemia, sedentary living habits, psychosocial tension, and a positive family history of early atherosclerotic disease are also correlated with increased risk of atherosclerosis. The more risk factors the patient has, the more likely it is that he will develop coronary heart disease.

Fatty streaks in the coronary arteries have been linked strongly to the development of coronary heart disease; these streaks may be present in children beyond 10 years of age. Fatty streaks in the aorta, which are less clearly related to the development of coronary heart disease, may be present as early as fetal life.

Primary familial hypercholesterolemia type II-A hyperlipoproteinemia) is the most commonly recognized form of familial hyperlipidemia in children. It is considered the most significant of the hyperlipoproteinemias with regard to the later development of premature cardiovascular disease. It is thought to be inherited as an autosomal dominant trait. The incidence is estimated to be as high as 1 in every 200 persons in the United States.

Patients who are homozygous for type II familial hypercholesterolemia may develop premature coronary artery disease, with myocardial infarction occurring as early as the first decade of life. This form of the disease is rare.

Children who are heterozygous for familial hypercholesterolemia may be asymptomatic during childhood, though a shortened life span from coronary artery disease is likely. Laboratory tests usually show an increase in low-density lipoprotein (LDL) which may or may not be accompanied by a cholesterol and triglyceride elevation. These tests should be performed at about 1 year of age on children who have a positive family history of premature cardivascular disease (myocardial infarction in males under age 50) or hyperlipidemia. These determinations also should be obtained early in infancy for children born to parents who are heterozygous for the familial hypercholesterolemia trait. Screening for cholesterol and triglyceride determinations in normal children should be performed after 2 years of age and repeated at about 16 years of age. All siblings of hyperlipoproteinemic patients should be tested regardless of their age. A fasting serum cholesterol above 230 mg/100 ml represents the 95th percentile for lipid levels of children in the United States. Treatment consists mainly of a prudent diet and the control or elimination of risk factors associated with cardiovascular disease, such as hypertension, obesity, smoking, and use of oral contraceptives. Other significant risk factors may be modified or eliminated through careful medical treatment, counseling, and patient teaching. The nurse plays an invaluable role in motivating the patient to reduce risk factors.

Bacterial Endocarditis

Bacterial endocarditis is a febrile illness which is frequently difficult to diagnose. It usually occurs as a complication of congenital or rheumatic heart disease or after a systemic infection. Bacterial endocarditis has been classified as acute or subacute; however, the former is seldom seen in pediatric patients. When it occurs, the acute form is usually fatal; therefore, the subacute type of endocarditis will be discussed.

Subacute bacterial endocarditis (SBE) is an infectious disease caused by *Streptococcus viridans* in a majority of cases with other types of streptococci, staphylococci, or gram-negative organisms implicated in the remainder. The infection involves abnormal heart tissue, especially rheumatic lesions or congenital heart defects. It may develop wherever turbulent blood flow exists, particularly where mechanical stress or jet streams are present. It is associated with episodes of bacteremia which may occur with sepsis, dental infections or surgery, or other intrusive procedures.

Lesions consist of vegetations composed of fibrin, leukocytes, and bacteria which adhere to the valvular or endocardial surface. As a result of the turbulent blood flow, portions of these vegetations may dislodge and embolize either to the lungs or to the coronary vessels, spleen, kidneys, or brain.

The signs of SBE are subtle and may be overlooked. There is an insidious onset with a fever, lethargy, general malaise, and anorexia. Splenomegaly and retinal hemorrhages may be present. *Splinter hemorrhages* (longitudinal black splinter-shaped hemorrhagic areas involving the distal third of the nail) and *Osler's nodes* (reddish-purple raised nodules with white centers found in the distal pads of fingers or toes) are evidence of embolic phenomena. Pericarditis and myocarditis may also be present.

An ECG reveals a prolonged PR interval and changes in the T wave. Cardiomegaly is evident on x-ray. Laboratory studies indicate an elevated erythrocyte sedimentation rate, leukocytosis, anemia, albuminuria, and sometimes microscopic hematuria. A new or altered murmur may be present and changeable in character, and the heart action is forceful and rapid with an occasional gallop rhythm.

It is essential to identify and treat the causative organism; therefore, multiple blood cultures are obtained routinely. While the treatment depends on the organism cultured out, it generally involves the administration of large doses of antibiotics for a prolonged period. For example, if *S. viridans* is the culprit, penicillin may be given intravenously for up to 6 weeks. Combinations of drugs, such as streptomycin and penicillin, may be used. The causative agent determines the selection, and an individualized treatment schedule is devised for each patient.

Long-term follow-up care is imperative, and blood cultures are a part of each subsequent examination. If a repairable cardiovascular anomaly is present, corrective surgery is considered. In children with a congenital heart defect or prior rheumatic infections, antibiotics should be administered routinely when a dental procedure or surgery is performed or when an acute respiratory infection is present.

Nursing Management

The hospitalization of a child with bacterial endocarditis is long term because of the need of parenteral antibiotic therapy to eradicate the underlying infection and avoid additional cardiac damage. Adequately preparing the child for an intravenous line and venipunctures for subsequent blood cultures is critical if cooperation is to be achieved. Once therapy is started, the rate of intravenous fluid administration is monitored closely, the insertion site is checked for any sign of infection, and the child's response to the drugs used is noted. It is imperative for antibiotics to be administered at proper intervals.

Since the child may be confined to bed until the acute infection is controlled, the nursing care plan should incorporate stimulating, age-appropriate diversionary activities in order to avoid the boredom which an otherwise active child may experience. When mobility is possible, a nurse may evaluate the need to continue the mode of treatment (e.g., suggesting to a physician the use of a heparin lock, which is less confining for the child).

While nurses play a vital role in teaching both the child and parents about the disease, the medications being used, and the procedures being done in the course of treatment, future use of prophylactic measures must be emphasized. Antibiotics should be prescribed for these children before tooth extractions and before genitourinary or gastrointestinal surgery and/or instrumentation since these procedures increase the possibility of infection and recurrence.

Nurses need to stress the importance of complying with follow-up visits. Aggressive use of parenteral antibiotics has improved the prognosis; however, SBE continues to be a serious inflammatory process. The outcome depends on the length of time the infection is present before diagnosis and the severity of the associated heart failure. If valvular endocarditis causes repeated emboli or persistent and/or severe CHF, the child ultimately may require cardiac valvular replacement.

Pericarditis

Pericarditis is an inflammation of the pericardium which may be caused by rheumatic fever, collagen diseases, pyogenic microorganisms, trauma, and certain severe hereditary anemias. The cause also may remain unknown. The involvement of the pericardium may be of the dry and fibrinous type or one in which an effusion develops. The latter may be serous, exudative, hemorrhagic, or purulent in nature. If the infection is acute, the exudative effusion may initiate the development of fibrosis and chronic constrictive pericarditis, which compresses the heart and restricts returning blood flow and cardiac contractility.

In pericarditis without effusion there is an acute sharp pain which is relieved by sitting up, turning to the side, or leaning forward. It is made more intense by moving, coughing, or laughing. Pain is identified in the infant by his persistent crying and restlessness. Older children complain of referred pain to the tip of the shoulder, the neck, or the left arm. A friction rub may be heard at any point over the precordium, and it varies in intensity according to changes in position.

With pericardial effusion there is pain, a cough, and possible dyspnea. X-rays reveal cardiac enalargement. While a friction rub is present, the heart sounds are usually muffled. On x-ray the lung fields may be congested if the patient is in heart failure. A complications of pericarditis with effusion in addition to chronic constrictive pericarditis is *cardiac tamponade.*

Cardiac tamponade occurs if there is compression of the heart by fluid within the pericardium which hinders venous return, restricts the heart's ability to fill properly, and produces increased systemic and pulmonary venous pressure and decreased cardiac output. When fluid accumulates slowly, a compensatory measure allows the walls to stretch gradually, and cardiac tamponade is avoided.

A nurse who observes a patient with a rapid accumulation of pericardial fluid sees an acutely ill child who appears to be very anxious and has cold and clammy extremities indicative of decreased cardiac output. There is systemic venous engorgement, the neck veins probably are distended, and the pulse is rapid and difficult to palpate. *Pulsus paradoxus,* a fall in the systolic blood pressure during inspiration greater than 5 to 10 mmHg, is an important but late indication of tamponade.

Significant pericardial fluid must be removed by means of pericardicentesis. The nurse must gather appropriate resuscitation equipment, including the defibrillator, for

utilization if the need arises. The patient is monitored continually during the procedure and for a period of time after the aspiration. As the fluid is removed, the patient's status improves dramatically; however, the condition may recur. These patients frequently are placed in intensive care units where careful observation and monitoring of vital signs, especially blood pressure and venous pressure, can be done easily. The fluid which is removed is studied to determine the cause of its accumulation and prevent its recurrence. The chemotherapy which may be instituted is determined by the causative organism or precipitating factor.

Nursing Management of the Child Undergoing Heart Surgery

Preoperative Period

To prepare children and parents adequately for cardiac surgery, children usually are admitted to the hospital approximately 1 to 3 days before the surgical procedure. The presurgical evaluation includes a history, a physical examination, and diagnostic tests. The diagnostic procedures include an ECG, echocardiogram, chest x-rays, cardiac catheterization, angiocardiography, and possibly pulmonary function tests (see Diagnostic Tests above).

The results of blood tests are used for preoperative assessment and as a basis for comparison in postoperative nursing and medical management. Essential tests include a complete blood count, hemoglobin, hematocrit, bleeding and clotting studies, prothrombin time, blood urea nitrogen, serum electrolytes, and blood typing and cross match. Several units of blood are reserved for use in the operative and postoperative periods. The white blood cell count is checked to help determine the absence of infection. The preoperative urinalysis, and the pH and specific gravity in particular, provide important reference criteria for comparison in the assessment of postoperative kidney function.

Preoperative Nursing Assessment

This assessment begins with the admission procedures and is an essential component of the total preoperative evaluation. Measurements of length or stature, weight, and vital signs are made upon admission. Thereafter, the temperature, pulse, respirations, and blood pressure are measured and recorded three or four times a day. The child's preoperative vital signs will be used as a standard of reference in evaluating the child's physiological status during and after surgery. Since the child must be free from fever and infection before surgery, any elevation in temperature or other symptoms of infection should be reported promptly to the surgeon.

The nurse should ensure that the child is weighed daily, on the *same scale,* and at the same time each day. Early morning is preferred for recording daily weight. The length or stature and weight measurements are used to calculate the child's body surface area in determining dosage of medications and anesthesia and to identify the child's fluid, blood, and nutritional requirements during and after surgery. Because any existing fluid and electrolyte imbalance must be corrected before surgery, the preoperative record of intake and output is an essential assessment tool which much be complete and accurate.

The nursing history provides information necessary to plan individualized pre- and postoperative care. Pertinent factors such as the child's level of understanding, usual routines, preferences, and special needs should be discussed during this interview. The initial interview and history also allow the nurse to assess the child's and parents' behavior and the patterns of parent-child interaction. These nursing observations often provide an indication of the degree of the child's and parents' anxiety concerning the anticipated surgery.

Preparation of the Child and Parents

Preparation for the preoperative, operative, and postoperative periods is a mandatory nursing responsibility. The teaching, counseling, and emotional support of the child and parents initiated by the nurse during the first contact with the family are essential throughout the child's hospitalization. Intensive care nurses also do preoperative teaching and orientation to the intensive care unit.

Preparing the Parents

The nurse should provide opportunities for the parents to discuss the child with the nurse at a time when the child is not present in order to establish a rapport with the parents. The nurse can use this time to assess the *parents'* needs in relation to the child's hospitalization and surgery.

The nurse should recognize that anticipation of the child's surgery, with its benefits and risks, is likely to be very stressful for the parents and that they may need the nurse's assistance to verbalize their questions and feelings. Despite overwhelming concern, many parents are reluctant to ask the nurse to answer their questions. Rather than assume that parents do not need to confer with her because they seem informed, the nurse should initiate conferences with them as often as necessary. The nurse needs to provide ample time, privacy, and a relaxed atmosphere for the discussions. Parents should be encouraged to ask questions, and questions should be answered succinctly, accurately, and in sufficient depth.

In preparing parents for the child's surgery, the nurse should ask them what they already know and what they have told the child about the hospital and the operation. The nurse then can elaborate on what the parents already know and correct any misinformation or misunderstanding that they might express. Visual aids should be used whenever possible because the parents' anxiety interferes with their accurate perception of the nurse's teaching.

When the nurse thinks that the parents are ready, details of all pre- and postoperative procedures the child will experience can be explained. If the nurse and parents plan and carry out the child's care together, the benefit to the child is likely to be greater than will be the case if the parents and nurse support the child independent of one another. The nurse should encourage parents to participate in the child's preparation for surgery as much as possible if they feel comfortable taking part.

It is important to assure the parents that a nurse will always be with the child in the operating room and after his operation. In many hospitals, the nurse who cares for the child before surgery accompanies him to the operating room and remains with the child until he is under anesthesia. This practice is considered to be effective in reducing the parents' and child's apprehension. It is also beneficial for the family to meet the operating room, recovery room, and special care unit nurses before the day of surgery. The preparation of children and parents should include a visit to these special areas.

The nurse must explain thoroughly all postoperative treatments and procedures the child is likely to receive as well as the complex machines, tubes, drainage apparatus, and infusion bottles that will surround the child after the operation. Parents should be given as much detail as they are ready to accept. Photographs and diagrams should be used when the parents cannot see the actual equipment. If the nurse does not prepare the parents with a realistic version of the child's postoperative appearance, they may be stunned or unduly frightened when they first see the child. The nurse should tell the parents that although the child may appear very ill when surrounded by all the equipment, he will be having frequent postoperative treatments and exercises which are essential to his recovery (Fig. 24-18). The nurse should explain to the parents that preparation for surgery is geared to the child's level of understanding and paced according to his readiness to learn. It is important for the child's physical and emotional well-being before the operation and his successful recovery after surgery.

Preparing the Child

The child's preparation for cardiac surgery begins a few days before the operation. Initiating preparation early tends to promote the child's cooperation during the actual procedures because the child has had a chance to "practice" what he will do and the routines and equipment will be somewhat familiar to him.

All preoperative instruction is individualized according to the child's informational and emotional needs. His age, previous knowledge of his condition, and previous experiences with hospitalization and surgery must be considered by the nurse in planning a teaching approach. Principles which should govern teaching-learning activities for the child include (1) building on the child's previous information, (2) proceeding from the simple to the complex, (3) presenting nonthreatening activities before those which might be threatening to the child, (4) utilizing short teaching and practice sessions, (5) pacing the introduction of new information in accordance with the child's readiness, (6) giving reasons for treatments and activities in simple but truthful terms, and (7) using miniature models, dolls, diagrams, photographs, and actual equipment when appropriate.

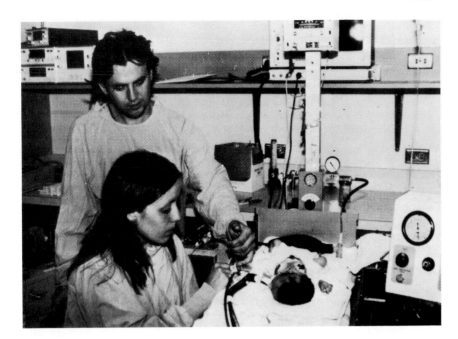

FIGURE 24-18   Infant and parents postoperatively. The child's appearance postoperatively may be overwhelming for the parents; prior preparation is essential. Parental visitation and, when possible, participation in care are frequently beneficial for the parents and the child. The nurse's support of the parents is important during this time. *(Courtesy Irwin Weinfeld.)*

Turning, Coughing, and Deep Breathing

The nurse should explain that after the child awakens, a nurse helps him turn from his back to his side and he is asked to take deep breaths and cough deeply. The nurse can demonstrate each exercise for the child and then ask the child to imitate each one. The child probably will need to repeat the exercises several times during the first session, and he should "practice" them every day with the nurse or his parents. Blowing bubbles and blowing up balloons make deep breathing fun for the child.

The nurse may need to spend time teaching the child to cough *deeply,* not just in his throat. If the child coughs only in his throat, he is not able to raise mucus which accumulates in the bronchi and trachea after anesthesia. In order to teach him to cough properly, the nurse can tell the child to take a deep breath and to make the cough come from "down deep inside" while he lets the air out. During practice sessions, the child should sit upright and lean forward slightly (the position which will be assumed for coughing postoperatively) and the nurse should place both hands on the child's chest as if "splinting" the chest. If the child is coughing properly, the nurse should feel the chest expansion during inspiration and the thoracic wall vibrations during the cough. The child should be told that it is harder to cough deeply after the operation because his chest hurts, but nurses will help him by holding their hands or a pillow against his chest.

Chest Physical Therapy

Chest physical therapy and postural drainage often are used to promote adequate respiratory function postoperatively. The treatments frequently are initiated 2 or 3 days preoperatively in order to improve respiratory function before surgery and to familiarize the child (and parents) with the procedure. If chest physical therapy is planned for the child after the operation but not initiated before

surgery, the nurse or physical therapist should demonstrate the techniques at least once during the preoperative period. The reader is referred to the section on chest physical therapy in Fig. 10-17.

Inhalation Therapy

The child is likely to receive humidified oxygen via face tent, mist tent, croupette, or, if the child is older, mask. The child should see and handle the respiratory equipment. The machines should be turned on for a short time so that the child can become accustomed to the sound and the feeling of the oxygen flow. If the child is placed in a mist tent, the fog in the tent will diminish his ability to see out. The presence of mist can be extremely frightening for the child upon awakening, and it may also cause the child to become disoriented or restless. It is advisable to set up a tent with mist and encourage the child to explore sight and sound from inside the tent during the day or evening before surgery.

Some children require mechanical ventilation postoperatively. These children should be prepared to wake up to the ventilator with an endotracheal tube in place. They should be told that while the tube is in place they will not be able to talk. The nurse should emphasize that this treatment is only temporary and that the tube is used to help the child get better.

Water-Seal Chest Drainage

The child should be informed that when he awakens there will be a large bandage on his chest and one or two drains which will come through the bandage from his chest. The child should be told that the drains should never be pulled until the doctor says they may come out. The nurse should explain that the drains will be attached to special bottles that collect air and blood but that the drainage tubing will be long enough for him to sit up and turn in his bed. It should be emphasized that the chest drains are temporary and will be removed by the doctor a few days after the operation. The nurse can give the child a simple explanation of the removal of the drains if he asks how the drains will come out.

Infusions and Angiocatheters

In explaining the cutdown or angiocatheters that will be used for infusions and to measure arterial and central venous pressures, the nurse can tell the child that he will have small soft tubes in his arms and legs when he wakes up and that the doctors and nurses will give him sugar water and medicines through the tubes until he is allowed to eat again. The nurse should tell him that the tubes will not hurt and will be removed when he starts to get better.

Cardioscope

The ECG leads may be familiar to most children because of repeated preoperative tests, but the child should be informed that he will awaken with lead wires on his chest. The nurse should show the child the monitor that will be used and demonstrate the alarms. Because the cardioscope-pacemaker-defibrillator monitor is much larger and louder than the usual ECG machine, its size may be threatening for the child.

Immediate Preoperative Preparation

In most hospitals, routine preoperative preparation is not extensive and is best done on the day or evening before surgery. Explanation of the skin prep, if the surgeon prescribes one, can be done a short time before the nurse does the treatment.

The child should be told that he will not be able to eat anything after a specified time during the night. The nurse should explain that as soon as the tube is removed the child will have a sore throat but will be able to speak. The child should know that he will not be able to eat or drink because of the danger of aspiration. The nurse should explain to the child that before he goes to the operating room he will receive injections that will make him feel sleepy. The means of transport to the operating room (e.g., stretcher or the child's own bed) and who will accompany him should be discussed. The child should be told if he must wear a hospital gown instead of his own pajamas. If a child is determined to wear his own clothes to the operating room, arrangements may be made with the surgical staff to honor this request. The parents should be encouraged to see the child on the morning of surgery. If they plan to be present, the child should be told that he can see them in the morning. The nurse should tell the child that he probably will feel sore when he wakes up and that he should tell the nurse when he feels sore so that she can give him medicine to take the "hurt" away.

The *skin preparation* of children who have cardiac surgery varies with institutions and surgeons. In some hospitals, skin preparation is limited to a scrub with an antibacterial skin cleanser which is done in the operating room. Some surgeons prefer to begin skin preparation on the evening before surgery or a few days before surgery.

The nurse is responsible for ensuring that the proper number of scrubs, baths, or showers, usually with an antibacterial agent, have been carried out as specified by the surgeon.

Solid food and most liquids usually are withheld for 12 hours prior to the induction of anesthesia, but the child should be permitted to have water up to 6 or 8 hours before induction in order to maintain adequate hydration. Because the ratio of water to total body size is very high in young infants, neonates and infants up to 6 months of age should be given feedings of clear glucose water until 4 hours before induction.

The nurse caring for a child undergoing cardiac surgery will be responsible for the administration of certain *medications*. Children usually are placed on a series of prophylactic doses of antibiotics in order to prevent postoperative infection, especially endocarditis. In order to achieve a satisfactory blood level of the antibiotic, the first dose of a broad-spectrum antibiotic or two antibiotics, one for gram-positive and one for gram-negative organisms, usually is administered intramuscularly on the evening before surgery or intravenously at the beginning of the procedure. Therapy is continued for 2 to 5 days postoperatively.

Digitalis, a drug commonly used to treat infants and children in CHF, is known to affect cardiac rhythms adversely during surgery. The usual dose of digitalis is withheld on the day of open-heart surgery. If necessary, therapy may be resumed postoperatively.

Infants and small children receive minimal or no *preanesthetic medication* prior to cardiac surgery to avoid inducing the side effect of cardiorespiratory depression. Infants receive a small intramuscular dose of *atropine sulfate* which helps minimize production of secretions and prevents bradycardia, which can occur as an adverse effect of endotracheal intubation. In addition to atropine sulfate or *scopolamine,* older children may be given a small dose of a mild barbiturate sufficient to make them quiet and relaxed when arriving in the operating room. It is very important that the nurse administer these preoperative medications at the time designated. The anesthesiologist usually times the administration of the preanesthetic medications so that anesthetic induction can be performed when the actions of the medications are at their peak.

Intraoperative Period

Surgical treatment of congenital heart defects are usually performed on infants and young children. Cardiovascular surgery may be either corrective or palliative. *Corrective surgery* is aimed at restoring a normal sequence of blood flow in the heart and great vessels. *Palliative surgery* is performed on a child with a complex heart disease which is not amenable to immediate surgical correction because of the complexity of the defect or because of the child's size or clinical condition. The objective of palliative surgery is to improve the existing hemodynamics sufficiently to allow the child's survival until the corrective surgery can be performed. Examples of palliative surgery are (1) creation of a shunt to the pulmonary artery from the sub-clavian artery for severe tetralogy of Fallot, (2) atrial sep-tectomy (Blalock-Hanlon operation) for transposition of the great vessels, and (3) pulmonary artery banding for single ventricle or complex VSDs. Children who had pal-liative surgery as infants usually are scheduled for correc-tive surgery when they reach 1 to 5 years of age.

Patent ductus closure, coarctation repair, and most palliative procedures generally are performed without the use of cardiopulmonary bypass. Most complex lesions re-quire the use of cardiopulmonary bypass during correc-tion.

Extracorporeal circulation, also called cardiopulmo-nary bypass, is a system used in open-heart surgery in which a heart-lung machine oxygenates venous blood which has been removed from the body and returns the freshly oxygenated blood to the arterial circulation. The use of extracorporeal circulation diverts blood from its usual route through the heart and lungs to permit the sur-geon to correct intracardiac defects. Extracorporeal circu-lation is established by inserting a cannula in the inferior and superior venae cavae through a small incision in the right atrium; the cannulae divert venous blood to the ma-chine. Oxygenated blood from the machine is returned to circulation by an arterial cannula. Hypothermia also is used during the repair of many cardiac lesions.

Postoperative Period

After the incision is closed and the wound is dressed, por-table monitoring is established to provide continuous dis-play of ECG and arterial pressure during transport to the recovery room or intensive care unit. Some children may be extubated in the operating room if their general condi-tion is good; however, if respiratory function is weak, the endotracheal tube will not be removed until later.

In hospitals where there is a special care nursery, the neonate usually will go directly to that unit after surgery. Before transfer to a special care or intensive care unit, in-fants and older children may go the recovery room.

Continuous, astute observation and meticulous atten-tion to supportive care measures characterize the postop-erative nursing management of children who have had cardiovascular surgery. As soon as the child returns to the postoperative care unit, priority must be given to reestab-lishment of controlled ventilatory support and careful monitoring of cardiorespiratory function. During the stay in the intensive care unit, the nurse carefully monitors the child's appearance, airway status, vital signs, central venous pressure, blood gases, chest tube function, fluid and electrolyte balance, and intake and output.

Complications of cardiac surgery include shock as a result of hypovolemia, hemorrhage, cardiac tamponade, myocardial failure, and arrhythmias; CHF; pneumothorax; and pulmonary edema. Frequent monitoring and close ob-servation allow early detection of problems and rapid in-tervention.

The length of stay in the intensive care unit varies with the child's preoperative status, the complexity of the surgery, and postoperative complications. Tubes and lines are usually removed over a period of a few days, and the child then returns to the pediatric unit.

Convalescent Period

After the early postoperative period, nursing management is focused largely on helping the child gain strength and in preparing the entire family for his discharge from the hospital. If the child has an uneventful postoperative course, he may be discharged about 5 to 10 days after sur-gery and allowed to resume full activity in 1 or 2 months.

Planned activity and rest periods and visits from sib-lings as well as parents are important for the convalescent child. It is also advisable to allow older children to have occasional short visits from schoolmates and peers. These activities are helpful in easing the child's transition to home and community after a long hospitalization.

The convalescent period should be one during which the child starts to move from the dependent role he nec-essarily assumed during hospitalization to one of more in-dependence. Many of the child's former limitations are re-moved by the surgery, and most activity limitations even-tually are lifted. The child and parents need the nurse's as-sistance in becoming comfortable in dealing with the child's newly acquired capacities. They need to learn how to help the child pace his activities in order to prevent fa-tigue. The child who formerly had many restrictions needs much encouragement and support from the nurse and parents as he attempts new activities.

The nurse should confer with the parents concerning their plans for the child after discharge. They are likely to need some assistance in comfortably allowing the child to engage in new activities and exercise the amount of inde-pendence appropriate for his age. The hospital nurse can also facilitate the child's transfer to home and community by initiating a referral to the community health nurse and providing the school nurse with a summary of the child's hospitalization and present condition. The nurse also might suggest that the parents investigate the informal parents' discussion groups which are sponsored by the American Heart Association in some communities as a helpful resource for them after the child goes home.

Independent Study Activities

The student can best learn to recognize the signs and symptoms of cardiovascular distress by taking every op-portunity to observe children with cardiovascular prob-lems throughout their hospitalization. In addition, obser-vations of these children in an outpatient setting will pro-vide valuable information about the child's adaptation to his cardiovascular disease and the child's and family's in-terpretations of the disease process and medical therapy.

1. Obtain a pediatric health history and perform a basic cardiovascular assessment on several pediatric patients. Discuss any abnormalities or concerns with the child's primary nurse or your clinical instructor.
2. Whenever caring for a pediatric patient, listen to the child's heart sounds at each of the major auscultatory areas (apex, aorta, etc.).

3. Whenever a physician notes that a child demonstrates abnormal heart sounds or pulses, listen to the child and palpate the child's pulses until you are able to recognize the abnormality.

4. Be present during the preparation of a child and parent for cardiac catheterization and attend the catheterization. Compare the description that the child was given of the catheterization with the events as you observed them. Develop a teaching plan for a preschool child and a school-age child to prepare a child at an age-appropriate level for what he will see, hear, and feel.

Study Questions

1. The clubbing of fingernails which is often seen in children with cyanotic heart disease is a result of chronic:
   A. Arterial oxygen desaturation.
   B. Venous oxygen desaturation.
   C. Decreased capillary filling time.
   D. Impaired tissue oxygenation.

2. When admitting a patient who is thought to have a coarctation of the aorta, a nurse identifies the characteristic:
   A. Excessive clubbing of the toes.
   B. Lower blood pressure in the lower extremities.
   C. Bounding femoral pulses.
   D. Thready, poor-quality radial pulses.

3. Children with cyanotic heart disease instinctively squat in an effort to:
   A. Rest during exercise.
   B. Increase pulmonary blood flow.
   C. Decrease systemic arterial pressure.
   D. Avoid a syncopal episode.

4. After cardiac catheterization, weak arterial pulses, unusual coolness, blanching, or mottling in the extremity should alert a nurse to:
   A. Venous obstruction.
   B. Cardiac perforation and tamponade.
   C. Hemorrhage.
   D. Aterial thrombosis.

5. Children who have congestive heart failure can experience some relief from dyspnea and respiratory distress by being placed in:
   A. Knee-chest position.
   B. High Fowler's position.
   C. Semi-Fowler's position.
   D. Supine position.

6. An effective nursing intervention which decreases the energies expended by an infant with cyanotic heart disease is:
   A. Limiting his physical activity.
   B. Developing a consistent plan of care.
   C. Feeding the infant more frequently.
   D. Allowing the infant to "have his own way."

7. When working with the parents of children with cyanotic heart disease, it is important for nurses to stress the need for prophylactic antibiotics to decrease the likelihood of:
   A. Congestive heart failure.
   B. Infections.
   C. Pneumonia.
   D. Bacterial endocarditis.

8. In acute rheumatic fever, the structure which is most susceptible to damage is the:
   A. Mitral valve. C. Myocardium.
   B. Pericardium. D. Annulus.

9. A child with acute rheumatic fever who complains of nausea and tinnitus and also has stools which are guaiac-positive is demonstrating the toxic manifestations of:
   A. Erythromycin. C. Prednisone.
   B. Penicillin. D. Aspirin.

10. On the morning of the cardiac surgery, a nurse knows that the digitalis preparation is:
    A. Withheld.
    B. Doubled.
    C. Given as usual.
    D. Administered 4 hours before surgery.

11. The loss of consciousness or the "tet" spells demonstrated by an infant with tetralogy of Fallot can be relieved by:
    A. Placing the infant in the knee-chest position.
    B. Keeping the baby prone.
    C. Maintaining a high Fowler's position.
    D. Elevating the head of the crib 30 degrees.

References

Behrman, R.E., and V.C. Vaughan: *Nelson Textbook of Pediatrics,* 12th ed., Saunders, Philadelphia, 1983.
Fink, B., and W.J. Mandel: "Supraventricular Arrhythmias," in N.K. Roberts and J. Gelband (eds.), *Cardiac Arrhythmias in the Neonate, Infant, and Child,* 2d ed., Appleton-Century-Crofts, New York, 1983.
Fyler, D.C. (ed.), "Report of the New England Regional Infant Cardiac Program," *Pediatrics,* 65 (suppl.): 377-461, 1980.
Hazinski, M.F.: "Critical Care of the Pediatric Cardiovascular Patient," *Nursing Clinics of North America,* 16(4):671-697, 1981.
——: "Cardiovascular Disorders," in *Nursing Care of the Critically Ill Child,* Mosby, St. Louis, 1984a.
——: "Cardiac Catheterization," in B.C. Johanson et al., (eds.), *Standards for Critical Care,* 2d ed., Mosby, St. Louis, 1984b.
National Heart, Lung, Blood Institute: "Report of the Second Task Force on Blood Pressure Control in Children—1987," *Pediatrics,* 79:1-25, 1987.

Bibliography

Cloutier, J., and C. Measel: "Home Care for the Infant with Congenital Heart Disease," *American Journal of Nursing,* 82:100-103, 1982.
Hayman, L.J., V.C. Weill, N.E. Tobias, E.E. Stashinko, and J.C. Meininger: "Which Child Is at Risk for Heart Disease?" *MCN: The American Journal of Maternal/Child Nursing,* 13:328-333, 1988.
Rushton, C.H.: "Preparing Children and Families for Cardiac Surgery: Nursing Interventions," *Issues in Comprehensive Pediatric Nursing,* 6:235-248, 1983.

25

The Hemopoietic System

The editors wish to acknowledge the review and revision of the Leukemia section of this chapter by Kathleen Krumm, R.N., M.S.N., clinical nurse specialist. Pediatric Hematology, Oncology, at Rhode Island Hospital, Providence, R.I.

Objectives

After reading this chapter the student will be able to
1. Describe the functions of the hemopoietic system.
2. Identify the basic subjective and objective data to be obtained in assessing the child.
3. Understand the purpose of diagnostic tests and medical treatment.
4. Describe general nursing measures appropriate for pediatric clients who have problems involving the hemopoietic system.
5. Delineate specific nursing interventions appropriate for pediatric clients who have problems involving the hemopoietic system.

Anatomy and Physiology

The circulating blood consists of two portions: the liquid plasma and the formed elements. The formed elements are the *erythrocytes,* or red blood cells, the *leukocytes,* or white blood cells, and the *thrombocytes,* or platelets. These elements perform most of the functional activities of the blood. The erythrocytes function primarily in the transport of oxygen and carbon dioxide between the lungs and the tissues of the body. The leukocytes form one of the most significant parts of the body's defense against infections, while the thrombocytes, along with portions of the plasma, provide a mechanism for coagulating blood.

Erythrocytes

The erythrocytes are the blood's circulating red cells or corpuscles (Fig. 25-1). The early red cell, the erythroblast, is a large, nucleated cell which undergoes a series of changes bringing it to the functioning, nonnucleated, biconcave disk form of the mature erythrocyte. The erythroblast, produced in the bone marrow, gives rise to the reticulocyte and the erythrocyte. The reticulocyte is nearly as mature as the erythrocyte and is normally present in the circulation in small numbers. Erythrocytes live about 120 days. Their production in bone marrow is determined by the oxygen tension of blood. The release of erythropoietin stimulates red blood cell production in response to the body's need for increased oxygenation.

The main function of erythrocytes is the transport of

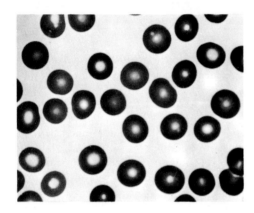

FIGURE 25-1   Normal erythrocytes as they appear under magnification. The hemoglobin is evenly centered in the biconcave disk of the cell. *(From A.M. Masuer, Pediatric Hematology, McGraw-Hill, New York, 1969, p. 25.)*

oxygen from the lungs to the tissues and the transport of carbon dioxide from the tissues to the lungs. This activity is contingent upon the most important component of the erythrocyte, hemoglobin. The outer membrane of the red cell functions to maintain the homeostasis of the cell by the transport of water and electrolytes.

An indicator of the number of erythrocytes is the *hematocrit* level, a reading of the percentage of red cells occupying the blood volume, measured after the blood sample has been spun down in a centrifuge. Hemoglobin and hematocrit are directly proportionate to each other.

A depression of the number of circulating red cells concurrent with a decreased hemoglobin is known as *anemia*. The average normal blood values at different ages are listed in Table 25-1.

Hemoglobin

Hemoglobin is composed of a simple protein, *globin*, attached to an iron-containing pigment, *heme*. Heme is the substance which gives the red coloration to the oxygenated erythrocytes, gives hemoglobin the ability to bind with oxygen and carbon dioxide for transport. At birth, 45 to 90 percent of the newborn's hemoglobin is of the fetal type. Adult hemoglobin is present in increasing amounts, replacing the fetal type by the first year of life. Some fetal hemoglobin may be present through the entire lifetime of a person.

When red cells are destroyed, iron is salvaged from the hemoglobin and returned to the bone marrow for storage and for production of new hemoglobin. The remainder of the hemoglobin, the globin and the iron-free particles, is excreted into the reticuloendothelial system, spleen, lymph nodes, bone marrow, liver, and connective tissues, where separation into the globin protein and degradation to bilirubin occur.

TABLE 25-1   Average Range of Normal Blood Values at Different Ages*

Component	Preterm	Full Term	2 days	7 days	14 days	2 mo
Hemoglobin, g/100 ml	13-18	13.7-20	18-21.2	19.6	13-20	13.3
Red blood cells/mm³, in millions	5-6	5-6	5.3-5.6	5.3	5-5.1	4.5
Nucleated RBC, %	5-15	1-5	1-2	0†		
Hematocrit, g/100 ml	45-55	43-65	56.1	52.7	30-66	38.9
White blood cells/mm³, in thousands	15	9-38	21-22	5-21	5-21	5-21
Neutrophils, %	40-80	40-80	55	40	36-40	36-40
Eosinophils, %	2-3	2-3	5	5	2-3†	
Lymphocytes, %	30-31	30-31	20	20	48-53	48-53
Monocytes	6-12	6-12	15	15	8-9	8-9
Immature white blood cells, %	Over 10	3-10	5	0*		
Platelets/mm³, in thousands	50-300	100-350	400	400	300-400	300-400
Reticulocytes, %	Up to 10	4-6	3	3	0.5-1.6‡	

*Compiled from a variety of sources.
†Not normally found in the circulating blood after this age.
‡Remains approximately the same for succeeding age levels.

Source: G. M. Scipien et al. (eds.), *Comprehensive Pediatric Nursing,* 3d ed., McGraw-Hill, New York, 1986, p. 986.

Hemoglobin in the cord blood of the newborn has a concentration of 16.6 to 17.1 g/100 ml of blood. Around 3 to 6 months, the hemoglobin level normally drops to its lowest point, creating a state of *physiologic anemia,* which is less than 10 g/100 ml. This occurrence is normal and simply represents the body's process of adjusting to improved oxygenation, requiring the bone marrow to work more rapidly. With the rapid rate of growth, iron is used, decreasing the hemoglobin. For the preterm infant, this decrease occurs early and is lower. It is called *anemia of prematurity* rather than *physiologic anemia.* This level of about 10 to 12 g/100 ml remains fairly constant until later in the second year of life. The hemoglobin concentration averages between 11 and 13 g/100 ml of blood for females and 16 g/100 ml of blood for males.

Bilirubin is a waste product formed from the hemoglobin. The two types of bilirubin are the *direct type,* or *conjugated bilirubin,* which becomes elevated in the blood following intra- or extrahepatic obstruction of the bile ducts, and the *indirect type,* which rises as a result of degradation of the erythrocytes and excessive destruction of hemoglobin, such as occurs in the hemolytic anemias. When the bilirubin level in the blood becomes elevated, a condition known as *hyperbilirubinemia,* the pigment stains the body tissues, skin, and sclera, producing a tinge of color referred to as *jaundice.* A normal amount of circulating bilirubin is 0.2 to 1.4 mg/100 ml of blood.

Leukocytes

Classification

The *leukocytes,* or white blood cells, are nucleated cells, larger in size than the erythrocytes. There are five kinds of white cells, each serving distinct functions for the body and each identifiable by particular characteristics. The leukocytes are classified into granular and agranular types by the presence or absence of granular substances in the cytoplasm. *Granulocytes* are of three types: neutrophils, eo-

sinophils, and basophils. *Nongranular leukocytes* are of two types: monocytes and lymphocytes. Immature white cells (precursors) are found in the circulating blood in certain disease states and have diagnostic significance. The lymphocytes and the granulocytes form in the lymphatic tissue of the lymph nodes and spleen, tonsils, thymus, bone marrow, and Peyer's patches of the gastrointestinal tract and liver. Monocytes originate and develop in the myleloid tissue of the red bone marrow, in the lymph nodes, and in the spleen.

The most important function of the leukocytes is to protect the body against infection. *Phagocytosis* is the process by which the leukocytes ingest and consequently destroy foreign particles and bacteria which invade the body, as well as fragmented cells in the bloodstream. Phagocytosis is the function of the neutrophils, concentrating on bacteria. The neutrophils are known as *microphagocytes* in contrast to *macrophagocytes,* the monocytes which concentrate on the ingestion of larger foreign particles and fragmented cells. The eosinophils are active and elevated in allergic states, such as asthma. When the basophils undergo degranulation during an anaphylactic reaction, heparin and histamine, contained in the cytoplasm of the cells, are released. Lymphocytes active in the formation of antibodies, are closely associated with *gamma globulin,* one of the proteins of the blood plasma. Gamma globulin, a substance formed in the lymphatic tissue and in the liver, is released during inflammatory reactions by the degradation of the lymphocytes. (In Table 25-2 types of leukocytes and their individual functions are listed.)

Severe depression of the white cells, *leukopenia,* is seen in certain viral infections, aplastic anemia, and leukemia. *Leukocytosis,* an increase in the number of white cells, frequently accompanies bacterial infections. The average normal values are listed in Table 25-1.

The life span of the leukocytes is generally unknown.

3 mo	6 mo	1 yr	2 yr	4 yr	8-12 yr	Adult	
						Male	Female
9.5-14	10.5-14	11-12.2	11.6-13	12.6-13	11-19	14-18	12-16
4.3-4.5	4.6	4.6-4.7	4.7-4.8	4.7-4.8	4.8-5.1	5.4	4.8
28-41	33-42	32-40	34-40	36-44	39-47	42-52	37-47
6-18	1-15	4.5-13.5	9-12	8-10	8	5-10	5-10
30-35	30-45	40-50	40-50	50-55	55-60	35-70	35-70
						2-3	2-3
55-63	48-60	48-53	48-50	40-48	30-38	30-35	30-35
7	5	5	5-8	5-8	5-8	5-8	5-8
360	250-350‡					250-350	250-350
						0.5-1.6	0.5-1.6

TABLE 25-2 Types and Functions of Leukocytes

Type of Leukocyte	Percent in the Blood	Major Function of the Cell	Disorders Causing Alteration from Normal
Granulocytes			
Neutrophils	4-5 (nonsegmented0 60-65 (segmented)	Microphagocytosis; phagocytosis of bacteria	Splenectomy, bacterial infections
Eosinophils	1-4	Phagocytosis of animal parasites (trichinae)	Splenectomy, eosinophilic leukemia, or leukemoid reaction, Hodgkin's disease, acute infectious lymphocytosis (recovery phase)
Basophils	0.-0.5	Release of heparin and histamine	Splenectomy, Hodgkin's disease, chronic myeloid leukemia, polycythemia vera, chronic hemolytic anemia
Nongranular leukocytes			
Lymphocytes	20-35	Antibody formation and release of gamma globulin	Infectious mononucleosis, leukemia (ALL), infectious lymphocytosis
Monocytes	5-10	Macrophagocytosis; phagocytosis of foreign particles and fragmentd cells	Infectious mononucleosis, Hodgkin's disease, acute infection, or bacterial invasion (recovery phase)

Source: G. M. Scipien et al. (eds.), *Comprehensive Pediatric Nursing,* 3d ed., McGraw-Hill, 1986, p. 989.

Some granulocytes live for 24 hours, others as long as 30 days. It is known that leukocytes survive both in the intravascular area of the circulating blood and in the extravascular tissues. The pulmonary circulation also serves as a reservoir for the leukocytes.

Thrombocytes

The *thrombocytes,* or blood platelets, are the smallest of the blood's formed elements. These nonnucleated, granular bodies function in homeostasis and in the storage of certain metabolic substances; in addition, they have some role in the process of phagocytosis and an integral role in the *coagulation process.* When the integrity of the vessel wall is destroyed, platelets adhere to the inner surface, forming a plug which slows and stops the flow of blood, thereby minimizing blood loss. In addition, degradation of the platelets causes the release of a platelet factor which interacts with other substances in the blood plasma to form a fibrous clot at the site of the injury (Fig. 25-2). Fibrinogen and prothrombin are essential to coagulation. The platelets simultaneously release serotonin, a vasoconstrictor, which further contributes to the slowing of the blood flow from the injured site. The normal quantity of platelets at various ages are listed in Table 25-1. A level of platelets below 25,000 to 50,000 cells per mm^3 is characteristic of *thrombocytopenia.* When the level of platelets is below 25,000 cells per mm^3, spontaneous bleeding can occur.

Plasma

The liquid portion of the blood, *plasma,* is the medium by which the formed elements are transported in the blood vessels. Constituents of plasma function in the maintenance of homeostasis by transport and distribution of nutrients, hormones, certain chemicals, and waste materials. About 90 percent of the plasma is water. When needed, the plasma can draw from the body tissues storing excess water. Approximately 6 to 8 percent of the plasma is the protein substances, albumin, gamma globulin, fibrinogen, and prothrombin. Albumin serves an osmotic function in the regulation of the volume of plasma in the blood vessels. The remaining 1 to 2 percent of glucose, amino acids, inorganic salts, gases, waste materials, and hormones.

Blood Volume

The volumes of plasma and of formed elements determine blood volume. A preterm newborn has a blood volume of about 89 to 105 ml/kg of body weight. A newborn at term has a volume of 50 to 100 ml/kg, with a mean of 85 ml/kg. Factors producing such a wide variation include methods of cord clamping, time of sampling, technique, and previous history, such as intrauterine transfusion. The difference in the blood volumes is due to the increased amount of plasma in the preterm newborn.

Lymph

Lymph, a fluid closely interrelated with the circulation of the blood and the lymphocytes, is derived from the blood plasma and has a similar content of water and solutes. Lymph plays an integral role in the body's defense against infections, since the concentration of leukocytes may be as high as 40,000 cells per n.m^3. These cells are mostly lymphocytes formed in the lymphoid tissue. An increased production of lymphocytes, as in the leukemia disorders, produces an enlargement of some lymph nodes where the lymphocytes are formed. The lymphatic system is anatomically interrelated with the cardiovascular system.

FIGURE 25-2   Coagulation process.

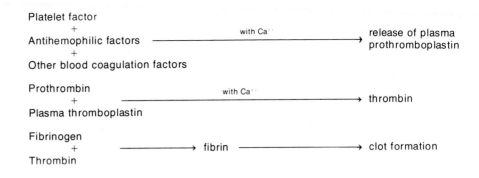

TABLE 25-3 Antigen-Antibody Compatibility

Blood Group	Antigen	Antibody	Compatibility	
			Can be Donor to Type	Can Receive from Type
A	A	Anti-B	A or AB	A or O
B	B	Anti-A	B or AB	B or O
AB	A and B	No antibodies	AB	A, B, AB, or O
O	No antigen	Anti-A and anti-B	A, B, AB, or O	O

Source: G. M. Scipien et al. (eds.), *Comprehensive Pediatric Nursing,* 3rd ed., McGraw-Hill, New York, 1986, p. 991.

Blood Groups

The erythrocyte is singularly important in the blood groups and the Rh factor. A substance on the surface of the red cell is responsible for *agglutination,* or clumping, of red cells in the presence of an *antibody,* or an *agglutinin.* This substance is known by its characteristics as an *agglutinogen,* or an *antigen,* which makes possible the agglutination of red cells.

The ABO System

In this system there are four blood groups: A, B, AB, and O. The blood group is determined genetically by pairing of parental genes. There are six possible genotypes: AA, AO, BB, BO, AB, and OO. It is impossible to distinguish between the AA and AO and BB and BO genotypes of the A and B groups, respectively.

Blood from two persons is considered compatible when agglutination does not occur in the presence of the antibody. The antibody in the plasma enables plasma to agglutinate or cause clumping of the red cells. The A blood group has the A antigen and the anti-B antibody, while the opposite B antigen and the anti-A antibody are present in the B blood group. The AB blood group has both the A and B antigens and neither antibody; thus it is compatible with any other blood group when it is the recipient. The O blood group contains both the anti-A and anti-B antibody but neither antigen. The O blood group is considered a universal donor because it is compatible when given to any other blood group (see Table 25-3).

The Rh Factor

Landsteiner and Weiner in 1940 discovered the Rh factor from their experiments with rhesus monkeys, from which the name *Rh* is derived. The *Rh factor* is an antigen contained in the outer membrane of the erythrocyte. Its function and nature are generally unknown. There are several antigens in the Rh system, the most important being the D antigen. The presence or absence of this antigen gives rise to the Rh-positive or Rh-negative identification. Formerly, when a woman who was Rh-negative carried an Rh-positive fetus, the result was the leaking of Rh antigens into maternal circulation, where antibodies formed against Rh-positive antigens with serious consequences for the neonate. However, Rh incompatibility has become almost an historic disease as a result of RhoGAM. This preparation of anti-Rh antibodies is administered to unsensitized Rh-negative women after the termination of a pregnancy to prevent development of antibodies that would cause erythroblastosis fetalis in subsequent pregnancies.

Assessment

A child suspected of having a hemopoietic problem presents the nurse with a tremendous challenge because these disorders have many etiologies. They can develop from an extensive, acute blood loss, long-term nutritional deficits, and a variety of acute or chronic systemic diseases, as well as being acquired genetically. It is important for the pediatric nurse to know the common types of hematologic problems which occur at specific stages of childhood in order to assess these infants, children, and adolescents most expeditiously. Assessments are made based on subjective and objective data.

Subjective Data

1. Age, sex, race
2. Onset and symptoms
    (a) Pallor
    (b) Bruises, petechiae, hematomas, jaundice
    (c) Irritability
    (d) Easy fatigability
    (e) Anorexia
    (f) Shortness of breath on exertion
    (g) Tiring easily when fed
    (h) Edematous hands and feet
    (i) Weak cry
    (j) Weight loss
    (k) Lethargy
    (l) Hematuria
    (m) Prolonged bleeding episodes
    (n) Muscle weakness
    (o) Behavioral changes
3. Neonatal history
    (a) Apgar score
    (b) Bleeding episodes
    (c) Blood incompatibility (ABO)
    (d) Type of feeding (formula, breast)
    (e) Problems, such as jaundice, cephalohematoma, sepsis
    (f) Length of hospital stay
4. Nutritional history
    (a) Type of foods taken
    (b) Problems eating
    (c) If an older infant, the amount of milk consumed in a 24-hour period, to the exclusion of solid food
    (d) Vitamin and iron supplements taken
    (e) Any changes in eating patterns
5. Past medical history
    (a) Hospitalizations
    (b) Transfusions received, especially reactions
    (c) Congenital blood disorders such as sickle cell trait or disease, thalassemia
    (d) Chronic problems such as plumbism, pica, iron-deficiency anemia
    (e) History of drug ingestion
    (f) Recent exposure to infection (viral)
6. Family history
    (a) Bleeding tendencies
    (b) Inherited diseases such as hemophilia, thalassemia, sickle cell trait or disease

Objective Data

1. *Complete physical examination* (specific observations follow)
    (a) The skin is inspected for petechiae, bruises, ecchymosis, hematomas, pallor, and jaundice.
    (b) The joints are examined for swelling and pain.
    (c) The conjunctivae, sclerae, and mucous membranes are inspected for color.
    (d) The nail beds are assessed for capillary refill.
    (e) The lymph nodes are palpated for enlargement.
    (f) The heart is auscultated for tachycardia and arrhythmias, and the pulses are assessed.
    (g) The lungs are auscultated for signs of congestive failure.
    (h) The abdomen is palpated for hepatosplenomegaly, tender areas, and masses.
2. *Laboratory data* (Pertinent laboratory data specific to the symptoms presented are reviewed. Several screening and diagnostic tests are discussed in the following section.)

Common Screening and Diagnostic Tests

Since anemia is the most common blood disorder found in the pediatric population and iron stores are naturally depleted by 4 to 6 months of age in full-term infants, a complete blood count (CBC) is a routine procedure performed in the second half of the first year of life during well-baby visits. In some settings, a CBC is done between 6 and 9 months of age and in others between 9 and 12 months of age. A CBC yields the following information: total red blood count (RBC), hemoglobin, hematocrit, mean corpuscular volume (MCV), mean corpuscular hemoglobin (MCH), mean corpuscular hemoglobin concentration (MCHC), platelet count, total white blood cell count (WBC), and percentages of lymphocytes, monocytes, and granulocytes. The normal values, with the exception of MCV, MCH, and MCHC, are found in Table 25-1.

The MCV reflects the average size of each red blood cell (microcytic, normocytic, or macrocytic). Estimated normal values are as follows:

6 months to 4 years: 72 to 86 femoliters (fl) (mean 80)
5 to 10 years: 75 to 95 fl (mean 83)
11 to 14 years: 77 to 97 fl (mean 85)
15 to 19 years: 79 to 100 fl (mean 88)

The MCH is an expression of the average hemoglobin content in each red blood cell. Estimated normal values are as follows:

6 months to 4 years: 24 to 30 picograms (pg) (mean 28)
5 to 10 years: 25 to 33 pg (mean 29)
11 to 14 years: 26 to 33 pg (mean 29)
15 to 19 years: 27 to 35 pg (mean 30)

The MCHC represents the average concentration of hemoglobin in each red blood cell. This red cell index is normally between 33 to 34 g/dl. The MCHC is not as helpful in the diagnostic process as are the other two red cell indices (MCV and MCH).

If iron deficiency is suspected based on the results of RBC, hemoglobin, hematocrit, and red cell indices, additional blood tests that are needed are reticulocyte count (Table 25-1), peripheral blood smear, serum ferratin, percent saturation of transferrin, total iron-binding capacity (TIBC), free erythrocyte protoporphyrin (FEP), and a stool for occult blood. Through the peripheral blood smear, abnormalities in the shape and size of red blood cells can be identified (e.g., variations in size, irregular shapes, clumping of red blood cells, and basophilic stippling).

Serum ferritin (the major iron-storage protein) is measured to assess the adequacy of iron reserves. The normal value is 30 ng from 6 months to 15 years. The percent saturation of transferrin (the iron-transporting plasma protein) is normally 15 to 55 from 6 months to 3 years and 20 to 55 thereafter. The TIBC yields information on the amount of available transferrin for binding more iron. The normal value is 250 to 400 μg/dl.

Iron combines with protoporphyrins to form heme. The normal FEP is less than 60 μg/dl. (When FEP is used as a screening test for lead poisoning, values > 35 μg/dl warrant determination of lead level.) Protoporphyrins accumulate in the blood if insufficient iron is present. To rule out chronic bleeding, a stool for occult blood is done when iron-deficiency anemia is suspected.

A laboratory test that is used for both screening and diagnostic purposes is the hemoglobin electrophoresis. Either cord blood or capillary blood may be used. This test is useful for early identification of sickle cell disease and thalassemia minor by differentiating the various types of hemoglobin (Hb). Normal values are as follows:

HbF (average):	75 percent	Newborn (remainder mostly HbA)
	20 percent	4 months
	2 percent	1 year
HbA	80 percent	4 months
	95–98 percent	After 6 months
HbA$_2$	Small fraction	Newborn
	1.5–3.5 percent	After 6 months

Methods of obtaining blood samples are found in Chap. 10, Table 10-4, and Figs. 10-23, 10-26, 10-28, and 10-29. Collection of a stool sample is discussed in Chap. 26, Table 26-1.

A bone marrow aspiration is used to evaluate peripheral blood, especially the production of erythrocytes, leukocytes, and platelets, since they are found in the marrow in various stages of development. This procedure is not necessary for diagnosing iron-deficiency anemia, sickle cell disease, or β-thalassemia; however, it is important for leukemia, aplastic anemia, and malignancies.

The site selected is usually the posterior iliac crest, and so the child is placed on one side. Since it is a surgical technique, the area is washed thoroughly with an iodine solution (which is allowed to dry) and alcohol. The area is draped with sterile towels. A local anesthetic is injected into the skin, subcutaneous tissue, and periosteum. The bone-marrow needle is in place, the stylet is removed, and 0.2 ml of marrow is withdrawn with a 20-ml syringe.

It is important to explain the purpose and the procedure to the parents and/or child. Honesty is crucial. The nurse should tell the child that there is pain when the periosteum is penetrated and aspiration occurs; however, if there is cooperation, it can be done quickly. It is important for the child to lie immobile in a specific position, and parents or the nurse may help the child in maintaining that position. The child needs to know that he can express his anger by screaming or crying. Certainly, talking

about the procedure later is helpful. After the marrow has been removed, it may be necessary to apply a pressure dressing to prevent a hematoma from forming. Sterile technique is utilized. The results of this test are usually available within 24 hours.

General Nursing Measures
Nursing Diagnoses
A hematologic problem in childhood may be the result of cancer or a genetic deficiency, or it may be acquired in any number of ways. Some examples of nursing diagnoses for children with blood disorders are

Potential for injury (and bleeding)
Altered nutrition: less than body requirements
Impaired gas exchange
Social isolation
Pain
Fluid volume deficit (actual or potential)
Potential joint contractures
Diversional activity deficit
Knowledge deficit related to disease, management
Noncompliance
Fear
Anxiety

Blood Loss
Problems in any aspect of the coagulation process result in blood loss of different degrees. Any active bleeding requires prompt action.

Ecchymoses, purpura, petechiae, and a complaint of bruising easily are all causes for concern. Unfortunately, bleeding is not always easy to detect, as in the child with hemophilia who may be bleeding into a joint (hemarthrosis). While active blood loss necessitates immediate replacement, direct pressure on the site, cold compresses, and ice, as well as nasal packing for epistaxis, are all efforts directed toward stopping the flow of blood. Whenever possible, a nurse should record the amount of blood lost so that replacement can be more accurate. When involved, extremities are usually elevated and splinted to relieve the pain and swelling, as well as to decrease the likelihood of further injury.

Children who are actively bleeding need to have their vital signs monitored frequently until they have stabilized. The intake and output volumes are recorded, a dipstick test for hematuria is done, and the specific gravity is noted. Such children should be in a quiet environment, and they should be kept as comfortable as possible. Any changes in position need to be made slowly and as tolerated by these young clients, who are weak, irritable, and disinterested in everything. In addition, the beds of these children should be padded to protect them from injury, and thought should be given to providing safe, soft toys. The bed rails should be in the up position at all times.

The skin of such children needs to be examined for evidence of increasing ecchymosis or petechiae. Mucous membranes and gums should be inspected for bleeding. It may be necessary to use a very soft toothbrush to decrease the likelihood of damage.

In many health care facilities, these children are put on "hematology precautions," which include no rectal temperatures, no rectal medications, no injections, and no visits to the playroom with specific platelet counts, among other criteria. If an injection must be given, a nurse must apply pressure to the site for at least 10 minutes or until the bleeding stops. It is imperative for a nurse to monitor the blood counts of these children and to know the implications of a low platelet count or neutropenia.

These children are assessed frequently for such complications as congestive heart failure, hypotension, and changes in behavior that may indicate low hemoglobin levels. Peripheral perfusion can be evaluated by pulses, skin temperatures, and capillary refill. Any delay in capillary refill may indicate decreased tissue perfusion. Unfortunately, congestive heart failure may develop in the child with a severe anemia. The anemia decreases the oxygen-carrying ability of the blood, and as a result, the cardiac output increases in an effort to correct the deficit.

Shock can be associated with or secondary to the decreased peripheral perfusion. A nurse needs to know the signs of impending shock: tachycardia, pallor, agitation, thirst, and confusion. As shock progresses, a child becomes less and less responsive.

While it is important to restore circulatory volume, the choice of fluid depends on the cause of the hypovolemia. Whatever intravenous solutions are ordered, it is critical to run them at the rates ordered, taking care to record the amounts infused at least hourly. The specific care involved in a transfusion is described below.

These children and their families are frightened and anxious, regardless of the amount of blood lost. They need explanations and reassurance.

The most trying time for parents comes when their toddler with a blood dyscrasia begins to walk. They need to be advised about the use of a helmet and knee and elbow pads whenever such a child is out of bed. Once he has mastered this skill and remains upright, then these protective devices can be discarded. Parents also appreciate being reminded about the advantages of supervising a toddler at play on grass or a rug rather than cement/asphalt or wooden floors.

Nutritional Needs

Children with hematologic disorders require certain foods and fluids which may exceed normal requirements in order for recovery to occur. Children who are weak and anorexic are not interested in eating, which requires the nurse to be innovative in overcoming their apathy.

The nursing history should include a complete description of the child's eating patterns, especially his food preferences. These children are on calorie counts, which necessitate observing and recording exactly what is consumed so that it can be reviewed by the nutritionist. Such children are usually weighed every day, on the same scale, at the same time. The results are plotted on a weight chart. Nutritional assessments are critical regardless of the blood disorder.

While it is important for all children to be hydrated adequately, for some, such as those with sickle cell anemia, it is imperative. In most instances, these children in crisis may need as much as twice their normal fluid requirements. Although such children receive intravenous fluids, oral fluids also need to be consumed. The average adolescent understands and cooperates; however, some adolescent females obsessed about their weights may be problematic. Some successful strategies for a nurse to use include popsicles, jello, ice cubes made of a variety of fruit juices, and puddings. While it is best to perform stressful, invasive procedures at least 1 hour before meals, thought also needs to be given to the environment in which such children eat. Sitting at childsize tables, surrounded by other children, and supervised by nurses and other adults can enhance the intakes of these children.

For some children whose anemias developed as a result of the absence of certain foods, their intake usually consists of foods that are high in iron (meats, fish, eggs, poultry, green leafy vegetables, cereals, breads). Since fresh juices are high in vitamin C (which enhances the absorption of iron), they are offered freely. To supplement iron intake, often these infants and children are given prescribed iron preparations. The nurse who administers an oral preparation needs to remember that it cannot be given with milk because this dairy product interferes with iron absorption. In addition, liquid iron preparations can stain teeth, so they should be given with a straw. Brushing the teeth following iron administration will lessen the stain.

As the iron levels rise and the hemoglobin increases, the behaviors of these anemic children change. They resume their normal activity levels, and their eating patterns change dramatically.

Infections

Infection control is a major problem in children with blood dyscrasias. When these children are neutropenic, they are vulnerable. When normal flora are suppressed, opportunistic organisms flourish.

Again, the environment is critical, occasionally requiring a private room. While conscientious hand washing is imperative for everyone, there is also a need to screen all visitors and health care providers for any sign of infection. If the child is not in a private room, his roommates also should be examined carefully for infections. While the immediate environment can be controlled, when a child leaves his room, it is more difficult to prevent exposure to some infections in the playroom or other areas of the hospital.

Vital signs need to be taken routinely and, in the presence of an elevated temperature, more frequently. For older infants and children, a rising temperature is a good indicator of infection. If an infection is suspected, urine, blood, and nasopharyngeal cultures should be done.

Rest periods need to be encouraged because they decrease a child's oxygenation needs. For the infant who is weak for nutritional anemia, activity is limited easily. The child in sickle cell crisis is in pain, and so his tolerance level is extremely low.

A child's oral mucous membranes and gums need to be examined for any signs of infection. It is essential for a nurse to assess and maintain a child's skin integrity because it too is a critical measure of avoiding infection. Cutting a child's fingernails and toenails is another effective method of avoiding a major problem.

On occasion, it is important to place a child in protective isolation. In such instances, it is critical for everyone to know and respect the need for maintaining that form of isolation. With gown, gloves, and masks required for entry, the numbers of visitors decrease and sensory as well as social isolation result. Nursing interventions need to be directed toward lessening this deprivation.

Parents need to be taught basic hand-washing techniques and methods of avoiding infection as well as identifying its presence. On discharge, parents need to be instructed about avoiding crowded shopping malls, markets, and people who have colds or other forms of infection.

Transfusions

A *transfusion* refers to the intravenous administration of red blood cells to the child who is anemic; however, other blood components, such as white cells, platelets, and cryoprecipitate, also can be given when needed. The child who as a severe blood loss can receive a *packed red cell infusion,* a preparation from which most of the plasma has been removed. Sometimes *white cell transfusions* are given to children with a hematologic malignancy, such as leukemia. Granulocytes are the primary components administered. *Platelet transfusions* may be required for those children who cannot produce adequate numbers of platelets. They are especially helpful in treating certain thrombocytopenic problems, and they are also administered to children who are immunosuppressed. *Cryoprecipitate,* a fresh-frozen plasma product containing the missing factor VIII, is given intravenously to children with hemophilia who are bleeding.

The nursing responsibilities to a child receiving a transfusion are great. The child should be monitored closely for signs and symptoms of a transfusion reaction. Most reactions will occur within 10 minutes. The signs and symptoms and nursing interventions for transfusion reactions are listed in Table 25-4. When a reaction is suspected, the transfusion should be stopped at once and the physician should be notified. It is advisable to administer transfusions with a double setup in which both blood and an intravenous solution are connected by a stopcock. With this arrangement, fluid is available to maintain the patency of the intravenous line in the event that the transfusion must be stopped. The untransfused blood should be saved and returned to the blood bank.

If possible, a parent should remain with the child during this procedure. The nurse should explain the procedure to the parent and elicit his or her assistance during the preparation, if it is appropriate to do so. The infusion site should be securely immobilized in a position that is comfortable for the child. He should be provided familiar comforting objects and diversionary activity during the procedure.

Infusion of the blood may be difficult and tedious, but transfusions should be administered slowly to prevent volume overload and to protect the child's small, fragile veins. The cells may clog the tubing, and it may be necessary to flush the tubing with an intravenous solution intermittently.

Hematologic Problems in Infancy and Toddlerhood

Acquired Immune Deficiency Syndrome

Pediatric acquired immune deficiency syndrome (AIDS) encompasses those children who are under 13 years of age. Adolescents are grouped with adults. The causative organism is believed to be a retrovirus, called *human immunodeficiency virus* (HIV). Current evidence suggests that HIV is transmitted through blood and blood products and through semen during intimate sexual contact, particularly anal intercourse.

The risk groups that are pertinent to pediatric HIV infection include parents who are intravenous drug users, mothers who have had multiple sexual partners or whose partners have had multiple sexual contacts, and children who received transfusions of blood or blood products between 1978 and 1985. Most children with HIV infection are under 2 years of age, and the infection was acquired during the perinatal period.

In 1985, the provisional case definition of pediatric AIDS adopted by the Centers for Disease Control (CDC) was a child who has had

1. A reliably diagnosed disease at least moderately indicative of underlying cellular immune deficiency [same as in adult AIDS plus chronic lymphoid interstitial pneumonitis coupled with a positive test for HIV, toxoplasmosis, or herpesvirus *after 1 month of age* and cytomegalovirus (CMV) *after 6 months of age*).
2. No known cause of underlying cellular immune deficiency or any other reduced resistance reported to be associated with that disease (CDC, 1985).

Pursuant to the belief held by physicians who cared for HIV-infected children (whether symptomatic or asymptomatic) that only about 50 percent of these children fulfilled the strict CDC criteria, the CDC convened a consultant panel to develop a classification system more pertinent for children under 13 years of age (CDC, 1987a). The CDC surveillance case definition for all AIDS patients was revised and published in 1987. The new pediatric AIDS classification system was incorporated into this document. For a complete revised definition, the reader is referred to the August 14, 1987, *MMWR* supplement (CDC, 1987b). Some highlights from this publication applicable to pediatric AIDS include the 1985 definition plus:

TABLE 25-4 Transfusion Reactions

Hemolytic Transfusion Reaction

Prevention

Identify patient and blood product to ensure proper match. Double-check all blood products with another nurse or health professional.

Begin infusion at a slow rate, and remain with patient for first 15 minutes. Severe reactions tend to begin soon after initiation of transfusion.

Signs and Symptoms

Immediate onset, usually. Delayed onset may be observed when an Rh incompatibility is involved.

Burning sensation along the vein.

Facial flushing.

Fever, chills, temperature may be 105°F or higher.

Chest pain; rapid, labored respirations.

Headache.

Lower back pain.

Shock.

Nursing Actions

Stop transfusion immediately to reduce further risk. Severity of reaction is related to amount transfused.

Treat stock if present. Administer oxygen, fluids, epinephrine as ordered by physician.

Recheck blood slip with unit of blood and patient to determine if error was made.

Obtain two blood samples from a vein distant from infusion site. One specimen is sent for centrifuge (pink or red plasma indicates hemolysis); other specimen is sent to blood bank with remainder of transfusion.

Obtain first voided urine to test for hemoglobinuria. Specimen may be red or black, indicating potential renal damage.

With suspected renal involvement, physicians initiate prompt treatment with mannitol to promote diuresis and prevent renal tubular damage. Monitor fluid and electrolyte balance as soon as diuresis begins.

Allergic Reaction

Prevention

Determine whether patient has history of allergy, particularly a previous allergic reaction to transfused blood products.

Administer antihistamine, for example, diphenhydramine (Benadryl) orally or parenterally 15 to 20 minutes before starting infusion.

Signs and Symptoms

Urticaria (hives), pruritus.

Facial and/or glottal edema (rare).

Asthma (rare).

Pulmonary edema with infiltrates (rare).

Analphylaxis.

Headache, flushing, tachycardia, and general discomfort may be present.

(Symptoms may persist for 8 to 10 hours; most are more transient.)

Nursing Actions

Stop transfusion immediately.

Treat life-threatening reactions (edema, anaphylaxis) immediately.

Administer antihistamine parenterally.

Bacterial Reaction

Prevention

Maintain aseptic collection techniques.

Change transfusion equipment frequently.

Do not allow blood to stand at room temperature unnecessarily, even while infusing.

Do not use blood that has been heated to above room temperature.

Do not prewarm infusions.

Inspect all blood for evidence of hemolysis.

Signs and Symptoms

Shaking fever.

Severe hypotension.

Dry, flushed skin.

Pain in abdomen and extremities.

Vomiting and bloody diarrhea.

Nursing Actions

Stop transfusion immediately.

Administer broad-spectrum antibiotics as ordered immediately, by most rapid route.

Treat shock aggressively.

Monitor vital signs, fluid and electrolyte balance.

Circulatory Overload

Prevention

Give packed cells to persons susceptible to circulatory overload (eldery, infants, persons with cardiac or respiratory disorders).

Administer infusion slowly, with patient in a sitting position.

Signs and Symptoms

Tightness in chest, labored breathing.

Dry cough.

Rales at base of lungs.

Pulmonary edema.

Nursing Actions

Stop—or slow—transfusion, depending on severity of symptoms.

Have patient sit up.

Monitor vital signs.

Treat severe overload with rotating tourniquets or phlebotomy.

Administer diuretics as ordered.

Febrile Reaction

Prevention

Keep patient covered and warm during transfusion.

Administer antipyretic medication to presons known to have this reaction.

(Transfusion with leukocyte-poor red blood cells or frozen washed packed cells may prevent this reaction in persons susceptible to it.)

Signs and Symptoms

Chills and fever, usually beginning about 1 hour after start of infusion.

Nursing Actions

Stop transfusion immediately.

Treat symptomatically.

Air Embolism

Prevention

Avoid introducing air into system.

If air is introduced, stop the infusion.

Signs and Symptoms

Cyanosis.

Dyspnea.

Shock.

Cardiac arrest.

Nursing Actions

Lower patient's head and turn patient on left side. Air will collect in right atrium, where it can be released gradually to the lungs.

Treat shock and/or cardiac arrest immediatley if these events should occur.

Source: L. C. Callins, "Preventing and Treating Transfusion Reactions," *American Journal of Nursing,* 79:936, May 1979.

1. Children under 15 months of age whose mothers are not thought to have had HIV infection during the perinatal period; however, these infants/children are repeatedly reactive for HIV antibody by enzyme-linked immunosorbent assay (ELISA) with a subsequent positive Western blot or immunofluorescence assay.

2. Children under 15 months of age whose mothers are thought to have had HIV infection during the perinatal period; the infant/child is repeatedly reactive for HIV antibody, has elevated serum immunoglobin levels, has a positive Western blot or immunofluorescence assay, and has at least one of the following:

   (a) Decreased absolute lymphocyte count.

   (b) Depressed T-helper lymphocyte count.

   (c) Decreased T-helper to T-suppressor lymphocyte ratio.

   (In this group of children, a positive ELISA alone may reflect passively acquired maternal antibodies. Thus additional evidence as noted is necessary.)

3. Children 15 months or over who are repeatedly reactive for HIV antibody by ELISA with subsequent positive results from Western blot or immunofluorescence assay.

4. Children less than 13 years of age who have multiple or recurrent serious bacterial infections, lymphoid interstitial pneumonia, or pulmonary lymphoid hyperplasia (these entities *do not* apply to adults) and laboratory evidence of HIV infection. (A presumptive diagnosis may be made in the absence of laboratory evidence for lymphoid interstitial pneumonia or pulmonary lymphoid hyperplasia.)

5. Children who have a progressive loss of behavioral/developmental milestones not related to any other known condition and laboratory evidence of HIV.

6. Children who fail to thrive and have laboratory evidence of HIV.

The highest percentage (about 75 percent) of AIDS in the pediatric population is in infants born to mothers infected with HIV (estimated risk of transmission is 30 to 50 percent). AIDS prevalence is greater in black and Hispanic infants, and HIV infection is seen more frequently in the Northeast, California, and Florida than in other parts of the United States. Prior to 1985, infants and children who needed transfusions of blood or blood products were at risk. Since 1985, donor blood has been subjected to screenings for HIV antibody and has been heat-treated to inactivate the virus. Even with this advance, some adolescents who need transfusions (e.g., those with sickle cell anemia, thalassemia, and hemophilia) may refuse these procedures because of fear of AIDS. Nurses need to help them overcome this fear.

Treatment for infants and children with pediatric AIDS is supportive. There is no known cure. The greatest need for children who have HIV infection is prevention of the occurrence of opportunistic infection. Intravenous gamma globulin therapy (once or twice each month) has had a impact on the reduction of bacterial infections, particularly in children under 2 years of age. This costly procedure requires 2 to 3 hours to complete.

Symptomatic HIV infection is often first seen as failure to thrive, which has various causes. Vigorous nutritional support is needed. If oral routes fail, then hyperalimentation may be necessary to achieve adequate weight gain. The treatment of infections that occur varies according to the specific entity.

Immunization status is an important consideration for infants and children who have HIV infection, whether symptomatic or asymptomatic. All these young patients can receive DTP and MMR at the specified times (Chap. 4). However, inactivated poliovirus vaccine must be substituted for OPV. *Hemophilus influenzae* type b conjugate vaccine is considered for administration at 18 months of age. If the child is asymptomatic, neither pneumococcal nor influenza vaccine is given; however, if the child is symptomatic, both are recommended as preventive measures (CDC, 1988).

Nursing Management

Nurses caring for HIV-infected children need to direct their energies toward prevention of opportunistic infection, nutritional support, and education. It is imperative that blood and body fluid precautions be observed. Gloves and a gown are worn whenever there is direct contact with blood, secretions, or excretions. Hands are washed thoroughly when nurses, other health care personnel, or parents enter and leave the room. If parents or others come to visit, gloves and gowns are not necessary unless they anticipate coming in contact with the child's blood or body fluids. Personnel or parents who have open skin or mucous membrane lesions should wear gloves, however. The published hospital regulations for decontaminating and/or disposing of needles, syringes, and linen and for removing and transporting specimens should be followed.

Contaminated surfaces are washed with a 1:10 bleach solution. If clothing comes in contact with blood or body fluids, it also can be washed in a bleach solution.

Nursing assessments, interventions, and evaluations vary depending on the child's specific problems. However, vital signs, skin care, nutrition, and enhancing the child's growth and development are overriding nursing concerns.

Vital signs and temperature measurements are done frequently to determine if there is any evidence of sepsis. Examining the skin and mucous membranes for fungal infections is also important.

Nutrition is of concern. Careful recording of intake and output and plotting of length, weight, and head circumference are imperative in assessing nutrition and in evaluating the outcome of the current diet, whether oral or parenteral. Hydration status is ascertained by determining the condition of the oral mucosa (moist or dry), the lips (moist or dry and cracked), tears (present or absent), skin turgor, anterior fontanelle (soft or depressed), and urine output and specific gravity. Aseptic technique is of prime importance in preventing infection for those children who are receiving hyperalimentation.

Parents may have questions about the child's attendance at day care or school. No reported cases of AIDS have been transmitted in these settings. The main danger is transmission of infection from other children in these settings to the HIV-infected child. If a child has bowel and bladder control, does not bite others, has no open lesions, and does not mouth objects, the child poses no problem to other children or to day care center or school personnel. The parents and the physician need to assess the risks for the HIV-infected child's attendance at day care or school on an individual basis. In general, no restrictions are placed on school-age children who have the approval of their personal physician.

Day care and school administrators should develop and adopt guidelines for handling blood and body fluids from any child. These guidelines should be available to all personnel who work in the setting, including those in housekeeping. Personnel who have open skin or mucous membrane lesions should not come in contact with the blood or body fluids of children who have HIV infection.

Prevention of pediatric HIV infection is a part of the national effort supported by the surgeon general. If responsible sexual practices were adopted by all sexually active people, drug addition were curtailed, and sexual abuse were eliminated, this dread disease could be contained. Nurses can help by becoming involved in education regarding sexual transmission, drugs, sharing needles and syringes, and having multiple sexual partners or partners who have multiple sexual contacts.

In relation to the total number of AIDS cases, the percentage of children is small, about 1.5 to 1.6 percent. With the adoption of the new case definition as of September 1, 1987, this percentage may increase. These children and their families have to contend with multiple psychosocial issues as well as the physical problems the child may suffer. Isolation, fragmented family life, violence, drug addiction, hardship, and loss may feed into the stresses experienced by the child and family. Thus the approach to care requires a multidisciplinary team effort to be effective.

Anemia

Anemia, the most common hemopoietic disorder of childhood, results from a reduction in the number of red blood cells, a lowered concentration of available hemoglobin, or both. The anemias may be divided into two categories: those resulting from impairment in production of red blood cells and those resulting from increased destruction or loss of red blood cells.

Clinical features of anemia are related to the decrease in the oxygen-carrying capacity of the blood. Signs and symptoms may be nonspecific: pallor, irritability, weakness, anorexia, decreased exercise tolerance, and lack of interest in surroundings. When the hemoglobin level falls below 7 to 8 g/100 ml, cardiac compensatory adjustments occur and pallor of the skin and mucosa may develop. When anemia is severe, the skin may assume a waxy, sallow appearance. Cardiac decompensation occurs, and congestive heart failure may develop with symptoms of tachycardia, tachypnea, shortness of breath, dyspnea, edema, and hepatomegaly. A peculiarity of infants is their ability to adjust to the stress of anemia unusually well. It is not uncommon for an infant to maintain a hemoglobin as low as 4 or 5 g/100 ml and manifest few signs or symptoms. Older children also demonstrate an ability to tolerate low hemoglobin levels, particularly if their anemia develops gradually.

The nursing assessment should include determination of the child's current functional level. An estimation of his exercise tolerance and level of frustration should be made. Factors which may contribute to the disease process should be investigated. A thorough dietary history (Chap. 7) should be taken. Possible toxic agents in the environment, such as chemicals and drugs, should be identified. Close observation of the interaction of family members may reveal what influence they have on the child's adjustment to the limitations of his disease. Do family members automatically assist the child when he needs assistance, or must he ask for help? Is he allowed to participate in activities when he is able, or is he restricted?

Anemia is diagnosed from a decreased hemoglobin and examination of other factors such as red blood cells indices, reticulocyte count, iron studies, hemoglobin electrophoresis, and bone-marrow aspiration. Through these tests, the specific type of problem can be determined.

Treatment varies with the cause. Specific therapy will be discussed later in the chapter when specific disorders are described. Transfusion of packed cells may be used with several types of anemia. When cardiac compensatory adjustments occur, the blood volume is increased to enhance perfusion of tissues. The volume of whole blood required to supply the necessary quantity of red blood cells may overload the child's circulatory system. When packed-cell transfusions are prepared, the erythrocytes are spun down and the bulk of fluid and other formed elements are left behind. This type of transfusion enables the child to receive a high concentration of erythrocytes in a small volume.

Nursing Management

The nurse who is attuned to early signs of irritability, fatigue, and frustration in the child should be prepared to make necessary adjustments in the environment. The irritable infant must have his needs met promptly. Crying may cause further fatigue. Disruptive treatments and procedures should be scheduled together to allow for uninterrupted periods of rest. In the case of an older child, careful selection of activities in which he can engage without frustration is essential. When he begins to show signs of fatigue, sedentary activities such as handicrafts and coloring should be presented. When possible, he should be given several alternatives and allowed to choose. A short attention span should be anticipated.

Fear of hospitalization can be exaggerated by fear of separation from mother. Allowing the mother to participate actively in the child's care may reduce his fear. Explanation of procedures and exploration through play may reduce anxiety and fear in the older child. When intrusive procedures are necessary, allowing him to participate in the preparation for the procedure by wiping the area with alcohol and applying the adhesive cover may help him maintain some control of the situation.

Anemic children are often anorectic. Infants should be fed slowly and offered frequent small feedings if necessary. The child should be rewarded for positive attempts to eat. The older child may wish to participate in the selection and preparation of the food. Simple tasks, such as helping younger children prepare their meal trays, may stimulate their eating. Tiring activities and unpleasant procedures and treatments should not be scheduled at mealtime.

Depending on the type of anemia and treatment modality, the child may require a transfusion. The nursing responsibilities have been described above under Common Nursing Measures.

Iron-Deficiency Anemia

Iron-deficiency anemia is the most common type of anemia in childhood. It occurs most commonly between the ages of 6 and 24 months. Prior to this time, the child's iron requirements are usually met by the reserves acquired during fetal life. A positive iron balance in childhood is dependent on several factors. Possible causes of iron deficiency include

1. Insufficient supply: dietary deficiency; inadequate stores at birth—low birth weight, preterm birth, twins, iron-deficient mother, prenatal fetal blood loss.
2. Impaired absorption: chronic diarrhea: malabsorption syndrome; gastrointestinal abnormalities
3. Excessive demands: growth requirements, particularly prematurity and adolescence
4. Blood loss: chronic or acute hemorrhage; parasitic infection
5. Vitamin E deficiency

In adolescence, the incidence of mild iron deficiency increases with acceleration in the rate of growth and onset of menstrual loss in girls and androgen-related increase in hemoglobin concentration in boys. Diet is characteristically low in iron. This deficiency continues until the early twenties in both sexes.

The clinical features of iron deficiency are similar to those mentioned in the general discussion of anemia. When children with iron deficiency acquire infections, their condition is aggravated by a decreased absorption of iron. *Pica*, a hunger for and ingestion of unsuitable substances, such as clay or starch, may result from and contribute to iron deficiency. The nursing assessment should focus on the child's dietary habits. Information should be obtained regarding the type and quantity of food eaten, the methods of feeding used, the child's reaction to eating, and the parents' understanding of dietary requirements and nutritional value of foods. The clinical findings of pallor combined with the history of an iron-deficient diet are suggestive of iron-deficiency anemia.

The characteristic appearance of the stained blood smear is that of many small red cells or *microcytes* that are pale or *hypochromic*. This central pallor of the cells indicates the marked deficiency of hemoglobin. MCV and MCH are decreased (microcytic, hypochromic anemia), as

are serum ferritin and transferrin saturation. FEP and TIBC are increased.

Iron-salt preparations are administered orally in most cases. Ferrous sulfate is most often used because it is both inexpensive and effective. A rapid response in the hemoglobin is expected when therapy is begun, but the child is continued on oral iron for 4 to 6 weeks after normal blood values are established to replenish body stores. If insufficient dietary supply is the cause of the deficiency, a change in dietary habits is essential. Milk is a relatively poor source of iron. Many infants and children who drink large quantities of milk do so to the exclusion of other foods which contain more iron. When this situation pertains, milk intake should be limited to ¾ qt per day. Foods high in iron, such as meat, fortified cereal, vegetables, and fruit, should be introduced to the diet. Additional information on dietary treatment is in Chap. 7.

Nursing Management

The best approach to management of iron deficiency is prevention. In preterm infants, iron supplementation is begun no later than 2 months of age, and in full-term infants, no later than 4 months of age. In high-risk groups (e.g., the poor, those of AFDC, those who are enrolled in WIC programs), newborns who are bottle-fed are placed on iron-fortified formulas immediately rather than at 2, 4, or 6 months of age. In low-risk groups, bottle-fed infants are given iron-fortified formulas between 2 and 4 months of age. Parents are advised to continue with these formulas until the infant is at least 9 months of age, preferably until 12 months of age. When breast-fed infants are weaned, iron-fortified formula is recommended as with bottle-fed infants. Once solid foods are begun (between 4 and 6 months), iron-fortified rice cereal is the first food introduced.

In those children who do develop iron deficiency, ferrous sulfate is prescribed, and treatment will last for at least 3 months and possibly as long as 5 months. With severe anemia, an elevated reticulocyte count in response to iron therapy may be seen as early as 3 days. In milder anemia, the increase occurs in 7 to 10 days. A hemoglobin rise is noted by 3 weeks. Nurses working with these families need to stress the importance of giving the anemic infant or toddler the prescribed amount of iron (usually in three divided doses) between meals. Taking the medication with orange juice or other citrus juices (source of ascorbic acid) enhances iron absorption in the small intestine. Absorption is decreased by cow's milk. Liquid iron preparations may stain the teeth. Parents should be assured that the stain is temporary. The iron changes the color of the bowel movement to a tarry green. Only 1 month's supply of the iron preparation is kept in the home to reduce the risk of accidental poisoning.

On follow-up visits, the nurse can inquire about stool color. If it has not changed to the expected color, the reason may be that the infant or child is not absorbing an adequate amount or is not being given the prescribed amount. Stool color, dietary intake, and follow-up laboratory studies provide means for evaluating interventions.

NURSING CARE PLAN

25-1 *The Child with Iron Deficiency Anemia*

Clinical Problem/Nursing Diagnosis	Expected Outcome	Nursing Interventions
Pallor Anemia Altered tissue perfusion (anemia) related to decreased iron stores	Given appropriate nursing care, child will achieve adequate iron stores, tolerate iron-enriched diet, tolerate supplemental iron medications without side effects, and demonstrate improvement in color of vascular beds (increase in pink color) After 7 to 10 days of the prescribed iron-replacement preparation, child will demonstrate increased reticulate count and upward trend in hematocrit and hemoglobin measurements	Assess color of mucous membranes and nailbeds; monitor for increased pink color in relation to treatment Assess baseline vital signs: note presence of tachycardia, murmur, regularity of heart rate, quality and equality of breath sounds, and presence of tachypnea and/or dyspnea and note respirations (rate and depth); monitor blood pressure for hypertension and/or hypotension; monitor changes in vital signs in response to treatment Note baseline hemoglobin/hematocrit (HgB/Hct), reticulocyte count, and FEP; monitor trends in these values in response to treatment Administer prescribed iron replacement preparations; administer iron supplements with meals to minimize gastric irritation; prevent contact of teeth with liquid iron supplements by using a straw; observe for side effects from iron supplements (constipation, nausea, change in color of stool to black); teach parents proper medication administration and possible side effects for which to observe child
Fatigue Weakness Irritability Decreased activity level Activity intolerance related to anemia and alteration in oxygen transport mechanisms	Child will demonstrate increased interest in play activities and progressive increase in activity tolerance, energy level, alertness, and overall behavior	Provide quiet, restful environment to promote rest Limit participation in strenuous, stressful, energy-consuming activities until child benefits from effective treatment Conserve energy reserves; suggest participation in quiet play activity: art, painting, reading, coloring, modeling with clay, and building projects Support active play with adequate rest periods Teach and assist child with deep breathing and relaxation techniques Provide adequate opportunities to express feelings and fears through play or art expression to reduce emotional stressors Assess child's ability to gradually tolerate increased amounts of activity as HgB and Hct are corrected with treatment
Developmental delay Altered growth and development related to anemia	Child will demonstrate progressive improvement in accomplishing various developmental milestones	Assess neurological status; assess level of activity, motor and sensory function, strength of reflexes, muscle tone, behavioral changes, level of alertness, and response to environment Assess areas of developmental delay with age-appropriate developmental assessment tool (DDST) Communicate identified areas of delay to physician; facilitate referral for developmental evaluation and intervention for follow-up care
Pica Lead poisoning Potential for injury (lead poisoning) related to exposure to toxic substance and pica	In presence of coexisting lead intoxication, child will excrete toxic substance after treatment and return to safe, lead-free environment	See care plan for lead poisoning Observe for abnormal behavioral patterns relating to ingestion (pica) Document FEP and lead levels; administer chelation therapy as ordered Contact agencies to investigate home for lead Ensure return to safe lead-free environment

Clinical Problem/Nursing Diagnosis	Expected Outcome	Nursing Interventions
Gastrointestinal blood loss	Child's stools will remain normal	Observe stools for evidence of blood; note presence of melena Note guaiac stools and/or emesis and document results Assess type, color, amount, and consistency of gastrointestinal output
Potential for injury related to blood loss		Send stools to laboratory for ova and parasites Evaluate presence of cow's milk allergy; eliminate cow's milk and milk products from diet and evaluate clinical response
Congestive heart failure	Child will maintain cardiopulmonary homeostasis	Monitor trends in daily weights; note weight gain Monitor child for tachypnea, tachycardia, rales, diaphoresis, poor peripheral perfusion, cool mottled extremities, and decreased urine output
Decreased cardiac output related to alteration in oxygen transport mechanisms		Provide humidified oxygen therapy as needed Administer diuretics as ordered Monitor and correct electrolyte imbalances Properly administer ordered blood transfusions as dictated by child's clinical status
Diet poor in iron-enriched foods and protein	Child will tolerate high-protein, iron-enriched diet	Obtain detailed nutritional history: determine daily dietary intake of iron and protein prior to therapy; note report of excessive intake of cow's milk
Excessive intake of cow's milk		Provide infant with iron-fortified formulas (through the first year of life) and cereals
Altered nutrition: less than body requirements related to inadequate intake of iron-enriched foods; excessive intake of cow's milk		Encourage children and adolescents to increase dietary intake of iron-rich foods, i.e., iron-enriched breads and cereals, organ meat, poultry, fish, egg yolk, dark green leafy vegetables, dried fruits, and ascorbic acid-rich juice to improve iron absorption Suggest high-protein snacks (peanut butter and cheese crackers and sandwiches) Collaborate with nutritionist to assist parents and child with meal planning for a high-protein, iron-enriched diet
Increased susceptibility to infection	Child's vital signs will remain within normal range, indicative of absence of infection	Monitor for changes in vital signs: tachycardia, tachypnea, hypotension and/or hypertension, and elevated temperature Frequently monitor temperature for elevations Report temperature 38.5°C to physician
Potential for infection related to increased susceptibility with iron deficiency		Obtain blood, urine, and tracheal aspirate for culture Assess focal sites for redness and swelling Administer antibiotics and antipyretics as prescribed and evaluate effectiveness of treatment Practice strict hand washing techniques: prevent exposure to visitors and friends with symptoms of infection

The nurse should stress to parents the importance of continuing iron therapy according to the physician's plan. Many parents are tempted to discontinue therapy when a good response is obtained.

Diet teaching can be a delicate matter. The nurse must be aware that dietary habits are influenced by cultural and socioeconomic factors. In some cultures, a fat, chubby baby is considered a reflection of good mothering. Babies fed nothing but milk and carbohydrates for the first year of life may be fat and appear healthy to the mother. It is difficult for her to appreciate the need for a change in dietary habits. Mothers may resist including iron-containing foods in their babies' diet because they are more expensive or are unfamiliar.

It is important to explain the reasons for diet change to the parents in language they can understand. Visual aids and pictures may be helpful. Explanations and suggestions may need to be repeated several times. The nurse may investigate with the parents sources of inexpensive iron-containing foods which are available in their community. A plan should be implemented to introduce new foods to the baby's diet. The baby may tolerate frequent small feedings better. The environment should be free of stress at feeding time, and the infant should be fed in the presence of other children or family members if possible. It is important that the nurse be accepting of the family's cultural habits and patterns but stress the rationale for the change in a nonjudgmental way.

The infant may resist transferring from an exclusive milk diet to one that includes new, unfamiliar foods. It is important to limit consistently the amount of milk offered and to continue gently offering foods even if the infant rejects them. He will eventually turn to the new foods to satisfy his hunger.

Sickle Cell Disease

The *sickle cell hemoglobinopathies* are hereditary disorders characterized by the presence of an abnormal type of hemoglobin in the red blood cell. The basic defect in hemoglobin S is a substitution of valine for glutamic acid in the sixth position of the beta polypeptide chain of the hemoglobin molecule. This structural change facilitates the sickling phenomenon. In the presence of deoxygenation, a stacking of sickle hemoglobin molecules occurs and the cell assumes an irregular shape. The abnormally shaped cells increase blood viscosity, and viscosity results in stasis and sludging of the cells and further deoxygenation. Deoxygenation leads to further sickling, eventual occlusion of small vessels, and tissue ischemia, with infarction and necrosis occurring.

The sickling phenomenon takes place when oxygen tension in blood is lowered. Decreased oxygen tension may be triggered by infection, dehydration, exposure to cold, or physical or emotional stress (Fig. 25-3).

Sickle trait is a heterozygous occurrence of the sickle gene resulting in a combination of normal adult hemoglobin and sickle hemoglobin in the red blood cell. *Sickle cell anemia* is a homozygous occurrence of the sickle gene resulting in a severe hemolytic anemia (Fig. 25-4). Two other more common forms of sickle cell disease are sickle hemoglobin C disease (doubly heterozygous with equal amounts of S and C hemoglobin) and sickle

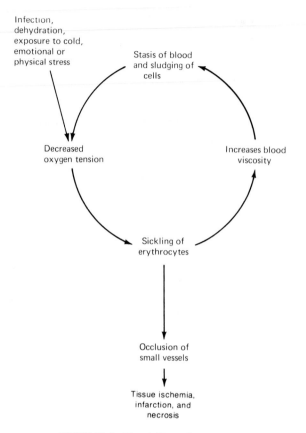

FIGURE 25-3   The sickling phenomenon.

FIGURE 25-4   The inheritance pattern of sickle cell disease.

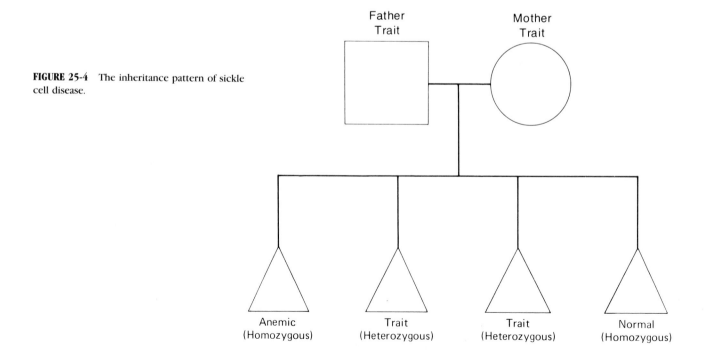

β-thalassemia (more S than A and F hemoglobins). According to Lubin and Mentzer (1987), fewer complications are seen in children who have sickle hemoglobin C disease and sickle β-thalassemia: however, the severity of a vasoocclusive crisis may be comparable to that seen in sickle cell anemia.

Clinical manifestations of sickle trait are rare. Discovery of the trait is often incidental or a result of a screening effort. Occasionally, severe hypoxia resulting from shock, exposure to low oxygen content, or surgery may result in discovery of sickling.

Clinical manifestations of sickle cell anemia occurring in infancy include frequent infections, failure to thrive, irritability, pallor, hepatosplenomegaly, jaundice, and growth retardation. Periods of well-being may be interrupted by periods of sickling crisis. Manifestations rarely occur before 4 months of age (F hemoglobin concentration is greater than 20%, so sickling does not occur) and may not occur until the child is 2 to 3 years of age. Older children complain of joint, back, and abdominal pain, headache, nausea and vomiting, and frequent infections, particularly of the respiratory tract.

Vasoocclusive or thrombotic crises, the most common complications of the disease, are responsible for a majority of defects acquired by the child with sickle cell disease. The thrombotic crises may involve any area of the body. Soft-tissue swelling and pain result from vascular occlusion in the area of a large joint. The "hand-foot" syndrome (Fig. 25-5) is a complication seen in children under 2 years of age. Characteristically, this syndrome is accompanied by pain, fever, swelling of soft tissue of the hands and feet, and infarction of underlying bones. The complication is self-limiting, and complete healing can be expected. Vital organs such as the lungs, kidneys, liver, brain, and eye may be involved, and serious complications can result.

Aplastic or anemic crises may be associated with a bacterial or viral infection. A transient decrease in the rate of red blood cell production coupled with the short life span of circulating red cells can produce a profound anemia of rapid onset.

A splenic sequestration crisis is characterized by a rapidly enlarging spleen which traps a large portion of the red cell mass. Profound anemia and shock may result.

Sickle cell disease is found primarily in the black population. The occasional appearance in Caucasians is thought to be the result of distant intermarriages or a new genetic mutation. It also occurs is some people of Mediterranean ancestry.

The incidences of the most common forms of sickle cell disease in the United States are as follows:

Sickle cell anemia (SS): 1 : 600
Sickle hemoglobin C (SC): 1 : 800
Sickle β-thalassemia: 1 : 1700
Sickle cell trait (AS): 1 : 12

It is important to obtain parental permission to screen black neonates before discharge from the newborn nursery. A hemoglobin electrophoresis may be done on either

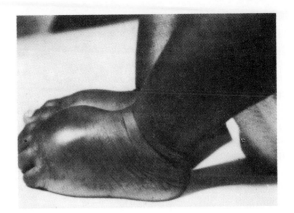

FIGURE 25-5   The appearance of the feet in the "hand-foot" syndrome in infants with sickle cell disease. *(From A.M. Mauer, Pediatric Hematology, McGraw-Hill, New York, 1969, p. 94.)*

cord blood (obtained in the delivery room) or on peripheral blood to identify the various hemoglobins. If F and S hemoglobin are present but no A, then the newborn most likely has either sickle cell anemia or sickle β°-thalassemia. In sickle β⁺-thalassemia, the concentration of A hemoglobin is reduced but not absent. If F, S, and C hemoglobins are found, then the newborn has sickle hemoglobin C disease. With sickle trait, A, S, and F hemoglobins are present, with A greater than S. A confirmatory hemoglobin electrophoresis is done after 6 months of age when the hemoglobin F concentration has reduced naturally.

Children who were not tested during the first year of life can be screened with a hemoglobin electrophoresis. Examination of a stained blood smear in sickle cell anemia may reveal a few sickled cells. Hemoglobin and hematocrit are decreased, and the reticulocyte count is elevated. The bilirubin level is increased owing to the fragility of the red blood cells. The life span of a sickle cell is shortened in contrast to the normal red blood cell's life span of 120 days.

The basic objectives of detection of sickle cell hemoglobin states are (1) early diagnosis and anticipation and prevention of severe complications and death, and (2) informed genetic counseling. If benefits are to be gained from early diagnosis, testing must be done early in infancy, since the disease is usually manifest during the first year of life.

If screening is not done early in infancy or early childhood, it is appropriate to introduce it with the onset of adolescence. At that time, children are readily available in a school setting, developmentally prepared to understand the genetic implications, and fast approaching the point in their lives when decisions about marriage and family planning will be made. In any screening program, whether for infants, children, adolescents, or adults, the cornerstone must be a well-organized, effective counseling program.

Administration of oral and intravenous fluids is essential. Dehydration causes decreased blood volume, sludging, increased blood viscosity, and further sickling. Fever, which may accelerate dehydration, can be controlled with antipyretics. Crises are usually accompanied by severe pain which persists for several days. Analgesics should be used appropriately to control the pain.

Hyptertransfusion of packed cells may be used during vasoocclusive crises when involvement of vital organs may be life-threatening. Raising the hemoglobin to high levels diminishes bone-marrow production of additional sickle cells and dilutes the existing sickle cells with normal transfused erythrocytes. The viscosity of the blood, thereby, is decreased, but the complications of long-term hypertransfusion contraindicate using this approach routinely.

Well-child care and immunizations are very important as means of preventing infection. Since both *S. pneumoniae* and *H. influenzae* are frequent causes of infection in these children, early immunizations with pneumococcal vaccine (at 1 year, booster at 2 years, and boosters every 4 years thereafter) and with the *H. influenzae* conjugate vaccine (at 18 months) are important. In children and infants who have sickle cell anemia, prophylactic penicillin is given b.i.d. from 3 months to 5 years. Children who receive multiple transfusions should have a hepatitis B vaccination.

Prognosis for patients with sickle cell anemia is generally grave. Death may occur in childhood or early adult life. Most deaths in childhood occur during the first 10 years and are due to bacterial infection or sequestration crises. Death in adult life is usually caused by dysfunction of affected organ systems. Occasionally patients with sickle cell anemia experience only few and minor complications. Patients with sickle trait can expect to live a normal life span uncomplicated by the defect.

Nursing Management

If sickle cell disease is diagnosed in the newborn period, it is important to teach parents the early signs of infection. Anytime the child's temperature is above 38.9°C (102.2°F) the physician should be notified immediately.

All too often, efforts are focused on episodic treatment of crises, and the more general aspects of continuing care are overlooked. The astute nurse should incorporate the principles of nursing in health maintenance and chronic illness when managing the sickle cell patient. When the child is experiencing a crisis, nursing assessment should be used to determine the source of pain, if possible and measures which may comfort an irritable infant or child. Measures to be considered include holding or rocking the infant, singing to him, or reading stories. Providing familiar objects or persons may be helpful. Bathing the child in warm water or applying local heat or massage may reduce the pain.

In many situations, measures which may comfort the patient must be selected by trial and error. When effective measures are identified, they should be recorded and shared with the entire nursing staff.

It is important to assess the environment to identify factors which may aggravate the sickling process and to provide optimal surroundings for the patient. He should be warm, well hydrated, free from stress, and protected from infection.

An evaluation of the patient's parents' understanding of the disease and the genetic implications is essential. The goal of genetic counseling is to inform the child's parents of the genetic implications of the disease. If they request information about birth control methods, it should be made available to them.

β-Thalassemia (Cooley's Anemia or Mediterranean Anemia)

β-thalassemia is a hereditary disorder of hemoglobin synthesis in which there is an impaired ability to form adult hemoglobin. Red cell production is affected, and consequently, the individual red cells contain markedly diminished amounts of hemoglobin. The erythrocytes produced are fragile, abnormally shaped, and easily destroyed. The erythropoietic system compensates for the defect by producing abnormally high amounts of fetal hemoglobin. Found primarily in persons of Mediterranean descent, it may affect individuals in most racial groups. The heterozygous state, *β-thalassemia minor,* is associated with mild anemia. Children carrying this trait are usually asymptomatic.

β-thalassemia major, or *Cooley's anemia,* the homozygous form of the disease, results in a severe progressive hemolytic anemia which is seen after the first 6 to 12 months of life when the normal physiologic anemia of the infant becomes progressively worse. The signs and symptoms of severe anemia discussed earlier accompany this disease. Children who receive chronic transfusions develop hypersplenism within 5 to 8 years. This event will have several additional effects, including a further decrease in the ability of the red cells to survive, thus necessitating more frequent transfusions. Hypersplenism also will result in an increased rate of iron accumulation. Marked splenomegaly causes a protrusion of the child's abdomen. In an attempt to compensate for the hemopoietic defect, the bone marrow becomes hyperplastic, the marrow space enlarges, and skeletal changes result. The most prominent example of this process is the characteristic "mongoloid" or "rodentlike" appearance of the child's facies (Fig. 25-6). Growth retardation resulting from chronic anemia becomes apparent in later childhood. There is delayed or absent sexual maturation in both sexes.

A combination of the cardiac decompensation associated with anemia and the myocardial fibrosis caused by hemosiderosis produces cardiac failure in the older child. *Hemosiderosis* is an accumulation of the iron-containing substance *hemosiderin* following the phagocytic digestion of erythrocytes. This deposit of iron is an inevitable complication of frequent transfusions. The characteristic muddy yellow complexion seen in these children results from a combination of jaundice, hemosiderosis, increased gastrointestinal absorption, and pallor.

The diagnosis of thalassemia major (β-thalassemia) is suspected in a severely anemic child of Mediterranean extraction between 6 months and 1 year with the character-

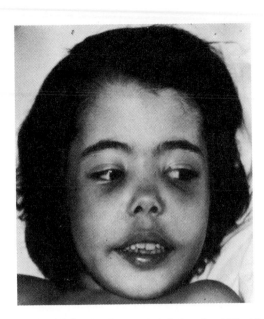

FIGURE 25-6 The characteristic facies of a child with thalassemia major. *(From A.M. Mauer, Pediatric Hematology, McGraw-Hill, New York, 1969, p. 137.)*

istic clinical findings and blood picture. The diagnosis is confirmed by the child's electrophoretic pattern, which reveals predominance of fetal hemoglobin and no or small varying amounts of normal adult hemoglobin. Hemoglobin A_2 may be decreased, normal, or increased and so is of little diagnostic value.

In the newborn, the hemoglobin electrophoresis may reveal either reduced hemoglobin A (β^+-thalassemia) or no hemoglobin A (β^0-thalassemia). In β-thalassemia, hemoglobin F is always increased. With β-thalassemia trait, A $_2$ hemoglobin is elevated.

The treatment objectives for thalassemia major are (1) to control the chronic anemia (repeated blood transfusions), (2) to treat the side effects of iron accumulation (repeated subcutaneous injections of deferoxamine), and (3) to reduce effects of chronic anemia (hypersplenomegaly; with abnormal sequestration of red blood cells and increased demand for transfusion, a splenectomy may be necessary).

Nursing Management

To control chronic anemia, the child is placed on a regimen of transfusions to maintain an adequate hemoglobin. This therapy may necessitate admission to the hospital or to the short-stay unit every 3 to 4 weeks. Nursing care of the child receiving a transfusion is discussed earlier in this chapter.

Treatment to increase iron excretion consists of repeated subcutaneous infusions of deferoxamine (Desferal) over an 8- to 12-hour period. Dosage varies from 20 to 50 mg/kg/day, based on the amount of iron excreted in the urine over a 24-hour period.

Desferal helps to reduce the consequences of iron deposition and to decrease the rate of iron accumulation in the body. It is infused through a small, portable infusion pump attached to the child's leg or worn on a belt. If the infusion is started during the day, the child can engage in many normal activities; however, if it is started at bedtime and infused throughout the night, the child's activities will not be disturbed during the day. (In Table 25-5, administration of Desferal is described, and in Fig. 25-7 is a picture of an infusion pump.)

The nurse's main responsibility is to plan a teaching program and demonstrate the technique of administration of Desferal so that the parents and child can continue with this treatment at home. The older child may be able to do this procedure himself with support from his parents.

Before beginning te teaching program, the nurse must assess the readiness of the child and parents to learn the procedure. It is helpful to provide them with a step-by-step outline of the procedure for later reference. The parents also need adequate supplies for home treatment. The technique used by the child and parents can be assessed periodically by the nurse during the child's visits to the health care facility for transfusions and immediate re-education can be provided, as needed.

The main consequences of long-term transfusion therapy for chronic anemia in children who have β-thalassemia is hypersplenomegaly. If the enlarged spleen begins to sequester red cells abnormally and the demands for transfusion are increased, a splenectomy may be indicated. Pre- and postoperative nursing care of the child having a splenectomy is discussed in the preschool/school-age section. Pneumococcal vaccine and prophylactic antibodies are given after splenectomy to decrease the risk of infection.

The incidence of overwhelming infeciton following splenectomy is very high. A major aim of nursing care is to prevent nosocomial infection. Fever and dehydration should be treated as soon as possible. The discharge plan must include teaching the child and the parents the importance of avoiding situations that could cause an infection.

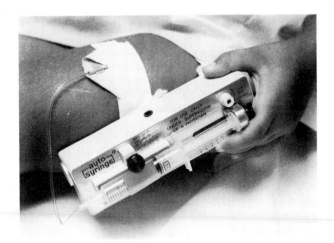

FIGURE 25-7 Portable continuous infusion pump for the administration of subcutaneous deferoxamine.

TABLE 25-5 Administering Deferoxamine (Desferal) Using a Subcutaneous Route

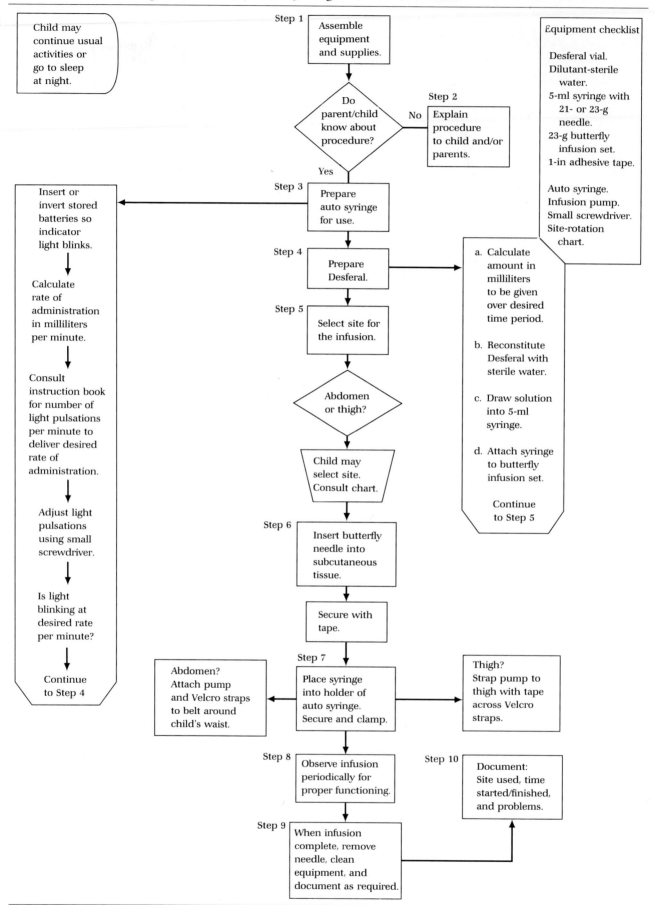

Source: G. M. Scipien et al. (eds.), *Comprehensive Pediatric Nursing*, 3rd ed., McGraw-Hill, New York, 1986, p. 1014.

The prognosis depends on the severity of the disease. Some patients do relatively well with few transfusions. Others require transfusions with increasing frequency. If the child lives to adolescence, his disease may become less severe. Most children succumb to complications of anemia, infection, or frequent transfusion before adolescence.

Hemophilia

Hemophilia is an inherited coagulation disorder. The most common forms of the disease, classic hemophilia (hemophilia A, or factor VIII deficiency) and Christmas disease (hemophilia B, or factor IX deficiency), account for 95 percent of the hemophilias, with classic hemophilia accounting for 85 percent of the total.

Classic hemophilia and *Christmas disease* are transmitted in a sex-linked recessive manner, generally from an asymptomatic carrier mother to an affected son. The disease is due to deficient activity of the coagulation factor involved. Children with less than 1 percent of the plasma factor are considered severe hemophiliacs. Children with 1 to 4.9 percent or 5 to 39.9 percent of the factor activity may have respectively, a moderate to mild form of hemophilia. These children may be free of spontaneous bleeding and require replacement therapy only with surgery or trauma. In Fig. 25-2 the role of antihemophilic factors in blood coagulation is depicted.

The disease, characterized by recurrent episodes of hemorrhage, may be spontaneous or caused by slight injury. Specific manifestations depend on the area involved. Certain types of bleeding are characteristic of particular age groups. In infancy, prolonged hemorrhage may occur following circumcision. As the child progresses to the toddler stage and experiences frequent falls, bleeding into soft tissues and from mucous membranes becomes more common. Injuries of the nose and mouth cause most of these bleeding episodes.

The school-age child with severe hemophilia must cope with the most debilitating complications of the disease, *hemarthrosis,* or bleeding into the joint. Early signs are stiffness, warmth, tenderness, pain, and limitation of motion. As bleeding progresses, the joint becomes swollen. Muscle spasms and changes in soft-tissue structure occur, resulting in the formation of flexion contractures. Recurrence causes further degenerative changes which may lead to permanent damage of the joint.

Hematuria and gastrointestinal bleeding are more common in the adolescent. School-age children and adolescents may experience frequent episodes of epistaxis. Fortunately, bleeding within the central nervous system is a rare complication.

A history of congenital bleeding disorder in a male child that appears in other maternal male relatives should lead the physician to a diagnosis of a coagulation disorder. However, hemophilia may appear without a history of affected family members. A number of coagulation studies, including screening tests and specific factor assays, can be done to determine which clotting factor is deficient. An essential part of the diagnosis is the establishment of the severity of the disorder, which is related to the level of the affected factor.

Protection from injury is an important aspect of treatment. With infants, the crib and playpen may be padded. Pacifiers may aggravate frenulum trauma. When the child begins to walk, the environment should be as free of hazards as possible. Removal of large, hard toys and sharp pieces of furniture such as end tables provides a much safer area to explore. Aspirin and other drugs that interfere with platelet function should never be used. Deep intramuscular injections should be avoided, and pressure should be applied for 5 minutes after an intravenous puncture or a subcutaneous injection for immunizations.

When bleeding episodes occur, local and systemic measures are employed to arrest the process. Local measures include ice bags and pressure to the affected area. When bleeding occurs in the mouth or nose, the area may be packed with hemostatic agents. The child is at complete rest with the affected part immobilized. Joints should be elevated and supported in a slightly flexed position.

Plasma replacement therapy should be started immediately. Infusion of appropriate sources of the deficient factor will raise the plasma factor level sufficiently to allow hemostatis. Cryoprecipitate is often the treatment of choice, is less expensive than commercial concentrates, and is easily prepared in the blood bank from fresh plasma. Commercial concentrates can be stored at 41 to 50°F for long periods and at room temperature for 2 to 4 weeks and are, therefore, more convenient for home transfusion and when traveling. Hemarthroses may require continuation of replacement therapy for 3 to 4 days.

When bleeding into a joint has been controlled, active range of motion to the level of pain should be instituted. Motion of the joint facilitates absorption of the blood and may prevent contracture of the tissues. Cautious ambulation may begin in 48 hours. Surgical management of the affected joint may be necessary. Aspiration of residual blood under sterile conditions and application of traction with splints and casts are two orthopedic approaches.

Epsilon-aminocaproic acid (EACA) (Amicar) may be administered in conjunction with factor replacement to control mouth bleeding. EACA is an inhibitor of the fibrinolytic enzyme system, which is particularly active in mucosal tissue. Suspected renal bleeding usually is a contraindication for administration of Amicar.

Approximately 10 percent of patients will develop an immunoglobin G (IgG) antibody to factor VIII. This inhibitor in the patient's plasma results in the inactivation of factor VIII in normal plasma. The development of an inhibitor calls for an alteration of the plan for treatment of bleeding problems. Alternative approaches to management are currently being investigated.

The cost and inconvenience of frequent infusions have promoted the development of home management programs. In these programs, patients and their families are taught to admininster their own infusions. The goals of

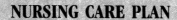

NURSING CARE PLAN

25-2 The Child with Hemophilia

Clinical Problem/Nursing Diagnosis	Expected Outcome	Nursing Interventions

Impaired function of coagulation process
Increased tendency to bleed into joints, tissue, muscles, skin, and mucous membranes
 	
Potential for injury related to deficiency in clotting factors; increased risk of hemorrhage
	Child will be protected from injury by being provided with safe environment, which decreases likelihood of bleeding episodes	*Prevention*
		Parents provide safe environment for child while maintaining opportunities for normal play activities which promote developmental growth; measures include
		   Thick layers of padding on bottoms of cribs and playpens
		   Purchasing toys that *do not* have sharp edges, points, or features which can injure child
		   Encourage play with soft toys, foam balls, clay or dough, coloring and painting sets, soft rubber building blocks
		Keep nails short to prevent bleeding from scratching skin or mucous membranes
		Promote good dental hygiene: use soft-bristled toothbrush and soft foam swabs; use soft "jelly" type teething rings; caution parents about child chewing hard, sharp foods such as potato chips and hard candy
		Pad clothing at knees and elbows for toddlers learning to walk; such measures cushion skin and protect joints from trauma
		Encourage use of flexible, well-fitting shoes for toddler beginning to walk
		Remove environmental hazards (pointed tables with sharp edges, glass items); pad table edges
		Supervise safe, diversional play activities (Discourage participation in contact sports (football); guide toward archery and swimming
		Encourage adolescents to use padded clip-on earrings and electric razors
		Stress wearing medical identification bracelet
		Avoid use of intramuscular medications; coordinate administration of immunizations following factor replacement infusions
		Apply pressure to puncture sites for at least 5 min
		Do not administer drugs which alter platelet function (aspirin and antihistamines)
		Evaluate need for prophylactic infusion programs to prevent bleeding and/or decrease severity of bleeding episodes by maintaining adequate levels of clotting factors
		Ensure administration of clotting factor infusions proplylactically prior to dental work or surgical procedure
		Control and treatment of bleeding episodes
		Teach parents and child how to detect and manage bleeding episodes
		Observe for evidence of active bleeding: locate all cuts and abrasions; inspect skin for bruises, soft tissue bleeding, pain, and swelling
		Apply pressure and ice immediately; immobilize affected extremity
		In presence of mucosal bleeding, pack nose or oral area with prescribed hemostatic, fibrinolytic-inhibitor agents; for epistaxis, apply pressure and insert gel foam saturated with bovine thrombin into nares to restore hemostasis; report hematuria or blood in stools promptly
		Observe for changes in child's level of consciousness and/or altered neurological function
		For severe injury, trauma, and deep cuts, *apply pressure and ice immediately;* immobilize affected extremity; replace clotting factors immediately; promote rest
		Assess child for active bleeding into joints (hemarthrosis): limp and/or decreased movement of affected extremity; pain, tenderness, restrictd joint movement, and altered sensation in affected extremity
		Apply ice directly to affected joint; apply pressure using elastic bandage; immobilize joint using splint for support
		Immediately institute factor replacement therapy, administering fresh-frozen plasma (FFP), cryoprecipitate, and/or factor VIII concentrate (lyophilized concentrates of factor VIII); need to be reconstituted and given immediately

Clinical Problem/Nursing Diagnosis	Expected Outcome	Nursing Interventions
		Advocate use of heat-treated concentrates to reduce risk of exposure to AIDS
		Allow children in home care management programs to help manage bleeding episode: starting IV, applying ice, or applying elastic bandage (participating in self-care promotes independence)
		Monitor laboratory values: clotting studies such as clotting times and factor VIII levels
Pain	In addition to being	Assess all joints and muscles for stiffness, swelling, deformities, pain, warmth, limited movement, or contractures
Agitation	free of joint and	
Bleeding into joints or muscles	flexion contractures, child will be	Monitor for altered sensory and/or motor function secondary to nerve compression from blood accumulation
Joint and/or muscle swelling and/or stiffness	relieved of pain as demonstrated by improved joint and	Obtain serial measurements of swollen joint to assess progress and/or deterioration
Muscle spasms	muscle mobility	Identify early signs of hemarthrosis (limpness, pain, tenderness, and limited movement; note progression); swollen, warm joints, with skin over joint tense and shiny; altered sensation in affected extremity
Therapeutic joint immobilization	and increased tolerance to range of	
Flexion contractures	motion exercises	Apply pressure immediately with splints and elastic bandage; apply ice to area (splints immobilize joint)
Impaired physical mobility related to bleeding into joints, muscles, and tissue		Encourage active range of motion exercises and ambulation when bleeding has been controlled
		Explain need for orthopedic care and follow-up
		Collaborate with physical and/or occupational therapist to develop individual exercise program for use at home or in hospital
		Consult physical therapist about splints, crutches, etc.
		Teach parents and child how to apply splints and elastic bandages on affected extremity
		Support child through all procedures such as aspiration of joint
		Provide parents and child with written instructions for daily exercise regimen and home care
Irritability	Child's pain will diminish with prompt	Create quiet, calm, controlled environment conducive to rest
Agitation	detection and management of bleeding episode	Immobilize affected extremity and/or body part during active bleeding episodes and apply ice
Restlessness		
Crying, moaning, and grimacing		Administer analgesics ordered and evaluate
		Do not apply heat to joints and/or muscles
Localized discomfort		Do not administer salicylates or medications which alter platelet function
Verbal description of pain		
Warm, swollen, stiff joints and/or muscles		Encourage independence in hospital setting after episode has ceased
		Develop diversional activities which distract child
Bruising over affected areas		Support child during joint aspirations to relieve pain and/or pressure from accumulation of blood
Pain related to acute bleeding into tissue, muscles, and joints		

Continued.

NURSING CARE PLAN 25-2 The Child with Hemophilia— cont'd

Clinical Problem/Nursing Diagnosis	Expected Outcome	Nursing Interventions
Request for information about hemophilia and treatments Lack of prior experience with illness and hospitalization Knowledge deficit related to disease, management, complications of therapy, home and follow-up care	Parents and child will verbalize and demonstrate understanding of hemophilia, strategies for preventing injury, methods of detecting and controlling bleeding, and details of home management and follow-up care	Teach parents and child about hemophilia and its management Review signs of bleeding, measures to take to control blood flow, and procedure for obtaining medical attention Evaluate extent of learning and understanding that took place See interventions for control of bleeding episodes Explain need to share information with all caregivers, including baby-sitter, so that everyone knows how to manage acute bleeding episode Instruct parents to compile list of phone numbers to be kept near phone for reference; should include physician, primary nurse, ambulance, and emergency room Advise parents to keep extra supplies of ice in plastic bags in freezer Review with parents methods of making home safe See nursing interventions for potential for injury and prevention Support and reassure parents as they are informed about disease and potential complications of therapy (antibodies to factor VIII, chronic arthritis secondary to hemarthrosis, chronic hepatitis and/or AIDS contracted from innumerable transfusions) Reassure parents about refined techniques for screening blood for hepatitis and AIDS; discuss heat treatment of blood, which reduces risk of AIDS Collaborate with family and physician in providing choices for factor replacement therapy (avoid pooled concentrate preparations) Evaluate child and family's strengths in relation to knowledge about care, preparing and administering factor replacements, self-infusions, and all efforts directed at promoting sense of control in child and family Facilitate communication with school system Arrange meeting with child and parents, teacher, school nurse, and physical education teacher to ensure their understanding of disease and measures to implement in bleeding episode and to encourage exercise activities Provide written instructions at discharge Encourage child's participation in summer camps for hemophiliacs and parental involvement in National Hemophilia Foundation at local level or attendance at support group for parents of children with hemophilia Explain to parents interdisciplinary team approach to which they will be exposed; provides experts who deliver the most comprehensive care possible, including nurse, hematologist, orthopedist, dentist, physical and/or occupational therapist, psychologist, and social worker Arrange and facilitate follow-up care in hematology and orthopedic clinics and other specialties as necessary
Feelings of guilt, resentment, and anger Living with stress of potential injury and/or hemorrhage Restrictions on family activities Altered family processes related to chronically ill child	Family will adapt to presence of member with chronic, potentially life-threatening illness and function optimally utilizing effective coping mechanisms	Discuss and arrange for genetic counseling for family members Familiarize family with health care facility and team members available to support child and family and meet new needs as they emerge Provide opportunities for child and parents to express feelings, fears, and concerns Support and help mother express feelings of guilt and responsibility for child's illness Assist child and family in developing plan of care which promotes child's independence and increases self-help responsibilities Help parents identify overprotective behaviors which may affect child's confidence and self-care activities Support family members through feelings of anger and resentment related to interruptions in family and/or individual normal activities as result of chronic illness Encourage family to maintain regular activities and interests Assist family in mobilizing support systems Identify and address family stressors Discuss with parents what child *can do*

Clinical Problem/Nursing Diagnosis	Expected Outcome	Nursing Interventions
		Identify family strengths and incorporate them into plan of care
		Involve all family members in planning creative, safe activities for child
		Refer family to community resources such as local chapter of National Hemophilia Foundation
		Facilitate meetings with peers so that child can share experiences of living with hemophilia
		Encourage participation in support groups for parents of children with hemophilia and siblings of children with hemophilia

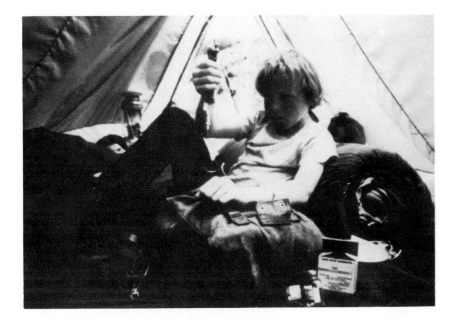

FIGURE 25-8   A child administering his cryoprecipitate. *(Courtesy of Cutter Laboratories, Inc.)*

the program are prompt and effective control of bleeding episodes and greater independence for the patient from the hospital and the health care team.

Patients soon learn to recognize the earliest symptoms of bleeding. Home care programs allow them to institue therapy minutes after they are aware of bleeding. Early institution of therapy permits earlier control of bleeding, fewer complications, and less interruption of normal activity. In some cases where the disease is severe and frequent transfusion are required to control bleeding, the patients are placed on prophylactic infusion programs. They are instructed to administer therapy routinely two or three times a week. The goal is maintenance of adequate levels of the clotting factor and prevention of bleeding. The prophylactic approach may be used to eliminate the risk of bleeding when the patient is participating in aggressive rehabilitative physical therapy programs and must be able to engage in active exercise. In some situations, children as young as 5 and 6 years of age are administering their own replacement therapy (Fig. 25-8).

The team approach to the treatment of hemophilia is essential. Ideally, the team should consist of the child and his family, a pediatrician, a hematologist, an orthopedist, a dentist, a physical therapist, a psychologist, a social worker, and a nurse. Coordination of the efforts of all members of the team should provide smooth, comprehensive management of this complex disease and afford the patient the opportunity to function as a healthy, independent individual.

Nursing Management

The child's functional ability may vary considerably from time to time. During bleeding episodes, he may be in extreme pain and any movement may cause more pain and possibly more bleeding. When the bleeding has been controlled, his range of motion can be established by trial and error. Anemia caused by blood loss may decrease his activity tolerance. Through nursing assessment the nurse

NURSING CARE PLAN

25-3 *The Child with Acute Leukemia*

Clinical Problem/Nursing Diagnosis	Expected Outcome	Nursing Interventions
Increased susceptibility to infection Altered immune function: neutropenia and/or lymphopenia Effects of chemotherapy on immune function Risk of superinfection from antibiotic therapy	Child will remain free of infection In presence of infection, child will be isolated and treated promptly to ensure its resolution	Practice strict hand washing techniques; prevent exposure to other ill or potentially infectious children Monitor child's absolute neutrophil count (ANC); normal range 3500-7500 mm^3 Provide child with private room when ANC <500 mm^3 Coordinate majority of care in outpatient setting (oncology clinic) to avoid exposure to nosocomial infections Monitor vital signs; observe for signs of infection: temperature >38.5°C (axillary); monitor apical for tachycardia and bradycardia; blood pressure for hypo/hypertension and widened pulse pressure; auscultate breath sounds for quality and equality of aeration; notify physician promptly of evident alterations in signs Detect early signs of respiratory infection or distress (tachypnea, labored respirations, elevated distress with feeding and/or activity)
Potential for infection related to treatment-induced immunosuppression; impact of leukemia on immune function Ecchymoses Petechiae Complications associated with multiple blood transfusions		Obtain cultures of blood, urine, open wounds, and secretions Monitor viral, bacterial, and fungal cultures to identify presence of opportunistic infections Maintain patent airway; promote adequate oxygenation (O$_2$ saturation >95 mmHg); provide oxygen; perform chest physical therapy Properly administer systemic antibiotics and antifungal agents Monitor IV for patency and signs of infiltration (redness, swelling, tenderness); assess integrity of vein; with infiltration, D/C infusion, elevate extremity and notify physician; assess need for injection of antiinflammatory drug around infiltration site and observe site for tissue breakdown and infection Take only axillary temperatures to prevent injury to rectal mucosa Examine anal area for tears in mucosa and early signs of rectal abscess formation Prevent constipation by administering stool softeners and providing fluids Assess oral activity for signs of infection, irritation, erythema, and bleeding; ensure meticulous oral hygiene (soft-bristled brush in the absence of lesions; rinse mouth with normal saline and H$_2$O$_2$ at comfortable temperature 4 times a day; avoid irritating mouthwash preparations) Maintain skin integrity; examine skin for signs of breakdown, open sores, and infected areas; cleanse open skin areas with H$_2$O$_2$; apply antimicrobial ointment and protective barrier Cleanse skin with povidine-iodine before skin punctures Provide meticulous care to central venous catheter sites Closely monitor child during granulocyte transfusions and note presence of elevated temperature, chills, hives, laryngeal edema, respiratory distress, and hypotension (immediately D/C infusion and notify physician; keep O$_2$ and antihistamines at bedside) Administer all medications and chemotherapeutic agents properly (know side effects, contraindications, and potential complications) Teach parents how to prevent, recognize, and promptly report signs of infection or changes in child's clinical status to oncologist; see interventions under Knowledge Deficit Ensure appropraite immunization prophylaxis (preparations containing killed virus) modified for immunocompromised children Communicate to child, family, schoolteacher, and nurse critical importance of preventing exposure to communicable diseases, especially varicella, and to immediately report exposure to oncologist to ensure prompt intervention

Clinical Problem/Nursing Diagnosis	Expected Outcome	Nursing Interventions
Anemia, pallor, increased fatigue, and dizziness Coagulopathies Thrombocytopenia: increased potential for hemorrhage and blood loss Potential for injury (alteration in bone marrow function) related to effects of chemotherapy	Any bleeding which occurs in child will be controlled promptly Child will be protected from injury	Monitor vital signs for evidence of blood loss (tachycardia and hyper/hypotension) Limit excessive blood drawing; monitor CBC, homoglobin (HgB), hematocrit (Hct), and platelet values Maintain Hct and platelet count in optimal range Administer blood products as ordered and monitor child for untoward reactions: anaphylactic shock (tachycardia, change in blood pressure, respiratory distress), fever, chills, rash, hives Monitor for signs of fluid overload Assess vital signs and note changes from baseline data Notify physician of reaction to transfusion and D/C IV; administer antihistamines as ordered; maintain patent airway (Advocate for heat treatment of blood products to reduce risk of AIDS infection) Do not administer aspirin or other salicylate medications Limit invasive procedures and avoid administering medications intramuscularly Prevent excessive drying of nasal mucous membranes and discourage use of force in blowing nose Assess child for evidence of bleeding: check for hematuria/hemaglobinuria; hematest stools/emesis; examine body for increased bruising and/or petechiae; monitor for behavioral changes and level of consciousness; notify physician promptly of any of the above Adhere to isolation precautions as needed (protective isolation; blood and body fluid precautions)
Dysuria Frequency Urgency Hematuria Altered patterns of urinary elimination related to effects of chemotherapy (rapid cell destruction and hyperuricemia)	Child's urinary output will remain adequate (>1 ml/kg/h), and renal function will be optimized While maintaining fluid and electrolyte balance, child will be free of uric acid neopathy	Monitor intake and output q 1-2 h Report output <1 ml/kg/h promptly Perform specific gravity q 4-8 h and maintain between 1.005 and 1.020 Dipstick urine and note presence of hematuria, glucosuria, proteinuria, and ketonuria; maintain pH ≥7.0 Promote alkalinization of urine: administer alkalinizing agents [acetazolamide (Diamox), NAHCO₃] Administer allopurinol as ordered Monitor all renal function studies (BUN, creatinine, electrolytes) Promptly correct electrolyte and/or acid-base imbalances Optimize hydration with oral and/or parenteral fluids
Dysphagia Sensation of choking Fear and anxiety Gagging and coughing Potential ineffective airway clearance related to airway obstruction	Child's airway will remain patent, providing adequate oxygenation to all body cells	Monitor vital signs; assess presence and degree of respiratory distress Observe for difficulty in swallowing or gagging and choking on small pieces of food Monitor for signs of respiratory distress (labored respirations, tachypnea, retractions, inspiratory stridor, grunting, nasal flaring, persistent cough, and changes in color) and notify physician Provide humidified O₂ Create calm, quiet, restful environment Assist child in maintaining comfortable position to support patent airway; maximize lung expansion; elevate head of bed; sit up and over bedside table on a pillow
Nausea and vomiting Lethargy Headache Increasing irritability	Child will be treated promptly to prevent development of neurological deficits	Obtain detailed preillness assessment of child's developmental and cognitive level of functioning and baseline neurological assessment Monitor child for signs of increased intracranial pressure, seizure activity, and meningeal irritation or infection Inform parents of need to contact physician for any changes in affect, behavior, level of activity, increased irritability, or persistent headache

Continued.

NURSING CARE PLAN 25-3 The Child with Acute Leukemia—cont'd

Clinical Problem/Nursing Diagnosis	Expected Outcome	Nursing Interventions
Potential cognitive-impairment related to neurophysiological pathology (leukemic invasion of CNS; infection)		
Chronic pain Irritabiity	Child will experience pain relief as evidenced by increased interaction with environment and increased interest in other activities	Assess child's pain and note type, location, duration, and severity
		Identify patterns of pain and events that increase pain
Pain related to leukemic involvement of bone and soft tissue		Identify interventions that are effective or not effective in controlling pain
		Provide consistent caretakers as much as possible to establish trusting relationships
		Support family participation in comforting role to increase sense of control
		Maintain calm, quiet, pleasant environment
		Assist child in seeking comfortable positions; move child slowly and gently
		Utilize imagery, deep breathing execises, tension-releasing activities, therapeutic massage, whirlpool therapy, and music to control or alleviate discomfort
		Evaluate effectiveness of interventions used for pain control
		Administer analgesics as prescribed
Insufficient sleep and/or rest Fatigue Weakness Malaise	Given nursing care provided, child will experience uninterrupted, restful sleep, free of pain	Promote frequent rest periods and provide long periods of sleep by organizing and coordinating medical examinations and blood work and limiting activities which interrupt sleep
		Provide comfort measures which reduce pain and stress and enhance relaxation (see interventions under Pain)
	Child will experience minimized noxious effects of treatment	Premedicate child before treatment to decrease noxious side effects
Activity intolerance related to disease process and/or treatment regimen		Prepare child, family, teacher, and school nurse for possible side effects of chemotherapeutic agents (overall weakness and decreased activity levels)
		Support child in selecting activities which are less demanding and tiring
		Encourage child's participation in activities he can enjoy without feeling different or fatigued; suggest bike riding or playing ball combined with periods of quiet activities such as reading, painting, and art: alternating endeavors decreases fatigue
Anorexia Nausea and/or vomiting Mucositis Altered taste sensations	Child will tolerate diet rich in protein and caloric value, remain in positive nitrogen balance, and maintain weight appropriate for age and height	Obtained detailed nutritional assessment which includes preillness weight, muscle mass, dietary habits, favorite foods, and eating patterns
		Monitor trends in weight loss and/or gain using the same scale in every clinic visit or admission
Altered nutrition: less than body requirements related to decreased food intake; increased metabolic demands and effects of disease as well as treatment protocol		
Irritation of mucous membranes Dysphagia Weight loss		Nausea
		Promote pleasant environment; remove noxious smells, sights, and sounds
		Maintain positive attitude about eating

Clinical Problem/Nursing Diagnosis	Expected Outcome	Nursing Interventions
		Encourage parents to offer praise for eating
		Teach parents to avoid foods when child is nauseated and nagging about poor intake
		Discuss with parents need to offer food attractively, in small portions, perhaps more fequently
		Encourage meals high in protein and calories, to be eaten slowly
		Assist with meticulous oral hygiene measures and determine need for topical analgesics to relieve pain present with oral fungal infections (see interventions under Potential for Infection)
		Administer antiemetics, sedatives, and tranquilizers as ordered prior to chemotherapy
		Document child's response to each medication, especially its effectiveness in alleviating nausea
		Collaborate with health care team to develop plan to optimize control of nausea and comfort during treatments
		Avoid providing liquids with meals to decrease sensation of fullness
		Encourage oral liquids frequently throughout day rather than during meals
		Offer chilled oral fluids
		Identify patterns of nausea (precipating factor, specific smell or sight)
		Encourage low-fat foods and cold foods during nauseated periods (avoid fat, greasy, hot, spicy, fried foods and foods with strong odors)
		Vomiting
		Promote comfortable, safe position for child
		Delete noxious sights, sounds, and smells
		Change clothing and linens promptly after child vomits
		Assist with oral hygiene; help child rinse mouth with cool water to remove bad taste
		Offer hard candy to older children to suck on to remove unpleasant taste of emesis
		Clean sore gums and teeth with soft swabs saturated with water and H_2O_2; encourage frequent rinsing of mouth to remove food and bacteria and promote healing
		Promote regular dental care, use of soft-bristled toothbrush, and rinsing of mouth
		Advance diet slowly to regular intake
		Offer soft, tender, pureed foods; cut food into small pieces
		Offer foods that are cold or at room temperature
		Add bland gravies and sauces or butter to ease swallowing and increase caloric value
		Avoid acidic, spicy, salty, rough, coarse, and dry foods
		Encourage intake of ice cream, milk shakes, and bananas (parents can be told to freeze quantities of milk shakes in small containers so they are avaialble when child desires one)
		Encourage parents (during hospitalization) to bring home-cooked favorites for child
		Prepare parents for increased appetite of child who is on prednisone (optimize nutritious caloric intake but limit salt)
		Maximize child's food intake in absence of nausea or vomiting
		Include parents in meal planning
		Consult with and involve nutritionist in helping family plan meals; offer suggestions for maximizing nutritious, tasty, high-calorie intake
		Provide parents with resources, e.g., *Diet and Nutrition: A Resource for Parents of Children with Cancer,* from American Cancer Society

Continued.

NURSING CARE PLAN 25-3   The Child with Acute Leukemia—cont'd

Clinical Problem/Nursing Diagnosis	Expected Outcome	Nursing Interventions
Frequent loose stools Diarrhea related to effects of treatment on GI tract; infection; malabsorption	Child's bowel patterns will remain normal, with adequate absorption of nutrients to maintain fluid and electrolyte balance	Obtain history of child's elimination patterns Encourage bed rest to reduce intestinal contractions Supply small, frequent feedings Provide clear liquid diet for short-term diarrhea; slowly advance diet to full liquids, then soft foods which are low in roughage and bulk Offer liquids at room temperature during day; do not supply with meals Assess for presence of lactose intolerance; evaluate effect of eliminating milk products on bowel patterns Provide foods high in fiber and avoid fatty, greasy, and fried foods
Constipation Constipation related to effects of treatment	Through high-fiber, high-bulk foods, child will have more normal bowel habits	Obtain history of child's bowel habits Maximize high fluid intake Offer hot beverages in morning and evening to stimulate bowel movements Provide diet high in fiber and bulk Administer stool softeners or laxatives as ordered Observe and record responses to treatment
Alopecia Cushingoid features Fluctuations in weight Broviac catheter placement Body image disturbance related to effects of treatment	Child and family will be prepared for effects of treatment Child and family will be assisted in coping with changes in body image Child will feel dignified and respected, and sense of self-esteem will be maintained	Explore feelings of child and family regarding changes in child's appearance which result from treatment Encourage child to verbalize concerns and express them through storytelling, drawings, and other therapeutic play activities Provide explanations based on child's developmental level Prepare child and family for anticipated body image changes such as hair loss, weight fluctuations, swollen face, and catheter placement Encourage older children to think of creative ways to deal with loss of hair (scarfs, hats, caps, wigs) Teach older children to care for central lines; this increases their sense of control (suggest loose, baggy, nonrestrictive tops for those with Broviac catheters) Instruct child and parents about care and dressing for central line Prepare child for hair loss (on pillow, when brushing or washing hair) Suggest short haircut to ease adaptation to loss of hair Prepare child and family for reactions of neighbors, friends, and peers to loss of hair Help child and family express their anger and emotions and teach them how to cope with painful encounters Utilize diverse methods in teaching child about disease and treatments (puppet show, coloring book, storytelling, art) Support child through reactions of peers to loss of hair and encourage verbalizations of feelings Arrange meetings with other children who have cancer so they can share similar experiences
Invasive procedures Pain Effects of chemotherapy Fear related to serious illness; treatment; alteration in daily activities Developmental and cognitive abilities may restrict ability to process and understand experiences	Child will express fears and demonstrate effective response to psychological support Child will verbalize and demonstrate increase in psychological and physiological comfort	Identify age-related fears and anticipate relationship of fears to potential experiences Identify actual or potential stressors for child (loss of control, fear of illness or death) Help parents promote open communications; provide honest answers to child's questions Provide opportunities for child to express feelings through art therapy, storytelling, and role-playing Identify effective and ineffective coping measures Include parents in planning coping strategies Suggest the child read *You and Leukemia* and *What Happened to You, Happened to Me*, available from American Cancer Society (they may facilitate meaningful expressions of child's feelings) Encourage child's socialization with peers who have cancer

Clinical Problem/Nursing Diagnosis	Expected Outcome	Nursing Interventions
Shock, denial, guilt, and anger Difficulty accepting diagnosis Fear of illness and death Stressors of chronic illness Changes in daily family experiences Physical and/or emotional fatigue Communication breakdowns Feelings of resentment over extra attention directed to ill child Siblings struggling with feelings of guilt and jealousy Altered family processes related to seriously ill child in family	Family will function optimally, utilizing effective coping strategies	Assess psychological impact of illness on all family members Approach family with compassion, respect, and support for their individual feelings and responses Provide opportunities for child and family to express fears and concerns; clarify questions Identify, enhance, and utilize family's strengths Encourage parents to participate in providing care (acknowledging their level of comfort in doing so) Support all family members in their individual roles Facilitate family's sense of control in coping with illness Encourage parents to normalize family's activities (meals together, play time, discipline, school activities) Involve peers in play, relaxation, and support Maintain open communication system for child and family, encouraging exchange of information about diagnosis, prognosis, and treatment plans (any changes in treatments must be shared with siblings) Discuss support systems available to child and family (oncologist, primary nurse, social worker, and nutritionist) Inform parents about other community support systems such as those for parents of children with cancer, peer support groups, and various camps for children and adolescents with cancer as well as support groups for siblings of a brother or sister with cancer Suggest the following books from American Cancer Society: for parents—*Emotional Aspects of Childhood Cancer and Leukemia: A Handbook for Parents* and *Childhood Leukemia: The Family Disease;* for siblings—*When Your Brother or Sister Has Cancer*
Lack of information about leukemia, its treatment, and its effects Home care Follow-up care Lack of information about sources of information, support, and assistance Knowledge deficit related to disease, treatment, and effects; follow-up care; sources of information, support, and assistance	Parents and child will verbalize understanding of information provided to promote confidence and enhance delivery of comprehensive care to child	Arrange and coordinate meeting with health care providers (physician, primary nurse) to share information with family about acute leukemia, routine diagnostic tests, and invasive procedures as well as proposed treatment plans Provide family with written instructions for treatments, tests, and schedule of clinic visits Supply parents with resource books from American Cancer Society Teach parents about medications to be taken at home (times, proper dose, route, side effects, and administration techniques) Evaluate family's knowledge about all medications prescribed for administration at home Prepare child and family for side effects of chemotherapy and radiation Review child's nutritional requirements with parents; seek assistance of nutritionist (see interventions under Altered Nutrition) Teach parents to recognize signs of infection and prevent exposure to infection (temperature >38.5°C, low WBC, increased bruising, labored respirations, difficulty feeding, diarrhea, vomiting, headache and pain anywhere in body, alterations in mucous membranes, blurred vision, pain on urination or bowel movement, and evidence of bleeding (nosebleed, blood in stools, hematuria, blood in emesis); notify physician immediately Emphasize to parents, teacher, and child importance of reporting and/or preventing exposure to communicable diseases, especially varicella; advise physician to ensure prompt medical intervention Familiarize child and family with oncology clinic and outpatient services Provide family with specific phone numbers of health care team members to ensure contact in presence of a problem in child Review community support systems and resources: American Cancer Society, Leukemia Society of America, Candlelighters, Ronald McDonald houses

can define the amount and kind of activity and exercise the child can tolerate and what assistance those caring for him should supply.

The young child who may not be familiar with the hospital may be frightened by the strange new environment. He may be in pain or frightened by a bleeding episode. His parents' fear and anxiety are easily communicated to him. Supporting the child's parents and making it possible for them to remain with the child are essential nursing functions at this time. The first objective may be to prepare for and administer the infusion as soon as possible, but the nurse should never be too rushed to explain what is happening. If restraints are necessary, they should be explained, and the child should be made as comfortable as possible.

Optimal positioning is essential. During a bleeding episode, the child is at rest and comfortable with the site of bleeding immobilized. The child can tell the nurse how he will be most comfortable and direct those moving him accordingly. When the bleeding is controlled and mobilization has begun, the child may need considerable encouragement and positive reinforcement for his efforts. He may hesitate to move for fear of increasing his pain. The nurse should *never* forcefully move a joint.

An assessment of the child's environment is made to identify hazardous objects. Removing toys from the path of an unsteady toddler may prevent unnecessary falls. Mothers are advised to sew padded patches into the knees and elbows of clothing to protect joints during falls. Helmets provide head protection. Tight clothing should be avoided.

Success in a home transfusion program is dependent on the family's attitude. The nurse is often in the best position to assess the family's readiness to approach this endeavor. By allowing parents to assume increasing responsibility in caring for the child and observing their reaction to this responsibility, the nurse can evaluate the parent-child interaction and adjustment to the situation. The nurse may delegate to the parent some of the preliminary procedures of the transfusion, such as preparing the area with alcohol and applying a tourniquet.

When the family is ready to learn the techniques for transfusion, detailed instruction and support is needed. The nurse should anticipate repeating instruction several times and should convey acceptance of the parents' fears and hesitancies. The family must be alerted to notify some member of the medical team if any questions or unexpected complications arise. It is advisable to provide them with a pamphlet explaining in detail the transfusion procedure, indications for transfusion, and the complications.

The process of adjusting to hemophilia as a chronic illness is a complex one for the child and his family. Genetic aspects of the disease have obvious implications. Many mothers feel responsible and guilty. Maternal overprotection may be a component in the development of the two behavior patterns commonly seen in hemophilic children: passive-dependent and risk-taking behaviors. A fine balance between meeting the child's needs for protection from injury and allowing independence must be established. Fathers and siblings resent the child's limitations. The constant threat of hemorrhage interferes with many family activities and stands between the child and his peers who are able to lead active lives. Fortunately, home transfusion programs have afforded the hemophiliac and his family a degree of independence from the hospital that was never possible before.

Hematologic Problems in Preschool and School-Age Children

Leukemia

Leukemia is a malignancy of unknown cause affecting the blood-forming organs. The disease, characterized by a replacement of normal marrow elements with abnormal accumulation of leukocytes and their precursors, is subclassified according to the type of white blood cell which is predominant in the bone marrow and peripheral blood. Approximately 80 percent of the cases of childhood leukemia are classified as *acute lymphocytic,* or *lymphoblastic, leukemia* (ALL). The majority of the remaining cases are *acute myelocytic,* or *myeloblastic, leukemia* (AML). Myeloblastic leukemia is less responsive to therapy, and the patients have a graver prognosis. Results of recent investigations suggest that other factors, such as immunologic cell-surface characteristics and clinical features as well as leukemia cell cytogenetics, should be considered in classifying acute leukemia. Leukemias which possess surface markers suggesting a T-cell or B-cell origin appear to have a poorer prognosis than those in which the cell of origin cannot be identified (null cell).

Common signs and sypmtoms of leukemia include fever, abdominal and bone pain, anorexia, lethargy, pallor, hepatosplenomegaly, lymphadenopathy, malaise, petechiae, and ecchymoses. These findings may be present at the time of diagnosis and may recur periodically as the disease progresses. The clinical features may be related to the disease process itself or to the therapy used. Those related to the disease fall into four main categories: anemia, infection, hemorrhage, and leukemic invasion.

Anemia results from eyrthropoietic failure and from blood loss. The complications of anemia are similar to those discussed earlier.

Infection results from immunosuppression caused by the disease and the effects of treatment. Replacement of normal marrow elements with leukemic cells reduces the production of normal white blood cells. A serious consequence is *neutropenia,* which interferes with the patient's ability to cope with bacterial infections. *Lymphopenia* is also common and interferes with both humoral and cellular immunity, placing the child at high risk for viral and fungal infections and those caused by other opportunistic pathogens. Impaired chemotaxis or decreased migration of cells to the site of infection has been observed in patients with Hodgkin's disease and AML. Also, the bactericidal activity of leukocytes is diminished in children with acute leukemia.

Many of the chemotherapeutic agents listed in Table 25-6 cause myelosuppression. Antibiotic therapy, used to treat infections, destroys normal flora as well as pathogenic organisms. Thus other pathogenic organisms which were previously controlled by the normal flora are able to grow, and superinfection may develop.

Hemorrhage is the result of an insufficient number of platelets. Preexisting thrombocytopenia may be worsened

TABLE 25-6 Commonly Used Leukemic Drugs

Drug	Uses	Storage/ Stability	Supply/ Reconstitution	Administration*/ Dosage	Side Effects/ Toxicity
Vincristine (Oncovin)	Induction, reinforcement	Refrigerate before and after reconstitution, use within 14 days after mixing	1- and 5-mg vials, reconstitute with 10 ml supplied diluent; 195 mg ready-mix vials	IV, avoid extravasation 1.5 to 2mg/m^2 (max. 2 mg) IV weekly × 2 to 6 weeks	Alopecia, peripheral neuropathy, constipation, SIADH, hyponatremia, mild myelosuppression, jaw pain, bone pain, sore throat
Prednisone	Induction, reinforcement	Store at room temperature	2.5-, 5-, 20-, and 50-mg tablets	PO, is bitter to taste 40 to 60 mg/m^2 for 14- to 28-day course	Cushing's syndrome, fluid retention, muscle wasting, hypertension, hyperphagia, immunosuppression, diabetes, gastrointestinal tract ulceration, striation, psychosis, irritability sleep problems, erratic behavior
L-Asparaginase (Elspar) (Erwinia†)	Induction, intensification	Refrigerate, use immediately, discard unused portion	10,000-U vials, reconstitute with 2 to 5 ml unpreserved sterile water or sodium chloride	IV or IM; observe for hypersensitivity reaction, have epinephrine and resuscitation equipment available Various dosage schedules	Hypersensitivity reaction, pancreatitis, nausa/vomiting, anorexia, weight loss, lethargy, somnolence, fever, hepatotoxicity, coagulopathy, hyperglycemia, convulsions
Adriamycin	Induction	Store at controlled room temperature, discard unused portion	10- and 15-mg vials, reconstitute with 5 or 25 ml normal saline	IV, avoid extravasation† 90 mg/m^2 in divided doses (usually 3); total cumulative lifetime dose 400 to 500 mg/m^2	Nausea/vomiting, alopecia, mucositis, myelosuppression, cardiotoxicity, (continuous infusion less cardiotoxic) red urine, hives at injection site
Daunomycin Cérubidine	Induction	Store at controlled room temperature, discard unused portion	20-mg vials, reconstitute with 4 ml sterile water	IV, avoid extravasation† Various dosage schedules. Total cumulative lifetime dose 400 to 550 mg/m^2	Cardiotoxicity, myelosuppression, nausea/vomiting, abdominal pain, alopecia, fever, skin rash, red urine

*IV, intravenous; IM, intramuscular; IT, intrathecal; PO, by mouth; SC, subcutaneous
†Investigational agent.

Source: Adapted from G. M. Scipien et al. (eds.), *Comprehensive Pediatric Nursing,* 3rd ed., McGraw-Hill, New York, 1986, pp. 1020-1021.

TABLE 25-6 Commonly Used Leukemic Drugs—cont'd

Drug	Uses	Storage/ Stability	Supply/ Reconstitution	Administration*/ Dosage	Side Effects/ Toxicity
Hydrocortisone (Solu-Cortef)	Central nervous system (CNS) treatment, prophylaxis, induction, maintenance	Store at controlled room temperature	100-mg plain (reconstitute with 2 ml sterile water) and 100-, 250-, 500-, and 1000-mg Mix-O-Vials (as directed)	IT, do not enter vial twice. Should be diluted with preservative-free vehicle --- 15 to 30 mg/m²	Same as Prednisone
B-Cytosine arabinoside (Cytosar) (ARA-C)	CNS prophylaxis, induction, maintenance; systemic induction, maintenance	Store at controlled room temperature; after reconstitution, store at room temperature, for 48 h, discard if haze appears	100- and 500-mg vials, reconstitute with 5 to 10 ml supplied diluent	IV, IM, SC, or IT; may require premedication with antiemetics. Do not enter vial twice for IT use --- IV, IM, SC; various dosage schedules; IT once or twice weekly	Nausea/vomiting myelosuppression, mucositis, hepatotoxicity, immunosuppression, fever, rash, conjunctivitis
Methotrexate	CNS prophylaxis, induction, and maintenance systemic maintenance; intensification	Store at room temperature	2.5-mg tablets, 5-mg and 50-mg/ 2-ml vials in solution, 20-, 50-, and 100-mg vials of cryodesiccated powder	PO, IV, IM, IT; IT preparations should be diluted with preservative-free vehicle. Do not enter vial twice for IT use --- 10 to 15 mg/m² IT once or twice weekly × 6 weeks (maximum dose 15 mg); 5 to 20 mg/ m² once or twice weekly, IV, IM, or PO	Nausea/vomiting, mucositis, myelosuppression, hepatotoxicity, pneumonitis, osteoporosis, hyperpigmentation, dermatitis, diarrhea, renal toxicity (calcium leucovorin antidote)
6-Mercaptopurine (Purinethol)	Maintenance	Store at room temperature	50-mg tablets	PO --- 50 mg/m² daily	Nausea/vomiting, myelosuppression, anorexia, dermatitis, stomatitis, hepatotoxicity, abdominal pain.
Cyclophosphamide (Cytoxan)	Intensification, maintenance	Store at room temperature, refrigerate after reconstitution	25- and 50-mg tablets, 100-, 200-, and 500-mg vials, reconstitute with 5 to 25 ml sterile water	PO, IV; maintain liberal hydration 48 h after weekly dose and continuously when given daily --- 2.5 to 5 mg/kg daily PO; various IV-dosage schedules	Nausea/vomiting, myelosuppression, alopecia, hemorrhagic cystitis, mucositis, infertility, immunosuppression, hyperpigmentation
(OFFER HARD CANDY DURING ADMINISTRATION TO COMBAT METALLIC TASTE)					
6-Thioguanine (Thioguanine)	Induction, maintenance	Store at room temperature	40-mg tablets	PO --- 80 to 100 mg/m²/day	Nausea/vomiting, stomatitis, myelosuppression, liver function abnormalities, dermatitis

TABLE 25-6 Commonly Used Leukemic Drugs—cont'd

Drug	Uses	Storage/ Stability	Supply/ Reconstitution	Administration*/ Dosage	Side Effects/ Toxicity
Etoposide (VP-16)	Reinforcement, relapse	Room temperature; stable for 48 h in glass and plastic containers	100 mg/5 ml vial (ready to use)	IV over 30 min $\overline{\quad}$ 50-100 mg/m^2 per day; schedule varies	Hypotension with rapid infusion, myelosuppression, alopecia, nausea, bronchospasm
Tenoposide (VM-26)	Reinforcement, relapse	Room temperature	50 mg/5 ml ampule	Slow IV drip over 45 min; benadryl given before administration $\overline{\quad}$ 60-80 mg/m^2 q 21 days	Myelosuppression, hypotension, anaphylaxis, alopecia, nausea, dizziness, erythema

by infection. Occasionally, a child with a low platelet count may not manifest signs of bleeding until he develops an infection. In most cases, thrombocytopenia alone may account for the bleeding.

Leukemia invasion of any organ in the body can result in alteration or failure of that organ system. Disease occurring in an organ other than the bone marrow is termed *extramedullary.* The central nervous system is a common site of leukemic infiltration. Children affected with central nervous system leukemia show signs and symptoms of increased intracranial pressure and of meningeal irritation. The most common signs and symptoms are nausea, vomiting, lethargy, headache, and irritability. Convulsions, cranial nerve palsies, papilledema, pain on neck flexion, hyperphagia, and blindness may occur. Infiltration of the liver, spleen, lymph nodes, lungs, kidneys, testicles, ovaries, and bones may also occur.

When therapy is instituted and large numbers of cells are rapidly destroyed, large amounts of uric acid are produced. If there is crystallization of the uric acid in the kidney, obstruction of the renal tubules and impaired renal function may result. *Hyperuricemia* usually can be effectively controlled with increased fluid intake, alkalinization of the urine with intravenous sodium bicarbonate, and admininstration of allopurinol.

The untreated disease progress rapidly, with death occurring within weeks to months after diagnosis. However, utilization of chemotherapeutic agents enables greater than 90 percent of children with newly diagnosed ALL to achieve an initial *remission.* When a child is in remission, he is free of signs and symptoms attributable to leukemia, and his bone marrow shows evidence of adequate function (reasonable numbers of red blood cells, white blood cells, and platelets) and less than 5 percent abnormal blast cells. As many as 40 to 50 percent of children are being maintained in their initial remission states in excess of 5 years. Current recommendations have been to discontinue therapy after 3 years if the child has remained in continuous complete remission. Most children who reach

this point will never experience a relapse. Males have a slightly increased rate of relapse due to testicular recurrence.

In spite of this optimistic outlook for many children, a significant number are not able to experience long-term control of their disease. A number of prognostic factors evaluated at the time of diagnosis seem to be predictive of the likelihood of disease eradication: the classification of the disease based on cell-surface markers, cell cytogenetics, the age of the patient at the time of diagnosis, the initial white blood cell count, the degree of organomegaly, and the presence of detectable extramedullary disease. Generally, a child with null-cell leukemia between the ages of 2 and 10 years with a white count of less than 10,000 cells per mm^3 and no significant extramedullary disease has a much better prognosis. If the child's leukemic cells become resistant to the drugs being used or the leukemic-cell population is not totally eradicated, the abnormal cells return and a *relapse* occurs. In boys, testicular relapses are occurring more frequently as more reach the point of long-term survival. Appearance of abnormal cells in the spinal fluid, an indication of central nervous system invasion, is termed a *central nervous system relapse.* Extramedullary relapses are frequently followed by *bone-marrow relapses.* The duration of remissions becomes more difficult to obtain and remissions are progressively shorter. A child may experience several remissions and recurrent relapses before he succumbs to complications of the disease.

The diagnosis of leukemia is established by a stained smear of peripheral blood and bone-marrow aspirate which reveals the typical picture of replacement of normal marrow elements with abnormal cells. The child's course is followed closely with frequent evaluations of his peripheral blood. The policy for reexamining the child's bone marrow at specific time intervatls varies from one institution to another. Bone marrow aspiration is discussed above in Common Screening and Diagnostic Procedures. Children are most often concerned with the po-

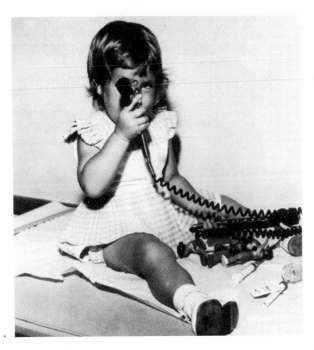

FIGURE 25-9 A child using play as a means of exploring traumatic hospital procedures.

sition they will have to assume and the number of injections that will be necessary. Providing a means of talking about the experience through play, storytelling, or role playing may be helpful (Fig. 25-9).

The goal of therapy is eradication of leukemic cells and restoration of normal marrow function. The drugs included in Table 25-6 can be used in a variety of combinations to induce and maintain a remission. Side effects are experienced by all children, but the severity of these side effects varies from one child to another. Those entities most often encountered include appetite fluctuations, alopecia, development of cushingoid features, nausea, vomiting, myelosuppression, infection, mucuous membrane ulceration, and transient peripheral nervous system effects such as decreased deep-tendon reflexes, weakness or numbness and tingling in the arms and legs, and constipation.

The *induction* course of therapy is designed to reduce the leukemic cell population sufficiently to achieve a complete remission. It is thought that at the time of diagnosis approximately 1 trillion (10^{12}) leukemic cells are distributed throughout a child's body. To achieve a clinical remission, the leukemic cell population must be reduced to 1 billion (10^9) or less, a thousandfold reduction.

Certain drugs are more effective in inducing a remission than others. The chemotherapy most commonly given in this phase is a combination of prednisone given daily, vincristine given weekly, and a third agent such as daunomycin or L-asparaginase.

Generally, after 4 to 6 weeks of induction therapy, a remission is achieved. Current methods of evaluation may fail to detect up to 10^9 leukemic cells. Thus a complete

remission should not be equated with toal eradication of all leukemic cells. Therefore, many treatment programs include a course of *consolidation* or *intensification* chemotherapy designed to reduce the number of leukemic cells further. This reduction can be accomplished by administering single agents, such as methotrexate or L-asparaginase, in intensive courses or multiple agents in cyclic or combination therapy.

The central nervous system is apparently shielded from systemic chemotherapy by a physiologic barrier termed the *blood-brain barrier*. Standard doses of antileukemic agents, with the exception of prednisone, do not effectively cross this physiologic barrier. As a result, leukemic cells that infiltrate the central nervous system early in the disease in essence exist in a sanctuary protected from therapeutic doses of agents that are effective against leukemia in the bone marrow and viscera. At least 50 percent of children can be expected to develop central nervous system leukemia within the first 36 months after diagnosis unless some form of central nervous system prophylaxis is administered early in the disease.

At the present time, the general trend is to avoid cranial radiation in all children except those who have T-cell ALL or overt central nervous system disease at the time of diagnosis. It is presumed that *all* children have microscopic CNS disease. Hence they are all treated with intrathecal agents. The CNS triple therapy consists of methotrexate (12 to 15 mg/m^2), hydrocortisone (15 to 30 mg/m^2), and ARA-C (15 to 30 mg/m^2). They are given intensively in the beginning, and then they are administered every 8 weeks for the total duration of treatment.

Treatment to prevent central nervous system relapse early in the course of illness generally consists of cranial irradiation, plus intrathecal methotrexate. The dose of radiotherapy is administered to the whole brain in 12 fractions through two opposing lateral ports. Twelve to 15 mg/m^2 of methotrexate is given weekly or twice weekly for five to six doses.

Initial intensive intrathecal therapy with methotrexate alone or in combination with ARA-C and hydrocortisone followed by intrathecal treatment every 2 months may be as effective as whole-brain irradiation and intrathecal drugs and may be associated with fewer acute side effects. Further investigation in this area is ongoing.

For those children who receive cranial irradiation, the consistent acute side effect is alopecia. The severity and duration of alopecia vary from patient to patient, but generally children lose all their hair before the completion of therapy. Hair grows back within several months but may be of a different color and texture. The IQs of these children drop 5 to 10 points as a result of this irradiation, especially in those who are less than 2 years old. Learning disorders, endocrine changes, and CAT scan changes also occur (Freeman, 1984).

Side effects of meningeal irritation due to intrathecal methotrexate may be prevented by diluting the drug with a preservative-free vehicle (nonpreserved sterile saline, sterile water, or Elliott's B solution), filtering it through a

0.22-mm millipore filter, and bringing it to room temperature before administration. After a well-placed atraumatic lumbar puncture is performed, a volume of spinal fluid is removed that is equivalent to the volume of drug. Without aspiration, the medication is injected in a continuous infusion, the stylet is reinserted, and the needle is removed. Usually children do not develop a postinjection headache. For the purpose of ensuring optimal circulation of medicated spinal fluid throughout the central nervous system, some investigators recommend having the child remain in the Trendelenburg or supine position for 30 minutes after intrathecal injections.

The goals of *maintenance* or *continuation* chemotherapy are to maintain remission and to continue reducing the residual leukemic cell population toward zero. A combination of 6-mercaptopurine administered daily and methotrexate administered weekly is effective continuation therapy and is associated with minimal complications of drug toxicity. To increase the duration of remission, some investigators have employed *reinduction* or *reinforcement* therapy. With this approach, prednisone alone or prednisone plus vincristine "pulses" are given every 3 to 4 months for 2 to 4 weeks.

When a relapse occurs, induction therapy with vincristine and prednisone may be administered. When these agents are no longer effective, L-asparaginase, Cytosar, daunomycin, adriamycin, and other investigational agents may be used as single agents or in combination. After the remission has been reinduced, maintenance therapy is administered. Usually the occurrence of a single relapse, whether in the bone marrow or in an extramedullary site, means that permanent control of the disease is more difficult to achieve. However, more and more children who have relapses now can be cured.

AML is less responsive to therapy. Combination of drugs such as vincristine, prednisone, adriamycin, cyclophosphamide, daunomycin, Cytosar, and thioguanine are effective for remission induction in approximately 50 to 80 percent of children with AML. Some of these agents, particularly Cytosar and thioguanine, are used for maintenance also, but the duration of remission is usually short—less than 1 year. Four- to five-year disease-free survival is seen in only 20 percent of children with AML.

Bone-marrow transplantation is now being used more extensively. It is the treatment of choice for patients with AML, providing remission is achieved and a matched donor, usually a sibling, is available. It is also being used in relapsed ALL children, especially those with the T-cell form of disease. Both autologous and allogenic transplants are available to children who meet the criteria of transplant centers.

Supportive therapy is essential during periods of intesive treatment. Early recognition of infection and prompt institution of appropriate measures can be lifesaving. Antibodies are used aggressively to combat infection. Tranfusions counteract the complications of bone-marrow suppression. Packed red blood cells are generally transfused in place of whole blood to avoid volume overload. The use of platelet concentrations has helped to control the hemorrhagic manifestations of thrombocytopenia. Granulocyte transfusions have been studied for use during profound neutropenia, but the benefit remains controversial and the expense and difficulty of preparation limit their use.

Another measure to combat complications of leukopenia is to place the child in a germfree laminar-airflow unit and administer white blood cell transfusions. While such units clearly reduce the infectious complications during intensive treatment, most studies have failed to show improved patient survival.

Nursing Management

A child with leukemia can experience extreme changes in his state of well-being within a short period of time. At the moment of diagnosis he may be asymptomatic or have a few minor complaints, or he may be critically ill. When therapy is begun, the disease process may be reversed with surprising rapidity. As the disease progresses, the child may or may not experience severe toxicity to the drugs used. The nursing assessment must be extensive to determine the effects these factors have on the child's functional level. Frequent reassessments are necessary to detect changes in the patient's needs.

During periods of intensive treatment, the nurse should examine the patient several times each day for early signs and symptoms of infection and toxic reactions to treatment. The mouth and skin should be inspected for signs of infection, such as redness, swelling, drainage, and tissue warmth. Any evidence of toxicity or infection should be reported to the physician at once.

Certain problems are common in childhood leukemia and should be considered when planning for nursing care. All families are faced with the task of understanding and adjusting to a chronic, fatal illness. The nursing implications of this aspect of the disease are discussed in Chaps. 15 and 16.

Normal eating patterns are often interrupted by fluctuations of appetite and mechanical difficulties with chewing and swallowing. One of the side effects of steroids is a marked increase in appetite. The child and family generally welcome this change from the previous anorectic state. When steroids are discontinued, the child's appetite tapers off rapidly before it returns to preillness levels.

When the child is experiencing a loss of appetite, a behavior-modification approach may be helpful. All too often the child's hesistation to eat becomes a focus of the entire family's attention. If attention is paid to the child's attempts to eat and not to his refusal to eat, he may respond to the positive reinforcement and make a greater effort to eat. High-caloric preparations which are available commercially provide an excellent means of supplementing daily requirements. These preparations are available in assorted flavors and supply as much as 1.5 kcal/ml.

A pleasant environment can encourage the anorectic child to eat. Eating in a group, either with the family at home or with other children in the hospital, may be desirable. Preparing the child and family for changes in appetite may reduce their anxiety about this phenomenon. Oral intake of food has long been associated with well-being and survival. Family members who have not adjusted to the implications of the illness feel helpless and frustrated. The child's refusal to eat accentuates these feelings of helplessness, particularly for the mother, who may identify providing nourishment as an essential part of her role. When possible, the anorectic child should be allowed to participate in the selection of his diet. He will need supervision, but allowing him some form of control may stimulate his interest in eating.

Painful mouth ulcers or infections of the oral cavity may prevent the child from chewing or swallowing. Children taking methotrexate and adriamycin may develop lesions of the oral and gastrointestinal mucosa. The lesions may become infected and necrotic, and large portions of tissue may be sloughed. When thrombocytopenia and hemorrhage develop, there may be oozing from the gums. The child is discouraged from eating by the pain and unpleasant taste in his mouth (Fig. 25-10). When oral lesions are present, soft foods and cold foods may be tolerated better. Foods such as yogurt and milk coat the mucous

membranes and make consumption easier. While the addition of gravies and sauces may entice some children to eat, blenderizing certain foods may increase the oral intake of others. A slightly brewed, cooled tea bag applied to the bleeding site may aid in hemostasis.

The nurse must accurately assess the patient's oral hygiene and make an appropriate plan for mouth care. Several approaches are possible. A soft-bristled toothbrush should be used. It can be made softer still by rinsing in hot water. If lesions are neither extensive nor painful, the child can continue to use a toothbrush but should avoid brushing the lesions. When brushing is contraindicated, rinsing the mouth with a hydrogen peroxide and saline solution may be substituted. If the mouth is severely affected and the solution will not be tolerated, rinsing with water will be of some help. The child may specify the water temperature he desires. Mouthwash can be used to leave a fresh taste in the mouth. Some commercial preparations may cause irritation and should, therefore, be used with caution. When oral lesions are present, the use of straws and other sharp eating utensils should be avoided.

Many children develop constipation while taking vincristine. If the child is very ill, measures which facilitate normal bowel function such as exercise and intake of foods high in bulk may not be realistic. It is important that the child maintain an adequate fluid intake. Stool softeners are generally admininstered routinely; laxatives, if constipation develops. The physician should be notified if there is any indication that a child taking vincristine is becoming constipated. If not managed properly, constipation can progress to obstipation and ileus.

Rectal ulcers may develop. They may result from mucosal damage by chemotherapy or infection, particularly with *Pseudomonas* organisms. The ulcers may begin as small, tender erythematous areas and progress to large necrotic lesions. It is important to examine the neutropenic child's perirectal area routinely for any early signs of these lesions. The policy at many institutions is to avoid taking rectal temperatures on leukemic patients to prevent trauma to the gastrointestinal mucosa and the possible introduction of bacteria into a neutropenic child's bloodstream. The perianal area should be washed well to remove any feces or urine. It is not advisable to apply ointments to the area if skin breakdown has occurred, because these agents tend to trap bacterial organisms. Positioning the child so that there is no pressure on the lesion and applying a heat lamp four times a day may promote healing.

Maintenance of skin integrity is most important for the neutropenic child. When punctures must be done, the area should be cleansed with an iodine solution and alcohol. In Fig. 25-11 a cellulitis resulting from a finger puncture is shown.

Prevention of infection is imperative. A large percentage of infections are caused by a patient's flora, so good personal hygiene should be emphasized. Because the child is most likely to contract an infection while he is hospitalized, every effort is made to carry out treatment

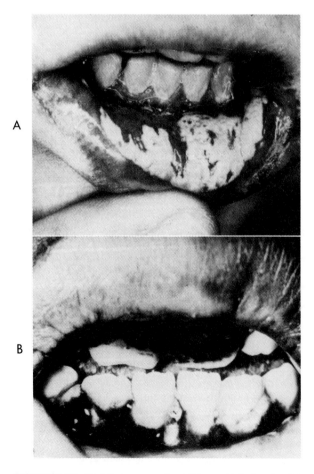

FIGURE 25-10 Oral lesions seen in children with leukemia. *(A)* Oral candidiasis or thrush. *(From W.T. Hughes and S. Feldman, Hospital Medicine 8[12]:68-69, 1972.)*

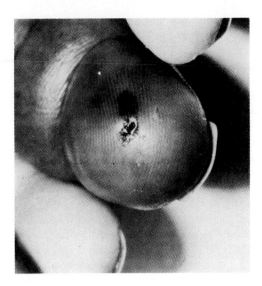

FIGURE 25-11   Cellulitis resulting from a finger puncture. *(From W.T. Hughes and S. Feldman, "Infections in Children with Leukemia." Hospital Medicine, 8[12]:68-69, 1972.)*

programs on an outpatient basis. The nurse must ensure that the parents are well-informed about measures to prevent exposure and the signs and symptoms of infection that require medical treatment. An episode of fever, rash, increased respiration, diarrhea, headache, and inability to bend the neck forward or alteration of mucous membrane should be reported to the physican immediately.

Varicella (chickenpox) presents a particular threat to children with leukemia. In normal children it is a benign disease confined to the skin, but in the immunosuppressed child it may become a life-threatening disease. Pneumonitis, hepatitis, pancreatitis, meningoencephalitis, and bacterial infection of skin lesions may occur as complications for the leukemic child. There is some controversy about modifying or stopping chemotherapy with exposure to varicella. Such action is thought to be a greater risk to relapse than the varicella. Prednisone is thought to worsen the course of the disease if it is given in the early incubation period. Chickenpox has become more manageable with the use of acyclovir. This antiviral agent is almost always administered intravenously when a leukemic child contracts varicella. If it is started within 48 hours of the first lesion's appearance, the disease does not disseminate.

Pneumocytis carinii is a widespread organism which causes diffuse pneumonia in immunosuppressed children. Early diagnosis enhances the child's chances of a favorable response to treatment. In most hospitals, these patients are placed on prophylactic Bactrim b.i.d. 3 days a week.

Thorough hand washing is the single most useful technique to reduce contamination of any child who is in the hospital. The nurse should communicate this precaution to the child and parents verbally and through example.

If granulocyte transfusions are used, the child may experience untoward reactions. The most common reaction is shaking chills and temperature elevation. Generally this reaction is not serious, and it can be treated symptomatically. Hives may occur as an allergic response to plasma proteins and can usually be treated with an antihistamine. When hives appear on the face or neck, the nurse should be alert for signs of laryngeal edema.

A severe hypotensive or anaphylactic reaction requires immediate interruption of the transfusion and emergency medical treatment. Symptoms similar to those seen in pulmonary embolism may herald a respiratory reaction. This response is caused by white cells migrating to the lungs, where agglutination may cause a virtual embolism. The reaction is most common in patients with pulmonary infections. When it does occur, it usually resolves within an hour. The transfusion is discontinued, oxygen is administered, and the patient is kept at rest.

Bleeding is a frequently encountered complication. The child may have numerous ecchymoses and petechiae which can appear in any area of the body. Bleeding into soft tissue provides an excellent medium for infection. Efforts must be made to prevent bleeding, and so protecting the child from injuries is essential. Intramuscular injections are avoided during this period of time. Those children who are receiving IM L-asparaginase (25-gauge needle) must have pressure applied to the site. The nasal and oropharyngeal mucosae are frequent sites of external bleeding. In many institutions, salt pork packs or bacon strips have been used to control anterior nasal bleeding. They are cut to size and packed snugly into the nostril to provide an astringent pack and pressure at the point of bleeding. Removal of this pack may cause less damage to the mucosae that does removal of conventional packs.

Physical changes in appearance are inevitable. Some changes are related to the side effects of medications; others are caused by the weight loss and wasting of chronic illness. It is important for the nurse to prepare the child and his family for these changes and assist them in coping with their feelings as they arise. Young children may cope with their feelings through play and storytelling. The nurse should facilitate play activities for the child and take advantage of opportunities to communicate with him through play. Older children, concerned about hair loss, may be interested in selecting and wearing a wig, cap, or scarf. Many parents of young children are more concerned about these changes than the child himself. They may be embarrassed by comments made by friends and strangers and feel guilty about their reactions. Reassuring the family that these feelings are shared by other parents and that the nurse understands and accepts their feelings is most helpful.

During periods of exacerbation, the child is often irritable and in pain. Those caring for him should move him gently. Bone and soft-tissue involvement may make any sudden movement painful. Careful positioning can relieve tension of these areas. The use of analgesics is important in controlling pain. Providing a quiet, pleasant environment may promote comfort and rest. The nurse should support the family members and enable them to remain with the child as much as possible. Fear of separation from parents is of major concern to the preschooler.

If the child is able to participate in diversions, he may enjoy selecting the activities in which he is most interested. The nurse should take advantage of every opportunity to allow the child to control his environment. It is important to avoid exposing him to activities he will be unable to accomplish.

When the disease is controlled, the child should return to normal activities. His family should be encouraged to treat him as a normal child when possible. It is difficult for parents to discipline and make demands of the child who has a potentially terminal illness, but the child feels most secure in an atmosphere that approaches the one with which he was familiar before he became ill. This lesson is, perhaps, the most difficult one for parents of a leukemic child to learn. The experience of participating in a parents' group has helped many. In this setting, parents can share their feelings and ideas and exchange comfort and experience.

The nurse may be in contact with persons in the community who will be involved with the child as he returns to normal activities. Teachers and ministers are frequently in close contact with the child. They often have fears and misconceptions about the illness which the nurse can dispel.

Return to school is an essential part of rehabilitation that should be anticipated from the time of diagnosis. The nurse should facilitate ongoing communication between the child and the school and plan measures which will aid the child in returning to school.

Implementation of an appropriate nursing care plan is a joint effort of the child, his family, and the nurse. Truth telling and accurate information are critical components in providing care to these children and their families. Family members should be allowed to participate in the care and to assume as much responsibility as they comfortably can. Suggesting specific tasks that they can do may reduce their feelings of helplessness and anxiety.

The nursing care plan should include provisions for meeting the nurse's needs. There should be adequate opportunity for the nurse to explore her feelings about death with members of the staff who are able to offer support. The nurse's feelings of helplessness may be reduced by the development of a structured nursing care plan which specifies concrete solutions to nursing problems.

The availability of effective chemotherapy and supportive therapy has made long-term survival a reality for many children with leukemia. In addition to the joy and hope that accompanies long-term survival, there is increasing concern about the possibility of late effects of disease and treatment. There is new evidence to suggest that young children, in particular, may have neuropsychological deficits as a late effect of cranial irradiation and intrathecal methotrexate for prophylactic treatment of the central nervous system for leukemia (Fergusson, 1981). One also must wonder what effect 3 years of antineoplastic therapy will have on the child's liver, kidneys, and other organs as he encounters the usual physiologic stresses of life for 70 or more years.

The difficulties encountered in measuring and evaluating medical consequences of disease and treatment are only magnified when one attempts to measure and evaluate psychosocial effects. *The Damocles Syndrome,* by Koocher and O'Malley (1981), is a report of a 4-year investigation into the psychological, medical, and practical life problems of 120 children who were successfully treated for cancer.

To summarize briefly some key findings of the study, it does appear that psychosocial effects may be another major consequence of survival. When well-adjusted survivors were compared to those with evidence of problems, a number of variables seemed to contribute to the discrepancy. Children whose cancer is discovered in infancy or early childhood, whose treatment is short, who do not have relapses, and whose families are supportive and communicate openly have the best psychological prognosis.

Survivors who were judged to be poor copers reported more depression, more anxiety, and more problems with self-esteem. These findings seem to reflect the chronic continuing uncertainty faced by all cancer survivors, which is especially important to those who are not able to cope effectively. Denial and suppression of stressful feelings appeared to be important defense mechanisms.

Divorce rates among parents of survivors were lower than in the general population. In fact, many parents described the cancer experience as having had a positive effect on their marriages, drawing them closer together and helping them become more sensitive to each other's needs. Siblings frequently experienced feelings of being "left out," jealousy, resentment, guilt, and worry about their own health. They were particularly vulnerable when the family failed to communicate openly.

Visible physical impairment did not seem to be related to long-term psychosocial adjustment. However, the females who were never married were more likely than married females to have more severe visible impairments. Married males had more visible impairments than the males who had never married.

The spouses of married survivors did not think that the cancer experience had left residual negative effects. Many of the survivors had become parents and all of the children were in good health. Forty percent of the adult survivors reported some form of employment or insurance problem linked directly to their cancer history. Life insurance was particularly difficult to obtain.

Of particular interest is the finding of a higher frequency of adjustment problems among those who were not told their diagnosis until late in treatment or those who found out independently rather than from their parents or physicians. This finding may relate as much to open patterns of family communication as to the actual telling of the diagnosis. Nurses caring for patients with cancer should be very alert to the signs of physical or psychological effects of treatment in both children undergoing treatment and those who are long-term survivors.

Aplastic Anemia

Aplastic anemia is a disease of the bone marrow characterized by a profound depression of the production of the formed elements of the blood: red blood cells, white blood cells, and platelets. This disease may be congenital or acquired. *Fanconi's anemia* is the eponym given to the congential form of the disease. Abnormalities of the skeletal and renal structures, the central nervous system, and the skin pigmentation are associated with the syndrome.

In some cases, acquired aplastic anemia is related to drug, radiation, or chemical exposure. Chloramphenicol, sulfonamides, phenylbutazone, DDT, benzene, radiation, and chemotherapeutic drugs are considered to be possible causative agents. In a signficant number of situations, no cause is discovered.

The clinical features of the disease are related to the degree of marrow depression. They may closely resemble the complications of myelosuppression seen in the leukemic patient. Hemorrhagic manifestations of thrombocytopenia are often the first signs of the disease. Bacterial infections and severe anemia subsequently develop. Those with severe acquired aplasia have a particularly grave prognosis; median survival is usually less than 67 months, and 80 percent die within 1 to 2 years (Gale et al., 1981). When a patient responds to therapy, the progressive course of improvement may take from several months to several years. The first sign is an increase in the production of red cells. Next, the white count increases and returns to normal. Platelets are the last cells to respond, and thrombocytopenia may persist for several months to years.

A first step in controlling the disease is recognition and removal of any toxic agent with which the child is in contact. Essential supportive measures include transfusion of packed red cells and platelet concentrations and administration of appropriate antibiotics.

Bone-marrow transplantation has evolved as the preferred therapy for selected patients. Unfortunately, most potential transplant candidates lack sibling donors with identical homologous leukocytic antibodies (HLAs). Unrelated donor transplants are not successful because of complications of graft rejection. When transplantation is done, multiple marrow aspirations are taken from the donor under general anesthesia. The patient receives the marrow by intravenous infusion.

Nursing Management

Many of the complications of anemia, infection, and bleeding seen in the child with leukemia are also seen in the child with aplastic anemia. He is irritable, weak, listless, and anorectic. His normal patterns of eating and elimination may be interrupted by painful oral and rectal lesions. Hemorrhagic and infectious lesions may appear on any part of his body. Many of the skin-care, mouth-care, and comfort measures described above for the care of the child with leukemia can be used.

The task of adjusting to aplastic anemia is complicated by the uncertainty of the prognosis. During the first few months of the illness, it is impossible to determine whether the child will respond to therapy or fail to respond and die of complications. The child and his family anxiously await the results of each blood test. This uncertainty reinforces the feelings of denial experienced by many family members who are accepting a chronic, potentially fatal illness. It is important to avoid encouraging the family unrealistically. The greatest harm in denying the possiblity of eventual death is that the child and his family may not feel free to discuss their feelings of fear and anger in an atmosphere of unquestionable hope.

When bone-marrow transplantation is done, sibling donors are preferrerd. All potential donors are typed for compatibility. This event can create a number of stressful situations. Incompatible family members as well as compatible donors may blame themselves for treatment failure. Parents are faced with another difficult decision. Many express hesitation to subject a well sibling to the trauma of marrow extraction in the face of possible treatment failure.

When the child returns to school and peers he must cope with their curiosity. It may be helpful for the nurse to contact the child's teacher. Explaining the physical changes and complications of the disease and therapy may allay the teacher's fears and correct misconceptions.

The Purpuras

The group of disorders known as the *purpuras* is characterized by bleeding into the skin. Bleeding from mucous membranes and other organs and tissues also may occur. Purpuras can be classified as *nonthrombocytopenic* (normal platelet count) or *thrombocytopenic* (a reduced number of platelets). Nonthrombocytopenic bleeding is related to a deficit of small-vessel or platelet function. *Anaphylactoid purpura*, or *Henoch-Schönlein syndrome*, is the most common nonthrombocytopenic purpura. The syndrome is an acute allergic response of unknown cause characterized by a confluent purpuric rash on the extensor surfaces of the arms and lower legs and the buttocks, pain and swelling of the joints, abdominal pain, and renal involvement.

Idiopathic Thrombocytopenic Purpura

Idiopathic thrombocytopenic purpura (ITP) the most common form is an acute, self-limited disease characterized by a reduction of the number of peripheral platelets, usually to less than 40,000 cells per mm^3. The onset is sudden and often follows a viral infection. Approximately 80 to 90 percent of children with acute ITP have an uneventful recovery. The length of time from diagnosis to remission varies from a few weeks to 1 year. Most children recover within the first 6 weeks. Approximately 10 percent of children develop a chronic form of the disease, but most eventually recover.

The most common hemorrhagic manifestations are petechial and ecchymotic lesions of the skin and bleeding from the nose and mucosal tissue. Rarely, intracranial hemorrhage may occur.

Transfusions of fresh blood may be administered to replace blood loss. Platelet transfusions may be administered to arrest active bleeding, but the survival of transfused platelets is brief. Corticosteroid therapy is employed to reduce the severity of the hemorrhagic manifestations and hasten remission. If thrombocytopenia persists beyond 6 months, a splenectomy may be performed. Approximately 75 percent of children with chronic cases of the disease recover after splenectomy.

Nursing Management

During periods of active bleeding, the child should be observed closely for signs and symptoms of shock and intracranial hemorrhage. Bleeding is frightening for the child and his family. The nurse should reassure them that the blood loss can be controlled with transfusions. Epistaxis may be persistent and troublesome. When routine compression and packing measures are not successful at controlling the bleeding, the nose may be packed with a hemostatic substance or a small wedge of salt pork.

Protection from injury is important during periods of thrombocytopenia. Slight falls precipitate hemorrhage into internal organs. The child may return to school, but he should avoid body-contact sports. It is generally advisable that he not participate in physical education.

Aspirin and other drugs which interfere with platelet function are never used. Deep intramuscular injections are avoided, and pressure is applied for 5 minutes after an intravenous puncture or subcutaneous injection for immunizations.

Spleen Trauma and Splenectomy

Traumatic laceration of the spleen, causing intraperitoneal hemorrhage, is the most common reason for splenectomy in childhood. Occurrence increases with age, as the child's involvement in sports and more adventuresome play increases. A blunt blow to the abdomen can occur in auto accidents, fights, falls from trees or playground equipment, contact sports, and sledding accidents. Children with bleeding disorders are prone to such accidents. The blow may produce symptoms and perhaps other injuries, such as bruises and bone fractures. Often, though, the injury is mild, with no external signs, and almost overlooked until symptoms develop.

Abdominal pain and tenderness in the upper left quadrant are accompanied by nausea and vomiting. Pain in the left shoulder may occur. Additional symptoms are those of blood loss: increased pulse, perspiration, pallor, and falling blood pressure. A slowly falling hemoglobin may be indicative of splenic trauma if not readily diagnosed. The spleen may be enlarged and palpable as a mass in the left upper quadrant.

A peritoneal tap will produce blood, but a negative tap does not mean laceration is not present. Abdominal and chest x-rays assist in differential diagnosis. A serum amylase test will be high in pancreatitis (which produces similar symtpoms) but normal in lacerated spleen.

Nursing Management

Preoperative preparation for splenectomy depends largely on the illness of the child, on the urgency of the situation, and on his history. The most important measure is evaluation of the child's condition, to which perceptive nursing observations may contribute greatly. Blood transfusions may be necessary to stabilize the condition of the child with splenic laceration. The child may have other injuries which must be considered in preparation for surgery. Platelets and fresh whole blood can be used during surgery performed for ITP to maximize hemostasis. Gastric compression is the other measure required preoperatively.

Regardless of the reason for the surgery, it is usually simple and without complications. The postoperative course follows closely that of uncomplicated appendectomy.

Although not confirmed by immunologic studies, many clinical studies show a high incidence of serious, overwhelming infection following splenectomy. Infants and young children, in particular, are susceptible to septicemia and meningitis. When infections do occur, the mortality rate is higher than might be expected.

Hematologic Problems in Adolescence
Hodgkin's Disease

Hodgkin's disease is a malignancy of the lymphoid system characterized by the occurence of solid tumors in the lymph nodes; they may appear in many nodes in distant areas of the body. A variety of histologic patterns of malignant cells can be identified, but the occurrence of a unique type of cell, termed a *Reed-Sternberg cell,* is considered by most pathologists to be essential for the diagnosis of Hodgkin's disease. Though the disease is uncommon in early childhood, it may occur in children between the ages of 4 and 12 years. There is a significant increase in the number of cases in children 11 years of age and older, with the peak incidence occurring between 15 and 29 years of age.

The manifestations of the disease are generally related to lymph node enlargement. The nodes are characteristically painless, firm, and movable in the surrounding tissue. The most serious complication of node enlargement is tracheobronchial compression and subsequent airway obstruction when the mediastinum is involved. Compression of the esophagus may inhibit swallowing.

Splenic involvement occurs early. Infiltration of nonlymphoid organs may produce a wide variety of symptoms. In advanced stages, the disease may involve the liver, lungs, kidneys, bones, and rarely, the central nervous system. Systemic reactions are common and include fever, pruritus, rash, night sweats, anorexia, lethargy, weakness, and general malaise.

Anergy, a diminished sensitivity to specified antigens, accompanies the disease, particularly in the later stages. Infection is a major complication of this phenomenon. Viral, bacterial, and fungal infections may be widely disseminated and overwhelming.

Accurate treatment is dependent on an accurate diagnostic evaluation of the disease. A surgical biopsy of an affected node is done to determine the type of cell involved. A lymphangiogram may be done to detect metastatic nodal involvement. An exploratory laparotomy and splenectomy may be done. Multiple biopsies are done at the time of surgery. A staging system is used to classify the extent of the disease. (Criteria commonly used for staging Hodgkin's disease are found in Table 25-7.)

A histopathologic classification is used to describe Hodgkin's disease. Four types have been identified: lymphocytic predominance, nodular sclerosis, mixed cellularity, and lymphocytic depletion. Nodular sclerosis is most common in children.

The selection of therapy depends on the stage of disease. It may consist of radiation (either localized or total nodal), chemotherapy, or a combination of both. MOPP is commonly used. *MOPP* includes mustargen, vincristine (Oncovin), procarbazine, and prednisone. Another combination of drugs includes vincristine, bleomycin, and vinblastine. These combinations are not cross-resistant, and one may be used if the other fails.

Therapy can cause the side effects discussed earlier, such as appetite fluctuations, peripheral neuropathy, constipation, alopecia, nausea and vomiting, and bone-marrow suppression. The response to therapy varies with the stage of disease. With pathologic staging and treatment, it is common for two out of three patients to be disease-free 5 years after diagnosis.

Nursing Management

Caring for an adolescent with a chronic and potentially fatal illness is a difficult task for many nurses. The adolescent is accustomed to assuming the responsibility of planning his activities and caring for himself. With Hodgkin's disease he must cope with the limitations of the disease itself as well as the toxicities of the therapy. Many of his previous activities are too strenuous. The side effects of therapy impose embarrassing changes of appearance on his already rapidly changing body. A major developmental task of adolescence is establishment of emotional and physical independence. The limitations of the disease force the adolescent to rely on family members and medical and nursing personnel for assistance with basic activities of daily living. The task of facing this change of life-style and possible death force him to turn to others for emotional support as well. The nurse frequently is uncomfortable in this situation. The patient's hesitancy to ask for help is often met with the nurse's hesitancy to offer help.

It is more difficult to talk about illness and death with the adolescent. Thought he may have a realistic understanding of death, his family may feel the need to protect him from the truth to prevent him from worrying.

It is usually most helpful if the nurse conveys to the adolescent a willingness to talk about his illness if he

TABLE 25-7 Stage, Treatment, and Prognosis of Hodgkin's Disease

Stage	Extent of Involvement	Treatment	Prognosis
I	Limited to one anatomic region or two contiguous anatomic regions on same side of diaphragm	Irradiation to an extended field.	With a favorable histology, long-term disease-free control (more than 10 years) can be achieved in 90% of patients.
II	Present in more than two regions or two noncontiguous regions on same side of diaphragm	Irradiation to an extended field. Physicians in some centers may institute chemotherapy.	With a favorable histology, long-term disease-free control can be achieved in about 80% of patients.
III	Present on both sides of diaphragm but not extending beyond involvement of lymph nodes, spleen, or Waldeyer's ring	Irradiation therapy to an extended field and/or total nodal (mastoid to groin); may be given chemotherapy: a. Mustargen, Oncovin, prednisone, and procarbazine (MOPP); Cyclophosphamide, Oncovin, prednisone, and procarbazine (COPP); or a combination of the above agents, also including vincristine, bleomycin, and vinblastine	With a favorable histology, about 60% of patiens can expect long-term disease-free control.
IV	Involvement extends to bone marrow, lung parenchyma, pleura, liver, bone, skin, gastrointestinal tract, or any tissue or organ in addition to lymph nodes, spleen, or Waldeyer's ring	b. With evidence of recurrence, BCNU, Adriamycin, or DTIC may be used effectively.	About 25 to 40% of patients survive for about 5 years.

Subdivisions
A: No symptoms at the time of diagnosis
B: Symptoms at the time of diagnosis, including unexplained fever, weight loss, and night sweats

Source: Phillip Lanzkowsky, "Diseases of the Blood and Childhood Malignancies," in Robert A. Hoekelman et al. (eds.), *Principles of Pediatrics,* McGraw-Hill, New York, 1978, p. 1049.

wishes to do so. He will feel more secure if his questions are answered honestly and directly.

When possible, the adolescent can plan activities around his therapy schedule. Many patients receiving therapy in the morning can expect a few hours of nausea and vomiting immediately following the treatment but will recover by afternoon. If chemotherapy is given on the same day each week, he can leave that day free in his schedule in anticipation of side effects.

At the time of diagnosis, the adolescent should be approached in a direct, open manner. The diagnostic procedures such as the biopsy, lymphangiogram, and exploratory laparotomy may be much less stressful if he knows what to expect.

The adolescent is encouraged to take part in his care as much as possible. If he is experiencing night sweats, it may be advisable to supply him with a change of bed clothes at night so that if he awakens with moist clothing, he can solve the problem himself and not have to call the nurse for assistance.

Infectious Mononucleosis

Infectious mononucleosis is an acute infectious disease now thought to be caused by a member of the herpesvirus group called *Epstein-Barr virus,* or *EB virus.* Epidemiologic and laboratory observations suggest that the organism is transmitted with oral contact and exchange of saliva rather than casual exposure. However, studies of families and students in college dormitories indicate that infectious mononucleosis does not spread primarily from case to case. The incubation period is between 4 and 14 days. The age peak incidence is between 17 and 25 years.

Examination of peripheral blood reveals an increase in the number of lymphocytes and the appearance of an atypical form of lymphocyte called a *Downey cell.* During the course of infectious mononucleosis, patients acquire a high titer of heterophil antibodies. Clinical symptoms include fever, sore throat, malaise, headache, fatigue, and lethargy. Lymph node enlargement and splenomegaly are common. Symptoms may last for 2 weeks or longer.

The disease is self-limiting, and no specific therapy has been shown to be effective in controlling the uncomplicated disease process. Symptomatic relief of pain with analgesics and fever with antipyretics is indicated. Bed rest during the acute febrile stage of the disease may be required by the patient, but there is no evidence that it will shorten the course of the illness. The patient's activity should be governed by his fatigability. He should be observed closely for evidence of superinfection, so that appropriate antibiotics may be administered.

Nursing Management

An important goal of nursing care is to make the patient as comfortable as possible. Coordination of feedings and administration of analgesics make it easier for the patient with a sore throat to swallow and help him rest more comfortably after eating. Maintenance of an adequate fluid intake is often difficult. The patient is uncomfortable, irritable, and not eager to swallow. Cool, bland fluids which are often best tolerated may not be available to the college-age patient recovering in a dormitory room. If student volunteers are available, it is advisable to have someone visit the patient as often as possible to replenish his supply of liquids.

The adolescent is often involved in numerous school and extracurricular activities. The nurse may help him rest more comfortably by assisting him in making necessary arrangements to continue his activities in bed or to return to them when he recovers.

Learning Activities

1. Obtain from a hospital special hematology laboratory transparencies of the following: stained slides of peripheral blood and aspirated bone marrow from a normal patient, a patient with aplastic anemia, a patient with hereditary spherocytosis, and a patient with sickle cell anemia (peripheral blood only for the last two). Have students compare and contrast the slides.
2. Obtain, from the local American Cancer Society office, the following films for viewing with students: *When a Child Has Cancer—Helping Families Cope, #4562,* and *Blood Components in Cancer Therapy, #3792.*
3. Obtain from the hospital blood bank outdated packaged blood products (whole blood, packed red cells, platelets). In the student learning laboratory provide administration equipment and allow students to practice assembly.

Independent Study Activities

1. Visit the local community blood center or the hospital blood bank. Observe the procedure for collecting, fractioning, and processing blood products. You may choose to donate a unit of blood in return for the staff's time and cooperation.
2. Ask the hospital radiologist to show you the results of a lymphangiogram done on a patient with Hodgkin's disease before and after treatment.
3. Observe a bone-marrow aspiration done on a school-age child. After the procedure, ask the child to describe his perception of the event.
4. Assess the nutritional status of an infant or child who has iron-deficiency anemia. Then consult the nutritionist to determine possible dietary treatment.

Study Questions

1. Bilirubin levels, which need to be monitored closely in certain newborns, identify a waste product of
   A. Erythrocytes.
   B. Platelets.
   C. Hemoglobin.
   D. Thrombocytes.
2. Pediatric AIDS encompasses only those children who are under age
   A. 2 years.
   B. 6 years.
   C. 13 years.
   D. 18 years.
3. When providing nursing care to HIV-infected children, the nurse
   A. Must always wear a gown and gloves.
   B. Must always wear gloves only.
   C. Must observe precautions only when giving IV or IM medications
   D. Must always wash her hands upon entering and leaving the child's room.
4. Iron-deficiency anemia is not evident before 6 months of age because
   A. The iron needs of infants under 6 months are minimal.
   B. Formulas with iron additives are used.
   C. Bone-marrow cellular production is high after birth.
   D. Iron requirements are met by reserves acquired in utero.
5. The best source of iron which should be included in the diet of a breast-fed anemic infant is
   A. Orange juice.
   B. Fortified cereal.
   C. Egg yolks.
   D. Applesauce.
6. A clinic nurse teaching parents of children with sickle cell disease stresses the need to
   A. Encourage participation in physical activities.
   B. Provide high-iron foods.
   C. Push large amounts of fluids.
   D. Administer all medications as ordered.
7. In order to prevent sickle cell crisis, a nurse should emphasize the need to
   A. Encourage a normal level of activities.
   B. Avoid individuals with infections.
   C. Prepare nutritious meals and snacks.
   D. Maintain an adequate fluid intake.
8. Daily continuous infusions of deferoxamine in the child with thalassemia reduces the consequences of
   A. Chronic lead ingestion.
   B. Ammonia accumulations.
   C. Hemosiderosis.
   D. Hepatomegaly.
9. For children with thalassemia who have had splenectomies for this disorder, a nurse teaches the parents to assess their offspring for
   A. Hypostatic pneumonia.
   B. Bleeding episodes.
   C. The presence of anemia.
   D. Overwhelming infections.
10. Cryoprecipitate is a form of transfusion which provides a child with
    A. Platelets when his count is below 150,000.
    B. The missing factor VIII.
    C. Necessary blood components except granulocytes.
    D. An equal amount of platelets and red blood cells.
11. A route used frequently to administer a combination of chemotherapeutic drugs to prevent CNS involvement in children with leukemia is
    A. Oral.
    B. Intravenous.
    C. Intramuscular.
    D. Intrathecal.
12. After working with parents of a toddler with hemophilia, a nurse can conclude that the teaching done was effective when a home visit reveals
    A. That parents encourage active exploration.
    B. That parents have assumed responsibility for administering cryoprecipitate.
    C. That a plan has been developed for responding to a bleeding episode.
    D. That a large protective environment is available for exploration.
13. A major nursing problem emerges when children with leukemia develop oral and gastrointestinal lesions from
    A. Methotrexate.
    B. Prednisone.
    C. Vincristine.
    D. Daunomycin.
14. When a leukemic child is receiving vincristine, it is most important for a nurse to
    A. Examine urine for blood.
    B. Monitor stools.
    C. Maintain a high protein intake.
    D. Increase the fluid intake.
15. The most difficult issue with which the parents of a leukemic child must deal is
    A. Overprotection.
    B. Normality.
    C. Discipline.
    D. Overindulgence.
16. The drug which can cause the development of aplastic anemia if used for an extended period is
    A. Amoxicillin.
    B. Nafcillin.
    C. Gentamycin.
    D. Chloramphenicol.
17. A major problem with which children suffering from aplastic anemia and their parents must cope is
    A. The uncertainty of its prognosis.
    B. Acceptance of its remissions and exacerbations.
    C. The complexity of treatment protocols.
    D. The devastating side effects of treatments.

Information for Patients and Professionals
Sickle Cell Disease

National Association for Sickle Cell Disease, Inc., 945 South Western Avenue, Suite 206, Los Angeles, Calif. 90006.

Leukemia

American Cancer Society, Inc., 261 Madison Avenue, New York, NY 10016, (212) 599-3600 (For state and metropolitan divisions, see listing in *CA–A Cancer Journal for Clinicians*)

Candlelighters, 1901 Pennsylvania Avenue, N.W., Washington, DC, 20006, (202) 659-5136 (a support group for parents)

Leukemia Society of America, Inc., 733 Third Avenue, New York, NY 10017, (212) 573-8484

National Cancer Institute, Office of Cancer Communications, Building 31, Room 10A17, Bethesda, MD 20014

References

Centers for Disease Control: "Immunization of Children Infected with Human Immunodeficiency Virus–Supplemental ACIP Statement," *MMWR: Morbidity and Mortality Weekly Report,* 37:181-183, 1988.

Centers for Disease Control: "Classification System for Human Immunodeficiency Virus (HIV) Infection in Children Under 13 Years of Age." *MMWR: Morbidity and Mortality Weekly Report,"* 36:225-230, 1987a.

Centers for Disease Control: "Revision of the CDC Surveillance Case Definition for Acquired Immunodeficiency Syndrome," *MMWR: Morbidity and Mortality Weekly Report,* 36(Suppl. 1S):3S-14S, 1987b.

Centers for Disease Control: "Revision of the Case Definition of Acquired Immunodeficiency Syndrome for National Reporting–United States," *MMWR: Morbidity and Mortality Weekly Report,* 34:373-375, 1985.

Fergusson, J.H.: "Cognitive Late Effects of Treatment for Acute Lymphocytic Leukemia in Children," *Topics in Clinical Nursing,* 2:21-29, 1981.

Freeman, A.I.: *Childhood Acute Lymphocytic Leukemia: Progress and Prospects,* Lederle Pharmaceutical Co., Pearl River, N.Y., 1984.

Gale, R.P., et al.,: "Aplastic Anemia: Biology and Treatment," *Annals of Internal Medicine,* 95:477-491, 1981.

Koocher, G.P., and J.E. O'Malley: *The Damocles Syndrome,* McGraw-Hill, New York, 1981.

Lubin, B.H., and W.C. Mentzer: "Sickle Cell Disease," in A.M. Rudolph and J.I.E. Hoffman (eds.), *Pediatrics,* 18th ed., Appleton-Lange, Norwalk, Conn., 1987.

Bibliography

Byrd, R.L.: "Late Effects of Treatment of Cancer in Children," *Pediatric Annals,* 12:6, 1983.

Fochtman, D., and G.V. Foley, (eds.): *Nursing Care of the Child with Cancer,* Little, Brown, Boston, 1982.

Gradof, B.: "Sickle Cell Anemia in Children," *Issues in Comprehensive Pediatric Nursing,* 6(5-6):295-306, 1983.

Ruccione, K.: "Acute Leukemia in Children: Current Perspectives," *Issues in Comprehensive Pediatric Nursing,* 6:329-363, 1983.

Stark, R.: "Bone Marrow Transplantation: Progress and Problems," *The Journal of Pediatrics,* 105(9):414-418, 1984.

U.S. Department of Health and Human Services: *Report of the Surgeon General's Workshop on Children with HIV Infection and Their Families,* USDHHS, Rockville, Md., 1987.

Yasko, J., and P. Greene, "Coping with Problems Related to Cancer and Cancer Treatment," *CA—A Cancer Journal for Clinicians,* 37(2):106-125, 1987.

26

The Gastrointestinal System

Objectives

After reading this chapter, the student will be able to:
1. Describe the functions of the gastrointestinal system.
2. Identify appropriate subjective and objective data to be elicited from the child and family.
3. Understand the purpose of diagnostic tests and medical treatments.
4. Explain general nursing measures appropriate for pediatric clients who have gastrointestinal problems.
5. Delineate specific nursing measures appropriate to the care of clients who have various gastrointestinal problems.

Anatomy and Physiology

Alimentary Canal

The gastrointestinal system (digestive tract, alimentary canal) has the major function of moving food through the body. The process includes *ingestion* (the intake of food controlled by various physiological and psychological factors), *digestion* (the physical and chemical breakdown of foods into simpler molecular units), *absorption* (the passage of digested foods into the body circulation), and *elimination* (the passage of undigested and/or undigestible substances from the body). The alimentary tract includes the mouth, esophagus, stomach, and small and

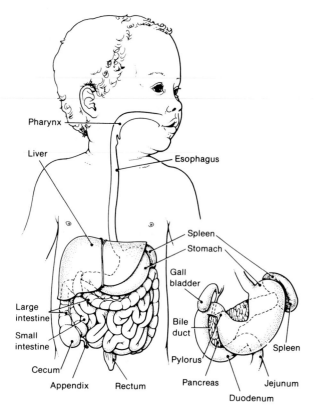

FIGURE 26-1   Anatomy of the gastrointestinal system.

large intestines (Fig. 26-1). The liver, gallbladder, and pancreas are considered accessory digestive organs, and they perform a variety of functions which will be described later.

Once food enters the mouth, *mastication,* or chewing, occurs, which changes food into minute particles (mechanical digestion) and breaks down protein, carbohydrates, and fats into absorbable substances (chemical digestion). *Deglutition,* or swallowing, and peristalsis are the mechanisms which propel the bolus of food down the esophagus and into the stomach.

The entrance to the stomach, controlled by the cardiac sphincter, prevents the reflux of stomach contents back into the esophagus. The stomach is a reservoir for food. Its mucous lining is arranged in longitudinal folds called *rugae* which allow it to distend. Glands in gastric mucosa secrete gastric juices (mucus, enzymes, hydrochloric acid) which act on its contents. The stomach (1) serves as a reservoir for food until it is partially digested and moved on, (2) secretes gastric juices and the unknown intrinsic factor responsible for Vitamin B_{12} absorption, (3) by contracting its musculature churns food into small particles which become the mass known as *chyme,* and (4) absorbs a very limited amount (water, alcohol, and some drugs). The churning action of the stomach mixes the food and digestive juices thoroughly in preparation for its exit. Once the pyloric sphincter, which controls the exit of food from the stomach by an enterogastric reflex relaxes, the highly acidic chyme begins to pass

into the small intestine.

As gastric contents liquefy, small amounts are ejected into the duodenum by peristaltic waves at approximately 20-second intervals. Emptying of the stomach takes 1 to 4 hours for an average meal. For the most part, the small intestine completes the digestive process. Its inner mucosal layer has microscopic projections called villi which greatly increase the surface area available for digestion and absorption. While digestive enzymes are being secreted, clusters of lymph nodes called *Peyer's patches* and solitary lymph nodes facilitate the entry of absorbed nutrients into the lymphatic circulation. The small intestine has three main functions: (1) completing the digestion of foods, (2) absorbing the end products of digestion into the blood and lymphatic systems, (3) secreting hormones which control the flow of bile and intestinal and pancreatic juices. Chyme takes about 6 hours to move through the small intestine.

Once this mass reaches the large intestine, very little or no digestion occurs. Substances which have not been absorbed in the small intestine are indigestible and will be excreted. Peristalsis and contractions move the waste matter through the ascending colon, the transverse colon, and the descending colon to the sigmoid colon and rectum. As waste matter accumulates, emptying of the rectum, or *defecation,* occurs as a reflex action. The distending rectum stimulates receptors in the rectal mucosa which affect the anal sphincters and, together with colonic peristalsis and voluntary straining, result in the expulsion of feces.

Glands and solitary nodes also are located in the submucosal layer of the large intestine. Three thick bands of smooth muscle run along this section of the alimentary canal; because they are shorter than the colon itself, they pucker the walls of the colon, form pouches along its length, and give it a scalloped appearance. These pouches are called *haustra.* The main functions of the large intestine are the absorption of water, an undetermined role in the absorption of fats, and elimination of waste.

Accessory Digestive Organs

The *liver* is a vital organ and the largest gland in the body. Its functions include secreting bile (a pint a day), which facilitates digestion and absorption of fat; removing some waste products; and metabolizing all three food types. In carbohydrate metabolism the liver carries on the processes of glycogenesis, glycogenolysis, and gluconeogenesis, all of which are essential in the homeostasis of blood sugar. Liver cells also carry out fat catabolism. Liver cells perform an essential function in protein anabolism by synthesizing blood proteins—prothrombin, fibrinogen, albumins, and many globulins—which are important in blood clotting, water balance, and maintenance of normal blood pressure and circulation.

The *gallbladder* stores and concentrates bile, which enters the hepatic and cystic ducts. During digestion, the gallbladder contracts, ejecting the concentrated bile into the duodenum.

The *pancreas* (1) secretes the digestive enzymes found in pancreatic juice, (2) from beta cells secretes insulin, the hormone with major control over carbohydrate metabolism, and (3) from alpha cells secretes glucagon, which is important in carbohydrate metabolism.

Digestive Juices

Complicated reflex and chemical (hormonal) mechanisms control the *flow of digestive juices* so that they are secreted when needed and in the needed amounts. Chemical, mechanical, olfactory, and visual stimuli initiate reflex secretion of saliva. Gastric secretion is initiated partly by the same reflex mechanism. The hormone gastrin, released by gastric mucosa in the presence of partially digested proteins, controls the gastric secretion, while enterogastrone, which is stimulated by fats and sugars, inhibits the secretion. Pancreatic secretion is controlled chemically by the hormones secretin and pancreozymin and by some reflex action. Secretin is released when hydrochloric acid, protein, and fat digestion products act on the duodenal mucosa and stimulate the pancreas. Pancreozymin stimulates enzyme production by the pancreas.

Secretin also stimulates the liver to secrete bile. The ejection of bile from the gallbladder is controlled by a hormone, cholecystokinin, which is formed by the intestinal mucosa when fats are present in the duodenum.

Regulation of the secretion of intestinal juice is not fully understood. It is thought that hydrochloric acid and food products stimulate the intestinal mucosa to release a hormone, enterocrinin, into the blood, which stimulates intestinal secretion. Neural and reflex mechanisms also may play a part.

Chemical Food Changes

The body's use of the food it takes in is an impressive orchestration of all the organs which make up the gastrointestinal system. The biochemical breakdown which occurs in the carbohydrates, proteins, and fats ingested allows the utilization of the nutrients which sustain the body. The enzymes which are present play a critical role in the preparation of food for absorption and utilization.

Carbohydrate digestion varies according to the complexity of the compound, since carbohydrates are saccharides. Polysaccharides, starches, contain many saccharide groups and must be hydrolyzed to disaccharides by enzymes known as *amylases,* which are found in saliva (ptyalin) and pancreatic juice (amylopsin). Disaccharides are hydrolyzed to monosaccharides by sucrase, lactase, and maltase, which are found in intestinal juice (succes entericus). Monosaccharides (glucose, fructose, and galactose) are absorbed directly.

Protein digestion is facilitated by enzymes called *proteases* which catalyze the hydrolysis of the large protein molecule into intermediate compounds (proteases and peptides) and then into amino acids. The main proteases are pepsin in gastric juice, trypsin in pancreatic juice, and peptidases in intestinal juice.

Fat digestion must be facilitated by *emulsification* of fats since they are insoluble in water. Bile emulsifies fats since they are insoluble in water. Bile emulsifies fats in the small intestine. The main fat-digesting enzyme is pancreatic lipase.

Vitamins, minerals, and water are absorbed in their original form. Residues of digestion (cellulose, undigested fats, and undigested connective tissue and toxins from meat proteins) resist digestion and are eliminated from the body.

Assessment of the Gastrointestinal System

History

Systemic disease can produce alterations in the gastrointestinal system, or problems can result from congenital or acquired entities of the alimentary tract. It is critical to obtain baseline data on the child's normal health state before the significance of symptoms can be determined. An accurate health history is beneficial to both the child and health care providers.

A prenatal and birth history are particularly important for infants. Formula intolerances should also be noted. The child's usual diet, appetite, food preferences, and meal schedule are included. Any previous history of gastrointestinal problems should be recorded. Elimination patterns of the child, stool characteristics, and toileting habits are additional factors of importance. Any recent changes within the family unit are essential to note as children often develop gastrointestinal symptoms as a response to stress within the family.

The child's general appearance and nutritional state are observed and documented by the nurse. The distinction between an acute illness and a chronic illness can sometimes be inferred by the child's overall physical state. Height and weight are recorded and compared with previous data. Symptomatology onset and duration are discussed after baseline information is obtained.

Physical Assessment

The physical examination starts with inspection of the oral cavity for any condition that could interfere with sucking, swallowing, or chewing. Bleeding or ulcers of the mucous membranes, dental caries, and congenital anomalies (cleft lip or palate) potentially can hinder oral intake and consequently nutritional status. Dysphagia or an enlarged tongue may also curtail solid intake. A sore throat must be differentiated from dysphagia.

The abdomen is inspected for color, distention, turgor, and contour. If pain is a complaint, its location is pinpointed as accurately as possible. Children poorly articulate the source of pain; thus, the nurse must observe the child's facial expression during gentle palpation of the abdomen. Any abdominal masses are noted at this time. The abdominal girth should also be measured.

Auscultation of the abdomen reveals the presence or absence of peristalsis. Some alterations result in hyperperistalsis, while others produce a paralytic ileus. The abdomen should also be inspected for visible peristalsis,

TABLE 26-1 Common Diagnostic Procedures

Purpose	Procedure	Nursing Implications
Cellulose tape smear Determine presence of oxyuriasis (pinworm) ova	At night or early morning, press piece of cellulose tape over anal and perineal areas for less than a minute; tape to clean glass slide; label; send to lab	Explain purpose and procedure to parent and/or child: discuss female pinworm's proclivity for migrating at night down the intestine and depositing eggs on the perineum; explain relationship among pruritus, scratching, and carrying eggs to mouth; discuss personal hygiene and need for treating all family members.
Stool culture Diagnose causative agent in diarrhea (e.g., pathogenic *Escherichia coli, Salmonella sp., Shigella sp.*)	For infants and children not toilet trained, scrape freshly expelled bowel movement, using wooden tongue depressor, from diaper to stool specimen container; label; send to lab; for older child, instruct child to use bedpan for next bowel movement; remove specimen from bedpan; place in container; label; send to lab.	Explain purpose and procedure to parents and/or child: collect specimen; send to lab: if results are positive, control measures implemented until repeat culture negative; in hospital, isolation technique must be used; observe strict hand washing; maintain special handling of diapers, stool, food, formula; explain regimen to parents and/or child; observe other infants and children for symptoms; at home, teach family about hand washing and handling of diapers, stool, food, formula; explain common modes of transmission.
Rectal swab Same as stool culture; if diarrhea so severe that no solid specimen can be obtained, rectal swab may be done	Position as for rectal temperature; taking care not to contaminate equipment and remove cotton plug and sterile swab from test tube; gently insert swab into rectum (as with rectal thermometer), rotate around rectal wall, remove, replace in test tube, insert cotton plug in tube; label; send to lab	Same as stool culture; when explaining procedure, tell child it is similar to having rectal temperature taken; if necessary, parents may be asked to help restrain child.
Barium swallow Evaluate esophageal structure and function, determine presence of pyloric stenosis in absence of palpable tumor, evaluate abdominal mass, demonstrate varices, determine presence of gastric or duodenal ulcer	Infant or child given prescribed amount of contrast medium by mouth; amount to be swallowed determined by radiologist; course of medium from esophagus to duodenum and sometimes through small intestines is followed via fluoroscopy and cine	Explain purpose and procedure to parents and/or child; if child is less than 18 mo, he is NPO* for 3 h; a bisacodyl suppository is given 90 min before barium swallow and repeated in 45 min if the child does not have a large bowel movement; if child is 19 mo or older, 1 bisacodyl tablet (below 40 kg in weight) or 2 tablets (above 40 kg in weight) is/are given hs (at bedtime); must be swallowed whole (not chewed or crushed and not taken within 1 h of ingesting antacids or milk; suppository may be given in place of tablets hs*; child is NPO 4-6 h; both tablets and suppositories are contraindicated in children who have an acute surgical abdomen or ulcerative colitis; a bisoacodyl suppository is given 90 min prior to barium swallow and repeated in 45 min if no results

Source: Martha Underwood Barnard et al., *Handbook of Comprehensive Pediatric Nursing*, McGraw-Hill, New York, 1981.

*NPO = nothing by mouth; hs = at bedtime.

TABLE 26-1 Common Diagnostic Procedures—cont'd

Purpose	Procedure	Nursing Implications
Barium enema Determine presence of low obstruction (e.g., ileal or colonic atresia, meconium ileus, Hirschsprung's disease, intussusception)	Infant or child given prescribed amount of contrast medium by rectum; course of the medium from rectum through large intestine is followed via fluoroscopy and cine	Explain purpose and procedure to parents and/or child; child is given a clear liquid diet for 24 h prior to barium enema; milk and dairy products are excluded; bisacodyl in form of tablets or suppository as for barium swallow given hs; infants NPO for 3 h and older children for 4; bisacodyl suppository 90 min prior to barium enema with repeat in 45 min if no results

which is found in infants with pyloric stenosis and in very thin children.

If the child is vomiting, the characteristics should be noted and the vomitus should be tested for the presence of blood. Similarly, any nausea occurring prior to or after vomiting is recorded.

Parents can be of aid during the physical examination, especially with infants and small children. They should be encouraged to assist the nurse and to provide support to the child during this time.

Common Diagnostic Tests

The most commonly performed procedures employed in the diagnosis of gastrointestinal disorders can be found in Table 26-1. The nursing responsibilities are also included. In addition to these tests, biopsies of selected areas may be indicated to confirm or differentiate the diagnosis.

Liver biopsy is performed frequently in children when deterioration of liver tissue is suspected, as in biliary atresia, portal hypertension, and neoplasms of the liver. The child does not receive food or fluids immediately before the procedure and is usually given a sedative or analgesic. Immobilization is imperative for a safe, successful procedure, but it may be difficult to achieve in the young child. Older children usually cooperate if the procedure is explained fully. The child may be asked especially to hold his breath when the needle is inserted. Manual immobilization of the abdomen must usually be done with infants and very small children. If all the equipment is prepared in advance, the nurse can concentrate on supporting or positioning the child. Hemorrhage, a most frequent and dangerous complication, can be avoided if the patient is properly restrained and if moderate pressure is applied for 5 to 10 minutes after the procedure has been completed.

Biopsy of the *small intestine* is seldom necessary unless it is done as part of an operative procedure to identify obscure enteropathies. A *large intestine* biopsy is important in the diagnosis and differentiation of ulcerative colitis, Crohn's disease, tumors, or Hirschsprung's disease. Except when performed during abdominal surgery, a lower intestinal biopsy is done through a sigmoidoscope. It is

done most commonly by rectal biopsy (pinch) forceps. Nothing, including a thermometer, is inserted into the rectum for approximately 3 to 5 days afterward.

Other Types of Procedures

Dilations

The purpose of dilating either the *esophagus* or the *anus* is to prevent scar tissue contractions which form strictures or to stretch already contracted tissue. The esophagus may contain scar tissue at the anastomotic lines of a tracheoesophageal fistula repair and colon interposition. Scarring may be an aftermath of lye ingestion. The anus may require dilation because of stenotic or membranous imperforate anus or as a postsurgical procedure following a pull-through operation for an imperforate anus or Hirschsprung's disease.

Esophageal dilation is accomplished by using Tucker or mercury dilators. *Tucker dilators,* hard rubber tubes tapered at both ends, have nylon cord loops (about 20 in long) attached to each tapered end. A gastrostomy must be present since a thin nylon cord is threaded through the nostril, toward the stomach, and the end leaves the stomach through the gastrostomy. The gastrostomy end of the nylon cord is knotted to the end entering the nostril, making a complete circle. During dilation, the knot is untied and the string at the nostril is tied to the well-lubricated dilator while a new length of string is tied to the other end. When the dilator is pulled down through the esophagus emerging through the gastrostomy, the new string remains in place. The ends are knotted as before, and the string is used for the next dilation. These dilations are done on a regular basis (every few days) for minor strictures until a large-sized dilator passes easily.

Mercury dilators are long, nontapered rubber tubes weighted with mercury on the insertion end. They are used for dilation when no gastrostomy is present. In many cases, anesthesia is necessary to perform the procedure because of fear, uncooperativeness, discomfort, gagging, and coughing by the child. However, when support and assistance are given during these procedures, the patient may learn to swallow the tube with a minimum of fear and discomfort. The dilator is threaded down slowly and withdrawn immediately. This type of dilation may need to be carried out for long periods of time, especially after severe lye burns of the esophagus. The child is able to eat soon after these procedures.

Hager dilators, used for anal dilation, are smooth, conical metal instruments varying from size 2 to 32. The ends are rounded, with each end a different size so that the dilator increases in diameter as it is inserted. Efforts should be made during the procedure to prevent tension and subsequent tightening of the anus by the child. The dilator is warmed and lubricated. When in position, it is held in place for a few minutes or longer. The next largest size is used when no resistance is encountered. This procedure may be necessary on a daily basis up to 2 weeks postoperatively. It may be continued at home by finger dilation or with a wax candle of appropriate diameter.

Endoscopy

Esophagoscopy is a diagnostic aid and a treatment tool. It is necessary diagnostically to determine the extent of esophageal varices and in treatment to sclerose the varices. The procedure is used to determine the extent of scarring after surgery for lye ingestion and the presence of stenosis or esophagitis. Dilation with mercury dilators for scarring and stricture can be done through an esophagoscope. Since the procedure is done under general anesthesia, preoperatively the child is given nothing by mouth for 6 to 8 hours and is medicated accordingly. Usually a normal diet is resumed after the child has recovered from anesthesia.

Proctoscopy and *sigmoidoscopy* are used as diagnostic aids in some diseases of the bowel such as Hirschsprung's disease and rectal polyps. Repeated examinations may be necessary in evaluating treatment, as with patients with ulcerative colitis.

The instruments used are rigid hollow tubes with illumination within the unit. Adult sizes are used with larger children, while the size used for infants is only 14 cm in length. A flexible sigmoidoscope is used for viewing beyond the rectum. Biopsy can be done with this instrument. The knee-chest position is desired, although the infant may be placed on his back with his thighs abducted to his flanks. The nurse holding him should stand at his head. Efforts are directed at relaxing the child to make the procedure less painful and to make visualization successful. An older child needs a complete explanation of what is to be done. Most children do not need analgesics. Bowel preparation is avoided because it may cause mucosal changes, negating the diagnostic value of the examination. The discomfort disappears as soon as the procedure is over, and the child returns to his previous activity and diet.

Gastric Intubation

A nasogastric tube may be necessary in order to instill medication or feedings, remove gastric contents, obtain gastric secretions for diagnostic tests, remove amniotic fluid in the neonate, and decompress the stomach pre- and postoperatively. Extensive content relating to the insertion of a nasogastric tube, gavage tube feedings, gastric lavage, and nasogastric decompression can be found in Chapter 10, "Common Pediatric Nursing Procedures."

Surgical Openings (Ostomies)

Cervical esophagostomy is a procedure performed for types of esophageal atresia where a proximal blind esophageal pouch exists. It enables definitive surgery to be postponed until later. The end of the pouch is exteriorized at the base of the neck so that naso- and oropharyngeal secretions drain to the outside. The left side is preferred because of the approach used for subsequent anastomosis of the colon.

Initially, a plastic catheter may be placed into the stoma to facilitate drainage for the first few days or longer. After removal, a soft piece of toweling or absorbent material is placed over the opening to collect the secretions. Saliva is not irritating to the skin, and excoriation does not occur if the area is cleansed regularly and the toweling is changed frequently. Ointment may be applied to the peristomal area to prevent skin breakdown.

An accompanying gastrostomy is necessary to provide nutrition. The child should be introduced to oral fluids (formula, if an infant), which drain from the esophagostomy after fluids are swallowed. Some physicians prefer to give only sugar water. These oral "feedings" are given concurrently with the gastrostomy feedings so that the child can relate satiation of hunger and fullness in his stomach to the sensations of swallowing. Oral feedings have been found to relax the pyloric sphincter, promoting digestion. If this concurrent feeding is not done, the child will need to relearn the eating process, which he often resists. Description of the technique which may be used to resume oral feedings when resistance is encountered is included in the discussion of esophageal atresia below.

Gastrostomy is a common component of surgical management of gastrointestinal diseases. It provides a means for earlier postoperative nutrition and for gastric decompression. A gastrostomy eliminates the potential hazards of prolonged nasogastric intubation and prevents esophageal reflux. It acts as a safety and outlet valve when vomiting occurs. Reflux of air and gastric contents when the infant cries or strains prevents additional pressure in the stomach. See Chapter 10.

Colostomy and *ileostomy* are stages in the treatment of specific pediatric intestinal diseases. They are most often temporary, enabling definitive treatment to be delayed until the child grows and more complex procedures may be done, as with imperforate anus and Hirschsprung's disease. Extensive ulcerative colitis may require a permanent ileostomy, while a temporary ileostomy may be done for meconium ileus. As with adults, either may be necessary when widespread malignant tumors or irreparable intraabdominal trauma is present.

Sigmoid colostomy with a single stoma is the most common procedure. A colostomy for Hirschsprung's disease is placed in the transverse colon when the diseased portion is large. Divided or loop colostomy is done when the distal bowel segment must be available for preparation for definitive surgery or when an outlet for drainage is needed, as in Hirschsprung's disease.

Since most ostomies are done on smaller children, irrigation is not a factor in management, but prevention and treatment of skin excoriation around the stoma are problems. A collection bag must be used as soon as an ostomy begins to function to prevent skin breakdown, which appears quickly as a result of the large amounts of digestive enzymes found in the liquid stool. The bag must fit snugly around the stoma and prevent stool contact with the skin. For even the tiniest infant, a small fistula pouch with the smallest adhesive possible is used. The adhesive area can be reduced further by using powder or paper tape. The procedure is as follows: (1) The stoma is fitted to the pattern, (2) the adhesive area is matched to the pattern, (3) the excess exposed area is blocked out, and (4) protective cream is placed over the exposed area, and then the bag is applied. It should be washed daily with soap and water, but the seal should last 2 to 3 days longer with larger children.

A variety of products or combinations of products are used to prevent as well as heal skin excoriation. The most frequently used are a form of karaya and Silicote ointment and a protective cream made especially for ostomies. Although exposure to air and a treatment light are successful interventions for colostomy-induced breakdown, they will only produce further excoriation with ileostomies. Changes of either bag or dressing must take place more frequently with infants for several reasons: Skin breakdown is more frequent; the bag or dressing does not stay in place as well; and infant elimination is more frequent than with older children.

Preoperatively, the parents and child must be informed about the purpose of a colostomy or ileostomy. They need to know about the appearance of the stoma and its location. Prior teaching by nursing personnel is essential. Older children are capable of comprehending broader and more detailed explanations than are preschoolers. Nurses must adapt their teaching methods to the cognitive level of clients.

If parents will have the primary responsibility for ostomy care, they must be given time postoperatively to demonstrate their capabilities. Multiple sessions may be required, depending on the parents' level of anxiety. Prior to the child's discharge, parents must be secure and comfortable in the care they will provide.

School-age children and adolescents are very concerned with peer acceptance and body image. They need to know that normal activities and social life are not precluded by ostomies. Nurses need to be sensitive to individual needs and provide time for clients to address their particular concerns.

General Nursing Measures

The nurse has many responsibilities in caring for an infant or child with a gastrointestinal problem. They include tak-

ing a careful history, identifying how the child responds to pain, and monitoring the client after surgery or teaching parents procedures which need to be continued in the home. The parents of all infants and children need to become involved in the care being provided, especially in the case of newborns who are separated from parents by transport to medical centers early in life.

Nursing Diagnoses

Fluid and electrolyte problems are common in this segment of the pediatric population, and they must be identified early. The reader is urged to review the information in Chap. 11. With the variety of procedures available for treatment, it is important for the nurse to serve as a resource for parents and children who need information. Teaching, then, is a major nursing function.

Many nursing diagnoses may be developed for these young children and their families, including the following:
Diarrhea
Knowledge deficit of parents or child in relation to the particular problem
Potential altered parenting related to impaired parent-infant attachment
Pain
Potential impaired skin integrity
Fluid volume deficit
Altered nutrition: less than body requirements
This list is not all-inclusive. The diagnoses depend on the status of the infant or child and must be revised as the child is monitored and his condition changes.

Gastrointestinal Problems in the Neonate

Surgical Emergencies

Congenital Diaphragmatic Hernia

This defect involves hernation of abdominal contents into the thoracic cavity and represents one of the most acute emergencies in the newborn period. The most common area of herniation is on the left side through the foramen of Bochdalek, which results in a hypoplastic left lung (Fig. 26-2). There is no predilection of either sex or race. Mortality rises rapidly in treatment of the youngest and smallest infants and is highest in the first 24 hours after birth.

The neonate has a large (barrel) chest in comparison to his scaphoid abdomen. Breath sounds may be absent on the affected side, heart sounds are displaced to the opposite side, and chest movements are asymmetrical. The thorax on the affected side is dull to percussion. Severe respiratory distress and cyanosis are present in these babies. Classic signs of intestinal obstruction may accompany this defect. Death is usually due to severe oxygen deprivation.

Diagnosis is confirmed by chest x-ray. Gas-filled bowel and stomach can be seen in the thorax, with a collapse of the lung and displacement of the mediastinum toward the unaffected side.

Nursing Management

Immediate relief of respiratory distress is attained through gastric and endotracheal intubation. The nasogastric tube,

FIGURE 26-2 Comparison of pathological anatomies of diaphragmatic malformations.

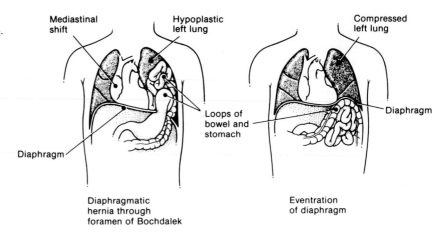

attached to suction, decreases the amount of air and fluid in the herniated bowel and thereby reduces respiratory compromise. Endotracheal intubation and positive pressure ventilation oxygenate the infant and aid in reducing carbon dioxide levels (PCO_2). Respiratory and metabolic acidosis are present and need to be stabilized prior to surgery. Preoperatively, the nurse should elevate the infant's head and thorax (semi-Fowler's position) to displace abdominal contents downward. The baby should also be placed on the affected side to allow expansion of the normal lung.

Surgery is performed as soon as the neonate's respiratory status and acid-base status are stabilized. A subcostal incision is used to expose the diaphragm and replace the abdominal contents into the peritoneal cavity.

Postoperatively, the neonate may have an endotracheal tube in place while on a ventilator. The nurse must monitor his status closely and suction when needed. Chest physical therapy should be performed as frequently as ordered, with documentation of the results of the treatment. Bilateral chest tubes are in place because of the increased incidence of a pneumothorax on the unaffected side. It is important to observe the type and amount of drainage, and it may be necessary to "milk" both tubes to ensure patency. If the surgeon elects to perform a gastrostomy, it is attached to gravity drainage (Chap. 10). A nasogastric tube with intermittant suction is maintained till peristalsis occurs; therefore, intravenous therapy must be used.

Nursing focus must be on the respiratory effort of the baby. The nurse is alert to signs of complications and to the possibility of hemorrhage. In addition to maintenance of treatments noted previously, the nurse makes frequent changes in the infant's position and carries out nasopharyngeal and endotracheal suctioning at necessary intervals to assist him in reestablishing normal respiration. Many postoperative problems, acute and chronic, are due to poorly functioning lungs.

In the recovery period, the focus of nursing care shifts to feeding problems. Frequently, these newborns are lethargic and disinterested in eating. If coaxed, they gag easily and vomit. A flexible schedule which takes advantage of the infant's readiness to eat and his appetite at each feeding (with a maximum limit) is best. The nurse uses feeding techniques which eliminate air swallowing and compression of the infant's stomach by poor positioning of the arms. Frequent burping is essential.

The neonate's parents can be overwhelmed, particularly by the speed with which surgery must be done, the severity of the symptoms, the high mortality rate, and the mass of mechanical aids which they see surrounding the small infant. The parents are encouraged to participate in his care, especially feedings, so that they can learn the best technique and achieve success prior to his discharge.

Esophageal Atresia with Tracheoesophageal Fistula

Rapid diagnosis is vital to the newborn with esophageal atresia. The types of esophageal atresia, with particular characteristics of each, are shown in Fig. 26-3. The largest percentage are type III. Complications occur often; the prognosis depends directly on the speed of treatment, which frequently has a prolonged and tortuous course.

The classic picture of an infant with this anomaly is one who has excessive amounts of mucus, sometimes bubbling from his nostrils, and is choking, sneezing, and coughing. Cyanosis occurs particularly at his first feeding (of diagnostic importance). The feeding is often expelled through the nostrils immediately. Respiratory difficulty and cyanosis are relieved temporarily but noticeably by suctioning the nasopharynx. Because air travels in and out of the stomach through the fistula, progressive recurrent abdominal distention may be present.

Type III, atresia of the esophagus with a fistula from the lower pouch and a blind upper pouch, is described as a "classic picture" of the disease. Aspiration takes place through overflow of the upper pouch (as in type I) but also results from reflux of gastric secretions through the fistula into the bronchi, which can be more serious. The reflux occurs when intrathoracic pressure is increased (from crying, for example), causing air to rush into the lower esophagus via the fistula and into the stomach, which becomes distended and produces vomiting. Gastrostomy and constant drainage of the upper pouch may

FIGURE 26-3 Types of esophageal atresia.

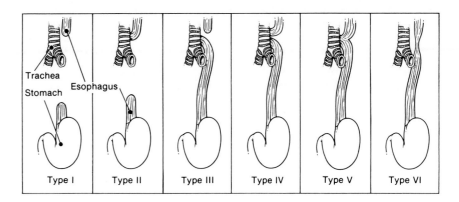

Trachea
Stomach Esophagus

Type I Type II Type III Type IV Type V Type VI

be used to postpone more definitive surgery in preterm neonates and in newborns who are too ill for complex surgery.

Confirmed diagnosis of the presence of esophageal atresia and differentiation of types depends on x-ray examination. A radiopaque catheter is inserted into the blind pouch which shows on film. Radiopaque contrast material is not used unless absolutely necessary because of aspiration dangers. Fistulas are not constantly patent, making the diagnosis more difficult.

The wide variation and combinations of approaches in treatment reflect the differences in the six types and also the accepted philosophy of treatment of this defect, known as *staging* (repeated operations separated by periods of time, waiting for growth). Staging is the approach for preterm and critically ill infants, those who have major associated anomalies, and those in which a wide disparity between the blind ends of the esophagus in size or in distance exists. The severity of aspiration pneumonia may also be a determinant. Ligation of the fistula must always take place immediately. If possible, primary end-to-end anastomosis of the esophagus is performed at the same time. Some surgeons do a gastrostomy as a supportive measure, while others do not.

If the surgery is deferred, there are three methods to prevent the oral secretions from accumulating in the blind pouch. Most common is the use of a double-lumen nasogastric tube which ends in the blind pouch and is attached to suction. The tube is changed daily to ensure patency. A less known method is an *esophageal frame*, a metal frame used with a canvas cover which contains an opening for the baby's face, shoulder rests, and canvas restraint straps. The baby is placed face downward in Trendelenburg's position so that mucus drains by gravity. Gastrostomy feedings are used in both methods. The time interval allows for growth of the esophageal blind segments so that primary anastomosis may be possible, although esophageal reconstruction may still be the final outcome. When the patient's condition is stable, a surgeon may attempt elongation of the proximal pouch by *bougie* treatment, using mercury-weighted dilators or firm catheters inserted briefly each day to stretch the esophagus.

The third method used is cervical esophagostomy, which is done when the child's respiratory problems are too severe, when the need for esophageal reconstruction is unavoidable, or when the first two methods of management prove unsuccessful in controlling secretions. A stoma is placed on the neck to drain mucus and saliva. Tracheostomy may be an additional supportive operation the child must endure if respiratory complications are too severe.

Reconstruction of the esophagus (esophageal replacement, colon transposition, or colon transplant) is performed when there is too wide a gap between the proximal and distal pouches of the esophagus in esophageal atresia without fistula or when a leak occurs in the primary anastomosis. A child tolerates this procedure better over the age of 24 months; however, it is a surgeon's choice. Until that time, he must be maintained by cervical esophagostomy to handle saliva and by gastrostomy feedings, with sham oral feedings if at all possible. Preoperatively, a clear liquid diet and succinylsulfathiazole are used to clean the colon, but enemas or laxatives are avoided because of possible adverse effects.

Postoperatively, water-seal chest drainage is continued for 7 to 10 days, the most common time for anastomotic leaks to occur. The nasogastric catheter decompresses the stomach for 2 to 3 days to prevent strain on the suture line. The gastrostomy tube is open and elevated even after the catheter is removed, and oral fluids are begun in gradually increasing amounts and strengths. Ischemia, which causes total breakdown of the transplant, is the most common complication.

The colon has a propulsive action but adapts soon to functioning in unison with the esophagus, which has peristaltic action, thereby accounting for the large amounts of burping the baby does in the first few weeks and the uncomfortable sensations he seems to feel which cause him to be fussy without obvious reason. His breath often has a strong stool odor in the first postoperative month.

Nursing Management

Immediately upon diagnosis, intermittent suction through a double-lumen catheter ending in the blind pouch should begin. Close observation of respiratory behavior demonstrates any need for additional suctioning of the nasopharynx. The nurse should be especially alert for indications of respiratory effort: retraction, circumoral cyanosis, "fussing," open mouth, and nasal flaring. Oxygen, humidity, and warmth via open warmer are important preoperatively and for several weeks postoperatively. Intravenous fluids are begun before surgery and are often changed to hyperalimentation.

The best position for the baby varies, but generally, the infant is continually elevated in a semi-Fowler's position. The physician may determine the position to be used when a fistula opens from the upper pouch. The baby also may be placed flat or very slightly prone in Trendelenburg's position. He should be kept *flat* after anastomosis but should be *elevated* if catheter drainage of the pouch is being done (to promote pooling of secretions at the catheter tip) or after cervical esophagostomy. Hyperextension of the neck should be avoided since it places tension on any existing suture line.

For nasopharyngeal suctioning postoperatively the nurse must use a catheter marked so that it will not be inserted too near the anastomosis. Suctioning as frequent as every 5 to 10 minutes may be necessary the first day. Nursing judgment must be acute in determining the need since suctioning may increase the edema already present from the surgery. Regular oral hygiene prevents bacterial growth in the abundant secretions.

In catheter drainage of the pouch, the nurse must observe its patency and maintain suction at a low, intermittent level. Depending on the procedures of the hospital, the nurse may be responsible for changing the tube. When the esophageal frame is used, the face needs to be wiped and cleaned frequently.

The nursing care plan must consider the physical restrictions placed on the baby with this defect as well as the social and emotional opportunities he lacks. The treatment for esophageal atresia extends over the entire first year, a crucial time in development.

After anastomosis, gastrostomy feedings are instituted after determination of the volume of gastric contents by aspiration with syringe. Feedings should be given slowly or dripped in every 2 to 3 hours. Oral feedings are begun 8 to 10 days postoperatively. They should be given slowly so that the baby expends as little effort as possible and may be completed by gastrostomy if the baby tires. The nurse should use techniques which prevent coughing or choking from too much or too rapidly delivered milk or from excess air. Some infants may be slow, lethargic eaters, although others are vigorous. A slightly elevated position is usually best for feeding. Developing complications may become evident during feedings.

Initial oral feedings are difficult, since the baby has never experienced eating. The process may take 2 to 4 or 5 weeks for older children to establish. Emphasis must be on patient, gentle, frequent, and pleasant feedings rather than on a rigid schedule of certain amounts. The most effective nursing action is to develop and follow a written care plan built around the child's reactions to and behavior during attempts at oral feeding. The baby then has a chance to use his energy to adapt to the feeding experience rather than a "hodgepodge" of various approaches. His mother can be especially effective if she is encouraged and helped to feel at ease in feeding.

Complications are common and often severe enough to require extended treatment. Most frequent in occurrence is *stricture* at the sites of anastomosis in the months after primary esophageal anastomosis or esophageal reconstruction. One or two dilations under anesthesia may be sufficient to eliminate it; regularly scheduled dilation with Tucker dilators will be necessary if the stricture is persistent. Signs of stricture (refusal of feedings, pronounced coughing, and dysphagia) should be reviewed with the parents prior to discharge after anastomotic surgery.

The prognosis for eventual complete recovery or even for recovery at all depends on innumerable factors. Infants may have a frequent "brassy" cough and a lowered resistance to respiratory infections in the first 6 months to 2 years of life.

Imperforate Anus

Anorectal malformation is a more accurate term than *imperforate anus.* This anomaly occurs equally in both sexes and is seen infrequently in nonwhites. Other major anomalies occur in 40 to 50 percent of cases. Esophageal atresia with tracheoesophageal fistula is associated more frequently with imperforate anus than with other gastrointestinal tract anomalies.

There are four types of imperforate anus (Fig. 26-4). There may be normal outward anal appearances, abnormal anal musculature, inadequate innervation of the area, and associated fistulas of the agenetic type because development of the rectum is minimal or nil. A dimple exists at the site where the anus should be, and there may be puckering of the surrounding skin, an indication of the presence of sphincter muscles. However, there may be neither puckering nor dimple; the anal area may be rather flat between the buttocks. In severe cases the buttocks may be completely flat, indicating poor levator ani development. There is a high incidence of fistular development between the rectum and genitourinary tract in males and between the vagina and rectum in females.

Diagnosis is often made by an observant nurse on newborn examination. The neonate may pass meconium through the fistula or develop symptoms of intestinal obstruction because of an inability to pass meconium.

Definitive diagnosis is made by x-ray. The infant is held upside down while the abdomen is filmed. Gas in the colon rises to reveal an outline of the rectal pouch, giving an indication of its position in relation to the anal membrane. A small catheter inserted into any fistula present and injected with contrast material also aids in the diagnosis.

In surgical management of low agenetic types, corrective surgery is an anoplasty done under general anesthesia. A Hager dilation regimen is instituted as soon as initial healing takes place.

FIGURE 26-4 Different types of imperforate anus.

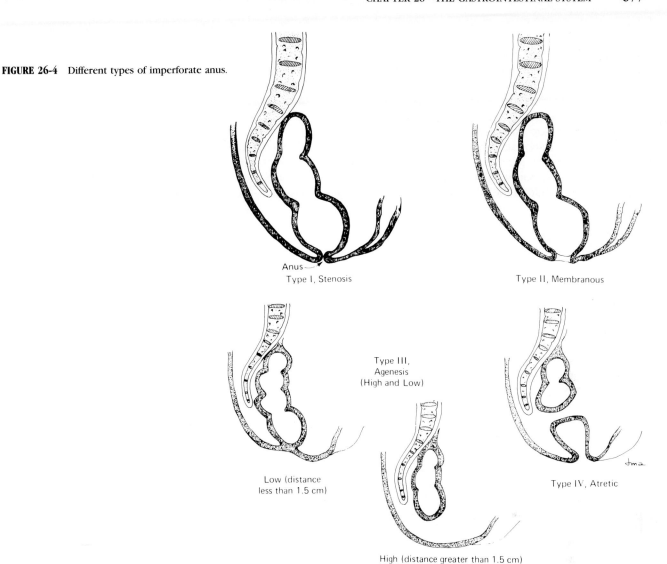

Anus
Type I, Stenosis

Type II, Membranous

Type III,
Agenesis
(High and Low)

Low (distance
less than 1.5 cm)

Type IV, Atretic

High (distance greater than 1.5 cm)

In surgical management of high agenetic and atretic types, a transverse, divided colostomy or sigmoid colostomy is done immediately. Later, at age 6 to 12 months, the infant has a sacroabdominoperineal pull-through operation. The location of the blind pouch of the rectum in relation to the pubococcygeal line, seen on roentenogram, is important in determining the surgical approach.

As far as a prognosis is concerned, normal bowel control is realized after surgery for the stenotic membranous and low agenetic types of imperforate anus. The success of a pull-through procedure depends on the rectum within the puborectalis sling and the status of the sphincters postoperatively. Additional treatment may be necessary.

Nursing Management

If an anoplasty has been done, nursing activities focus on the prevention of suture line infection and the promotion of healing. Generally, the diaper is left off and the suture line is cleaned, using cotton-tipped applicators and hydrogen peroxide or the solution chosen by the physician after each stool. *Nothing* is inserted into the rectum. The

baby's position is changed from side to side to decrease tension on the suture line. Feedings are started a day or two after surgery.

Nursing care postoperatively is the same for both colostomy and pull-through operations. Intravenous fluids and nasogastric suction are necessary until feedings are begun. The infant rarely needs oxygen and nasopharyngeal suctioning longer than 1 or 2 days postoperatively. After a colostomy, the baby is fed when stooling has started. Oral feedings following a pull-through are not begun until peristalsis resumes, stooling occurs, and initial healing has taken place. The baby usually eats eagerly, and vomiting is unusual. Parents need to learn both colostomy care and the rectal dilation procedures they will use after the pull-through operation. Their anxiety, which may increase because of a wait of months or years for final assurance that normal bowel function has been achieved, requires understanding from the nurse.

Even though assured of complete bowel control, the parents approach toilet training with trepidation. They need a great deal of support during this period. Attitude is more important than anatomy. If the child has less than optimum control, toilet training may be unsuccessful or very stressful for both parents and child. The family then faces uncertainty as to when and whether the child will achieve control. Constipation leading to fecal impaction and overflow diarrhea can be avoided by having the child defecate at a regular daily time. Cleanliness, odor, and perineal breakdown are continuing problems for some children. It is most important for the nurse to focus on specific measures which parents may use to maintain skin integrity. Inability to control bowel movements is a serious handicap to the child in regard to socialization and school attendance.

Intestinal Atresias

Atresia along the intestinal tract is the most common cause of intestinal obstruction in the newborn. The incidence of *duodenal* and *ileal* atresias is highest, but the *jejunum* is affected frequently, the *colon* least frequently (Fig. 26-5). Atresia of the bowel is an interruption in continuity which can consist of stenosis, complete atresia of varying lengths, separated blind ends of bowel, or multiple atresias.

Classic symptoms of newborn intestinal obstruction are vomiting of green bile, abdominal distention, and absence of stooling in the first 24 hours.

In the presence of *duodenal atresia,* abdominal distention may be less than with other atresias or may be absent. However, the reflux of duodenal secretions may cause distention in the epigastric area, and there is much more vomiting than in other types. These newborns may pass normal stool.

Surgically, a duodenoduodenostomy (joining the proximal and distal portions of the duodenum) is done whenever possible. A gastrostomy is created during surgery, although some surgeons prefer to use TPN. Both forms of nutritional support allow the anastomosis to heal.

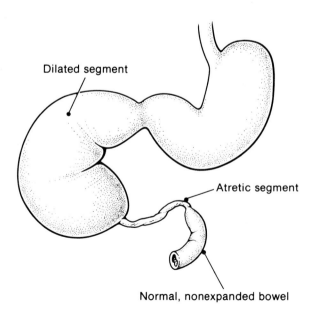

Dilated segment

Atretic segment

Normal, nonexpanded bowel

FIGURE 26-5 Jejunal atresia.

When a newborn has a *jejunal* or *ileal* atresia, stool will occur in the former but be absent in the latter. X-rays confirm the diagnosis. In a surgical correction, the atretic section is excised and a portion of the bowel proximal to the atresia also is removed because it lacks adequate perstalsis. A direct anastomosis is done.

Nursing Management

Vomiting and *aspiration of vomitus* are the greatest dangers in both preoperative and postoperative periods. The nurse must take preventive measures such as positioning, maintaining patency of nasogastric or gastrostomy tubes, nasopharyngeal suctioning, and observation for aspiration. Intravenous fluids are begun prior to surgery and continued afterward. For many, especially preterm infants, those in critical condition, and those requiring extensive resection, hyperalimentation is used. Oxygen with humidity may be required after surgery.

Gastric decompression is done by nasogastric catheter before surgery and, in most cases, by gastrostomy after surgery. The gastrostomy tube is clamped and removed later, often after discharge. Resumption of feedings is gradual. Feeding problems consist of vomiting, low intake, lack of interest in feeding, abdominal distention after feedings, and sometimes diarrhea. The infant may need special formulas which are predigested or nonallergic in content.

If a feeding tube is present in the infant, the nurse must use careful handling and slow feeding to prevent slipping the tube in the intestine or pulling the tube out of place completely. During and after the feeding, the nurse observes for signs which indicate that the tube is out of position, such as vomiting, unusual distention, milk seepage, and milk in the gastrostomy tube.

Episodes of diarrhea occur intermittently and may be severe enough to necessitate intravenous therapy for a few days. The nurse must observe stool size, frequency, and consistency, particularly in relation to increases in feedings. Stool monitoring for protein content and sugar absorption is also routinely done. Guaiac testing determines the presence of bleeding.

Prior to the infant's discharge, parents need to demonstrate comfort and competency in feeding. If special formulas are required, the nurse should inform the parents where to obtain them and how to prepare them if necessary.

Necrotizing Enterocolitis

Necrotizing enterocolitis (NEC) primarily affects preterm infants weighing between 1200 and 2000 g who have sustained a period of stress or hypoxemia. Necrotic lesions are most frequently found in the ileum or proximal colon, although they may be present in any part of the intestine. Hypoxia in the stressed neonate leads to bowel ischemia, which permits bacterial proliferation and subsequent mucosal injury. NEC is characterized by frequent mucosal ulcerations, pseudomembrane formation and inflammation, pneumatosis intestinalis (extraluminal or intramural air bubbles), and perforation.

Early enteral formula feeding may play a major role in NEC. Hydrogen gas is a major component of the intramural bubbles and is formed by a carbohydrate substrate and enteric bacteria. Formula feedings increase the production of hydrogen gas and therefore contribute to the development of NEC.

The onset, which usually occurs during the first few days of life, is marked by abdominal distention, increasing gastric residuals, lethargy, temperature instability, and vomiting. Apnea, gross or occult blood in stools, and metabolic acidosis are other manifestations. An abdominal x-ray showing intramural bowel gas confirms the diagnosis of NEC.

Medical management of NEC consists of supportive measures. A nasogastric tube is inserted and attached to low suction. Intravenous hydration is essential. Stool and blood cultures are obtained, and antibiotics are started because sepsis occurs concurrently. All enteral feedings are stopped, and parenteral alimentation is started. Blood studies include electrolyte values, prothrombin time (PT), partial thromboplastin time (PTT), white blood cell count, and platelet count. The abdominal girth is measured often, and x-ray films are obtained every 4 hours to monitor the progress of the disease. Medical management continues for 7 to 10 days.

Surgical intervention is necessary when acidosis is progressive and persistent, x-rays show free intraperitoneal air, disseminated intravascular coagulation occurs, or symptoms do not abate with medical management. Resection of the perforated bowel is done along with the creation of proximal and distal stomas. Reanastomosis is performed at a later time, when the infant's condition is vastly improved. Parenteral nutrition and antibiotic therapy are continued postoperatively for 7 to 10 days.

Nursing Management
Astute, continuous nursing observation is essential, and minute changes in the neonate's appearance or behavior should be reported. At-risk infants are monitored for abdominal distention and tenderness. Prior to feeding, the abdominal girth is measured, along with the gastric residual contents. If NEC is detected early, the prognosis is significantly better.

Nursing responsibilities include accurate intake and output measurements, frequent assessment of vital signs, accurate infusion of intravenous fluids, antibiotic administration, and continual assessment of the infant's condition. Awareness of the electrolyte and blood gas values is also important. Endotracheal intubation and ventilator support may be required for some infants, particularly those who have undergone surgery. Stoma care is necessary for surgically treated infants.

Parental support is a major nursing intervention. Parents need frequent contact with the baby, honest information, and reassurance. Preterm delivery is a stressful event in itself for parents, and NEC contributes to their anxieties. If surgery is indicated, the parents need to be informed as to the purpose of the procedure.

Enteral feedings are restarted 10 days after treatment, whether surgical or medical. Feedings given are in small amounts, and the nurse must carefully observe and record the infant's response, since NEC can recur. Stools should be tested for the presence of blood and glucose. It is most important for the parents to participate in providing care whenever possible.

Complications of NEC include stricture formation at the involved site. Short bowel syndrome may occur in some babies who have had major bowel resections. Early recognition and more effective treatment modalities have decreased the mortality rate for this disease entity.

Short Bowel Syndrome
One type of acquired malabsorption problem in newborns and infants occurs as a result of the removal of a portion of the small intestine. NEC, a variety of intestinal atresias, or another gastrointestinal condition may necessitate such a massive resection. Although as much as 50 percent of the small intestine can be removed without a devastating long-term effect, another determinant of the prognosis is the location of the resection. If the distal portion is involved, the absorption of fat-soluble vitamins, bile salts, and vitamin B_{12} is affected. Removing the jejunum results in the malabsorption of calcium, iron, and folic acid as well as decreasing the availability of lactase, sucrase, and maltase, If the proximal section of the small bowel is removed, an overgrowth of bacterial flora, overproduction of intestinal gas, and diarrhea occur.

With the infant unable to digest and absorb essential nutrients, his nutritional status is a major concern. The medical management is aimed at providing an intake the infant can absorb, replacing the substances lost, and maintaining fluid and electrolyte balance. Vitamin, mineral, and electrolyte levels are monitored closely. It may be necessary for the physician to order supplemental vitamins and trace elements.

Hyperalimentation (TPN) may be necessary for the first 6 to 12 months. Some infants thrive on the slow and progressive advancement to Portagen, carbohydrate-free, or Pregestimil preparations. The prognosis depends on the amount of small bowel intact. While their dietary intake will be lowfat, there are no other restrictions, and those who survive can become asymptomatic within a year and a half or 2 years. However, the use of TPN contributes to complications and infections, resulting in a long and difficult hospitalization.

Nursing Management
These neonates and infants are critically ill initially, and so nutritional as well as elimination assessments are crucial nursing actions. If hyperalimentation is instituted, it is imperative to observe the site for evidence of infection (redness, drainage). Sepsis also can develop; therefore, vital signs are monitored closely, especially the body temperature, because it can be elevated *or* subnormal (Chap. 17).

A nurse must observe the infant closely for any indication of a deficiency. For example, the presence of a rash may indicate a trace element deficit, while muscle twitching or a seizure can occur because of a mineral deficit. Although blood is drawn frequently to monitor electrolytes, vitamins, and minerals, observations provide a significant amount of information about the neonate's overall status.

If the infant is advanced to one of the special formulas used in nutritionally treating short bowel syndrome, it is essential to document its tolerance. Abdominal distention, changes in the frequency and character of stools, and diarrhea may be signs of intolerance. It may be necessary to dilute the formula, change it, or stop all oral feedings. In any circumstance, the physician needs to be told of the infant's response to feeding.

Precise measurement of an infant's intake and output cannot be overemphasized. Every single cubic centimeter must be accounted for in these infants. Diapers are always weighed. The specific gravity of urine is done, as are tests for protein, glucose, ketones, etc. Stool may be tested for pH or blood. In addition, the infant is weighed every day, at the same time, on the same scale, with the same items (nude but with armboard, nasogastric tube, etc).

Whenever a significant weight change is noted, the nurse needs to identify why. Often the weight fluctuation relates to the removal of an armboard or dressing since the last weight was done. Sometimes it may be necessary to weigh some infants at more frequent intervals, such as once a shift.

Meticulous skin care is another important nursing responsibility. The elimination of enzymes and bile salts results in a rapid breakdown of skin, and efforts need to be directed toward maintaining its integrity. Diapers should be changed frequently, and the skin must be cleansed and dried thoroughly before application of a new diaper. It may be necessary to expose the perineal area to circulating air to speed the healing process. Proper positioning is essential to maintain maximum exposure. In some cases a *Candida* infection develops, necessitating the conscientious use of antifungal creams. They should be applied only after complete cleansing and drying of the surface area.

Hospitalization is lengthy, and physical as well as psychosocial development can be affected. These infants need stimulation and a colorful environment with mobiles and soft animals as well as nurses who talk with them while feeding or holding them (Chap. 9). Whether the infant meets normal developmental milestones depends on the efforts of nurses, who play a vital role in enhancing the infant's overall development.

Parents need to be involved in caring for the infant. Initially, there is some hesitation; however, as explanations are made and they feel comfortable, they assume more responsibility, even in the presence of hyperalimentation (Chap. 17).

Omphalocele and Gastroschisis

Both omphalocele and gastroschisis are defects immediately apparent at birth in which abdominal viscera protrude through an abdominal wall defect and are lying out on the abdomen (Fig. 26-6). A gastroschisis is located below, to the right of, and separate from the umbilicus, and no membranous sac encompasses the viscera. An omphalocele is centrally located, includes the umbilicus, and is covered by a sac or its remnants.

Omphalocele results from failure of intestines to reenter the abdominal cavity and failure of abdominal lateral folds to fuse in utero. *Gastroschisis* is due to the failure of embryological tissue to mature in the abdominal layers, leaving a full-thickness abdominal-wall defect. An underdeveloped abdominal cavity also is present. The sac of omphalocele (a transparent avascular membrane) is easily ruptured either in utero or during birth, causing an immediate emergency and high mortality. If rupture occurs, the intestines become thickened, matted, and edematous, a primary cause of other complications. There may be respiratory difficulty, pneumonia, signs of sepsis, or peritonitis.

When a small defect is present, complete closure is possible with the placement of the bowel within the abdominal cavity. In most instances, the defect is too large and requires several stages of repair. A gastrostomy is done in almost all instances.

Creating an artificial coelom (sac) has become the choice for larger defects as well as ruptured omphaloceles. The sac, which consists of Dacron polyester sheeting coated with Silastic and sometimes with knitted Telfa, is sutured to the skin. A shortening of the sac takes place, under sterile conditions, every day or two, although about half the mesh can be removed after 24 hours. A final closing of the abdomen and removal of the mesh can be done in 7 to 14 days.

FIGURE 26-6 Baby with an omphalocele: *(left)* before surgery; *(right)* after surgical repair.

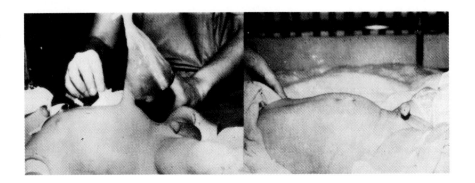

Nursing Management

Infection control is instituted immediately after birth by covering the sac or exposed abdominal organs with sterile towels or sponges saturated with warm normal saline. These coverings are kept wet, covered with dry sterile towels to maintain sterility of the inner dressings, and changed when loosened for examination. A newer transport technique consists of immersing the lower part of the baby in a clear bag of warm sterile physiological solution. Solutions must be warm; hypothermia is a constant and major concern. Sterile gloves are always used. Antibiotic therapy is begun before surgery and continued until the danger of infection has passed.

Another primary consideration is to prevent tension on the area. Positioning, turning, and restricting behavior (arm restraints) must be done cautiously. Since it may be necessary to do treatments and take x-rays in the warmer, handling may be awkward, and two people may be necessary. Supportive therapy, such as gastric decompression, is begun immediately. A nurse needs to assess its patency and carefully document the amounts of saline used to irrigate the nasogastric tube. The exposed viscera increase heat and fluid losses of the neonate. Nursing care should minimize further losses. Dressings must be changed quickly to reduce evaporative losses and to reduce exposure of abdominal contents. The dressings applied should not constrict the intestinal blood supply.

In the presence of a large defect, the potential for infection is very high. Choice of local infection control varies according to physician preference and includes an antibiotic solution or silver nitrate by continuous drip on Xeroform gauze dressings and Betadine ointment applied to sheeting edges. Parenteral antibiotics are given in either situation. Sterile handling and basic supportive care are required. Feedings via gastrostomy may be started before the skin flap procedure if the child's condition is stable. Supportive measures such as intravenous fluids, nasopharyngeal suctioning, and the use of humidity as well as oxygen, are crucial in some instances. Hyperalimentation has been increasingly valuable in maintaining nutrition, rapid healing, and resistance to infection.

Infants who undergo primary closure for very small omphaloceles usually tolerate full-strength formula feeding within a few days postoperatively. Ileus is prolonged in infants with either gastroschisis or a large or ruptured omphalocele. Therefore, feedings may be delayed, necessitating parenteral nutrition for a longer period. Mortality rates have decreased with the use of staged repairs, adequate alimentation, and antibiotic therapy both pre- and postoperatively.

Other Newborn Problems

Cleft Lip and Cleft Palate

Occurring together or separately, with many variations, cleft lip and cleft palate require a long-term interdisciplinary approach for optimum treatment. These defects create problems with feeding, upper respiratory and ear infections, speech, dental formation, and self-image.

The defects are generally considered hereditary, although no exact pathogenesis has been found, and the defect may appear without a familial history. The two anomalies are not always present together. Cleft lip with or without cleft palate has a higher incidence in males, while cleft palate alone is more common in females.

The *complete* cleft involves the alveolus to some degree, and the nostril is distorted to one side. The floor of the nose and upper gum may also be deformed. Any combination of these malformations may occur.

The defects of a cleft palate are usually diverse. The cleft may involve the *soft palate* with the tissues of the uvula, or it may include the *hard palate* and sometimes the nose. The cleft occurs in the midline of the soft palate, but it may exist on one or both sides of the hard palate. It always extends front to back. The cleft palate forms a passageway between the nasopharynx and the nose, causing feeding and respiratory difficulties and susceptibility to infection. It is more difficult to repair than is the lip.

Surgery to close the lip is usually performed when the infant is 3 to 4 months old. Palate surgery is postponed until about age 9 to 12 months. Too early a repair may harm tooth buds; with a late repair, undesirable speech patterns may be established and the palatal structure may be too rigid. Surgery for revisions of repair, correction of nose deformities, and reconstruction of the nasopharynx for speech improvement (*a velopharyngeal flap operation*) are frequently necessary at a later time.

Nursing Management: Cleft Lip

Feeding is the most immediate and most apparent problem. The infant cannot maintain closed suction around the nipple in his mouth or use mouth movement adequately to pull on the nipple because of the open palate. However, he has a strong desire to suck, and sucking motions are present, providing success in nipple feeding before lip closure. A soft but regular crosscut nipple is best, although a nipple of the type for preterm newborns may be needed for very small babies. The nipple is placed in the usual position in the mouth, not in the cleft, so that the newborn can use his sucking muscles as strongly as possible. For some babies, a Breck feeder (an Asepto syringe with an attached rubber tip) may be necessary. Because sucking and swallowing are an integrated process in an infant's feeding, this method prevents choking, coughing, and other difficulties in feeding.

Since the baby swallows more air than normal, burping must be frequent. Being fed in a sitting or semisitting position adds to the baby's success in swallowing and prevents choking and aspiration. Caution must be taken to refrain from constantly removing the nipple from his mouth because of the noises he makes or the fear of choking. The baby becomes more upset and crying adds to the problem. He takes longer to feed than most babies. A small amount of water should be given after a feeding to rinse the mouth. Once the nurse has instituted a successful feeding pattern, the process should be taught to the infant's parents.

Precautions against infections are required. Ear and respiratory infections are frequent because the pharyngeal opening of the eustachian tube is often in an abnormal position. Feeding in an upright position and not allowing the infant to lie on his back for long periods decreases ear infections. The baby breathes through his mouth, and care is taken to prevent dry, cracked lips.

The presence of an unsightly defect causes guilt, fear, misunderstanding, and at times revulsion on the part of parents. The hereditary factor may lead parents to believe that they caused the defect. They need accurate, emphatic reassurance that the defect causes no malfunctioning of the remaining gastrointestinal tract. Parents need emotional support as well as teaching from nurses during this time. Parent-infant bonding is of major importance. The visible anomaly is extremely upsetting to the parents. The nurse should encourage parents to hold the infant and participate in his care and should allow them to verbalize their feelings and concerns. Both parents should demonstrate their comfort and ability to feed the infant prior to discharge.

After surgery the baby may be restless, irritable, and fussy, wanting to be held much of time in the first few days. He has a difficult time adapting to the small airway and to the excess mucus which may be a temporary result of the surgery, especially during feedings. The nurse must evaluate the respiratory distress and observe for swelling of the tongue, mouth, and nostrils. Crying adds to the infant's distress and puts a strain on the suture line. Often, a mist tent is used postoperatively to minimize respiratory distress and hemorrhage, which constitute the two greatest complications after cleft-lip closure.

A second area of nursing concern involves the positioning and restraining required after surgery. The suture line must be protected from blows, rubbing, pressure, and sucking. A curved metal Logan bow, taped down on either side of the suture line and over the lip, is put in place after surgery. The baby must wear elbow restraints at all times to prevent him from putting hands or objects into his mouth. These restraints should be removed every 4 hours so that the arms can be exercised. Since the baby can lie only on his back, it is best to seat him in a plastic infant seat as much as possible for variety, comfort, and entertainment. He also may have difficulty sleeping if he is accustomed to sleeping on his abdomen. Measures such as placing him out where there is activity, holding him when he is fussy, and hanging toys within his sight and within reach of his restrained arms help alleviate the effects of all these restrictions.

Feedings must be given with a flexible medicine dropper, which is always placed on the side of the mouth and away from the suture line. The baby is prevented from sucking on the dropper. This method of feeding is continued for about 3 weeks until the lip is completely healed and breast or bottle feedings are resumed. Dropper feeding is often a frustrating, tiring effort for the baby, especially at first. He cannot suck, he cannot get the formula as fast as he would like, and he swallows more air. Small, frequent feedings may help. Clear liquids are given on the first postoperative day, and then milk feedings are resumed. The nurse should feed at the pace at which the baby would suck, adding to his contentment at feeding time and preventing suture line stress. After a feeding, sterile water should be utilized to rinse out the mouth.

Immediately after feedings, the suture line is cleaned with cotton-tipped applicators and half-strength hydrogen peroxide. Prevention of crusts (with prevention of strain on the suture line) is a major nursing focus. They can cause uneven healing and scarring of the suture line. A collection of exudate and milk on the suture line may also lead to infection and separation of the line, marring the lip repair. The Logan bow serves to hold a narrow strip of fine mesh gauze over the suture line. This material is constantly moistened with normal saline until all sutures are removed, thereby preventing crust formation. The gauze is removed before feeding, and a new strip is applied after feeding so that it does not lie on the suture line saturated with milk. The tapes which hold the Logan bow must be kept clean and dry.

Parents need to be taught how to feed with the medicine dropper because this feeding method will be required at home. It may be beneficial to demonstrate the technique preoperatively when the child is not likely to be fussy and irritable. Suture line care is essential for good cosmetic results, and parents should be instructed in this care.

Nursing Management: Cleft Palate

Closure of the palate is done before speech begins, if possible, because if it is not, the nasal tone due to the open palate may remain even after repair, when normal speech is possible. The palate may require one repair, as in the case of a soft-palate defect, or a two-stage repair, when a severe defect is present. Preoperatively, in addition to basic preparation, bleeding and clotting times are determined as hemorrhage or excess bleeding is a frequent postoperative complication.

Postoperatively, the child is placed on his abdomen or side to facilitate the drainage of mucus and blood. He must be observed closely for signs and symptoms of hemorrhage. Mist tents are used to humidify the environment and prevent drying of the mucous membranes. The child must be monitored for signs of respiratory distress because mucus, blood clots, and surgical packs can cause airway obstruction. Since the child is older than one who has had surgery for cleft lip, he is more active and aware of his pain and restraints. Analgesics are given as prescribed to relieve the child's discomfort.

After the first day, the child may be up with elbow restraints in place. Techniques which make feeding more enjoyable are utilized. Paper cups are used. Straws, plastic cups or glasses, and eating utensils are never used because they may harm or even perforate the suture line. Sterile water rinses are done after feedings. The infant resumes a full diet in 3 to 4 weeks. Closure of the palate is more difficult and subject to more strain and infection than is closure of cleft lip.

Elbow restraints will be required after the child is discharged, and parents must know the reason for this measure. The child must be prevented from putting any objects in his mouth. Activities involving sucking and/or blowing are not permitted because injury to the operative site can result.

Even after cleft palate repair, long-term care and follow-up for associated problems are essential. Almost without exception, the palatal defect crosses the alveolar ridge and interferes with tooth formation in that area. Orthodontic care is required to realign malpositioned teeth and to provide prosthetic devices for missing teeth.

Speech development may be severely hindered by palatal defects. The palatal and pharyngeal muscles may not function adequately enough to foster proper speech and word pronunciation even after repair. Speech therapy helps these children overcome the nasal tone and remedy speech problems.

Otitis media is a common recurrent problem which can lead to hearing impairment. The coexistence of otitis media with speech impairment puts these children at a disadvantage in relation to communication. Audiological examinations are done annually or more often if the child exhibits signs of decreased hearing acuity. Tubes may be inserted in the tympanic membranes if otitis media persists and results in accumulation of fluid. Children with cleft palates require years of follow-up care. Revisions of lip repair, nasal correction, or the velopharyngeal flap may need to be done when the child is of school age. Since several disciplines are involved, parents may feel bewildered and confused as to whom to ask for information and direction. Nurses play a central role in providing information and guidance to families. The child's psychosocial adjustment depends to a large extent on parental acceptance and support. The rehabilitation phase of cleft palate repair necessitates cooperation and communication among disciplines if the child and family are to derive the benefits of an interdisciplinary approach.

Gastrointestinal Problems in Infancy

Diarrhea and Gastroenteritis

Diarrhea is one of the symptoms most frequently seen in pediatrics. It is a disturbance in intestinal motility and absorption, interfering with water and electrolyte absorption and accelerating the excretion of intestinal contents. The most important criteria for identification are an increase in frequency of stooling, a change in consistency (watery), and the appearance of green-colored stools. Diarrhea may be a primary disease entity or an associated symptom of another disease (Table 26-2). The majority of diarrhea conditions are classified as infectious. The incidence of all infectious diarrheas is affected by health, nutrition, hygiene, climate, and seasonal variation.

Acute nonspecific gastroenteritis or viral gastroenteritis is highly contagious and may be widespread. Often, since the disease is brief, self-limiting, and mild, the causative agent is presumed to be viral and the virus is not actually identified by laboratory methods. Onset is sudden, usually beginning with vomiting for 6 to 24 hours, accom-

TABLE 26-2 Causes of Diarrhea in Children

Acute Diarrhea	Chronic Diarrhea
Otherwise well child	Otherwise well child
Antibiotics	Carbohydrate intolerance
Contaminated foodstuffs	Dietary indiscretions
Dietary indiscretions	Irritable colon syndrome
Parasites	Milk protein allergy
Poisons	Parasites
	Polyposis
Sick child	
Enteral	Sick child (not thriving)
Appendicitis	Abetalipoproteinemia
Bacterial gastroenteritis	Acrodermatitis
Carbohydrate intolerance	enteropathica
Hirschsprung's disease	Carbohydrate intolerance
Inflammatory bowel	Carcinoid tumors
disease	Celiac disease
Milk protein allergy	Chronic pancreatitis
Nonspecific gastroenteritis	Cystic fibrosis
(viral)	Enterokinase deficiency
Necrotizing enterocolitis	Exocrine pancreatic
Pseudomembranous	hypoplasia
enterocolitis	Familial chloride diarrhea
	Ganglioneuroma
Parenteral	Hyperthyroidism
Upper respiratory tract	Immune deficiencies
infection (otitis media)	Inflammatory bowel disease
Urinary tract infection	Lymphangiectasis
	Maternal deprivation
	Polyposis
	Protein calorie malnutrition
	Short bowel syndrome
	Stagnant loop syndrome
	Whipple's disease
	Zollinger-Ellison syndrome

panied by fever. Diarrhea, which follows, lasts 3 to 10 days, often producing a distended abdomen, crampy severe abdominal pain, and increased bowel sounds. Symptomatic treatment is usually all that is necessary in this type of diarrhea.

When diarrhea occurs in infants, the gram-negative bacteria *Escherichia coli* is suspected immediately as the causative agent. Attacks are sporadic and often are identified with frequent, rapid-spread outbreaks of diarrhea in newborn nurseries and in infant areas of institutions.

The organism grows in the entire intestinal tract, and diagnosis is made by stool culture. The onset may be gradual or sudden—the latter is usually more severe. Infants with mild disease may have green, liquid diarrhea with fever and irritability for only a few days. In the majority of cases, projectile vomiting and explosive, green liquid diarrhea are the presenting symptoms. Abdominal distention is marked. Because of the rapid loss of fluid into the gastrointestinal tract, the infant may be very ill, displaying the following signs of dehydration and acid-base imbalance: high fever, rapid and shallow breathing, hollow eyes, and a depressed fontanel. The length of the illness depends on the promptness of treatment, but it may linger for weeks.

The disease is carrier-passed, and prevention is extremely important. In newborn nurseries or pediatric infant areas control measures must be implemented immediately and should include (1) isolation of an infant with diarrhea or a history of diarrhea followed by stool culture, (2) observation of other children as symptoms occur, and (3) strict hand washing techniques and special handling of diapers, stool, food, and formulas. Such procedures need to be in effect until stool cultures are negative.

Bacterial gastroenteritis caused by *Salmonella* or *Shigella* organisms occurs sporadically or in epidemics. It is a mild, self-limiting disease affecting children under 5 years of age. The most common mode of transmission is food, especially eggs, meat, shellfish, and milk. During preparation, one contaminated food may infect another. The food itself may be contaminated, initially by the handler in a meat-packing plant, canning factory, poultry plant, restaurant, home, or institution kitchen. Direct transmission can occur from household pets such as dogs, cats, turtles, and parakeets. *Salmonella* organisms have been found in water traps, air, and dust.

The mucosa of the stomach and small intestine is inflamed and edematous. *Peyer's patches* show edema and superficial ulceration. Gastroenteritis begins with vomiting, fever, and diarrhea, the latter being watery, with large amounts of pus and mucus. There may be nausea with severe abdominal pain. Symptoms are gone in several days. Salmonellosis and shigellosis are diseases reportable to the health department. Household contacts must be investigated because of its frequency in other family members. Younger children are especially vulnerable. A carrier—one who has been asymptomatic or has recovered from the disease—still excretes microorganisms for 3 to 4 weeks or as long as 2 months. Teaching the family about stool handling, food handling, and common modes of transmission must be thorough and immediate. Stool cultures and medical examinations should be done conscientiously at intervals.

With the *Shigella* bacterium responsible for shigellosis or bacillary dysentery, the clinical picture for transmission, manifestations, incidence, and control is identical to that of salmonellosis. Shigallae can be transmitted by carrier flies as well as the modes already mentioned. The incidence is higher in warm months and in warm climates. One strain of *Shigella* is neurotoxic, and others produce endotoxins which have neurotoxic activity. Therefore, a child with even milder disease may have convulsions, and meningismus may be present. Convalescence is longer than that for salmonellosis. A picture of low fever, intermittent diarrhea, and failure to thrive may last for weeks.

Nursing Management

Once the child's status deteriorates rapidly, the most immediate need is replacement of fluid and electrolyte losses. The patient is not given anything to eat in order to rest the bowel. Readiness for oral fluids is determined by a decrease in the number of stools or progress toward firmer consistency. The baby is given clear fluids initially, usually in satisfying amounts.

An oral electrolyte solution (Pedialyte) may be used to replace loss and to maintain electrolyte balance even if diarrhea has not subsided. With improvement, the infant is advanced to half-strength formula and then full strength over a period of 1 to 3 days in most cases. The physician may choose to use a *BRAT* diet, the letters standing for *b*ananas (fresh), *r*ice cereal, *a*pplesauce (canned), and *t*oast. It is nonirritating to the bowel and is used if diarrhea continues sporadically. A soy formula is the choice for several weeks after diarrhea to avoid reactions to milk proteins. In a young baby or one with severe diarrhea, a lactose-free formula is ordered to avoid disaccharide intolerance, which is sometimes present temporarily. Older children are given full fluids and then return to a full diet within a few days.

Medications are not usually prescribed because they mask symptoms. A short-term course of cholestyramine has proved successful in controlling persistent or chronic diarrhea, used with a lactose-free, hypoallergenic diet. The drug is capable of binding cathartic bile acids and endotoxins.

Parenteral fluids are required in the majority of hospitalized infants. Because of a reduction in plasma volume secondary to water and electrolyte loss, the child may exhibit signs of shock. Normal saline or a balanced lactate solution is given intravenously to correct volume. The rate and composition are changed so as to maintain normal hydration and correct the electrolyte deficit (based on an estimate of weight loss). If the child is in severe acidosis, sodium bicarbonate is given initially.

Some commonly used parenteral solutions are listed in

TABLE 26-3 Composition of Parenteral and Oral Solutions

Solution	Na^+, meq/liter	K^+, meq/liter	Cl^-, meq/liter
0.9% NaCl and water	154	—	154
0.33% NaCl and water	56	—	56
3% NaCl and water	513	—	513
Lactated solution			
Ringer's and water	130	4	109
D5W.45NS	77	—	77
Ringer's Solution	147.5	4	156
Pedialyte (oral)	30	20	30
Lytren (oral)	50	20	30

Table 26-3. The degree of dehydration and the signs and symptoms accompanying the level of dehydration are given in Table 26-4.

Nursing observations must be accurate when monitoring infants with fluid and electrolyte loss. The baby should be weighed daily or twice daily in severe cases. Additional fluid loss is determined by weighing the infant's vomitus and used diapers. Labstix, guaiac test, and Clinitest tablets on stools provide further data on the status of the patient.

Isolation should be instituted for all cases of bacterially caused diarrhea. The family needs to be taught the necessary hospital measures for isolation, especially of the stool.

Recovery, even in a severely ill baby, is rapid and is evident in his behavior. The baby or child becomes active, alert, and playful, and his appetite returns.

Intractable Diarrhea

A puzzling, irreversible, self-perpetuating diarrhea develops in some infants beginning soon after birth. The onset may be gradual or rapid. The mortality rate is high, and often the child deteriorates despite hospital treatment. Repeated negative stool cultures and diarrhea of more than 2 weeks' duration point to the diagnosis.

The pathology is that of widespread inflammation and necrosis of intestinal mucosa the entire length of the bowel, with thinning (rather than the more common inflammatory reaction of thickening) of the bowel wall. It may appear secondary to any one of the causes of diarrhea noted in Table 26-2. Screening studies include abdominal x-rays; barium enema x-ray; blood, urine, and stool cultures; stool test for ova and parasites; a sweat test, blood smear; stool fat absorption, serum electrophoresis, and blood acid-base tests; elimination of cow's milk from the diet; repeated testing of stool for pH and reducing substance (to rule out disaccharide intolerance); and repeated guaiac tests for blood.

The child may have other gastrointestinal signs such as vomiting and abdominal distention. A continuous untreated condition results in shock and death. The baby has malnutrition with continued weight loss. Treatment consists of a long period of rest for the bowel until normal functioning resumes with accompanying supportive measures. Immediate restoration of fluid and electrolyte losses and acid-base balance by intravenous fluids and drugs are essential. Albumin, plasma, and whole blood are given intermittently. Hyperalimentation makes it possible to maintain the baby nutritionally when no oral fluids or feedings are allowed and cautiously to resume feedings tailored to the infant's daily response (levels of diarrhea and vomiting). Oral feedings begin with glucose water and progress through one-fourth, one-half, and three-fourths strength of lactose-free formula, with each strength given for a period of up to a week or more. At times the diet must be lowered one "step" in strength if the baby's symptoms recur. If these symptoms persist intermittently, a carbohydrate-free formula may be used with specifically ordered and gradually advanced carbohydrate. Oral feedings other than formula are contraindicated until complete intestinal

TABLE 26-4 Assessment of Dehydration

Mild dehydration
 Infants, 5% loss (50 ml/kg)
  Decreased skin turgor
  Dry mucous membranes
  Pallor
  Slight oliguria
  Normal blood pressure
  Normal or slightly increased pulse
 Children, 3% loss (30 ml/kg)
  Decreased skin turgor
  Dry mucous membranes
  Pallor
  Slight oliguria
  Normal blood pressure
  Normal or slightly increased pulse

Moderate dehydration
 Infants, 10% loss (100 ml/kg)
  Moderately decreased skin turgor
  Very dry mucous membranes
  Gray color to skin
  Oliguria
  Normal or slightly decreased blood pressure
  Tachycardia
  Depressed anterior fontanel
  Cool extremities
 Children, 6% loss (60 ml/kg)
  Moderately decreased skin turgor
  Very dry mucous membranes
  Gray color to skin
  Oliguria
  Normal or slightly decreased blood pressure
  Tachycardia
  Cool extremities

Severe dehydration
 Infants, 15% loss (150 ml/kg)
  Cyanosis or mottling
  Oliguria and azotemia
  Sunken eyeballs
  Decreased blood pressure
  Pronounced tachycardia
  Shocklike symptoms
 Children, 9% loss (90 ml/kg)
  Cyanosis or mottling
  Oliguria and azotemia
  Sunken eyeballs
  Decreased blood pressure
  Pronounced tachycardia
  Shocklike symptoms

recovery is ensured. The course of treatment often becomes erratic owing to the baby's unpredictable response. Antibiotics and gastrointestinal drugs are not used routinely, with the exception of cholestyramine.

Nursing Management

Nursing responsibility focuses on the prevention of physical and emotional deprivation. Care is directed toward (1) conserving the baby's energy (schedules, rest, stable environmental temperature), (2) preventing fractures, contractures, hemorrhage, and bruising, (3) providing hu-

NURSING CARE PLAN

26-1 *The Child with Diarrhea*

Clinical Problem/Nursing Diagnosis	Expected Outcome	Nursing Interventions
Fever Hyperthermia (axillary temperature > 38.5°C) related to infection	Given appropriate antibiotics and/or antipyretics, child will attain normothermia as evidenced by axillary temperature of 37°C	Monitor vital signs with temperature measurements q 1 h while febrile Obtain stools for culture; send stool for ova and parasites Administer antibiotic therapy as ordered for bacterial infections (salmonella and shigella) Administer antipyretics as ordered; evaluate effects on control of fever; document child's response
Frequent loose watery stools with associated vomiting Fluid volume deficit and electrolyte imbalance related to gastric losses	Given appropriate nursing care, child will experience restoration of fluid and electrolyte balance, cessation of diarrhea, and normalization of bowel patterns	Accurately assess stool output (volume, color, frequency, and consistency); guaiac stools for presence of heme and clinitest stools for presence of sugar; observe stool for mucus and pus Accurately assess urine output (volume, pH, protein, glucose, blood, and specific gravity) Obtain accurate daily weights to monitor child's fluid status Monitor intake and output volumes Assess hydration status (sunken fontanel, moisture of mucus membranes, sunken eyeballs, presence of tears, and skin turgor); monitor urine specific gravity with every void Monitor electrolyte (Na^+, K^+, and Cl^-) values; promptly report and correct evidence of acidosis or electrolyte imbalances While child is NPO perform mouth care Administer intravenous fluids with electrolyte replacement calculated for gastric losses as ordered; assess placement, patency and site of intravenous catheter Gradually advance diet as stool consistency improves and stool frequency decreases; administer fluids PO beginning with pediatric glucose/electrolyte solutions, gradually advance with diluted formula, then full-strength formula, and gradually introduce age-appropriate "BRAT" diet (Banana, Rice cereal, Applesauce, Toast)
Weight loss and malnutrition Altered nutrition: less than body requirements related to diarrhea	Through adequate nutritional intake, child will receive caloric requirements appropriate for promotion of growth and development	Enforce bowel-rest regimen as outlined above; gradually advance diet Obtain accurate daily weights; monitor food intake; document calorie counts Assess and document amount, frequency, color, odor, character, and consistency of stools in response to feeding While child is NPO, provide pacifier to encourage sucking and perform mouth care Consult physician and nutritionist to evaluate caloric needs and source of intake (hyperalimentation) Prepare child and family for diagnostic tests (upper GI, barium enema, and bowel biopsy) to assess presence of bowel disease Support child and family through all aspects of care
Red, excoriated buttocks Impaired skin integrity related to irritation from frequent loose, watery stool	Child will experience alleviation of skin irritation as evidenced by decreased redness and excoriation and prevention of skin breakdown	Frequently change child's diaper; keep skin clean and dry Wash skin with mild soap; dry skin thoroughly and avoid vigorous rubbing Avoid taking rectal temperatures Apply nonirritating cream to affected areas (petrolatum) Keep buttocks open to air for periods of time Monitor vital signs; observe for tachycardia, hypotension, and fever
Systemic infection Potential for infection related to bacterial invasion	The child will remain free of systemic infection through early detection and prompt treatment of focal infection	Assess neurological status; look for changes in behavior Assess for signs of decreased peripheral perfusion (cool, mottled extremities and diminished pulses) Assist with blood culture and obtain stool cultures Administer antibiotic therapy as ordered Promptly report signs of sepsis to physician for treatment

Clinical Problem/Nursing Diagnosis	Expected Outcome	Nursing Interventions
Infectious loose watery stools Potential for infection (transmission) related to infectious diarrhea	Through enteric isolation and enforcement of strict handwashing, the child will be protected from secondary infection and from transmitting diarrhea to others	Maintain enteric isolation procedures; enforce strict hand washing practices; dispose of linen, food, and supplies properly; teach parents importance of hand washing even after child is asymptomatic (shigella may be shed in stool for significant period of time)

man and sensory stimulation, (4) observing for neurological defects and signs of fatty acid deficiency, and (5) decreasing the possibility of infection.

A major area of nursing care is monitoring the baby's condition by use of the stool tests mentioned above and careful output measurement in addition to routine nursing procedures and astute observation. The nurse can prevent later complications in the feeding and developmental areas by providing stimulation and human contact essential to the baby's well-being. Otherwise the infant becomes inactive and withdrawn, loses the ability to make eye contact, and stops cooing or smiling. Without nursing intervention, the child spends most of the time "curled in a ball," sucking voraciously on his fingers. When oral feeding is resumed, it is extremely difficult to entice him to suck on a nipple because he prefers the fingers.

There are several other *causes* of diarrhea of which a nurse should be cognizant. Staphylococcal food poisoning causes symptoms similar to infectious diarrhea; however, it is self-limiting. Diarrhea may also occur as a response to several antibiotics. Malnutrition may lead to altered mucosa, abnormal motility, changed bacterial flora, defective disaccharidase activity, and ultimately diarrhea. Dietary diarrhea may occur from overfeeding, a change in the composition of a baby's formula, a transition from breast to bottle feeding, the introduction of new foods, and in older children the ingestion of spices or irritating foods. In allergic diarrhea, the incitant may be milk protein or lactose.

Hirschsprung's Disease

Also termed *megacolon* or *aganglionosis* of the large intestine, Hirschsprung's disease is identified and treated in infancy. It appears more frequently in males than in females. The aganglionic segment is most frequently located in the rectosigmoid area.

The specific defect of Hirschsprung's disease is a congenital absence of the parasympathetic nerve ganglion cells in the mesenteric plexus of the distal bowel. Affected bowel is unable to transmit coordinated peristaltic waves and to pass fecal material along its length. The *normal* portion of intestine proximal to it becomes hypertrophied and greatly dilated (megacolon) from the effect of peristalsis and the fecal mass which accumulates. The fecal mass impedes reabsorption of water and essential minerals through the colonic mucosa.

The usual presence of a transition area containing normally and abnormally innervated areas between the dilated bowel and the unused, narrow bowel creates a *conical* or funnel-shaped appearance, a diagnostic sign of the disease (Fig. 26-7). The transitional segment is often narrow, uneven, or "patchy," skipping areas of bowel. Defecation is controlled by the parasympathetic nervous system, to which the internal and external sphincters, the anus, and the lower colon respond in a coordinated manner.

In the neonate, delay in the passage of meconium or the signs of intestinal obstruction are primary clinical manifestations. In older infants, who constitute a majority of cases, the initial symptom is *obstinate constipation*. Intermittent, progressively increasing abdominal distention is present, and large fecal masses may be palpated. The undiagnosed older infant has anorexia, malnutrition (due to protein-losing enteropathy), muscle wasting, nausea, and lethargy. The abdomen is protuberant, and bowel movements are infrequent. The foul odor of breath and stool is striking. The presence of diarrhea may indicate enterocolitis and a rapidly worsening condition, accompanied by dehydration and electrolyte imbalance.

Barium enemas and abdominal x-rays are done before treatment is initiated. A definitive diagnosis requires a full-thickness rectal biopsy.

A temporary colostomy is the initial treatment for most children with Hirschsprung's disease. It serves to deflate and clean the bowel prior to other procedures and avoids the development of enterocolitis. In older, newly

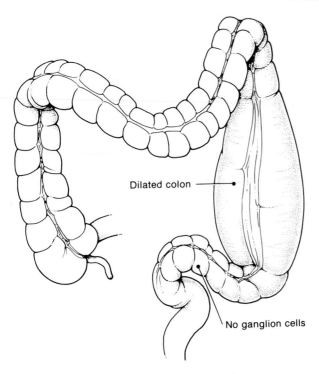

FIGURE 26-7   The affected bowel in Hirschsprung's disease.

diagnosed children, a delay in the operation allows their nutritional and general health status to improve. The major corrective procedures optimally are done when the child is at least 6 months old. Frozen-section biopsy at the colostomy site and in selected areas of the colon is done to gain more accurate knowledge about the extent of the problem. Prior to the colostomy procedure, the child receives stool softeners, liquid diet, and neomycin by mouth and instillation rectally. Removal of stool is done manually and by colonic irrigations. Basically, each of the major definitive operations consists of dissection of the dilated (not functional) bowel and the segment of aganglionic bowel and then anastomosis.

Nursing Management
Rehydration and the improvement of nutrition, although based on the physician's orders, are largely functions of nursing persistence preoperatively and postoperatively. After diagnosis of Hirschsprung's disease, intravenous fluids may be administered. These fluids are continued postoperatively until the operative area and/or bowel are ready for feedings, a few days after colostomy and 10 days or more after a pull-through procedure. Gastric decompression by nasogastric tube is done postoperatively. The replacement of electrolytes in the fluid is always necessary because of the loss due to intestinal dysfunction and vomiting.

Prior to pull-through procedures, the infant is put on a clear liquid diet and the bowel is prepared by means of colonic irrigations to which neomycin or another medication is added to decrease intestinal flora. Postoperatively,

a nasogastric tube is used for decompression. Intravenous therapy with electrolyte additives is required for several days. The anal area must be kept clean and dry to promote the infant's overall comfort. It is not unusual for small amounts of bloody drainage or mucus to be eliminated.

Liquid stools resume approximately 4 to 5 days after surgery. The nurse carefully must record the number, frequency, and characteristics of stools. Fluid and electrolyte losses can be high because of frequent liquid stools, and intravenous replacement therapy may be necessary.

The child may be irritable and fussy owing to discomfort, immobilization, and the numerous tubes. The nurse should spend time holding him and encourage parents to do the same. Deprivation of oral feedings contributes to his discomfort. Pacifiers for infants are not encouraged as they can produce abdominal distention from swallowed air.

Sudden abdominal distention, irritability, and fever may indicate anastomotic disruption or leakage. The child must be monitored for these complications. Intermittent distention may occur as a result of the child's inability to evacuate. A rectal tube may be inserted carefully to relieve this problem.

A clear liquid diet is given initially and advanced gradually according to the child's individual tolerance. Nursing observations during this time focus on any difficulties with elimination, abdominal distention, and the child's behavior during feeding. A primary area of concern is reestablishment of normal elimination. Accurate descriptions of early stools or alterations are important in determining whether the child is progressing toward formed stools. Testing for the presence of sugar and blood are continued until stools are considered normal. If diarrhea develops, the precipitating food is eliminated from the diet temporarily.

Parents may be concerned about toilet training and whether continence will be attained. Most children achieve bowel control. The nurse should instruct the parents to approach toilet training in a relaxed manner to facilitate the child's mastery of this task. If anal dilatations are required at home, the nurse must instruct parents in this procedure.

Intussusception
Intussusception is the invagination or telescoping of a portion of the small intestine (usually the terminal ileum and colon are involved) or colon into a more distal segment (Fig. 26-8). It is rare in infants under 6 months of age and occurs equally in infants between 6 and 12 months and children between 1 and 2 years of age. If affects white males most frequently.

The onset is sudden in an otherwise healthy child. The symptoms are vomiting, paroxysmal colicky abdominal pain, and stools which resemble "currant jelly" (brown, bloody, mucoid material). The infant responds to the pain by loud, shrill crying, paleness, and pulling his legs up sharply. A sausage-shaped mass along the course of the ascending or transverse colon can be palpated, and an x-ray of the abdomen confirms the diagnosis. The cause is unknown, but it may be related to disturbances in intestinal motility such as cystic fibrosis, infection, and recent abdominal surgery or injury.

Nursing Management

A barium enema is used to reduce the telescoped bowel by hydrostatic pressure. It cannot be used if bowel perforation has occured or if signs and symptoms of peritonitis are present. If the barium enema is successful, normal feedings are resumed within 24 hours and the infant is discharged within 48 hours. However, he must be observed during this period of hospitalization for signs of recurrence.

Surgery is indicated when the barium enema is unsuccessful or when small bowel obstruction is evident. The invaginated intestine is reduced manually by the surgeon. Intestinal resection is necessary only if irreparable damage is evident. Pre- and postoperatively, the nurse is responsible for managing gastric decompression and intravenous fluids. The child is positioned to prevent strain on the suture line. Feedings are resumed when peristalsis returns.

Pyloric Stenosis

This condition occurs predominantly in male infants, particularly the firstborn. The incidence is high in the offspring of mothers who had the problem as infants. Vomit-

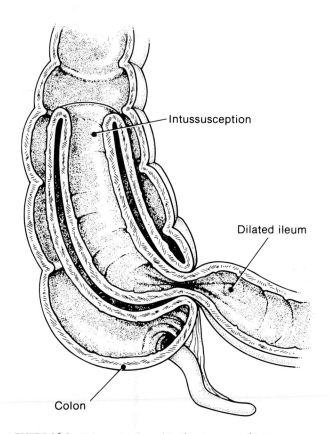

FIGURE 26-8   Telescoping bowel in the presence of intussusception.

ing begins soon after birth or in the following 3 to 4 weeks. It may be gradual and intermittent or sudden and severe. The vomiting becomes projectile in nature, it occurs generally within 30 minutes after feeding, and the infant will eagerly suck, even after vomiting.

Peristaltic waves passing from left to right are visible during or immediately after feeding. In the majority of cases, the hypertrophied pylorus can be palpated in the upper right quadrant as an olive-sized mass. Dehydration, malnutrition with weight loss, and alkalosis can result if the vomiting is not treated. A conclusive diagnosis is made by barium x-ray, which demonstrates gastric retention with an elongated and narrow pylorus.

The definitive treatment for pyloric stenosis is the Fredet-Ramstedt operation. The procedure is done immediately if the infant is well hydrated and in electrolyte balance. Intravenous fluids and often gastric decompression are begun prior to surgery and continued for 1 or 2 days postoperatively. In moderate to severe cases, preoperative treatment also includes monitoring blood gas and blood electrolyte levels at 4- to 8-hour intervals until the infant's condition is stable enough for surgery. After surgery, oral feedings are introduced slowly, beginning with 5% glucose and water. After progression from quarter strength to full-strength formula, amounts are increased every few feedings up to a normal amount for age. Some vomiting may occur postoperatively.

Nursing Management

Pre- and postoperative nursing emphasis should be on careful control of intravenous fluids, gastric decompression, and observations of the baby's response to treatment. Besides aspiration pneumonia, hypoglycemia is an emergency postoperative complication caused by a depletion of hepatic glycogen preoperatively. However, a major nursing responsibility involves reinstitution of oral feedings. A nurse's observations help the physician determine the baby's readiness for increases in the amount and strength of feedings. The nurse should burp the baby frequently, and the nipple selected for use should not allow the flow of milk to be too fast. Positioning after feeding is not a major factor in retention of the formula.

Since the mother may have become negatively conditioned to the baby's constant vomiting, she is hesitant and nervous about feeding him, which may contribute to a higher postoperative incidence of vomiting. It is important that she participate in feeding the infant in order to become more comfortable in her caretaking ability.

Anal Fissure

Anal fissure, a common acquired lesion in infants and children up to 2 years of age, is a frequent cause of constipation and/or rectal bleeding. It is variously described as a cut, tear, slit, or crack at the mucocutaneous line of the anus. It may be secondary to vigorous cleansing of the anal area, constipation, persistent diarrhea, or some type of perianal condition such as oxyuriasis. The infant may experience pain on defecation and subsequently refuse to defecate. Occasionally, bright red blood is noted on the stool surface, or the parent may report bleeding after defecation. In an ambulatory setting, whenever the parent states that the infant or toddler is constipated, the primary provider should inspect the anus.

The infant or child is placed on his abdomen. The buttocks and the margins of the anus are gently separated. The lower end of the fissure can usually be visualized. If not, the examiner places a finger cot over the fifth finger, lubricates it, and gently inserts it into the rectum. The mucosal folds are then examined for fissures. To decrease pain on defecation, stool softeners are given until the stools become soft. A lubricant containing a local anesthetic is applied several times a day and is continued for a short time after healing. If the sphincter is tight, parents are taught gentle digital stretching with the use of a finger cot over the fifth finger and adequate lubrication. Sitz baths several times a day may also be helpful. The lesion usually heals in 1 to 2 weeks. Early treatment is important in preventing chronic constipation and acquired megacolon with their psychological problems.

Gastroesophageal Reflux (Chalasia)

Gastroesophageal reflux (GER), which is seen in newborns or very young infants, occurs when the cardiac sphincter of the stomach does not function properly and allows gastric contents back into the esophagus (reflux). The most commonly symptom is excessive vomiting, but recurrent aspiration pneumonia and weight loss also are seen. If the reflux is severe, the gastric acid can erode the distal esophagus and cause bleeding (hematemesis or melana). The reflux mechanism can be confirmed by a barium esophagogram and monitoring of the esophageal pH, which identifies the level of reflux in the lower portion of the esophagus.

In a majority of cases, thickened feedings, given slowly and in small amounts, frequent burping, and remaining in an elevated prone position for an hour or more after feedings result in an improvement. The old position (upright, propped with blankets and pillows) may result in increased intraabdominal pressure; hence, the use of a slant board is being advocated. The desired position is maintained more effectively. Some pediatricians have the infant remain elevated 24 hours a day. A small percentage of infants do not respond to conservative positional treatment and may require surgical intervention. At that time, surgeons create a more efficient cardiac sphincter, which prevents the gastric reflux; the procedure is called a fundoplication.

Nursing Management

It is important to identify these newborns and young infants in order to ensure an adequate nutritional intake, decrease the frequency of these reflux episodes, and help parents deal with what they perceive to be a difficult problem. A nurse needs to thicken the formula to the consistency of a milkshake/frappe, feed slowly, and burp frequently (every 1-1½ ounces). When the slant board is used, the infant's perineal area needs to be examined for pressure areas. They can develop as the baby straddles the padded peg projecting from the board, thereby maintaining proper position. These infants must be assessed for edema of the hands and feet, which can be avoided by exercising the extremities and raising as well as lowering the board between feedings. With the baby restrained on the slant board, his head needs to be turned from side to side to prevent torticollis. Attention also needs to be given to age appropriate developmental activities. Toys should be placed at eye level. These babies need to be cuddled and caressed while positioned on the board.

If vomiting occurs, the type and character as well as the time at which it occurs need to be recorded. It is most important to keep an accurate intake and output. Occasionally, the physician may write an order to refeed the infant after vomiting; however, it depends on the volume vomited.

An infant who is irritable and is crying, vomiting, and sucking on his fists may lead his parents to question their abilities to care for someone totally dependent on them. They are frustrated by the bouts of vomiting and may feel guilty about the baby's weight loss. They need to be reassured and supported during this interval. Getting them involved in feeding and caring for the infant with the nurse as role model and supervisor can result in more effective parenting skills and coping patterns.

Biliary Atresia

Atresia of the bile ducts may be the result of fetal malformations and an extensive inflammatory process or an underlying metabolic defect. The bile ducts fail to develop completely, are ribbonlike and unopened, or end in a blind pouch. Bile builds up in the liver because it lacks a passageway to the intestines. The incidence of biliary atresia is higher in females than in males and is rare in preterm infants.

Jaundice in the neonatal period, which becomes progressively worse, is the primary symptom. Initially the direct bilirubin level may not be abnormal, but it becomes elevated as the problem persists. The infant's stools are white or clay-colored, and the urine is extremely dark owing to the presence of bile salts and bilirubin. Hepatomegaly is present and progresses. Splenomegaly develops later. In early stages, the infant appears healthy and content despite his jaundice. After 6 months of age, irritability, cachexia, and lethargy are manifested.

An exploratory laparotomy with a liver biopsy and cholangiography at the time of operation confirms the diagnosis and differentiates biliary atresia from neonatal hepatitis. The Kasai procedure, or *hepatic portoenterostomy,* an anastomosis of the end of the duct to a section of jejunum, relieves the jaundice and offers an extension of life for these infants. When no evidence of patent ductular strictures can be found, treatment is supportive. Repeated episodes of ascending cholangitis remain the most persistent complication following the anastomosis. It develops as a result of intestinal secretions refluxing into

26-2 *The Child with Gastroesophageal Reflux (GER)*

Clinical Problem/Nursing Diagnosis	Expected Outcome	Nursing Interventions
Poor weight gain and malnutrition Vomiting ———— Altered nutrition less than body requirements related to vomiting and/or reflux	Through proper positioning during and after feedings and through thickened feedings, the child will receive adequate nutritional intake to promote growth and development	Assess and document tolerance of feedings; timing of emesis in relation to feeding and type of vomiting (projectile, nonprojectile); observe amount, color, and consistency of emesis Monitor trends in daily weights; obtain baseline data and plot on graph Thicken feedings with rice cereal provide small frequent amounts (q 2-3 h) Maintain upright position during feedings; prone on slant board elevated, 30° after feedings Administer cholinergic drugs 20 to 30 min *before* feedings Prepare parents for diagnostic studies (barium swallow, manometry, and esophagoscopy) Prepare infant and parents for possible surgical intervention (fundoplication)
Aspiration ———— Potential for injury related to aspiration of gastric contents causing respiratory compromise	Through appropriate nursing care, the child will maintain a patent airway, as evidenced by either prevention of aspiration or minimization of effects of aspiration	Provide small *thickened* feedings of formula Maintain upright positioning during feedings and 30° after feedings; promote quiet, restful environment immediately after feedings Assess respiratory status; note presence of tachypnea, labored respirations, retractions, flaring nostrils, and color changes Auscultate breath sounds for quality and equality of aerations; note presence of crackles and diminished breath sounds (note past history in regard to chronic cough, frequent respiratory infections, pneumonia, wheezing and asthma symptoms) Administer humidified oxygen as needed Administer vigorous physical therapy (q 2 h) (facilitate removal of secretions with nasopharyngeal or bulb sunctioning) Prepare and support infant and parents through diagnostic studies (chest x-ray and arterial blood gases) Promote adequate periods of uninterrupted rest Administer antibiotics as ordered
Reflux of gastric contents Irritation of mucosal lining of esophagus: upper abdominal pain and/or burning bleeding ———— Pain related to esophageal irritation; reflux of gastric contents	Through appropriate observations and interventions, the child will experience alleviation of discomfort related to esophagitis	Assess child for increased irritability during feeding and decreased interest in feeding Note reports of upper abdominal pain or burning discomfort from older children Identify successful comfort measures; record in Kardex Monitor for hematemesis, blood in stool, and guaiac emesis and/or stool Administer antacids as ordered Monitor complete blood count, HgB, and hematocrit values; admininster blood replacement with severe loss as ordered Prepare parents and child for esophagoscopy to determine cause of pain and bleeding
Apneic episodes and bradycardia ———— Ineffective breathing pattern and/or heart rate related to reflux of gastric content	Through control of gastroesophageal reflux, child will have decreased episodes of apnea and bradycardia	Monitor cardiovascular and respiratory status of infants with apneic episodes; note presence of bradycardia with apnea Document episodes of apnea and bradycardia on bedside chart: note duration and frequency of apnea, degree of bradycardia, stimulation requirements, effects on perfusion, and presence of changes in color Provide supplemental oxygen with frequent apnea and/or bradycardia Prepare child and parents for diagnostic monitoring (apnea testing and thermister study)
Parents request information regarding GER and home care ———— Knowledge deficit related to GER, management, home care, and follow-up care	Parents will verbalize and/or demonstrate understanding of GER, management, home care, and follow-up care	Evaluate need to teach parents caardiopulmonary resuscitation; home monitoring of apnea and bradycardia Develop teaching plan which will inform parents about GER, its management, and potential complications Teach parents to thicken feedings; review positions in which to place child during and after feedings; also suggest bathing and dressing before feedings; adhere to giving cholinergic medications 30 min before feeding; home monitoring of apnea and bradycardia Encourage parents to use methods of promoting growth and development (talking with child; using brightly colored toys, mobiles, musical toys, etc.)

the liver. Cirrhosis and intrahepatic disease develop in most children who have been treated surgically. However, if the diagnosis is made and surgery is performed prior to the second month of age, the prognosis is better. The Kasai procedure does not correct the biliary atresia. The only alternative is liver transplantation. However, this organ is not readily available, and an extremely high rejection rate makes this option an extremely poor one.

Nursing Management

Nursing observation can help greatly in diagnosis. The nurse observes and records the color and consistency of stools, tests them for bile, and may need to save them for examination by the physician or the laboratory. The nurse must bear in mind that the urine's dark pigment can discolor the stool. Preoperatively, the baby is fed orally and maintained on intravenous fluids. Injections of vitamin K are given to prevent excess bleeding.

Postoperatively, nasogastric decompression and intravenous fluids are necessary until feedings are resumed. The risk of pulmonary infection is higher with biliary atresia, and the nurse must reposition the infant frequently and do nasopharyngeal suctioning when needed. Pruritus can be severe in the older infant but should decrease postoperatively. The nurse may need to cover the baby's hands with mittens and keep his fingernails short to prevent scratching and resultant skin excoriation. These infants may be very irritable and uncomfortable. They require extra comfort, holding, and gentleness from the nursing staff.

Children who are not surgical candidates need measures such as vitamins K and D, antihistamines to relieve pruritus, and diuretics for the edema due to hypoproteinemia. This group of affected children usually die by 2 years of age. Ascites, infections, and esophageal varices necessitate repeated hospitalizations.

Surgery is a palliative measure, not a curative one. Parents need to understand this important distinction, and nursing support on a long-term basis is essential.

Gastrointestinal Problems in the Toddler and Preschooler

Foreign Bodies

During the inquisitive years of toddlerhood, children frequently ingest objects which cannot be digested. Pins, parts of toys, coins, and buttons are the items most commonly swallowed. Most objects pass spontaneously from the gastrointestinal tract, but objects which are long or sharp may present serious difficulty. The child should be hospitalized for ingestion of any sharp object.

After ingestion, the child does not necessarily experience dysphagia, although the object remains in the esophagus. The most common areas in the gastrointestinal tract where objects lodge are the esophagus at the cricopharyngeal level, the aortic level, and the upper diaphragmatic area. These objects can be removed easily by esophagoscopy under general anesthesia after being visualized

on chest roentgenogram. After 24 hours of observation, the child is usually discharged.

Foreign bodies in the esophagus may also be removed by means of a Foley catheter, which is inserted into the esophagus to a point below the object. Under fluoroscopy the balloon is inflated and then slowly removed with the foreign body ahead of it. The child is sedated for this procedure, but the risks of general anesthesia are avoided.

If the object lodges in the stomach, the child can be observed for passages. It should pass through the pylorus in 5 days or less. Bobby pins and long objects have particular difficulty passing through the duodenum because of the U shape. Coins and other large objects may remain at the pylorus or the ileocecal valve. The appendix and the rectum are two other common areas of difficult passage. Objects in the rectum are accessible to proctoscopy. The child's stool should be checked carefully during this time. Repeat roentgenograms monitor the passage. Surgical intervention is necessary when perforation has occurred, abdominal pain is present, or the object does not progress along the gastrointestinal tract for a significant period of time.

Nursing Management

Many times, especially since the predominant age group is under 5 years, the hospitalization and procedures are more upsetting than the object itself, a fact that should guide the nurse in caring for these children. Preparation before surgery and care afterward are largely according to the operative procedure, and observation for complications plays an important role. Humidity by croup tent or mask may be needed if esophagoscopy is done. After abdominal surgery, intravenous fluids and nasogastric tube for gastric decompression are used for 1 to 3 days, followed by rapid progression to a normal diet. Resumption of normal activity is fairly rapid. The child's parents often feel guilty, and they need to know that medical personnel do not consider it their fault. Since the child is well to begin with, recovery is fast and complete.

Hernias, Inguinal and Umbilical

An *indirect inguinal hernia* is the most common surgical problem in children, affecting mostly males. About 50 percent occur in infants under 1 year of age, while the remaining 50 percent are seen in children between 1 and 5 years of age. The hernia may be unilateral (the right side is more common) or bilateral. Undescended testicle and/or hydrocele may be accompanying problems. Loops of intestine prolapse through a congenital weakness or lack of closure at the inguinal ring above the scrotal sac. Often, hernias are asymptomatic and are found on a routine examination. The symptoms, if present, are colicky pain at the site, general discomfort, irritability, and slight tenderness of the groin and scrotum.

A hernia becomes strangulated or *incarcerated* when a portion of the intestine becomes so tightly caught in the hernial sac that its blood supply is cut off. Reduction must be done immediately to prevent bowel necrosis. The child is sedated and placed in Trendelenburg's position, and ice is applied to the scrotum. It is then possible to reduce the hernia by gentle manipulation.

Surgery, the treatment of choice, is brief and is done in a "day surgery" unit. Emergency surgery is necessary if the strangulated hernia cannot be reduced or has been present too long. Ideally, it is postponed for 24 to 48 hours until the edema subsides.

When tissue does not close at the umbilicus, *umbilical hernia* occurs as a small bulge or a larger protuberance. It is essentially asymptomatic and rarely incarcerates. The majority close spontaneously, but elective surgery is sometimes performed by 4 to 5 years of age if the hernia persists. Parents are assured that generally as the child begins to use his abdominal muscles more vigorously through crawling and walking, the defect will become smaller and eventually will close.

Nursing Management

Preoperative nursing care of the child with an inguinal hernia is directed toward keeping the infant from straining, as he does when he cries or attempts to pass a constipated or an irritatingly loose stool. Straining may aggravate or induce strangulation; therefore, diet should be geared to regulating stools, and the child should be kept as happy and as quiet as possible. Playing strenuously or crying because he cannot have anything to eat before surgery may precipitate dehydration in the child. Generally, an infant can be allowed clear fluids until approximately 4 hours before surgery, although this practice varies. The nurse must ensure that the infant receives some fluid 4 hours before surgery to prevent dehydration, provided that fluids are not otherwise contraindicated.

Preoperative teaching is directed toward the parents to relieve their anxiety. They should understand that the surgery is far less complicated in the infant than in the adult and that the infant will be awake and playing a few hours after surgery. Postoperatively, the child may have his diet as tolerated and be as active as he desires.

If surgery is performed on a child with an umbilical hernia, a pressure dressing is applied over the operative site. It is most important that the dressing be kept in place as well as be kept dry and clean. The nursing care is otherwise essentially the same as that for inguinal hernia, and recovery is extremely rapid in an otherwise healthy child.

Intestinal Parasites

The intestinal parasites are found commonly in North America, with southern areas having the highest incidence. Preschoolers seem most susceptible to all types, with the exception of pinworms. Fecal contamination of food, soil, water, and hands begins each infestation, although cycles differ with different types. Hospitalization occurs infrequently.

Nematodes (Roundworms)

In general, roundworms cause symptoms of gastroenteritis. *Ascariasis,* which occurs mainly in southern areas, starts with the eggs present in topsoil contaminated with feces. After the eggs are ingested, they hatch in the duodenum. The larvae pass through the intestinal wall into the bloodstream, are carried via the portal system to the liver, are carried to the lungs, and migrate up to the epiglottis. After they are swallowed, they remain and develop into adults in the small intestine, causing colicky and recurrent abdominal pain. The child may eliminate a pencil-size worm in vomitus or stool. Complications are rare but may develop because of the bulk of the roundworm (intestinal obstruction, acute appendicitis, intussusception, or intestinal perforation). Treatment with piperazine citrate daily for 3 days eliminates the parasite.

Oxyuriasis, or pinworm infection, is found most commonly in schoolchildren. After initial infestation, the 2- to 12-mm worm attaches itself to the mucosa of the cecum and appendix. Females migrate at night down the intestine, crawl outside, and deposit their eggs on the perianal area and perineum. Since the most common and persistent symptom is anal pruritus, the eggs are carried back to the mouth, are ingested, hatch in the duodenum, and pass to the cecum. Local perianal infection, vaginitis, and urinary tract infections may accompany infestation. Diagnosis is confirmed by collection of pinworms with the clear cellulose tape method (placing the tape on the perianal area less than a minute, preferably at night or early morning), then examination on a slide covered with toluene under a microscope. All family members must be treated and need to carry out thorough personal hygiene measures. The mother may help the child refrain from scratching by frequent washing of the anal area and using a spray to prevent itching. Pyrvinium pamoate is used in one dose and another dose 2 weeks later, or piperazine citrate is used daily for 7 days and then repeated for 7 days after a week's rest.

Cestodes (Tapeworms)

When human beings ingest meat infected with encysted larvae of the beef tapeworm (*Taenia saginata*) or the pork tapeworm (*T. solium*), they develop *taeniasis.* The ingested larvae hatch in the small intestine, where they attach themselves to the wall. Clinical manifestations are diarrhea, "hunger pain," increased appetite, loss of weight, and eosinophilia. The tapeworms are very long and may cause obstruction if they mass in the intestinal lumen. Segments may break off and obstruct the appendix.

The drug quinacrine is administered either by mouth or by duodenal tube, which gives a greater concentration of the drug in the intestine. Two doses are given 1 hour apart. A saline cathartic follows 2 hours after the last dose. Another drug, niclosamide, in a single dose may be used for treatment of beef tapeworm. Mebendazole is effective against both *T. solium* and *T. saginata.* It is the drug of choice for pediatric patients. It is given twice a day for 4 days, 200 mg per dose. Prevention relies on thorough cooking of meat and adequate sanitation. The nurse's role, especially that of the office nurse, public health nurse, and school nurse, is one of teaching good personal and environmental hygiene, emphasizing the reasons for its importance.

Lye Ingestion and Corrosive Esophagitis

The ingestion of any highly acidic or alkaloid material will cause immediate inflammatory reaction or damage (burns, ulcerations) to the mucosal lining of the upper gastrointestinal tract. Oral and gastric burns are the result of acid ingestion. Alkali ingestion produces esophageal burns.

Nursing Management

Immediate treatment is to neutralize the action of the chemical. Large amounts of water or, preferably, milk are given to dilute the acid or alkali. Forced emesis and gastric lavage are contraindicated. Admission to the hospital is necessary to determine the extent of burns. The child is given pain medication and placed in a humidified tent. Food and fluids are withheld until an esophagostomy can be done. This procedure is performed within 12 to 24 hours. Esophageal burns may be present even though oral burns are absent. If burns are not extensive, antacids are given frequently and regularly. Steroids are used to decrease inflammation and scarring. The length of steroid treatment varies with the severity of the burns but usually covers a 3-week period.

If the child can eat, he is allowed only fluids, clear or full liquid, until inflammation is under control. Then he is advanced to soft, nonabrasive foods or to a normal diet. Bed rest is not necessary. If the child is unable to swallow, he must be positioned so that saliva runs out, and he may need careful suctioning. Soothing ointments and creams may be used on external burns of the mouth.

Dilation is instituted to prevent esophageal stricture as soon as inflammation has subsided. In severe burns, regular dilation may continue for months or years to combat unpreventable stricture. A gastrostomy may be necessary in severe cases. Colon interposition, as used for esophageal atresia, is done when other treatment proves unsuccessful.

In most children, the burns are not extensive and treatment is limited to the immediate treatment with perhaps a short course of dilation. Even in mild cases, the child is frightened, the parents are guilt-ridden and shocked, and both need understanding.

Celiac Disease

Gluten enteropathy, commonly called *celiac disease*, or *sprue*, is a symptom complex resulting from generalized malabsorption. It is most common in children between 9 and 18 months of age. The inability to absorb rye or wheat gluten may be hereditary, or it may result from a constitutional tendency, may be environmentally caused, or both. Theories of the cause range from an enzyme deficiency to an immunologic response to the gliaden fraction of gluten.

The two most common symptoms are diarrhea and failure to thrive. The stools are huge, pale, bulky, foul-smelling, and greasy. They often *float* in water, whereas normal stools sink. The combination of calorie loss from diarrhea and anorexia produces a rapid deceleration in height and weight parameters. The child has a grossly distended abdomen and muscle wasting of the limbs and buttocks, in contrast to a rounded face. Abdominal pain and vomiting are part of the complex in some children. The chronic illness produces an irritable, difficult to handle child. The child may have peripheral edema and finger clubbing due to anemia and hypoproteinemia.

A battery of tests establish the diagnosis. Barium x-ray of the small intestine shows changes in the intestine and mucosa. Bone age is retarded on x-ray or may show deficiency changes.

Stool examination for volume, consistency, and odor, and density is a most important test. Stool cultures, stool smears, and chymotrypsin test on stool are all normal. A 3-day fecal fat collection shows a high degree of fat malabsorption with over 5 g a day of fat eliminated. Liver function tests and sweat test (for cystic fibrosis) are normal. Glucose tolerance and D-xylose tolerance tests show poor absorption because of the overall malabsorptive ability of the bowel. Blood test results include low serum protein, low hemoglobin and serum iron. Definitive diagnosis is made by small intestine biopsy.

Nursing Management

A gluten-free diet is prescribed, and lactose is omitted until repair of the intestinal mucosa takes place. Since the child is severely malnourished and anorexic, small frequent meals are most successful. It is most important for the nurse to create an environment which is pleasant and conducive to eating. Symptomatic treatment may include vitamin injections, iron preparations, and magnesium and calcium gluconate for tetany. Electrolyte imbalances are corrected. In severe disease, corticosteroids are used to hasten mucosal repair.

The chronic illness, irritability, and anorexia present problems for nursing. The nurse must use time, patience, and ingenuity to provide increased calories and protein and to help the child gain the developmental milestones he may lack. In teaching parents, emphasis on the cause of the problem and the need for maintaining the specific diet are imperative issues for successful management.

A gluten-free diet must be maintained for life. Some children, particularly during adolescence, may experience an asymptomatic period while off the diet. However, intestinal mucosa remains abnormal, and adherence to the dietary regimen is advocated.

Gastrointestinal Problems in the School-Age Child and Adolescent

Appendicitis

Inflammation with infection of the vermiform appendix is one of the most common conditions requiring surgery in children from age 2 years and older. It is very common in school-age children and adolescents. Males are affected in higher numbers than are females.

The appendix is a vestigial remnant located on the

cecum just beyond the ileocecal valve and has no recognizable function. The lumen becomes blocked, causing inflammation of the walls of the appendix and stasis of fecal material within, and infection develops. The obstruction is common, usually caused by a fecalith. As the infection progresses, pressure within the appendix may cause perforation. When the appendix ruptures, generalized peritonitis occurs in younger children, and a more localized or walled-off abscess is seen in older children (because of a larger omentum, which aids in preventing spread).

Early recognition prevents rupture and its complications. Pain is *always* present so that any child with abdominal pain is immediately suspected of having appendicitis. The disease may begin with the child's complaint of a "stomachache." The pain is periumbilical, persistent, and progressive and quickly localizes in the right lower quadrant, midway between the umbilicus and the iliac crest (McBurney's point). Pain progresses from tenderness to rebound tenderness. After the onset of pain, nausea and vomiting may be accompanying signs. Fever is mildly increased usually.

An elevated white blood cell count may be present but is not a definitive diagnostic tool. The child may assume a "bent-over" posture while walking or a knee-chest position when in bed. The right thigh may be flexed (psoas sign) to relieve abdominal pain. Abdominal x-rays are not obtained routinely except in infants and small children. Diagnosis of appendicitis in these age groups is difficult, and usually perforation has occurred. X-rays demonstrate an abnormal gas pattern or free peritoneal air or fluid. Infants and small children generally have higher temperatures, have diffuse abdominal tenderness, and appear extremely ill.

NURSING CARE PLAN

26-3 The Child with Appendicitis or Appendectomy

Clinical Problem/Nursing Diagnosis	Expected Outcome	Nursing Interventions
Fear and anxiety Lack of prior experience with hospitalization and surgery Knowledge deficit related to hospitalization, surgery, postoperative and follow-up care	Parents and child will cope effectively, with adequate preparation for hospitalization experiences Parent and child will verbalize and demonstrate understanding of teaching specific to preparation for surgery, postoperative and home care	Identify the child and parents' previous experience with hospitals, surgery, and health care Provide adequate opportunities for parents and child to express fears and concerns Clarify questions and misconceptions Design explanations and/or teaching to child's developmental and cognitive level *Preparation for surgery* Use doll to explain location of appendix and reasons for pain Use therapeutic play with doll to explain need for nasogastric (NG) tube and IV and IM medications Teach child deep breathing exercises (with purpose) and use of incentive spirometry Describe transportation to operating room and appearance of staff (gown, mask, cap) as well as recovery area where child will 'wake up" Reassure child about location of area where parents will wait during operation Advise child that he may take security item, stuffed animal, or toy with him *Postoperatively* Provide opportunities through therapeutic play to work through experiences and fears regarding IV, dressing changes, and injections Read stories that address child's fears of hospitalization to encourage free expression of feelings to help process painful events Provide opportunities for art expression (drawing self in hospital, what he experienced) *Preparation for home care* Review with parents wound site care, signs of infection, and procedure for changing dressing Encourage preparation of well-balanced high-protein diet for wound healing Identify activity levels and project date for returning to school Provide written instructions for home care Arrange follow-up visit to pediatric surgery clinic

Continued.

NURSING CARE PLAN 26-3 The Child with Appendicitis or Appendectomy—cont'd

Clinical Problem/Nursing Diagnosis	Expected Outcome	Nursing Interventions
Fever Hyperthermia (rectal temperature > 38.5°C) related to infection	Child's temperature will remain in normal range (37.0-37.5°C)	Monitor temperature q 2 h while febrile Administer antipyretics as ordered and evaluate effectiveness in controlling child's temperature Support child during blood-drawing procedures and obtaining cultures Administer intravenous antibiotics properly pre- and postoperatively Examine IV site to ensure placement and patency of line
Nausea Vomiting Loss of appetite Altered nutrition: less than body requirements related to infection	Child will experience decrease in nausea, cessation of vomiting, and nutritional intake which promotes wound healing	Monitor color, amount, and consistency of emesis Perform guaiac test on all emesis Administer antiemetics as ordered Assess child for abdominal distention, firmness, and tenderness and perform serial abdominal girths q 4h Ensure patency and placement of NG tube attached to low intermittent suction for stomach and bowel decompression Irrigate NG tube q 2h and record amount instilled and amount removed; use normal saline solution Auscultate abdomen for bowel sounds; note presence of flatus Monitor for bowel movement; record type, color, and amount Admminister clear liquids after removal of NG tube; evaluate child's response; advance diet to full liquids, soft foods, and ultimately a regular high-protein, high-caloric diet
Gastric content losses via NG tube Fluid volume deficit (fluid and electrolyte imbalance) related to pre- and postoperative fluid losses	Child wil return to and maintain fluid and electrolyte balance	Monitor intake and output Assess placement and patency of NG tube Monitor NG drainage for amount, color, and consistency; test for pH and blood; report presence of pH > 5 and blood Replace NG drainage with IV fluids as ordered Assess child's hydration: skin turgor, mucous membranes, and tears Perform specific gravity on urine once per shift Monitor IV rate, solution, and patency according to doctor's orders, especially in correcting any deficiency
Abdominal pain Pain related to infection and surgery	Child will demonstrate pain relief as evidenced by increasing participation in age-appropriate activities	Assess child for peritoneal signs (rigidity, pain in lower right quadrant) Determine character of pain (location and intensity) Observe for events which exaggerate pain (coughing, deep breathing, changing positions) Observe for signs of pain in young children: knee-chest position, splinting and/or guarding abdomen Perform and record measurement of abdominal girth preoperatively *Postoperatively* Monitor abodminal girth q 4-8 h Assess patency and placement of NG tube; function of low, intermittent suction Examine integrity of surgical wound: pain at incision, presence of drainage, erythema Assess child for evidence of pain: guarding, grimacing, increasing irritability, tachycardia, hypertension Acknowledge child may deny presence of pain for fear of injection; use therapeutic play to increase child's understanding of and ability to cope with injections Utilize variety of relaxation techniques: deep breathing, massage, music Administer analgesics as ordered; premedicate for dressing changes, prior to ambulation, deep breathing exercises Evaluate child's response to analgesics to ensure effective pain control

Clinical Problem/Nursing Diagnosis	Expected Outcome	Nursing Interventions
Fever Erythema Purulent drainage from incision	With use of antibiotics and meticulous dressing changes, child's wound will heal without evidence of infection	Assess child's vital signs for alterations (elevated temperature, tachycardia) Examine wound for signs of infection (redness, swelling, pain, presence of purulent drainage with odor); take culture of drainage and send to lab
Potential for infection related to surgical wound		Perform sterile dressing changes as ordered: assess patency of drains present; record type of drainage and amount and color Administer IV antibiotics as ordered and evaluate child's response to treatment Provide diet high in protein and calories to promote wound healing
Child communicates fear of moving, walking, and performing deep breathing exercises	Child's pulmonary function will remain normal	Auscultate breath sounds for quality and equality; note presence of crackles, diminished breath sounds, labored respirations, and elevated temperature; promptly report alterations to physician Premedicate child prior to dressing changes, ambulation, and breathing exercises Evaluate child's response to analgesics
Potential ineffective airway clearance related to fear of pain and decreased mobility		Splint abdomen with pillow and/or hands during incentive spirometry or deep breathing (encourage exercises q 2h) Assist child in ambulation, getting out of bed, etc. Encourage progressive increase in frequency and duration of ambulation Assess child's tolerance of activities

Nursing Management

Appendectomy is the definitive procedure. Preoperatively, the child is allowed nothing to eat or drink. Vomiting may be controlled by a nasogastric tube attached to suction. Lavage of the stomach will be necessary if the child has eaten recently. Narcotics are given for pain, or the preoperative medication for surgery will be pain-relieving if surgery is imminent. The haste of hospitalization and surgery combined with the pain is frightening. Short, simple explanations about what is being done with an opportunity for questions is most reassuring, along with the knowledge that the pain will be eliminated. The parents are often very apprehensive, sometimes out of proportion to the "simple" surgery being done, because they have had no opportunity to prepare themselves and because they often fear there is something more seriously wrong.

Postoperative recovery is rapid and usually trouble-free. Intravenous fluids, gastric decompression, and nothing by mouth are continued until peristalsis is established in 1 to 2 days. The child is usually allowed out of bed soon after surgery or the next day. Diet and activity rapidly return to normal. After discharge, the child may return to school in 1 to 2 weeks. Sports and strenuous activity such as bicycle riding are restricted for several more weeks. Antibiotics are given routinely. Besides general assistance and encouragement in his progression to recovery, nursing observations for the development of abscess or peritonitis are most important. The signs may be vague

and variable, such as irritability, reluctance to move, prolonged complaints of postoperative pain, and poor appetite rather than definite pain, fever, and more apparent illness, which develop later in abscess formation. Therefore, this behavior should be recorded and reported as it is noticed.

If the appendix has ruptured, the child will be sicker and the course of recovery longer. Penrose drains are placed in the incision at the time of surgery to drain the exudate and prevent abscess formation or to drain the abscess if one is present. The child should lie in a semi-Fowler's position so that the exudate collects in the lower abdomen. Frequent positioning on his right side facilitates drainage through the drains. If drainage is successful, the drains will be "advanced" regularly till they can be removed. It is the nurse's responsibility to maintain sterile, dry dressings to prevent further complications and to minimize discomfort and odor.

If an abscess develops, an incision and drainage by laparotomy must be done after it localizes. The Penrose drain procedure must be utilized again, and the physician may order irrigations of the incision, using antibiotic solutions if the infection is persistent. In very severe cases, an abscess develops more than once and requires repetition of the entire course of treatment. During this time, antibiotic therapy with more than one drug by intravenous fluid drip is maintained. The nurse should be aware of the many reasons for the depression and irritability which the child displays. He begins to feel he will never get better; this psychological effect alone requires much patience and support from the nurse.

Chronic Inflammatory Bowel Disease (Ulcerative Colitis)

Ulcerative colitis generally occurs between the ages of 10 and 19 years. Genetic and environmental factors seem to contribute to its development. Frequently other family members have a history of bowel disease as well as rhinitis, asthma, eczema, and other allergies.

Emotional factors may exacerbate ulcerative colitis in some cases. Affected children tend to be dependent and emotionally fragile and to have personality disturbances. This situation is probably due to the chronicity of the disease rather than the psychogenic factors.

Suspicion that an inflammatory bowel disease is present is verified by upper gastrointestinal barium x-ray study and barium enema x-ray. A rectosigmoidoscopy is necessary, with either a mucosal section or full-thickness biopsy. Anemia due to blood loss is present. Decreased serum albumin reflects the presence of chronic inflammation and protein-losing enteropathy. Colon malabsorption in ulcerative colitis causes an abnormal fecal fat test.

Ulcerative colitis may have an insidious onset or an acute one. Attacks may be mild, moderate, or severe. With an insidious onset, arthralgia, arthritis, peripheral edema, clubbing, and chronic malnutrition, may be evident.

Findings on x-ray early in the disease include superficial ulcerations and thickening of the bowel wall. The colon is affected in all cases, generally along with the rectum. Chronic disease is noted by a complete disappearance of haustral markings, shortening of the colon, and thickening of the bowel wall to a degree that a diagnostic feature of the disease is "lead-pipe" colon.

The risk of carcinoma is significantly high in children who have ulcerative colitis before 20 years of age and in patients who have had the disease 10 years or more. The highest risk occurs in those in whom the total colon is involved, and suceptibility increases with the length of the disease. Since these carcinomas are poorly differentiated and metastasize early, the child should receive frequent x-ray and endoscopic examinations.

Nursing Management

Hospitalization during acute exacerbations is necessary if the attack is severe or dehydration and signs of complications occur. The time during hospitalizations can be used by a nurse to help child and family adjust to and understand the illness. Communication between doctor and nurse must be constant to provide consistent information and approach and thus decrease stress.

A high-protein, high-carbohydrate, normal-fat, high-vitamin diet is preferred. If malabsorption is a problem, a lactose-free diet may be used in addition. During acute attacks, the child may need fluid or blood volume replacement. The child is given nothing by mouth if he is vomiting. Hyperalimentation improves the child's nutri-

tional condition and rests the bowel. Small frequent meals, flexibility in times of meals, allowing the child to choose his own foods, and use of appropriate snack or "fun" foods are successful nursing interventions in combating anorexia.

Bed rest is required in acute attacks, although activity is allowed according to the child's ability. Children with ulcerative colitis may engage in normal play and school activities during remissions. They may need encouragement in self-help and in participation in play. The nurse must be alert to opportunities for acceptable amounts of activity and provide a variety of these opportunities. Progress in increasing activity, interest, and participation is never sudden and full but slow and fluctuating.

A number of drugs may be used with many variations in combinations. Antidiarrheal agents, opiates, anticholinergic drugs to reduce rectal spasm, and aspirin for discomfort are supportive drugs. Salicylazosulfapyridine relieves symptoms in acute attacks and is a deterrent to further exacerbations but produces many gastrointestinal side effects, and the dosage must be adjusted. Adrenocorticotropic hormone (ACTH) and parenteral corticosteroids are given to reduce the inflammatory reaction and may be given by enema in acute rectal involvement. They are discontinued when clinical improvement occurs. Immunosuppressive drugs may be used. Broad-spectrum antibiotics are used after surgery.

Psychotherapy in conjunction with medical and surgical treatment has influenced the success of treatment. Its value is becoming recognized increasingly. When medical management is not enough to control ulcerative colitis, when the bowel has carcinomatous degeneration, or when there is total colonic involvement, a total colectomy may be necessary. The ileostomy created may add further complications.

The complexity of medical and surgical treatment requires close continuous observation, monitoring, and reporting as a major nursing emphasis. Response to treatment and drugs, development of complications, and his emotional response to his environment are all interrelated factors requiring astute judgment by the nurse.

About one-half of children with ulcerative colitis may lead relatively normal lives with mild or infrequent exacerbations. A severe, initial attack or total colon involvement may produce a guarded prognosis. Extension of the disease to nonaffected colon occurs very early in the development of the disease if it occurs at all.

Crohn's Disease (Regional Enteritis)

This entity is also known as *regional enteritis* and is distinctly different from ulcerative colitis (Table 26-5). Fibrosis and destruction of the intestinal muscle layer occur as a result of inflammatory changes. It is not uncommon for granulomas to form. Major symptoms are abdominal pain and diarrhea. Weight loss, anemia, and growth retardation may precede the onset of gastrointestinal manifestations.

Several areas of bowel are affected concurrently, producing a "cobblestone" pattern on barium swallow x-ray

TABLE 26-5 A Comparison of Clinical Manifestations of Ulcerative Colitis and Regional Enteritis

Manifestations	Ulcerative Colitis	Regional Enteritis
Initial symptoms	Good health till onset Painless passage of blood stools, often in early morning Change in bowel habits with constipation	Growth retardation often before gastrointestinal signs Resembles gastroenteritis or acute appendicitis Early systemic signs: arthritis, uveitis, stomatitis, erythrema nodosum Fever, often of unknown origin
Most frequent symptoms	Severe diarrhea Abdominal pain: less severe, crampy, sensation to defecate induced by eating, relieved by defecation Anorexia in acute stage Dehydration Malnutrition, retarded maturation, includes secondary sex characteristics Mucocutaneous lesions of skin, eyes, joints Signs of inflammation (chills, low evening fever, leukocytosis)	Abdominal pain, crampy, severe, induced by eating, relieved by defecation if colon involved: periumbilical, often in right lower quadrant Anorexia: may be severe Diarrhea: not always present, acute, severe; mucopurulent indicates severe rectosigmoid disease; bleeding is rare; early morning or nocturnal urge to defecate Chronically ill, muscle wasting Peripheral edema, early, if present
Symptoms indicative of severe disease	Nausea and vomiting Nocturnal urge to defecate Abdominal distention (toxic megacolon or impending perforation) Anal fissure Chronic hepatitis Fatty infiltration of liver due to chronic malnutrition	Nausea and vomiting Clubbing of fingers Perirectal disease: abscess, fistula

examination. Surgery is indicated in the presence of obstruction, perforation, or fistula formation. Recurrences are common after surgery.

Sulfasalazine may be used in the treatment but does not always produce the same benefits it does with ulcerative colitis. A high-carbohydrate, high-protein, low-residue diet is used. Anemia is treated with iron. Nursing care is similar to that for ulcerative colitis.

Independent Study Activities

1. In the clinical setting, interview a child with a colostomy or ileostomy and evaluate the adjustment the child has made to it.
2. In the clinical setting, perform a complete assessment of a child with a gastrointestinal alteration.
3. Devise a teaching plan for parents whose infant has a new gastrostomy which will be necessary for a prolonged period of time.
4. Interview the parents of a child with a cleft lip and palate. Identify the needs and concerns of the parents and the child. Assess their adjustments and methods of coping.
5. In the clinical setting, assess the factors that surrounded the incidence of a child's accidental ingestion of a corrosive substance. Then devise a teaching plan for parents to prevent future accidents.

Learning Activities

1. Assign clinical students to infants and children who have a variety of gastrointestinal problems.
2. Invite the parents of a neonate with NEC to the classroom so that they can share their experiences in dealing with this problem.
3. Invite an adolescent with celiac disease to share his thoughts about having this problem with students in the clinical setting.
4. Rotate students through the pediatric gastroenterology clinic so that they may better understand the scope of problems which occur and see "firsthand" how parents cope with them.

Study Questions

1. To prevent hemorrhage after a liver biopsy, an infant's abdomen is immobilized manually during the procedure. After the procedure:
   A. Slight pressure is applied to the biopsy site for 5 to 10 minutes.
   B. Moderate pressure is applied to the biopsy site for 5 to 10 minutes.
   C. A pressure bandage is applied for 1 hour.
   D. Deep pressure is applied for 3 to 5 minutes.

2. In confirming the presence of pinworms, the cellulose tape smear procedure is done at night or in the early morning because:
   A. The female pinworm migrates at night and deposits ova on the perineum.
   B. The child is groggy and therefore less afraid.
   C. When the child is wide awake, he may carry the eggs to his mouth.
   D. The stool is more moist at that time.

3. During the acute postoperative period after the surgical repair of a diaphragmatic hernia, the nursing focus is on:
   A. The neonate's respiratory effort.
   B. The baby's feeding problems.
   C. Relieving the respiratory acidosis.
   D. Rotating positions.

4. Ten days after surgery for NEC, a neonate is started on enteral feedings in small amounts. In addition to observing and recording the baby's response to the feeding, the nurse should:
   A. Do chest physical therapy.
   B. Determine urine pH values.
   C. Include pancreatic enzymes in the formula.
   D. Test stools for blood and glucose.

5. An infant who has had a surgical repair of a cleft lip is in elbow restraints, and his parents have asked why he has a chain of safety pins from the wrist of the restraints to the diaper pins. The nurse should explain that the pin chain prevents the infant from:
   A. Sucking his hands.
   B. Putting objects in his mouth.
   C. Rubbing his lips with his arms.
   D. Dislocating his shoulders.

6. In addition to preventing any strain on the suture line of a newly repaired cleft lip, a nurse implements measures which:
   A. Prevent speech defects.
   B. Prevent crust formation.
   C. Deter hemorrhage.
   D. Discourage the use of straws or plastic cups.

7. A BRAT diet for diarrhea consists of:
   A. Bananas (fresh), rice cereal, applesauce (canned), and tea (weak).
   B. Baked potatoes, rice cereal, applesauce (canned), and toast.
   C. Bananas (fresh), rice cereal, applesauce (canned), and toast.
   D. Bananas (fresh), rice cereal, applesauce (infant), and toast.

8. The parents of an infant with intussusception ask the nurse what it is. The nurse explains that:
   A. It is the twisting of the bowel upon itself.
   B. It is a telescoping of the bowel.
   C. It is similar to an inflamed bowel.
   D. The bowel is greatly dilated.

9. The mother of a toddler who has just ingested a copper penny asks the nurse why it is necessary to examine the child's bowel movements for the next 5 or 6 days. The nurse explains that:
   A. She really needs to observe the stool only for 24 hours.
   B. She needs to check for any blood in the stool.
   C. It takes about 5 days for the coin to pass from the stomach into the small intestine.
   D. The physician needs to know whether the bowel has become irritated.

10. The most likely diagnosis for a school-age child with a history of pain which is periumbilical, persistent, and progressive and which quickly localized to McBurney's point is:
    A. Regional enteritis.   C. Appendicitis.
    B. Megacolon.   D. Umbilical hernia.

Bibliography

Boyd, C.W.: "Postural Therapy at Home for Infants with Gastroesophageal Reflux," *Pediatric Nursing, 8:*395-398, 1982.

DeBenham, B.J., M. Ellet, R.C. Perez, J.H. Clark: "Initial Assessment and Management of Chronic Diarrhea in Toddlers," *Pediatric Nursing, 11*(4):281-285, 1985.

Gantt, L. and C. Thompson: "Short-gut Syndrome in the Infant," *American Journal of Nursing, 85*(11):1263-1266, 1985.

Gryboski, J. and W. Walker: *Gastrointestinal Problems in the Infant,* 2d ed., Philadelphia, Saunders, 1983.

Harris, J.A.: "Pediatric Abdominal Assessment," *Pediatric Nursing, 12*(5):355-362, 1986.

Hartwig, M.: "Sticking to a Gluten-free Diet," *American Journal of Nursing, 83:*1308-1310, 1983.

Hegenah, G., J. Harrigan, and M. Campbell: "Inflammatory Bowel Disease in Children," *Nursing Clinics of North America, 19*(1):27-39, 1984.

Henley, M. and J. Sears: "Pinworms: A Persistent Pediatric Problem," *MCN The American Journal of Maternal-Child Nursing, 10*(2):111-113, 1985.

Moynihan, P.J. and A.B. Gerraughty: "Diaphragmatic Hernia: Low Stress-High Survival," *American Journal of Nursing, 85*(6):662-665, 1985.

Myers, S.: "Overview of Inflammatory Bowel Disease," *Nursing Clinics of North America, 19*(1):3-9, 1984.

Paarlberg, J. and J.P. Balint: "Gastrostomy Tubes; Practical Guidelines for Home Care," *Pediatric Nursing, 11*(2);99-102, 1985.

Perez, R.C., L. Beckom, L. Jebara, M.A. Lewis, and Y. Patenaude: "Care of the Child with a Gastrostomy Tube: Common and Practical Concerns," *Issues in Comprehensive Pediatric Nursing, 7*(2-3):107-119, 1984.

Plapp, P.R.: "Nursing Considerations in Early Recognition of Necrotizing Enterocolitis," *Issues in Comprehensive Pediatric Nursing, 4*(2):77-81, 1980.

Silverman, A., and C. Roy: *Pediatric Clinical Gastroenterology,* 3d ed., St. Louis, C.V. Mosby, 1983.

27

The Urinary System

Objectives

After reading this chapter, the student will be able to:
1. Describe the functions of the urinary system.
2. Identify appropriate subjective and objective data to be elicited from the child and family.
3. Understand the purpose of diagnostic tests and medical treatment.
4. Explain general nursing measures appropriate for pediatric clients who have urologic problems.
5. Delineate specific nursing measures appropriate to the care of pediatric clients who have various urologic problems.

Anatomy and Physiology

The urinary system consists of the kidneys, ureters, bladder, and urethra. In children, the kidneys are slightly lower than they are in adults. With less protection from the rib cage and less perinephritic fat for padding, the kidneys in children are more susceptible to injury. The ureters are composed of mucosal, muscle, and fibrous layers. Urine is propelled along by the peristaltic waves produced by the muscle layer. The bladder is the resevoir for urine. Interference with innervation to the bladder muscles can result in a neurogenic bladder and a lack of bladder control. If the ureters are implanted incorrectly or lack normal valve function, urine can be forced upward toward the kidneys; this reflux can cause kidney damage. The urethra is shorter in children than it is in adults. This difference allows for easier passage of bacteria from the outside to the bladder. Children, and young girls in particular, are susceptible to cystitis and bladder infections.

The kidney removes wastes from the body, maintains body fluid homeostasis, secretes hormones, and plays a role in metabolism. The kidneys of a healthy newborn are qualitatively able to perform these functions despite renal immaturity. However, when illness of a newborn or preterm infant intervenes, special considerations must be taken into account in regard to the functional limitations of the kidney with drug therapy, formulas prescribed, and administration of parenteral fluid.

Urine Production and Maintenance of Fluid and Electrolyte Balance

The three discrete processes involved in the formation of urine are glomerular ultrafiltration of plasma, selective tubular reabsorption of water and solutes, and selective tubular secretion of solutes. The formation of urine initially begins at the glomerulus through ultrafiltration of plasma.

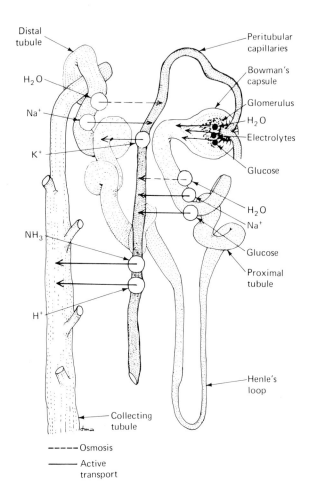

FIGURE 27-1 Diagram of glomerular filtration, tubular reabsorption, and tubular secretion.

Ultrafiltration occurs when the hydrostatic pressure within the glomerular capillary exceeds the colloid osmotic pressure of the plasma proteins. This pressure forces a filtrate of plasma through the walls of the glomerular capillaries. The capillaries function as ultrafilters which allow small molecules to pass but restrain larger protein molecules. When the pressures are equal, filtration ceases.

About 99 percent of the glomerular filtrates is reabsorbed from the tubular lumen into the peritubular interstitial fluid and then into the blood (Fig. 27-1). This process is selective since substances that are essential for homeostasis are recaptured. The reabsorption of water, glucose, sugars, amino acids, and electrolytes occurs primarily in the proximal tubules; urinary concentration of solutes is determined at more distal sites.

Tubular secretion refers to the movement of substances into the tubular lumen. This process helps in the elimination of compounds that are foreign to the body and are not disposed of by metabolism alone.

Sodium and Water Balance

The balance between the intake and output of water and sodium depends on tubular reabsorption since the amount filtered far exceeds intake. From 60 to 65 percent of the filtered sodium and water is reabsorbed in the proximal tubules and another 20 to 25 percent in Henle's loop. The amount of water reabsorbed in the distal collecting tubules is related to the blood concentration of antidiuretic hormone.

Water reabsorption can be regulated independently of sodium balance. Antidiuretic hormone alters the amount of water that is reabsorbed from the distal tubules and collecting ducts. When there is a high concentration of antidiuretic hormone, the permeability of the nephron to water is increased, and vice versa. Consequently, this process affects the concentration and dilution of urine.

Potassium Balance

All potassium in the glomerular filtrate is reabsorbed in the proximal tubule. The greatest percentage of potassium secretion is thought to occur because of passive transfer rather than as a result of the amount of sodium reabsorption in the distal tubule. The transfer of potassium into the distal tubule is facilitated by increased levels of intracellular potassium. Sodium may facilitate potassium secretion by increasing the tubular flow rate (thus maintaining a concentration gradient for potassium) and by creating a favorable electrochemical gradient in the tubule (which enhances potassium transfer). Other factors which regulate potassium excretion are alkalosis and high levels of aldosterone. Conversely, acidosis and low levels of aldosterone can reduce potassium secretion. The function of potassium in advanced renal disease is discussed later in this chapter. Fluid and electrolyte balance is in Chap. 11.

Acid-Base Balance

The pH of the plasma and interstitial fluid is maintained by the kidney's regulating the bicarbonate level of the plasma as well as the respiratory system's stabilizing the carbonic acid level. When an acid-base imbalance occurs that is not corrected by the chemical buffers of cells, bone, extracellular fluid, or the respiratory system, the body is dependent on the renal excretion of acid or alkali.

Production of Hormones

There is increasing evidence that the kidney has a function in the production of several hormones (Richards, 1986). It is a primary site for the production of erythropoietin and in the synthesis of prostaglandins. The juxtaglomerular cells store and release renin, which in turn functions as an enzyme that converts angiotensinogen to angiotensin I. Angiotensin I is converted in the lung to angiotensin II, a potent vasoconstrictor.

Assessment of the Urinary System

The nursing assessment of a well child or a child with suspected urinary system disease requires a systematic approach. In Tables 27-1 and 27-2 subjective and objective data pertinent to the urinary system are outlined. The information is obtained during routine well-child visits as indicated by the age of the child (Chap. 4).

Other extremely important factors to be considered in routine well-child care are the sex and age of the child. These factors determine when and what kind of screening tests are to be done as well as the content of the anticipatory guidance. Age or developmental level may also influence the ways in which a child is found to have urinary system disease. Often young children have vague and unrelated symptoms which do not focus on the urinary system (see Urinary Tract Infections below.) Also, age is a major factor in determining when various diseases are most likely to occur.

Diagnostic Procedures

The nurse should be well versed in the diagnostic procedures that are included in a urinary system workup. She not only is responsible for the collection of specimens and assisting in the performance of some procedures but also plays a vital role in preparing the child for various tests. In addition, parents may be confused and anxious over the barrage of procedures scheduled for a child. Although the physician may initially explain each diagnostic test and its purpose, the nurse is in an excellent position to reiterate and expand upon those explanations. By including details regarding the child's anticipated feelings and sensations, she can help prepare the child and parents for these encounters with unfamiliar techniques, equipment, and personnel. Diagnostic tests are summarized in Table 27-3.

Urinalysis

The nurse should be familiar with the purposes of the routine urinalysis and the factors which affect its reliability. A routine urinalysis is helpful in identifying the presence of urinary abnormalities and screening for the adequacy of renal function. Proper collection and storage of urine samples is vital so that increased patient cost and delay in diagnosis can be avoided. Urinalysis results can be influenced by a variety of factors, including fluid intake, diet, level of physical activity, menstruation, and masturbation. Ideally, the urine specimen is the first-voided specimen of the morning, which ensures an accurate detection of abnormalities. A child should not be given an excessive fluid intake in order to obtain a urine specimen quickly, as this excess can cause dilution of the urine. Very dilute urine is unsuitable for examination because white and red cell casts may be disintegrated, accurate information about the concentrating ability is lost, and abnormalities may be obscured. For example, a 2+ reaction for protein in a concentrated urine may appear as only a trace reaction in dilute urine, or in dilute urine, bacteria may fail to meet accepted significant values.

The nurse should describe the color, odor, and appearance of the specimen and document the method by which it was obtained. Urinalysis includes determination of pH and specific gravity; tests for the presence of protein, blood, glucose, and ketones; and microscopic examination for cells, casts, bacteria, and crystals.

TABLE 27-1 Nursing Assessment of Urinary System, Subjective Data

---

I. Past history (data to be collected on initial visit)
  A. Prenatal history
    1. When did prenatal care begin?
    2. Were any medications taken during the pregnancy? Alcohol? Other drugs?
    3. Were cigarettes smoked during the pregnancy? If so, how much?
    4. Were there any complications to the pregnancy?
  B. Labor and delivery
    1. Length
    2. Medications
    3. Problems
  C. Family history
    1. Kidney disease
    2. Diabetes
    3. Urinary tract infection
    4. Enuresis
  D. Past medical history
    1. Kidney disease
    2. Urinary tract infection
  E. Illness or injuries
    1. History of trauma to back
    2. Venereal disease
    3. Vaginitis
  F. Hospitalization for urinary system disease
  G. Review of urinary system
    1. Polyuria
    2. Dysuria
    3. Oliguria
    4. Nocturia
    5. Edema (periorbital, scrotal, pedal, ankle, and hand)
II. Present history (data to be collected on each well-child visit)
  A. Urinary habits
    1. Characteristics of urine: color, odor, number of voidings or of wet diapers per day, description of stream
    2. Toilet training when appropriate
  B. Sexual activity when appropriate

TABLE 27-2 Nursing Assessment of Urinary System: Schedule of Well-Child Visits with Outline of Appropriate Objective Data and Anticipatory Guidance to Be Done

Age	Measurements	Physical	Anticipatory Guidance	Procedures
1 mo	Lg, Wt, HC*	Complete	Discuss good perineal hygiene; discuss cleaning of uncircumcised penis	
2 mo	Lg, Wt, HC	Complete		
6 mo	Lg, Wt, HC	Complete		
9 mo	Lg, Wt	Complete		
12 mo	Lg, Wt, HC	Complete	Encourage water in diet; discuss time to begin toilet training (Chap. 4)	
15 mo	Lg, Wt	Complete	Review signs of readiness for toilet training; encourage cotton underwear for females	
18 mo	Lg, Wt	Complete	Review toilet training	
2 yr	Lg, Wt, HC		Review correct wiping procedure for females; discourage use of bubble bath	
2½ yr	St, Wt	Complete		
3 yr	St, Wt, HC, BP	Complete	Review good perineal hygiene	Urinalysis
4 yr	St, Wt, HC, BP	Complete	Encourage water in diet	
5 yr	St, Wt, HC, BP	Complete	Review good perineal hygiene	Urinalysis
6 yr	St, Wt, HC, BP	Complete	Encourage cotton underwear for females	
7 yr	St, Wt, HC, BP	Complete		
8-9 yr	St, Wt, HC, BP	Complete	Review good perineal hygiene	Urinalysis
10-12 yr	St, Wt, BP	Complete	Encourage cotton underwear and ventilated pantyhose	
13-15 yr	St, Wt, BP	Complete	Discourage use of feminine hygiene sprays; encourage water in diet	Urinalysis
16-21 yr	St, Wt, BP	Complete	Review good perineal hygiene; discuss voiding after intercourse for females	

*Lg = length; Wt = weight; HC = head circumference; St = stature; BP = blood pressure.

Source: Adapted from American Academy of Pediatrics, Schedule for Preventive Child Health Care.

TABLE 27-3 Summary of Common Renal Diagnostic Tests

Test	Nursing Implications	Normal Values
Urinalysis (pH, specific gravity, glucose, protein, ketones, casts, cells, crystals, and bacteria)	An early morning specimen is optimal for evaluating formed elements Fluids should not be forced because dilute urine may mask results	pH: 5.0-7.0 Specific gravity: 1.010-1.030 Negative: for glucose, protein, casts, cells, and crystals Bacteria: zero to two colonies
Urea and/or creatinine clearance tests	First specimen is discarded and urine is collected for an exact period of time, ending with child emptying his bladder; urine loss affects the resulting laboratory value and must be reported	Creatinine clearance: 110 ml/min per 1.73 m^2 Urea clearance: 70 ml/min per 1.73 m^2
Urine concentration test	Hydration status of patient during fluid deprivation should be monitored	Specific gravity: above 1.030
Serum creatinine		Newborn: 0.8-1.0 mg/100 ml Infant: 0.2-0.4 mg/100 ml Child: 0.3-0.8 mg/100 ml
Serum urea nitrogen	Value is affected by hydration status	Newborn: 3-10 mg/100 ml Child: 5-20 mg/100 ml
Intravenous pyelogram (IVP)	Child is NPO* 3-8 hours before test, depending on age; bowel evacuation is needed using suppository or castor oil; clear liquid diet is given night before procedure for older children; for infants last feeding given before procedure is clear liquids	Structural normality of upper urinary tract
Voiding cystourethrogram (VCUG)	Measures are similar to those for IVP Teaching regarding catheterization and need for child to void on x-ray table is included	Structural normality of bladder and urethra and absence of reflux
Cystoscopy	Child is NPO, and test is performed under general anesthesia	Structural normality of lower urinary tract

*NPO = nothing by mouth.

Urine Specimen Collection

Pediatric nephrologists generally recommend that all samples for urinalysis be obtained using the clean-catch midstream method. If parents collect the first sample of the morning and refrigerate it until the sample is brought to the office or laboratory for examination, a high degree of reliability for routine screening is attained and the sample can be used to check for asymptomatic bacteriuria. The collection of clean-catch specimens is described below. If the sample is obtained at home, it is important to provide the parent with specific instructions and reasons for each step.

Infants

Commercially available sterile collection bags are used to collect specimens from infants of both sexes. After the preliminary cleansing and drying of the infant, the bag is applied. In males, the penis is inserted into the opening of the bag and the adhesive backing is applied to the skin. In females, the labia are spread and the bag is applied (Fig. 27-2). As soon as the baby voids, the bag should be removed. The sample is aspirated by syringe and placed in a sterile container. If the infant does not void within 30 minutes after the bag has been applied, the cleansing procedure needs to be repeated and a new bag applied.

Girls

A child of 3 years or older cooperates in voiding into a container. If the child is cooperative and toilet trained, the nurse explains that the child's help is needed to collect some urine (noting from the nursing history the child's term for urine, such as "pee-pee"). Because of modesty, the child may wish to obtain the sample alone or with the assistance of the parent. In the latter instance, the procedure is explained carefully to the child and/or parent and equipment is provided. The child is asked to assume her normal sitting position on the toilet or bedpan and spread her legs widely. Next the labia majora are spread apart, and the vulva and meatus are cleansed with a soapy solution on sterile cotton balls. Cleansing strokes are from front to back, using a new cotton ball for each stroke (generally, three cotton balls are used—one for each side of the labia and, lastly, one down the center). This procedure is repeated using sterile cotton balls saturated with water to rinse the area. The cleansed area is then dried carefully with sterile gauze. Careful drying is important, as infecting bacteria may not grow if the urine specimen is contaminated with an antiseptic. Keeping the labia spread, the nurse or parent should encourage the child to begin to void. Only after the stream has started and while the stream is continuing should one attempt to catch the midportion of urine in a sterile wide-mouthed container so that it does not touch the child's skin or clothing. Upon collection of the specimen, the child is thanked for her help and cooperation. The sample should be taken to the laboratory or refrigerated immediately.

Boys

Using similar preliminaries and normal voiding posture, the nurse or parent should cleanse the glans penis and meatus from the distal end to the base in the same fashion as described above. In uncircumcised male children the foreskin must be retracted and the glans gently cleansed. It may be impossible to retract the foreskin in newborn infants or in boys with phimosis, and force should not be used; the physician should be notified. With the foreskin remaining retracted, the boy is requested to void, and the urine specimen is obtained. The child should receive praise for his cooperation. Adolescent boys can collect their own midstream specimen adequately, given a sufficient explanation.

Alternate Sample Collection Methods

Properly collected bag specimens often yield unclear results, and it may be necessary to gain the specimen by

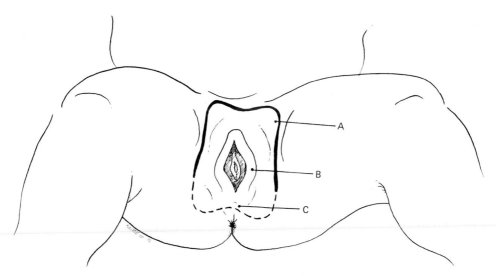

FIGURE 27-2 Application of a pediatric urine bag for female infants. (A) Pediatric urine bag. (B) Labia Majora. (C) Pelvic floor (in female infants, it is important to attach the bag securely at this point). *(Courtesy of Nancy E. Westcott.)*

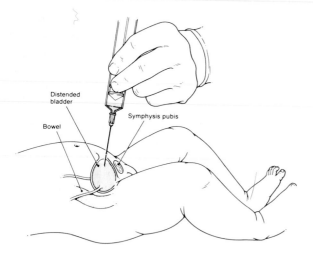

FIGURE 27-3 Suprapubic bladder aspiration.

means of either catheterization or suprapubic bladder tap. These procedures offer more definitive results since contamination is less of a problem.

In preparing the infant for a suprapubic tap, the nurse should place the child in a supine, frogleg position. The abdomen is scrubbed with a betadine solution. A 22-gauge 2-cm sterile needle is inserted at a 30° angle directly into the bladder, and urine is aspirated (Fig. 27-3). This procedure involves little risk to the patient but should be avoided if the child has abdominal distention. Timing of the procedure can influence successful obtainment of the sample. Therefore, 30 minutes to 1 hour should elapse after the child has voided and before the tap is done. Parents should be given explanations of the procedure, as they may be unnecessarily concerned.

When a urine specimen must be obtained and clean catch and suprapubic tap are not viable alternatives, catheterization using a red rubber straight catheter may be ordered. The nurse should exercise care to avoid introducing bacteria through the urethra by using careful cleansing and proper aseptic technique of catheter insertion. Trauma during the procedure can be minimized through the appropriate selection of catheter size (No. 8 to 15 French catheter generally is used) and proper restraint of the patient. Instructions for catheterization of male and female children can be found in a pediatric procedure manual.

pH

The acidity of the urine specimen can be determined using a dipstick; however, a pH meter is employed in the laboratory when a more precise pH measurement is needed. The dipstick contains nitrazine indicator paper, which changes through a range of colors from yellow to dark blue over the usual urine pH range of 4.0 to 8.2. The pH is usually acidic, 5.0 to 6.0, in the fasting state. It becomes more alkaline with the ingestion of dairy products. Alkalinity beyond 8.0 or 8.2 suggests that the patient has a urinary infection due to a urea-splitting organism, such as *Proteus,* or that the specimen has been allowed to stand at room temperature for several hours, permitting a luxuriant growth of contaminating bacteria in the container. Control of urine pH is an important factor in obtaining maximum therapeutic value from certain antibiotics and urinary disinfectants.

Specific Gravity

The specific gravity provides an estimation of the kidney's concentrating ability, a function which frequently is compromised in children with renal disease. The specific gravity of a concentrated specimen collected in the early morning is normally 1.024 to 1.030 and is measured roughly by a hydrometer or more accurately by a total solids meter that utilizes a single drop of urine. During diuresis, the specific gravity may fall to 1.000 or 1.001. Conversely, large particles such as protein, glucose, and radiographic dyes will greatly increase the value.

Dipstick

The dipstick test for blood, glucose, and ketones is very convenient for screening specimens, for testing at home, and for testing when the available urine volume is small. Reagent strips may deteriorate and hence provide inaccurate results if they are not stored in a tightly capped, moisture- and light-protected bottle. The nurse should recheck the specimen if unusual color reactions are present.

Proteinuria is frequently an initial sign of renal disease in asymptomatic children. The dipstick detects protein concentrations above 30 mg/100 ml and turns green-blue when abnormal amounts of albumin are present in the urine. Normal children have had documented orthostatic proteinuria with activity, so if a positive specimen is obtained, it should be rechecked using the first specimen collected in the early morning after the child has been supine through the night. Transient proteinuria has also been found in children suffering febrile illnesses.

The presence of sugar in a urine sample is an abnormal finding. It can be detected using a dipstick which will react with an amount of 100 mg of glucose per deciliter of urine. The dipstick, however, does not recognize other reducing substances, such as galactose and fructose. False-positive reactions may be seen when the child is receiving medications, such as streptomycin and certain tetracyclines.

Dipsticks also are used to screen urine samples for free hemoglobin released from lysed red cells. Hematuria can be a transient, benign phenomenon such as with male joggers or after urethral instrumentation or menstruation. Conversely, it can be a significant indication of a renal pathological condition, as in glomerulonephritis.

Ketones may also be identified utilizing a dipstick; however, the dipstick tests for only one of the three types of ketone bodies, acetoacetate. Positive reactions are seen in a variety of situations, including children with weight loss, dehydration, infection, and renal disease. It is important to use a fresh or refrigerated urine sample when checking for ketones, because standing urine promotes bacterial growth, thus increasing the amount of ketones.

Microscopic Examination

The sediment of a centrifuged urine specimen should be examined for cellular elements within an hour of collection. The presence of white blood cells (WBCs) in urine is a common indicator of infection, although WBCs also are found with dehydration, stress, and urinary tract irritation. Red blood cells also may be detected. They can signify blood dyscrasia, urinary bleeding, trauma, or the presence of infection. Casts formed in the lumen of the nephron may be observed on the microscopic examination. The appearance of most types of casts is indicative of renal disease. Crystal formation may be insignificant or can provide clues to the existence of kidney stone formation or metabolic disease.

Bacteriuria Screening

These screening tests for urinary infections are inexpensive and accurate. Positive results of these tests can be confirmed with a quantitative culture.

The nurse may be responsible for "planting" clean-voided urine on Testuria, a handy screening medium. A commercial adaptation of the filter paper dipstick is used to inoculate a small agar plate, which is then incubated at 37°C (98.6°F) overnight. Although actual identification of bacterial type is not possible, Testuria provides a screening test for bacterial presence and for colony count. A range of zero to two colonies is considered negative or minimal contaminant. A range of 3 to 25 colonies is suspicious, corresponding to the range of 10,000 to 100,000 bacteria per milliliter, and the culture should be repeated. A finding of more than 25 colonies is considered positive, equal to or greater than 100,000 or 10^5/ml of urine. All positive Testurias are forwarded to the main clinical laboratory for identification and various antibiotic sensitivity tests. Other rapid, reliable screening methods in current use are Culturia (a dip-slide method with two-growth media for gram-positive and gram-negative bacteria) and Bacturcult (a test tube-pour method).

Chemical reagent dipsticks provide simple methods of screening for bacteria. The nitrite strip, which indicates the presence of bacteria when the strip turns pink as a result of the chemical reaction, is commonly used. Since enough time may not have elapsed for the bacteria to convert nitrite to nitrite, the first morning specimen provides the most accurate result.

12- or 24-Hour Urine Collections

A diagnostic urine collection of 12 or 24 hours may be ordered. The nurse should explain collection techniques to the child, parents, and other nursing staff members to ensure proper collection. These lengthy collections are often required to determine (1) quantitative protein excretion (any amount in excess of 200 mg/24 h is considered abnormal), (2) the rate of excretion of red cells, white cells, and casts in urine, known as an Addis count (normal values are 600,000/12 h for red blood cells, 1 million/12 h for white blood cells, and 10,000/12 h for casts), and (3) urine electrolyte concentrations for sodium, potassium,

and chloride. The nurse should know of any dietary and/or fluid alterations which are necessary before urine collection begins as well as the specific procedure for collection (e.g., whether the specimen should be kept on ice or whether buffered formalin is to be added to the container as a preservative). Situations which hinder collection should be anticipated and discussed with the child and parents. For example, a child who needs to have a bowel movement during the collection period should be asked to urinate first so that the specimen is not contaminated or discarded with the stool.

The collection period is begun just after the child has voided (this specimen being discarded) and is completed with the collection of the specimen voided 12 or 24 hours later. Timed collections always begin and end with the bladder empty. Infants and young children rarely void "by the clock," and so the nurse should know that a 13-hour or 22-hour specimen is satisfactory provided the dates and exact times of starting and ending the collection period are recorded on the collection bottle and accompanying identification cards. If any of the urine from the collection period is lost, the estimated amount lost should be recorded and the laboratory should be consulted to determine whether the collection should be restarted. Since the results are based on the amount of a particular substance present in the volume of urine produced during a specific time period, any urine lost can yield inaccurate values.

Collecting 12- or 24-hour specimens from active infants is difficult; It is more feasible if the nurse adheres to certain guidelines. When not being held by a nurse or parent the infant may need to be mildly restrained in the supine position, using soft cotton wrist and ankle restraints (Chap. 10). After the skin around the meatus and perineum has been cleansed and thoroughly dried, a 24-hour collecting bag is applied in the same way as a urinalysis bag. Special care is needed to ensure that the adhesive surface is pressed firmly onto the skin posteriorly to avoid leakage and fecal contamination especially in female infants. The topical application of tincture of benzoin on the perineal surface prior to application may help keep the bag in place.

The infant should then be diapered to prevent him from pulling on the bag or loosening it as he kicks. In order to remove individual specimens collected during the 12- or 24-hour period without removing the bag each time, a syringe is attached to the bag's tubing and individual voidings are aspirated and added to the specimen bottle. The collection device should be checked every 30 minutes throughout the collection period to avoid the loss of any specimens. Informed parents are invaluable in the successful collection of these timed specimens.

Renal Function Tests

Blood urea nitrogen (BUN) and *serum creatinine* tests measure the concentration of nitrogenous wastes in blood. Concentrations increase with impaired kidney function. Creatinine is derived from skeletal muscle as an end produce of creatine metabolism. Normal plasma concentration is age-related and increases as the child develops more muscle mass. Levels of 0.2 to 0.4 mg/dl are typical during infancy, and levels of 0.4 to 0.8 mg/dl are seen in the preadolescent period. The BUN (normally less than 10 mg/dl in infants and less than 20 mg/dl in children) is influenced by a protein and fluid intake, liver function, gastrointestinal absorption, and hemorrhage. Its sensitivity to variables other than renal perfusion make it a less specific index of changes in renal function than is the plasma creatinine.

Clearance tests express the rate of urinary excretion of urea or creatinine in terms of a certain volume of plasma: the volume of plasma that contains the same total amount of the substance as appears in the urine in 1 minute. Urea and creatinine are normally present at relatively stable concentrations in plasma and can be measured in timed urine specimens using simple chemical methods. Both determinations may result in wide errors if the nurse is not careful to ensure complete emptying of the bladder with each voiding, especially if collection periods are short. Credé techniques (using the hand to apply external pressure on the bladder to express urine) and temporary catheterization may be indicated in a child with neurogenic bladder or an ileal conduit. Strict adherence to time is also vital.

A urine concentration test determines the maximum specific gravity that the child can achieve after fluid deprivation. While the inability to concentrate urine can be a sign of either renal or metabolic disease, this test does not differentiate between them. After 12 hours of fluid deprivation, the specific gravity of the urine of a normal child usually exceeds 1.024 and the osmolality is above 800 mOsm/kg. As renal function deteriorates, there is a tendency to lose normal concentrating and diluting ability, so that urine from a patient with severe renal deficiency has a relatively fixed specific gravity (around 1.010).

A concentration test is conveniently run overnight, although fluid restriction for infants is generally less than 12 hours. It is important for the child to be hydrated adequately prior to the test. If the child is in a diuresing stage, the test is postponed. For an older child, fluids are withheld after supper; the child voids, discards the specimen, and notes this time. Twelve or more hours later or whenever the child awakes for the day, the first specimen obtained is suitable for a concentration determination, but the second specimen of the morning prior to any fluid intake is more accurate in determining concentration because the urine is definitely not residual.

Nursing care includes careful assessment of the child for signs of dehydration. An accurate weight needs to be obtained prior to starting the test. A child should be reweighed during the test if there is any question about dehydration. If the child loses more than 3 percent of his body weight, the test should be terminated. The child should be given adequate fluids to restore his hydration status.

Common X-Ray Procedures

In general, x-ray studies are used to determine the size, shape, and position of the kidneys and details of their blood supply. In addition, kidney function can be roughly determined according to how well each kidney concentrates and excretes contrast media.

Intravenous Pyelogram

The *intravenous pyelogram* (IVP) is used to study the upper urinary tract. It is especially valuable in diagnosing suspected structural anomalies in the collecting system, assessing the extent of pyelonephritis, and identifying masses causing obstruction of the urinary tract. A radiopaque dye is injected into an antecubital vein, circulates through the bloodstream, is identified as a foreign substance by the kidneys, and is filtered out in the urine. X-ray films taken at intervals outline the renal collecting systems and ureters. Preparation procedures vary from one facility to another but generally involve food and fluid restriction for a period of time and laxatives or enemas for bowel emptying. The major contraindication to an IVP is a previous severe sensitivity reaction to the contrast material; such reactions are rare. A preliminary test dose of 1 ml of contrast medium is injected intravenously and the child is observed for 30 to 60 seconds. If there are no adverse signs, the full dose is injected. The nurse should be careful to observe for signs of a sensitivity reaction in any child who has had an IVP. Urticarial hives and wheezing can be well controlled with intravenous diphenhydramine hydrochloride (Benadryl), which should be kept readily available.

Voiding Cystourethrogram

The voiding cystourethrogram (VCUG) is used to study the lower urinary tract, visualize the bladder and the contour of the urethra during voiding, and demonstrate the presence of vesicoureteral reflux. The patient is chateterized, and the bladder is slowly filled with contrast material so that its size and outline can be determined. Bladder capacity ranges from 75 ml in newborns to 300 ml in older children. In older children, the catheter is removed and the patient is encouraged to void. Small infants urinate spontaneously whenever bladder filling reaches the point of discomfort. X-ray films are taken at intervals to outline the urethra for evidence of obstruction and to demonstrate vesicoureteral reflux, evident either when the bladder is filling or during urination. A final film is taken to demonstrate if the bladder has emptied completely and if there is evidence of refluxed contrast medium in the renal pelvis.

The purpose of the procedure and how it is performed is explained to the child and his parents. The child is told about the sensation of being catheterized and is given the opportunity to handle the catheter. The importance of voiding after the catheterization is emphasized, because it is embarrassing for the child to urinate on the examining table. For a young child who has been recently toilet trained, it is important for parents to reassure the child that it is indeed all right and a part of the test. A VCUG is contraindicated in the presence of acute urinary tract infection because of the risk of spreading infection to the kidney by reflux.

The nurse can help the child relieve postcatheterization discomfort by forcing fluids and applying cold compresses to the urinary meatus as necessary. The nurse may also suggest to the parent that the child be placed in a tub of warm water and be allowed to void for the first time in the tub. The nurse should assess the child's ability to void, document the time and, if possible, the amount of urine initially voided after the VCUG.

Imaging Procedures

Recent advances in radiological technology have added a series of imaging tests which can provide helpful information in the detection of certain renal abnormalities. These tests are utilized selectively and depend on the type of renal problem suspected. They are especially helpful in evaluating abdominal masses, which are frequently renal in origin. Ultrasonography is a noninvasive test which identifies the location of the mass and differentiates between solid and cystic lesions. It is useful with infants suspected of having multicystic kidney disease. The renal scan involves an injection of a radiopharmaceutical agent which provides a better visualization of the child's kidney function than does the IVP. It reveals important data about the presence of congenital anomalies, vascular problems, and hydronephrosis of the kidneys. Nuclear cystograms identify reflux. Computerized axial tomography is an expensive procedure utilized to diagnose solid masses, such as a follow-up to cancer therapy, or to evaluate trauma. This procedure can be noninvasive or contrast material can be injected. Explanations of the purpose and procedure should be provided prior to each event.

Cystoscopy

A urologic procedure done under general anesthesia, cystoscopy remains the most direct means of studying the anatomy of the lower urinary tract and is a prerequisite to retrograde pyelography. Cystoscopic findings are related to ureteral orifice size, shape (normal, cone, stadium, horseshoe, golfhole), and location (lateral or proximal in trigone of bladder) and to abnormalities of function such as reflux. Some major indications for cystoscopy and possible retrograde pyelography include the following:

1. Absent or imperfect visualization of one or both collecting systems by IVP
2. Unexplained hematuria, to determine bleeding and its cause, for example, cystitis, stone, or tumor
3. Suspected ectopic opening of the ureter, persistent reflux, or suspected ureterocele
4. Unexplained anuria with suspected bilateral ureteral obstruction
5. Suspected unilateral renal or renal vascular disease where the urine from each kidney must be examined separately

6. Recurrent urinary tract infection with a normal or doubtfully abnormal IVP and cystogram

Because this procedure involves general anesthesia, the nurse preoperatively should coach the patient in deep breathing and coughing techniques; colorful balloons at the bedside are excellent reminders. Early ambulation is an added plus. The physician will order frequent checking of blood pressure and pulse throughout and forced fluids upon full recovery from the anesthesia; comfort measures similar to those used after catheterization (discussed in the section on VCUGs above) may be employed.

Renal Biopsy

Percutaneous needle biopsy of the kidney often provides critical information on which the physician can base a diagnosis or prognosis in children with clinically established renal disease. Several biopsies, along with clearance tests of renal function, assess the progress of children with persistent nephritic processes and help in determining the choice of therapy and its value. Diagnostic renal biopsy is generally recommended in the following situations:

1. Unexplained hematuria or proteinuria
2. Nephrotic syndrome that is unresponsive to steroid therapy
3. Systemic lupus erythematosus
4. Persistent glomerulonephritis
5. Acute renal failure of unexplained cause
6. Unexplained hypertension

The biopsy procedure itself may be explained to parents and children as a diagnostic study involving the removal of a small piece of kidney tissue (about the size of a pencil lead) for examination under the microscope and for special staining. These techniques are helpful in determining the type and severity of disease within the kidney and may be helpful in guiding appropriate treatment. The nurse should stress that although the child remains awake, lying on his abdomen during the procedure, his back is "put to sleep" so that only distinct deep pressure will be felt at the moment of securing the tissue itself. For young, highly anxious children, however, the physician may request that supplemental anesthesia be available.

Prerequisites to biopsy include signed parental consent and x-ray evidence of the location and configuration of both kidneys. Laboratory studies verifying a normal red blood cell count and blood-clotting mechanisms and baseline data on serum creatinine levels and urinalysis are collected. Contraindications for a renal biopsy are a solitary kidney, small kidneys, severe hypertension, polyarteritis, bleeding disorders, and perinephric abscesses.

The child is premedicated usually with a lytic cocktail (promethazine 1 mg/kg, chlorpromazine 1 mg/kg, and meperidine 0.5 mg/kg of body weight). After careful cleansing of the skin, a solution of 1% lidocaine (Xylocaine) is used intradermally and deeply to numb the biopsy site. Fluoroscopy is an extremely useful adjunct in guiding placement of the biopsy needle after initial localization of the kidney cortex. Although a sterile pressure bandage may be applied afterward, the incision through which the biopsy needle passes is just a nick—less than 2 mm.

After the biopsy, strict bed rest with no exceptions is maintained for at least 12 hours; the chid may lie on his back or abdomen. The nurse checks regularly and frequently for bleeding from the bandage site and monitors pulse and blood pressure as ordered (every 15 minutes times 8; every half-hour times 4; every hour times 4; then every 3 hours). The child is requested to force fluids to a specified amount, depending on body weight, and to save all voided urine at the bedside so that it can be checked visually and with reagent dipsticks for bleeding. Some flank tenderness and guarding is common for 24 to 48 hours after the biopsy and may reflect a small amount of perirenal bleeding. The physician may order a mild analgesic to relieve this discomfort. The nurse should immediately report to the physician any gross hematuria, severe pain, or hypotension, because these symptoms are indicative of active bleeding. It is also important to be sensitive to and supportive of the child and parents' probable anxiety as they await the test results (Table 27-3).

General Nursing Measures

Nursing Diagnoses

Because of the variety of urologic anomalies and dysfunction, many nursing diagnoses can be developed. The following represent some possible common diagnoses:

Altered patterns of urinary elimination related to dysuria and frequency, retention or obstruction, neurogenic bladder, or acute renal failure

Potential or actual electrolyte imbalance related to fluid retention or renal failure

Potential for infection related to edema, immunosuppressive drugs, indwelling catheters, or dialysis procedures

Altered growth and development related to poor appetite

Anxiety related to tests and procedures

Body image disturbance related to real or perceived change in body structure or function, i.e., nephrectomy, urostomy, edema, renal transplant

Nursing Management

In addition to assessment information discussed earlier, there are several important general nursing measures. Proper collection and storage of specimens are vital in obtaining accurate results. The nurse also may be responsible for testing urine for protein, blood, specific gravity, or other components.

Accurate measurement and recording of length/stature, weight, and blood pressure provide parameters for the child's overall health status. Atypical growth patterns or abnormal blood pressure may be indicative of renal pathology.

Frequently a child hospitalized with urinary system disease requires accurate record keeping of intake and output. Precise measurement and recording of all fluid intake and urine output are of prime importance. Accurate measuring of output with children who are not toilet trained or are in the process of being toilet trained can present a challenge. Parents can be of great assistance in these situations. Diapers must be weighed before being put on the child and again after the child has voided. If the young child is toilet trained, a potty chair by the bedside can serve as a remainder of the importance of collecting all voidings.

Proper labeling of the Kardex and the patient room and even taping an intake and output (I & O) sign on the child's clothing can be of assistance to all personnel in obtaining accurate intake and output measurements. Educating older patients and parents about the procedure as well as showing them how to measure and record intake and output can be of great benefit in successfully obtaining an accurate intake and output record.

Many of the same principles can be applied to obtaining a routine intake and output. However, it does not require the exactness that an accurate record does. For example, recording the number of diaper changes and voidings will suffice as will an appropriate estimate of fluid intake. In Table 27-4 the average 24-hour urine outputs for children of different ages are presented.

There are times when the nurse is responsible for caring for a patient with an indwelling catheter. It is of prime importance to maintain continuous free drainage. Tubing is arranged so that urine flows downhill into the drainage bag; the tubing is inspected for kinks, twists, or pressure from resting body parts; and the tubing is not allowed to hang below the drainage bag.

If catheter irrigations are ordered, the procedure should be done with strict aseptic technique since there is a high risk of contamination. Encouraging fluids is another means of flushing the catheter. Fluids that promote an acidic urine such as cranberry juice, prune juice, and tea can serve as a protective mechanism to inhibit bacterial growth.

An important nursing measure is good perineal hygiene. The area surrounding the urethral meatus and the catheter should be cleaned at least twice a day with a bacteriostatic agent such as aqueous benzalkonium chloride solution or a bactericidal solution such as povidone-iodine.

The drainage bag or collecting container should be emptied every 8 hours or more frequently if needed. The importance of following strict aseptic technique cannot be stressed enough.

Since many drugs are excreted via the kidneys, the

TABLE 27-4 Average 24-Hour Urine Output

Age	Output, ml
<6 mo	400-500
6 mo-2 yr	500-700
2 yr-5 yr	600-800
6 yr-8 yr	700-1200
9 yr-14 yr	1000-1500
>14 yr	1500 or more

nurse needs to be aware of those which are, particularly when a patient has any form of kidney disease. In addition, certain drugs are known to be nephrotoxic and should not be used when kidney function is compromised. Parents need to be informed of this aspect, especially when the child is being treated for other health problems by other physicians who may not be aware of the kidney disease. Making the parent a partner or member of the health team can prove invaluable in such instances.

Another important nursing measure to be considered is evaluating the hydration status of a child. One way of determining this status is to weigh the patient daily. Weighing should be done at the same time each day and on the same scale, and the results must be recorded on the patient's chart. Other ways to assess the hydration status are discussed in Chap. 11.

Urinary Problems in the Newborn and Infant

According to several authorities, 5 to 10 percent of all infants are born with a malformation of the urinary tract. Fortunately, many urinary tract deformities are clinically unimportant and many others are surgically correctable.

The majority of urinary tract anomalies are asymptomatic; however, some may be detected because of the significant correlation between anomalies of the urinary tract and other congenital anomalies. The following anomalies are commonly associated with urinary tract malformations:

1. Low-set malformed ears
2. Chromosomal disorders, especially D and E trisomy
3. Absent abdominal muscles
4. Anomalies of the spinal cord and lower extremities
5. Imperforate anus or genital deviation
6. Wilms' tumor
7. Congenital ascites
8. Cystic disease of the liver
9. Positive family history of renal disease (hereditary nephritis, cystic disease)
10. Widely spaced nipples

The anomalies which are symptomatic present a challenge to the nurse since early diagnosis is needed to prevent renal damage. Important symptoms to observe in the infant are:

1. Abdominal mass in the neonatal period
2. Unexplained dehydration, acidosis, anemia, or failure to thrive

Wilms' Tumor

Wilms' tumor occurs in approximately 1 of every 10,000 births, with 75 percent of patients being less than 5 years of age and most being 2 to 3 years of age at the time of diagnosis. This embryonic tumor, rarely found in neonates or adolescents, is most frequently unilateral, involving a mass which replaces normal renal tissue.

Initial signs of the tumor are commonly discovered by the parents as they note an enlarging abdomen and have difficulty fastening the child's clothing. A firm, nontender mass may be reported in the upper quadrant. Other signs and symptoms may include abdominal pain, hematuria, fever, anorexia, and malaise. If the tumor has gone undetected, its increased size may cause abdominal pain, vomiting, or constipation because of gastric compression.

Nursing Management

When Wilms' tumor is suspected, care should be taken to limit the number of abdominal palpations done because they can increase the danger of metastasis. Posting a sign at the head of the crib serves to alert other health team members. Daily abdominal girth measurements are obtained and noted to provide baseline data for later evaluation.

Diagnostic tests common in the workup of a child with Wilms' tumor include a flat plate of the abdomen, chest x-ray, IVP, and often a computerized axial tomography scan. Additional information is provided by the following laboratory tests: complete blood count, urinalysis, renal function tests, and coagulation studies. It is important to provide both child and parent with all the information necessary for understanding. This teaching needs to be at an appropriate level for both child and parents. Often the hospitalization is sudden and parents are fearful of outcomes; therefore, explanations need to be repeated frequently.

Current therapy combining surgery, chemotherapy, and radiotherapy has resulted in increased survival rates. Prognosis and treatment protocols are based on the extent of tumor involvement and the age of the patient. Generally a radical nephrectomy is performed; then radiation to eradicate any residual tumor is begun after the return of bowel function. If the tumor is large and invasive, radiotherapy may be employed preoperatively to decrease the size of the tumor. Chemotherapy is introduced postoperatively to eradicate any occult systemic micrometastasis. Vincristine and actinomycin D are the chemotherapeutic agents most commonly used, and the nurse should be aware of their normal mode of action, dosage, and common side effects. Maintenance therapy is usually continued for 15 to 18 months. During that time, laboratory studies are performed periodically to follow the child's response to therapy and to detect disease recurrence (pulmonary metastasis is the most common occurrence). Throughout the induction and maintenance therapy, the nurse should be alert to common problems encountered by children receiving radiation and chemotherapy. Parents and children need teaching and support as they adjust to the various phases of treatment.

Congenital Deformities

Obstruction of the urinary tract can occur anywhere in the system. Chronic obstructive disease causes hydronephrosis and can result in irreversible destruction of the nephrons if treatment is delayed. The most common site for obstruction is at the ureteropelvic junction. Obstruction may be due to pressure from an aberrant blood vessel, narrowing of the ureter, or abnormal insertion of the ureter into the renal pelvis. Other sites for obstruction are at the ureterovesical junction, at the bladder neck, and in the urethra. The child may be asymptomatic or may present with abdominal pain, nausea, vomiting, elevated blood pressure, or recurrent urinary tract infections. Duplication of the collecting system, ectopic ureters, ureteroceles, and posterior urethral valves are other anomalies which may cause obstruction.

Nursing Management

Nursing care for congenital renal conditions is aimed at monitoring the child's renal function for progressive dysfunction. If surgical intervention is indicated, nursing management will include general postoperative care, monitoring of renal function, and support and teaching of parents.

Exstrophy of the Bladder

Exstrophy of the bladder is a urinary tract anomaly seen in 1 out of 30,000 live births. In this condition the bladder, instead of being a closed container, has an anterior surface opening on the lower abdomen. The closed surface appears bright red and is sensitive because of nerve exposure. This defect is commonly associated with other lower urinary tract anomalies: epispadias, undescended testes, shortened penis, cleft scrotum, and bifid clitoris. Pelvic musculoskeletal formation is also affected and results in rectal prolapse, inguinal hernias, and hip malformations.

Upon delivery, parents are faced with several psychological dilemmas, including adjustment to a disfiguring congenital defect, adaptation to a less than perfect child, and the accompanying grief reaction. They do not always receive adequate support because of a lack of general knowledge concerning this condition. They are also faced with a lack of initial information as to the sex of the child, having to wait 1 to 2 weeks for the results of chromosome tests.

Nursing Management

Preoperative care is aimed at preventing infection, preserving renal function, avoiding trauma, and promoting infant attachment and normal developmental needs. Because of the bladder eversion, there is continuous bathing of the mucosa and surrounding abdominal skin with urine. This condition requires immediate and meticulous nursing intervention to prevent skin breakdown and ulceration of the bladder mucosa. Fine-mesh gauze impregnated with petrolatum or a layer of Saran Wrap can be applied to prevent irritation and to promote comfort to the sensitive bladder mucosa, and various barrier creams can be applied to the surrounding skin for protection. Frequent diaper changes and meticulous skin care, particularly after each stool, also aid in preventing skin breakdown and infection. The baby is bathed daily using a mild soap, and diapers should be applied loosely. Twice a day

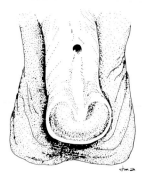

FIGURE 27-4 Penile epispadias with dorsal chordee.

the area is exposed to warm room air or sunlight to promote thorough drying. These neonates have typical newborn needs; however, they have a tendency to be irritable and fussy. Causes of their fussiness need to be identified since this behavior aggravates their hernias and predisposes them to rectal prolapse.

Until surgery is performed, the parents assume responsibility for the baby's care. Seeing the defect, cleaning the affected area, and feeding the baby are psychologically difficult procedures for them. They need encouragement, support, and time in which to assimilate and demonstrate the teaching that is done. Surgical intervention varies among institutions. Some physicians recommend urinary diversion surgery since bladder reconstruction has had limited success. However, other physicians favor a reconstructive surgery which occurs at 12 to 18 months of age in two stages: (1) pelvic reconstruction and (2) urethra and bladder reconstruction with abdominal closure.

Epispadias

Epispadias, a congenital anomaly in which the urethral meatus is located on the dorsal surface of the penis, rarely occurs as an isolated condition. It is more commonly seen as a component of exstrophy of the bladder. The condition in males should be repaired between 2 and 3 years of age for functional and cosmetic reasons.

Epispadias is classified according to the position of the urethral meatus. In the least severe form the meatus is located in the dorsum of the glans. When the meatus is located along the dorsum of the penis, epispadias is considered to be more severe (Fig. 27-4). In this type the penis is curved dorsally, is flattened, and is smaller than usual. In the most severe type, the penis is short and blunt and the urethral meatus is present at the penopubic junction. Incontinence accompanies this degree of epispadias, the prepuce hangs from the ventral surface, and the symphysis pubis is widened.

Hypospadias

Hypospadias is an anomaly in which the urethral meatus is located on the ventral surface of the penis (Fig. 27-5). The meatus most frequently ends in the shaft of the penis or near the glans. Less common forms in which the meatus is found in the scrotum or in the perineum are most severe.

Chordee accompanies most types of hypospadias and results from normal tissue being replaced by a tough band of fibrous tissue, which bends the penis ventrally.

Hypospadias is treated surgically by a multi- or single-stage procedure. In the one-step procedure, an extension of the urethra is formed from a skin graft and the chordee is released initially and urethroplasty is done in one or

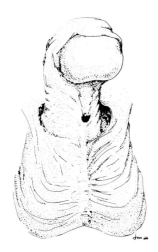

FIGURE 27-5   Midpenile hypospadias and chordee.

more future operations. Assessment for these problems includes observation of the physical appearance of the genitalia, the voiding pattern, and the straightness of the urine stream.

Nursing Management

Nursing management for hypospadias and epispadias varies depending on the severity and the surgical intervention required. It is important not to circumcise these infants as the foreskins may be needed to elongate the urethra. Preoperatively, the surgical field is scrubbed carefully with an antiseptic soap to reduce the incidence of infection. Nursing care postoperatively includes monitoring for wound infection and urinary tract infection. Edema is a common postoperative problem and needs to be controlled to avoid wound separation; thus, positioning is important in avoiding dependency edema. Postoperative nursing management includes careful maintenance of urethral and suprapubic catheters, restraining the patient as needed, and monitoring the appearance and amount of urinary flow. Adequacy of fluid intake is ensured. Pain medication is administered to provide for patient comfort and relief from bladder spasms.

The repair frequently occurs during an age period where fears about body integrity are common; the proce-

 NURSING CARE PLAN

27-1 The Child with Hypospadias

Clinical Problem/Nursing Diagnosis	Expected Outcome	Nursing Interventions

Dysuria; frequency; retention; urgency; hesitancy; incontinence; urethral trauma secondary to surgery
 	
Altered patterns of urinary elmination related to hypospadias requiring surgical repair
	The child will void a minimum of 1 cc/kg/h 24 h postoperatively and the color of the child's urine will progress from red (bloody) to clear by discharge	Monitor amount, color, consistency, and appearance of urine continually
		Document strict intake and output volumes hourly
		Properly administer ordered IV/po fluids dictated by child's electrolyte values and clinical status
		Maintain proper placement and patency of urinary catheter; protect from infection, dislocation
		Assess child for signs of abdominal distention
		  Measure abdominal girth q 4 h
		  Palpate bladder for distention
		Assess child for signs of increased pain (note location, quality, precipitating factors)
		Notify physician of changes in color or consistency of urine
		Note and record urine output/cc/kg/h; note and report increased abdominal distention
		Assess patency of urinary drainage tubes and presence of clots every hour
		Consult urologist immediately if obstruction to urinary flow via catheter is noted
		Avoid irrigation of urinary catheter if possible
		Prevent dislocation of urinary catheter
		  Secure catheter by taping to abdomen
		  Assess catheter placement q h; report dislocation of catheter/trauma to surgical site immediately

Continued.

NURSING CARE PLAN 27-1 The Child with Hypospadias—cont'd

Clinical Problem/Nursing Diagnosis	Expected Outcome	Nursing Interventions
		Apply extremity restraints as necessary to ensure safety of catheter placement and surgical site; restrain cautiously; explain purpose to child and parents
		Assess child for presence, frequency, duration of bladder spasms
		Prevent pressure on penis from bed linens (use bed cradle or overbed warmer without covers)
		Prevent increased edema to surgical site
		Position child to protect wound integrity
		Use Bellevue bridge (folded sheepskin) for penile and scrotal sac support
	The child will urinate spontaneously within 6-8 h after catheter clamping or removal	Notify physician of absence of urinary void within 8 h after catheter clamped or removed
		Observe quality of urinary sytream for color, amount, force, and line of flow first several voids after catheter removal
		Assess presence and degree of pain associated with voiding
Pain Pain related to surgical repair	The child will experience control of pain as evidenced by ability to rest and interact with environment in comfort	Assess child for signs of pain: restlessness, increased irritability, tachycardia, diaphoresis, facial grimacing, guarding, inability to rest, or day tugging at groin
		Assess type, location, quality, duration of pain; note precipitating and relieving factors q 1-2 h
		Properly administer pain medications, bladder analgesics, and antispasmodics as ordered
		Document and assess effectiveness of analgesics and antispasmodics
		Provide comfort through proper positioning; avoid pressure on penis
Fever Cloudy urine; infected wound site Potential for infection related to surgical trauma	Given the necessary nursing interventions, the child will have a temperature of 37.5°C	Preoperatively cleanse surgical area with antiseptic soap as ordered
		Obtain preop urinalysis and urine culture results preoperatively
		Monitor vital signs for increased temperature, tachycardia
		Monitor temperature q 2 h while febrile
		Notify physician of temperature ≥ 38.5°C
		Institute antipyretic measures as ordered and document effectiveness
		Encourage coughing, deep breathing, use of incentive spirometer postoperatively: note quality of breath sounds in all lung fields
	The child will experience wound healing without infection	Assess surgical wound for increased edema, erythema, purulent drainage, quality of wound healing, and tissue integrity
		Prevent increased edema to wound site to prevent incisional separation: Avoid pressure from bed linens on surgical site; avoid positions that promote dependent edema
		Use folded sheepskin roll to elevate scrotal sac/penis (Bellevue bridge)
	The child will have negative urine cultures	Assess urine for clarity or cloudiness, presence of sediment, clots
		Maintain patency of urinary catheter and urinary flow
		Prevent backflow of urine to the bladder
		Do not place urinary collection bag on siderail
		Maintain a closed sterile drainage system
		Utilize strict aseptic technique if system is opened (changing of IV bladder irrigation tubing)
Nausea; vomiting; surgical losses Potential fluid volume deficit and electrolyte imbalance	The child will attain adequate hydration status as evidenced by urine output of at least 1 cc/kg/h; specific gravity of 1.025; electrolyte balance	Monitor vital signs every hour for first 12 h postoperatively
		Assess child for presence of tachycardia, hypo or hypertension, dyspnea, and/or tachypnea
		Monitor serum electrolyte values, CBC
		Continually assess urine output for increased bleeding, presence of clots
		Assess surgical dressing for amount and color of drainage, note for bleeding q 2 h
		Assess hydration status: note quality of skin turgor, presence of tears, moist mucous membranes; check fontanel; measure urine, and specific gravity
		Note quantity of intake and output

Clinical Problem/Nursing Diagnosis	Expected Outcome	Nursing Interventions
Fearful behavior; restlessness; frequent nightmares; persistent withdrawal; regressive behavior	The child will attain mastery of hospitalization and surgical procedure without long-term psychological sequelae	Familiarize child and parents with hospitalization experiences through therapeutic play appropriate to age (include preparation for Foley catheter, IV, O$_2$ mask, going to the OR)
		Encourage use of proper terminology when referring to body parts (may need to identify the child's penis using words he is familiar with to ensure adequate communication; document this information on nursing care plan)
Fear related to developmental concerns with body integrity		Reassure the child that he is a good boy and is not being punished in any way
		Show the child his penis immediately when awake postoperately; reassure him that his penis is still present, intact, and whole
	The child will maintain developmental milestones that were present prior to hospitalization	Provide opportunities for the child to have choices and control
		Provide play activities that enhance child's strengths, allow the child to work through fears in hospital play and art therapy
		Encourage parents to verbalize feelings about the defect and required surgical repair
		Provide parents with information and support:
		Along with physician, address fears about child's future appearance and sexual function
		Address concerns and questions about surgery, post-op recovery, chld's psychological response to experience of hospitalization
		Teach parents how to assess for signs of infection, proper administration of medications, care of surgical site
		Facilitate follow-up care with urology clinic

dure needs to be explained in simple terms, and the child must be reassured that his penis will remain intact. It is important that the nurse let the child see his penis as soon as possible postoperatively. Parents may have fears regarding future appearance and sexual function, and these fears need to be addressed.

Renal Problems in the Toddler

Nephrotic Syndrome

The term *nephrotic syndrome* refers to a clinical entity with a primary symptom of proteinuria associated with hypoalbuminemia, hyperlipidemia, and edema. This disease may appear in the course of various systemic disorders, such as sickle cell disease and lupus, and then is designated as the secondary form. However, in children nephrosis is most frequently of the primary variety with an unknown cause. Previously diagnosed children may develop a chronic recurrent form of this disease (Vehaskari and Robson, 1981).

Regardless of the underlying cause, nephrotic syndrome has certain distinguishing clinical and pathophysiological features. The underlying defect is increased glomerular membrane permeability to large molecules so that considerable quantities of plasma proteins escape into the urine. Albumin is lost in greatest quantity because of its high plasma concentration and relatively low molecular weight. The loss of albumin disrupts the pressure gradient which monitors the filtration and absorption of water and electrolytes across the peripheral vascular beds. Intravascular fluid is transferred to the interstitial spaces, thus producing edema.

The nephrotic child is usually brought to the pediatrician because of "swelling." Parents first notice periorbital edema which does not subside; they may say that the child's shoes or trousers have been difficult to fasten or that the child has shown a sudden weight gain. Edema usually develops initially either in areas with low interstitial pressure (periorbital tissue) or in areas with the highest intracapillary pressure; thus it is seen in the dependent areas of the child's peritoneal cavity, legs and external genitalia (labia or scrotum). As the disease progresses, the extracellular fluid volume is expanded and the child has generalized edema. The skin over his abdomen may become stretched and shiny, with veins prominent; the devitalized skin in this region and other edematous areas has a characteristic waxy pallor and frequently breaks down because of increased interstitial fluid pressure and poor tissue tone. The child may have rectal prolapse, herniation, and/or hydrocele for similar reasons. Peripheral edema may be accompanied by fluid accumulations in pleural and pericardial cavities. A child may demonstrate symp-

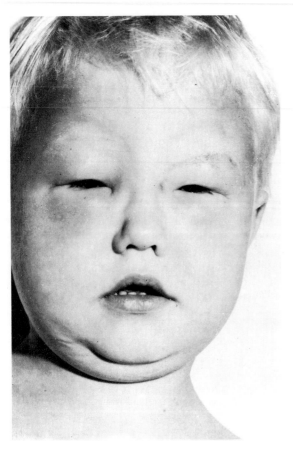

FIGURE 27-6   Child with active nephrosis. Note the severe periorbital and facial edema. *(Courtesy of S. Hellerstein.)*

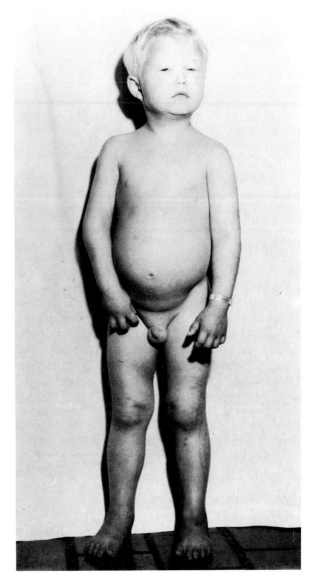

FIGURE 27-7   Full-length view of the child in Fig. 27-6. Note edema of the abdomen, scrotum, arms, legs, and feet. *(Courtesy of S. Hellerstein).*

toms of respiratory embarrassment due to pulmonary edema or because the ascites causes diaphragmatic elevation.

Progressive wasting of skeletal muscles may take place because of the continuous, voluminous drain of plasma protein nitrogen. Like the child who is suffering exclusively from protein malnutrition, the chronic nephrotic patient's wasted, sticklike extremities and prominent rib cage are in sharp contrast to his distended abdomen (Figs. 27-6 and 27-7). His hair may appear to lack luster because of this continuous protein drain. The loss of protein can influence immunoglobulin G (IgG) and IgA plasma levels, and the child may demonstrate an increased susceptibility to infections.

The parent notices a decreased frequency of the child's urination and foamy- or frothy-looking urine. Despite his appearance, the child with nephrosis appears to feel relatively well, although he tires easily and his appetite is poor. His blood pressure is normal or slightly lower than average. He may be anxious and embarrassed by his edematous, unattractive appearance; nurses, doctors, and other health care workers should avoid thoughtless remarks concerning the child's unusual appearance.

Parents' questions deal with "cause of this" and "the difference between nephritis and nephrosis." Clinical symptoms and laboratory tests can assist in differentiating between these two disease entities (Table 27-5).

Having received the diagnosis, parents next question the natural course of nephrosis: "How long will it last? Will my child remain this severely affected?" Parents need to know that childhood nephrosis is a chronic disease; they should think of the condition in terms of months or years rather than days or weeks. Regardless of initial treatment success, parents must understand that medical supervision will have to be continued for years because of the risk of exacerbation.

The duration and severity of any child's clinical course are variable. At one extreme is the child who undergoes spontaneous or steroid-induced diuresis after one edematous episode and experiences no relapse; at the other extreme is the child who remains persistently swollen, fails to respond to steroids and other drugs, and dies of progressive renal disease in 2 to 3 years. The majority of nephrotic children lie between these extremes, experi-

TABLE 27-5 Comparison of Acute Glomerulonephritis and Nephrosis

	Acute Glomerulo-nephritis	Nephrosis		Acute Glomerulo-nephritis	Nephrosis
Cause	Antigen-antibody reaction to group A beta-hemolytic streptococci	Unknown	Radiology	Cardiac enlarge-ment and pulmo-nary vascular congestion on chest x-ray	
Laboratory find-ings			Physical signs and symptoms	Periorbital edema Hypertension	Ascites Normal blood pressure
Urine	Gross hematuria Decreased output Proteinuria, rarely more than 3 g/24 hours	Proteinuria 2-10 g or more per 24 hours	Prognosis	In young children, 90-100% cure In older children, possibility of chronic renal disease	Remissions and exacerbations lasting up to 1-5 years
Blood	Blood urea nitro-gen and creati-nine: moderately increased in 50% Antistreptolysin titer: increased in 80% Complement: usually C_3	Hypoalbuminemia Hyperlipidemia			

 NURSING CARE PLAN

27-2 The Child with Nephrosis

Clinical Problem/Nursing Diagnosis	Expected Outcome	Nursing Interventions
Edema (increased H$_2$O); oliguria; hy-poalbuminemia; hypokalemia; hy-poproteinemia; pro-teinuria Fluid volume deficit and Electrolyte im-balances related to edema	The child will reach intravascular vol-ume homeostasis and electrolyte acid-base balance	Monitor strict intake and output volumes hourly Record urine specific gravity and pH; check urine for protein, glucose, blood, ketones q 4 h Assess urine for amount, odor, color, presence of foamy froth character-istics Monitor serum sodium, potassium, bicarbonate, BUN, creatinine, ammo-nia, protein, albumin values Assess changes in renal function values with corresponding treatment Obtain daily or BID weights; weigh child at the same time of day, docu-ment the scale used Assess location and severity of edema (periorbital, scrotal) Measure and record abdominal girth for increased ascites, assess for presence of fluid waves Monitor vital signs for symptoms of intravascular depletion (tachycardia, hypotension) and reporting findings to physician Properly administer ordered crystalloid and colloid solutions based on lab and clinical findings Properly administer salt poor albumin (.5-1g/kg) IV as ordered (usually followed by a diuretic); monitor vital signs, urine output, weights, lab values to assess effectiveness of therapy Properly administer steroids (e.g., prednisone 2 mg/kg/day); assess di-uretic response, decrease in weight, decrease in proteinuria Assess child for side effects or adverse reactions to medications such as steroids or immunosuppressive drugs (Chlorambucil) ordered to treat edema

Continued.

NURSING CARE PLAN 27-2 The Child with Nephrosis—cont'd

Clinical Problem/Nursing Diagnosis	Expected Outcome	Nursing Interventions

Edema; hypoproteinemia
 	
Potential impaired skin integrity related to edema; nutritional deficits
	Given the necessary nursing care, the child will avoid skin breakdown related to edema	Present pressure and excoriation injuries to skin from tape burns, sheet burns, temperature and pulse oximetry, probe burns
		Promote increased mobility through position changes q 1 to 2 h
		Protect skin from exposure to urine and stool:
		  Change diaper frequently and thoroughly wash affected skin and skin-fold areas with mild soap and H_2O (Keri bath oil)
		  Dry skin area thoroughly, avoid vigorous rubbing, apply cornstarch or non-perfumed powder to skinfold areas to decrease irritation
		  Provide scrotal support to decrease pressure and edema of scrotal sac: place a folded roll of sheepskin (Bellevue Bridge) under scrotum
		Limit venipunctures (especially to femoral site)
		Avoid intramuscular injection sites for route of medication administration
		Promote diet high in protein and nutritional value
		Assess skin areas susceptible to ulceration (scrotum, perineum, buttocks); check bony prominences for reddened areas
		Cut out foam pillows to protect bony prominences from pressure injury
		Provide sheepskin directly under child's skin
		Provide water mattress, water pillow to decrease pressure on skin

	Given the necessary nursing care, the child will be free of infection secondary to loss of skin integrity	Child with skin breakdown: Discontinue the use of powder or lotions; continue thorough washing and drying of skin; expose affected skin areas to air
Anorexia; diarrhea; negative nitrogen balance Altered nutrition: less than body requirements related to edema, anorexia, fatigue	With the appropriate meal plan, the child will reach positive nitrogen balance, have decreased tissue wasting, and tolerate a diet high in protein and low in saturated fats	Incorporate child's favorite food and snacks appropriately into meal plan Encourage frequent small feedings of high-protein, calorie enriched snacks (e.g., protein and calorie packed milkshakes) Promote diet high in protein (milk, meat, eggs) with a minimum intake of 2 to 3-g protein/kg/day Promote diet low in saturated fats and restricted in sodium (i.e., 1-2 gm daily for moderate restriction and 300 mg daily for severe restriction) Encourage rest, vitamin-enriched juices, fruits (oranges, bananas, grapes) Prohibit foods high in salt or the addition of table salt to foods Consult dietician to ensure adequate caloric, protein, vitamin intake in relation to age, weight, disease process Limit energy expenditure Prevent hypermetabolic states (promote adequate rest; maintain normothermia)
Ascites; dyspnea; tachypnea; rales Ineffective breathing pattern related to restricted chest expansion from ascites, edema	Given the appropriate nursing care, the child will realize adequate gas exchange and adequate oxygenation (O_2 sat 95 mmHg)	Monitor vital signs q 2 to 4 h Note changes in baseline HR, RR, BP, temperature, neurological status Immediately report changes to physician Monitor child for clinical signs of pulmonary edema and pleural effusion; assess for increased respiratory distress (note for presence of tachypnea, rales, retracting, flaring, grunting, hemoptysis, productive cough) Note color of nailbeds and mucous membranes Measure oxygen saturation values via pulse oximeter (notify physician for O_2 desaturations 95 mmHg) Properly institute oxygen therapy as indicated Promote positions that decrease pressure of abdominal contents on thoracic cavity from ascites (elevate head of bed; avoid prone position) Measure and record abdominal girth q 4 h Encourage coughing and deep breathing, incentive spirometry q 1 h Perform chest physical therapy with stable platelet counts

Clinical Problem/Nursing Diagnosis	Expected Outcome	Nursing Interventions
Fatigue Potential activity intolerance related to fatigue	The child will have adequate rest with appropriate balance of play and school activities	Provide increased rest periods during rapid diuresis phase of disease process Organize care to optimize prolonged periods of uninterrupted sleep
Edema Impaired physical mobility related to edema, fatigue Decreased interest in social play Body image disturbance related to edema (pharmacologic)	The child will gradually increase activity to prevent complications of immobility The child will participate in social interaction with self-confidence and self-esteem	Assess degree of limitation with fine motor skills due to edema Encourage range of motion exercises Promote gradual increase in toleration of activity Prevent child from having complication of immobility with meticulous attention to skin care and pulmonary hygiene Provide play and school activities that enhance child's strengths Explore child's perception of body image through expression in art therapy Provide opportunity to work out fears of altered body image through therapeutic play Explain presence of edema and Cushing's syndrome in terms appropriate to developmental level
Drug-induced immunosuppression Potential for infection related to hypoproteinemia; drug therapy	Given adequate protection the child will remain free of infection	Monitor for temperature elevations with vital signs: notify physician for temperature 38.5°C Institute antipyretic measures as indicated Protect child from contact with staff, visitors, patients with signs of infection Practice strict handwashing Promote toleration of diet high in protein and calories Use strict aseptic technique with invasive procedures; keep catheter sites clean and dry Do not administer vaccines during steroid treatment Teach parents that immunizations are not given until one year of remission from illness; school-age children will need protection from outbreaks of infectious disease, i.e., home tutoring
Knowledge deficit Potential ineffective family coping related to stressors of chronic illness, knowledge deficit	The family will be able to utilize appropriate coping mechanisms and achieve optimal family functioning given proper redemonstrating of established learning needs: medication administration (dose, time, side effects); dietary plan; verbalization of signs of infection; signs of increased proteinuria, by the time of discharge	Recognize and understand individual family responses to illness and individual coping mechanisms Explore parental understanding of child's illness and required treatments Clarify factual information concerning illness and required treatments Assist parents to participate in child's care Teach parents proper administration and side effects of steroids and immunosuppressive medications Prepare parents and child for symptoms of Cushing's syndrome (rounding of face, flushing, increased appetite) and that symptoms disappear 2 to 3 months after steroid therapy is discontinued Teach parents how to test first morning urine specimen for protein with reagent strip and to record daily outcomes Instruct parents to notify physician for results of +1/+2 protein content in urine for two consecutive days Teach parents to notify physician for increased edema, headaches, nausea, vomiting, fever Provide emotional support during stress of hospitalization and coping with a long term illness Assess the need for a visiting nurse or other support personnel to enhance comprehensive care for the child and family

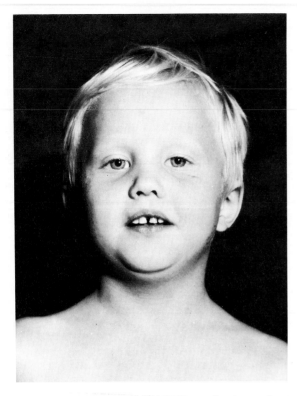

FIGURE 27-8 The child shown in Figs. 27-6 and 27-7 after 1 month of corticosteroid therapy. *(Courtesy of S. Hellerstein).*

encing any number of remissions (Fig. 27-8) and exacerbations over a period of years. These children generally recover but may have compromised renal function for life. Prognosis and treatment generally depend on the cause and type of glomerular lesion. In most instances the type of nephrotic syndrome present is best determined by renal biopsy.

Minimal-Change Nephrosis

Idiopathic or primary nephrosis is the most common form of the syndrome in children in the United States; of these patients, approximately 70 percent have minimal-change nephrosis. The most common age of onset is between 1½ and 2½ years of age, with the peak period being between 2 and 3 years.

It is impossible to predict the prognosis of minimal-change nephrosis by the patient's responses to steroids or by laboratory data. A favorable sign in patients is responsiveness to adrenocorticosteroids with loss of proteinuria at the onset. Lack of responsiveness to steroids when infection is not present is usually indicative of more serious renal disease.

Active nephrosis can have its complications. The child with generalized edema is unusually susceptible to intercurrent infections; this susceptibility is not solely attributable to reduced serum gamma globulin. Prophylactic treatment with extraneous gamma globulin does not seem to reduce the frequency of infection significantly. Edema fluid in living tissue is an excellent culture medium which offers little resistance to the spread of infection.

Deaths from bacterial infection in nephrotic patients are now rare, thanks to intensive, appropriate antibiotic treatment when necessary. Furthermore, children can be maintained edema-free with steroid therapy. However, the nephrotic child is as susceptible as any child to the common viral respiratory infections, and these infections frequently appear to precipitate exacerbations of edema.

Complications related to edema buildup may include ascites and respiratory distress. Diuretic therapy is usually effective in relieving this massive edema, and paracentesis is rarely needed. A common problem may be loose bowel movements, probably resulting from intestinal malabsorption secondary to edema of the bowel wall. Nursing management includes (1) reassuring the child that the frequent bowel movements are "not his fault" and subside as his edema decreases and (2) maintaining immaculate skin care to prevent excoriated buttocks and perineum.

Nursing Management
Activity and Diet

The nephrotic child, considering his age and developmental level, generally paces his own activity and sets his own limits satisfactorily. Dietary restrictions, except for the exclusion of salty foods, are not necessary (McEnery and Strife, 1982). Added salt in cooking and at the table is not allowed, but regular foods (bread, butter, milk) rather than salt-free are allowed. Once diuresis has occurred, an occasional cracker, piece of bacon, or other salty treat may be allowed.

A high-protein diet (much milk, meat, and eggs) would be desirable in nephrotic children to offset their persistent negative nitrogen balance and tissue wasting due to heavy proteinuria, but toleration for such a diet is a problem. A compromise diet containing 2 to 3 g of protein per kilogram of body weight per day is satisfactory. Protein intake may need to be monitored if the child shows signs of renal dysfunction and altered glomerular filtration rate. Low-saturated fats are included in the diet.

Edematous nephrotic children retain sodium and excrete potassium and ammonia as the principal urinary cations. Their diet therefore includes extra potassium in the form of juices, fruits (oranges, bananas, grapes), and milk. Fluid restriction is imposed only in extreme edematous phases; restriction is based on the child's previous day's urine output plus estimated insensible losses by way of the skin and lungs. When careful monitoring of fluid intake and urine output is desired, the nurse often can enlist the aid of the young patient by means of a simple bedside picture chart; the child feels he is actively participating in his care and exercising some control over his own restrictions. The child should be weighed daily to evaluate the progress of treatment, with care being taken to ensure accuracy.

Infection

A common complication of the nephrotic syndrome is infection. Clean technique with frequent hand washing is used by hospital personnel and visitors. Persons with obvious infection should not come in contact with the child. General recommendations now are that the young nephrotic child be kept away only from large gatherings (parties, Sunday school classes), especially during periods of increased respiratory infections. For the older nephrotic child, the benefit of attending regular school classes generally outweighs the risk of increased exposure to infection, but this decision must be made on an individual basis by the physician. Prior to the child's discharge from the hospital, the nurse and parents begin to plan for his being tutored at home if he is unable to resume regular schooling. Routine immunizations are omitted until the child has been in remission for 1 year, as live vaccines should not be used in conjunction with steroids. During outbreaks of infectious diseases in school, the school-age child may need to remain at home.

Skin Care

Potential skin care problems of edematous nephrotic children have been mentioned. Ulceration occurs most readily over the scrotum, perineum, and buttocks, where deterioration is aided by pressure, immobility, and exposure to urine and the proteolytic action of loose stools. Prevention of breakdown of the skin is the key word for the nurse in planning a meticulous program of skin care which includes frequent diaper changes, careful washing and drying of the exposed skin and skinfolds with mild soap and water, the liberal use of nonallergenic powder or cornstarch. Improvisation of a nonconstricting scrotal or labial support from soft cotton batting may be needed. If, despite precautions, the skin breaks down, powder and ointment should be discontinued; careful washing should continue, and the skin should be exposed to freely circulating air. Heat lamps should be used with utmost care to avoid burns. Some physicians favor the use of zinc oxide paste on resistant denuded areas to protect the skin against further irritation by urine and stool. Until the precipitating state of edema is relieved through diuresis, healing of severely ulcerated areas will usually not occur.

Support for Parents and Patients

Confronted with explanations of the child's disease and the many details of his daily management whether in the hospital or at home, parents understandably may appear bewildered and overwhelmed, requiring continuing psychological support and education from the nurse, physician, and other team members. Parental behavior and verbal expressions denoting excessive feelings of guilt, denial, overindulgence, and other potentially harmful attitudes should be recognized, respected, and approached honestly by the nurse and physician. Empathy, respect, and a willingness to become involved to assist parents in working through their own solutions to problems are prerequisite skills for any nurse associated with the parents of children with chronic disease. While the outlook for recovery is reasonably good, parents and children may express frustration over the slow response to treatment and the unpredictable pattern of disease recurrence.

Psychological support for the child is provided by parents and nurse on a daily basis. Behavioral or verbal expressions of anxiety over hospitalization and separation, depression, change in body image, and fear of a permanent disease state and death are likely in various forms from all nephrotic children. To pretend these factors do not directly influence the child's progress is to deny the child that progress. The nurse must practice listening and observational skills, respect the child's right to his feelings, and allot sufficient time and energy to demonstrate caring daily. The child often suggests ways to solve his own problems and to facilitate independence and participation in his own care. Dietary restrictions, urine testing, frequent testing and doctor visits, and the treatment side effects are all sources of concern for the child and his family.

Corticosteroid Treatment

Corticosteroids have become the mainstay of medical management, offering a brighter prognosis for the child and cooperative responsibilities for the nurse and parents. The goal of corticosteroid therapy is to decrease the amount of proteinuria, reverse the sequence of events which results in the syndrome, and promote excretion of edema fluid. The exact mode of action of corticosteroids in nephrosis is unknown. Though all corticosteroid preparations (cortisone, hydrocortisone, prednisone, prednisolone, triamcinolone, dexamethasone, and others) are equally effective in inducing remissions when given in an equivalent dosage, prednisone is generally the drug of choice because it has less of a tendency to induce salt retention and potassium loss.

Prednisone initially is given in divided doses on a daily basis. This schedule continues for 10 to 14 days after diuresis occurs and the urine is protein-free. This outcome is usually accomplished in about a month. The prednisone regimen is then changed to an alternate morning schedule for 1 month (McEnery and Strife, 1982). Treatment is tapered off gradually over another 2 months. Family members are instructed in the use of a protein reagent strip to test urine and are told to record the results once or twice weekly.

Steroid therapy has its common, bothersome, but not serious side effects; it also has some severe but rare complications (Table 27-6). The nurse should remember to reassure patients and parents that nearly all persons treated with steroids develop Cushing's syndrome to some degree. Children may be alarmed by the flushing and rounding of the face (moon facies), appearance of a pad of fatty tissue over the base of the neck (buffalo hump), abdominal distention, striae, liver enlargement, greatly increased appetite with accompanying weight gain, and increased body hair (hirsutism). Acne may be aggravated in adolescents. Though cushingoid features cause distress and embarrassment, they tend to become less prominent when intermittent maintenance therapy is begun and often disappear entirely within 2 to 3 months after steroid treatment is stopped.

TABLE 27-6 Side Effects of Corticosteroids

Body System	Common	Uncommon
Cardiovascular	Plethora	Thromboembolism
Hematologic	Leukocytosis	Hypertension
Gastrointestinal	Hepatomegaly	Peptic ulceration
	Abdominal distention	Pancreatitis
Endocrine	Adrenal suppression, sometimes persistent	Diabetes mellitus (reversible or irreversible)
Eye		Cataracts
Skin	Poor healing, striae	Panniculitis
	Moniliasis	
	Hirsutism	
Central nervous		Pseudotumor
		Seizures
Psychiatric	Depression	Psychosis
	Hyperactivity	
Skeletal	Osteoporosis	Compression fractures
	Delayed growth	
		Avascular necrosis
Immunologic	Decreased resistance to infection	Exacerbation of tuberculosis
	Decreased febrile response to infection	Fatal chickenpox
General	Obesity	Edema
	Increased appetite	Hypokalemia and alkalosis
	Azotemia if renal function impaired	

Serious side effects and uncommon complications of steroid therapy include the "masking" of infections, particularly gram-negative bacillary infections and staphylococcal infections (chickenpox, could prove fatal), peptic ulceration (less common than previously thought), growth suppression, cataracts, precipitation of diabetes mellitus, osteoporosis, thromboembolism, intracranial hypertension, and adrenal suppression and insufficiency. The latter factor is most worrisome because the frequency of permanent adrenal suppression in children who have received long-term steroid therapy for nephrosis is unknown. Parents should thus be alerted to this "stress factor" and should never discontinue the child's steroid therapy without the physician's knowledge and consent.

Monitoring during Recovery

While the child is under the close supervision of the physician, the nurse advises the parents of symptoms to report: additional weight gain, headaches, nausea, fever, or evidence of infection. The nurse carefully monitors the child's weight and blood pressure (using the appropriate size cuff and noting the child's posture, standing or recumbent) during the hospitalization or frequent office or clinic visits. The nurse, in conjunction with the physician, also monitors serum sodium, potassium, bicarbonate, and BUN at the beginning of therapy and at regular intervals

thereafter, noting major changes. If the child develops evidence of infection, hypertension, or electrolyte imbalance, he will no doubt be admitted to the hospital without delay; advance preparation for these eventualities is helpful to parents.

There may be periods of proteinuria for 2 to 3 days which are usually associated with respiratory infections but may occur without any obvious cause. If they do not persist, therapy is not reintroduced. Relapses usually occur within the first 3 months of treatment. The child is given the full dosage of daily prednisone until the proteinuria clears, then continued for 1 week, and then instituted every-other-day as stated above. The latter therapy may be continued for 4 to 6 months after proteinuria has cleared. No data indicate that this regimen decreases frequent recurrences. Wider recognition of the steroid-dependent group of children, increasing concern about the side effects of long-term steroid therapy, and the advent of cytotoxic drug therapy have combined to swing the pendulum back toward short courses of steroid therapy.

Unresponsiveness to Steroids

Unfortunately, steroids cannot be hailed as the "miracle drugs" of nephrosis since not all children respond favorably to steroid therapy. On the basis of therapeutic response, patients with the nephrotic syndrome may be classified into three groups:

1. *Steroid-sensitive:* Children may respond to a single short course of steroids without evidence of relapse after cessation of therapy. Less than 10 percent of children with idiopathic nephrotic syndrome fail to undergo a remission during the initial course of steroid therapy. Up to 40 percent of such children may be in this group.
2. *Steroid-dependent:* Some children respond incompletely; proteinuria is decreased but not absent, and edema subsides somewhat. These children tend to relapse on lowered doses of steroids and require further supportive treatment (diuretics, diet). They tend to have frequent relapses over many years and therefore receive large amounts of steroids, resulting in cushingoid features and growth retardation.
3. *Steroid-resistant:* Approximately 10 to 25 percent of children and a much higher percentage (70 to 80 percent) of adults become resistant to steroid treatment or cannot be maintained in remission without developing serious side effects from steroid therapy.

For the latter group, recognition of long-term toxic effects of corticoids, as well as therapeutic failures, has prompted a revival of interest in immunosuppressive drugs [chlorambucil, cyclophosphamide (Cytoxan), methotrexate]. Immunosuppressives in conjunction with steroids have proved promising in providing longer remissions. The nurse should be aware of toxic reactions to cyclophosphamide: suppression of bone marrow (white blood cell count below 3000 cells/mm^3), intercurrent fulminating bacterial or viral infections (measles and chickenpox), ulceration of gastric mucosa, alopecia, hemorrhagic cystitis, and others. Severity of the toxic effects of chlorambucil, particularly in regard to testicular injury in prepubertal boys, has been documented in several studies.

In children who have late relapses, the nephrosis usually is brought under control quickly with a short course of steroid therapy. It is justifiable to be moderately optimistic about the future if the child remains free of all signs of the disease for longer than a year. In any event, the nurse should expect to share with the child and his family the ups and downs of a chronic condition that will, it is hoped, eventually resolve.

Urinary Tract Infections

The seriousness of urinary tract infections (UTIs) in children is best appreciated when potential long-term effects are considered (Fig. 27-9). The nurse in a pediatrician's office or in a pediatric outpatient clinic cannot fail to be impressed by the sheer number of children diagnosed as having "UTI." The staff nurse or clinical specialist cannot fail to be impresssed by the tenacity of infection in children with chronic, recurrent pyelonephritis and the crippling sequelae. Traditionally, the responsibility for the care of children with UTIs has been shared by the general practitioner, pediatrician, and urologist. Today the nurse is assuming an expanded role in the care of these patients by carefully collecting specimens, planting "screening" cultures, interpreting growth results, helping supervise home medication regimens, screening, and educating parents about the importance of long-term follow-up care. The radiologist provides important additional information in determining whether kidneys are functioning normally and whether there is an unobstructed flow of urine throughout the urinary tract. Thus, nurse, pediatrician, urologist, radiologist, and parent must communicate continually and consistently against a background of change and conflicting recommendations to ensure optimum care for the affected child.

In order to understand UTIs one must become familiar with current terminology. *Bacteriuria* means simply growth of bacteria in the urine. Since bladder urine is normally sterile, a positive urine culture implies that (1) there is active bacterial growth in the urinary tract or (2) contamination has occurred after passage through the urethra.

Urine containing bacteria of the same pathogen in a concentration of 100,000 bacteria per milliliter or 10^5 by culture is indicative of a UTI. If two specimens collected under aseptic precautions contain 100,000 bacteria per milliliter of the same pathogen, a diagnosis of UTI is made. The patient may or may not be symptomatic. However, smaller numbers may be significant due to dilution of the urine or suppression by chemotherapy. Bacterial counts of 10^3 to 10^5 are considered suspicious and deserve further investigation (Durbin and Peter, 1984). However, finding the same bacteria in the urine, regardless of number, obtained from a noncontaminated suprapubic bladder tap is always indicative of UTI.

Clinically, the nurse may see patients whose diagnoses utilize traditional terminology, which attempts to localize symptoms. The patient having bacteriuria with urgency, frequency, and dysuria has symptoms suggesting infection in the lower urinary tract (cystitis). Patients with bacteriuria and back pain, chills, fever, and vomiting have symptoms suggesting infection of the *upper* urinary tract (acute pyelonephritis). Chronic pyelonephritis refers to actual renal disease *believed* to be caused by bacterial infection in the kidney, either past or present. Because of the difficulties in localizing the site of infection from clinical findings alone and because infection spreads easily within the tract, many authorities prefer to use the general term *urinary tract infection* without further qualification.

Bacteria commonly responsible for infection in the urinary system are *Escherichia coli,* one or more species

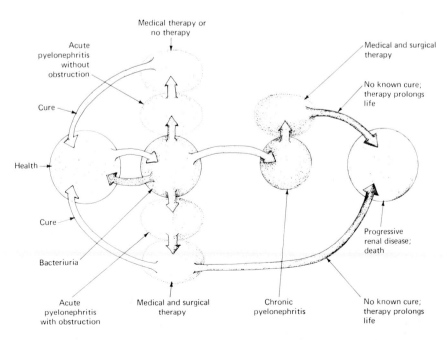

FIGURE 27-9 Schematic diagram demonstrating the seriousness of urinary tract infections in children.

of *Klebsiella, Enterobacter, Proteus, Pseudomonas,* and various enterococci, all normal constituents of the fecal flora. *Escherichia coli* is the causative organism in about 80 percent of first infections and 75 percent of recurrences. The *Klebsiella* and *Enterobacter* organisms account for 10 to 15 percent, and the remaining are due to *Proteus, Staphylococcus,* and *Pseudomonas.* These patterns occur in patients in whom no obstruction exists and neither antimicrobial agents nor instruments have been used. In contrast, patients who have been treated with antimicrobial drugs or who have been subjected to urologic procedures are more likely to have *Proteus, Pseudomonas, Klebsiella,* or *Enterobacter* as the offending organisms.

Urinary tract infection in children is often closely asso-

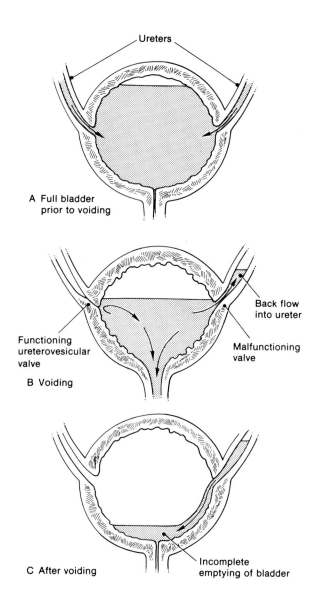

FIGURE 27-10 Vesicoureteral reflux. (A) Note the incompetent valve on the right and the competent valve on the left. (B) During voiding, urine is refluxed into the right ureter. (C) After voiding, the urine returns from the right ureter to the bladder.

ciated with *vesicoureteral reflux;* this term refers to the retrograde flow of bladder urine up into the ureters, a phenomenon which can be demonstrated radiologically. The reflux implies that the valve mechanism normally guarding the vesicoureteral (bladder-ureteral) junction is incompetent, possibly owing to the edema and inflammation caused by infection (Fig. 27-10). When reflux occurs, urine goes up the ureters during voiding and returns to the bladder when voiding has stopped. Therefore, residual urine results, and a pool for further infection exists. Reflux may be slight or gross, transient or persistent, unilateral or bilateral depending on clinical evidence of infection and/or radiological evidence of obstructive uropathy. The natural history of nonobstructive vesicoureteral reflux in children is to improve or cease with age (Hellerstein, 1982).

Other anatomic and physiological factors have been identified relating to susceptibility and/or resistance to UTI. Protective factors include the periodic removal of bacteria by urination and maintenance of an acidic urine. The bladder mucosa also has been demonstrated to have an ability to lyse bacteria with which it is in close contact. However, if much residual urine is present, this lysis cannot take place. Factors which increase susceptibility to UTI include catheterization and instrumentation, obstruction to the flow of urine, and the short female urethra.

Nursing Management
The clinical manifestations of UTI have already been discussed in part and vary greatly depending on the age of the child, the site of infection, and the chronicity of the infection. The neonatal period and the first year of life appear to have special significance in the prognosis of UTI. Nonspecific symptoms of poor feeding, slow weight gain, vomiting, diarrhea, irritability, and lethargy predominate. However, bacteremia occurs in approximately one-third of newborns with UTI and can lead to life-threatening sepsis and meningitis (Durbin and Peter, 1984). In infants 1 month to 2 years of age nonspecific symptoms still predominate. Sepsis and severe illness become somewhat less common. A 6 percent incidence of bacteremia was noted in infants 3 to 8 months of age compared with 31 percent of neonates and 18 percent of infants 1 to 3 months of age (Ginsburg and McCracken, 1982).

Acute pyelonephritis in toddlers and older children has an acute onset with high fever, unilateral or bilateral costovertebral angle (CVA) tenderness, vomiting, and dysuria. Febrile convulsions are not unknown. A history of vomiting, anorexia, and loose stools may lead to a probably diagnosis of gastroenteritis. In actuality the child may have a UTI. Therefore, in cases of unexplained illness in a young child, a urinalysis with microscopic examination should be routine.

Peak incidence for asymptomatic and recurrent UTI is in 6- to 13-year-old females. Symptoms include pallor, listlessness, and anorexia over a period of time. Exacerbations of infection may cause the child to pass cloudy, odorous urine; complain of burning and discomfort during urination; and relapse to nocturia or enuresis. It is important to follow the assessment guidelines outlined in Tables 27-1 and 27-2 so chronic kidney disease can be prevented.

The child with cystitis more often will complain of severe lower abdominal pain, burning on urination, and urgency or enuresis but will lack signs of systemic disturbances such as fever and vomiting. Frank hematuria may occur. During the nursing history the parent or child may recall these symptoms, which are common in the 2- to 5-year old since this age group is the peak period for symptomatic UTI. In Table 27-7 the ages at which various clinical symptons are most likely to occur are outlined.

The aims of treatment of children with UTI are to identify and clear the infection, to correct surgically any congenital or acquired obstruction in the urinary tract, and to reduce by means of long-term follow-up the number of clinical or bacteriologic exacerbations. Nursing care encompasses and furthers these goals and nurses provide supportive, symptomatic care for the child and parents.

One of the nurse's most important functions in the identification and management of a child with a UTI is the proper collection of a clean-catch urine specimen for a urine culture. After the specimen has been collected, the urine either introduced to a cultural medium in a petri dish within 30 minutes or refrigerated. The urine may be refrigerated for as long as 48 hours without changing the bacterial count. Since antibacterial drug therapy is the mainstay of treatment, the nurse should become familiar with bactericidal or bacteriostatic agents most frequently used, the dosages, their common side effects, and adverse reactions. Antibiotic treatment should be guided by the results of urine culture and sensitivities and by the clinical response to treatment. The nurse assists in obtaining initial and follow-up urine specimens for culture and relays pertinent information about the child's response to drug therapy. Initial symptoms generally disappear 2 to 3 days after the start of treatment. A repeat urine culture is done 48 to 72 hours after the start of drug therapy and should be negative if an effective antibacterial agent has been selected.

The hospitalized child may require intravenous fluid therapy until the infection and fever are brought under control. If "forcing fluids" is prescribed not only to prevent dehydration but also to ensure frequent flushing of the bladder, an oral fluid plan (specified in milliliters per 8-hour period) may be worked out with the child's cooperation and posted at the bedside. Allotments for waking hours take precedence, and equivalent measures for the child should be shown (for example, one large drinking glass = 240 ml).

After 10 to 14 days of treatment for an acute infection, the following approach may be instituted:

1. Two to three days following treatment, urine culture is repeated.
2. Two to three weeks after therapy, urine culture is repeated; thereafter it is done at 3-month intervals for 1

year. If there are no recurrences, the cultures can be discontinued.
3. Urine cultures need to be done at 4-month intervals the second year. If there are no recurrences, the cultures can be discontinued.
4. Three to five weeks after an infection has cleared, an IVP and VCUG need to be done. Renal ultrasound and radionuclide voiding cystography, if available, may be used (Durbin and Peter, 1984). Current research supports doing the x-ray studies after the initial infection because of the high recurrence rate in females and be of the high incidence of reflux in patients under 2 years of age.
5. Patients with frequent recurrences may be placed on prophylactic therapy for 3 to 6 months following the acute therapy. After treatment is discontinued, urine cultures need to be repeated every 3 to 4 months (Hellerstein, 1982).

Recommendations made by the nurse to the patient and/or family may have value in helping to keep the patient free of bacteriuria. The nurse instructs the child or adolescent to do the following as appropriate to age, development, and life style:

1. Wipe from the front to back after urination and bowel movements to avoid contamination from the rectum
2. Urinate frequently
3. Maintain an adequate fluid intake, particularly water, to promote flushing of the bladder
4. Avoid constipation since there seems to be a correlation between constipation and urinary retention
5. Avoid chemical irritants such as bubble bath soap
6. Take short tub baths, showers, or sponge baths
7. Avoid prolonged sitting in infant swimming or wading pools
8. Avoid feminine hygiene products, which can cause irritation
9. Wear cotton underwear and pantyhose with a cotton crotch to avoid perineal irritation

The nurse can play a primary role in helping patients and families understand the importance of proper follow-up. Often it is difficult for parents to comprehend the long and costly follow-up, particularly when the child seems to be fine. Perhaps the use of self-administered dipsticks could help defray the costs and ensure proper medical follow-up.

Ureteral Reimplantation

Surgical intervention may be necessary in children to relieve severe obstructive or nonobstructive uropathy so that ensuing renal damage from reflux, inadequate urinary drainage, and infection be prevented. Reimplantation of the ureters is performed to correct vesicoureteral reflux. Normally the ureters pass obliquely through the muscle of the bladder wall so that a flap valve is formed to prevent any backflow of urine into the ureters when the bladder contracts and empties. Reflux of urine into the ureters and renal pelvis on one or both sides during voiding indicates that the ureterovesical valve mechanism is incompetent.

TABLE 27-7 Clinical Manifestations of Urinary Tract Infection

Age	Symptoms	Comments
Neonate	Poor feeding, vomiting, diarrhea, fever, respiratory distress, CNS* symptoms of irritability	Child may be septic, have CNS disease, or have structural anomalies of urinary system as underlying causes
Infant	FTT,* anorexia, vomiting, irritability, fever, malaise	FTT is sign of chronic infection with kidney involvement
Toddler and preschooler	Fever, dysuria, urgency, frequency, enuresis, abdominal and loin pain	Classical picture of acute UTI* is seen in these age groups; peak incidence occurs in these age groups
School-age child and adolescent	Asymptomatic child Chronic nocturnal enuresis Dysuria, frequency, urgency	Peak age for recurrent or asymptomatic infection occurs in this age group Classical symptoms may be due to sexual activity— "honeymoon cystitis," vaginitis, or veneral disease

*CNS = central nervous system; FTT = failure to thrive; UTI = urinary tract infection.

 NURSING CARE PLAN

27-3 The Child with a Urinary Tract Infection (UTI)

Clinical Problem/Nursing Diagnosis	Expected Outcome	Nursing Interventions
Fever Chills — Potential for infection related to bacteremia Potential for recurrent urinary tract infections	Given antibiotic therapy, the child will have a normal temperature in 48 h	Monitor vital signs for signs of infection (tachycardia, hypotension) Monitor temperature for elevations q 2 h: notify physician for temperature 38.5°C, institute antipyretic measures as ordered Properly obtain clean catch urine specimen for culture and sensitivity; prevent contamination of specimen; rapidly transport specimen to laboratory and refrigerate immediately Properly administer prescribed antibiotics Flush bladder; encourage PO fluids: properly administer ordered intravenous solutions to optimize hydration status Check urine cultures 48 h after treatment
	Given the proper instructions, the child will remain free from recurrent UTIs.	Instruct child/parents how to prevent recurrent UTIs, appropriate to age: Teach to wipe from front to back after urinating or stooling to decrease fecal contamination from rectum Encourage frequent urination: teach to prevent holding in need to void Promote flushing bladder with frequent PO intake of H₂O, cranberry juice (especially in summer months) Teach to control constipation with a diet high in fiber, bulk, and fruits Teach to avoid use of bubble bath, chemical irritants Teach to limit tub baths; to shower Teach to avoid sitting in children's pools and to limit time wet swimming suit is worn Teach to eliminate feminine hygiene products Teach to wear cotton crotch to avoid perineal irritation Teach to report early signs of UTI (dysuria, low-grade fever) promptly to physician Teach proper administration of pharmacologic prophylactic therapy in children with frequent recurrences Provide written instructions of prevention plan Assess client/parent compliance with preventive regimen
Urgency Frequency Dysuria — Altered patterns of urinary elmination related to bacteriuria	After taking antibiotics for 48 to 72 h, the child will be free of urgency, frequency, and dysuria	Properly administer prescribed antibiotics Properly administer urinary tract analgesics (phenazopyridine hydrochloride) and antispasmodics Assess degree of pain, burning on urination, bladder spasms Assess presence of lower UTI signs (urgency, frequency, dysuria) Assess for signs of upper UTI: back pain, uni/bileraretal costovertebral angle tenderness, chills, fever, vomiting, abdominal pain Assess voiding pattern and urinary stream

NURSING CARE PLAN 27-3 The Child with a Urinary Tract Infection (UTI)—cont'd

Clinical Problem/Nursing Diagnosis	Expected Outcome	Nursing Interventions
Pain related to UTI		Monitor urine output; note amount, color, odor, presence of sediment; check specific gravity; dipstick for pH; blood glucose; protein, ketones q 4 h
		Note presence of nocturia/enuresis
		Change diaper frequently
		Wash perineum with mild soap and H_2O; cleanse thoroughly; dry well
		Properly obtain urine culture 48-72 h after antibiotic therapy
		Monitor serial urine culture, CBC
		Support child and parents through procedures, interventions, x-ray studies (IVP, cystourethrogram)
		Assess comfort status for effectiveness of analgesics and antispasmodic medication
Anorexia; nausea; vomiting; abdominal pain; diarrhea	Given the necessary nursing interventions, the child will have an adequate nutritional intake	Encourage foods and fluid that acidify urine (cranberry juice)
		Promote caloric value of food and fluid intake
Altered nutrition: less than body requirements related to anorexia and abdominal pain		Properly administer ordered intravenous solution to optimize hydration status, flush bladder

Armed with such diagnostic findings from a VCUG and cystoscopy, the pediatric urologist may intervene surgically to reimplant the ureter(s) more obilquely into the bladder and to lengthen the submucosal tunnel. Surgical reimplantation of one or both ureters may be performed at that time. The urologist defers surgery until (1) the urinary tract has been adequately drained by means of an indwelling catheter, a suprapubic cystotomy, or nephrostomy tubes, (2) the urinary tract has been cleared of infection, if possible, by the use of appropriate antibiotics, and (3) kidney function has improved to the greatest extent possible.

Nursing Management

Most commonly this surgery is undertaken during the preschool period. Preoperative teaching includes basic explanations of the procedure and equipment which the child will encounter. Special attention is paid to fears about body integrity, which are common and are likely to be intensified by the presence of invasive equipment.

Postoperative care of the child with a ureteral reimplantation includes not only the general nursing measures implemented for any child who has undergone a major surgical procedure but also some unique measures particular to this type of surgery. The child returns from surgery with a suprapubic catheter in the bladder. Depending on the surgeon, he may also have bilateral ureteral

splints in place and a urethral catheter. Each tube is attached to separate closed drainage systems, with the character and amount or absence of urine from each tube noted and recorded separately. The tubes must be kept free of any obstruction or compression. The physician must be notified of clots which may obstruct urine flow so that irrigation can be ordered to maintain patency. Small amounts of urine may leak around the ureteral and suprapubic catheters. Dressing covering these areas should be changed frequently to prevent skin irritation and infection. Antibiotics frequently be administered to reduce the risk of infection.

Postoperatively the nurse must take care to prevent tension on the catheters when turning and positioning the patient. The tubing should be manipulated to allow gravitational flow of urine. The patient may need to be restrained, especially during the early postoperative period, to prevent displacement of catheters. Frequent turning, coughing, and deep breathing are important to prevent postoperative complications. The nurse should monitor hydration status to ensure adequacy of fluid intake. During the early postoperative period the child is given intravenous fluids and then gradually advanced to oral intake. Because of lack of activity and discomfort, the child may eat sparingly.

During the postoperative phase pain due to the child's bladder spasms. Restlessness, irriability, crying, and withdrawal are frequent signs of pain in young children. Bladder spasms should be treated with antispasmodics. Belladonna and opium suppositories provid relief as they relax the bladder wall. Early ambulation is a challenge for both nurse and child, but it can and should be accomplished with proper care and assistance.

Unfortunately, not all problems of infection and inadequate drainage can be completely solved by ureteral reimplantation, since normal drainage depends on the normal peristaltic activity of the ureter and pelvis. This drainage is usually impaired to some degree by previous infection, tortuosity, and scar tissue. The child will be watched closely and will have repeated IVPs and VCUGs to monitor his progress for 3 to 5 years.

Hemolytic-Uremic Syndrome

Hemolytic-uremic syndrome (HUS) is distinguished by a triad of feature: hemolytic anemia, thrombocytopenia, and azotemia. This disease most frequently affects young children and has a high rate of mortality; however, the prognosis improves with early diagnosis and intervention.

In most cases no specific causative agents have been identified; the potential causes most frequently suggested include an antigen-antibody reaction and a viral infection. Genetic factors may also be involved (Fong et al., 1982). This disease commonly affects previously healthy children who have had an episode of gastroenteritis 1 to 10 days before the appearance of acute symptoms. The child then begins bleeding from various sites: gums, nares, vagina, gastrointestinal tract, and urinary system. Because of the bleeding, the child is pale, weak, and anemic. Frequently, the neurological system is involved and symptoms of irritability, lethargy, convulsions, stupor, or coma are present. Renal failure may be present with either oliguria or anuria; however, nonoliguric acute renal failure may occur. Hypertension and edema are also accompanying signs. If the renal failure progresses, the child may develop congestive heart failure, pulmonary edema, and respiratory distress.

The child with HUS demonstrates a number of laboratory abnormalities including elevated BUN, creatinine, and serum potassium. The white blood cell count is frequently increased, and platelets may be low. Anemia is always present, and reticulocytosis is evident. The urinalysis demonstrates hematuria, proteinuria, and increased cast cells.

Nursing Management

The nursing management for HUS is primarily supportive. Acute renal failure protocol is instituted and the child is usually placed on peritoneal dialysis or hemodialysis. Common patient problems which the nurse should anticipate include hypertension, fluid and electrolyte disturbances, and infection. HUS has also been treated using dialysis in combination with exchange transfusions. Another form of treatment commonly used is the administration of heparin to prevent fibrin from being deposited in the glomeruli. Careful monitoring of dosage and patient re-

sponse is vital. It is also important that the nurse provide supportive psychological care for the child and family, (e.g., exploring parental feelings of helplessness and threat of death, talking in a reassuring tone to the child even if he is in coma, providing pre- and postprocedural play and/or discussion sessions for the child who is conscious). The disease occurs as an acute, life-threatening process, and the child and family need adequate information and support in coping with this situation.

Renal Problems in the Preschool and School-Age Child

Glomerulonephritis

Acute immune complex-mediated glomerulonephritis may result from one of several agents, including bacterial, viral, and parasitic sources (Jordan and Lemire, 1982). *Poststreptococcal glomerulonephritis* is the most common form of glomerulonephritis in children. It is more prevalent during the school-age years, with an average age at onset of 6 to 7 years. While most series report a 2:1 ratio of boys to girls, analysis of patients affected during epidemics of poststreptococcal glomerulonephritis show a 1:1 male to female ratio (Jordan and Lemire, 1982).

Streptococcal infections of the upper respiratory tract or skin most often precede poststreptococcal glomerulonephritis. A latent period occurs between the infection and the onset of nephritis (1 to 2 weeks for pharyngitis, 2 to 3 weeks for skin infections). The disease results from deposits of antigen-antibody complexes within the glomeruli. With electron microscopy the deposits can be seen in the glomeruli and basement membrane. Diagnosis is based on (1) the presence of glomerular injury (hematuria and proteinuria), (2) identification of a nephritogenic strain of group A beta-hemolytic streptococcus, and (3) a rise in antibody titers to streptococcal products after the latent period (Jordan and Lemire, 1982).

Acute Phase

The onset is usually abrupt, with the most common clinical manifestations being hematuria and edema. Periorbital edema (Fig. 27-11) is often present, and edema of varying degrees is found in individual patients. Gross hematuria, described as reddish-brown or Coke-colored urine, is present in a majority of children, and microscopic hematuria is found in nearly all children with the disease. The child appears lethargic and pale and has a poor appetite. Hypertension is usually mild to moderate but can be severe enough to cause hypertensive encephalopathy. The hypertension is most likely secondary to the increased sodium and water retention.

Circulatory congestion due to increased extracellular fluid may result in dyspnea and cough. Pulmonary congestion or pleural effusion may occur. Oliguria is common, but anuria is rare. Occasionally systemic symptoms such as nausea and vomiting, abdominal pain, and mild fever are present. The acute symptoms usually fade in 1 to 2 weeks.

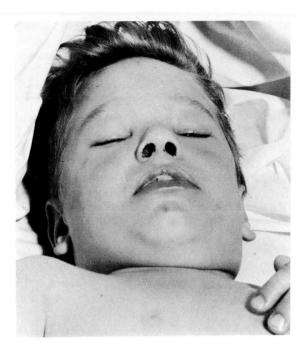

FIGURE 27-11 A child in the acute phase of poststreptococcal glomerulonephritis. Note the periorbital edema. *(Courtesy of S. Hellerstein.)*

Convalescent Period

The convalescent period begins at the completion of diuresis and the resolution of hypertension. During this phase the child feels well and wants to be active. Three or four days before discharge the child is observed closely for gross hematuria and weight gain. At discharge the child is permitted indoor activities, and he will be able to return to school in 2 weeks if there is no recurrence of hematuria or hypertension. Since microscopic hematuria and proteinuria may persist for a year or more, it is generally recommended that the child participate in ordinary activities since the course of nephritis does not seem to be adversely affected by activity.

Poststreptococcal acute glomerulonephritis in young children is a benign disease, and the prognosis is considered to be good. However, children in the older age groups do not share this excellent prognosis, as a significant percentage develop chronic renal disease.

Nursing Management

The treatment for acute glomerulonephritis involves management of the child's acute symptoms and complications that develop. Many children can be treated at home if the symptoms are mild and the family can provide close observation and care. The family needs to be able to monitor vital signs, intake and output, and weight. The clinic nurse and/or visiting nurse can teach the family these skills as well as signs of reduced renal function. Regular visits or telephone calls from the nurse can be a great support to the family and provide the nurse with the opportunity to evaluate the child's progress. Recovery is spontaneous in almost all cases if in the acute phase there is intelligent use of dietary and fluid restrictions and drug therapy.

The amount of activity allowed is proportional to the severity of the clinical manifestations. Children with gross hematuria, edema, circulatory congestion, or moderate to severe renal failure are encouraged to remain on strict bed rest to decrease the risk of cardiac failure. These children generally feel ill and limit their activity voluntarily. The nurse can suggest to the child and family quiet activities that can be carried out in bed.

Dietary restrictions depend on the severity of the clinical signs and symptoms. With edema and hypertension the intake of sodium is restricted to 1g, and with mild hypertension a no-added-salt diet is allowed. Potassium intake is limited until the child is voiding an adequate amount. A low-protein diet may be advised if the BUN is elevated above 75 to 100 mg/ml. Fluid intake also is limited if oliguria and renal failure are present.

The aim of treatment is to increase urinary output and may be accomplished through diuretics. The nurse must monitor blood pressure and intake and output carefully. If the diastolic blood pressure rises above 100 mmHg, antihypertensive therapy is required in addition to the diuretics. All patients should be weighed daily at the same time and on the same scale. Weight change is the best index of overall fluid balance. Increased urinary output and a subtle decrease in body weight alert the nurse to the first signs of improvement. Within several days, urine volume increases greatly and may be as much as 3 liters/24 h. As diuresis progresses, the blood pressure begins to drop and the child's appetite and sense of well-being return to normal (Fig. 27-12).

Treatment of patients with acute glomerulonephritis

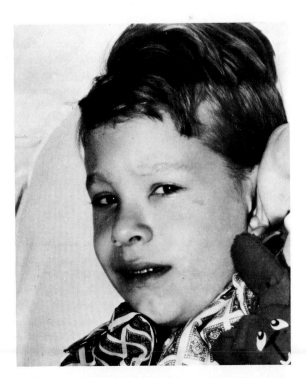

FIGURE 27-12 The child shown in Fig. 27-11 after several days of diuresis. Note the decrease in periorbital edema. *(Courtesy of S. Hellerstein.)*

usually includes an adequate course of penicillin unless the patient has been treated prior to admission. During the convalescent period penicillin therapy is not recommended. However, throat cultures need to be obtained from all immediate family members, and treatment must be given for all positive cultures.

Renal Trauma

Accidents are a common problem in the pediatric population. Renal trauma can involve the upper urinary tract, including the kidney and ureter, or the lower tract, involving the bladder and urethra. Renal injury is frequently seen in children suffering major multiple trauma, but it has also been documented in some children with minor trauma.

Damage to the kidney as a result of blunt trauma from an automobile accident or sports injury usually is indicated by the presence of hematuria and flank pain. Often these symptoms are indicative of a contused kidney, and surgery is rarely necessary. Penetrating kidney injuries or kidney rupture can result in extensive hemorrhage with blockage of the ureter with clots. These conditions require immediate surgery. Close follow-up after discharge is necessary for the evaluation of renal function.

Bladder injuries are more frequently seen in the child because of the intraabdominal positioning of the bladder. Signs indicative of bladder injury include pain, inability to void, and abdominal tenderness. Contusions and small tears may be treated using continuous urinary drainage. Large tears and urethral injuries may require operative intervention and then continuous urinary drainage via a suprapubic tube.

Nursing Management

Bed rest, supportive care, and monitoring of renal function are aspects of nursing care for the patient with a renal contusion. For injuries requiring surgical intervention, postoperative care should include monitoring for signs of shock and adequacy of renal function in addition to the usual postoperative management. Careful attention to catheters for patency and description and measurement of output must be implemented and documented. The parents and child need teaching and supportive care which may have been delayed because of the suddenness of the injury and subsequent surgery.

With bladder trauma, nursing care is aimed at providing adequate fluids, maintaining catheter security, monitoring the quality of renal function, and providing relief of bladder spasms. Teaching and adequate follow-up after surgery are needed. Also, the nurse should discuss the importance of protection to prevent renal trauma, such as proper fitting of abdominal protectors for children playing football.

Neurogenic Bladder

Neurogenic bladder is caused by impairment of the motor and/or sensory nerve supply to the bladder. Urinary incontinence and/or retention occur, and infection, reflux,

and renal failure can result if treatment is not implemented. Social problems resulting from incontinence become a concern as the child enters the preschool and school-age years.

The cause is most often a spinal defect such as a myelomeningocele, but this condition also can be due to spinal cord injury, tumors, or other congenital anomalies or neurological diseases. Initial assessment, whether at birth or after injury or disease onset, includes observation of voiding patterns (stream, dribbling, frequency), color and odor of urine, abdominal palpation to check for retention and careful output measurement. Signs and symptoms of a UTI may be present. Skin breakdown may be a problem, with constant wetness. Further delineation of renal status, bladder capacity and pressures, and residual urine volumes are accomplished through radiological procedures, cystoscopy, and urodynamic studies performed by the urologist.

Goals of Management

The four clear objectives in the treatment of a child with urinary tract dysfunction are to (1) salvage and preserve renal function, (2) provide for adequate urinary drainage, (3) keep the patient free of infection and (4) optimize the child's social condition (Mitchell and Rink, 1985). Over the past several years both surgical and nonsurgical treatment of neurogenic bladder problems has been developed and refined.

Clean Intermittent Catheterization

The procedure of clean intermittent catheterization (CIC) is a method to achieve retention of urine and decrease the problems of infection, vesicoureteral reflux, and incontinence. In a study of 53 children with myelomeningocele managed with intermittent catheterization for 5 years or more, 43 were dry, 8 were incontinent only at night, and 2 had some daytime wetness. The incidence of UTI was decreased, and 46 patients had stable or improved renal status (Uehling et al, 1985). This clean procedure can be taught to the parents of a young child and to the child when he is old enough. A mental age of about 5 years and child readiness are prerequisites to the child's learning self-catheterization. The degree of disability, amount of bracing, and other factors will also influence how soon and how readily the child can accomplish the task.

Urinary Diversions

While CIC has proved beneficial in the management of neurogenic bladder problems, it is not successful in all patients. Some children require a diversion on at least a temporary basis.

A *cutaneous vesicostomy,* to open the bladder into the abdominal wall via a stoma, is a temporary diversion in the young child. It is not functional for older children or adults as stomal problems and problems of appliance adherence are common.

The *colon conduit* (diversion into a loop of colon) has been used over the past 10 to 15 years, but more

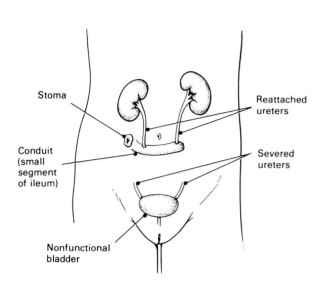

FIGURE 27-13 Anatomic drawing of a conduit.

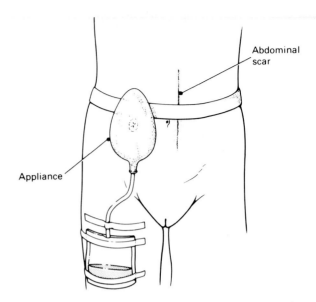

FIGURE 27-14 Position of the permanent appliance after a conduit procedure.

long-term data are needed. In this operation a small segment of the colon (a few inches) is resected. The colon ends are rejoined to retain a normal digestive tract. One end of the small segment is sutured closed. The other end is brought through a small opening in the child's abdominal wall, folded back, and attached to the outside of the abdominal wall to form a stoma (Fig. 27-13). The ureters are severed near the bladder and attached to the segment of colon. They can be implanted in a manner that prevents reflux of urine back into the ureters. The urine then drains from the colon segment through the stoma into a pouch worn over the stoma (Fig. 27-14). The pouch is emptied at intervals during the day, connected to dependent drainage at night, and changed every 4 to 7 days or more often if needed.

Other Surgical Procedures

Bladder augmentation procedures enable a child to stay dry on CIC or avoid diversion. A segment of ileum, sigmoid colon, or cecum is used as a patch to enlarge the small high-pressure bladder and increase storage capacity.

Undiversion, or the takedown of previous conduits, is being performed on some older children. The use of bladder augmentation procedures and artificial urinary sphincter implants has made undiversion more feasible. However, careful patient selection and evaluation are necessary before these procedures are undertaken (Mitchell and Rink, 1985).

The *artificial urinary sphincter* has been improved over the past several years and is now used in both children and adults to achieve continence. Careful evaluation of the child's urinary status and the patient and family's ability to manage the device and maintain appropriate follow-up is necessary before undertaking this surgery. Long-term prognosis is still unknown (Mitchell and Rink, 1985).

Nursing Management

Preoperative teaching of the child and family helps them understand changes in body function, postoperative care and needs, and long-term follow-up care. Immediate postoperative nursing care of a child who has had conduit surgery, bladder augmentation, or undiversion includes monitoring of intravenous fluids, nasogastric tube function, urinary output, incisional care, and coughing and deep breathing. The sphincter implant does not require the nasogastric tube, and recovery is generally faster as the surgery is not as long and complex. If a stoma is present postoperatively, the nurse should be alert to cues from the child and family indicating readiness to view the stoma.

The conduit surgery results in a major change in body structure. There may be reluctance on the part of both parents and child to accept the change in body image. Prior to discharge, it is the responsibility of the nurse to assist the child and parents in learning the techniques involved in the child's individual management program.

Renal Problems in the Adolescent
Chronic Glomerulonephritis

Chronic glomerulonephritis is any idiopathic, progressive form of renal disease in which the clinical picture of proteinuria, hematuria, and hypertension indicates major involvement of the glomeruli. There may be no history of an attack of acute glomerular disease or there may be a history of recurrent episodes. Since it may not be associated with any other disease process, it is possible for significant renal destruction to occur before symptoms become evident. The adolescent with chronic nephritis may show varied symptoms. He may feel entirely well with proteinuria detected on a routine physical, or he may present with gross hematuria, hypertension, edema, or unexplained renal failure. Laboratory values indicate deteriorating renal function.

The natural progression of the disease is highly individual. The renal insufficiency may extend over many years or may progress rapidly over 1 to 2 years.

Nursing Management

In addition to assisting with the diagnostic aspects such as specimen collections, the nurse plans care to revolve around his daily activities and needs. Normal activity and school attendance are advocated versus bed rest, except during flare-ups with edema and hypertension. The clinic nurse may need to help the adolescent boy or girl find viable substitutes for strenuous competitive and/or contact sports (such as managing a team or playing in a band).

The need for hospital admission in chronic glomerulonephritis is similar to that of acute glomerulonephritis and nephrotic syndrome (i.e., when the patient has severe edema, acute or uncontrolled hypertension, oliguria, severe electrolyte imbalance, and severe intercurrent infection). Usually no dietary restrictions are imposed unless the patient is edematous, hypertensive, or azotemic. For edema and hypertension, a no-added-salt diet (1 to 2 g sodium/d) is prescribed; if the BUN exceeds 50 to 60 mg/100 ml (normal 8 to 15 mg/100 ml), a protein-restricted diet similar to that used for chronic renal failure (0.5 to 1 g protein/kg body weight with protein-containing essential amino acids) may be indicated. Supplemental vitamins and essential minerals need to be included.

Intercurrent infection often causes exacerbations of edema, hematuria, and electrolyte imbalance in adolescents with chronic nephritis. Vigorous antibiotic therapy may be instituted to prevent further deterioration of the kidneys. The nurse needs to reassure the adolescent that the transient edema altering his or her appearance is often a function of intercurrent infection and/or hypertension and may subside with appropriate drug treatment. Thiazide diuretics along with reserpine and hydralazine are generally the drugs of choice. Additional drug therapy may include corticosteroids in combination with cytotoxic drugs. Dialysis and transplantation may restore health and make it possible to manage more effectively the patient whose disease has progressed to chronic renal insufficiency.

The psychological aspects of management are extremely important. Any existing weaknesses or strains in the parent-child relation will no doubt surface. While parents may exhibit guilt, denial, and overindulgence, the adolescent may react with aggression and/or withdrawal. Depression over the illness and the possibility of death may be dealt with overtly or covertly by the adolescent and his parents; confrontation with these issues may be wished for and feared at the same time. By merely giving verbal recognition to the existing state of tense ambivalence, the nurse can initiate open communication between parents and child and between medical personnel and child, thereby enabling all concerned to cope more effectively with the energy and resources available.

Systemic Lupus Erythematosus

One other condition which has renal complications in adolescence as part of the overall systemic disease process is lupus erythematosus (SLE). Of unknown cause, SLE is characterized by the development of numerous autoantibodies directed toward components of the patient's tissues, and reactions involving these antibodies are responsible for most of the clinical and laboratory findings. The disease is more common in girls and is generally seen in children over 6 years of age. A majority of these children have renal involvement.

Upon biopsy, focuses of necrosis and hypercellularity are found within the glomeruli. The systemic symptoms of lupus (skin rash, joint pains, and fever) can be greatly suppressed with high-dose corticosteroid therapy, but the effectiveness of steroids in controlling the progression of the renal lesions is less pronounced. Currently, azathioprine is the alternative drug of choice, often in conjunction with prolonged low dose steroids. Diuretics and antihypertensives may be added to the regimen in light of edema and high blood pressure. Because patients with lupus appear to be unusually susceptible to infections, prolonged treatment with steroids and azathioprine, which suppress the body's resistance to systemic infection, is not without hazard. Lupus erythematosus carries a more serious prognosis in the child than in the adult, largely because of the elements of renal failure and infection. Each child's progression is variable, and experience with cytotoxic drugs in lupus is still too limited to allow assessment of prolongation of survival time.

Acute Renal Failure

Acute renal failure, a potentially reversible condition, is evidenced by a sudden reduction in urine output and BUN retention, usually due to renal ischemia. Common causes in children include severe dehydration, poisonings, transfusion reactions, HUS, acute glomerulonephritis and obstruction.

Two pathophysiological events are responsible for the occurrence of most signs and symptoms. First, the kidney is no longer able to regulate the balance of fluid and electrolytes, thus producing certain metabolic imbalances including hyperkalemia, acidosis, hyperphosphatemia, and hypocalcemia. Second, urea is retained, a condition which causes alteration in the central nervous system function and metabolic balance. The usual course of acute renal failure is divided into three basic phases.

1. In the oliguric phase, urine output is greatly reduced and fluid-electrolyte imbalance is present. This phase can last days or weeks. Major patient risks are water overload, acidosis, hyperkalemia, uremia, and infection.
2. The diuretic phase usually begins 10 to 14 days after the onset of the oliguric phase. Urine output is gradually increased, and then large amounts suddenly appear. The BUN level continues to rise, as few nephrons are functional. Major risks to the patient are loss of sodium and potassium.

3. The recovery phase lasts several months until the ability of the kidney to concentrate and filter returns thoroughly. Anemia and electrolyte disturbances are primary patient problems.

Nursing Management

Nursing measures for acute renal failure include care for the underlying cause of the failure and careful attention to the child's renal state. Monitoring of fluid and electrolyte balance and the hypertension, reduction of the buildup of uremic waste products, prevention of infection, and provision of an adequate caloric intake are all considerations in care. Support and reassurance for parents and child are major nursing responsibilities during this stressful and potentially life-threatening time.

Chronic Renal Failure

Chronic renal failure may occur when the acute episode fails to resolve or the patient experiences progressive kidney deterioration. This disease process can be divided into early- and end-stage, or terminal disease. In the early stage the renal compensatory mechanisms are decreased but still functioning, whereas in the end state disease compensation has ceased and extrarenal support is needed. Before end stage, care is needed so the patient can be maintained with a medical and nursing regimen to prevent complications and preserve remaining kidney function (Table 27-8). The patient with progressive, chronic renal failure, whatever the cause, may reach a point in the course of his disease when conservative management fails and more aggressive treatment is indicated. Such treatment may be medical or surgical.

Dialysis

Dialysis can be an effective procedure for correcting body fluid homeostasis and preserving life in the child whose renal function is so severely limited that he would otherwise die. For the child in acute renal failure due to sudden illness or trauma, poisoning, drug intoxication, or other cause, dialysis may be the supportive interim treatment of choice, used to tide him over the period of oliguria. For the uremic child in chronic renal failure, however, dialysis may represent a more permanent commitment to the full gamut of treatment available: long-term dialysis and preparation for homotransplantation.

Dialysis is based on the physical principle that small molecules (crystalloids) in a volume of fluid will diffuse through a semipermeable membrane from an area of greater concentration to an area of lesser concentration of that solute. Undesirable solutes, such as urea and potassium, are removed through this process.

In peritoneal dialysis the abdominal cavity acts as the semipermeable membrane through which water and small molecule solutes move by osmosis and diffusion. The child is given an analgesic prior to catheter insertion. The bladder is emptied before the insertion of the catheter. The abdomen is prepared for surgery, and the insertion site is anesthetized with a local anesthetic. Unless ascites

TABLE 27-8 Supportive Nursing Care in Chronic Renal Failure

Common Problems	Common Interventions
Abnormality in salt and water hemeostasis	Monitoring of hydration
	Monitoring of intake and output
	Daily weights
	Sodium restriction
	Fluid restriction
Hyperkalemia	Dietary restriction of high potassium foods
	Kayexalate if potassium level above 6 meq/L
Acidosis	Sodium bicarbonate orally
Hypertension	Sodium restriction
	Antihypertensive agents
	Diuretics
Anemia	Oral iron supplement
	Folic acid
	Limited number of blood transfusions
Uremia	Protein restriction when blood urea nitrogen is above 100 mg
	High-calorie diet including pure carbohydrates
	Phosphorus restriction
Growth inadequacy	High-calorie diet; frequent dental exam for caries
	Vitamin D and calcium supplements
Infection	Early detection and treatment of infections
	Avoidance of crowds and infectious individuals
Psychological maladaptation	Provision of variety in diet as feasible
	Promotion of normal development as feasible
	Counseling to assist parents and child in dealing with progressive renal dysfunction

is present, the peritoneal cavity is filled with dialysis fluid (about two-thirds of the exchange volume) using an 18-gauge needle inserted near the midline. This step of the procedure allows for safer placement of the peritoneal catheter. After placement, commercially prepared dialysis fluid warmed to room temperature flows by gravity into the cavity, remains for equilibration, and then flows out by means of gravity drainage. Each pass requires about 1 hour and continues for 36 to 48 hours. Automated peritoneal dialysis machines are available.

In hemodialysis, blood is circulated outside the body through a cellophane coil or membrane in the artificial kidney or hemodialyzer. Hemodialysis usually is reserved for children in end-stage renal disease. It requires the placement of an arteriovenous shunt which may be external or subcutaneous. The internal shunt requires venipunc-

NURSING CARE PLAN

27-4 The Child with Acute Renal Failure

Clinical Problem/Nursing Diagnosis	Expected Outcome	Nursing Interventions

Edema; weight gain; oliguria; dyspnea
 	
Fluid volume excess with electrolyte and acid-base imbalance related to compromised renal regulatory mechanisms
	The child will attain fluid, electrolyte, acid-base homeostasis	Monitor vital signs q 1-2 h; note irregularities in heart rate, breathing pattern, blood pressure, perfusion, neurological status
		Assess child for signs of congestive heart failure, pulmonary edema (increased respiratory distress, rales, decreased urine output, poor peripheral perfusion)
		Monitor strict intake and output volumes hourly
		Insert Foley catheter as ordered during acute phase
		Document the type of intake (e.g., PO apple juice, IV albumin) and the type of output (urine, stool, emesis) in *exact* amounts
		Obtain accurate weights BID using the same scale at the same time
		Monitor for clinical signs of metabolic acidosis (hyperventilation) poor perfusion, tachycardia, obtundation
		Closely monitor lab reseults:
		  Serum electrolyte values (sodium, calcium, potassium, and phosphorus)
		  Arterial blood gas values (metabolic acidosis)
		  CBC
		  Renal function values (BUN, creatinine, phosphate, uric acid levels)
		Properly administer ordered fluid and electrolytes to maintain balance

Oliguria/anuria
 	
Altered patterns of urinary elimination related to renal failure
	The child will eliminate uremic waste products through urination or dialysis and will gradually increase urine output during diuretic recovery phase of disease	Measure and record strict intake and output hourly
		Insert Foley catheter using strict aseptic technique
		Obtain urine for electrolytes, creatinine clearance, urinalysis, urine culture
		Document BID weights with consistency in time, scale
		Monitor renal function values closely (BUN, Cr, phosphate, uric acid)
		Document response of urine flow to diuretic therapy
		Institute prompt replacement of fluid and electrolyte deficits during rapid diuretic phase to maintain equilibrium
		Child with peritoneal dialysis:
		  Protect peritoneal dialysis catheter from infection or dislocation; ensure patency
		  Assess catheter site for signs of infection (increased redness, purulent drainage); check for bleeding, leakage
		  Provide clean, dry sterile dressing over catheter site
		  Warm dialysis fluid (37-37.5° C)
		  Accurately monitor and record infusions, exchanges, and fluid balance
		  Weigh child pre and post dialysis
		  Properly administer dialysate solution based on clinical and lab findings
		  Monitor vital signs q 30 minutes during dialysis (assess child for tachycardia, arrhythmias, hypotension) for significant changes in baseline vital signs
		  Assess child for abdominal pain, muscular weakness, cramping, dizziness, nausea, and vomiting
		  Monitor child for clinical signs of fluid depletion and overload and for electrolyte and acid-base imbalance
		  Promptly report temperature elevations 38.5°C to physician; monitor for signs of peritonitis (severe abdominal pain and rigidity)

Lethargy; drowsiness; lack of interest in play; fatigue Altered thought processes related to impaired excretion of waste products	The child will be alert with appropriate mental status The child will have increased energy for play/school activities	Monitor child's neurological status with vital signs q 1-2 h; assess for increased irritability or lethargy; note changes in behavior or level of consciousness; report signs of CNS depression immediately to physician Avoid use of narcotic sedation to prevent masking CNS depression Prepare child's bedside for seizure precautions to support prompt intervention Conserve child's energy reserves; organize care to promote optimal periods of quality sleep and rest

Clinical Problem/Nursing Diagnosis	Expected Outcome	Nursing Interventions
Hypertension; circulatory congestion; anemia; coagulopathy	The child will attain intravascular homeostasis, be normotensive for age, and have adequate cardiac output as evidenced by increased peripheral perfusion, pink color, warm extremities, strong peripheral pulses, brisk capillary refill, decreased circulatory congestion, stable vital signs for age, adequate oxygenation (pulse oximetry O_2 saturation 95 mmHg)	Monitor HR, PR, BP, temperature, neurological status q 1-2 h; report irregularities in rhythm, rate, quality
Decreased cardiac output related to hypertension, fluid imbalance, altered hemodynamics		Measure blood pressure with proper cuff for child's size and age
		Document position of child and extremity used with BP measurement
		Note complaints of headache, blurred vision, dizziness, nausea and vomiting
		Properly administer antihypertensives as ordered, check accuracy of dose/kg, frequency (note side effects of all medications)
		Assess peripheral perfusion: note strength of pulses, color and warmth of extremities, and quality of capillary refill bilaterally
		Assess for clinical signs of circulatory congestion (rales, tachypnea, dyspnea, jugular neck vein distension, productive cough for pink frothy sputum)
		Monitor CBC, platelets, pt/ptt lab values
		Limit number of venipunctures; avoid IM injections; administer chest vibration, not vigorous chest percussion, with decreased platelets and elevated ptt values
		Monitor hemoglobin/hematocrit values and assess effect on oxygenation via PAO_2 or O_2 saturation monitor
		Assess child for presence of bruising, petechiae, prolonged bleeding from puncture sites
Fever; compromised skin integrity secondary to edema, uremic waste; pulmonary congestion secondary to immobility, increased abdominal girth	The child will be free of infection secondary to impaired skin integrity	Enforce strict handwashing before visitors and staff enter child's room
		Prevent child contact from visitor and staff with URIs or signs of infection
		Protect child from exposure to infectious diseases, from other children on unit
		Provide meticulous skin care; prevent skin breakdown:
		Wash and dry skin thoroughly especially in skinfolds
		Use sheepskin; no bed linen directly under child's skin
		Change child's position q 2 h
Potential for infection related to compromised physical invasive procedures		Administer circular massage to skin
	The child will be free of pulmonary congestion secondary to immobility	Promote pulmonary hygiene measures:
		Encourage coughing, deep breathing
		Encourage use of incentive spirometry (age appropriate)
		Administer chest vibration
		Elevate head of bed
		Change position frequently
		Encourage ambulation when possible
		Facilitate positions that promote maximal lung expansion
		Maintain strict asepsis with invasive equipment, e.g., IV tubing, dialysate setup
		Ensure patency and security of peritoneal dialysis catheter
		Assess child for signs and symptoms of sepsis, peritonitis (elevated temperature, abdominal pain, alteration in vital signs); report findings immediately to physician
		Obtain cultures as ordered
		Administer antipyretic measures as indicated

Continued.

NURSING CARE PLAN 27-4 The Child with Acute Renal Failure—cont'd

Clinical Problem/Nursing Diagnosis	Expected Outcome	Nursing Interventions
Nausea and vomiting; diarrhea; restricted diet Altered nutrition: less than body requirements related to therapeutic dietary restrictions; diarrhea	The child will accept a diet low in protein, Na, and K as one means of tolerating renal failure	Promote diet low in protein, Na, and K high in calories and carbohydrates Eliminate intake of foods high in potassium (bananas, citrus fruits, potatoes, chocolate, nuts) Document type, amount, caloric value of food intake every shift Provide child with favorite foods in accordance with dietary plan, allow choices by child and family in diet plan as much as possible to support compliance Consult medical team for IV (TPN) nutritional supplementation as indicated Consult dietician for suggestions to enhance nutritional value of intake Reinforce child and family teaching of therapeutic dietary restrictions
Anxiety Fear related to knowledge deficit, sudden illness, hospitalization	The child will master stressors of hospitalization; child will maintain developmental milestones with self-esteem	Provide child with favorite security object (blanket and pillow from home) Encourage parents to bring in family photograph, tape recording of siblings, parents reading stories, singing songs Utilize passive hospital play (while acutely ill) to explain treatments and procedures as appropriate to age Utilize active hospital play to encourage child to work out fears, stresses with traumatic experiences (e.g., needle play with doll and play with medical kit (stethoscope, thermometer, BP cuff) Explore child's feelings, perceptions of self, through art therapy Encourage parents to read books about "going to the hospital" when child is stable Assist parents to verbalize concerns about child's illness and treatments; address needs to increase parental effectiveness in supporting child through stressors of hospitalization

ture to allow entry into the shunt for access to the artificial kidney. Hemodialysis is usually performed two to three times weekly for periods of 6 to 8 hours.

With appropriate education and training in the use of equipment, either peritoneal dialysis or hemodialysis can be carried out at home. The most recent development has been the technique of continuous ambulatory peritoneal dialysis (CAPD). A double-cuffed soft catheter is sutured in place in the abdomen. The warmed dialysate solution is placed in a plastic bag and flows in by gravity. The line is clamped, and the bag is attached to the body for 4 to 8 hours of equilibration before draining. After draining by gravity flow, another bag is hung to keep fluid in the abdomen at all times.

CAPD appears to offer improved control of uremia. Children undergoing this technique are permitted a more liberal diet and minimal fluid restrictions. Patients and families experience a better quality of life because of increased freedom associated with less frequent need for medical supervision (Salusky et al., 1982).

Nursing Management

The nurse's chief responsibility in peritoneal dialysis lies in monitoring infusions and exchanges, charting accu-

rately, and assessing the child's comfort. Vital signs and weight also are monitored.

Because of the possibility of nausea and vomiting, it is wise to limit oral intake to ice chips and a very little fluid during the first 24 hours of dialysis. Later, sour ball candy may help satiate the child. Mouth care and lemon swabs to keep lips moist make the child feel better. Complications of peritoneal dialysis include bleeding and leakage, inadequate fluid return, puncture of the bowel or bladder, and infection (peritonitis).

Hemodialysis, because of its long-term use, puts unusual stress on the child and family. In addition to coping with the diagnosis of chronic renal failure, this treatment requires transportation to the dialysis center and time away from usual activities several times a week. Shunts and fistulas can clog up, and infections can occur.

The advent of CAPD has allowed for much greater freedom. Children remain in school, and parental time away from work or other activities is greatly diminished. The nurse working with these children and their families is responsible for much of the teaching. This education includes the technical aspects of the procedure as well as information about the disease, the treatment plan, and the monitoring required to detect or prevent problems.

Kidney Transplantation

Finally, when extended hemodialysis and homotransplantation are offered to pediatric patients, surgical intervention is ultimately part of the picture. The maximum time usually allowed on dialysis is 4 years. In actual surgery, the donor kidney is removed and perfused with cold saline to clear it of blood and to reduce the temperature of the graft to 4 to 10°C (39.2 to 50°F). It is then implanted without delay into the iliac fossa of the recipient; the main renal artery and vein are connected to the iliac vessels, and the ureter is implanted into the bladder of the recipient. Bilateral nephrectomy is carried out on the recipient before or during the transplantation procedure when there is severe hypertension or when the underlying disease is polycystic disease or chronic pyelonephritis. The recipient must be maintained on dialysis until urine formation in the transplant begins, which may be hours or weeks. The child is monitored carefully and put into strict isolation. The first 2 weeks are the most critical time period for serious complications to develop, including rejection, kidney infection, and sepsis.

Immediately after surgery the child is started on immunosuppressive drug therapy, usually a combination of prednisone and azathioprine, to counteract the major threat of rejection. Cyclosporin A (CS-A) has significant immunosuppressive characteristics. Its potential importance in pediatric transplantation rests with its successful use with little or no concomitant corticosteroid administration (Gradus and Ettenger, 1982). Signs of rejection may occur immediately or be delayed for some months; such signs are falling urine output, fever, rising BUN and creatinine, graft pain, and, on biopsy, infiltration of the kidney with lymphocytes. Some physicians are including a lymphocyte depletion regimen in order to prevent rejection which also further reduces the child's ability to fight infection. Many patients have difficulty with regulation of blood pressure, and the medication diazoxide may be given to maintain normal levels. One should also avoid abdominal palpation since kidneys are transplanted in the middle of the abdomen.

Concomitantly, the child receiving large doses of steroids and immunosuppressives is a prime candidate for generalized infection, especially of fungal and viral origin. (More transplant patients succumb to infection than to rejection processes.) The child may also be maintained on broad-spectrum antibiotics to assist in infection prevention.

Transplantation has been undertaken successfully in children ranging from 3 months through 21 years of age. The most successful transplants are those between identical twins, since the problem of rejection does not arise. The next most successful are those in which kidneys are transplanted between related individuals. In general, it appears that siblings are most likely to be the best match, parents are somewhat less compatible, and more removed relatives even less. Transplants from unrelated donors and from donor cadavers, performed immediately after death of the donor, are even less likely to be successful, although there is evidence that a good match from an unrelated donor has a 70 to 80 percent chance to be functioning after 2 years. There are many moral and ethical issues surrounding homotransplantations. One issue concerns the alternatives available to a child recipient whose potential donor parent or mature sibling [both in age (21 years or older) and outlook] either is medically unsuitable or is unwilling to donate a kidney.

Nursing Management

Children and their families need to understand the procedures and tests required as preparation for transplantation. Play sessions provide an opportunity for preschool and school-age children to act out the transplant and postoperative care activities. The acute postoperative period involves reverse isolation for several days; careful monitoring and documentation of output, fluid replacement, electrolyte balance, weight, and vital signs; and observation for signs of infection or transplant rejection. Acute rejection usually occurs between a few days and 6 months after transplantation. Signs of rejection include fever, hypertension, a swollen tender kidney, oliguria, weight gain, and increased BUN or creatinine.

Long-term support and guidance are necessary as the child and family cope with ongoing immunosuppressive therapy and care needs. Noncompliance can be a problem. Promoting normal life patterns for the child and family while maintaining needed vigilance to detect serious complications is a difficult task. Helping the child cope with a changed body image, return to school, and achieve appropriate independence is a challenge for the nurse caring for children who have had kidney transplants (Hollander, 1985).

Learning Activities

1. Assign students to observe an IVP and/or VCUG. Critique the preparation and support given to the child and family prior to and during the procedure.
2. Invite a member of a local ostomy association to discuss problems of care and psychosocial adjustments with the class. Also include an enterostomal therapist or nurse clinician.
3. Demonstrate to students how to take a history to rule out renal disease as well as the necessary physical examination. Also outline what laboratory work may be done.

Independent Study Activities

1. Visit the local kidney foundation and see what types of literature, services, and support groups are available to patients and families.
2. Contact an organ bank and obtain criteria for donor candidates. List nursing measures to ensure organ survival prior to transplantation.

3. Interview a family with a child who has chronic urinary tract infections to obtain information about changes in life-style brought on by the disease as well as problems with the long-term follow-up.

Study Questions

1. In assessing a very young child admitted with a urinary system disease, a nurse needs to know that:
   A. Flank pain is a common complaint.
   B. Hematuria is commonly present.
   C. Symptoms depend on the child's age.
   D. Vague, unrelated symptoms are common.
2. Ideally, a urine specimen which ensures the accurate detection of abnormalities is one collected:
   A. After fluids have been forced.
   B. Just after bedtime.
   C. On rising in the morning.
   D. After the order has been noted.
3. If a suprapubic tap is to be done on an infant, it is most important for a nurse to:
   A. Explain the procedure to the parents.
   B. Prepare the area properly.
   C. Identify the time of last voiding.
   D. Force fluids beforehand.
4. A procedure which can be done on urine to measure the concentrating ability of kidneys is called:
   A. Dipstick.   C. Dextrostix.
   B. Specific gravity.   D. Hydrometer.
5. An intravenous pyelogram is a radiological procedure used in diagnosing:
   A. Structural anomalies of the urinary tract.
   B. The presence of vesicoureteral reflux.
   C. A renal vascular disease.
   D. A urinary tract infection.
6. A voiding cystourethrogram is contraindicated in children who have:
   A. Urinary reflux.
   B. Acute urinary tract infections.
   C. Polycystic kidneys.
   D. Epispadias.
7. The head of the bed of a child who is being evaluated for a Wilms' tumor frequently has a sign on it which:
   A. Identifies urine collection times.
   B. Encourages the intake of fluids frequently.
   C. Limits abdominal palpation.
   D. Restricts fluid intake.
8. The parents of a child with nephrotic syndrome frequently relate that they have observed:
   A. Increased urination.
   B. Frothy, foamy urine.
   C. Increased appetite.
   D. Listlessness.
9. In comparing acute glomerulonephritis and nephrosis, children with nephrosis have:
   A. Gross hematuria.
   B. Normal blood pressure.
   C. Hypertension.
   D. Decreased output.
10. A common but possibly fatal disease for a child with nephrotic syndrome who is receiving steroids is:
    A. Parotitis.   C. Rubella.
    B. Rubeola.   D. Varicella.
11. A urinary tract infection in a child often is closely associated with:
    A. Toilet training.
    B. Difficulty in urination.
    C. Vesicoureteral reflux.
    D. Hydronephrosis.
12. The nurse needs to know that a common occurrence following a ureteral reimplantation is:
    A. The development of constipation.
    B. Pain due to bladder spasms.
    C. Increased urinary output.
    D. Improved oral liquid intake.
13. Postoperatively, care of a child who has had a urinary conduit procedure includes all of the following actions except:
    A. Monitoring intravenous fluids.
    B. Coughing and deep breathing.
    C. Determining the patency of the nasogastric tube.
    D. Maintaining a side-lying position.
14. The most common infection which precedes glomerulonephritis is:
    A. Group A beta-hemolytic streptococcus.
    B. Group A alpha-hemolytic streptococcus.
    C. Group B beta-hemolytic streptococcus.
    D. Group B alpha-hemolytic streptococcus.
15. A major problem of hemodialysis in children is:
    A. Shunt removal.
    B. Impaired shunt functioning.
    C. Clotting of the shunt.
    D. Infection.

References

Durbin, W.A., and G. Peter: "Management of Urinary Tract Infections in Infants and Children," *Pediatric Infectious Diseases,* 3(6):564-574, 1984.

Fong, J.S.C., et al.: "Hemolytic-Uremic Syndrome," *Pediatric Clinics of North America,* 29(4):835-855, 1982.

Ginsburg, C.M., and G.H. McCracken: "Urinary Tract Infections in Young Infants," *Pediatrics,* 69:409-412, 1982.

Gradus, D., and R.B. Ettenger: "Renal Transplantation in Children," *Pediatric Clinics of North America,* 29(4):1013-1038, 1982.

Hellerstein, S.: "Recurrent Urinary Tract Infections in Children," *Pediatric Infectious Disease,* 1(4):271-281, 1982.

Hollander, L.A.: "Renal Transplantation in School Age Children: Beyond Physiologic Care," *ANNA Journal,* 12(4):252-254, 264, 1985.

Jordan, S.C., and J.M. Lemire: "Acute Glomerulonephritis," *Pediatric Clinics of North America,* 29(4):857-873, 1982.

Lapides, J., et al.: "Clean, Intermittent Self-Catheterization in the Treatment of Urinary Tract Disease," *Journal of Urology,* **107**:458-461, 1972.

McEnery, P.T., and C.F. Strife: "Nephrotic Syndrome in Childhood," *Pediatric Clinics of North America,* **89**(4):875-893, 1982.

Mitchell, M.E., and R.C. Rink: "Urinary Diversion and Undiversion," *Urologic Clinics of North America,* **12**(1):111-122, 1985.

Richard, C.J.: *Comprehensive Nephrology Nursing,* Little Brown, Boston, 1986.

Salusky, I.B., et al.: "Continuous Ambulatory Peritoneal Dialysis in Children," *Pediatric Clinics of North America,* **29**(4):1005-1012, 1982.

Uehling, D.T., et al.: "Impact of an Intermittent Catheterization Program on Children with Myelomeningocele," *Pediatrics,* **76**(6):892-895, 1985.

Vehaskari, V.M., and A.M. Robson: "The Nephrotic Syndrome in Children," *Pediatric Annals,* **10**(1):42-63, 1981.

Bibliography

Brem, A.S., et al.: "Long-Term Renal Risk Factors in Children with Myelomeningocele," *Journal of Pediatrics,* **110**(1):51-55, 1987.

Dracopoulos, D.T., and J.B. Weatherby: "Chronic Renal Failure: The Effects on the Entire Family," *Issues in Comprehensive Pediatric Nursing,* **6**(2):141-146, 1983.

Frauman, A.C., and L. Lansing: "The Child with Chronic Renal Failure: I. Change and Challenge," *Issues in Comprehensive Pediatric Nursing,* **6**(2):127-133, 1983.

————: "The Child with Chronic Renal Failure: II. Developmental Habilitation," *Issues in Comprehensive Pediatric Nursing,* **6**(2):135-139, 1983.

Light, J.K.: "The Artificial Urinary Sphincter in Children," *Urologic Clinics of North America,* **12**(1):103-109, 1985.

28

The Endocrine System

Objectives

After reading this chapter, the student will be able to:
1. Describe the functions of the endocrine system.
2. Identify the basic subjective and objective data to be obtained in assessing the child.
3. Understand the purpose of diagnostic tests and medical treatment.
4. Describe general nursing measures appropriate for pediatric clients who have problems involving the endocrine system.
5. Delineate specific nursing interventions appropriate for pediatric clients who have problems involving the endocrine system.

Functions of the Endocrine System

The endocrine system regulates metabolic processes governing energy production, fluid and electrolyte balance, stress responses, personality development, growth, and sexual reproduction. Hormones are intracellularly synthesized substances secreted by the endocrine glands into the circulation, where they are transported to various sites of action. They act as agents for the transfer of information from one set of cells to another, producing effects on the total cell population. Since hormones are operative in low concentrations, they may function as stimulators, regulators, pacemakers, or catalysts for metabolic processes instead of being direct participants in biochemical reactions. The endocrine and nervous systems are closely linked, as they both influence bodily functions and regulate homeostasis. Neurotransmission at synapses in the central and peripheral nervous systems and neural activity in peripheral tissues are affected by the release of various substances, including acetylcholine, norepinephrine, and dopamine, regarded as local hormones (Greenspan and Forsham, 1986). General hormonal activity, which is mediated by the blood, is similar to neurotransmission, except that these hormones exert their influence at a distance.

Three basic components constitute the endocrine system: (1) an endocrine cell which delivers a particular chemical message to other cells by means of a hormone, (2) the target cells that receive the chemical message, and (3) the environment through which information is transported. The major channels of hormone transport are the blood, lymph, and extracellular fluids, which carry hormones from the site of synthesis to sites of cellular action and eventually to sites of metabolic inactivation. A summary of the endocrine glands is provided in Table 28-1.

The secretions of most endocrine glands are governed

TABLE 28-1 Summary of the Major Endocrine Glands

Gland	Hormones	Target Area	Action	Clinical Disorders
Pituitary Anterior lobe	GH (growth hormone, somatotropin)	Bones, soft tissue	Promotes protein anabolism; bone and soft tissue growth; promotes fat mobilization and catabolism	Hypopituitarism Gigantism Acromegaly
	TSH (thyroid-stimulating hormone)	Thyroid	Promotes secretory activity	Hypothyroidism Hyperthyroidism
	FSH (follicle-stimulating hormone)	Ovaries, seminiferous tubules	Promotes development of ovarian follicle and seminiferous tubules; estrogen secretion; sperm maturation	Delayed sexual maturation, precocious puberty
	LH (luteinizing hormone) ICSH (interstitial cell-stimulating hormone in male)	Graffian follicle, interstitial cells (testes)	Promotes ovulation and formation of corpus luteum; secretion of estrogen and progesterone; secretion of testosterone	Delayed sexual maturation, precocious puberty
	Prolactin (luteotropic hormone)	Corpus luteum, breasts	Maintains corpus luteum and secretion of progesterone during pregnancy; stimulates milk secretion	Inadequate lactation
	ACTH (adrenocorticotropic hormone)	Adrenal cortex	Stimulates secretion of glucocorticoids	Addison's disease Cushing's syndrome
	MSH (melanocyte-stimulating hormone)	Skin	Promotes skin pigmentation	Increased skin pigmentation
Posterior lobe	ADH (antidiuretic hormone, vasopressin)	Distal tubules of kidneys	Enhances reabsorption of water	Diabetes insipidus
	Oxytocin	Uterus, breasts	Stimulates uterine contraction; milk ejection into breast ducts	

Continued.

TABLE 28-1 Summary of the Major Endocrine Glands—cont'd

Gland	Hormones	Target Area	Action	Clinical Disorders
Thyroid	Thyroid hormones (thyroxine, triiodothyronine)	Widespread	Controls growth rate of body cells; regulates metabolic rate; promotes gluconeogenesis and fat mobilization; influences exchange of water, electrolytes, and protein	Hypothyroidism Goiters Thyroiditis Hyperthyroidism Thyroid hyperplasia of adolescence
	Calcitonin	Skeleton	Promotes calcium and phosphorus metabolism	
Parathyroids	PTH (parathyroid hormone)	Bone, kidneys, gastrointestinal tract	Promotes calcium reabsorption and excretion of phosphorus; bone calcification	Hypoparathyroidism Hyperparathyroidism
Adrenal gland Cortex	Mineralocorticoids (aldosterone)	Primarily kidneys	Maintains fluid/electrolyte balance; reabsorbs sodium; excretes potassium	Adrenogenital syndrome Adrenocortical insufficiency Aldosteronism
	Glucocorticoids (cortisol)	Widespread	Promotes fat, protein, and carbohydrate metabolism; mobilizes body response to stress; promotes gluconeogenesis; suppresses inflammation	Addison's disease Acute adrenocortical insufficiency Cushing's syndrome
	Sex hormones (androgens, estrogens, progesterone)	Gonads	Influences secondary sex characteristics; bone development; development of reproductive organs	Adrenogenital syndrome Ambiguous genitalia
Medulla	Epinephrine, norepinephrine	Widespread	Produces vasoconstriction with increased blood pressure; increased blood sugar via glycolysis; stimulates ACTH production; activates sweat glands; inhibits gastrointestinal action	Pheochromocytoma Neuroblastoma Ganglioneuroma
Pancreas	Insulin	Widespread	Promotes glucose transport into cells (decreased blood glucose); increases glucose utilization and glycogenesis; promotes lipogenesis; and protein synthesis	Diabetes mellitus Hyperinsulinism
	Glucagon	Widespread	Acts as antagonist to insulin, increasing blood glucose concentration via glycogenolysis	Hypoglycemia
Gonads Ovaries	Estrogens	Widespread	Promotes development of secondary sex characteristics and sexual function; promotes protein anabolism and epiphyseal closure of bones; breast development; stimulates water and sodium reabsorption in kidney tubules	Precocious puberty Delayed puberty Premature closure of epiphyses
	Progesterone	Uterus, breasts	Prepares for and maintains pregnancy; inhibits myometrial contractions; promotes development of mammary gland secretory tissue; aids salt and water retention in endometrium	
Testes	Testosterone	Widespread	Promotes development of secondary sex characteristics and normal sexual function; promotes epiphyseal closure; increases protein anabolism for growth	Delayed sexual development Precocious puberty Premature epiphyseal closure

by a feedback mechanism by which the production of a hormone is activated when its action is needed and inhibited when the effect has been achieved. The most common relationship is *negative feedback* (Fig. 28-1). A hormone that has a direct effect on a particular tissue is released. The secreted substance circulates and returns to the gland to inhibit further production of the original hormone, for example, insulin-plasma glucose and parathyroid hormone-plasma calcium.

Sometimes, direct control of the secretory gland is removed through mediation by enzyme activation (Fig. 28-2). An example is the relationship of sodium to aldosterone, which is mediated by the enzyme renin. Renin catalyzes production of angiotensin, which in turn stimulates secretion of aldosterone by the adrenal cortex.

Most of the systems of endocrine control are closed-loop systems (Fig. 28-3), by which the output influences the behavior of the system and its response to an input. Multiple paths are involved. (Solomon, 1980):

1. The controller of hormone release (hypothalamus)
2. Stimulators to and inhibitors of hormone release
3. A target organ or gland on which the stimulators and inhibitors act and which may secrete additional hormones
4. Response of peripheral tissue
5. Signal feedback to the controller

In addition to negative feedback, a positive feedback system may exist. In positive feedback, an adequate level of one hormone is necessary to stimulate secretion of another. An example is the release of estrogens from the ovarian follicle. Elevated blood estrogen levels stimulate a midcycle peak in the pituitary luteinizing hormone (LH) and follicle-stimulating hormone (FSH) secretion necessary for ovulation.

Organism homeostasis is maintained by the integrated endocrine and nervous systems. Neuroendocrine control

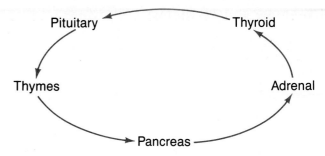

FIGURE 28-3 Closed-loop system. (*From K.M. Van de Graaff and R.W. Rhees, Schaum's Outline of Theory and Problems of Human Anatomy and Physiology, McGraw-Hill, New York, 1987.*)

is centrally maintained. The axis of control is central nervous system—hypothalamus—anterior pituitary—target gland. The hypothalamic-pituitary relationship is an important dimension of the neuroendocrine system. The hypothalamus, which is part of the brain and is under the influence of the higher nervous centers, participates in the regulation of many autonomic functions and bodily rhythms: It contributes to regulation of body temperature, blood pressure, heart rate, respiration, mood reactions, food and fluid intake, sleep, gastrointestinal peristalsis, bladder contraction, and sexual activity. The hypothalamus contains cells which combine neural and secretory activity, and it is functionally designated as the endocrine hypothalamus. It directly controls the anterior pituitary gland (adenohypophysis) and indirectly (via the pituitary) controls the adrenal cortex, the gonads, and part of the thyroid. A portion of the hypothalamus extends into the posterior pituitary (neurohypophysis) to form a single unit. Hypothalamic hormones play an important role in the release or inhibition of release of various pituitary gland hormones. They display rapid action, have a brief half-life, and are principally transported to the anterior pituitary gland by a portal system. The followign factors or hormones have been identified: thyrotropin-releasing hormone (TRH), corticotropin-releasing hormone (CRH), gonadotropin-releasing hormone (GRH) (follicle stimulating hormone, FSH/LH-releasing factor), prolactin release-inhibiting hormone, somatotropin-inhibiting hormone (somatostatin, growth hormone), and melanocyte-stimulating hormone (MSH-releasing factor). The hypothalamus is also responsible for production of the neurohypophyseal hormones, oxytocin and vasopressin.

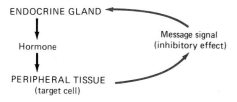

FIGURE 28-1 A simple negative feedback system.

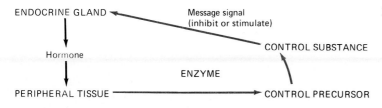

FIGURE 28-2 Feedback control with enzyme release.

Anatomy and Physiology

Pituitary

The pituitary, or hypophysis, is a small organ which is housed in the sella turcica in the sphenoid bone at the base of the brain. Its two lobes—anterior (adenohypophysis) and posterior (neurohypophysis)—are connected to the hypothalamus by a hypophyseal stalk. The anterior lobe secretes six hormones important in the control of metabolic functions of the body: growth hormones (GH); adrenocorticotropic hormone (ACTH); thyrotropin, or thyroid-stimulating hormone (TSH); FSH and LH in females and interstitial cell-stimulating hormone (ICSH) in males; and prolactin. Several peptides (β-lipotropin, α and β-melanocyte-stimulating hormone, and the endorphins) with structural similarities to ACTH exist in the anterior pituitary (Kannan, 1986). The posterior lobe secretes two hormones: vasopressin (antidiuretic hormone, ADH) and oxytocin.

Somatropin, or growth hormone, promotes protein synthesis or anabolism, fat mobilization and catabolism, and growth of soft tissues and bones. Its action on carbohydrate metabolism is not clear, but it appears to cause a rise or a decrease in blood glucose (Davidson, 1987). Secretion of growth hormone is regulated by a somatropin-releasing factor (SRF) that originates in the hypothalamus. Corticotropin (ACTH) is responsible for controlling the secretion of glucocorticoids by the adrenal gland. The hypothalamus controls ACTH secretion with the corticotropin-releasing factor (CRF) and thyrotropin (thyroid-stimulating hormone, TSH) with a thyroid releasing factor (TRF). Gonadotropic hormones (LH, FSH, ICSH, and prolactin) are governed by a complex interaction of the central nervous system, the hypothalamus, and effects of gonadal estrogens and androgens. They foster growth and development of the gonads at puberty and guide reproductive activities throughout life.

The posterior pituitary hormones—vasopressin and oxytocin—formed in the supraoptic and paraventricular nuclei of the hypothalamus, are stored and released from the neurohypophysis. Vasopressin causes the distal and collecting tubules of the nephron to become permeable to water, leading to increased reabsorption. Oxytocin stimulates the pregnant uterus to contract after delivery. It also triggers the letdown reflex in the breast by facilitating ejection of milk from alveoli into the breast ducts.

Thyroid Gland

The thyroid, composed of two lobes (right and left) that are connected by an isthmus, is located immediately below the larynx on either side of and anterior to the trachea. It secretes three hormones: thyroxine (T_4), triiodothyronine (T_3), and calcitonin. T_4 and T_3 have a profound effect on the metabolism of the body, whereas calcitonin is important in balancing serum calcium levels. TRH from the hypothalamus stimulates secretion of pituitary thyrotropin (TSH), which then activates the synthesis and secretion of thyroid hormones. A negative feedback mechanism leads to increased thyroxine and triiodothyronine levels and subsequent suppression of TSH secretion. In

TABLE 28-2 Effects of Thyroid Hormones

Metabolism or Target Tissues	Physiological Effects
Carbohydrate metabolism	Increases uptake of glucose by cell
	Enhances glycolysis and gluconeogenesis
	Increases rate of absorption from gastrointestinal tract
	Increases insulin secretion
Fat metabolism	Increases lipid mobilization from fat tissue
	Increases oxidation of free fatty acids by cells
Blood and liver fat	Decreases cholesterol, phospholipids, and triglycerides
	Increases free fatty acids
Protein synthesis	Increases rate of protein formation from ribosomes
	Increases RNA synthesis by genes
Vitamin metabolism	Increases quantities of enzymes, thereby increasing need for vitamin intake
Basal metabolic rate	Increases metabolism of most cells of the body
Cardiovascular system	Promotes vasodilatation for increased heat elimination
	Increases heart rate
	Increases strength of heartbeat
	Increases blood volume
Respiration	Increases utilization of oxygen
	Increases formation of carbon dioxide
	Increases depth and rate of respiration
Gastrointestinal tract	Increases appetite
	Increases rate of secretion of digestive juices
	Increases motility of gastrointestinal tract

Source: A. Guyton, *Textbook of Medical Physiology,* 6th ed., Saunders, Philadelphia, 1981.

the gland, thyroglobulin combines with iodine to form T_3 and T_4. Calcitonin decreases calcium ion concentration in order to maintain proper blood calcium levels. The thyroid hormones increase the body's metabolic rate and stimulate growth in children (Table 28-2).

Parathyroid Glands

The four parathyroid glands, two superior and two inferior, are located on the posterior aspect of the thyroid gland, two on each side. Parathyroid hormone (PTH) is secreted by the glands, and its function is to maintain a stable serum calcium level through three mechanisms. It promotes absorption of ingested calcium in the gastrointestinal tract, increases reabsorption of calcium and promotes phosphate excretion in the kidneys, and facilitates the resorption of bone, releasing calcium. Secretion of PTH is controlled by negative feedback from serum calcium levels. When serum calcium levels rise, secretion of PTH is suppressed.

Adrenal Glands

The adrenal glands lie retroperitoneally at the upper pole of each kidney and consist of two parts: the cortex, or outer layer, and the medulla, or inner core. The adrenal cortex has three anatomic layers (zona glomerulosa, zona fasciculata, and zona reticularis) that secrete several steroid hormones. The zona glomerulosa, the outer layer, secretes primarily mineralocorticoids, of which the most important is aldosterone. The zona fasciculata and the reticularis of the cortex secrete sex steroids (primarily androgens) and glucocorticoids (cortisol and corticosterone) (Table 28-3).

Endocrine Pancreas

The pancreas, located behind the stomach, is made up of two specialized tissues, (1) the acini, or exocrine pancreas (secrete digestive juices) and (2) the islets of Langerhans, or endocrine pancreas (secrete insulin and glucagon). Only the endocrine function is discussed here.

The islets of Langerhans contain three types of cells: alpha, beta, and delta. The beta cells synthesize insulin which affects carbohydrate metabolism. Insulin increases the rate of glucose metabolism, decreases blood glucose concentration, and increases glycogen stores in the tissues. An increase in blood glucose stimulates insulin secretion. When glucose levels return to a normal fasting level, insulin levels drop quickly. The alpha cells secrete glucagon, which causes a rise in the glucose level through stimulation of glycogenolysis in the liver and other body cells. The control mechanism for glucagon is the exact opposite of that of insulin; its release is triggered by a low blood glucose level and is inhibited when glucose levels reach a normal level. The delta cells produce gastrin and/or somatostatin. Somatostatin is thought to have the capability of inhibiting secretion of both insulin and glucagon; however, not all of its important functions are known (Guyton, 1987).

TABLE 28-3 Actions of Adrenal Steroids

Steroids	Actions
Mineralocorticoids	Maintenance of electrolyte equilibrium
Androgens	Initiates adrenarche
Glucocorticoids	Regulates protein, carbohydrate, and lipid metabolism
	Fights stress
	Catabolic effect on many tissues
	Anabolic
	Enhances gluconeogenesis and glycogenolysis
	Insulin antagonist
	Pressor effect

Source: Adapted from Kannan, 1986, p. 237.

Assessment of Endocrine Function in Children and Adolescents

The diagnosis of an endocrine disorder relies on findings from a thorough history, physical examination, and laboratory testing. Many endocrine disorders are not acute. A detailed past medical history of family and child is important in considering the possibility of an endocrine problem. Areas of particular concern are each parent's current height and weight and the age at onset of puberty; complete maternal menstrual history, including age at the onset of puberty, menarche, and menopause; each sibling's growth, development, and general health; occurrence of abnormalities or constitutional patterns of growth, such as tendencies to slowed or excessive growth in more distant members of the family; and any endocrine disorders in immediate or extended family members.

Special note is made of maternal abnormality during pregnancy (e.g., rubella, goiter). The birth history should be recorded, with attention directed to type of birth; weight, length, head circumference, and gestational age. The child's feeding history includes any digestive or nutritional disorders and atypical behavior during feeding, such as lethargy and poor eating (characteristic of hypothyroidism). The occurrence of a viral illness preceding the appearance of endocrine dysfunction can be significant, for example, prior to the onset of type I diabetes.

A detailed history of the child's growth and development is essential in identifying delays in physical maturation and mental processes, including the ages when the infant first held up his head, rolled over, sat alone, stood, and walked; when the child began talking; when the child began school and progress in learning. Sequential records of length/stature, weight, head circumference; age of fontanel closure; tooth eruption; and replacement of deciduous teeth with permanent teeth are relevant. Abrupt changes in growth progression can signal endocrine dysfunction. Sexual development is carefully documented. In boys, the onset of axillary and pubic hair growth, voice change, and gonadal enlargement is noted. Ages of sexual hair growth, breast development, and menarche are recorded in girls.

Physical Examination

As with other systems, a thorough physical examination is necessary to rule out endocrine disorders. Of particular importance are progressive changes in skeletal proportions with age and accurate sequential length/stature, weight, and head circumference measurements (for identifying deviations from the norm). Growth parameters will generally fall into a particular percentile (as in NCHS growth charts) and stay there throughout infancy and childhood. A child with a congenital endocrine condition interfering with growth shows a persistent deviation away from the normal curve at a very early age. Conversely, a child with an acquired endocrine aberration affecting growth follows a normal curve for a variable period of time and then begins to deviate from it. Head circumference measurements have a relatively narrow range of normal for any age group; an abnormally large or small value can be indicative of hypothyroidism or an intracranial lesion. The skeletal proportions most commonly used are the ratio of upper body segment to lower body segment and the relationship between arm span and height. Certain body proportions may help reveal an endocrine problem. For example, children with hypothyroidism have relatively short extremities compared with the trunk, whereas short children with nonendocrine disorders, such as constitutional delay in growth and familial short stature, are normally proportioned. Children with growth hormone excess have normal body proportions. Long extremities are found in patients with hypogonadal tall stature and specific genetic conditions (e.g., Marfans syndrome).

Other physical findings that aid in diagnosis are type of body build, shape and size of the head, and description of facies (spacing of the eyes, width and type of nose, and general facial expression). The shape and length of fingers and toes and the type and distribution of fat may be significant. The skin may be mottled, ruddy, gray, cool or warm, dry and scaly, or unusually pigmented. Seborrhea or acne may be present.

The pattern of tooth development can be slow or abnormal, and so a description of all deciduous and permanent teeth is needed. Since abnormalities in bone development may be endocrine-related, bone age determinations are often necessary. In a number of endocrine disorders (e.g., hypothyroidism and hypopituitarism), bone age is delayed compared with chronological age. A good description of the gonads is also valuable. In girls, assessment includes evaluation of a vaginal smear and measurement of breasts, nipples, areolae, and amount and distribution of sexual hair. In boys, the prostate is examined, the testes and penis are measured, and the location and amount of sexual hair are recorded. This information is then used to determine the Tanner stage (Chap. 29). Finally, psychometric evaluations may be indicated to determine approximate mental age. Such tools are carefully administered and evaluated by skilled professionals, allowing for individual ethnic, socioeconomic, and cultural differences.

Diagnostic Tests

Bone or skeletal age, a key index of osseous development, is usually obtained from roentgenograms of the left hand and wrist and occasionally the knee, where the appearance and union of the epiphyseal centers of ossification follow a fairly definite pattern from birth to maturity. Epiphyseal maturation may be delayed in all endocrine disorders which cause short stature. An excess of androgens may accelerate bone development and epiphyseal closure. Glucocorticoids in excess can cause osteoporosis and mild to moderate skeletal delay.

A number of assays are performed to determine the level of hormones in body fluids. The assay is determined by the disorder which is being diagnosed. Additionally, other hormones are measured to determine the treatment outcome (Felig et al., 1987).

Pituitary Function

Most tests of pituitary function measure the blood serum level of pituitary hormones or their hypothalamic releasing factors. Methods of obtaining blood samples are discussed in Chapter 10.

To obtain growth hormone (GH) levels, oral L-dopa and oral clonidine, which cause both central stimulation and release of GH, are administered during a fasting state. Serum GH levels are then determined. Somatomedin can also be measured. These intermediary hormones are peptides with molecular weights about one-third that of GH and appear to be synthesized in the liver and kidney. GH secretion is normally suppressed by the administration of oral glucose, as in a glucose tolerance test. GH levels are measured on an outpatient basis or for 24 hours on an inpatient basis. During this time, nighttime GH secretion is of special importance. Nausea and vomiting may occur during the GH stimulation test resulting from the hypoglycemia that may occur during testing.

ACTH is measured either directly through serum levels or indirectly through stimulation of adrenal glucocorticoid secretion. Levels of glucocorticoid end products (17-ketosteroids and 17-hydroxycorticoids) are assessed in a 24-hour urine specimen.

Normal pituitary response in secreting thyrotropin (TSH) is tested by administration of TRF. Levels of thyrotropin should rise.

The gonadotropins—LH, FSH, ICSH—can be measured by blood and/or urine assays. Simultaneous measurement of gonadal steroids such as estradiol and testosterone is often obtained for complete evaluation.

At the present time, ADH cannot be measured by direct serum radioimmunoassay. Use of a standard 8-hour water deprivation test shows whether the pituitary gland secretes ADH appropriately. When fluids are withheld, ADH secretion will normally concentrate and decrease urine output. Measurement of the urine/blood osmolalities ratio should be 1:1.9. These children require close observation of fluid output and weight loss. When diabetes insipidus is suspected, dehydration can easily occur. The child has free access to water the night before the test. Testing is done during the day. If the child loses more than 5 percent of body weight, the test is discontinued. The child needs explanations of why fluids are not being allowed and the reasons for periodic urine and blood samples.

Thyroid Function

Simple blood level concentrations of thyroid hormones are measured in protein-bound iodine (PBI), total and free thyroxine (T_4) and triiodothyronine (T_3), free T_4 index, and resin T_3 uptake. Tests that reflect hormonal regulation of the thyroid include TRF, TSH concentrations, TRF stimulation, and T_3 suppression testing.

Studies which indicate the metabolic effects of thyroid hormones include basal metabolic rate, bone age determinations, serum cholesterol, alkaline phosphatase, carotene, blood urea nitrogen (BUN), and hemoglobin concentrations. Antithyroid antibody levels, radioactive iodine uptake, thyroid scan, and ultrasonography are useful in identifying the etiology and pathophysiology of thyroid dysfunction.

Parathyroid Function

Serum levels of PTH are measured by radioimmunoassay. A simultaneous determination of serum calcium is needed to assess whether an abnormal PTH level is primary (from the gland) or secondary (from a target organ). Measurement of phosphate serum levels (4 to 5 mg/dl is normal in children) indicates dysfunction of PTH, since this electrolyte is retained or secreted in response to calcium blood levels. The phosphate level increases when calcium levels decrease.

A kidney function exam, the Ellsworth-Howard test, is designed to assess renal response to exogenous PTH. A standard dose of parathyroid extract is administered, and phosphate levels in urine are measured hourly for 3 to 5 hours. Adequate fluids are given to provide increased urine output. The normal response is a five- to sixfold increase in phosphate excretion. The nurse must gain the child's cooperation in drinking fluids and producing an hourly urine specimen. A urine-collecting bag is applied to infants.

Adrenal Function

There is diurnal variability in the blood cortisol levels of normal individuals. Blood is obtained for measurement of basal cortisol concentration usually between 8 and 9 A.M. Determination of basal plasma ACTH concentration, along with serum cortisol and/or 24-hour urine 17-hydroxysteroid excretion, improves the value of basal hormone estimates. Normal values are shown in Table 28-4.

The metyrapone (metopirone) test is a useful method of establishing cortisol deficiency. Metyrapone inhibits the last step of cortisol synthesis, the conversion of 11-deoxycortisol (compound S) to cortisol (compound F). The protocol is as follows:

1. Collection of a 24-hour urine sample for baseline 17-KGS and creatinine
2. Intravenous infusion of metyrapone (30 mg/kg) in 500 ml normal saline over a 4-hour period—started at the beginning of a second 24-hour urine collection the following day
3. Collection of blood samples at 0, 5, and 8 hours to determine compounds F and S plasma levels (compound F should be lower than compound S)

Children with manifestations of adrenal insufficiency are observed closely during the procedure. The nurse monitors vital signs and intravenous intake carefully, providing supportive treatment if hypotension or vomiting occurs.

The ACTH stimulation test offers additional information in the diagnosis of cortisol deficiency. Both short-term and long-term ACTH stimulation may be employed. The preferred diagnostic agent for short-term stimulation is cosyntropin (Cortrosyn). This substance contains the first 24 amino acids of the natural ACTH chain. Cosyn-

TABLE 28-4 Cortisol Function Tests and Normal Values

Basal tests	
Serum cortisol (A.M.)	5-15 μg/dl
24-hour urinary 17-hydroxysteroids	1-5 mg/m^2/d
Plasma ACTH (A.M.)	45-70 pg/ml
Diurnal variation	
Serum cortisol (P.M.) or plasma ACTH (P.M.)	≤50% of A.M.
Metyrapone test	
Plasma compound S	<7 μg/dl
ACTH stimulation tests	
Short-term cosyntropin test	Two- to sevenfold increase in serum cortisol concentration
Long-term ACTH-gel test	
24-hour urinary 17-hydroxysteroids	Five- to tenfold increase
Serum cortisol	Five- to tenfold increase
Dexamethasone suppression tests	
Overnight screening	
Serum cortisol	≤4μg/dl
Low-dose dexamethasone	
Serum cortisol	≤4μg/dl
24-hour urinary 17-hydroxysteroids	≤4 mg/24 h
High-dose dexamethasone	
ACTH dependent (serum cortisol and 17-hydroxysteroid excretion)	≤50% of baseline values
ACTH independent (serum cortisol and 17-hydroxysteroid excretion)	>50% of baseline values

tropin is administered intramuscularly after a baseline cortisol blood sample has been obtained. At 30 minutes, there is normally a two- to sevenfold increase in the serum cortisol concentration. Long-term ACTH stimulation is performed by giving ACTH-Gel intramuscularly every 12 hours for 4 days. Response is measured by the level of serum cortisol or 24-hour urinary 17-hydroxysteroids.

The dexamethasone suppression test determines if cortisol excess is present. Dexamethasone acts to suppress ACTH secretion. As an overnight screening test, dexamethasone is given in a single dose of 15 μg/kg up to a maximum of 1.0 mg at 11 P.M. Serum cortisol is measured the next morning at 8 A.M. The plasma cortisol level should fall, usually to less than 10μg/100 ml. A more prolonged dexamethasone test may be indicated. In a low-dose suppression test, dexamethasone is given every 6 hours for 48 hours. Serum cortisol and 24-hour urinary 17-hydroxysteroid excretion are measured before and during dexamethasone administration. A diagnosis of cortisol excess is confirmed if there is failure to suppress the ketogenic steroids formed by ACTH secretion after 2 days.

TABLE 28-5 Urinary Excretion Tests to Measure Adrenal Medulla Function

Compound	Disease Detection	Food/Drug Interference

Vanillylmandelic acid (VMA)	Adrenal medullary tumors	False *high* readings may result from
		  Foods
		    Coffee, tea, bananas, citrus fruits, nuts, vanilla, chocolate
		  Drugs
		    Nalidixic acid, aspirin, antibiotics, sulfonamides, methocarbamol
		False *low* readings may result from
		  Drugs
		    Clofibrate and monoamine-oxidase (MAO) inhibitors

Metadrenalines (metadrenaline and normetadrenaline)	Pheochromocytoma	False *high* readings may result from
		  Drugs
		    Chlorpromazine, MAO inhibitors, and methyldopa

Epinephrine and norepinephrine	Pheochromocytoma Neuroblastoma	False *high* readings may result from Coffee, salicylates, MAO inhibitors, antibiotics, methyldopa
Dopamine Homovanillic acid (HVA)	Ganglioneuroma Neuroblastoma Pheochromocytoma	

A high-dose suppression test may be used to establish whether cortisol excess is ACTH dependent or independent.

Urinary 17-Hyroxycorticosteroids constitute the end products of cortisol excreted in the urine. Their measurement is usually part of a dexamethasone suppression test. While most are excreted conjugated as cortisol metabolites, cortisol may also be secreted unchanged and unconjugated (free cortisol). Free cortisol in the urine is a useful test in Cushing's syndrome. The nurse should explain the method of urine collection to the child and parents and carefully supervise the procedure. The period of urine collection begins with the first voiding (this specimen is discarded) and ends with the last specimen 24 hours later. The dates and exact times of the collection period must be accurately recorded on the appropriate urine container and identification cards.

Aldosterone is measured in either blood or urine. Levels of serum aldosterone vary with time of day, age, sodium intake, and posture. The range of aldosterone in plasma tends to be higher in children than in adults and is especially high during the first year of life.

Adrenal androgens are excreted in the urine as 17-ketosteroids. Excretion of 17-ketosteroids does not, however, provide a measure of testosterone production. Testosterone is detected by specific methodology in either blood or urine. Urinary 17-ketosteroids are low prior to 8 to 10 years of age, although there is a gradual rise throughout adolescence until adult levels are reached.

Catecholamines are usually measured by 24-hour urine specimens. These specimens determine total excretion and are collected in dark bottles containing hydrochloric acid. Certain drugs and foods can interfere with tests results (Table 28-5). The nurse should be alert to such items and should take precautions to limit them before a test is begun.

Assessment of Pancreatic Function

Serum levels of insulin are measured by radioimmunoassay and are normally low when blood glucose is low. When an oral hypoglycemic agent such as tolbutamide is administered, insulin levels should remain unchanged whereas glucose levels should drop.

A normal fasting blood glucose level, taken at least 8 hours after ingestion of a meal, should be 80 to 100 mg/dl. Blood samples drawn 1 hour after eating (postprandial blood glucose) should not exceed 120 mg/dl.

The procedure for testing insulin response to increased levels of glucose is an oral or intravenous glucose tolerance test. In definitive testing, the patient eats a high-carbohydrate diet for 3 days prior to the examination to prime the pancreas (usually 25 g of carbohydrate a day). After an overnight fast, glucose is given (1.75 g/kg) and blood samples of glucose and insulin are drawn simultaneously at 0.30, 60.90, and 120 minutes and then hourly for a total of 1 to 6 hours. Normal response shows a drop in blood glucose to normal levels within the first 2 hours. Concurrent urine samples are checked for glucose and ketone levels. If a child has an elevated fasting blood sugar over 120 mg/dl or has glycosuria and ketonuria, the diagnosis of type I diabetes is made and an oral glucose tolerance test (OGTT) is not necessary to confirm the diagnosis. In fact it may result in ketoacidosis. Treatment with insulin should be started by a person familiar with the treatment of children with type I diabetes (Jackson and Guthrie, 1984).

Glucose is not normally found in urine, although a number of renal disorders or steroid treatments may result in glycosuria. A reducing test (Clinitest) or enzyme test (Tes-Tape, Clinistix) can reveal zero to 5 percent (negative to 4+) glucose levels in urine. These findings are often correlated with a high blood glucose reading.

General Nursing Measures

Nursing Diagnoses

A number of nursing diagnoses are applicable to children or adolescents with an endocrine disorder. Examples of some nursing diagnoses are:

Altered nutrition: more than body requirements (or exogenous obesity)

Altered patterns of urinary elimination

Alteration in heart rate, bradycardia

Knowledge deficit

Anxiety

In addition to the specific nursing measures for each individual diagnosis, there are several general nursing considerations that apply to the care of a patient with an endocrine disorder. Because growth is so strongly affected in children with endocrine disorders, the nurse is responsible for obtaining accurate length/stature and weight measurements. They should be plotted out on standardized growth grids and made a part of the child's permanent health record. In addition to these measures, accurate measurement of both intake and output is considered very important for the diagnosis of most endocrine disorders and is also important in determining the outcome of treatment strategies. Not only is volume important, but also specific gravity and/or urine dipstick can provide health professionals with valuable information necessary for the overall management of patients with endocrine disorders.

Vital signs are crucial when considering a diagnosis and/or determining treatment outcome. An example is monitoring heart rate in assessing thyroid function.

As with all disorders, patients and their families must have information regarding their diagnosis, treatment, anticipated treatment outcome, and anticipated emotional responses. Without education tailored to the individual and his family, optimum patient care and management will be not only less likely to occur but will probably be impossible. More specific nursing management strategies follow in the discussion of various disorders.

Anterior Pituitary Dysfunction during Infance and Early Childhood

Hypopituitarism

When there is decreased pituitary secretion, one or more hormones may be deficient. Idiopathic hypopituitarism generally is seen as a growth hormone deficiency. Occasionally thyrotropin, gonadotropin, and/or ACTH are also lacking. In the majority of patients with this condition, no identifiable cause is found. Familiar cases have been reported, suggesting an autosomal recessive inheritance pattern. Glandular destruction due to intracranial injury, infection, or surgery. Tumors of the hypothalamus and/or pituitary often lead to total pituitary deficit (panhypopituitarism).

The presenting problem in hypopituitarism is short stature. The child is usually of normal weight and length at birth. Growth retardation appears by age 1 year in many children. In others, a pattern of regular but slow growth is seen, with measurements falling below norms for the child's age. Because of good nutrition, weight gain may not be delayed as much as in stature gain, resulting in an overweight child. The skeletal proportions remain normal even though total bone length is greatly retarded. The facial structure is immature, and the teeth, which erupt late, are often crowded in the underdeveloped jaw. The child looks younger than the corresponding chronological age. The gonads develop normally but are often small, and puberty is delayed. Mental development is usually normal. These children may seem advanced in their learning abilities in view of their seemingly small size. A summary of symptoms is provided in Table 28-6.

Euthyroidism must be documented before growth hormone testing can be done (T_4 by radioimmunoassay and TSH). A growth hormone stimulation test reveals no response of increased GH to induced hypoglycemia or to central stimulation. Radioimmunoassay levels of somatomedin are low. Roentgenographic studies demonstrate delayed bone age; the centers of ossification appear late, and epiphyseal development is delayed. Skull x-rays can disclose an intracranial lesion such as a craniopharyngioma. Specific endocrine studies for deficits of thyrotro-

TABLE 28-6 Clinical Manifestations of Panhypopituitarism

Target Gland or Tissue Deficit	Clinical Manifestations
Thyroid (thyrotropin deficiency)	Infantile skeletal proportions Short stature Cool, dry, yellow skin Reduced body temperature Constipation Delayed dentition Bradycardia Dyspnea on exertion
Adrenal gland (ACTH deficiency)	Hypoglycemia Loss of appetite, weight loss Hyponatremia, hyperkalemia Hypotension, with possible circulatory collapse in adrenal apoplexy
Gonads (gonadotropin deficiency)	Lack of secondary sex characteristics Absence of gonadal development No menses and decreased spermatogenesis
Skin (melanocyte-stimulating hormone deficiency)	Decreased pigmentation
Kidney nephrons (ADH deficiency)	Increased thirst Fluid loss Increased urine output Low urine specific gravity
All body cells (growth hormone deficiency)	Slowed growth Short but proportionate bone size Delayed bone age

pin. ACTH, and gonadotropins may show decresed levels of these hormones.

Replacement of growth hormone is the most desirable treatment. It is given subcutaneously three times a week but may be given on a daily basis in the future. Most children respond well to the therapy, and growth is accelerated. However, some children develop antibodies to the replacement hormone. Certain anabolic agents, such as oxandrolone, may be useful substitutes. Because these agent tend to cause premature closure of epiphyses and advance bone age more quickly than they advance skeletal age, careful monitoring during treatment is needed. When other hormone deficiencies occur (e.g., thyroxine or sex hormone), replacement therapy is also indicated. Surgical intervention is recommended when a tumor is the causative agent in hypopituitarism. Cranial radiation may be required if tumor removal is incomplete.

Nursing Management

The nurse who works in an ambulatory care setting is often the first health professional to recognize signs of growth deficiency. Sequential weight, length/stature, and head circumference recordings can reveal progressive decline in normal growth. If past recordings are not available, the nurse should obtain a detailed history of the child's growth as it compares with that of siblings. Parents sometimes report that the child did not outgrow clothes as siblings did but tended to wear them for much longer periods of time. Because of their short stature, these children are teased by their peers and may become extremely shy and withdrawn.

If GH therapy is recommended, it is important to provide explanations of the triweekly injections. A thorough education should be provided so that parents can prepare and give GH. Since somatotropin is destroyed by the action of digestive juices in the stomach, it must be administered subcutaneously or intramuscularly. Subcutaneous injections result in less painful GH injections. The nurse can involve the child in designing an injection site rotation plan to allow the child some autonomy and control of the painful treatments. Injections are preferably given on the same days (Monday, Wednesday, and Friday or Tuesday, Thursday, and Saturday), at the same time each day, preferably in the morning so the child does not worry about the injection throughout the day; and in the same home environment if at all possible. Routines lessen the chances of delay and the potential for increased anxiety centered on the injection procedure. The family needs to understand that increased growth may occur at a slightly advanced rate. The child is likely to remain smaller than peers and to attain adult height at a later age. Psychological counseling may be required.

Anterior Pituitary Dysfunction in the School-Age Child and Adolescent

Pituitary Gigantism and Acromegaly

Primary hypersecretion of the pituitary is often associated with microadenomas that usually secrete growth hor-

mone, ACTH, or prolactin. If there is hypothalamic defect, the releasing factors for pituitary hormones are overproduced, leading to gigantism, hypercortisolism, hyperthyroidism, or precocious puberty.

The effects of hypersecretion of growth hormone are seen in the rapid but proportional overgrowth of the long bones. Muscle and visceral overdevelment also occurs. An increase in weight is usually not excessive but remains in proportion to the child's height. If GH excess occurs after epiphyseal shaft closure, the accelerated growth appears as enlargement of tissue (acromegaly), especially in the hands, feet, and face. The head circumference increases, the nose becomes broad, the lips are large, and all facial features become coarsened. The mandible enlarges, and the teeth may separate. Dorsal kyphosis can be present. Facial hair increases, and the skin thickens and appears deeply creased. Signs of increased intracranial pressure, including headache and visual disturbances, develop later.

Clinical features of craniopharyngioma, the most common pituitary tumor, involve growth retardation, signs of increased intracranial pressure, and vision difficulties. Headache and projectile vomiting may occur in the morning. As the tumor grows, memory loss, behavioral changes, seizures, or hemiparesis may develop. Decreased visual acuity and unilateral blindness can occur. In addition, any of a number of endocrine dysfunctions can become apparent, such as short stature, hypothyroidism, diabetes insipidus, and lack of gonadal maturation and development.

The main clinical manifestations of the diencephalic syndrome are severe emaciation, vomiting, hyperkinesis, inappropriate euphoria, pallor, nystagmus, and decreased visual acuity. Hydrocephalus may be present. Children with tumors leading to precocious puberty are often tall for their age and have all the signs of gonadal maturation (e.g., sexual hair and gonad enlargement).

In both gigantism and acromegaly, GH serum levels are elevated. Suppression testing with hyperglycemia does not reduce the level of GH. Since a hormone-secreting tumor can also affect other endocrine glands, excesses of thyroid, adrenal, and sex hormones are not unusual findings. X-rays of the skull may show enlargement of the sella turcica and paranasal sinuses with a tumor present.

When a tumor has been identified, surgery is indicated. The surgeon may be able to remove the microadenoma and leave functional pituitary tissue intact. Hormone replacement to maintain adequate thyroid, adrenal, and gonad function is necessary after total hypophysectomy and external irradiation therapy.

Nursing Management

The nurse who provides well-child care in an ambulatory setting is likely to encounter children with growth excess. Careful plotting of growth on appropriate growth charts will detect a child whose stature is above the normal percentiles for age. If signs of increased intracranial pressure are present, such as headaches, poor vision, and vomiting, the nurse should be aware of a possible tumor. The child and parents need clear explanations of the cause of growth excess and the rationale behind the various types of therapy. When surgery is recommended, the family and child require an adequate explanation of preoperative events. If the child is to receive irradiation without or after surgery, a visit to the nuclear medicine department prior to treatment can help acquaint the child and family with the equipment.

The favorable prognosis of pituitary tumor treatment can be emphasized when surgery is discussed. Psychological preparation for surgery is extremely important. The child should know what to expect in the postoperative period. The nurse can explain the site of the incision, the need for preoperative shaving, and the large dressing that will cover the head. Postoperative craniotomy care involves observations for bleeding, signs of increased intracranial pressure, and any indications of endocrine dysfunction. Close assessment for signs and symptoms of diabetes insipidus and/or ACTH deficiency is essential. The nurse instructs the parents in the medication therapy, including method of administration and side effects (see the section on diabetes insipidus and adrenal syndromes).

Posterior Pituitary Dysfunction during Infancy and Early Childhood

Diabetes Insipidus

The major dysfunction of the posterior pituitary is diabetes insipidus, resulting from decreased ADH secretion. This will occur with destruction of the ADH-producing cells in the hypothalamus, as happens with head injuries, tumors (especially craniopharyngiomas), histiocytosis, encephalitis, sarcoidosis, tuberculosis, and actinomycosis. Operative procedures in the region of the pituitary or hypothalamus can produce transitory or permanent diabetes insipidus. When ADH secretion is diminished, the distal tubules and collecting ducts of the nephron fail to reabsorb water, causing fluid loss.

Polydipsia and polyuria are the outstanding presenting symptoms of diabetes insipidus. Infants have increased irritability and crying which are relieved by water feedings. The infant is susceptible to rapid weight loss, hyperthermia, dehydration, and collapse. Toilet-trained preschoolers may become enuretic and constantly request drinks of water. Older children may not complain of any problem but satisfy their excess thirst with increased water intake. Water or fluids are given at room temperature. Small infants may have hypothermia and/or chills after ingesting large volumes of cold or ice water. The intense thirst and large water intake cause less formula and food to be ingested, and weight loss may occur until ADH replacement is started. This entity may be confused with diabetes mellitus clinically, but in diabetes insipidus there is no glycosuria.

Urine output is greatly increased in volume (4 to 10 liters a day), is pale and dilute, and has a specific gravity less than 1.005. When a water deprivation test is performed, the fluid restriction fails to decrease urine output. The patient has an elevated plasma osmolality, but the urine osmolality remains low and specific gravity fails to rise. When exogenous vasopressin is given, the urine osmolality and specific gravity both rise quickly. Skull x-rays may reveal evidence of an intracranial tumor.

There are several ways to replace the ADH deficit. Intramuscular injections of pitressin tannate in oil relieve symptoms for 24 to 72 hours. The medication is warmed and shaken sufficiently to resuspend the drug in oil. It is injected deep into the muscle with a long (at least 1 in) 20- to 22-gauge needle. Intranasal synthetic lysine vasopressin can be used, but its effects last only 2 to 6 hours and it may cause nasal mucosa irritation. An intranasal preparation, desmopressin (DDAVP), can be administered once or twice daily. DDAVP is absorbed more slowly from the nasal mucosa and persists in the plasma, increasing its effect on the kidneys.

Nursing Management

The alert nurse can identify the presence of diabetes insipidus by careful history taking. If a parent reports unexplained bedwetting in a previously toilet-trained child, the nurse can inquire about signs of unusual thirst and drinking. Close observations during the water deprivation test are required. Since dehydration and weight loss of up to 5 percent may occur in as little as 6 hours in children, hourly checks of urine volume output, specific gravity, and weight measurements are essential. Once the diagnosis has been made, an important nursing responsibility is to educate the family in the prescribed method of hormone replacement. When intranasal DDAVP is used, it comes with a special nasal tube for administration. If injectable Pitressin is considered, the child and parents are taught appropriate injection technique. The child and family must understand that the treatment for diabetes insipidus is lifelong. The child should carry extra nasal spray and should be instructed in its use when urine output increases. A Medic Alert tag can alert people to emergency care in case the child becomes unconscious. School officials are also informed of the child's special need for unlimited lavatory privileges and free access to water.

Thyroid Dysfunction during Infancy and Early Childhood

Hypothyroidism

There are two types of hypothyroidism, congenital and acquired. Most children with congenital hypothyroidism are born without sufficient or properly functioning thyroid tissue, as a result of faulty embryonic development, leading to aplasia or hypoplasia; dietary lack of iodine (endemic goiter); autoimmune thyroiditis; or hypopituitarism. Acquired hypothyroidism is most often related to chronic lymphocytic thyroiditis (Hashimoto's thyroiditis). It can also result from a hypoplastic thyroid gland which functions normally for several years but is later unable to meet the growing body's increased demands.

In the newborn period, few discernible signs and symptoms are noted. The infant may be the product of prolonged gestation, weigh more than average, feed

NURSING CARE PLAN

28-1 *The Child with Hypothyroidism*

Clinical Problem/Nursing Diagnosis	Expected Outcome	Nursing Interventions
Insufficient thyroid hormone Potential for injury (impairment of mental development) related to insufficient thyroid hormone	Through *early* identification and treatment of hypothyroidism, child will experience normal growth and development	Ensure accurate (T$_4$) screening in newborn period Obtain detailed history of newborn period; be alert to reports of prolonged gestation, prolonged neonatal jaundice, poor feeding patterns, constipation, and "weak" behaviors by baby Report concerns to physician; facilitate referral for endocrinology evaluation as indicated to ensure prompt treatment Participate in educating peers and children about screening for hypothyroidism and critical importance of early hormone therapy
Hard, small infrequent stools Constipation related to hypotonic abdominal muscles and decreased activity level	Through *early* identification and prompt treatment of constipation, child will have soft, regular bowel movements	Monitor frequency, color, shape, amount, and consistency of bowel movements Assess abdomen for distention, firmness, and tenderness Evaluate need for stool softeners; properly administer as ordered; evaluate effectiveness of stool softener preparation on stooling patterns; regulate dose and frequency of administration based on child's response Ensure adequate fluid intake in diet; administer increased volume of fluid as ordered Assist with passive range of motion exercises until child's activity level increases Teach parents to monitor stool patterns and consult physician for treatment to prevent complications from constipation; teach parents proper administration of prescribed stool softeners; provide written instructions on medication schedule, dose, and frequency
Weak suck Protruding tongue Fatigue Altered nutrition: less than body requirements related to difficulty with feeding	Given recognition of specific areas of developmental delay and subsequent referral to available developmental programs child will achieve optimal growth and development	Identify feeding difficulties, observe child during feeding, note strength of suck reflex, difficulty swallowing (gagging), and regulation; observe parental feeding techniques and support parental learning of feeding techniques; suggest to parents supporting infant's chin to enhance strength of suck, supporting child in upright position with head elevated to prevent aspiration, administering slow, small, frequent feedings; use a small, flexible, easy flow nipple; provide adequate rest periods between feedings; prevent aspiration—position child prone or on side after feedings
Developmental motor delay Delayed somatic growth Altered growth and development related to insufficient thyroid hormone production	Through early identification of need for and administration of hormone replacement, child will continue to grow and develop	Perform thorough neurological assessment; assess for presence of lethargy, slow deep tendon reflexes, hypotonicity, and delayed language and cognition; confirm suspicion of delay with Denver Developmental Screening Test or other age-appropriate developmental assessment tools Obtain detailed health history specific to milestones achieved or not achieved at home, behaviors, and level of activity; note age of onset and duration of time without treatment prior to diagnosis Refer to developmental stimulation programs Encourage developmental stimulation with bright colors, age-appropriate toys, and exercise to increase activity level and strengthen muscle tone Administer daily thyroid replacement as prescribed (dose is dependent on age and clinical response) Administer hormone replacement early in morning and on empty stomach; crush tablet preparation Observe for signs and symptoms of thyrotoxicity: tachycardia, tremors, weight loss, fever, dyspnea, and diarrhea Teach parents importance of daily hormone replacement for life, proper administration, and signs of toxicity Monitor response to hormone, behavior, and facial expression

Clinical Problem/Nursing Diagnosis	Expected Outcome	Nursing Interventions
Parents verbalize lack of information regarding hypothyroidism management and care	Parents will verbalize and redemonstrate understanding of daily hormone replacement and prescribed medications, feeding techniques, prevention of constipation, developmental stimulation exercises, and follow-up care	Teach parents feeding techniques (preventing aspiration and providing adequate rest) as outlined in care plan
		Teach parents to prevent and monitor for constipation as outlined in care plan
Knowledge deficit related to hypothyroidism; potential complications with home and follow-up care		Teach parents purpose and importance of daily hormone replacement and proper medication administration (dose, frequency, and preparation); teach parents signs of toxicity and how to report concerns to physician
		Teach and encourage parents in use of developmental stimulation activities and daily exercise regimens
		Provide written instructions specific to all aspects of home care needs
		Assist in arranging for ongoing follow-up care with an endocrinologist and/or pediatrician
		Stress importance of regular evaluations to regulate medications, monitor child's response to hormone replacement, monitor child's growth parameters and bone-age studies, and closely monitor serum protein-bound iodine levels
		Support parents with stressors associated with chronic management of hypothyroidism

poorly, have prolonged neonatal jaundice, seem quiet and sleep much, or have constipation.

As the child grows, more definitive manifestations are seen. Growth and development are obviously slowed, and the extremities become short in proportion to the body. The hypothyroid child has a characteristic facies: eyes spaced far apart, broad depressed nose, swollen eyelids, open mouth with protruding tongue, coarse features, and prominent cheeks (Fig. 28-4). Bone development is delayed, and muscles are hypotonic with umbilical hernia often present. Hair becomes coarse, scanty, and brittle. Tooth development is delayed and abnormal. The skin is dry, scaly, and cool to the touch as a result of the decreased metabolic rate. Carotenemia may cause a yellow discoloring of the skin as there is decreased conversion of carotene to vitamin A by the liver. Respiratory infections are frequent with profuse mucous discharge. The heart rate is slow, and cardiomegaly often occurs, leading to abnormal electrocardiogram (ECG) readings. Body temperature is low, often below 35°C (95°F). Developmental milestones are delayed, and if the diagnosis is not made early in the first *months* of life, permanent and severe mental retardation will result because of the lack of nervous system maturation. Most states by law require phenylketonuria (PKU) and T$_4$ screening in newborns. In the older child, myxedema of the skin appears and constipation is common. Increased sleepiness with decreased ap-

petite and physical activity occur, as well as general slowing of physical and mental development.

Typical laboratory findings show low serum T$_4$ and T$_3$ concentrations and elevated TSH values. X-rays demonstrate delayed and retarded osseous development, often with absence of the distal femoral epiphysis. Scintiscans with radioisotope of technetium (^{99m}Tc) may reveal little or no thyroid tissue. ECG findings may identify low-voltage P and T waves with diminished amplitude of QRS complexes. An electroencephalogram (EEG) frequently displays low-voltage readings.

Lifelong thyroid replacement therapy is used to reestablish normal growth and development in affected children. The drug of choice for thyroid replacement is synthetic sodium levothyroxine (T$_4$) calculated for body weight and slowly increased as the child grows. T$_4$ and TSH levels should be periodically checked to maintain a proper dosage. Growth rate measurements and bone age surveys indicate improved growth and development.

Nursing Management

The nurse is in a key position to identify hypothyroidism in its early stages. Careful attention to parents' descriptions of new babies' behavior in the first weeks of life can reveal early signs and symptoms. A young, inexperienced mother may think that her lack of knowledge is contributing to a baby who feeds poorly or is constipated. Careful

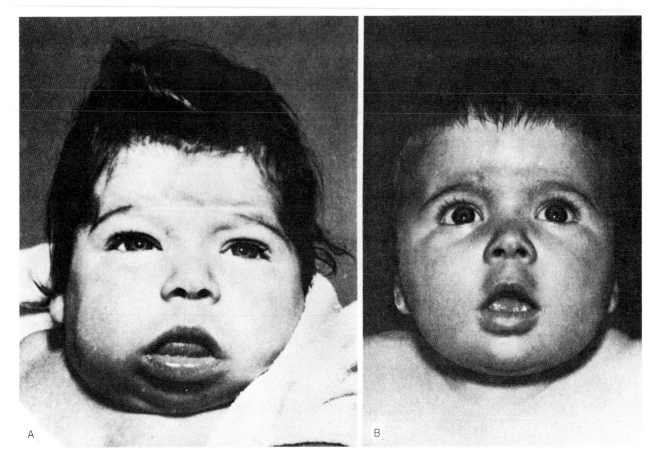

FIGURE 28-4   Congenital hypothyroidism in an infant 6 months of age. (*A*) Note puffy face, protruding tongue, and dull expression. (*B*) Four months after treatment with U.S.P. thyroid. Note decreased puffiness of face and alert appearance. (*From DiGeorge, 1979, p. 1637.*)

questioning and examination of the infant can disclose the thyroid deficiency. Once a diagnosis is established, parents need an explanation of the cause of the child's symptoms and of how replacement therapy will reverse them. Full effects of medication are observed in 1 to 3 weeks. It is important to teach the parents the signs of drug overdose, such as fever, sweating, insomnia, weight loss, irritabiity, rapid pulse, dyspnea, headache, diarrhea, nausea, and change in appetite.

If the condition is detected early and replacement therapy is introduced at once, normal mental development is enhanced. Mental retardation of varying degrees will occur if therapy is started after 3 months of age. Parents of children diagnosed late need emotional support and guidance in understanding the long-term implications of the child's mental capabilities. Overdosage with T$_4$ can by itself be neurotoxic and overdosage will not "reverse" prior damage due to hypothyroidism.

Goiters

A goiter refers to an enlarged thyroid gland and may be present in children with normal, hypo-, or hyperthyroid function. Goiters commonly result from increased levels of TSH secreted by the pituitary in response to decreased circulating levels of thyroid hormones. Increased TSH generates hypertrophy and hyperplasia of thyroid tissue and more hormone production. Any inflammatory or neoplastic process will increase thyroid gland size. The long-acting thyroid stimulator (LATS), found in thyrotoxicosis, also leads to goiter.

Goiters vary in size from those barely palpable to those easily visible with the neck in a normal position. While congenital goiter does not usualy interfere with breathing or swallowing, it occasionally can be massive enough to require surgical resection to facilitate respiration (Fig. 28-5). In infants with hyperthyroid-related goiter, there may be moderate exophthalmos and periorbital edema. These patients are irritable and hyperactive, and they lose weight and have tachycardia. Propranolol is used to block the peripheral actions of hyperthyroidism and to allow weight gain. Development of heart failure or thyroid storm can result in death.

Acquired goiters are more common than congenital goiters and often are caused by an underlying thyroiditis. This inflammation is usually of a chronic nature (Hashimoto's thyroiditis), and some patients have few observable symptoms. The child may complain of neck soreness, swallowing difficulty, or nervousness. The diagnosis is

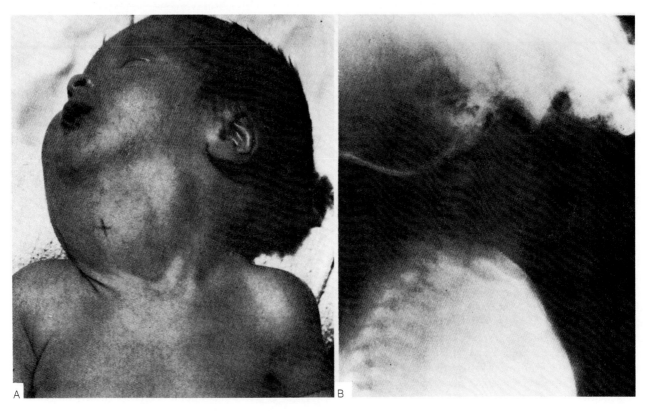

FIGURE 28-5   Congenital goiter in infancy. (*A*) Large congenital goiter in an infant born to a mother with thyrotoxicosis who had been treated with iodides and methimazole during pregnancy. (*B*) A 6-week-old infant with increasing respiratory distress and large goiter since birth. Note interior deviation and posterior compression of the trachea on x-ray. (*From DiGeorge, 1979, p. 1640.*)

confirmed by the presence of thyroid antibodies in the serum. Simple or idiopathic goiter occurs with no abnormal thyroid function and is frequently discovered during a normal physical examination. Toxic goiter is due to Graves' disease (hyperthyroidism).

When the underlying cause of a goiter is determined, appropriate therapy is begun. Congenital goiters due to lack of iodine are uncommon because of the widespread use of iodized salt; those resulting from an error in the synthesis of thyroid hormones require replacement therapy. Neonatal Graves' disease may require antithyroid therapy. Acquired goiter due to thyroiditis necessitates identification of the causative agent and, if indicated, specific antibiotic treatment.

Nursing Management

Nurses in ambulatory settings are often able to detect many of the goiters seen in young children. The clinician should be alert to the possible etiologies and need for further diagnostic evaluation. The parents and child require explanation of and preparation for the various examinations. Once a diagnosis is made, teaching is provided concerning the appropriate treatment. When replacement

therapy is necessary, parents must receive instruction in the dosage and frequency of medication.

Thyroid Dysfunction in the School-Age Child and Adolescent

Thyroiditis

Acute thyroiditis is due to bacterial infection of the thyroid and often progresses to abscess formation. Subacute thyroiditis is thought to be caused by a hypersensitivity reaction to a viral infection. Chronic lymphocytic (Hashimoto's) thyroiditis results from an autoimmune disorder in genetically susceptible individuals.

Both acute and subacute thyroiditis exhibit the classical symptoms of an infectious process. The thyroid area is swollen, warm, and tender. Chills, fever, and malaise are common. Myalgia, fatigue, and pain radiating to the jaw are present in subacute thyroiditis. Chronic lymphocytic thyroiditis often presents with asymptomatic, painless thyroid enlargement. Most patients have a positive test for antithyroid antibodies and normal thyroid function.

Once the causative agent is identified, appropriate therapy is initiated. Antibiotics for bacterial organisms are prescribed, and incision and drainage of abscesses may be necessary. Symptomatic treatment with salicylates and fluids is effective in managing subacute thyroiditis. Chronic thyroiditis may require hormone replacement, as a significant number of children with this disorder become hypothyroid. In others, the disorder is self-limited and therapy is not indicated.

Nursing Management

The nurse is responsible for managing the care of acutely ill children with thyroiditis. Intravenous antibiotic therapy must be monitored and coupled with simple explanations to the child and family. Since the child may protest violently when an intravenous catheter is inserted, the nurse should reassure him that it is used to deliver medication and is not punishment for any real or imagined wrongdoing. The child requires fever management until the infectious process responds to treatment. Increased fluid needs are met by offering the child a variety of juices or favorite drinks. If incision and drainage of an abscess are necessary, wound and skin isolation is instituted. Explanations are provided concerning the use of gowns and gloves, and the family is given special instructions about their contacts with the child. Subacute and chronic thyroiditis rarely necessitate hospitalization. The parents and child require support for and explanations of symptomatic treatment of fever and pain. If hypothyroidism develops, explanation and teaching about thyroxine replacement are essential.

Hyperthyroidism (Graves' Disease, Thyrotoxicosis)

Autoimmune factors are thought to contribute to the pathogenesis of Graves' disease (toxic goiter). Affected patients produce a genetically determined antibody which binds to a receptor for thyroid-stimulating hormone and activates thyroid function independent of the gland. This long-acting thyroid stimulator (LATS) leads to increased synthesis and secretion of thyroid hormones and gland hyperplasia. Tumors of the pituitary gland can also result in hyperthyroidism.

The symptoms tend to develop gradually and are less severe in children than in adults. Most bodily functions are accelerated. There is increased pulse, widened pulse pressure, and resultant cardiomegaly and systolic heart murmurs. Increased respirations and dyspnea on exertion occur. Appetite increases with unexplained weight loss. Increased bodily movements, irritability, restlessness, insomnia, and tremors are present. Linear growth and maturation of long bones are accelerated. Severe exophthalmos is infrequent, but prominence of the eyeballs, lid lag, infrequeng blinking, inability of convergence, and retraction of the upper eyelid may be noted. Heat intolerance is observed with flushed, warm skin and increased sweating. Goiter is often present. In a few cases, an abrupt release of thyroid hormone may occur; this "thyroid storm" causes severe hyperthermia, restlessness, tachycardia, vomiting, diarrhea, hypertension, and prostation. It can lead to delir-

ium, coma, and death. Thyroid storm is a medical emergency and demands prompt treatment with antithyroid drugs and iodine.

Serum levels of T_3 and T_4 are elevated, and TSH is usually low. Radioiodine uptake by the thyroid is increased. If hyperthyroidism is caused by a pituitary tumor, the TSH level is elevated as a result of inappropriate stimulation from the adenoma. A number of circulating antibodies may be present, LATS being the most common. Thyroiditis is differentiated from Graves' disease by normal T_3 and T_4 levels.

The preferred form of treatment for hyperthyroidism is medical management of the excessive levels of thyroid hormone. Drugs of choice include two thionamide antithyroids: propylthiouracil (PTU) and methimazole (Tapazole). Medication is generally continued for 1 to 2 years, when remission of the disease often occurs. Patients are carefully observed for reactions to drug therapy, including skin rash, urticaria, myalgia, loss of taste sensation, and enlargement of lymph nodes. The most serious side effect is agranulocytosis, which may occur in the first weeks of treatment.

Surgical intervention is usually suggested when drug therapy is ineffective or contraindicated. The patient receives preoperative preparation with an antithyroid agent in order to achieve a euthyroid state. Two weeks before surgery, iodine is administered either as Lugol's solution or as a saturated solution of potassium iodide (SSKI). These preparations inhibit secretion of thyroid hormone, augment the blocking of synthesis of thyroid hormone induced by antithyroid drugs, and diminish thyroid blood flow. The goiter is reduced in size, facilitating surgery and decreasing potential blood loss.

Nursing Management

The child with hyperthyroidism may first come to the attention of a school nurse or practitioner in an ambulatory setting. Complaints of behavior problems, short attention span, irritability, fatigue, or difficulty with fine motor skills, such as writing, are common. Once hyperthyroidism is diagnosed and drug therapy is initiated, much of the care and teaching for the family centers on minimizing the physical manifestations of the disease by providing a quiet, nonstimulating environment at home. Arrangements with school officials and teachers for at-home tutoring or a reduced school day may help in improving academic achievement.

Emotional outbursts related to nervousness are difficult for parents and families to understand. All parties concerned need an opportunity to discuss their reactions and find ways to deal with the situation. The child's increased appetite can be managed with five or six small meals a day. During the initial drug therapy, parents must understand that significant response to medication may not be observed for 6 to 8 weeks. They require reassurance that the symptoms will abate. Explanations of the possible side effects of antithyroid drugs are very important. If symptoms of agranulocytosis such as a sore throat and fever appear early in drug management, the child must see a physician immediately. Hypothyroidismlike symptoms can appear when the medication dose is too large, such as increased sleepiness or lethargy.

When surgery is recommended, the family needs preparation and support for the impending hospitalization. The child and parents require explanation of the drug regimen prior to surgery. Since oral iodine preparations have an unpleasant taste, they are generally mixed with fruit juice and administered through a straw. Allowing the child to help mix the medication in a strong-tasting juice increases awareness and understanding of treatment.

Preoperative psychological preparation is essential for all surgical procedures. Of special concern to a child facing thyroidectomy is the site of the incision. Many children have unspoken fears that they will have their throats cut during the operation. Assurance that the throat is not cut, only the skin to allow for gland removal, is emphasized. Showing an anatomic drawing of the gland's position can help an older child understand where the incision will be made. The child should also be prepared for the large postoperative dressing that will encircle the neck and the possibility of a "breathing" tube (endotracheal tube) after surgery.

Inspection for bleeding into the operative site is an important postoperative nursing responsibility. Blood may accumulate behind the neck and lead to asphyxiation. Slight flexion of the neck will prevent strain on the operative area. Observation for vocal cord paralysis is necessary in the early hours following surgery, since bilateral damage can cause airway obstruction. The nurse must be alert to signs of respiratory difficulties, especially the development of stridor. Emergency tracheotomy may be needed if an obstruction occurs. Hoarseness in the postoperative period signals unilateral laryngeal nerve damage and can result in permanent speech disability. The nurse observes for signs of hypothyroidism and hypoparathyroidism, both of which may occur with extensive gland excision. If hypoparathyroidism is present, the neuromuscular signs of calcium deficit appear. Any indications of paresthesia, tetany, or positive Chvostek's and Trousseau's signs alert the nurse to a drop in serum calcium. The lethargy and somnolence associated with hypothyroidism need laboratory confirmation (low T_3, low T_4, and elevated TSH levels). Both conditions will require lifelong hormone replacement. Parents should be informed as to their cause and treatment prior to the child's discharge from the hospital.

Thyroid Hyperplasia of Adolescence

Idiopathic, nontoxic goiters may develop when a child, usually a female, enters puberty. No evidence of inflammation or infiltration is present. The etiology of thyroid hyperplasia is unclear, although genetic factors may play a role. Many patients have a positive family history of thyroid disease. The greater demands of the body during puberty can cause the gland to enlarge in response to increased thyroxine need. Thyroid function tests are normal, and the gland is enlarged symmetrically. Some controversy exists concerning the treatment of nontoxic goiter. Use of thyroid hormone therapy is recommended by some physicians to avoid progression to a large multinodular goiter. Others, believing that spontaneous regression of the goiter is likely, recommend no treatment. Periodic and careful follow-up visits are suggestd to assess the condition.

Nursing Management

The nurse practitioner may be the first to detect a nontoxic goiter while performing a routine physical examination. The body-conscious adolescent girl will need careful explanation of this change in her appearance. If hormone therapy is not prescribed, the patient and family should understand why. Emotional support and reassurance of the adolescent are very important in dealing with the altered body image that accompanies a goiter. When medication is recommended, the patient and family need instruction in proper dosage, frequency, and possible untoward effects of hormone administration.

Parathyroid Dysfunction during Infancy and Early Childhood

Hypoparathyroidism

Hypoparathyroidism may develop following parathyroid removal or as a complication of thyroidectomy (surgical hypoparathyroidism). It also occurs commonly in the first 72 hours of life in preterm babies, infants with asphyxia, and those born to diabetic mothers. Transient hypoparathyroidism can be present in infants of mothers with hyperparathyroidism. Milk formulas with a high phosphate calcium ratio can produce this condition in children with immature parathyroid glands. Hypoplasia or aplasia of the glands causes congenital permanent hypoparathyroidism. Familial congenital hypoparathyroidism has been reported and appears to be transmitted as a sex-linked recessive trait. Idiopathic hypoparathyroidism is thought to result from an autoimmune phenomenon.

The classic symptom of hypoparathyroidism is tetany. Muscular pain and cramps are seen early, progressing to numbness and tingling of the hands and feet. There may be laryngeal or carpopedal spasms or generalized convulsions. Positive Chvostek's and/or Trousseau's signs are manifestations of latent tetany. The teeth are soft, erupt late, and have irregular enamel formation. Low calcium levels lead to decreased osteoclastic activity and stunted bone growth. The skin is dry and coarse, and the hair becomes brittle with areas of alopecia. Fingernails are thinned with smooth, transverse grooves. Cataracts can be present as well as other ocular disorders such as keratoconjunctivitis and photophobia. Nausea, vomiting, diarrhea, or constipation appear if the gastrointestinal system is irritated. If the condition is not diagnosed and treated early, mental retardation will develop.

Serum calcium is low (5 to 7 mg/dl), with phosphate levels rising to 6 mg/dl. PTH levels are low, and urinary phosphate excretion levels increase 10 times or more. Bone x-ray findings are usually normal, although some areas can have increased density. ECG readings reveal a prolongation of the QT interval, and EEG tracings show widespread slow-wave activity.

If tetany or convulsions are present, intravenous calcium gluconate is given. Concurrent administration of vitamin D increases calcium levels; however, dihydrotachysterol (DHT) acts more rapidly and has a decreased risk of causing hypercalcemia than does vitamin D, since it does not need hydroxylation by the liver and kidneys. Maintenance therapy includes calcium supplements and DHT or large doses of vitamin D. A high-calcium, low-phosphorus diet is recommended. Calcitriol may be used in older children. Successful therapy is evaluated with periodic determinations of the serum calcium level.

Nursing Management

A major nursing responsibility is recognition of hypoparathyroidism. The effects of acute hypocalcemia may necessitate emergency care, especially in infants with neonatal tetany or children who have had thyroid or parathyroid surgery. The following nursing measures in immediate treatment are related to the physical manifestations (i.e., signs of tetany or seizures): (1) observation for laryngospasm and signs of possible respiratory obstruction, (2) initiation of seizure and safety precautions, (3) reduction of environmental stimuli (private room, decreased lighting), and (4) placement of a tracheostomy tray and parenteral calcium gluconate at the bedside for emergency use if indicated.

Once a diagnosis of hypoparathyroidism is established, the nurse should teach the child and parents the proper medication replacement regimen. Parents must be able to recognize the side effects of vitamin D overdose, including abdominal cramps, nausea and vomiting, increased urination, dizziness, headache, photophobia, and tinnitus. Dairy products and eggs are restricted since the child is placed on a low-phosphorus diet. Infants require a formula with a high calcium/phosphorus ratio similar to that found in breast milk. Most commercially prepared formulas provide these levels.

Parathyroid Dysfunction in the School-Age Child and Adolescent

Hyperparathyroidism

Increased PTH production is most often compensatory, directed at correcting a hypocalcemic state in the target organs (secondary hyperparathyroidism). Major causes include chronic renal failure, malabsorption of intestinal calcium, and vitamin D-deficient rickets. Primary hyperparathyroidism is due to a parathyroid tumor or idiopathic hyperplasia of the gland.

Regardless of the cause, signs and symptoms of hyperparathyroidism are directly related to increased levels of calcium. In the kidneys, increased excretion of calcium and phosphorus lead to loss of renal concentrating ability, resulting in polyuria, polydipsia, urinary calculi, and pro-

gressive renal damage. Renal colic, hematuria, and dysuria are also present. Effects on the neuromuscular system involve hypotonicity, muscular weakness, cardiac irregularities and bradycardia, poor muscle tone of the intestines, constipation, nausea and vomiting, anorexia, and weight loss. Changes in bone composition produce pain (especially in the back and extremities), deformities, and spontaneous fractures.

In primary hyperparathyroidism, the parathyroid hormone level and serum calcium are elevated. Serum phosphorus levels may fall to as low as 3 mg/dl or less, and serum magnesium is also low. When renal disease is the causative agent, both phosphate and calcium levels will increase. Urine will show large amounts of calcium and phosphorus as well as a low and fixed specific gravity, because hypercalcemia blocks the action of ADH on renal tubules, causing diuresis and calciuria.

The recommended treatment for primary parathyroid hyperplasia is surgical removal of the gland. If hyperparathyroidism is secondary to any of a number of disease processes, treatment is directed toward remedying the underlying cause. The basic disorder, however, may be irreversible in some cases, such as in chronic renal failure. In this situation, drug therapy and diet modification aid in stabilizing serum calcium levels. DHT or vitamin D helps to mobilize calcium from bone, and calcium salts supplement dietary intake. A low-phosphorus diet (no dairy products or eggs) and aluminum hydroxide will decrease phosphate absorption, leading to a reciprocal rise in calcium levels. This in turn inhibits PTH secretion.

Nursing Management

Nurses are often able to detect the first manifestations of hyperparathyroidism. Since urinary symptoms are early presenting complaints, the nurse should be alert to reports of polyuria, polydipsia, and dysuria. In children with chronic renal failure, bone fractures or pain may signal the onset of secondary hyperparathyroidism.

The nurse plays an important role in administering specific care to relieve the physical symptoms of hyperparathyroidism. If skeletal complications occur, the child may need assistance in ambulation or application of corrective orthopedic devices. Providing a safe environment (e.g., siderails in place) is necessary to avoid falls due to muscle weakness and to prevent spontaneous fractures.

Increased fluid intake is encouraged to keep the child well hydrated and to decrease the occurence of renal calculi formation. Juices that lower the urine pH (e.g., apple or cranberry juice) are suggested, since the acidity of body fluids will increase calcium absorption. The family should receive instruction in diet modification and explanations of the elimination of dairy products and eggs. The nurse also instructs parents in the proper dosage and side effects of prescribed medications.

Heart function is carefully evaluated to detect irregularities or bradycardia. Apical pulse rates are taken for a full minute, and any abnormalities are reported. The child undergoing surgery for primary hyperparathyroidism requires care and preparation similar to that for a child with hyperthyroidism. These children are at risk for postoperative tetany due to hypocalcemia (see the section on treatment of hypoparathyroidism).

Adrenocortical Dysfunction during Infancy and Early Childhood

Acute Adrenocortical Insufficiency

Although this disorder is rare, a number of etiologic factors have been associated with the acute form of adrenocortical insufficiency (adrenal crisis). Common causes include destruction of the gland by hemorrhage, tumor, or calcification; severe systemic infection by meningococcus (Waterhouse-Friderichsen syndrome); abrupt cessation of corticotropin or corticosteroid administration; acute illness, surgery, or trauma; salt-losing forms of congenital adrenal hyperplasia; and pituitary or hypothalamic disease with inadequate ACTH secretion.

Clinical findings reflect an absolute or relative lack of adrenocortical hormones. Symptoms include anorexia, dehydration, nausea and vomiting, diarrhea, irritability, general weakness, fever, and abdominal pain. Other manifestations may involve hypoglycemia and hyperpigmentation of the skin, especially of the face, hands, genitalia, umbilicus, axillae, nipples, and joints. In the newborn, extreme hyperpyrexia, tachypnea, cyanosis, and convulsions can occur. Confusion, hypotension, circulatory collapse, metabolic acidosis, and coma may result as the condition deteriorates.

Laboratory data identify (1) decreased serum sodium, chloride, blood pH and blood volume, (2) elevated urinary sodium and chloride excretion, (3) elevated serum potassium, (4) increased circulating eosinophils, (5) lowered fasting blood glucose level, (6) decreased urinary 17-hydroxycorticosteroid excretion, and (7) decreased urinary 17-ketosteroid output except in cases due to congenital adrenal hyperplasia or cortical tumor.

Treatment requires cortisol replacement; restoration of fluid and electrolyte balance to correct dehydration, hypotension, and hypovolemia; administration of glucose solutions to combat hypoglycemia; and antibiotic therapy to treat infections. Isotonic saline solution (with 5% glucose) and intravenous hydrocortisone (Solu-Cortef) are initiated immediately. A salt-retaining hormone, desoxycorticosterone acetate (DOCA), may be given daily by the intramuscular route to maintain electrolyte balance. Newborn infants with adrenal hemorrhage may need vitamins K and C and whole blood transfusions. Vasopressors, such as levarterenol (norepinephrine, Levophed), phenylephrine (Neo-Synephrine), and isoproterenol (Isuprel), are used for vasoconstriction and maintenance of blood pressure. Many patients receive chronic replacement therapy for their deficiencies of cortisol and aldosterone. Cortisol is given in oral daily doses. Daily injections of DOCA can be replaced by oral preparations (e.g., fludrocortisone [Florinef]) or monthly injections of a longer-acting agent, desoxycorticosterone pivalate.

Nursing Management

This condition requires prompt recognition and intervention. The nurse assesses hyperpyrexia and a shocklike state closely by taking frequent vital signs and blood pressure. Seizure precautions are initiated, since febrile convulsions are not infrequent. The nurse carefully regulates intravenous therapy, records intake and output, and observes the child's response to fluid and cortisol replacement. Rapid administration of fluid and drugs is guarded against. Cardiac failure, hypotension, and abrupt drop in temperature can result from fluid overload or cortisol overdosage.

After the child is stabilized, oral fluids such as fruit juices or salted broth may be given. To prevent vomiting and subsequent dehydration, liquids are gradually reintroduced in small quantities. Soft foods are encouraged once the child is progressing well. The nurse must be sensitive and supportive to the family's psychological needs during the crisis period. Parents are informed of the child's progress and prepared for each procedure accordingly. Signs of improvement are emphasized (e.g., lowered temperature or increase in oral intake). Ongoing parental education and counseling are advised if treatment is to persist over a prolonged period.

Cushing's Syndrome

Cushing's syndrome is characterized by chronic excessive production of glucocorticoids. Generally, etiologies fall into one of four categories: Pituitary Cushing's syndrome with adrenal hyperplasia is due to excessive ACTH secretion (often termed *Cushing's disease*); adrenal Cushing's syndrome with excessive glucocorticoid secretion often results from adrenocortical neoplasms; ectopic Cushing's syndrome with autonomous ACTH elaboration is caused by extrapituitary neoplasms; and iatrogenic Cushing's syndrome occurs from administration of large quantities of glucocorticoids or ACTH. Prior to 7 years of age, adrenal tumors (adenoma or carcinoma) may be more frequent than hyperplasia (Fig. 28-6). Beyond this age, adrenal hyperplasia is more common. The principal physiological effect of Cushing's syndrome is loss of the typical diurnal variation of cortisol secretion. Depletion of body protein stores, abnormal carbohydrate and fat metabolism, and mineralocorticoid overproduction may also occur.

The primary feature is obesity, most noticeable in the trunk, face (moon-shaped), and cervicodorsal region (buffalo hump). The cheeks are often prominent and flushed. Signs of virilization frequently occur due to the androgen production of tumors. There may be generalized hirsutism, premature appearance of pubic and axillary hair, acne, and voice deepening. Growth is delayed, and length is often below the third percentile. Hypertension and increased susceptibility to infection are common. Other manifestations may involve purplish striae on the hips, abdomen, and thighs; pubertal delay; amenorrhea; muscle weakness; headache; emotional lability; hyperpigmentation; and renal calculi. Frank diabetes mellitus due to impaired carbohydrate tolerance can sometimes develop.

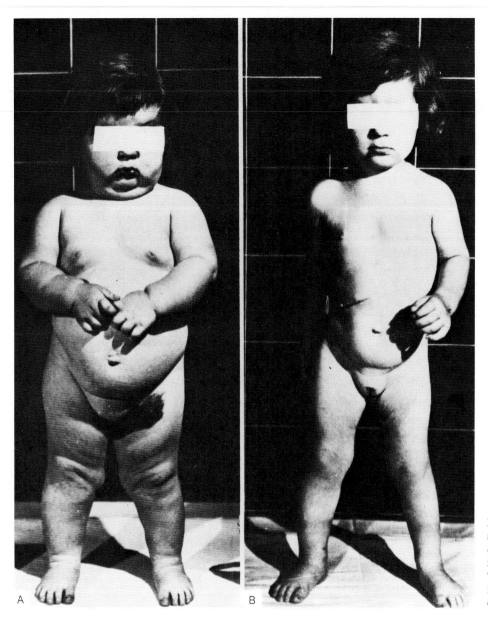

FIGURE 28-6 A child with Cushing's syndrome caused by adrenocortical carcinoma (*A*) prior to and (*[B]*) following surgical removal of tumor. The period between *a* and *b* was 3 months. (*From Kaplan, 1979, pp. 65-76.*)

Polycythemia, lymphopenia, and eosinopenia are usual. Additional data include elevated serum cortisol and 17-hydroxycorticosteroid levels, lowered serum chloride and potassium, elevated urinary 17-hydroxycorticosteroids and 17-ketosteroids, abnormal urograms, and osteoporosis (evident in spine roentgenograms).

The treatment of choice is surgical. Unilateral or subtotal adrenalectomy is indicated for benign cortical adenomas. Bilateral adrenal hyperplasia (Cushing's disease) is initially treated with pituitary irradiation and has induced remission in children. If irradiation is unsuccessful, bilateral adrenalectomy is performed and the patient takes replacement corticosteroids thereafter. The incidence of pituitary tumors following bilateral adrenalectomy is high.

Nursing Management

Postoperative complications of adrenalectomy, especially in infants, include sepsis, pancreatitis, thrombosis, poor wound healing, and sudden circulatory collapse. The nurse monitors vital signs closely and observes for signs of a shocklike state. Intravenous solutions are carefully regulated and urine output is recorded. Nasogastric decompression may be used to control anorexia, nausea, and vomiting. Supporting parental feelings and providing information both preoperatively and postoperatively are fundamental nursing responsibilities. Adequate explanations about diagnostic procedures and surgical treatment are needed. Parents should receive instruction on drug replacement during the postoperative period (see the section on Addison's disease). Physical changes (e.g., obesity, hirsutism, menstrual irregularities) that occur in females can alter body image. Efforts are thus made to encourage verbalization of feelings and facilitate coping abilities. Affected patients may also experience emotional disturbances that range from depression to euphoria. Parents are informed of the physiological basis of such symptoms in order to be supportive of the child. Other nursing measures involve the use of analgesics for muscle and joint pain, protection from the environment (e.g., assistance in ambulation) in view of muscle weakness and risk of fractures or soft tissue injury, and protection from undue exposure to infection.

Congenital Adrenal Hyperplasia

Congenital adrenal hyperplasia (CAH), also called adrenogenital syndrome, is an inherited deficiency ov various enzymes necessary for cortisol synthesis. Five different enzymatic defects are known, and each is transmitted as an autosomal recessive trait. Cortisol deficiency causes increased secretion of ACTH, which stimulates adrenal hyperplasia and overproduction of intermediary metabolites. As a by-product, there is excess androgen production, leading to premature virilization in the male or mascularization of the female.

21-Hydroxylase deficiency. This is the most frequent form of congenital adrenal hyperplasia. Both salt-losing and non-salt-losing varieties are identified. In the salt-losing form, the enzyme defect is complete with deficiencies of both cortisol and aldosterone. In the non-salt-losing type, a partial enzyme defect permits production of sufficient cortisol and aldosterone to prevent manifestations of salt loss.

11 β-Hydroxylase deficiency. This defect is characterized by cortisol deficiency and overproduction of mineralocorticoids and androgens. There is no salt loss. Hypertension and virilization are present.

17-Hydroxylase deficiency. The enzyme deficiency is found in both the adrenals and gonads. Hypertension results from increased production of salt-retaining hormones. Sex hormones are limited in amount. Gonadal defects include ambiguous genitalia in males and sexual infantilism in females.

3β-Hydroxysteroid dehydrogenase deficiency and lipoid adrenal hyperplasia. Both of these conditions are uncommon. Severe salt loss and varying degrees of ambiguous genitalia in both male and female infants are found.

Most patients with CAH have 21-hydroxylase deficiency. Because of fetal exposure to excess adrenal androgens, typical findings in newborn females include an enlarged clitoris, varying degrees of labial fusion, and a urogenital sinus. Breast development and menstruation may not occur unless the disease is adequately controlled. In the male, the main clinical picture is that of premature isosexual development. Enlargement of the penis, scrotum, and prostate; pubic hair appearance; acne; and deep voice are evident. Bone age may be advanced, and growth may be stunted permanently. Symptoms of the salt-losing form begin soon after birth. There is progressive weight loss, dehydration, vomiting, anorexia, and cardiac disturbances. Without treatment, circulatory collapse eventually develops within several weeks.

Elevated 17-ketosteroid levels are found in most types of CAH. In the 21-hydroxylase defect, urinary pregnanediol, testosterone, and 17-hydroxyprogesterone are ele-

vated. Children with the salt-losing form have low serum concentrations of sodium and chloride, elevated potassium levels, and increased plasma renin activity. Chromosomal analysis for accurate sex determination is usually done at birth. Affected females are chromatin-positive and have an XX chromosome pattern; males have a normal XY karyotype. Radiological examination consists of ECGs, vaginograms, abdominal plain films, bone age, and pyelography.

Intravenous fluids containing sodium, mineralocorticoid (DOCA), and cortisol are needed during salt-losing crises. Oral doses of cortisol or cortisone are given once the child is able to take fluids and nourishment by mouth. Parenteral DOCA can be replaced by oral administration of fludrocortisone (Florinef) in doses of 0.05 to 0.1 mg daily. In infants, smaller doses may be needed (e.g., 0.25 in the morning and 0.25 in the afternoon). Periodic follow-up is recommended in order to adjust drug dosage as well as evaluate signs of virilization, bone maturation, and steroid levels. Reconstructive surgery during the first 2 years of life may be indicated to correct clitoral enlargement and labial fusion, although clitorectomy is no longer commonly done, since it may later cause sexual dysfunction (e.g., anorgasmia). Surgery is often performed in stages, yields good results, and generally does not interfere with normal sexual activity or satisfaction. Genetic counseling should also be offered to parents.

Nursing Management

The nurse observes for evidence of adrenal crisis and monitors vital signs and fluid and electrolyte balance frequently. Parental education focuses on the use, side effects, and administration of medications; increased doses of steroids necessary during periods of stress (e.g., illness, vomiting, and surgery); free access to salt and water, particularly in hot weather and during periods of exercise; dietary supplements; and signs and symptoms of dehydration and salt-losing crises. Follow-up visits by a public health nurse are encouraged to answer questions and ensure that parents understand and comply with the prescribed treatment. Parent-infant bonding may be disturbed. The nurse should emphasize the child's attractive physical features and positive personality attributes. Healthy attachment behavior is facilitated by encouraging the parents to hold, feed, cuddle, and provide general care for the infant. Prior to diagnosis and sex confirmation, the infant should be referred to as "child" or "baby." Once gender assignment is made, it is important that the nurse use the child's name and refer to the infant as "he" or "she" (*not* "it"). Parents need to work through guilt feelings and fears about the child's condition. The nurse is in a key position to provide ongoing psychological assistance, including anticipatory guidance and supportive counseling in body image development. Older children may have difficulty relating to peers. Feelings of embarrassment and "being different" may be expressed because of stature, body size, or genital enlargment. The nurse may be involved in genetic counseling. Since CAH is an autosomal recessive condition, the clinician recognizes that both normal parents of an affected child are carriers, each parent possessing one normal and one defective gene. The chance for recurrence with each subsequent pregnancy is 1 in 4, or 25 percent. Both sexes are equally affected. Counseling should be offered to affected females who are capable of having children and to normal siblings who have a 50 percent chance of being carriers.

Adrenocortical Dysfunction in the School-Age Child and Adolescent
Chronic Adrenocortical Insufficiency (Addison's Disease)

Although tuberculosis was formerly a common cause of Addison's disease, congenital adrenocortical atrophy, hereditary enzymatic defects with congenital adrenal hyperplasia, and destructive lesions and neoplasms are current factors. A high percentage of patients with Addison's disease have circulating antibodies to adrenal protein antigens, suggesting an autoimmune phenomenon. Familial occurrence has been reported, although the genetics are not well defined. Addison's disease may also be associated with hypoparathyroidism, pernicious anemia, lymphocytic thyroiditis, diabetes mellitus, vitiligo, and chronic mucocutaneous candidiasis. Insufficient amounts of cortisol cause widespread physiological changes, including (1) hypoglycemic reactions, (2) decreased secretion of gastrointestinal digestive enzymes, (3) depletion of sodium and extracellular fluid volume, and (4) loss of diurnal cortisol variation.

The cardinal features are progressive weakness and hyperpigmentation. Glucocorticoid and mineralocorticoid insufficiency produce symptoms of hypoglycemia, anorexia, muscle weakness, dehydration, weight loss, hyponatremia, hyperkalemia, anemia, and hypotension. A small cardiac shadow is observed on chest x-ray. Pigmentary changes are due to elevated levels of circulating ACTH and peptides related to MSH. Pigmentation is marked in the palmar creases, nipples, operative scars, gums and buccal mucous membranes, and pressure points (elbows, knees). This hyperpigmentation is reversible after adequate steroid replacement.

Low serum sodium, high serum potassium, and low blood sugar are typical. Plasma ACTH levels are elevated, and the cosyntropin stimulation test shows inadequate responses.

Therapy involves administration of glucocorticoids and mineralocorticoids. Some children may only need oral supplements of cortisol (cortisone or hydrocortisone) along with a liberal salt intake. Cortisone should be administered with meals to reduce gastric irritation. The dosage is increased during periods of illness or stress (surgery) to accommodate the body's need for increased glucocorticoids. Mineralocorticoid treatment consists of administering oral daily doses of fludrocortisone, a synthetic salt-retaining steroid. During episodes of crisis, the mineralocorticoid desoxycorticosterone acetate is administered by intramuscular injection. Glucocorticoids such as hy-

drocortisone hemisuccinate can be given by the intravenous or intramuscular route.

Nursing Management

Parents need particular guidance and education on drug therapy. Continuous cortisol replacement is essential, and any sudden termination of the drug can precipitate an acute adrenal crisis. Parental instruction in the proper technique of intramuscular injection is advised, and a prefilled syringe of hydrocortisone should be available at home. Parents are informed about the various side effects of drugs. For instance, the side effects of cortisone are gastric irritation, excitability, sleeplessness, weight gain, and occasional behavioral change (depression, euphoria). Side effects of mineralocorticoids involve generalized edema (first apparent around the eyes), hypertension, headache, cardiac arrhythmias, and signs of hypokalemia (e.g., weakness, irritability). Continual follow-up is necessary to evaluate evidence of overdosage. The child's activities must be planned to allow for adequate exercise and rest periods. Stress situations should be avoided. Nursing measures during hospitalization include periodic weighing, hydration, regular monitoring of vital signs, measurement of intake and output, observation of electrolyte imbalance, prevention of exposure to infection, and supportive psychological care.

Pancreatic Dysfunction
Type I Insulin-Dependent Diabetes Mellitus

Multiple factors are involved in the etiology of type I diabetes or insulin-dependent diabetes. Specialists now consider type I diabetes mellitus to be a syndrome of several diseases with different causes and mechanisms of transmission (Barnard, 1986). The disease may be triggered by a combination of a viral infection and an autoimmune reaction. Genetic factors are important in diabetes causation, although there is little agreement about the exact mode of transmission. It is thought that affected children may inherit a recessive gene which is linked to the tissue-typing antigens, human leukocyte A (HLA). When a stress situation such as a viral invasion occurs, beta cells may suffer damage and activate an antigen-antibody response. The injured cells become the antigen, and the body produces islet cell antibodies to destroy them. The end result is death of the insulin-producing cells. Additional causative agents for this autoimmune inflammatory reaction include pancreatitis, growth hormone excess, steroid drugs, and pancreatic tumors.

When insulin is deficient, carbohydrates cannot be utilized for cell energy and excess glucose accumulates in the blood (Fig. 28-7). The hyperglycemic extracellular fluid exceeds the renal threshold (>180 mg/dl) for glucose and produces an obligatory osmotic diuresis, with subsequent dehydration. Large amounts of glucose, water, electrolytes, and minerals (sodium, potassium, calcium, phosphate, and magnesium) are excreted by the kidneys. The body turns next to metabolism of protein and fatty

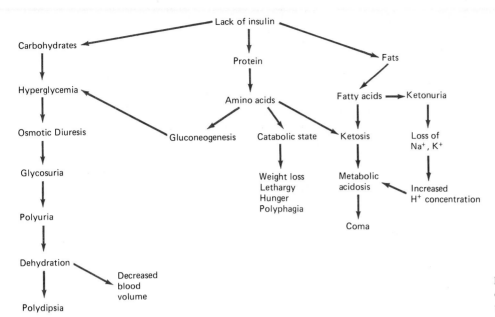

FIGURE 28-7 Effects of insulin lack on carbohydrate, protein, and fat metabolism.

NURSING CARE PLAN

28-2 The Child and Adolescent with Type I Diabetes Mellitus

Clinical Problem/Nursing Diagnosis	Expected Outcome	Nursing Interventions
Hyperglycemia Polydipsia Polyphasia Dehydration Electrolyte imbalance Metabolic acidosis Dry flushed skin Glucosuria Ketonuria Nausea and vomiting Abdominal pain Fruity breath odor Kussmaul's respirations Weakness Altered mental status	Child's blood glucose levels will be controlled between 70 and 110 mg/dl Child's blood gases will be normalized with pH between 7.35 and 7.45, PCO$_2$ 35-45, bicarbonate 24-32 meq/L	Maintain NPO (nothing by mouth) Assist in obtaining intravenous access for fluid and medication therapy; assess patency of IV; assess for signs of infiltration (pain, redness, and inflammation) Monitor blood glucose levels; promptly administer IV insulin as ordered; correct ketoacidosis; administer normal saline solution, sodium bicarbonate, and insulin intravenously as ordered or indicated by lab values and child response Monitor vital signs frequently; assess respirations for rate, depth, pattern, and regularity; report signs of respiratory distress (retractions, dyspnea, and fatigue) Administer oxygen therapy as needed Auscultate breath sounds for qualilty/equality or aeration Monitor heart rate for equality/rhythm Monitor for ectopy, tachycardia, and dysrhythmias; assess perfusion Monitor blood pressure for hypertension and hypotension Evaluate neurological status; assess pupils for size, equality, and reactivity to light; assess motor and sensory function, level of consciousness, and response to environment and stimuli Report alterations in vital signs to physician immediately
Potential for injury (diabetic ketoacidosis) related to insulin deficiency, impaired tissue utilization of glucose, and impaired fat and protein metabolism	Child's fluid and electrolyte balance will be restored	Monitor blood glucose levels, electrolyte values (potassium), and blood gases every hour and as necessary until stable Monitor for signs of hypo/hyperkalemia Maintain potassium levels between 3.5 and 5.0 meq/L; replace potassium needs when acidosis is corrected as ordered Identify and correct electrolyte acid-base imbalances promptly as ordered Insert a Foley catheter to maintain strict output volumes every 30-60 min

Continued.

Clinical Problem/Nursing Diagnosis	Expected Outcome	Nursing Interventions
		Test urine for glucose and ketones every 30-60 min
		Notify physician when urine is negative for glucose
		Monitor for signs of hypoglycemia
		Observe time when blood glucose levels decrease and notify physician
		Change intravenous fluid solutions and add dextrose to fluid therapy as ordered
		Inform parents and/or child to test urine routinely for presence of ketones, not to exercise as long as ketones are present in the urine, and to promptly consult physician to discuss management to assure early detection and treatment
Thirst and/or hunger		See interventions for diabetic ketoacidosis
Polyuria (bed-wetting in a toilet-trained child)		Encourage routine testing of blood and urine to adjust insulin needs to prevent hyperglycemia
Potential for injury (hyperglycemia) related to inadequate insulin, increased food intake, intake of improper foods, stress from illness or surgery, and emotional stress		
Nausea and vomiting	Child will achieve a balance between insulin replacement and nutritional intake	Discourage decreasing food intake
Abdominal pain		Encourage consistency with meal and snack intake; assist with adjustments in therapy related to changes in consistent daily meal and exercise regimens
Fatigue, weakness, drowsiness, headache, dizziness, and blurred vision		Encourage consistent exercise activities to help manage moderately high blood sugars; discourage exercise when blood glucose is greater than 300 mg/dl
Altered mental status, irritabiity		
Dehydration, cracked lips, dry skin, sunken eyes, and dry mucous membranes		
Elevated blood glucose level greater than 120-200 mg/dl		
Glucosuria		
Ketonuria		
Nervousness and/or irritability	When child is hypoglycemic, he will achieve adequate blood glucose levels of 70-100 mg/dl, given appropriate interventions	Administer a source of glucose by mouth promptly if alert (6-8 oz orange juice, 4-6 oz nondietetic soda, 1-2 glucose tablets, 2 large sugar cubes); follow with about 4 peanut butter/cheese crackers
Fatigue, weakness, and shakiness		Administer intravenous dextrose or glucagon as ordered in presence of altered neurological state
Diaphoresis, shivering, pallor, and cool clammy skin		Monitor blood glucose q 2 h until stable
Nausea		
Altered level of consciousness, dizziness, confusion, poor coordination, rapid pulse, and decreased blood glucose level <60 mg/dl		

Clinical Problem/Nursing Diagnosis	Expected Outcome	Nursing Interventions
Polyuria Polydipsia Nausea and/or vomiting, dry skin, and flushed cheeks Decreased elasticity or skin turgor, sunken fontanels, and sunken eyeballs Weakness	Child will achieve and maintain fluid, electrolyte, and acid-base balance, given the appropriate nursing care	Weigh child on admission and obtain daily weights Monitor vital signs every hour Monitor strict intake and output volumes every 30-60 min Administer calculated fluid replacement needs intravenously until stabilized Monitor CBC, Hgb, Hct, electrolyte values, glucose levels, and acid-base balance; identify and correct imbalances
Potential for injury (hypoglycemia) related to excessive insulin, decreased food intake, increased exercise level, and insulin dose higher than body needs Fluid volume deficit and electrolyte and acid-base imbalance related to impaired carbohydrate metabolism and altered protein and fat metabolism		Evaluate effectiveness of hydration therapy; assess moisture of mucous membranes, urine specific gravity, and skin turgor Prevent overhydration; monitor for signs of fluid overload (presence of crackles, edema, weight gain, and specific gravity less than 1.005) Titrate fluids; alter fluid solutions and electrolyte replacements based on laboratory values and clinical status as ordered
Improper balance between food intake and insulin regimen	Through appropriate interventions: Child will achieve optimum growth Child will have blood glucose levels between 70 and 110 mg/dl, child will maintain balance between food ingested and insulin regimen, parents will become actively involved in planning meals, the insulin regimen, etc., and parents will verbalize importance of maintaining program which is developed	Collaborate with nutritionist and physician to evaluate caloric requirements based on individual child's age, height, weight, activity level, and food preferences for balance with insulin dose regimen Consult with nutritionist to provide meal planning and nutrition counseling for diabetic child and family Promote a diet high in unrefined complex carbohydrates (vegetables, dried peas, beans, brown rice, whole grain flours and bread, and increased cereal and fiber intake) Calculate protein to 20-25% of total energy intake Limit intake of refined sugars and starches; prohibit intake of concentrated sugars (cakes, cookies, and candies) Limit fat and cholesterol from foods (fried food, sauces, and gravies) Communicate nutritional needs with a positive approach; emphasize what child *can* eat; stress fact that diet is a healthy one for entire family
Altered nutrition: less than body requirements related to inadequate insulin, impaired carbohydrate metabolism, and altered protein and fat metabolism		Monitor food choices and portion sizes to maintain a balance between food intake and insulin; teach child and family Ensure provision of balanced meals and snacks to maintain constant glucose levels Provide written instructions specific to developed meal plan to promote consistency in the amount of carbohydrate, protein, and fat consumed in child's daily diet; establish regular schedule for meals and snacks Inform parents and/or child about critical issue of matching food intake to insulin Teach parents and/or child importance of eating when insulin's blood-sugar-lowering action is strongest and explain that schedules of insulin depend on type and amount of insulin ordered, coordinated and balanced with meal planning

Continued.

Clinical Problem/Nursing Diagnosis	Expected Outcome	Nursing Interventions
		Refer child and/or family to resource books available from the American Diabetes Association: *Nutrition for Children with Diabetes,* the *American Diabetic Association Family Cookbook, Exchange Lists;* these resources for meal planning suggest a variety of nutrients appropriate for diabetic child while keeping calories, carbohydrate, fat, and protein intake constant
		Teach child and/or parents to always carry a form of concentrated sugar (fruit juices, sugar cubes, or glucose tablets)
		Inform child and/or parents to monitor frequency of hypoglycemic episodes
		Advise parents and/or child to consult nutritionist or physician to evaluate need to adjust meal planning
		Assist parents in planning for special events (birthday parties, eating out, etc.); inform parents that nutritionist can suggest preparing treats that are not high in sugar (birthday cake without icing) and evaluating need for extra insulin for special treats
		Teach child and/or parents importance of maintaining insulin and food intake during illness: advise parents and/or child to consult pediatrician or endocrinologist to evaluate need to alter insulin doses secondary to increased stress from illness
		Teach child and/or parents to test the blood and urine more frequently during illness and to follow nutritionist's guidelines for dealing with decreased appetite during illness
		Advise parents to promptly report vomiting and/or diarrhea to physician for management
		Consult nutritionist for food intake guidelines relative to increased activity periods (extra snacks), delayed meals (providing carbohydrate snacks to prevent hypoglycemia prior to regular scheduled meals), and periods of illness and/or decreased appetite
		Failitate communication to the schoolteacher regarding importance of consistent meal times
Lack of prior experience with diabetes Request for information regarding diabetes and required treatment	Child and/or parents will verbalize and demonstrate understanding of insulin administration, blood and urine testing, meal planning, and exercise program	I. *Administraiton of insulin*
		Teach parents and/ or child about diabetes and effects on the body; provide written instruction booklets available from the American Diabetes Association ("What You Need to Know about Diabetes and Your Child," for children; "What you Need to Know about Diabetes")
Knowledge deficit related to diabetes, long-term management, treatment of disease complications, home care, and follow-up care		Inform parents and/or child that a major treatment for type I diabetes is a combination of insulin by injection, diet with a balanced meal plan, and exercise on regular basis to control blood sugar levels
		Teach parents that injections are necessary because the body cannot make its own insulin so that insulin must be replaced; explain that normal blood sugar levels are 70-110 mg/dl or 100-140 mg/dl after meals
		Teach parents and/or child about different forms and sources of insulin (regular—short-acting; NPH and Lente—intermediate-acting) that differ in how long they act to lower blood sugar, how quickly they start working, and how soon after injection they work most effectively.
		Reassure parents and/or child that one or two types of insulin are prescribed to achieve adequate control
		Inform parents and/or child that insulin dosage depends on individual as determined by blood and urine glucose levels, urine ketone levels, food intake, and exercise activity level and that increased insulin needs may be required during illness, stress, trauma, surgery, infection, and periods of increased growth
		Familiarize parents and/or child with materials needed for injection, slowly and progressively handling parts of the syringe, drawing up insulin from a vial, maintaining aseptic technique
		Teach parents and/or child to inspect insulin for color, clarity, and consistency (free from clumps); avoid insulin exposure to heat, freezing, and light; avoid vigorous agitation by teaching them to roll the vial between their hands and not to shake the vial to avoid deactivation of insulin
		Refrigerate extra vials of insulin
		Teach parents how to draw up two types of insulin

Clinical Problem/Nursing Diagnosis	Expected Outcome	Nursing Interventions
		Demonstrate proper injection technique, ideally on self; inject at a 45- to 90-degree angle with skin and subcutaneous tissue pinched up; encourage parents and/or child to practice on a "sugar baby doll"
		Stress importance of rotating injection sites between upper arms, buttocks, abdomen (except a 1 in. border around the umbilicus), and upper thighs and keeping a record of size, insulin dose, time, date, and injection site used
		Teach parents and/or child how to promptly recognize complications from insulin (hypoglycemia, hyperglycemia—see nursing interventions under potential for injury: hypo/hyperglycemia); recommend the wearing of medical alert bracelets
		Encourage expression of feelings of fear, anger, frustration, and loss of control
		Provide opportunities for therapeutic play with "sugar baby doll" and role-playing process of giving injections to help child cope with stress and fear of injections
		Suggest that parents maintain consistent schedule and routine to assist child in adjusting to daily required injections
		School-age children need to be taught self-injections and daily care and shown how to assume control and responsibility for self-care
		II. *Meal planning*
		See nursing interventions under altered nutrition outlined in care plan
		III. *Blood and urine testing*
		Stress importance of balancing food, insulin, and exercise to maintain normal blood glucose levels and importance of evaluating diabetes control through testing
		Teach parents and/or child to test urine for sugar and ketones before meals and at bedtime using the double void method; instruct child to void once, then again approximately 30 min later; second specimen is to be tested using instruction of specific test method (reagent strips, ketostix); inform child that accuracy is maintained by protecting test strips from light and dampness
		Explain to parents and/or child method of measuring blood glucose
		Wash hands with warm water and soap; avoid use of alcohol; puncture periphery of finger; apply drop of blood on designated area of test strip; read test strip at designated time based on instructions for specific test; read blood glucose level with color comparison chart as specified
		IV. *Exercise*
		Help child and/or parents develop daily routine exercise program to aid in reducing blood sugar levels
		Encourage consistency in amount of daily exercise activity; inform them that changes in activity level may require changes in child's diet and insulin needs; insulin requirements and meal planning can be individually determined so children can participate in desired sports activity and exercise program
		Encourage regular exercise and active participation in school exercise programs and social events
		Inform parents and/or child about need for an extra snack before exercise and sometimes during or after exercise, especially strenuous exercise; suggest snacks such as peanut butter/cheese crackers
		Inform parent and/or child to consult physician or endocrinologist when exercise is prolonged or strenuous to make adjustment in insulin doses as needed
		Reassure parents and/or child that exercise need be avoided only when glucose levels are <60 mg/dl or >300 mg/dl and in presence of ketonuria
		V. *Education for schoolteachers and caretakers*
		Teach parents to educate caretakers, schoolteachers, and school nurse about basics of diabetes and management of low blood sugar, high blood sugar, ketoacidosis, meals and snacks, and exercise and activity level
		Suggest to schoolteacher ways to help child not feel singled out or different (allow all children to participate in snack time)

Continued.

NURSING CARE PLAN 28-2 The Child and Adolescent with Type I Diabetes Mellitus—cont'd

Clinical Problem/Nursing Diagnosis	Expected Outcome	Nursing Interventions
		Provide written information outlining what to do (pamphlet titled "A Word to Teachers and School Staff" is available from American Diabetes Association)
		Provide written list of emergency phone numbers for caretakers and schoolteachers; include numbers for parents, doctor, hospital, close relative, and ambulance
		VI. *Communicating with the health care team*
		Familiarize parents and/or child with support available from health care team members: diabetic nurse specialist, nutritionist, pediatrician, endocrinologist, and counselor
		Provide family with phone number list to facilitate communication with health care team
		Teach child and/or parents how and when to notify physician or diabetic clinic
		Teach parents and/or child to report vomiting, abdominal pain, diarrhea, shortness of breath, lethargy, signs of illness, temperature greater than 100°F, dehydration (dry mouth, thirst, dry skin, and decreased urination), large amounts of urine, ketones in urine, and high blood sugar level >200 mg/dl that is unresponsive to extra doses of insulin taken as ordered
		Inform parents and/or child that if they are unable to reach physician they must go immediately to local emergency room
		Inform parents and/or child to keep emergency phone numbers within easy access (physician, clinic, emergency room, ambulance, police, and pharmacy)
Anxiety Disturbances in daily routines Loss of control	Through the use of appropriate coping strategies, family will attain optimal family functioning	Familiarize family with health care facility and comprehensive health care team available to support child's and family's needs (pediatrician, endocrinologist, diabetic nurse specialist, nutritionist, diabetic clinic, social worker, and counselor); provide family with written list of names and phone numbers to facilitate contact when needed
Altered family process related to an ill child, stressors of a chronic illness, and daily management		Provide adequate opportunities for parents and/or child to express feelings of fear, disappointment, frustration, anger, resentment, and distress related to diagnosis of diabetes and daily management.
		Acknowledge parents' feelings of conflict between roles of comforter and inflictor of pain (injections)
		Identify parental strengths; emphasize strengths in parents' participation in care
		Encourage parents to maintain normality within family; support parents in understanding that special privileges and extra attention toward diabetic child can increase stress, tension, and resentment among family members
		Explore with parents feelings of other children in family (resentment, anger, and competition for attention)
		Encourage parents to maintain their interests and time for themselves
		Teach parents to treat injections, testing, and meal planning as daily routines to increase child's ability to learn to cope with diabetes as a part of life
		Encourage parents to promote increased independence and responsibility in the child (school age or older) for managing daily care; reassure parents that responsibility for care will increase child's sense of control and confidence
		Encourage parents to allow school-age children and older children to attend summer camp for children with diabetes for teaching of self-care and peer support
		Refer parents to community resources (Juvenile Diabetes Foundation and American Diabetes Association); assist parents and/or child with identification of local chapter support and local support groups for parents, children, and young adults

Clinical Problem/Nursing Diagnosis	Expected Outcome	Nursing Interventions
		Facilitate communication with other parents of children with diabetes and allow young adults to share feelings with peers who have diabetes
		Suggest professional counseling to increase family support systems as indicated
Anxiety, fear, and separation from family during hospitalization	Given appropriate interventions, child will preserve self-esteem and attain mastery of coping with diabetes and daily management in a manner which promotes optimal growth and development and participation in age-appropriate developmental activities	Explore child's feelings and fears about change in daily routines (injections, meal planning, and exercise)
Change in daily routines		Base preparation for procedures and experiences on child's cognitive and developmental level
Lack of experience with illness and daily management		Prepare preschoolers daily for insulin injections; reassure them that they are good and are not being punished; use therapeutic play to aid in explaining injection and procedures to encourage child's expression of fear
Fear related to loss of control and bodily injury		Encourage school-age children to develop increasing responsibility and control over daily care; acknowledge pain and fear of injections and praise them for responsibility in daily care (injections, blood and urine testing, and charting)
		Support adolescents through expression of anger, denial, and rebellion; assist them in understanding the reality of noncompliance; facilitate peer support with other adolescents dealing with diabetes
		Provide child or adolescent with control and choices; support active participation in daily care (insulin injections, testing urine and blood for sugar, meal planning, exercise, and record keeping of daily management)
		Facilitate opportunities for child to verbalize and express feelings, fears, and concerns through play, activities, and talk; read stories that depict fear of daily injections as well as addressing areas of diabetic management (story or coloring books that address a child's daily living with diabetes) to encourage meaningful expressions of feelings
		Provide opportunities for child to draw pictures about hospital experience or to make a story of what has been expeienced
		Support child's individual coping mechanisms
		Encourage attendance at summer camps for children with diabetes which include fun, promotion of independence and responsibility for care, increased education about diabetes, and peer support
		Encourage active participation in sports, school activities, and hobbies

acids to provide energy for cell activity. When body protein breaks down, gluconeogenesis increases and further hyperglycemia develops. With fatty acid utilization, ketone bodies are formed and oxidized for energy. These ketone bodies accumulate more rapidly than they can be used, and the excess is excreted in the urine. Sodium and potassium are lost as ketone bodies are transported out of the nephron tubules. The metabolic equilibrium of the blood is disrupted, causing increased hydrogen ion concentration and acidosis. The body is unable to compensate, and an elevated carbonic acid level dissociates into water and carbon dioxide, further lowering the blood pH. If this ketoacidosis progresses unchecked, coma and death occur.

The treatment of severe ketoacidosis requires intravenous fluids, volume expansion, insulin calculated for body weight, and glucose or calories to reverse the intracellular starvation. It also necessitates replacement of lost electrolytes and, if indicated, alkali and minerals. The most important nursing function is monitoring for complications such as shock, renal failure, hypoxia, thrombosis, paradoxical acidosis, underlying infection, cerebral edema, and hypoglycemia. Some of these complications can be caused by overly aggressive treatment. (Protocols for the management of mild, moderate, and severe acidosis may be found in Jackson and Guthrie, 1984).

The effects of abnormal carbohydrate metabolism lead to the classic "polys" of diabetes: *polyuria, polydipsia,* and *polyphagia.* Loss of body protein is reflected in weight loss, lethargy, and fatigue. Ketone accumulation in the blood can produce nausea, vomiting, or abdominal pain. These symptoms may mimic stomach flu or acute appendicitis in some children and can delay an accurate diagnosis. The stress of a viral illness or a bacterial infection may in fact be the final precipitating event of diabetes mellitus. One must always look for hidden infection, since these children may be hyperthermic on admission.

Urine glucose levels are high, and fasting glucose readings are above 120 mg/dl. Glycosuria and ketonuria are present. If ketoacidosis is present, urine ketones are positive and blood pH readings are below 7.35. Electrolyte levels of Na$^+$ and Cl$^-$ are decreased, and K$^+$ levels may be normal, elevated, or decreased depending on the amount of acidosis and dehydration.

Prediabetes describes the stage of the disease in genetically susceptible individuals before any abnormal metabolic findings are demonstrated. Tests of glucose tolerance may be normal or slightly abnormal.

Subclinical diabetes or chemical diabetes, is generally characterized by the lack of overt clinical symptoms. However, hyperglycemia may occur under stress, such as illness or trauma.

No classic symptoms are present in latent diabetes, but a glucose tolerance test reveals hyperglycemia. Urine glucose can also be present. Insulin treatment started at this stage prevents pancreatic decompensation and prolongs the honeymoon period.

Overt diabetes often occurs rapidly in children and is manifested by both fasting and postprandial hyperglycemia as well as glycosuria. Some patients progress to ketoacidosis and require emergency care.

The major objective in the treatment of juvenile diabetes mellitus is to maintain blood glucose levels in as close to a normal range as possible. The major objectives of medical and nursing care are to establish an insulin dose, meal plan, and exercise schedule that will support the child or adolescent in achieving blood glucose values within a normal range (Table 28-7). The child and his family are taught a self-treatment regimen that supports them in maintaining this degree of control. Jackson and Guthrie (1984) recommend a *physiological* management consisting of (1) at least two insulin injections of a combination of short, intermediate, and/or long-acting insulin per 24 hours, (2) a meal plan designed for the daily activities and insulin activity of the child or adolescent with diabetes, (3) an exercise program occurring five to seven times per week, about the same time each day, (4) daily blood glucose checks and, in the case of the very young, urine and/or blood checks three to four times a day, and (5) food, insulin, and exercise adjustment according to urine or blood glucose findings.

TABLE 28-7 Range of Blood Glucose Values for Self-Monitoring of Blood Glucose

	Preferred	Acceptable
Fasting	70-100 mg/dl	70-120 mg/dl
Premeals	70-105 mg/dl	70-130 mg/dl
Postmeals (1h)	90-160 mg/dl	90-180 mg/dl
Postmeals and bedtime (2h)	100-120 mg/dl	100-150 mg/dl

Nursing Management

Education and treatment go hand in hand in order to achieve the aforementioned goals of diabetes management. Like treatment, education and support should be provided by a diabetic team consisting of health professionals (physicians, nurses, dietitians, and social workers), the family, school personnel, ministers, and peers in the community. The nurse on the diabetic team is often the health professional who is responsible for coordinating the efforts of the individuals on the diabetic team, beginning with the initial diagnosis and continuing in the form of follow-up after the child is discharged from the hospital. Team conferences, patient rounds, and patient and family conferences are necessary and should be done on a daily basis to enhance the health team's and family's efforts toward the achievement of optimum diabetic control.

Education Process

After a careful nursing assessment is made and appropriate nursing diagnoses are made, an educational plan is developed based on the individual needs of the patient and members of the family. Objectives are written so that continued education is done to determine the outcome of the educational strategies. This evaluation is placed in the patient's chart so that all health team members can monitor the progress of the patient and family education, allowing them the opportunity to have feedback and to have input into the process.

Education is a continuous process for the child with diabetes and his family. It begins at the time of diagnosis and continues throughout the remainder of the hospitalization. After discharge, education continues with each subsequent phone call, clinic appointment, and hospitalization. Diabetic camps, diabetic organizations, and seminars also are essential for the education of the child and his family.

Initially, education should focus on answering the questions of the child with diabetes and his family along with helping them anticipate and understand the emotional responses of each individual in the familiy. Typically, the family learns technical skills best during this time of grief. Such things as blood glucose checks, urine checks, injection techniques, and treatment of hypoglycemia episodes are best learned 2 to 3 days after the initial diagnosis. More complex information (meal plan and insulin adjustment) is taught later in the hospitalization and throughout the follow-up outpatient evaluations. Because of the complexity of diabetes, too much information in the beginning may overwhelm the child and family, resulting in mistakes being made and diminished adherence to the recommended diabetes self-management routine.

Because the daily schedule of the child or adolescent and his family usually changes dramatically, a spontaneous lifestyle becomes difficult. During the first year after the diagnosis, guidance and support (phone calls and outpatient appointments) are needed by the family in order to adjust to the overwhelming task of reorganizing their lives.

Discipline

Each child and the child's siblings, depending on age, react differently to the new diagnosis and the ultimate lifestyle change. Each child and sibling bring unique challenges to the parents. Children with diabetes are children first, with their own developmental needs to be met. Like the child with diabetes, siblings also are youths with their own developmental needs to fulfill. Disregard for these children and their needs, lack of discipline, and lack of professional and family support result in noncompliance and a family whose members will experience emotional stress and problems (Barnard, 1986).

Insulin

Insulins are extracted from bovine and pancreatic tissue and are now being produced through DNA technology (biosynthetic human insulin). The use of beef and some less pure pork insulin is to be discouraged since these forms of insulin may result in the development of insulin antibodies which may cause (1) a diminished therapeutic insulin response, (2) a local or generalized allergic reaction, or (3) localized or generalized lipoatrophy. These effects are less likely to occur or can be treated with the use of biosynthetic human insulin or very pure pork insulin.

Insulin needs are greatest (up to 2 U/kg/d) when treatment is first initiated because of the body's need to replenish lost protein and fat stores, especially if the child has lost a significant amount of weight over a long period of time. Short-term weight loss is due to acute dehydration and is corrected by adequate rehydration. If the child, however, has been diagnosed early in the latent phase, the insulin dosage is low and in fact may need to be diluted (Jackson and Guthrie, 1984). Subcutaneous injections of insulin are administered three to four times a day in response to blood and urine glucose levels. If ketoacidosis is present, intravenous insulin and fluid and electrolyte replacement are necessary (see the section on diabetic ketoacidosis). When the child is stabilized, insulin requirements generally decrease slowly to 0.15 to 0.40 with a mean of 0.32 U/kg/d for preadolescent children. The 24-hour requirement for insulin can be supplied in a double- or multiple-dose injection schedule. When a two-dose schedule is used, the first injection (e.g., 2 parts NPH, 1 part Regular insulin) is given one-half hour before breakfast, providing two-thirds of the total daily requirement. The second dose (e.g., 2 parts NPH, 1 part Regular insulin) contains the final one-third requirement and is administered a half hour before dinner and in combination with three-meal, three-snack food distribution (Jackson and Guthrie, 1984). These combinations are thought to promote a normal glucose level (Guthrie, 1977).

The necessity for frequent insulin injections is likely to be the most difficult aspect of care for the child and family. Because the preschool child has tremendous fears related to injections, the nurse provides opportunities for needle play. The child then has a feeling of control and a chance to express the anger and frustration caused by daily injections. The older child generally learns quickly and takes pride in managing insulin administration. When teaching proper technique, the nurse promotes confidence in the parents and older child by having them practice first on an orange or doll. Allowing them to repeat the injection demonstration to the nurse is also helpful and the child may subsequently give the first injection on his/her own thigh.

Adequate instruction in mixing, diluting, injection technique, and storage of insulin is provided in the total teaching plan. When a child is receiving a 2:1 ratio of Regular and NPH insulins, the most advantageous method is to premix the insulins in larger amounts or to have the family order insulin already premixed by the pharmaceutical company. If Regular is mixed along with NPH, Lente, or Ultralente in a syringe, the injection should be given immediately after drawing up the insulins and not allowed to be in the syringe for more than 10 minutes (this may alter the action of the insulin.

Parents should be instructed in diluting insulin (only Regular and NPH can be diluted) to U50, U25, and U10 concentrations because of the very low insulin requirements. This education can be done under the direction of a nurse or physician. Diluting fluid is obtained from the pharmaceutical companies, not from the pharmacy. Using decreased concentrations allows the patient and parents to make insulin dosage adjustments in one-half, one-fourth, and one-tenth increments, which is usually necessary for the young diabetic patient who is in remission, thus requiring low doses of insulin.

Timing of insulin is often overlooked and seldom mentioned during the education process. It is not possible for insulin to act on food if the timing is inappropriate. For instance, the meal following an injection of Regular insulin should occur in 30 to 45 minutes. Without proper timing, hypoglycemia or hyperglycemia is likely to occur. *Timing can make a difference in diabetes control.*

In addition to timing, the rotation of insulin injections is discussed. Insulin is given subcutaneously over the arms, legs, hips, and abdomen. The legs are not used if the injection is given prior to participation in a sport involving the legs (e.g., swimming or track). A more neutral spot should be used for the injections, for example, the hips (Fig. 28-8).

The actual rotation pattern should be determined by the individual, keeping in mind that at least two finger breadths should be placed between two injection sites in the same area and that the same area should be used for a week at a time (Guthrie and Guthrie, 1982). Rotation is for the purpose of preventing hypertrophy or insulin injection pads. These pads are not as painful during the time of injection, thus resulting in an overuse of the same site. Unfortunately, insulin injected into an insulin pad is not absorbed properly, thus resulting in higher blood sugars. In addition, there may be a discrepancy of insulin amount

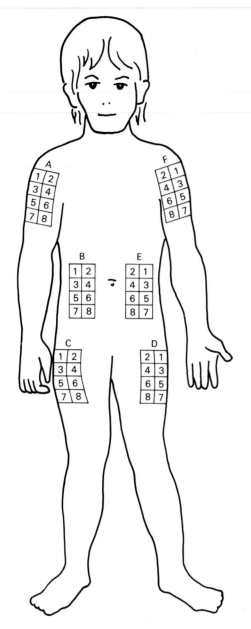

FIGURE 28-8   Injection site rotation plan. The child learns to administer insulin injections 1 inch apart at each site. The rotation plan involves use of the spaces in site A first, followed by sites B, C, etc. Site A is again returned to in approximately 1 month. (*Drawing courtesy of Steve Bittick.*)

depending on whether the insulin is injected into an insulin pad or into subcutaneous tissue.

Parents and older adolescents with diabetes are taught insulin dosage adjustment so that they can make appropriate changes outside the health care setting. These insulin changes are based on blood and urine glucose values, exercise, and meal plan. Illness or other stresses may precipitate either high or low blood glucoses, thus making it necessary to change the insulin dose or give supplemental doses of insulin. Education for insulin adjustment is closely supervised both in the hospital and by phone after discharge. Ideally, families have 24-hour access to the nurse and the doctor so that educational and emotional

needs can be met, especially in the first few months after the initial diagnosis.

Insulin requirements are likely to decrease 2 or 3 weeks after therapy has begun since some endogenous insulin secretion returns. This so-called honeymoon period (remission period) is the result of the healing and secretion of the remaining functional beta cells and can last a few months to several years depending on the degree of control and the stage of maturation the child is in. Insulin therapy is never discontinued during this honeymoon period. Because of the very low doses of insulin, the child or adolescent is closely monitored for adequate reduction in the insulin dose during the honeymoon or remission. Ideally the adjustment of the insulin dose is done in a hospital setting. However, in the majority of cases it is not possible, and so the nurse should have at least daily phone contact to assist the family in determining the insulin dose. All efforts should be made to avoid hypoglycemic episodes at this time.

In addition to adjusting the food for activity, parents must also be taught that as a child grows in size, both calories and insulin need to be increased. Increasing the insulin does not mean that the diabetes is worsening. The child's pancreas will secrete some insulin for years if good control is maintained. When puberty is reached, careful increases in insulin and blood glucose monitoring are necessary because of the large amount of sex hormones. After full maturation and menarche, insulin again must be diminished and stabilized at between 0.7 and 1 U/kg/d. Stress situations such as illness, surgery, and emotional upsets can increase insulin requirements. Types of insulin are shown in Table 28-8.

Meal Plan

Since children are active and require a continuous supply of energy, a small-portion, frequent-feeding pattern is commonly utilized. Three meals and one to three snacks are set up, with caloric intake adjusted to the daily activity schedule of the individual child and the pattern of growth. Times of increased physical activity are preceded by increased food intake. The diet often follows the exchange or point system designed by the American Diabetic Association. Some freedom is allowed in the foods chosen, but concentrated sugars are generally discouraged. A general rule is 50 to 60 cal/kg/d in growing children and 30 cal/kg/d after puberty. If the family is on the same type of meal plan as the child with diabetes, the child is more likely to adhere to the recommendations. This type of meal plan is usually a more healthy one for all the individuals involved.

Physical Activity

The exercise pattern of the child will vary somewhat on a daily basis; however, exercises ideally are done several days a week at about the same time each day. With planned exercise the child or adolescent can be taught about insulin adjustments (usually lowering) and caloric adjustments (usually increased) prior to, during, and even after the exercise. These additional calories can be in the

TABLE 28-8 Types of Insulin

Type	Onset of Action, hours	Peak Action, hours	Duration of action, hours
Fast-acting			
Regular	½-1	2-4	6-8
Semilente	½-1	2-4	10-12
Intermediate-acting			
NPH (isophane)	2	8-12	24-28
Lente	1-2	8-16	24-28
Globin zinc	1-2	8-16	18-24
Long-acting			
PZI (protamin zinc)	4-8	14-20	36+
Ultralente	4-8	16-18	36+

form of extra food (e.g., orange wedges), glucose solutions (e.g., half water, half Coke solution), or concentrated glucose (e.g., glucose tablets). Calories should be planned and carried out by the child.

Another type of exercise that is frequently encountered is unplanned exercise. If adequate calories are not provided, a hypoglycemic episode may occur. Because active children are confronted with unplanned exercise, they should be taught to carry glucose tablets or some type of fast-acting food. Parents, teachers, school nurses, and coaches should have these sources of calories in the event that they must treat the hypoglycemia.

Hidden exercise is often the cause of changes in blood glucose and may be hard to detect. Like unplanned exercise, hidden exercise can cause hypoglycemia and must be treated with additional calories. For example, young adults in college may fail to take into account that walking to classes is exercise (Barnard, 1986; Jackson and Guthrie, 1984).

Self-Monitoring

Insulin adjustments, meal plans, and physical activity indicate that self-monitoring is necessary and essential in the daily management of type I diabetes. Monitoring is done through self-monitoring of blood glucose, urine acetone, and/or urine glucose. The accuracy with which these procedures are carried out is positively correlated to the type of ongoing education and evaluation done. During every appointment, feedback and demonstration evaluations of the child's and parents' techniques must be included in the routine follow-up. The size of the drop of blood and the timing of the procedure must be accurate for the results of blood glucose monitoring to be reliable. In addition, the meter must be clean in order to produce accurate results.

Self-monitoring should be performed three to four times a day and more frequently by individuals involved in exercise and those who are ill. Overall patterns are determined after several days of monitoring. Insulin adjustments are made based on these patterns. The blood or urine glucose results along with insulin dosage, caloric intake, exercise, and any unusual stresses are recorded on a record sheet. The child, parents, and health team can use this information to identify patterns of blood glucose and its relationship to insulin dose, exercise, meal plan, and stresses. Thus, appropriate adjustments of food and insulin will be based on these patterns.

Special Problems of the Child with Diabetes Mellitus

Acute Complications

Diabetic Ketoacidosis In some children ketoacidosis may be the initial presentation of diabetes. In others, poor diabetic control, omission of insulin, increased food intake, illness, infection, or emotional stress will precipitate the condition. Some "brittle" diabetics who have wide fluctuations in blood glucose levels are prone to ketoacidosis and can require repeated hospitalization for treatment.

Ketoacidosis is treated with intravenous and subcutaneous insulin and fluid and electrolyte replacement. Continuous intravenous infusion of insulin in low doses (0.1 U/kg/h) has been very successful in lowering blood glucose levels quickly (Traisman, 1980). Frequent urine and blood checks are necessary to monitor response to therapy. Fluids containing electrolytes (Na^+, Cl^-, K^+) aid in reestablishing metabolic equilibrium by replacing volume electrolyte deficits and breaking the ketoacidosis cycle. The child may need cardiac monitoring if potassium loss is excessive. When blood glucose levels reach 250 mg/dl, glucose infusion is restarted to prevent hypoglycemia. Once stabilized, the child's previous insulin regimen is reinstituted.

Hypoglycemia Low blood glucose levels are not uncommon in type I diabetes. Skipping a meal, giving too much insulin, or excessive physical activity without added food intake can all lead to hypoglycemia. Manifestations of hypoglycemia are first noted in the brain and nervous system, since both require glucose for proper functioning. A comparison of hypoglycemia (or insulin reaction) and ketoacidosis is summarized in Table 28-9. Accurate diagnosis and prompt treatment are vital to prevent coma or brain damage. Most diabetics are able to recognize the signs of an impending insulin reaction, such as hunger, weakness, lethargy, and irritability. The reaction is easily avoided by eating a simple sugar. If a large drop in the

TABLE 28-9 Comparison of Hypoglycemia and Diabetic Ketoacidosis

Feature	Hypoglycemia	Diabetic Ketoacidosis
Onset	Rapid (15 min to 1 h)	Slow (2-3 days)
Causes	Delayed or missed meal Excessive insulin Excessive exercise	Overeating Insufficient insulin Stress (e.g., illness, surgery, emotional upset)
Manifestations	Weakness Sweating Blurred vision Mood change Hunger Pallor Rapid pulse Shock Coma	Polyuria Polydipsia Nausea and vomiting Abdominal pain Drowsiness Acetone breath Rapid, labored respirations Rapid pulse
Laboratory values Urine		
Sugar	Usually absent	Positive
Acetone	Negative	Positive
Blood		
Sugar	Decreased	Increased
Acetone	Negative	Positive
Treatment	Administration of glucose	Administration of insulin
Response to treatment	Rapid	Slow
Extra clues	Urine test not accurate at this time If ever in doubt, eat sugar	Urine test may show ketone spilling Flu-like symptoms

blood glucose level occurs, generalized sweating, dizziness, nausea, vomiting, and rapid pulse may appear with possible progression to convulsions and coma. Treatment consists of immediate glucose ingestion (Monojel or glutose) followed in 15 or 20 minutes with a simple carbohydrate meal. Intramuscular glucagon is given if loss of consciousness occurs or the child is uncooperative in eating the needed sugar. Vomiting may result, thus requiring intravenous dextrose solution until the patient is stabilized.

Hypoglycemia must be distinguished from Somogyi's phenomenon. This response develops when low blood glucose levels trigger epinephrine and corticosteroid release. The end result is a rebound and rise in blood glucose, although the initial symptoms mimic insulin reaction. Glucose is present in the urine. Somogyi's phenomenon is often observed after vigorous physical activity.

Long-Term Complications Patients with longstanding type I diabetes mellitus may show evidence of microscopic damage to the nervous and vascular systems. Affected organs can include the eyes, kidneys, heart, blood vessels, and peripheral nerves. Most investigators believe that such organ changes are due to the long-term effects of hyperglycemia and insulin deficit. Impaired glucose and fat metabolism may affect cell membranes, leading to destructive lesions in the small blood vessels (mi-

TABLE 28-10 HbA$_1$C Values and Degree of Control, Normals Vary with Lab Assay, and Values Need to be Established for Each Lab

HbA$_1$C Level, %	Degree of Control
<8.5	Excellent
8.5-9.5	Good
9.5-10.5	Fair
10.5-12.0	Fair to poor
>12.0	Poor

croangiopathy). The result can be blindness, neuropathy, and kidney damage (nephropathy). Changes in larger vessels can produce premature atherosclerosis, heart attack, and stroke. Good metabolic control of glucose levels has been directly related to minimizing the severity of these vascular changes.

Long-term control (over a 3-month period) can now be measured easily by a glycosylated hemoglobin (A$_1$C). Excess indicates constant hyperglycemia. Since the red blood cells are turned over every 120 days, the A$_1$C changes can be detected in 3 months. The goal is to keep A$_1$C in the *normal* range (Jackson and Guthrie, 1984). The use of home blood glucose monitoring can improve diabetic control as measured by A$_1$C (Table 28-10).

Psychologic Aspects In most families, the initial reaction to a diagnosis of diabetes is similar to the grief process which accompanies a major loss. Disbelief, anger, and a search for alternative answers are eventually replaced by a gradual acceptance of the condition.

Psychologic adjustment to diabetes is related to the child's age when the disorder is first diagnosed and to the family's attitude. Support from family members is very important during the adjustment period. Any chronic illness require modifications in the lives of the patient and family. The nurse supports the child and parents with helpful suggestions about disease management at home. The younger child is likely to accept insulin administration and urine testing as new activities in daily living. When parents are actively involved in the care, the child becomes confident in and comfortable with the therapeutic regimen. Problems arise when either the child or the parents refuse to accept responsibility for diabetes control. The nurse provides counseling and advice during follow-up visits, assisting with necessary changes in treatment when indicated.

The diabetic adolescent often feels different and estranged from his peers. In striving for sameness, insulin is skipped and diet modifications are ignored. If independency struggles exist with parents, the stress of emotional conflict can precipitate an episode of ketoacidosis. Some especially troubled teenagers require frequent hospitalizations and psychiatric counseling to aid in maintaining adequate control of their diabetes. Nursing responsibilities include promotion of a therapeutic environment and discussion of the difficulties of dealing with a complex chronic illness. Teenage support groups are useful in providing an important forum for sharing problems and solutions. A medical alert bracelet or tag is recommended for every patient with diabetes. With good diabetic control these children can do anything. They should be encouraged to become productive members of society and to lead a long and healthy life, free from the complications of diabetes.

Learning Activities

1. Present a case study of a young child who has a long-term endocrine disorder (e.g., hypothyroidism. Cushing's syndrome). Include history, physical examination, clinical manifestations, and treatment. Identify the major nursing problems and associated interventions pertinent to the care of the child.

2. Assume the role of a parent of a newly diagnosed neonate who has congenital adrenal hyperplasia. Have a second person assume the role of a primary nurse making the first contact during admission. Delineate the major parental concerns and immediate needs. Discuss the psychological impact of this diagnosis and its long-term implications.

Independent Study Activities

1. Compare and contrast the etiology, pathophysiology, clinical manifestations, treatment, and nursing management of diabetes insipidus and diabetes mellitus in children.

2. Design a teaching plan for an 8-year-old Mexican-American child newly diagnosed with diabetes mellitus. Include self-monitoring of blood glucose, urine testing, injection technique, diet planning, and treatment for hypoglycemic reactions. Special attention should center on the cultural influences that the child's background will have on management of this chronic disease.

3. Identify organizations and resource groups active in the community whose focus is the health care needs of children and families with endocrine disorders (e.g., American Diabetes Association and Juvenile Diabetes Foundation). Visit a local chapter or attend a group meeting to identify available services.

4. Take home urine glucose strips or blood-monitoring equipment, saline, and insulin syringes. Follow a diabetic self-management regimen for 1 week, including self-monitoring, record keeping saline injections, and meal plans.

Study Questions

1. Among their actions, thyroid hormones:
   A. Promote protein anabolism
   B. Control the growth rate of body cells.
   C. Promote bone and soft tissue growth.
   D. Control calcium reabsorption.

2. The ratio of upper body segment to lower body segment at birth is:
   A. 1:1.   C. 2:1.
   B. 1.7:1.   D. 2.5:1.5

3. The secretion of growth hormone is regulated by:
   A. Somatotropin-releasing factor.
   B. Corticotropin.
   C. Corticotropin-releasing factor.
   D. Thyroid-releasing factor.

4. Idiopathic hypopituitarism generally is seen as:
   A. Decreased thyrotropin.
   B. Growth hormone deficiency.
   C. Tumor of the hypothalamus.
   D. Tumor of the pituitary.

5. Somatotropin cannot be given orally because it:
   A. Causes gastroenteritis.
   B. Is inactivated by saliva.
   C. Cannot be absorbed in the duodenum.
   D. Is destroyed by the action of digestive juices in the stomach.

6. Diabetes insipidus is the result of:
   A. Decreased antidiuretic hormone secretion.
   B. Decreased insulin secretion.
   C. Decreased insulin production.
   D. Anterior pituitary dysfunction.

7. A newborn who is screened for hypothyroidism, as required by state law, is found to have a low T_4. Further testing confirms the diagnosis of hypothyroidism. The infant is treated with synthetic sodium levothyroxine. In order to maintain proper dosage:
   A. Periodic x-rays should be done.
   B. T_4 and TSH levels should be checked periodically.
   C. T_3 and TSH levels should be checked periodically.
   D. T_3 and T_4 levels should be checked periodically.

8. Infants with hypothyroidism can have difficulty with feeding because of:
   A. The incidence of diarrhea in these infants.
   B. A weak suck and protruding tongue.
   C. Thyroiditis.
   D. A decrease in ADH.

9. The nurse can confirm a suspicion of developmental delay in infants with hypothyroidism by:
   A. The use of age-appropriate developmental assessment tools.
   B. Referral to a pediatric neurologist.
   C. Referral to a pediatric psychologist.
   D. Examining the infant's sequential growth chart.

10. If a child has been diagnosed with insulin dependent diabetes early in the latent phase
    A. Insulin needs are great.
    B. Insulin needs are the same as in overt diabetes.
    C. Insulin dosage is low.
    D. Insulin needs are the same as in subclinical diabetes.

11. During the "honeymoon period" of insulin dependent diabetes
    A. Insulin therapy is discontinued.
    B. Insulin requirements decrease.
    C. Insulin requirements increase.
    D. Calories are increased.

12. The insulin dependent diabetic child who has hunger, weakness, lethargy, or irritability is instructed to
    A. Take glutose.
    B. Eat a simple carbohydrate meal.
    C. Ask his parents what to do.
    D. Eat a simple sugar.

13. If the diabetic adolescent if having independency struggles with her parents, the stress of emotional conflict can precipitate
    A. An insulin reaction.
    B. An episode of ketoacidosis.
    C. Frequent hospitalizations.
    D. A feeling of being different.

14. The time for teaching both parents and children about insulin dependent diabetes
    A. Begins on admission to the hospital and ends with discharge.
    B. Begins several days before discharge from the hospital.
    C. Is based upon psychologic state and readiness of the parents and/or child.
    D. Is governed by the physician's orders.

References

Barnard, M.U.: "Care of the Child with Type I Diabetes," *Pediatrics: Nursing Update,* 1(26):1-7, 1986.

Davidson, M.B.: "Effect of Growth Hormone on Carbohydrate and Lipid Metabolism," *Endocrine Reviews,* 8(2):115-131, 1987.

Felig, P., J.D. Baxter, A.E. Broadus, and L.A. Frohman: *Endocrinology and Metabolism,* 2d ed., McGraw-Hill, New York, 1987.

Greenspan, F.S., and P.H. Forsham: *Basic and Clinical Endocrinology,* 2d ed., Lange, Los Altos, Calif., 1986.

Guthrie, D.W.: "Exercise, Diet, and Insulin for Children with Diabetes," *Nursing,* '77, 7(2):48-54, 1977.

Guthrie, D.W., and R.A. Guthrie: *Nursing Management of Diabetes Mellitus,* 2d ed., Mosby, St. Louis, 1982.

Guyton, A.C.: *Human Physiology and Mechanisms of Disease,* 4th ed., Saunders, Philadelphia, 1987.

Jackson, R.L., and R. Guthrie (eds.): *Physiological Management of the Child with Insulin Dependent Diabetes,* Medical Examination Publishing Co., Chicago, 1984.

Kannan, C.R.: *Essential Endocrinology: A Primer for Nonspecialists,* 1st ed., Plenum, New York, 1986.

Solomon, B.L.: "The Hypothalamus and the Pituitary Gland: An Overview," *Nursing Clinics of North America,* 15(3):435-451, 1980.

Traisman, H.S.: "Treatment of Diabetic Acidosis," in *Management of Juvenile Diabetes Mellitus,* 3d ed., Mosby, St. Louis, 1980.

Van De Graaf, K.M., and R.W. Rhees: *Schaum's Outline of Theory and Problems of Human Anatomy and Physiology,* McGraw-Hill, New York, 1987.

Williams, J.A.: "Mechanisms in Hormone Secretion, Action, and Response," in F.S. Greenspan and P.H. Forsham (eds.), *Basic and Clinical Endocrinology,* 2d ed., Lange, Los Altos, Calif., 1986.

29

The Reproductive System

Objectives

After reading this chapter, the student will be able to:
1. Describe the functions of the reproductive system.
2. Identify appropriate subjective and objective data to be elicited from the child and family.
3. Understand the purpose of diagnostic tests and medical treatment.
4. Explain general nursing measures appropriate for pediatric clients who have various problems related to the reproductive system.
5. Delineate specific nursing measures appropriate to the care of pediatric clients who have various problems involving the reproductive system.

Anatomy and Physiology of the Reproductive System

The reproductive system consists of both internal and external structures in the male and female. It is important not only in the continuation of the human race but also in sexuality.

Male Anatomy

The internal organs of the male reproductive system lie in the pelvic cavity and consist of the seminal vesicles, the prostate, Cowper's gland, and a portion of the vas deferens. The seminal vesicles are just behind the urinary bladder. The ducts of these structures fuse with the vas deferens to form the ejaculatory duct. The prostate surrounds the neck of the urinary bladder and the beginning of the urethra (Chap. 27). Cowper's glands are anterior to the prostate. The vas deferens extends from the epididymal duct to the ejaculatory duct (Fig. 29-1).

The external male genitalia, inferior to the pelvic cavity, consist of the scrotum, testes, and penis. The scrotum is a pouch divided by a septum. Each side contains a testis. Within the testes are seminiferous tubules containing sperm in various stages of development. The epididymis, a reservoir for sperm, is a comma-shaped body posterior to each testis. The penis, the male organ of copulation, extends proximally into the perineal region. Its body, or shaft, terminates distally in the glans. Skin loosely attached to the body of the penis covers the glans. This flap of skin is called the prepuce or foreskin. The penile portion of the urethra is in the corpus spongiosum, the ventral body of the penis.

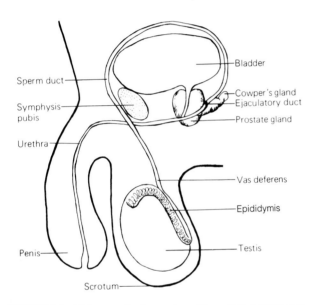

FIGURE 29-1 Male reproductive system. *(From G.M. Scipien et al. [eds.], Comprehensive Pediatric Nursing, 3d ed., McGraw-Hill, New York, 1986.)*

Female Anatomy

The internal organs of the female reproductive system lie in the pelvic cavity and consist of the uterus, fallopian tubes, ovaries, and vagina. The uterus, behind the urinary bladder, has three parts: the cervix, the body (or cavity), and the fundus. The fallopian tubes, on each side of the uterus, lie on the wall of the pelvic cavity. They extend laterally and downward. At the distal end of each tube are the fimbriae. The ovaries are on either side of the uterus, behind and below the fallopian tubes. The outer zone contains oocytes (immature ova). The vagina extends from its attachment at the cervix of the uterus to its outside opening on the perineum (Fig. 29-2).

The external genitalia of the female (the vulva), inferior to the pelvic cavity, consist of the vaginal orifice, the labia majora, the labia minora, the clitoris, and the mons pubis. (Also included in the vulva is the urinary orifice, discussed in Chap. 27.) The vaginal orifice contains the hymen, a thin membrane which changes the size of the opening. Some hymens are minimal. The labia majora are on the outer border of the vulva, while the labia minora are around the vaginal orifice and extend anteriorly to enclose the clitoris. The clitoris, which is usually covered by a prepuce, is anterior to the urinary meatus. The mons pubis lies over the pubic bone.

Hormonal Functions of the Male Reproductive System

Hormonal control of the reproductive system in both the male and the female is centered in the hypothalamus (Fig. 29-3). It is influenced by a number of elements such as heredity, environment, circulating reproductive hormones, and neural humors to increase or decrease its secretion of *gonadotropic hormone releasing factors.* These factors are the follicle-stimulating hormone releasing factor (FSHRF) and luteinizing hormone releasing factor (LHRF), and their action stimulates the anterior pituitary or adenohypophysis to release follicle-stimulating hormone (FSH) and luteinizing hormone (LH), respectively.

FSH in the male is responsible for the growth and de-

FIGURE 29-2 Female reproductive system. *(From G.M. Scipien et al. [eds.], Comprehensive Pediatric Nursing, 3d ed., McGraw-Hill, New York, 1986).*

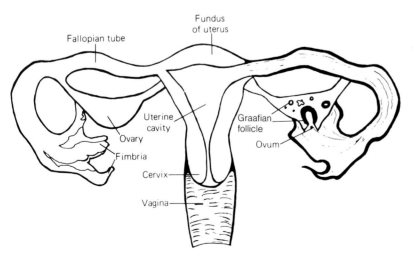

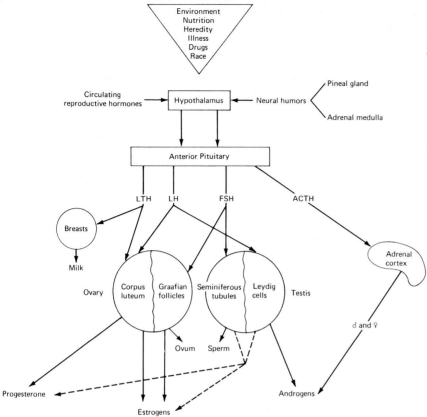

FIGURE 29-3 Hormonal factors influencing the reproductive system. *(From G.M. Scipien et al. [eds.], Comprehensive Pediatric Nursing, 3d ed., McGraw-Hill, New York, 1986.)*

TABLE 29-1 Action of the Gonadal Hormones

Hormone	Source	Action in the Male	Action in the Female
Androgens*	Leydig cells, adrenal cortex	Development of testes, scrotum, penis; voice change; pubic and axillary hair; seborrhea; skeletal and muscular growth; thickening of skin; deposits of melatonin in skin; increase in hemoglobin and red blood cell count; increase in basal metabolic rate	Development of clitoris and labia majora; pubic and axillary hair; seborrhea; skeletal and muscular growth
Estrogens	Graafian follicles, corpus luteum, seminiferous tubules, Leydig cells	Osteogenesis	Development of uterus, tubes, cervix, vagina, external genitalia; breast development (stromal tissue, fat deposits, ducts); distribution of body fat; osteogenesis
Progesterone	Corpus luteum, seminiferous tubules, Leydig cells	Acne	Endometrial secretions; breast development (lobules, alveoli); voice changes; increased body temperature; acne

*Action in female not clearly understood.
†Source and action in male not clearly understood.

Source: G. M. Scipien et al. (eds.), *Comprehensive Pediatric Nursing,* 3d ed., McGraw-Hill, New York, 1986.

velopment of the seminiferous tubules of the testes and for spermatogenesis. LH, sometimes referred to as *interstitial-cell stimulating hormone* (ICSH) in the male, is responsible for the development of the Leydig cells and the subsequent production of androgens and estrogens. LH is also required for the development of the seminal vesicles and the prostate and for their subsequent contribution to semen production and ejaculation.

Male sex hormones are called *androgens* whether they are produced by the testes or the adrenal cortex. *Testosterone* is considered to be the prime androgen because it is secreted in a much greater quantity than are any others that have been identified. Actions of gonadal hormones in males are listed in Table 29-1. The anterior pituitary produces a third gonadotropic hormone, luteotropic hormone (LTH), but at this time its function in the male reproductive system is unknown.

Pubertal Development

As a result of hormonal influences, structures directly involved in reproductive function mature. Secondary sexual characteristics—the physical signs distinguishing adults from children—appear according to a defined pattern (Figs. 29-4 and 29-5). The growth spurt precedes sperm emission by an average of 2 years.

While the external genitalia are changing, the interaction of FSH and LH results in tubular formation and enlargement of the testes, followed by the appearance of spermatogonia and, later, various stages of spermatogenesis. The prostate, seminal vesicles, and bulbourethral (Cowper's) glands enlarge and develop to form seminal fluid. Ejaculation, generally considered the first sign of adulthood by adolescent males, usually occurs spontaneously or by masturbation at the aproximate age of 14 years. Ejaculation generally precedes fertility by 1 to 2 years. The last secondary sexual characteristic to occur in the male is identation of the hairline.

Spermatogenesis

Spermatogonia (germ cells) are present at birth but are inactive. *Spermatogenesis,* or the production of spermatozoa from spermatogonia, actually begins at puberty. After puberty, under the influence of FSH, the germ cells, through rapid mitotic division, continue to proliferate through old age with little reduction in activity. Spermatogenesis may be divided into three stages: mitosis and mei-

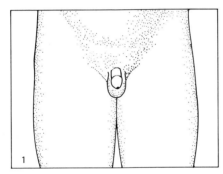
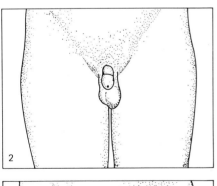
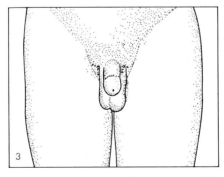
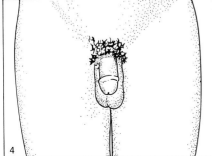
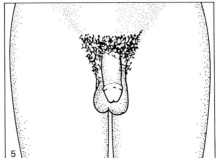

FIGURE 29-4 Stages of male genital development. Stage 1: childhood size. Stage 2: enlargement of scrotum and testes with reddening of scrotal skin. Stage 3: further enlargement of scrotum and testes and lengthening of penis. Stage 4: further enlargement of testes and scrotum and lengthening and broadening of penis. Stage 5: genitalia of adult size and shape. *(From J.M. Tanner, Growth at Adolescence, 2d ed., Blackwell, Oxford, 1962.)*

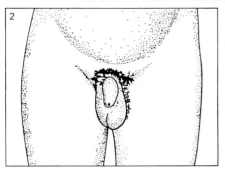
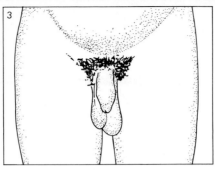
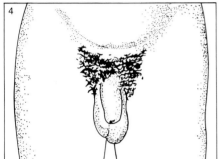
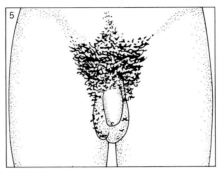

FIGURE 29-5   Stages of pubic hair development in males. Stage 1: none. Stage 2: sparse growth at base of penis of long, slightly pigmented downy hair which may be straight or somewhat curly. Stage 3: darker, coarser, curlier hair that is spread sparsely over junction of pubes. Stage 4: hair that is adult in type but over a smaller area. Stage 5: hair that is adult in type and quality. *(From J.M. Tanner, Growth at Adolescence, 2d ed., Blackwell, Oxford, 1962.)*

FIGURE 29-6   Stages of spermatogenesis. *(From G.M. Scipien et al. [eds.], Comprehensive Pediatric Nursing, 3d., McGraw-Hill, New York, 1986.)*

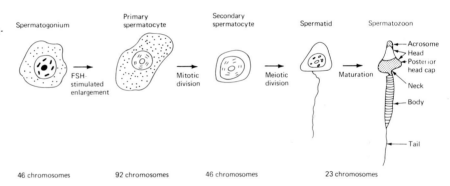

osis of the spermatocytes; maturation and storage of the spermatozoa; and emission, ejaculation, or degeneration of spermatozoa.

Spermatogonia increase in size to become *primary spermatocytes,* which reproduce their 46 chromosomes autocatalytically to 92 chromosomes; then, stimulated by FSH, they undergo mitotic division into *secondary spermatocytes* containing 46 chromosomes each (Fig. 29-6). Secondary spermatocytes divide through meiosis into *spermatids* containing 23 chromosomes each. In this fashion, each spermatogonium generates four spermatids.

After the meiotic phase, each new spermatid still has a simple epithelioid cell structure which matures into a highly differentiated spermatozoon by attaching to the *Sertoli* cells (sustentacular cells of the germinal epithelium). From the Sertoli cells, the new spermatids derive hormones or enzymes and nutrient material necessary to develop the head, neck, body, and tail of mature spermatozoa.

Once the spermatozoa develop from spermatids in the seminiferous tubules, they pass into the epididymis. At this point they are nonmotile and incapable of fertilization; yet within 18 hours they become mobile and capable of penetrating the ovum. A small number of spermatozoa are thought to remain in the epididymis, but most are stored in the vas deferens and its ampulla where they retain their fertility for as long as 42 days, though storage usually is not longer than a few days and sometimes a few hours.

During puberty and for some time thereafter, young males are prone to nocturnal emissions, which are thought to be the result of a buildup in the secretion of spermatozoa, seminal secretions, and prostate secretions which are released during sleep, possibly in connection with the normal erotic dreams of the adolescent male. In some normal adolescent males, masturbation is frequent enough to eliminate the need for nocturnal emissions.

Ejaculation is a complex process that results from reflex mechanisms integrated in the sacral and lumbar regions of the spinal cord and is initiated by either psychic or actual sexual stimulation. The first stage is erection, effected by parasympathetic impulses which dilate the arteries of the penis and constrict the veins. Arterial blood then enters the sinusoids of the erectile tissue under high pressure, causing the penis to become rigid and elongated. Penetration into the vagina is then possible. Intense stimulation of the glans penis, along with psychic stimuli, causes the release of sympathetic impulses from the spinal cord at the level of the 1st or 2d lumbar vertebra through the hypogastric plexus to the genitals. Peristaltic contractions are initiated in the testes, the epididymis, and vas deferens, causing the ejaculation of spermatozoa into the internal urethra. Rhythmic contractions of the prostate and seminal vesicles discharge fluid which, when mixed with spermatozoa, becomes semen. The process of ejaculation as described thus far is properly called *emission*. The pudendal nerve impulses sent from the cord to the skeletal nerves at the base of the penis cause rhythmic pressure increases and the eventual expulsion of semen out the urethra. This latter process is more appropriately termed *ejaculation*.

Once spermatozoa have been ejaculated into the vagina, their life span is 24 to 74 hours. With the assistance of myometrial contractions, they must ascend the uterus and enter the fallopian tubes in order to penetrate the ovum, which has traveled to the outer ampulla of the tube. Although over 100 million spermatozoa are deposited in the vagina, approximately 1 million manage to enter the cervix, and of these only a few thousand are able to navigate the uterotubal junction, so that 100 or fewer spermatozoa actually reach the tubal ampulla and the ovum. Only one spermatozoon is required to fertilize the ovum.

Spermatogenesis can be affected by a number of physical factors. Spermatogenesis will not take place in the absence of FSH. Orchitis secondary to mumps or gonorrhea may cause scarring of the seminiferous tubules and subsequent sterility if the infections are severe. Another factor is temperature. Optimum temperature for production and storage of spermatozoa is lower than the normal temperature of the abdominal cavity. Scrotal temperature averages 2.2°C lower than the abdominal cavity temperature, but it may range from 1.5 to 2.5°C lower. Substantially higher temperatures retard spermatogenesis temporarily and sometimes permanently. The body attempts to compensate for changes in temperature by relaxation and dangling of the scrotum away from the body in hot weather and retraction against the body in cold weather.

Hormonal Functions of the Female Reproductive System

The development and functioning of the female reproductive system are controlled by a complex, interacting system of hormones derived mainly from the hypothalamus, the anterior pituitary, and the gonads (Fig. 29-2). The same hypothalamic hormones in the female stimulate the anterior pituitary to produce three gonadotropic hormones: FSH, LH, and LTH. FSH stimulates the growth of the ovary itself and, more specifically, the growth of the primordial follicle. LH acts synergistically with FSH to cause rapid growth of the follicle with ovulation. LTH affects the development of the corpus luteum after ovulation. LTH also has a second effect, that of stimulating breasts to produce milk, and is often called *lactogen* or *lactogenic hormone*.

Stimulated by the gonadotropic hormones, the ovary produces two types of hormones: *estrogen* and *progesterone*. Their actions are listed in Table 29-1. Progesterone

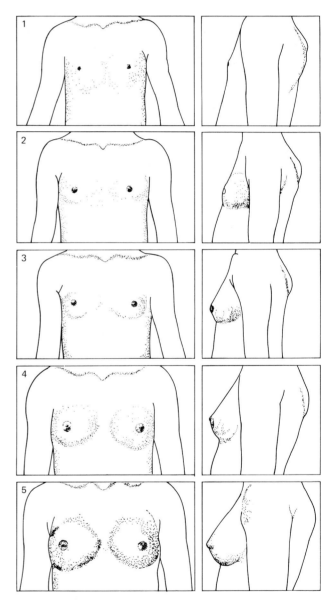

FIGURE 29-7   Stages of breast development in adolescent girls. Stage 1: elevation of papilla (preadolescent). Stage 2: breast buds with enlargement of areola. Stage 3: further enlargement of breasts and areola but without separation of contour. Stage 4: formation of secondary mound with projection of areola and papilla. Stage 5: recession of areola to general breast contour: resemble adult breasts. *(From J.M. Tanner, Growth at Adolescence, 2d ed., Blackwell, Oxford, 1962).*

also causes secretory changes in the breast, affecting the lobules and alveoli to make them capable of secreting milk. (Progesterone does not cause lactation, which is a function of LTH, but only develops the capacity for lactation.)

The interaction of the pituitary hormones and the ovarian hormones is affected by a feedback mechanism. Increasing levels of FSH stimulate the ovary to produce estrogen and the primordial follicles to develop into mature graafian follicles. LH enhances this development and promotes ovulation. After ovulation, the corpus luteum secretes large amounts of estrogen and progesterone. These circulating hormones exert a negative feedback effect on the anterior pituitary, causing a decrease in FSH and LH production. As the corpus luteum degenerates, decreasing levels of estrogen and progesterone are accompanied by increased secretion of FSH and LH. The third gonadotropic hormone, LTH, is not affected in this manner, but it acts in a reciprocal manner with FSH and LH: When the anterior pituitary secretes increased amounts of FSH and LH, secretion of LTH is decreased and vice versa.

Pubertal Development

Pubertal development in the female also follows a defined pattern, and physical changes can be anticipated at various stages (Figs. 29-7 and 29-8). The growth spurt precedes menarche by an average of 2 years. Hips increase in width and roundness, and the arms and legs become more shapely. The skin becomes thicker and coarser, and pores enlarge. Facial hair appears on the upper lips and cheeks. However, the first sign of significance to the adolescent female is the development of breasts. Axillary hair appears after pubic hair is present.

Approximately 2 years after the breast bud is present, menarche occurs. While the average age of menarche is 12.9 years, the range of normal is anywhere from 10 to 16.5 years. The first menstrual periods are erratic and anovulatory. As menstruation becomes cyclic in relation to gonadotropin and gonadal steroid production, ovulation occurs. Reproductive capacity is not present until menstruation is cyclic and ovulation has occurred.

The Menstrual Cycle

In the maturing female, a rhythmic cycle develops which results in the maturation and release of a single ovum from the ovary and in the preparation of the endometrial lining for the implantation of a fertilized ovum. The cycle repeats itself on an average of every 28 days (except during pregnancy), although it may vary from 20 to 45 days as a normal cycle.

The primordial follicle, begins to grow slowly under the stimulation of FSH. Initially, this growth involves the ovum itself and then growth of theca cells around the granulosa cells. The additional secretion of LH causes a more rapid growth of the follicle with a corresponding increase in the production of estrogen. With each cycle, as many as 20 primordial follicles may begin to mature; generally, one follicle supersedes the others and ovulates, while the others degenerate. In this mature graafian follicle, the ovum with surrounding cells has moved to one pole of the follicle and, on about the fourteenth day of the cycle, is expelled by the follicle, to be drawn in by the fimbriated ends of the fallopian tube.

In the next few hours, the cells of the follicle enlarge and acquire a distinctly yellow color, the whole becoming a corpus luteum. The corpus luteum is sustained by increased production of LTH from the anterior pituitary. It produces large amounts of estrogen and progesterone. About the eighth day after ovulation the corpus luteum begins to involute, and by about the twelfth day after ovu-

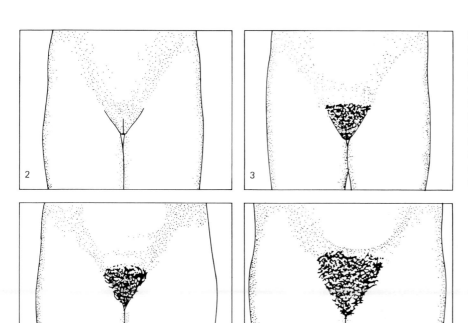

FIGURE 29-8 Stages of pubic hair development in females. Stage 1: none. Stage 2: sparse growth along labia of long slightly pigmented downy hair which may be straight or somewhat curled. Stage 3: darker, coarser, curlier hair that is spread sparsely over junction of pubes. Stage 4: hair that is adult in type but over a smaller area. Stage 5: hair that is adult in type and quantity. *(From J.M. Tanner, Growth at Adolescence, 2d ed., Blackwell, Oxford, 1962.)*

lation it has ceased functioning. Involution is associated with decreasing levels of LTH and decreasing production of estrogen and progesterone. With the decrease in the production of gonadal hormones comes an increase in the secretion of FSH to stimulate the primordial follicles and repeat the cycle.

At the beginning of the cycle, the uterine endometrium desquamates and becomes very thin. Estrogens produced by the developing follicle stimulate the endometrium to increase in number of cells. This *proliferative phase* continues until ovulation and the development of the corpus luteum. The endometrium enters the *secretory phase* and is affected by both estrogens and progesterone. Estrogens continue to affect cell proliferation. Under the influence of progesterone, epithelial glandular cells develop and secrete small amounts of epithelial fluid. With the involution of the corpus luteum and the rapid decrease of estrogens and progesterone, the epithelium again desquamates and menstruation occurs.

If the ovum released from the follicle is fertilized, the pattern of the cycle is interrupted. The early fertilized ovum develops trophoblastic cells which produce a hormone, chorionic gonadotropin. This hormone prevents the involution of the corpus luteum, which then continues to produce estrogens and progesterone. Gonadal hormones sustain the development of the endometrium, which is necessary for the development of the placenta and other fetal tissues, and neither menstruation nor follicular activity occurs.

Assessment

The assessment of the reproductive system can be a sensitive procedure for both the parent and the child. Initially, the examiner should establish an objective, nonthreatening atmosphere through appropriate phrasing of questions and discussion of concerns. In evaluating the younger child, most of the history is obtained from parents. However, the child should be included in the discussion according to his ability to communicate in order to identify level of understanding, evaluate parent-child interaction, and establish a rapport with the child before the physical examination. The examiner at this time can discuss specific concerns of the parent and child and provide relevant health teaching. During the physical examination, the parent can assist in reassuring the child; portions of the examination can be done with the parent holding the child if necessary.

Ideally, the adolescent is not accompanied by the parent during the history and physical examination, although the examiner interviews the parent when possible. The adolescent should be treated throughout the evaluation as an intelligent person with valid opinions. History-taking offers a valuable opportunity for discussing the normal concerns of adolescents regarding physiological changes which may be distressing. Such concerns can be alleviated by careful listening and discussion of what is normal for this developmental period. Many adolescents wonder if they are maturing at a rate similar to that of others and are self-conscious about their bodies and feelings. Confidentiality is maintained, and the adolescent is reassured that the provider will not discuss shared information with parents or others without permission.

History

Pertinent data related to the evaluation of the reproductive system include not only past and present changes or illnesses but also family, prenatal, and birth history; sexual development; sexual activity; and social history. History of changes or illnesses elicited on interview may include specific problems such as hypospadias, vulvovaginitis, and venereal disease. Also of concern are specific symptoms, including breast enlargement, masses, or discharge; genital enlargement, discoloration, lesions, itching, burning, or discharge; vaginal bleeding; and associated symptoms. Of particular importance in the family and prenatal history are medications, especially hormones, administered to the mother during pregnancy or family history of sterility, amenorrhea, inguinal hernia containing a gonad, and other reproductive disorders. These data indicate the need for further evaluation for possible intersex abnormalities in a newborn and follow-up evaluation for possible reproductive disorders in an older child. For example, footling or breech presentation at delivery may account for enlargement and discoloration of the genitalia in the newborn.

Evaluation of the child's sexual development addresses his sex-role identity, his level of knowledge and understanding of sexuality and sexual functioning, and sex education received. Of similar importance is the parents' attitude and response to the child's sexuality and the degree of assurance they feel in responding to his questions and to specific activities such as masturbation. Also included are age of onset of the various secondary sex characteristics: breast development, areola pigmentation, and appearance of pubic, axillary, and facial hair.

For the adolescent female, the reproductive history includes the age at onset of menses, the frequency and regularity of periods, the amount of menstrual flow, incidence of dysmenorrhea, and the date of the last normal menstrual period. Information is obtained regarding breast sensitivity, trauma, or change or asymmetry in size. Specific concerns regarding the breasts are elicited. The degree of sexual activity is determined. If the adolescent is sexually active, knowledge of contraception is assessed. The number of pregnancies (if any), pregnancy history, and history of miscarriage or therapeutic abortion are also included in the history. The presence of gynecologic complaints, including periods of amenorrhea, dysmenorrhea, and vaginal discharge or bleeding, is ascertained. Related pelvic pain is noted.

In adolescent males, the reproductive history includes information regarding the penis and testicles, the presence or absence of gynecomastia, and whether the teenager has been circumcised. Sexual activity and contraceptive use are determined. Concerns regarding normal developmental occurrences (e.g., nocturnal emissions or spontaneous erections) are discussed. Both males and females should be questioned about history of and exposure to venereal diseases.

Finally, eliciting an adequate social history can provide clues to possible sexual abuse. Sexual abuse is most likely to occur in a disordered family where unstable or disturbed marital relationships prevail. The child frequently responds with "problem" behaviors: anxiety of sudden onset (which may be expressed as insomnia, irritability, depression, sudden extreme weight loss or gain, or suicide attempts); unusual fears (especially of a particular person, usually noted by parents), night terrors, or clinging behavior; sudden, severe aggressive behavior and control problems, such as running away from home or serious rebellion, particularly against the mother; sexually precocious vocabulary and behavior, public or excessive masturbation, seductive behavior with adults and children of the opposite sex, sexual promiscuity in adolescents; school problems such as declining grades, truancy, poor peer relations, or social withdrawal; and sudden developmental regression, such as changed toilet habits or difficulty with eating or sleeping (Chap. 13).

Physical Examination

Physical examination of the reproductive system includes inspection and palpation of the breasts, abdominal examination, inspection and palpation of the external genitalia, and pelvic examination of females if indicated. Breasts are inspected for enlargement, symmetry, discharge, or discoloration and are palpated for masses or tenderness. Breasts in the newborn may be enlarged and may discharge milk because of placental transfer of maternal hormones. This engorgement disappears a few days after birth. The areola should be full, with a breast bud between 5 and 10 mm in size. The size can be determined by lightly grasping the bud between thumb and forefinger, lifting up slightly, and measuring the distance between thumb and forefinger. The intermammary index (distance between outside edges of right and left areolae) should be less than or equal to one-fourth of the newborn's chest circumference. A longer intermammary index may be indicative of Turner's syndrome or chromosomal anomalies. Asymmetry of the breasts in the school-age child or adolescent is not uncommon; one breast normally develops more rapidly than the other. Gynecomastia in the adolescent male should be noted. The stage of breast development in the female is recorded according to Tanner's stages (Fig. 29-7). The breast exam is an appropriate time to explain the need for breast self-examination and the proper procedure (Table 29-2).

In examining the external genitalia of the male, the stage of sexual development according to Tanner's stages is recorded (Figs. 29-4 and 29-5). The penis, scrotum, and testes are evaluated. The penis is inspected, keeping in mind that individual size and proportion may vary greatly. The foreskin is retracted and reduced. Any lesions or masses should be described with respect to both appearance and location. The pubic hair is described. The scro-

TABLE 29-2 Procedure for Self-Examination of Breast

1. Carefully examine your breasts before a mirror; check for symmetry in size and shape; note any puckering or dimpling of the skin; note if the nipple dents in
2. Raise your arms over your head and study the breasts during the motion for the same signs as in step 1
3. Lie down on the bed with a flat pillow or folded towel under your shoulder on the same side as the breast to be examined; this position distributes the tissues over a wider area
4. With the flattened surface of two or three fingers, gently palpate breast tissues, beginning at the upper outer area and proceeding in an orderly pattern around the breast
5. Carefully examine the area over the nipple for masses and/or discharge
6. Repeat procedure for other breast
7. Examine the area under your arm for masses or tenderness
8. If you find a mass or suspicious finding, *call your physician or nurse immediately and make an appointment!* Most breast lesions are not cancerous but do need to be checked

Source: G. M. Scipien et al. (eds.), *Comprehensive Pediatric Nursing*, 3d ed., McGraw-Hill, New York, 1986.

tum is inspected, and the contents palpated. Any unusual tenderness or masses should be recorded, describing size, tenderness, mobility, position, and character. The inguinal canal is palpated for hernia. If hydrocele or other masses are suspected, the scrotum is transilluminated and findings are recorded. The cremasteric reflex is elicited.

At birth, the penis of the male is approximately 3 to 4 cm (1.3 to 1.6 in) in length. A penis less than 2 cm in length raises questions of intersex anomalies, as does the presence of chordee, bifid scrotum, abnormal rugation, gonads above or below the inguinal ring, or hypospadias. A short penis is also associated with chromosomal anomalies 9, 15, 18, and 21. The prepuce (foreskin) in the newborn is adherent, not retractable, and cannot be retracted without trauma until about 3 years of age. Force should never be used. The urinary meatus of the newborn is generally not discernible at the tip of the glans. Therefore, the infant's voiding should be observed to ascertain the position of the meatus and to determine possible occlusion of the meatus by the prepuce. The scrotum of the newborn is symmetric, and the skin is thickened, wrinkled, and pigmented. Scrotal enlargement may be due to delivery trauma (breech or footling presentation) or to the placental transfer of hormones. However, it can also indicate hydrocele, orchitis, hernia, or hematocele. The testes usually can be palpated in the scrotum, and their size and consistency can be determined. However, *undescended testes* are not an uncommon finding on physical examination of the newborn. Although the testes generally migrate to the scrotum during the eighth month of fetal life, descent may not occur until 1 to 2 months after birth. If the testes are not present in the scrotum, they may descend when warm, moist compresses are applied to the infant's scrotum or lower abdomen or when he is put, sitting, into a warm basin of water. If the testes do not descend with warming, gentle pressure exerted on the lower abdomen may push them into the scrotum. Another technique is to grasp the inguinal canal between thumb and forefinger and gently "strip" it toward the scrotum.

To examine a young boy for descent of the testes, it is helpful to have him climb onto the examining table with as little help as possible and to assume a cross-legged "tailor" sitting position. Climbing causes abdominal pressure which forces normally retracted testes into the scrotum, and the tailor sitting position traps them by flattening the inguinal canal. Descent of the testes may also be achieved by having the child take a warm bath or cough and strain and then assume the tailor sitting position. Enlargement and discoloration of the scrotum in a young boy may be a result of trauma or torsion of the testes. Lesions, discharge, or bruising of the penis, scrotum, or perineal area should raise suspicion of abuse. In eliciting the *cremasteric reflex* (rise of the testes in the scrotum or even into the inguinal canal while stroking the inner aspect of the thigh), the examiner may occlude the inguinal canals by placing the fingers of one hand across the upper portion of the inguinal canal and eliciting the reflex with the other hand. Many adolescents have an extremely sensitive cremasteric reflex, where the testis is drawn into the inguinal canal as a result of cold, tough, or any number of stimuli. It should be explained that this reaction is not pathological and that the testis will resume its normal position.

Examination of the external genitalia of the female includes inspection for discharge, enlargement, discoloration, or lesions and palpation, including palpation of the abdomen, for masses. Pubic hair is described according to Tanner's stages (Fig. 29-8).

The clitoris in the normal female infant is only a few

TABLE 29-3 Screening Tests Frequently Used in Adolescent Gynecology

Test	Indication	Significance of Results	Comment
Papanicolaou's test (Pap smear)	Sexually active adolescent Oral contraceptive use After age 21 *Herpesvirus* genitalis	Grade I is negative Grade II indicates atypical cytology but no evidence of malignancy; may indicate dysplasia or chronic cervicitis Grade III is suggestive of but not conclusive for malignancy Grade IV is strongly suggestive of malignancy Grade V is conclusive for malignancy Cytological exam may also reveal *Herpesvirus* or *Trichomonas* organisms	Grade I results require annual repeat smears (semiannual smears in clients with herpes) Grade II results require correction of any preexisting condition (e.g., cervicitis, vaginitis) and a repeat smear in 1 month; if no preexisting conditions, a referral is made to gynecologist for further testing Grades III, IV, or V require referral to gynecologist for further testing
Acid phosphatase for prostatic fraction	Suspected rape or incest Perineal trauma in a pediatric or adolescent patient	Positive result indicates presence of semen in vaginal vault Result is accurate only if intercourse has occurred within 48 hours Penetration and ejaculation must occur for positive result	There should be no prostatic fraction in an adolescent who is not sexually active Findings should be documented and reported in suspected cases of rape or incest
Saline wet mounts of fluid from vaginal vault	Vulvovaginitis Any unusual vaginal discharge	*Trichomonas vaginalis* can be visualized microscopically if trichomoniasis is present	It is treated appropriately Wet mount is repeated after treatment to ensure eradication of organism
Potassium hydroxide wet mounts of fluid from vaginal vault	Vulvovaginitis Any unusual vaginal discharge	*Haemophilus vaginalis* and clue cells visualized indicate *H. vaginalis* vaginitis Candidiasis can be diagnosed if budding yeast and pseudohyphae are visualized	It is treated appropriately Repeat wet mount after treatment to ensure eradication of the organism

Source: G. M. Scipien et al. (eds.), *Comprehensive Pediatric Nursing,* 3d ed., McGraw-Hill, New York, 1986.

millimeters long. The labia minora are usually more prominent than the labia majora but will become smaller in the first few weeks after birth. The labia are symmetric and can be completely separated. Enlarged labia may be a result of placental transfer of hormones or of trauma from delivery. However, asymmetrical or enlarged labia should be palpated for masses (testes) associated with intersex anomalies. The urinary meatus is usually not visible, but the vaginal orifice is easily seen and normally appears reddened. *Pseudomenstruation,* a vaginal discharge of small amounts of bloody material, resulting from placental transfer of maternal, hormones which affect the endometrium of the infant's uterus, is transient and requires no treatment. In the young child, the labia minora are very small and flat, and the labia majora are puffy but proportionate to the perineum. The unestrogenized vaginal opening is more red than the rest of the genitalia. In later childhood, the labia minora fill out and the labia majora become more thickened; with puberty, these changes advance to adult status. Bruising of the genitalia may be the result of accidental trauma or may be associated with sexual abuse. *Physiological leukorrhea* may be present in the adolescent. An increase in circulating estrogen causes the cervix to secrete mucus and desquamated cells of the vaginal epithelium. If the secretions are heavy, a wet mount smear shows epithelial cells with no pus cells, blood cells, or bacteria. This normal physiological state does not indicate infection.

A complete pelvic examination is indicated in the presence of bleeding or other signs of a potentially serious condition and in any adolescent who complains of vaginal discharge, dysuria, pyuria, lower abdominal pain, irregular vaginal bleeding, or amenorrhea. Some of the screening tests frequently used in conjunction with the pelvic exam are listed in Table 29-3. In the absence of complaints, the pelvic examination should be conducted annually in any of the following circumstances: sexual activity, suspicion of sexual abuse, and suspected contact with or exposure to venereal disease. The pelvic examination is never done to satisfy the curiosity of a parent regarding the condition of the hymen.

The pelvic examination consists of four steps: (1) inspection and palpation of vulvar structures, (2) examination of extrapelvic sex areas, (3) bimanual pelvic and rectal examination, and (4) visualization of the cervix and vagina. In younger girls, examination under anesthesia may be required. However, rectal examination and visualization of the vagina frequently can be performed without anesthesia. The first pelvic examination often occurs in adolescence and can be a source of distress and fear for the girl. She may have heard distorted stories of what is to come. Since the first pelvic examination can set the stage for how conscientiously the female pursues her own health care, an approach that is not threatening is optimal. The adolescent should be prepared physically and psychologically for the examination. She should be well draped (Fig. 29-9), but it often helps to pull the drape down between her legs and raise the head of the table about 30 degrees so that she can see the examiner during the procedure. The girl should be allowed to inspect and touch any instruments which will be used. Illustrations of the pelvic organs help in describing the procedure. Explaining what is to be done and allowing time for questions before proceeding are helpful. It is often reassuring to have a mirror available so that the girl can observe what the examiner is doing. This maneuver also affords the practitio-

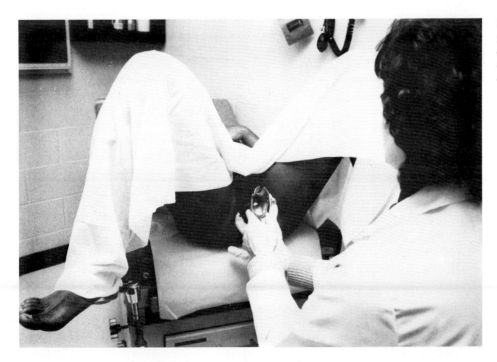

FIGURE 29-9 Proper draping for pelvic examination, *(From G.M. Scipien et al., [eds.], Comprehensive Pediatric Nursing, 3d ed, McGraw-Hill, New York, 1986.)*

ner an opportunity to explain the physiology and anatomy of the external and internal genitalia, the purpose of the pelvic examination, and the importance of regular Papanicolaou tests (Pap smears).

In the evaluation of the reproductive system, specific findings should alert the examiner to the possibility of sexual abuse. These findings include traces of blood on genitalia or underwear of preadolescents or younger children; venereal disease in preadolescent or younger children; chronic vaginitis, especially trichomoniasis; any injury, tear, bruising, or swelling near or on the genitalia, vaginal opening, or anus; recurrent urinary tract infections; semen in the vagina, anus, or mouth; and pain on urination and penile swelling or discharge in young boys (Chap. 13).

General Nursing Measures

Nursing Diagnoses

Serious disease involving the reproductive tract is relatively uncommon during childhood, primarily because of the anatomic and physiological immaturity of this system. Nursing care is therefore focused primarily on maintaining the cleanliness and integrity of the reproductive system, on health teaching related to the more frequently occurring minor illnesses, and on sex education. Sex education is discussed in Chapter 4.

Some examples of nursing diagnoses are:

Knowledge deficit related to hygiene of the reproductive system

Knowledge deficit related to menstruation

Knowledge deficit related to nocturnal emissions

Knowledge deficit related to minor illnesses related to the reproductive system and their treatment

Knowledge deficit related to response of the child to hospitalization for treatment of disorders related to the reproductive system and according to different developmental levels

The parents of the normal newborn are taught adequate hygienic measures for the infant, including thorough washing of the area after each urinary voiding or stool passage and separation of the labia in girls or gentle retraction of the circumcised prepuce in boys for cleansing. In conjunction with and following toilet training, the child is taught appropriate hygienic measures. Adolescent girls may have extremely limited knowledge about menstruation and need information about the physiology of the menstrual cycle as well as practical suggestions regarding hygiene, activity, and relief of attendant discomforts (see the section on dysmenorrhea). Nocturnal emissions may be both puzzling and embarrassing, and adolescent boys need to understand why they occur and to be reassured that they are normal.

When minor illnesses related to the reproductive system occur, it is important that both the condition and the treatment are explained adequately to parents and their child, according to level of understanding. Parents should be encouraged to approach the treatment in a casual man-

ner and to avoid unnecessarily frequent examination of the genitalia. Should the illness require hospitalization, the response of the child will be related to his age.

Developmental Considerations

Separation from his parents is interpreted by the child under 4 years of age as desertion or punishment and results in fears of attack and feelings of helplessness. However, the psychological meaning of illnesses and treatments seems to have greater potential effects on the 4- to 8-year-old than does separation from the parents. Anxiety, regression, and depression may result from fears of body mutilation (castration) and misinterpretation of painful treatments or surgery as punishment for real or imaginary transgressions. Nursing care must include reassuring the child that he is not being punished, explaining everything at his level of understanding, and if possible arranging for the parents to stay with him in the hospital.

Play may be useful therapy in preparing the child for surgery and helping him work through feelings about what is done to him. Preoperative teaching of the parents is more effective if all parents whose children are having surgery get together and learn as a group what to expect before and after surgery. It has been found that parents taught in groups ask more questions, have better rapport with the nurses, are more supportive of each other while the children are in surgery, are less anxious, and are more helful in keeping the child on his postoperative regimen.

Separation anxiety related to parents may not be a problem for a child in this age group, but some anxiety in relation to separation from peers is engendered when the child is hospitalized. Oedipal anxieties are usually dormant, and genital surgery is not usually as traumatic for him as it is for the preschooler or the adolescent. Castration fears are likely to be present, however, and careful explanation and repeated reassurances are important, even for the child who does not ask for them.

Postoperatively, the school-age child is not usually as active as the preschooler or as accepting of necessary procedures. He may react more aggressively and needs as much independence as possible. The school-age child is concerned about his body image. He fears genital inadequacy, loss of body control or mastery, and muscular weakness. Verbal reassurance is beneficial, but play which allows him to release pent-up energy and anxiety is more effective. It is important to the hospitalized child to be assigned to a room with others of the same age and sex.

Illness or surgery which involves the reproductive system can cause particular anxiety in the adolescent. He is very much aware of his developing sexuality, and anything which seems to impinge upon this awareness can be threatening to his self-image. It is important for the nurse to respect the characteristic shyness and need for privacy of this age group. Every procedure performed should be explained in detail to the patient, drapes should be used during examinations, and the nurse should remain in the room when the doctor performs a physical examination on an adolescent female. Findings should also be discussed, as the adolescent is prone to wild imaginings. Again, the nurse should not assume that the adolescent understands because he asks no questions.

The nurse must also be prepared to assist the adolescent with concerns about his developing sexuality. In order to do so, the nurse must first examine her own attitudes, feelings, and values. If she is uncomfortable with her own sexuality or with discussion of sexual questions, she will not be able to communicate effectively with the adolescent. The nurse must develop skill in teaching and counseling and possess accurate information about sexual development.

The nurse's objective is to help the adolescent identify values and make decisions. Therefore, the approach must be open, honest and nonjudgmental. With this approach, a nurse can create an atmosphere in which the adolescent feels comfortable in discussing concerns and feelings. The nurse must ensure confidentiality, especially in individual discussions. The adolescent needs to understand that these discussions will not be shared with parents or others but at the same time should know that, if the nurse believes that the adolescent is injuring himself or others, this information must be relayed to the appropriate people.

The nurse can assist parents in their relationships with their adolescents. Many parents are bewildered by adolescent behavior and unable to communicate with the adolescent. The nurse can help the parents understand the developmental problems which adolescents face and acquire the means to assist them in resolving these problems. Many parents are also uncomfortable in discussing sexual questions with their children regardless of age. The nurse can help the parents understand their children's sexual development and concerns at different ages and explore their own feelings about sex.

It is also the responsibility of the nurse to understand the legal aspects of the care of the adolescent. Laws were originally designed primarily for the *protection* of the minor; more recently, they are also taking into account the *rights* of the minor. However, laws vary from state to state. Most states permit physicians to diagnose and treat venereal disease without parental consent, and in all stages venereal disease must be reported to public health officials. Legislation in some states clearly and explicitly allows minors to consent to contraceptive services and in others does not specifically include or exclude minors. However, contraceptive services are in fact being provided in all states to minors without parental consent, and no judgment has yet been found against any health facility or physician for providing this service. Similarly, legislation relating to adolescents' seeking care for pregnancy or abortion differs greatly. All states have some form of legislation against incest and rape, but the age at which a girl may legally consent to sexual intercourse varies. The nurse should be familiar with the laws which affect her practice and will generally can acquire information through the state or local health department (Chap. 8).

Of more frequent concern to parents and child than illness related to the reproductive system are factors related to sexual development. A primary focus of the nurse's intervention is counseling and education related to sexuality. Adolescents who are sexually active or are pregnant should be referred to nurse clinicians, clinical nurse specialists, physicians, and counselors who have had special training in working with these teenagers and their families.

Diseases or Deviations in the Newborn and Infant

Phimosis

A tightening of the prepuce over the penis so that the foreskin cannot be retracted is termed *phimosis*. It is the normal condition in the newborn and, unless the urinary meatus is occluded, requires no treatment. The uncircumcised foreskin is not retractable for several years after birth. If the meatus is occluded or if phimosis occurs later in life, *circumcision,* surgical removal of the prepuce, is indicated. In the Jewish faith, ritual circumcision is performed on all male infants on the eighth day of life.

The routine circumcision of all newborn male infants is a much-debated procedure. Proponents believe that it is beneficial in providing for greater cleanliness as a prevention against future development of phimosis. They also note the decreased incidence of cervical carcinoma among women whose husbands have been circumcised. Opponents believe that after circumcision the penis is more prone to ulceration, which may lead to meatal stenosis. They also question the validity of the statistical evidence related to cervical carcinoma. Infants with congenital anomalies of the penis such as hypospadias or epispadias should not be circumcised routinely, because the prepuce skin may be needed for surgical repair at a later date.

Since circumcision is a surgical procedure, it requires the consent of parents. They should be given sufficient information to make an informed decision. Circumcisions are most commonly done with the Gomco clamp or a plastic circumcision device (Figs. 29-10 and 29-11). If the Gomco clamp is used, there may be some bleeding where the unnecessary prepuce or foreskin was excised. The penis is wrapped with petrolatum gauze or covered with petrolatum jelly to keep the diaper from adhering to the denuded glans and to promote blood coagulation and healing. The infant should be positioned and diapered in such a way that bleeding can be readily detected. Excessive bleeding should be called to the attention of the physician.

Nursing Management

The infant should be observed closely for adequacy of voiding, quality of the urinary stream, and presence of blood in the urine. The mother is taught to wash the entire glans penis carefully with soap and a moistened cotton ball each time the infant soils his diaper. She should not retract the prepuce. Cleansing motions are gentle and

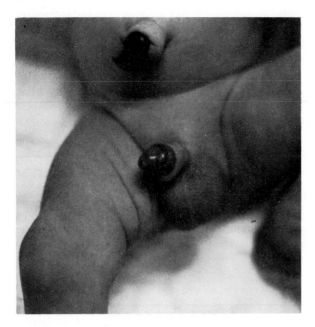

FIGURE 29-10   Penis of infant after circumcision with Gomco clamp. *(From G.M. Scipien et al. [eds.], Comprehensive Pediatric Nursing, 3d ed., McGraw-Hill New York, 1986.)*

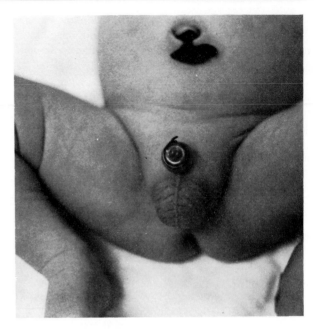

FIGURE 29-11   Penis of infant after circumcision with plastic circumcision device. *(From G.M. Scipien et al. [eds.], Comprehensive Pediatric Nursing, 3d ed., McGraw-Hill, New York, 1986.)*

not vigorous—no rubbing. The glans are then rinsed with water and patted dry gently with a soft material. The infant is not given a tub bath or in any way immersed in water until the prepuce is completely healed; healing usually occurs in 3 to 4 days. The mother is shown how to apply liberal amounts of petrolatum jelly to the glans. If petrolatum gauze is to be used, the mother is shown how to wrap the gauze gently without making it too tight. Keeping the denuded glans drenched in petrolatum jelly keeps the diaper from adhering to it and helps prevent contamination from fecal material. The mother is advised to call her physician if she notices excessive bleeding or swelling, pus, foul odor, or other signs of infection of the glans. Since mother and neonate may go home 24 to 48 hours after birth, the nurse should ensure that the parents understand postcircumcision care prior to discharge.

The plastic circumcision device is a small bell-shaped rim which is placed over the glans penis between the prepuce and the glans. A string is tied tightly around the prepuce at the coronal edge of the glans. The prepuce distal to the string becomes ischemic, atrophies, and falls off with the plastic bell attached, leaving a clean, well-healed line of excision.

The mother is informed that the plastic rim will usually drop off by itself within 5 to 8 days. The infant is treated as if he had not been circumcised. There are no special bathing, dressing, or diapering instructions. The mother is informed that a dark brown or black ring encircling the plastic rim is to be expected. This ring disappears when the plastic rim drops off. The mother is taught to observe for swelling. She should notify her physician immediately if swelling occurs. The physician should be called if the plastic rim does not fall off within 8 days, if the rim slips onto the shaft of the penis, or if healing fails to proceed as described.

If the infant is not circumcised, the mother is instructed in cleanliness of the area. The prepuce most not be forcibly retracted. Prolonged retraction of the prepuce can cause interruption of the blood supply to the glans.

Hydrocele

A *hydrocele* is a fluctuant mass of fluid within the processus vaginalis and is often associated with inguinal hernia. It may be communicating or noncommunicating and is sometimes difficult to differentiate from a hernia. It is a flexible but tense translucent mass below the spermatic cord.

A *noncommunicating hydrocele* occurs when peritoneal fluid is trapped in the testicular tunica vaginalis during closure of the processus vaginalis. No treatment is necessary because the fluid is usually reabsorbed slowly during the child's first year of life. A *communicating hydrocele* occurs when the processus vaginalis remains open, allowing peritoneal fluid into the spermatic cord or into the canal of Nuck in females. It may enlarge as the day progresses and the activity of the child forces peritoneal fluid into the cord or canal. Supine relaxation at night allows the fluid to flow back into the peritoneal cavity, making the hydrocele smaller in the morning. The hydrocele may be present at birth or may appear later. Since it is evidence of a patent processus vaginalis and an invitation for an inguinal hernia, surgery is the treatment of choice. The procedure involves opening the inguinal canal and removing the hernial sac. The nursing care for an infant or child with hydrocele and its repair is the same as that for an inguinal hernia (Chap. 26).

Disease or Deviations in the Toddler and Preschooler

Cryptorchidism

Failure of one testis or both testes to descend into the scrotum is termed *cryptorchidism*. It occurs unilaterally four times as often as it does bilaterally. The testis may be *internal* (within the inguinal tract or the abdomen) or *ectopic* (located superficially in the inguinal pouch, in the femoral area, or in the perineum at the base of the penis).

Undescended testes are present in 3 percent of the full-term male newborn population and in 20 percent of the preterm male population. By the age of 1 month, 50 percent have descended spontaneously, and by 1 year, 80 percent descend into the scrotum. Some testes that fail to descend in early childhood will do so spontaneously during puberty.

The cause of cryptorchidism is poorly understood. It is known that both the testes and the ovaries develop from the same point on the genital ridge, that the stimulus which causes the testes to move from the abdomen into the scrotum is the testosterone secreted by the male fetus, and that descent into the scrotum usually begins during the eighth fetal month. The known causes of nondescent are (1) mechanical interference with the passage of the testes into the scrotum, (2) a deficiency of gonadotropin, and (3) defective testes. The mechanical interference may be associated with undeveloped genital ducts or internal duct anomalies such as vaginal pouch remnants, fibrous bands, adhesions, or a short spermatic cord. When gonadotropins are deficient, there is not enough production of testosterone to stimulate or complete the descent.

Treatment of simple cryptorchidism is controversial and ranges from surgical intervention prior to the age of 6 years to no treatment at all. Conservative treatment is usually preferred to surgery, since the majority of testes descend spontaneously by puberty. The frequently recommended treatment is a short course of chorionic gonadotropin given intramuscularly. When the testes have not descended by the age of 8 and sometimes 10 years, chorionic gonadotropin is given for 6 to 8 weeks. If signs of testicular descent appear during the initial course, a repeat course may be given after 10 weeks. If there is no indication of improvement during the initial course of treatment, surgery is indicated.

Orchiopexy is the surgical procedure to correct cryptorchidism and consists of dissecting the testis and spermatic cord from the surrounding tissue and transplanting the testis through the inguinal canal. The testis is then secured in place with a suture to a rubber band attached to the thigh with adhesive tape. The rubber band serves to maintain the position of the testis in the scrotum, but it is not meant to apply pressure. There is as much risk of injury to the testes from surgical intervention as there is from no treatment, but some physicians believe that surgery should be performed before the age of 6 years because that is the age at which the testicular tubules begin to develop. Other physicians, however, believe that the damage to the tubules from the body temperature to which they are exposed is slight before the age of 8 or 10 years and prefer postponing surgery until then.

Abdominal testes are often defective and are associated with other genital abnormalities such as inguinal hernia and hypogonadism. Malignancy is common in testes that remain in the abdomen after puberty. Therefore, surgical removal of abdominal testes is indicated when biopsy reveals defective testes. However, undergoing orchiopexy does not protect the gonad from subsequent malignant changes. Sterility always exists when the testes remain in the abdomen, whether because of the associated abnormalities or because of the exposure of the testes to normal body temperature (2.2°C higher than the normal scrotal temperature) for an extended period of time. Higher temperatures retard spermatogenesis and may damage tubules to the extent that sterility is permanent.

Nursing Management

Case finding occurs with the older child during an examination or when anxious parents (or the child himself) approach the nurse. It is wise to reassure the child and his parents that testes present in the scrotum at birth or testes that descend at some point thereafter often ascend and may even reside out of the scrotum at intervals during childhood. A warm bath followed by coughing or straining will frequently achieve descent. In addition to the referral, the nurse must deal with the parents' anxieties, which usually center on concerns about sterility, homosexuality, or cancer. The parents may not feel comfortable verbalizing their concerns; they may even feel that the child is defective and inadequate and may not tell the child about his condition and pending treatment. In most cases, contrary to his parents' belief that he is ignorant of the problem, the child is aware that his scrotum is not normal, but he has a feeling that the problem should not be discussed. Sometimes he will deny its existence.

As soon as a child is admitted for orchiopexy, the nurse should assess what he knows about his condition and pending treatment and what his anxieties are. The attention that has been focused on his scrotum will heighten his concerns about genital mutilation. He is reassured that his penis will not be involved in the surgery, but only his scrotum. (The nurse should be sure that the child understands the terminology or should use the terminology with which he is familiar.) He is told to expect the rubber bands and informed that they will be removed within 5 to 7 days. He can expect some swelling of his scrotum after surgery and perhaps ice packs around the scrotum for several hours after surgery. His activity should be normal after anesthesia, and he should not have much pain. His fluid preferences are ascertained so that his favorite fluids can be offered after surgery to restore fluid balance. If the child is of school age, plans are made that will allow him an opportunity to see or converse by phone with his friends, as separation anxiety may be more closely related with peers at this age.

Postoperatively, attention is given to prevention of infection by keeping the suture line clean and free of fecal

NURSING CARE PLAN

29-1 *The Child with Cryptorchidism*

Clinical Problem/Nursing Diagnosis	Expected Outcome	Nursing Interventions
Undescended testicles<hr>Potential for injury (infertility and malignancy) and body image disturbance	Given the appropriate medical and nursing interventions, child will experience minimal complications associated with cryptorchidism, treatment, and surgical repair	*Preoperatively* Facilitate meeting with pediatric urologist, primary nurse, and family to explain cryptorchidism, required treatment, and surgical repair; provide time to clarify questions and concerns specific to issues of sexuality and sterility Administer human chorionic gonadotropin (HCG) therapy as prescribed (usual dose is 4000-5000 units IM 3-5 times per week for 2-3 weeks); rotate injection sites and document rotation schedule; assess injection sites for pain, redness, and swelling; assist child in coping with IM injections through use of play; follow effectiveness of HCG therapy (enlarging scrotum and testes) Prepare child (toddler or preschool age) and family for surgery and hospitalization experience
	Child will experience an uneventful postoperative course and be free of complications	*Postoperatively* Monitor child's vital signs; report temperatures >38.5°C; monitor for tachycardia, bradycardia, hypotension, and hypertension; auscultate breath sounds and note quality of aeration Monitor for signs of obstruction to testicular vascular supply: markedly tender testicles, increased severity of pain (slight elevation of testicles exacerbates the pain), marked edema, and erythema; report observations promptly Observe involved side or sides of scrotum for increased swelling, dark red discoloration, and edema; note degree, severity, and symmetry of testicular swelling; closely monitor scrotal sac for evidence of skin breakdown; keep perianal area clean and dry Place soft sheepskin under child's buttocks and scrotum postoperatively during period of scrotal edema to help maintain skin integrity
Pain<hr>Pain related to surgical repair	Child will be comfortable, as evidenced by increased interest in play activities	Assess child for signs of pain: restlessness, increased irritability, tachycardia, diaphoresis, facial grimacing, guarding, inability to rest or play, and tugging at lower abdomen or groin Administer analgesics postoperatively as prescribed; document and assess effectiveness of analgesics Promote a calm, quiet, restful environment Provide comfort through proper positioning; avoid pressure on scrotal sac Loosen diaper and encourage child to wear loose underwear as appropriate
Fever Infected surgical wound<hr>Potential for infection related to surgical trauma (orchiopexy)	Child will remain normothermic (37-37.5°C)	Monitor vital signs for elevated temperature, tachycardia, and changes in blood pressure; monitor temperature ever 2 h while febrile; report temperature >38.5°C Obtain cultures as indicated; institute antipyretic measures as ordered Evaluate effectiveness for fever reduction
	Child will progress in wound healing, without infection	Assess surgical wound (incision is usually made at lowermost abdominal skin crease), groin, and scrotum Inspect for evidence of edema, erythema, drainage, quality of wound healing, and tissue integrity Keep wound site dry and clean Prevent contamination with urine and/or feces

Clinical Problem/Nursing Diagnosis	Expected Outcome	Nursing Interventions
Child Fearful behavior Restlessness Frequent nightmares Withdrawal Regressive behavior Fear (child) related to developmental concerns with body integrity and separation from parents	Child will express fears about hospitalization and surgical procedure and will be without long-term psychological sequelae	Familiarize the child and/or parents with hospitalization experience through therapeutic play; prepare toddler as close to procedure as possible; use visual aids (doll or puppets) to role play anticipated toddler or preschool fears before and after surgery; provide child with time during play to become familiar with surgical masks and caps, oxygen masks, blood pressure cuffs, etc. Observe child's reaction and response during play; role play receiving IM injections; be honest about pain and reassure child that he is not being punished; support and comfort child during and after procedure (hold, hug, rock, and talk calmly to child)
Parents Verbalize concerns specific to sexuality, infertility, and psychological impact of hospital experience on child Fear (parental) related to surgery, child's sexuality, and psychosocial impact of hospitalization experience with child	Parents will support and comfort child through hospital experience Child will continue to master developmental milestones Parents will express their concerns and have questions clarified	Ask parents to share their experiences specific to measures which comfort the child; document individual comfort measures in the care plan Encourage parental participation in child's care, rooming-in if possible Provide child support from a favorite blanket, toy, or stuffed animal to enhance sense of security Encourage use of proper terminology when referring to body parts; may need to identify child's penis using words he is familiar with to ensure adequate communication; document this information in nursing care plan Show child his penis immediately upon awakening postoperatively; reassure child that his penis is present, intact, and whole Provide opportunities for child to have choices and control Provide play activities that enhance child's strengths; allow child to work through fears in play and art therapy Encourage parents to verbalize feelings about diagnosis of cryptorchidism and required treatment; assist in clarifying questions related to complications (infertility and/or malignancy) Reassure parents that trend toward surgical repair in infancy or early childhood aids in reducing complications Provide parents with information and support; address fears, concerns and questions about surgery, post-op recovery, issues of sexuality, and child's psychological response to hospitalization Reassure parents that surgical repair done before age 3 will protect child from embarrassment in comparing body parts with peers during school-age years Teach parents about assessment of surgical incision site for signs of infection, care of surgical site, and administration of prescribed medications Facilitate follow-up care with urology clinic

material. The child is taught to wipe posteriorly after bowel movements, and care is taken not to place too much pressure on the rubber band securing the testis in the scrotum. Antibiotics are sometimes administered to prevent infection.

Torsion of the Testis

Torsion is an idiopathic twisting of the vascular pedicle of the appendix testis or the spermatic cord, which interferes with the normally rich blood supply to the testis. There may be no symptoms during the neonatal period or there may be enlargement and tenseness of the testis with a unilateral red or bluish discoloration and swelling of the scrotum. The older child may complain of discomfort with the swollen testis. Later, there may be severe pain, exquisite tenderness, lower abdominal pain, fever, nausea, and vomiting—signs of infarction and necrosis of the testis. Surgical correction is the treatment. Unless it is necrotic, the testis is not removed but is attached to the scrotal tissue. If the testis is removed, a prosthesis may replace it for psychological reasons and for cosmetic effect.

Nursing Management

Nursing care is centered on relieving pain and distracting the child from his pain and discomfort both preoperatively and postoperatively. The mother's help is invaluable here, especially in relieving the excessive separation anxiety of the toddler. The nursing history should reflect the child's favorite pastimes and also indicate his terminology for his penis and scrotum.

Preoperative teaching is geared to the child's level of understanding. Support for the scrotum may be helpful in relieving the pain but may also be intolerable because of tenderness. Postoperative nursing care is directed toward relieving the discomfort now aggravated by surgery. Ice bags may be applied to the scrotum immediately after surgery to reduce swelling, but they may not be tolerable. Care is taken to prevent wound contamination, but the child may be as active as he desires.

Diseases or Deviations in the School-Age Child

Premature Thelarche and Adrenarche

Premature thelarche is the development of breast tissue, either bilaterally or unilaterally, in the young child before the onset of puberty but unaccompanied by the development of other signs of precocious puberty. Since the breasts begin normal development at about 8 years of age, premature thelarche must by definition appear before than and may occur in a child as young as 1 to 2 years of age.

Premature thelarche generally appears as disks of breast tissue around the nipple area, which may be associated with tenderness. The breasts may grow for a time, then arrest in development or even regress somewhat. There is, however, no development of the nipple and pigmentation of the areola.

Premature adrenarche (pubarche) is the development of pubic hair prior to the onset of puberty, unaccompanied by other signs of precocious puberty. Occasionally, the development of axillary hair is associated with pubarche.

When they occur in the absence of other signs of precocious puberty or organic disease, these conditions are benign and require no treatment. The nurse should help the parents understand these premature occurrences and treat their appearance calmly to avoid arousing undue concern in the child.

Vulvovaginitis

This inflammatory condition of the vulva and the vagina is common to both young girls and adolescents. The combined terminology is used because vulvitis rarely occurs without subsequent inflammation of the vagina, and vice versa. It is prevalent in young children because the unestrogenized vaginal mucosa has a neutral pH, is thin and taut, lacks glycogen and lactobacilli, and is therefore highly susceptible to infection.

The most common cause of vulvovaginitis is a bacterial infection which may result from poor hygiene, contamination by feces, urine, or unclean fingers; insertion into the vagina of such foreign bodies as hairpins, stones, nuts, pennies, and wads of toilet paper; and gonorrhea acquired from inadvertent indirect contact with discharge from an infected adult, attempted intercourse, or sexual abuse. Vulvovaginitis sometimes occurs when organisms associated with respiratory disease are transferred to the genital area by fingers contaminated by nose picking or finger sucking.

The vulvovaginitis resulting from poor hygiene is usually of nonspecific or mixed bacterial origin, but it may be caused by a virus, a fungus, or pinworms. Since isolating a single causative organism is difficult, the treatment of choice is good local hygiene. If necessary, local application of estrogen creams is instituted to reduce the susceptibility of the vaginal mucosa. A broad-spectrum antibiotic may be administered intramuscularly if the infection is severe or is associated with a respiratory infection.

When the condition continues, a foreign body in the vagina should be suspected. Once the foreign body is removed and the vagina is irrigated, no further treatment is necessary. The acute inflammation should subside within 3 days, and the infection should be gone within 1 to 3 weeks. Treatment of gonorrheal vulvovaginitis includes determination and elimination of the source of the infection and administration of antibiotics. For children who weigh less than 100 lb (45 kg), the regimen of choice is amoxicillin 50 mg/kg by mouth up to 3.5 g and probenecid 25 mg/kg by mouth up to 1 g. Instead of amoxicillin, procaine penicillin G 100,000 U/kg up to 4.8 million U may be given intramuscularly 30 minutes after the oral probenecid. For children who do not respond to these medications, spectinomycin hydrochloride 40 mg/kg up to 2 g may be given intramuscularly. Children weighing more than 100 lb who are allergic to penicillin may be given tetracycline hydrochloride 500 mg four times a day for 7 days by mouth. Other regimens include procaine penicillin G 3 g intramuscularly, amoxicillin 3 g by mouth, and ampicillin 3.5 g by mouth. With all three, probenecid 1 g is given.

Sexual interplay is the primary mode of transmission in children over 1 year of age, although nonvenereal transmission can occur. Therefore, the source of the infection must be determined and treated in order to prevent recurrence. The diagnosis of gonorrheal vulvovaginitis carries serious social, legal, and criminal implications and is treated discreetly.

Nursing Management

The nurse must be familiar with the symptoms of vulvovaginitis (see Table 29-4), being frequently the first health professional to discover it. The mother may approach the nurse because she has noticed a vaginal discharge; a red, swollen vulva; and excessive crying and irritability with one or more of the other signs and symptoms. If the child is old enough, she may complain of pain with walking, sitting, voiding, or defecating and a sensation of itching or burning. In the hospital, the nurse should be alert for vulvovaginitis in any child admitted with an infection, especially respiratory. Children contaminate their fingers with exudate and transfer the infection to the highly susceptible vulvovaginal area. Gonorrheal vulvovaginitis also spreads easily in institutions and is often not immediately diagnosed. Therefore, any child with vulvovaginitis should have her own thermometer and bedpan, and the personnel should be instructed to exercise extra care in hand washing.

Good local hygiene is the primary nursing goal and involves gentle but thorough cleansing of the area after each bowel movement and at least twice daily with a Castile soap. If the inflammation is severe, vegetable oil is preferable to soap. Since the mother is the best person to bathe the child who cannot bathe herself, the mother is taught to cleanse the area thoroughly from front to back, rinse well, and blot rather than rub dry. The area is left open to the air to complete drying, and cornstarch may be applied to reduce friction. Panties should be made of loose-fitting white cotton to avoid irritation from dye or constriction. As soon as she is old enough, the child is taught to wipe herself from front to back after voiding and defecating and during bathing. To prevent urine from flowing into the vaginal os and into the hymen, the child is instructed to sit forward on the toilet stool and spread her legs wide.

Poor health contributes to the child's susceptibility to vaginitis, and the nurse may have to work with both the child and her parents to improve nutrition and overall health status. It may be necessary to involve the dietitian to help the family with meal planning and the purchase of food.

Depending on age, both the child and her mother are usually concerned about the presence of a vaginal discharge. This event requires support, explanation, reassurance, and teaching by the nurse. The parents may need to know that their child is not a "bad girl" because she placed a foreign object in her vagina: She was simply indulging in ordinary childhood exploration and manipulation similar to placing objects in the ear or nose. However, if there is a recurrence, further investigation may be needed to rule out emotional disorders.

Acute Testicular Injury

Injuries of the scrotum and testes are common in young males over the age of 2 years. Falls on playground equipment and bicycle bars are the most frequent cause. There is exquisite pain at the time of the injury. Later there is usually pain and red or bluish discoloration of the scrotum where the injury occurred, sometimes accompanied by swelling. Pain and a history of injury are the essentials of diagnosis. Contusion is the usual result of such an injury, and no treatment is required. Ice may be applied immediately after the injury to decrease the contusion.

If the contusion is severe, necrosis may result. The symptoms resemble those of necrosis caused by torsion of the testis, and surgical removal of the affected testis is necessary.

Support of the scrotum is helpful, and warm baths may be soothing and increase the rate of absorption of the contusion after bleeding has stopped. Prolonged hot baths

TABLE 29-4 Vulvovaginitis in Children

Cause	Most Common Signs and Symptoms	Treatment
Nonspecific bacteria	Erythema; edema; excoriation; maceration; poor local hygiene; scratches; scant vaginal discharge	Good local hygiene, followed by local application of estrogen cream; if no response, broad-spectrum antibiotic intramuscularly
Foreign object	Erythema; edema; excoriation; profuse, bloody, foul, purulent vaginal discharge	Removal of foreign object; vaginal irrigation; good local hygiene
Gonorrhea	Erythema; edema; excoriation; maceration; profuse, purulent, yellow, creamy vaginal discharge; secondary urethritis and prostatitis are common	Elimination of source; aqueous procaine penicillin G intramuscularly

Source: G. M. Scipien et al (eds.), *Comprehensive Pediatric Nursing,* 3d ed., McGraw-Hill, 1986.

are contraindicated in a child who has reached puberty, since prolonged exposure to high temperatures may cause sterility. Parents are usually concerned that the child will become sterile as a result of the testicular injury, and so nursing care is designed to relieve this anxiety. In rare instances where surgery is required, the nursing care is the same as that for torsion of the testis.

Diseases or Deviations in the Adolescent

Menstrual Disorders

Amenorrhea

The absence of menses, or *amenorrhea*, may be either primary or secondary. *Primary* amenorrhea is defined as the delay of menarche past 17 years of age. In *secondary* amenorrhea, menses cease some time after menarche. Secondary amenorrhea is normal during pregnancy and lactation and after menopause. Excepting these instances, amenorrhea is a symptom of an underlying disorder which must be discovered and treated.

Since menstruation is related to delicate hormonal balance as well as to the integrity of the reproductive organs themselves, disorders which interfere with the functioning of the hypothalamus, the pituitary, the ovaries, or the uterus and vagina may produce amenorrhea. If primary amenorrhea is associated with the development of secondary sex characteristics, the absence of menarche suggests a defect in the anatomic structure of the uterus and/or vagina or an imperforate hymen. Primary amenorrhea associated with little or no development of secondary sex characteristics suggests disturbances in the hormonal interaction resulting from genetic defects such as adrenogenital syndrome, testicular feminization, and gonadal dysgenesis. Intracranial lesions and pituitary failure may also cause primary amenorrhea.

Secondary amenorrhea can be related to a variety of causative factors. Organic brain disease may be a cause, as may ovarian neoplasm or polycystic ovary. Nutritional (e.g., sudden weight gain, "crash" dieting) and psychological disturbances (e.g. emotional problems, psychiatric illnesses) apparently affect hypothalamic functioning, although the exact mechanism is unknown. Discontinuance of oral contraceptives that have been taken over a long period of time may produce amenorrhea.

Nursing Management

The adolescent with amenorrhea may be concerned and anxious about her continued failure to menstruate. Since amenorrhea is frequently a symptom of a physical disturbance, the nurse must encourage the girl to obtain a medical evaluation. The physical examination to evaluate primary amenorrhea includes a vaginal smear for estrogen, complete blood count, urinalysis, thyroid tests, and tests for diabetes. While it is common for an adolescent to have erratic periods for the first 2 to 3 years after menarche, evaluation for secondary amenorrhea should be carried out if there is an abrupt cessation of menstruation after regular cycles have been established or if there is a history of oligomenorrhea with subsequent amenorrhea.

Evaluation includes a thorough physical examination and pregnancy test. The nurse will be able to support the adolescent through the physical examination and necessary diagnostic tests. Subsequent nursing care will depend on the specific diagnosis.

Imperforate Hymen

The *hymen* is a membrane of epithelial tissue which develops at the juncture of the urogenital sinus and the vaginal plate. If the lumen fails to appear, the hymen is *imperforate*. The imperforate hymen usually is detected prior to puberty and generally causes no difficulty during early childhood. With menarche, however, the cyclical uterine discharge causes an accumulation of blood in the vagina (hematocolpos), in the uterus (hematometra), and eventually in the tubes (hematosalpinx). Initially, this problem may not cause noticeable discomfort but may present as a pelvic mass or, more rarely, with the initial complaint of flank pain due to urinary retention. However, the increase of accumulated blood may be accompanied by a gradual increase in pelvic discomfort.

Diagnosis is made by noting the bulging, intact hymen in a patient who supposedly has not reached menarche. Treatment consists of surgical incision of the hymen or, preferably, excision of a portion of the hymen, with release of the accumulated blood. There is no damage to the reproductive tract as a result of the accumulation.

Nursing Management

The adolescent girl is very conscious of her developing body and may be particularly concerned about surgical procedures involving the genital area. She should have a clear understanding of what is to be done and of the indications for the surgery. She should understand that after surgery she will menstruate in a relatively normal cycle and that this condition will not interfere with her ability to have satisfactory sexual experiences or to conceive and bear children. After surgery, mild analgesics or warm sitz baths relieve any transient discomfrot.

Dysmenorrhea

Painful menstruation, or dysmenorrhea, may be either primary or secondary. *Secondary dysmenorrhea* is a symptom associated with a specific organic cause, such as pelvic inflammatory disease or endometriosis, and the treatment is directed toward the primary disease entity.

Primary dysmenorrhea, seen more frequently in adolescent girls than secondary dysmenorrhea, is painful menstruation in the absence of obvious organic disturbance. It is associated with ovulatory cycles, as opposed to the usually painless bleeding of anovulatory cycles in dysfunctional uterine bleeding. The specific cause is not clear.

The symptoms of dysmenorrhea occur just prior to, at the time of, or following the onset of menses. The quality of pain may be sharp or dull, cyclic and cramplike, or steady and less intense. There may be associated anxiety symptoms (headache, fatigue, irritability) or gastrointestinal symptoms (nausea, vomiting). Evaluation includes a thorough history of menstruation, premenstrual signs and symptoms, the timing of the cramps, severity of the pain, and associated symptoms. If the physical evaluation is normal, treatment is symptomatic with analgesics or prostaglandin inhibitors.

Nursing Management

Simple means which may relieve dysmenorrhea include short periods of rest, nonstrenuous activities to occupy time and attention, and warm baths. Consideration at all times to good posture and general exercises to improve muscle tone helps decrease discomfort during menstruation. The nurse cautions the girl to take medications only as prescribed. Analgesics, if used, are taken before the pain becomes too severe. The adolescent should return to the practitioner after two menstrual cycles for evaluation of the effectiveness of treatment.

Dysfunctional Uterine Bleeding

For the purposes of this text, dysfunctional uterine bleeding in the adolescent is considered to be irregular, prolonged, or excessive bleeding not associated with disorders of the reproductive system, systemic disease, or pregnancy or its complications. In the adolescent, dysfunctional uterine bleeding is generally a result of idiopathic anovulation. Because ovulation fails to occur, there is no formation of a corpus luteum or production of progesterone. Consistent, elevated levels of estrogen maintain the proliferative phase of the endometrium until the endometrium can no longer support it and breakthrough bleeding occurs. The bleeding episodes may be irregular in occurrence, duration, and amount and are generally not accompanied by pelvic pain.

Diagnosis is generally made on the basis of history, physical examination, and diagnostic testing to rule out an organic cause. When the diagnosis has been established, treatment for the majority of adolescents may be primarily directed toward maintaining good health both physically and psychologically until the cycle readjusts itself. Anovulation is frequently associated with inadequate nutrition and psychological stress. Therefore, a well-balanced diet, rest, and relaxation are essential. Supplemental iron may also be given for associated borderline anemia.

Nursing Management

Health teaching is an important element in the nursing care of the adolescent with dysfunctional uterine bleeding. She must understand the normal menstrual cycle and the factors which may affect it. She must realize that adequate activity, exercise, and rest are important in maintaining a normal cycle. The adolescent can also be helped to understand factors which constitute good nutrition and to adjust her eating habits accordingly. She is encouraged to keep an accurate record of her menstrual cycle and assisted in distinguishing between normal and abnormal menstrual bleeding.

If the bleeding is particularly heavy, hormonal therapy may be introduced. A single course of progesterone ther-apy frequently will reestablish the menstrual cycle. If necessary, a more prolonged regimen involving progesterone administered over three or four cycles will be required. Once the cycle has been reestablished, the hormones are discontinued and the patient is observed closely in the expectation that the system will have regulated itself. The girl should understand the purpose of the hormonal therapy and should be encouraged to report any unusual side effects.

If an acute bleeding episode occurs, dilatation and curettage may be necessary to control hemorrhage. Following surgery, the girl should be checked closely for excessive bleeding from the vagina. If vaginal packing has been inserted after surgery, the girl may experience discomfort and difficulty in voiding. The discomfort is usually relieved with mild analgesics; more severe or persistent pain may indicate uterine perforation and should be reported immediately. The difficulty in voiding is usually overcome when the patient is able to get from the bed to the bathroom. The vaginal packing is generally removed within 24 hours after surgery, and the girl is again observed closely for excessive bleeding.

Breast Disorders

Most breast masses detected in the adolescent are benign, and breast cancer is extremely rare. Fibrocystic changes, the most frequent source of masses in this age group, are detected as diffuse, cordlike thickenings and lumps which may change in size and become tender before and during the menses. The adolescent is encouraged to check her own breasts frequently and to note any changes in masses, and the breasts should be examined frequently by a health care professional.

Breast contusions due to trauma are common in the adolescent period and are detected as poorly defined, tender masses which resolve within weeks. Remaining scar tissue from extreme trauma may be palpated indefinitely.

Breast infection is uncommon in nonlactating adolescents. A breast infection is typified by the sudden onset of a warm, tender mass with overlying skin redness. Breast infections are generally caused by staphylococcus and are treated with systemic antibiotics. Because of the recurrent nature of breast infections, follow-up is imperative.

Sexually Transmitted Diseases

The most common sexually transmitted disease (STD) in the United States is *Chlamydia trachomatis.* Classic venereal diseases, syphilis and gonorrhea, continue to be of major concern because of their prevalence in the population and their potential for severe and disabling consequences. The most recent STD is acquired immune deficiency syndrome (AIDS). However, the minor sexually transmitted diseases, such as trichomoniasis, are now being implicated in more serious conditions. Therefore, a discussion of sexually transmitted conditions must include these infections.

Some general points presented by Hatcher et al. (1981) must be considered in the management of sexually transmitted infections:

1. Usually both partners must be treated and, preferably, treated simultaneously.
2. Condoms should be used contraceptively throughout the duration of the treatment.
3. Patients must be urged strongly to continue taking medications throughout the prescribed course of treatment, even if symptoms subside, and follow-up should be aggressive and thorough.
4. Often patients with one sexually transmitted infection also have another. Case finding should include tests for all infections.
5. Long-term use of broad-spectrum antibiotics to treat sexually transmitted disease often predisposes women to overgrowth of *Monilia* in the vagina. Consideration of routine use of prophylactic antibiotics against *Monilia* is appropriate.
6. Patients should be encouraged to refrain from intercourse while symptoms from a sexually transmitted infection persist.
7. *Venereal disease* and *VD* are terms with negative connotations. The phrase *sexually transmitted infection* is less threatening, more accurate, and more desirable for use.

Chlamydia Trachomatis

In 1985, the Centers for Disease Control estimated that *Chlamydia trachomatis* infections would affect 3 to 4 million people in the United States (U.S. Centers for Disease Control, 1985). These gram-negative bacteria can cause neonatal inclusion conjunctivitis (Chap. 21), pneumonia in infants 2 to 14 weeks of age (Chap. 23), urethritis in both males and females, and cervicitis in females. Since cervicitis in females may be "silent," these infections often are not reported. Symptoms of urethritis may be absent or may include cloudy discharge, erythema around the meatus, or burning on urination. Cervicitis usually is asymptomatic. However, females may complain of urinary frequency, mild dysuria, and vaginal discharge. The incubation period is variable, from 7 to 28 days.

Isolation of the organism on tissue cultures provides a definitive diagnosis, but the results may not be known for 4 to 7 days. Direct immunofluorescence techniques for general screening purposes are processed in about 30 minutes. Enzyme immunoassay, another method used to detect the presence of chlamydial components, takes about 4 hours to complete. The diagnostic test employed depends on the practices followed at specific agencies.

Once the presence of *Chlamydia* has been confirmed, treatment is begun. Adolescents with uncomplicated genital tract infection are treated for 1 week with either tetracycline 500 mg by mouth four times a day or doxycycline 100 mg by mouth twice a day. For pregnant teenagers, an alternative is erythromycin. The adolescent is advised that thorough hand washing whenever hands come in contact with vaginal or urinary meatal secretions is necessary. It is recommended that sexual partners from the past 30 days be located, tested, and treated if presumptive signs are present. A follow-up visit is scheduled for 2 weeks after the initiation of treatment. Sexual contact should be avoided until follow-up laboratory tests are negative or treatment has been completed.

Nursing Management

Nurses working in ambulatory settings are the ones most likely to be working with these teenagers. The adolescent needs information regarding the causative organism, test results, and treatment. Written instructions following verbal ones are helpful. It is important to give the adolescent the name and telephone number of a contact person. Marvin and Slevin (1987) found that this practice increases compliance with the medical regimen and encourages locating contacts. If the adolescent cannot read, the nurse reviews the written material verbally. The nurse can also determine whether there is a support person available who can review this information with the teenager if questions arise. Examples include queries about the medication, dosage and schedule, and side effects; locating sex partners and informing them of the need for testing and treatment; ways of avoiding reinfection; and the need for follow-up visits. Such questions can also be asked of the telephone contact person before the scheduled follow-up visit. Evaluation of nursing interventions involves outcomes concerning compliance with recommended treatment, informing sex partners, keeping follow-up appointments, and following recommendations to avoid infection (Marvin and Slevin, 1987).

Gonorrhea

The incidence of gonorrhea continues to rise, with the greatest rate of increase occurring among adolescents and young adults. The causative agent, *Neisseria gonorrhoeae*, is becoming progressively more resistant to penicillin, although penicillin remains the drug of choice.

Diagnosis in the symptomatic male generally presents little problem. Symptoms include dysuria and a profuse yellow discharge. Gram-stained smear of urethral discharge shows gram-negative diplococci and is relatively (95 percent) accurate. However, about 5 percent of infected males are asymptomatic or have only a mild urethritis. The female is often asymptomatic. Nevertheless, it is increasingly evident that many women do have mild dysuria or nonspecific cystitis. Symptoms of mild pelvic inflammatory disease are also being recognized as gonorrhea in women. Other symptoms may include tenderness of lymph nodes in the groin, lower abdominal pain, fever, testicular pain in the male, and irregular and painful menses in the female. Pain on intercourse and postcoital bleeding may also occur.

Diagnosis is made by obtaining a sample of exudate for Gram's stain and culture on Martin-Lewis or modified Thayer-Martin medium (Table 29-5). In handling cultures, meticulous technique is required to avoid the likelihood of false-negative results.

Treatment is intramuscular injection of 4.8 million U of aqueous procaine penicillin at two sites, with 1.0 g of oral probenecid (a renal tubular blocking agent which helps maintain the initial high systemic level of penicillin). Because of the large dose of penicillin, injection is

TABLE 29-5 Screening Measures and Diagnostic Techniques for Syphilis and Gonorrhea

	Syphilis*	Gonorrhea
Screening measures	Serological reagin tests [venereal disease reaction level (VDRL) slide, unheated serum reagin (USR), rapid plasma reagin (RPR), and automated reagin (ART) tests] A reagin titer should be determined when the reaction is positive and a second specimen obtained to verify the reaction The same reagin test should be used after treatment to determine whether the treatment was effective	None currently satisfactory; diagnostic measures may be used for screening purposes but are expensive
Diagnostic tests	Treponemal tests [fluorescent treponemal antibody = absorption (FTA-ABS) test, microhemagglutination = *Treponema pallidum* (MHA-TP) test], and/or dark-field microscopy of lymph node or lesion aspirate for spirochetes Diagnosis from cerebrospinal fluid (CSF) is based on VDRL, cell count, and protein concentration of the CSF	Preadolescent male: urethral culture in modified Thayer-Martin (MTM) medium Preadolescent female: endocervical, anal, and oral cultures in MTM medium; Gram's stain is also reliable at this age Adolescent male: urethral culture in MTM medium Adolescent female: endocervical culture in MTM medium; Gram's stain smear is *not* reliable in postpubertal females

*The same screening measures and diagnostic tests are used for all age groups and both sexes.

Source: G. M. Scipien et al. (eds.), *Comprehensive Pediatric Nursing,* 3d ed., McGraw-Hill, New York, 1986.

performed by personnel trained in the treatment of anaphylactic shock, and the patient should be asked to remain in the clinic for 20 minutes after injection. Alternative oral treatment is ampicillin 3.5 g or amoxicillin 3.0 g with 1.0 g probenecid by mouth. Evidence, however, shows that these regimens are ineffective against pharyngeal and anorectal gonococcal infections. For patients sensitive to penicillin, tetracycline hydrochloride 0.5 g by mouth four times a day for 7 days is effective. However, a single dose of tetracycline is not effective. Other alternatives include ceftriaxone 250 mg intramuscularly and spectinomycin 2 g intramuscularly (Committee on Infectious Diseases, 1986).

Nursing Management
The client is instructed that notification and treatment of sexual partners is essential. The use of condoms until posttreatment negative cultures on both partners have been obtained is recommended to prevent reinfection. The client is instructed to refrain from oral-genital sex until negative cultures are obtained. Instructions are given regarding the possibility of *Monilia* infections or antibiotic-induced diarrhea. Follow-up cultures 4 to 7 days after completing treatment are mandatory. Cases of gonorrhea must be reported to the health department.

Syphilis
Three weeks after exposure, *primary syphilis* is manifested by a chancre, an indurated, painless, red-rimmed sore on the penis or on the edge of the vagina, cervix, or mouth, which disappears spontaneously in 2 to 6 weeks. *Secondary syphilis,* occurring approximately 6 weeks after healing of the chancre, is manifested by a rash (primar-

ily on the hands and soles of the feet), fever, sore throat, headache, arthralgia, sore mouth, anorexia, nausea, and/or inflamed conjunctiva. These symptoms usually disappear spontaneously without treatment. Moist, broad-based, flat-topped growths from 0.5 to 2 cm in diameter may appear on the warm, moist areas of the body. *Tertiary syphilis* indicates a long-standing infection of 10 to 30 years. Generally, tertiary syphilis includes heart disease, brain damage, spinal cord damage, or blindness. Serological examination is diagnostic for syphilis (Table 29-5).

For early syphilis, the treatment of choice is benzathine penicillin G 2.4 million U total by intramuscular injection at a single session. For patients who are allergic to penicillin, tetracycline hydrochloride 500 mg four times daily for 15 days or erythromycin 500 mg four times daily for 15 days is effective.

Nursing Management
The client is instructed that all sexual partners must be treated and that condoms should be used during intercourse for a month. After treatment, follow-up testing is done at 3, 6, and 12 months, since treatment failures or reinfections may occur (Hatcher et al., 1981).

Acquired Immune Deficiency Syndrome
Adolescents who have AIDS or AIDS-related complex (ARC) are classified according to adult criteria. The age range is 13 to 19 years as opposed to birth to 13 years in the pediatric AIDS group (Chap. 25). Since it is assumed that the topics of AIDS and ARC in adults have been covered in medical and surgical nursing texts, the material will not be repeated here.

To date, AIDS and ARC in adolescents constitute approximately 0.4 percent of all reported cases. These illnesses can be a consequence of sexual abuse, intravenous blood tranfusions (prior to 1985), intravenous substance abuse, and sexual encounters. To prevent the spread of AIDS in 13- to 19-year-olds, it is imperative that they be taught about risk behaviors. Since adolescents are apt to adopt an attitude of "It can't happen to me," this task may be difficult to accomplish. Nevertheless, health care professionals who have received special training in working with teenagers need to reach them.

There are no data concerning how the human immunodeficiency virus (HIV) affects adolescents during this second period of rapid growth. This question is of concern to the surgeon general. In April 1987, participants at the Surgeon General's Workshop on Children with HIV Infection and Their Families recommended that a group be conveyed "to focus on the specific problems of HIV infection in adolescents" (Silverman and Waddell, 1987, p. 53). More attention needs to be given to this vulnerable group. It is hoped that a report on adolescents with HIV infection and its prevention in nonaffected teenagers will be published soon.

Herpes Simplex Virus, Type 2

Herpesvirus infections have long been recognized, but only recently have the roles of sexual transmission and long-term consequences been noted. The primary lesions of *Herpesvirus* are multiple blisterlike vulvar, vaginal, or penile sores or ulcerations which are extremely painful. Dysuria, dyspareunia, vaginal discharge, pain and itching of the vulva and perineum may also be noted. Most viral shedding occurs when blistering lesions are present.

Diagnosis is made from the symptoms produced, viral cultures, and visualization of the lesions. Also, intranuclear changes produced by the *Herpesvirus* can be detected on a Pap smear. Treatment of herpes simplex virus, type 2 (HSV-2) is symptomatic. Some physicians may recommend topical anesthetics. Others prescribe acetaminophen with codeine by mouth every 4 to 6 hours for 2 days. Sitz baths may be soothing. The use of acyclovir ointment on *primary* lesions produces a slight benefit in the reduction of viral shedding and symptoms.

With recurrent HSV-2, acyclovir ointment may be prescribed. One to 2 days before the appearance of lesions, the adolescent will have a tingling sensation. The teenager is advised to begin the ointment at that time. Its use is thought by some physicians to lessen pain. However, many physicians believe that topical acyclovir is not beneficial in the treatment of recurrent HSV-2. Symptomatic treatment as described above will offer some relief once the lesions have reappeared.

Nursing Management

Spreading on the infection by autoinoculation and secondary infection with other agents can be decreased through daily bathing and thorough hand washing with mild soap and water before and after touching the affected areas. Methods of keeping the lesions dry include the use of a hair dryer (on low heat and held at a distance of 1 ft) to dry the lesions, washing or sitz baths, and wearing well-ventilated (loose) clothing and cotton-crotched underpants.

There is evidence to indicate that *Herpesvirus* antibody titers are higher in women with cervical cancer than in carefully controlled groups of women without cervical cancer, although the relationship is not conclusive. However, women with *Herpesvirus* infection should be cautioned to have annual or semiannual Pap smears to detect cancerous changes early (Baker, 1982).

Condoms should be used for at least 6 weeks and until all external signs of infection have disappeared in both partners. Abstinence from intercourse or use of condoms is recommended if lesions recur. If pregnancy is planned, the obstetrician should be notified of the history of *Herpesvirus* infection, since recurrence before delivery may infect the infant, causing disastrous results. The presence of active lesions prior to delivery is an indication for cesarean section. Disseminated herpes occurs at 9 to 10 days of age. Acyclovir may be helpful in treating affected neonates (Committee on Infectious Diseases, 1986).

The client should be informed that there is a possibility that the infection will recur (e.g., during periods of stress or with each menstrual period). However, subsequent infections are rarely as severe as the initial infection.

Minor Sexually Transmitted Diseases

Several diseases are classified as minor sexually transmitted diseases, including trichomoniasis, candidiasis, pubic lice, nonspecified vaginitis and urethritis, and condyloma. Although these conditions generally are contracted through sexual contact, they can be contracted in other manners. Differentiation and management of these conditions are included in Table 29-6. The drugs most commonly used in their treatment are described in Table 29-7.

Pelvic Inflammatory Disease

Pelvic inflammatory disease (PID) is an acute or chronic infection affecting the upper reproductive tract. The fallopian tubes (salpingitis) are most commonly affected, although the uterus (endometritis), ovaries (oophoritis), and peritoneal cavity (pelvic peritonitis) may also be involved. PID occurs most frequently as a secondary infection following gonococcal and/or chlamydial infection of the lower tract or external genitalia.

If the initial infection is untreated or inadequately treated, an ascending spread of the infection occurs, usually at the time of menstruation when the cervical mucous plug is absent and the menstrual blood is available as a medium for bacterial growth. The organism invades the mucosal surfaces of the tubes and the peritoneal serosa and produces a purulent exudate. In response to this bacterial invasion, normal defense mechanisms of the body are mobilized to localize and seal off areas of infection. This process results in fibrosis of the affected tissue with distortion of the structures and partial or total occlusion of the fallopian tubes, which can become the site of chronic low-grade infections.

A history of vaginal discharge prior to menstruation and the onset of bilateral, lower abdominal pain during or immediately following menstruation is helpful in establishing the diagnosis of acute PID. Frequently these symptoms may be the only ones noticed by the adolescent and may in fact be so mild that she does not seek treatment. Other symptoms may include abdominal tenderness and rigidity, elevated temperature, leukocytosis, nausea and

vomiting, and anorexia. The cervix is painful on motion, and adenexal thickening may be palpable. The symptoms vary widely in severity, but generally the adolescent does not appear to be acutely ill. (This finding is in contrast to PID caused by invasion organisms such as *Staphylococcus, Streptococcus,* or *Clostridium,* in which the appearance of marked toxicity is evident.) The organism may be cultured if vaginal discharge is present, provided that antibi-

TABLE 29-6 The Minor Sexually Transmitted Diseases

	Trichomoniasis	Candidiasis	Nonspecific Vaginitis	Pubic Lice	Condylomata Acuminata
Causative organism	Protozoa: *Trichomonas vaginalis*	*Candida albicans*	*Haemophilus vaginalis, Gardnerella vaginalis, Corynebacterium vaginale*	*Phthirius pubis* louse	Human papillomavirus
Subjective information	Intensive vulvar and vaginal pruritus Frothy, thin, greenish-white discharge Pain Frequency and dysuria Dyspareunia	Thick, white, cottage cheese-like discharge Intense pruritus Dysuria Dyspareunia Excoriation of genitalia and upper thighs (may or may not be present)	Thin, uniform, foul-smelling, grayish-white discharge; absence of pruritus and burning	Intense pruritus of the pubic area	Pruritus Chronic discharge at times Nonpainful lesions
Objective information	Vaginal discharge Punctate, red petechiae on cervix Visualization of motile, flagellated trichomonads on saline wet mount	Vaginal discharge Sometimes, beefy red or friable cervix Visualization of budding yeast and pseudohyphae on potassium hydroxide wet mount	Vaginal discharge, normal vaginal epithelium Clue cells on wet mount	Visualization of lice or eggs	Small to large, dry, fungating, wartlike growths of the vulva, vagina, cervix, or penis Biopsy results
Treatment	Metronidazole (Flagyl) 2 g by mouth stat *or* 250 mg tid for 7 days, Flagyl contraindicated in pregnancy; AVC dienestrol vaginal cream, one applicatorful nightly for 14 days	Miconazole (Monistat), one applicatorful nightly for 7 days	Metronidazole 500 mg by mouth bid for 7 days *or* ampicillin 500 mg by mouth qid for 7 days when metronidazole contraindicated	Liberal application of 10% gamma benzene lotion or shampoo (may repeat in 24 to 48 hours) Removal of lice and nits with a fine-toothed comb Washing of linens, undergarments, clothing in extremely hot water	Application of 20 or 25% podophyllin liquid or ointment to warts after protecting the surrounding area with lubricant jelly (e.g., Vaseline) Possible surgical excision of huge masses Weekly or biweekly application of podophyllin until lesions are gone
Complications	Cystitis Urethritis Prostatitis (male) Epididymitis (male)	Cervicitis	Cystitis Cervicitis Urethritis (male)	Secondary bacterial infection if scratching breaks skin	

Source: Adapted from G. M. Scipien et al. (eds.), *Comprehensive Pediatric Nursing,* 3d ed., McGraw-Hill, New York, 1986.

Continued.

TABLE 29-6 The Minor Sexually Transmitted Diseases—cont'd

	Trichomoniasis	Candidiasis	Nonspecific Vaginitis	Pubic Lice	Condylomata Acuminata
Nursing responsibilities	Emphasize that all medication must be taken even if symptoms subside Discourage use of alcohol as Flagyl may cause an Antabuse-like effect Treat both partners Use condoms throughout treatment to prevent reinfection	If chronic or recurring infection, rule out diabetes Teaching: use all of medication even if symptoms subside Preventive teaching: Wear cotton undergarments or pantyhose with a cotton crotch Avoid bubble bath Discontinue douching Use condoms throughout treatment to avoid reinfection	Treat partner as well Emphasize that all medication must be taken even if symptoms subside Use condoms during treatment to prevent recurrence	Emphasize that lotion or shampoo may not be used more than twice in 1 week as toxicity may result Treat both partners Teach perineal hygiene	Rule out syphilitic chancre Instruct to wash off podophyllin within 8 hours of application as toxicity may result Treat partner if symptomatic Use condoms until lesions are gone to prevent reinfection

otics have not been previously administered.

Treatment of acute PID consists primarily of administration of broad-spectrum antibiotics since more than one organism may be present. Additional treatment depends on the severity of the symptoms and includes administration of analgesics and antipyretics and adequate hydration and nutrition. If the symptoms are severe, the adolescent may be hospitalized for intravenous antibiotics, fluid therapy, temperature control, and activity restriction.

Chronic PID occurs infrequently, primarily because of the success of antibiotic treatment of the acute episode. Symptoms include persistent lower abdominal pain, backache, leukorrhea, and menstrual irregularities such as dysmenorrhea and menorrhagia. In addition, there may be periodic episodes of acute inflammation.

Conservative treatment including administration of antibiotics and corticosteroids is attempted with the first several chronic episodes. If treatment does not eliminate the chronic infection, surgical intervention may be the only means of preventing repeated and increasingly severe episodes. Hysterectomy and bilateral salpingectomy are then indicated; oophorectomy can be avoided in young women if the ovaries are not affected. If the chronic infection subsides without surgical intervention, infertility usually occurs as a result of tubal occlusion. If pregnancy occurs, the risk of ectopic implantation with subsequent tubal rupture is high.

Ruptured tuboovarian or peritoneal abscess can occur with acute or chronic PID and is a life-threatening emergency. The patient exhibits symptoms of acute abdomen (intense abdominal pain, abdominal rigidity, fever, nausea, vomiting, and symptoms of shock), and immediate surgical intervention is necessary.

Nursing Management

The nurse caring for an adolescent with PID must take into account not only the physical problem but also potential emotional and familial problems. It is important that the adolescent understand the basis for the medical regimen, particularly if she is receiving antibiotic therapy as an outpatient. She is encouraged to adhere to a well-balanced diet and to force fluids because of the frequent association of urinary tract infections with reproductive tract infections. She is given medication to relieve pain and control fever and, depending on the severity of the symptoms, is encouraged to limit her activity.

The diagnosis of PID, particularly if the episode is severe enough to require hospitalization, may generate many concerns in both the adolescent and her parents, and the nurse must provide an opportunity for them to discuss these concerns. For some parents, this diagnosis may be their first indication that their daughter has been sexually active. This discovery may be the source of guilt feelings or of conflict between the parents and the adolescent and must be discussed to be resolved constructively. If the nurse avoids making judgments on the behavior and response of either the parents or the adolescent and assists them in exploring their feelings and concerns, she can often be effective in helping the family resolve some of these problems. The adolescent and her parents are frequently concerned about the effects of this illness: Will the infection recur? Will the adolescent be able to resume normal sexual functioning? Will she be able to have children? Will she require surgical intervention? Together with the physician, the nurse must provide the adolescent and her family with accurate information which is presented clearly and understandably.

TABLE 29-7 Drugs Commonly Used in the Treatment of Minor Sexually Transmitted Diseases

Drug	Composition	Indication	Dose and Route	Side Effects	Nursing Care
Miconazole nitrate (Monistat)	2% miconazole nitrate	Local treatment of vulvovaginal candidiasis	One applicatorful intravaginally nightly for 7 nights	Vulvovaginal burning, itching, irritation Pelvic cramps (rare) Skin rash (rare) Headache (rare)	May use in pregnancy Stress importance of using all of medication even if symptoms subside Use sanitary napkin to prevent staining of clothing Stress importance of returning for follow-up exam to assess effectiveness of treatment
Betadine gel	Povidone-iodine	Possibly effective: *H. vaginalis* Candidiasis Trichomoniasis	One applicatorful intravaginally nightly, or local application	Local irritation Skin staining	Insert high into the vagina Notify if burning or itching Use a sanitary napkin to prevent staining of clothing
Metronidazole (Flagyl)	Metronidazole 250 mg per tablet	*Trichomonas* vaginitis	2 g in one dose by mouth *or* 250 mg tid for 7 days	Nausea and vomiting Headache Anorexia Moderate leukopenia Central nervous system manifestations Urticaria (rare)	Avoid alcohol, which may produce an Antabuse-like effect Take with food to avoid gastrointestinal upset Complete full course of therapy even if symptoms subside May cause darkening of the urine May cause an unpleasant metallic taste in the mouth Use concoms until infection subsides to prevent reinfection Treat partners as well

Source: G. M. Scipien et al. (eds.), *Comprehensive Pediatric Nursing,* 3d ed., McGraw-Hill, New York, 1986.

29-2 *The Adolescent with Pelvic Inflammatory Disease*

Clinical Problem/Nursing Diagnosis	Expected Outcome	Nursing Interventions
Fever and chills Hyperthermia (axillary temperature >38.5°C) related to infection	Adolescent will attain axillary temperature of 37.5°C	Monitor vital signs q 2 h while febrile; note presence of tachycardia, hypotension or hypertension, diminished pulses, and decreased peripheral perfusion (cool pale extremities with sluggish capillary refill) Administer antipyretics as ordered Evaluate effectiveness of antipyretic measures Properly administer antibiotic therapy as prescribed Provide adolescent with clean, dry sleepwear and bed linens during diaphoretic periods
Abdominal pain Pain related to infection	Adolescent will experience pain relief as evidenced by participation in daily care, adolescent activities, and ability to rest in comfort	Assess character of abdominal pain; note location (lower abdominal pain), intensity, presence of abdominal tenderness and rigidity, splinting, and guarding abdomen Administer analgesics as prescribed Assist adolescent with relaxation techniques: deep breathing, imagery, music (Walkman) Promote quiet, restful environment Prepare adolescent for surgery as indicated
Nausea Vomiting Loss of appetite Altered nutrition: less than body requirements related to infection and increased metabolic demands	Adolescent will cease vomiting, bouts of nausea will subside, and dietary intake will improve	Monitor amount, color, and consistency of emesis; guaiac emesis Administer antiemetics as prescribed Evaluate effect on controlling nausea and vomiting Progress diet as tolerated; encourage well-balanced diet high in protein and nutrients
Nausea Vomiting Fever Potential fluid volume deficit related to vomiting and fever	Adolescent's fluid and electrolyte balance will be maintained	Monitor intake and output volumes Assess hydration status; note skin turgor, moisture of mucous membranes, and presence of tears Monitor urine specific gravity Administer intravenous fluids as ordered Ensure patency and placement of IV Correct electrolyte imbalances as ordered Encourage generous po fluid intake
Adolescent and/or parents express need to discuss issues relating to adolescent sexuality and implications and management of pelvic inflammatory disease Knowledge deficit related to pelvic inflammatory disease (cause, management, and home care) and safe adolescent sexual practices	Adolescent will understand the cause of pelvic inflammatory disease	Obtain history of sexual practices in a compassionate, nonjudgmental manner, ask questions in direct manner; ensure privacy during history taking Encourage expression of feelings about sexuality, fears, and concerns; clarify myths and misinformation Provide pertinent information specific to safe adolescent sexual practices (birth control and prevention of AIDS and venereal disease) and importance of routine gynecological examinations; provide accurate clear explanations about cause of pelvic inflammatory disease and required treatment (antibiotic therapy, high-calorie, high-protein diet, and adequate rest, importance of high fluid intake to prevent urinary tract infection) Support adolescent through pelvic examinations Use a model or pictorial aid to explain anatomy of pelvic inflammatory disease; familiarize adolescent with the examination room, table, and instruments; prepare for sensations that may be experienced before and during exam Reassure adolescent that privacy will be maintained during exam; prepare for presence of a physician and nurse during exam Explain to adolescent exactly what is being done and what she may feel through entire examination Provide adequate opportunities for adolescent and/or parents to express concerns about diagnosis of pelvic inflammatory disease, required management, and potential complications

Clinical Problem/Nursing Diagnosis	Expected Outcome	Nursing Interventions
	Adolescent will understand issues encompassing sexuality (safe sexual practices, birth control, and prevention of venereal disease and AIDS)	Identify stressors and conflicts that may exist between adolescent and parents with regard to issues of sexuality and sexual activity Address conflicts in nonjudgmental direct manner; clarify questions and provide support to enhance effective family communication Encourage constructive expression of feelings (guilt and fear about working through conflicts) Assess need for ongoing counseling regarding issues of sexuality; facilitate referral to adolescent clinic and family counseling as indicated.

Learning Activities

1. Divide students into three groups. Assign each group the development of one of the following teaching programs for children ages 9 to 12 years:
   (a) Understanding the menstrual cycle
   (b) Understanding nocturnal emissions
   (c) Understanding fertilization
   Following completion of the assignment, have a group representative present each of the programs for discussion.
2. Present a case study of a 6-year-old child who has vulvovaginitis. Ask students to identify several nursing diagnoses, appropriate interventions, and outcome criteria to evaluate care.

Independent Study Activities

1. Based on concepts of development, devise a teaching plan concerning sexually transmitted disease for adolescents, both male and female.
2. With a classmate, role play as nurse and adolescent. Practice taking a reproductive history and recording findings in a systematic manner.

Study Questions

1. Once sperm have been ejaculated into the vagina, their life span is:
   A. 7 days.
   B. 42 days.
   C. 12 to 24 hours.
   D. 24 to 72 hours.
2. Luteotropic hormone:
   A. Stimulates growth of the ovary.
   B. Stimulates growth of the primordial follicle.
   C. Causes rapid growth of the primordial follicle with ovulation.
   D. Affects the development of the corpus luteum after ovulation.
3. When obtaining a history related to the child's sexual development, it is important to address sex-role identity, sex education received, and:
   A. Age at onset of menses.
   B. The presence of gynecomastia.
   C. Understanding of sexuality and sexual functioning.
   D. Family history of sterility.
4. In examining a 2-month-old male, the nurse is unable to palpate the left testicle. The right testicle is descended. The nurse shoud:
   A. Refer the infant to a genitourinary specialist.
   B. Tell the mother that testes often do not descend until the second year of life.
   C. Grasp the left inguinal canal between the thumb and forefinger and gently "strip" it toward the scrotum.
   D. Sit the infant in a basin filled with tepid water.
5. Phimosis, a tightening of the prepuce over the penis so that the foreskin cannot be retracted:
   A. Is normal in the newborn.
   B. Is abnormal at any age.
   C. Is abnormal in the newborn.
   D. Is an indication for newborn circumcision.

6. An important observation in differentiating noncommunicating from communicating hydrocele is:
   A. Change in scrotal size from morning to night to morning.
   B. The presence of a ventral hernia.
   C. The presence of a translucent scrotal mass.
   D. Flexibility of the mass.

7. Following an orchiopexy, the nurse should be aware of the amount of pressure placed on the rubber band extending from the scrotum to the thigh because:
   A. Its purpose is to apply pressure.
   B. Sterility can result.
   C. The band maintains the position of the testes in the scrotum.
   D. Scrotal temperature must remain constant.

8. Children who have had vulvovaginitis need to be taught to wipe themselves after voiding and defecating:
   A. With a warm moist cloth.
   B. From back to front.
   C. From back to front with voiding only.
   D. From front to back.

9. A 14-year-old boy in stage 3 of sexual development has sustained a contusion of the testicle resulting from a fall. Treatment will consist of:
   A. Prolonged hot baths twice a day.
   B. Immediate surgery.
   C. Application of ice immediately after the injury and support to the scrotum.
   D. Support to the scrotum and warm baths.

10. The mother of an 18-year-old girl in stage 6 of sexual development tells the nurse that her daughter has primary amenorrhea. She asks what that terminology means. The nurse explains that it is:
    A. The cessation of menses after menarche.
    B. The delay of menarche past 17 years of age.
    C. A sign of pregnancy.
    D. Normal in some girls.

11. Adolescents who have *Herpesvirus* infection of the genitalia are encouraged to have annual or semiannual Pap smears:
    A. To detect the presence of any cancerous changes early.
    B. To evaluate the effect of treatment.
    C. As a means of preventing recurrence.
    D. To determine antibody titers.

12. The nurse caring for an adolescent who has pelvic inflammatory disease encourages the teenager to force fluids because:
    A. She is receiving sulfonamides as part of the treatment.
    B. There is a risk of associated urinary tract infection.
    C. Of the possibility of fallopian tube occlusion.
    D. Her activity is limited.

References

Baker, D.: "Prospects for Treating Herpes," *Contemporary Ob/Gyn, 19:*179-187, 1982.

Committee on Infectious Diseases: *Report of the Committee on Infectious Diseases,* American Academy of Pediatrics, Elk Grove Village, IL, 1986.

Hatcher, R.A., et al.: *Contraceptive Technology,* 4th ed., Wiley, New York, 1981.

Marvin, C., and A. Slevin: "Chalmydia—Cause, Prevention, and Cure," *MCN: The American Journal of Maternal Child Nursing, 12:*318-321, 1987.

Silverman, B.K., and A. Waddell (eds.): *Report of the Surgeon General's Workshop on Children with HIV Infection and Their Families,* Department of Health and Human Services, Washington, D.C., 1987.

U.S. Centers for Disease Control: *Chlamydia Trachomatis Infections/Policy Guidelines,* U.S. Government Printing Office, Washington, D.C., 1985.

Appendixes

A

Denver Developmental Screening Test

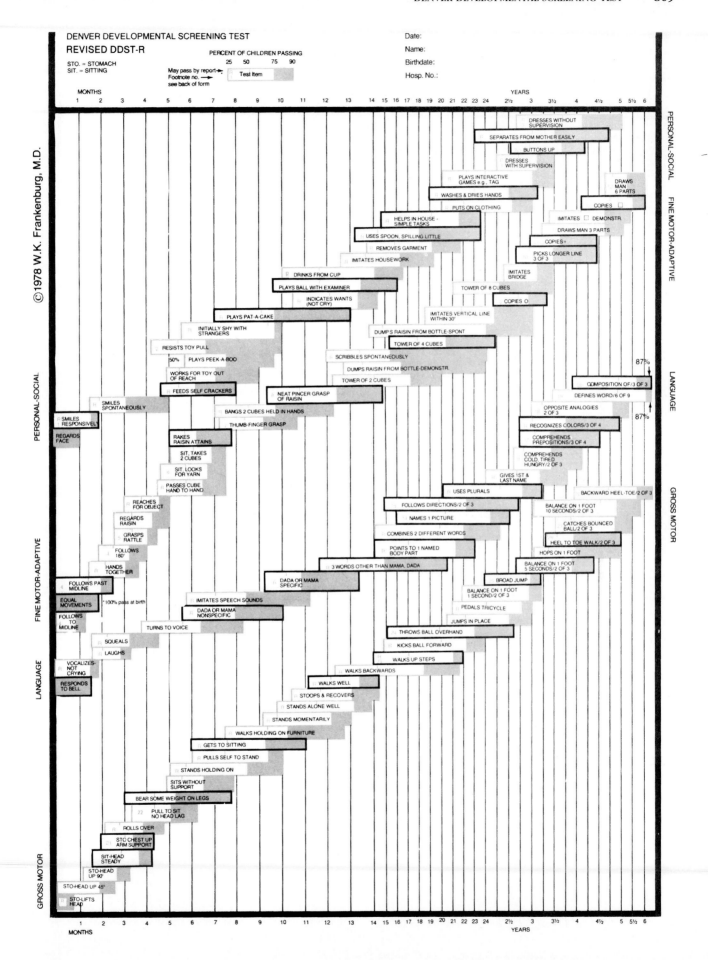

DATE

NAME

DIRECTIONS   BIRTHDATE

HOSP. NO.

1. Try to get child to smile by smiling, talking or waving to him. Do not touch him.
2. When child is playing with toy, pull it away from him. Pass if he resists.
3. Child does not have to be able to tie shoes or button in the back.
4. Move yarn slowly in an arc from one side to the other, about 6" above child's face.
   Pass if eyes follow 90° to midline. (Past midline; 180°)
5. Pass if child grasps rattle when it is touched to the backs or tips of fingers.
6. Pass if child continues to look where yarn disappeared or tries to see where it went. Yarn
   should be dropped quickly from sight from tester's hand without arm movement.
7. Pass if child picks up raisin with any part of thumb and a finger.
8. Pass if child picks up raisin with the ends of thumb and index finger using an over hand
   approach.

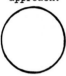 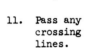 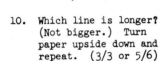

9. Pass any en-   10. Which line is longer?   11. Pass any   12. Have child copy
   closed form.   (Not bigger.) Turn   crossing   first. If failed,
   Fail continuous   paper upside down and   lines.   demonstrate
   round motions.   repeat. (3/3 or 5/6)

   When giving items 9, 11 and 12, do not name the forms. Do not demonstrate 9 and 11.

13. When scoring, each pair (2 arms, 2 legs, etc.) counts as one part.
14. Point to picture and have child name it. (No credit is given for sounds only.)

    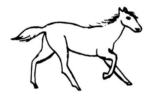 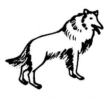 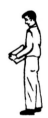

15. Tell child to: Give block to Mommie; put block on table; put block on floor. Pass 2 of 3.
    (Do not help child by pointing, moving head or eyes.)
16. Ask child: What do you do when you are cold? ..hungry? ..tired? Pass 2 of 3.
17. Tell child to: Put block on table; under table; in front of chair, behind chair.
    Pass 3 of 4. (Do not help child by pointing, moving head or eyes.)
18. Ask child: If fire is hot, ice is ?; Mother is a woman, Dad is a ?; a horse is big, a
    mouse is ?. Pass 2 of 3.
19. Ask child: What is a ball? ..lake? ..desk? ..house? ..banana? ..curtain? ..ceiling?
    ..hedge? ..pavement? Pass if defined in terms of use, shape, what it is made of or general
    category (such as banana is fruit, not just yellow). Pass 6 of 9.
20. Ask child: What is a spoon made of? ..a shoe made of? ..a door made of? (No other objects
    may be substituted.) Pass 3 of 3.
21. When placed on stomach, child lifts chest off table with support of forearms and/or hands.
22. When child is on back, grasp his hands and pull him to sitting. Pass if head does not hang back.
23. Child may use wall or rail only, not person. May not crawl.
24. Child must throw ball overhand 3 feet to within arm's reach of tester.
25. Child must perform standing broad jump over width of test sheet. (8-1/2 inches)
26. Tell child to walk forward, 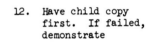 heel within 1 inch of toe.
    Tester may demonstrate. Child must walk 4 consecutive steps, 2 out of 3 trials.
27. Bounce ball to child who should stand 3 feet away from tester. Child must catch ball with
    hands, not arms, 2 out of 3 trials.
28. Tell child to walk backward, ◄━ ⊂◻⊃⊂◻⊃⊂◻⊃ toe within 1 inch of heel.
    Tester may demonstrate. Child must walk 4 consecutive steps, 2 out of 3 trials.

DATE AND BEHAVIORAL OBSERVATIONS (how child feels at time of test, relation to tester, attention
span, verbal behavior, self-confidence, etc,):

157. 10-70

NCHS Growth Charts

Adapted from the National Center for Health Statistics: NCHS Growth Charts, 1976. Monthly Vital Statistics Report, 25(3), Supp.(HRA)76-1120. Data from the Fels Research Institute. Charts prepared by Ross Laboratories, Columbus, Ohio, 1976.

GIRLS: BIRTH TO 36 MONTHS
PHYSICAL GROWTH
NCHS PERCENTILES   NAME_____   RECORD #_____

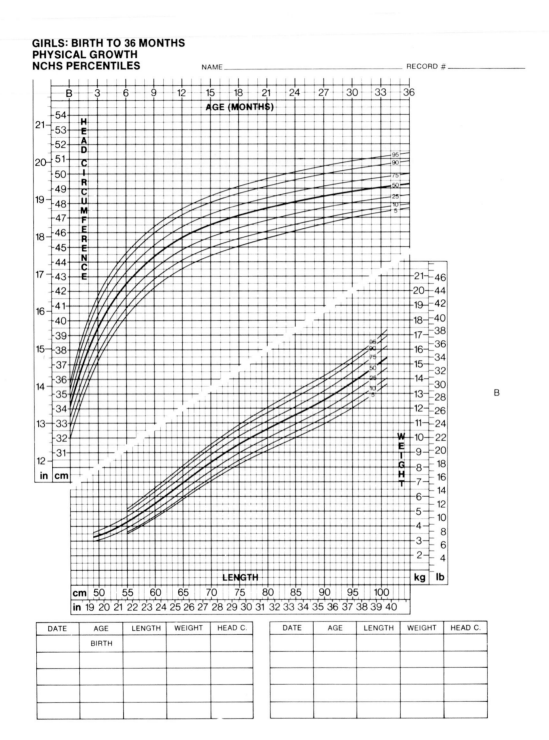

DATE	AGE	LENGTH	WEIGHT	HEAD C.
	BIRTH			

DATE	AGE	LENGTH	WEIGHT	HEAD C.

GIRLS: BIRTH TO 36 MONTHS
PHYSICAL GROWTH
NCHS PERCENTILES

NAME_____   RECORD #_____

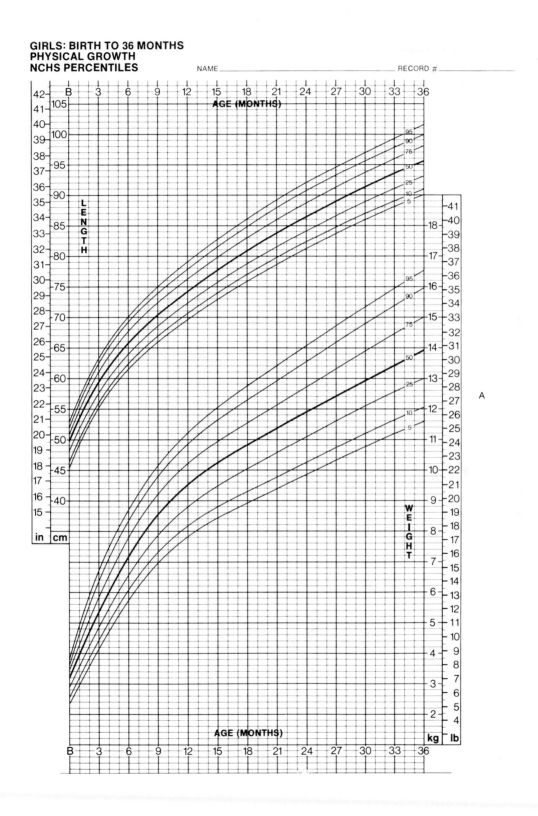

GIRLS: 2 TO 18 YEARS
PHYSICAL GROWTH
NCHS PERCENTILES

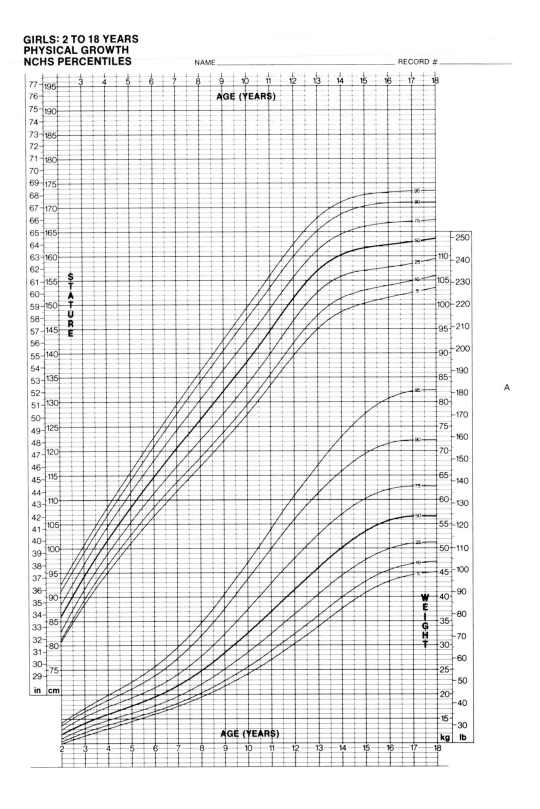

GIRLS: PREPUBESCENT
PHYSICAL GROWTH
NCHS PERCENTILES

NAME _____   RECORD # _____

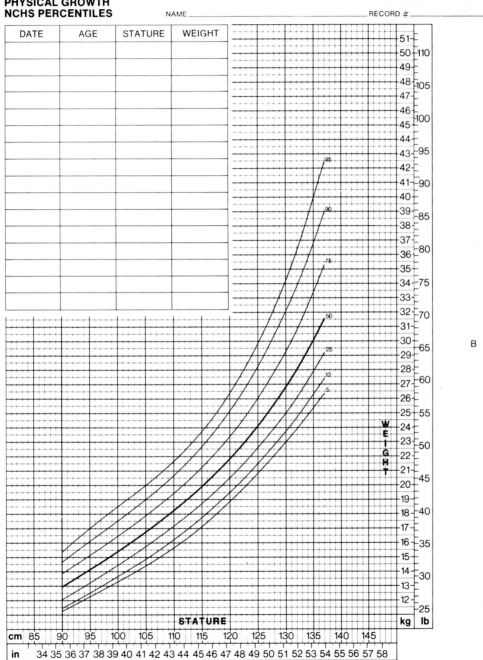

DATE	AGE	STATURE	WEIGHT

B

BOYS: BIRTH TO 36 MONTHS
PHYSICAL GROWTH
NCHS PERCENTILES

NAME _____   RECORD # _____

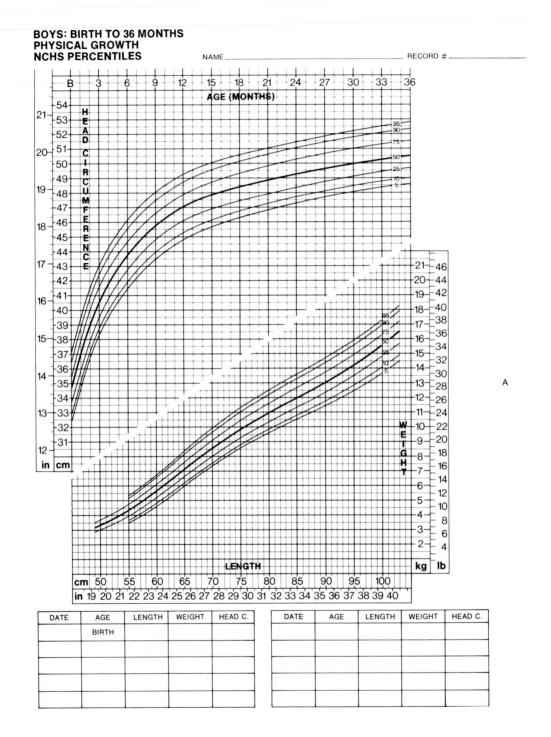

A

DATE	AGE	LENGTH	WEIGHT	HEAD C.
	BIRTH			

DATE	AGE	LENGTH	WEIGHT	HEAD C.

BOYS: BIRTH TO 36 MONTHS
PHYSICAL GROWTH
NCHS PERCENTILES

NAME _____   RECORD # _____

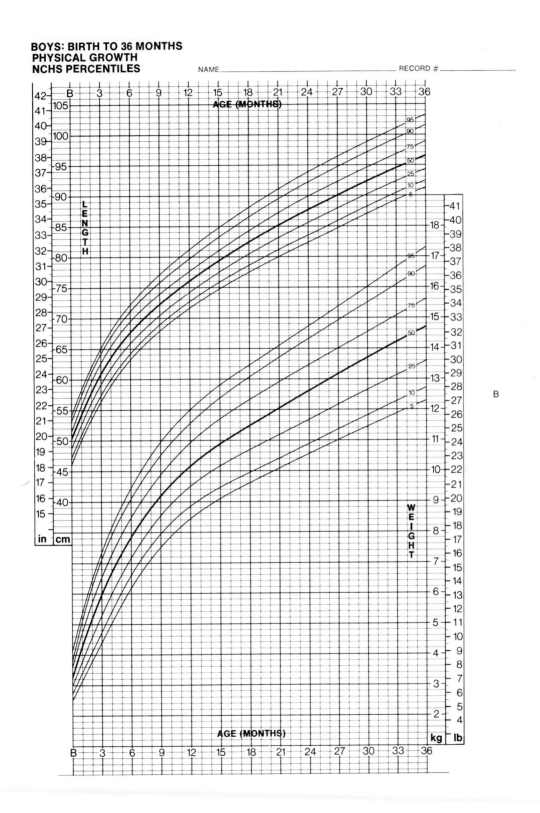

BOYS: 2 TO 18 YEARS
PHYSICAL GROWTH
NCHS PERCENTILES

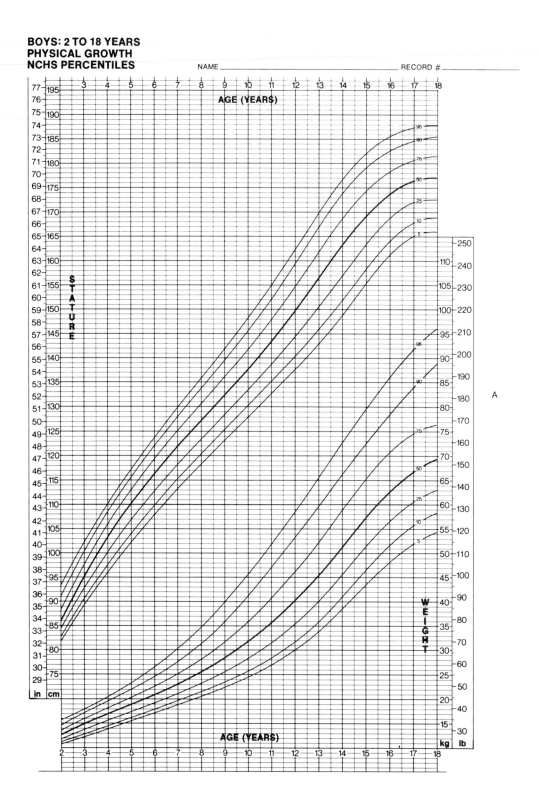

BOYS: PREPUBESCENT
PHYSICAL GROWTH
NCHS PERCENTILES

NAME _____   RECORD # _____

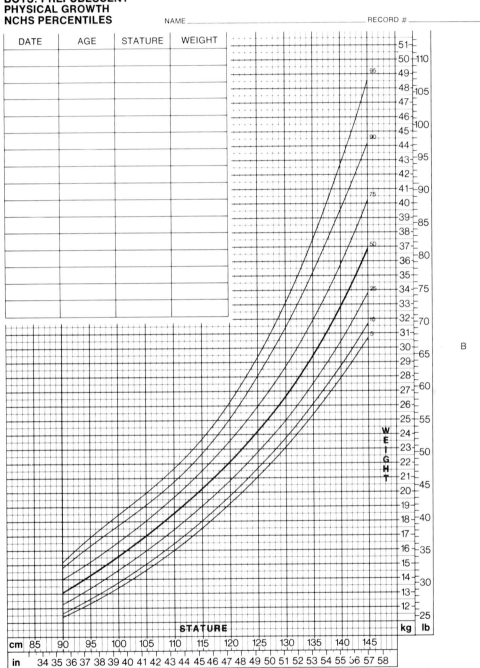

DATE	AGE	STATURE	WEIGHT

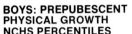

Functional Health Pattern Assessment: Infant and Early Childhood

Use a parent report until the child can answer the items. The following includes some screening items related to parent assessment or use adult assessment (Appendix E).

I. Health-perception–health-management pattern
   A. Parents' report:
      1. Pregnancy/labor/delivery history (this baby, child)?
      2. Health status since birth?
      3. Adherence to routine health checks? Immunizations?
      4. Infections? Frequency? Absences from school?
      5. If applicable: Medical problem, treatment, and prognosis?
      6. If applicable: Actions taken when signs/symptoms perceived?
      7. If appropriate: Been easy to follow things doctors or nurses suggest?
      8. Preventive health practices (diaper change, utensils, clothes, etc.)?
      9. Parents smoke? Around baby?
      10. Accidents? Frequency?
      11. Crib toys (safety)? Carrying safety? Car safety?
      12. Safety practices (household products, medicines, etc.)
   B. Parent (self): Parents'/family general health status?
   C. Observation
      1. General appearance of infant/child.
      2. General appearance of parent(s).

II. Nutritional-metabolic pattern
   A. Parents' report of
      1. Breast feeding/Bottle? Estimate of intake? Sucking strength?
      2. Appetite? Feeding discomfort?
      3. 24-hour intake of nutrients?
      4. Supplements?
      5. Eating behavior?
      6. Food preferences? Conflicts over food?
      7. Birth weight? Current weight?
      8. Skin problem: Rashes, lesions, etc.?
   B. Observation
      1. Height?
      2. Weight?
      3. Skin color, hydration, rashes, lesions.

*Source: M. Gordon, *Nursing Diagnosis: Process and Application,* 2d ed., McGraw-Hill, New York, 1987, pp. 443-445. Used with permission.

III. Elimination pattern
   A. Parents' report of
      1. Bowel elimination pattern (describe). Frequency? Character? Discomfort?
      2. Diaper change routine?
      3. Urinary elimination pattern (describe). Frequency of diaper change?
      4. Estimate of amount? Stream (strong, dribble)?
      5. Excess perspiration/Odor?

IV. Activity-exercise pattern
   A. Parents' report of
      1. Bathing routine? (When, how, where, type of soap?)
      2. Dressing routine? (Clothing, inside outside home)
      3. Crib or other? Describe.
      4. Typical day's activity (hours spent in crib, carrying, play, type of toys).
      5. Active? Activity tolerance?
      6. Perception of baby's/child's strength ("strong/fragile")?
      7. Child: Self-care ability (bathing, feeding, toileting, dressing, grooming)?
      8. Parent (self) child care, home maintenance activity pattern.
   B. Observation
      1. Reflexes (appropriate to age)
      2. Breathing pattern; rate, rhythm.
      3. Heart sounds; rate, rhythm.
      4. Blood pressure.

V. Sleep-rest pattern
   A. Parents' report of
      1. Sleep pattern: Estimated hours?
      2. Restlessness? Nightmares?
      3. Infant: Sleep position? Body movements?
   B. Parent (self): Sleep pattern?

VI. Cognitive-perceptual pattern
   A. Parents' report of
      1. General responsiveness?
      2. Response to talking? Noise? Objects? Touch?
      3. Following objects with eyes? Response to crib toys?
      4. Learning (changes noted)? What teaching baby?
      5. Noises/Vocalizations?
      6. Speech pattern? Words? Sentences?
      7. Use of stimulation: Talking, games, etc.?
      8. Vision, hearing, touch, kinesthesia?
   B. Child
      1. Name. Tell time, address, telephone number?
      2. Pain? Discomfort? (Describe)

VII. Self-perception—self-concept pattern
   A. Parent's report of
      1. Mood state?
      2. If child? Child's sense of worth, identity, competency?

   B. Child's report of
      1. Mood state?
      2. Many/few friends? Liked by others?
      3. Self-perception ("good" most of time? Hard to be "good"?).
      4. Ever lonely?
      5. Fears (transient/frequent?)
   C. Observation
      1. Child: Eye contact, speech pattern, posturing.
   D. Parent (self)
      1. General sense of worth, identity, competency?

VIII. Role/relationship pattern
   A. Parent's report of
      1. Family/household structure?
      2. Family problems/stressors?
      3. Family members/infant (or child) interaction?
      4. Infant/child response to separation?
      5. Child: Dependency?
      6. Child: Play pattern?
      7. Child: Temper tantrums Discipline problems?
      8. Child: School adjustment?
   B. Observation
      1. Smiling response (infant)?
      2. Social interaction (child)? Aggressive/withdrawn?
      3. Response to vocalizations? Requests?
   C. Parent (self)
      1. Role engagements? Satisfaction?
      2. Work? Social? Family? Relationships?

IX. Sexually-reproductive pattern
   A. Parents' report of
      1. Child's feeling of maleness/femaleness?
      2. Questions regarding sexuality? How respond?
   B. Parent (self)
      1. If applicable: Reproductive history?
      2. Sexual satisfaction/problems?

X. Coping-Stress tolerance pattern
   A. Parents' report of
      1. Child's pattern of handling problems, frustrations, anger, etc.? Stressors? Tolerance?
   B. Parent (self)
      1. Strategies for handling problems?
      2. Use of support systems?
      3. Life stressors? Family stress?

XI. Value-belief pattern Parent (self)
   A. Things important in life? Desires for the future?
   B. If appropriate: Perceived impact of disease on goals?

1988 North American Nursing Diagnoses Association Approved Nursing Diagnoses

Activity intolerance
Activity intolerance, potential
Adjustment, impaired
Airway clearance, ineffective
Anxiety
Aspiration, potential for

Body image disturbance
Body temperature, altered, potential
Bowel incontinence
Breastfeeding, ineffective
Breathing pattern, ineffective

Cardiac output, decreased
Communication, impaired verbal
Constipation
Constipation, colonic
Constipation, perceived
Coping, defensive
Coping, family: potential for growth
Coping, ineffective family: compromised
Coping, ineffective family: disabling
Coping, ineffective individual

Decisional conflict (specify)
Denial, ineffective
Diarrhea
Disuse syndrome, potential for
Diversional activity deficit
Dysreflexia

Family processes, altered
Fatigue
Fear
Fluid volume deficit (1)
Fluid volume deficit (2)
Fluid volume deficit, potential
Fluid volume excess

Gas exchange, impaired
Grieving, anticipatory
Grieving, dysfunctional
Growth and development, altered

Health maintenance, altered
Health-seeking behaviors (specify)
Home maintenance management, impaired
Hopelessness
Hyperthermia
Hypothermia

Incontinence, functional
Incontinence, reflex
Incontinence, stress
Incontinence, total
Incontinence, urge
Infection, potential for
Injury, potential for

Knowledge deficit (specify)

Mobility, impaired physical

822

Noncompliance (specify)
Nutrition, altered: less than body requirements
Nutrition, altered: more than body requirements
Nutrition, altered: potential for more than body requirements

Oral mucous membrane, altered

Pain
Pain, chronic
Parental role conflict
Parenting, altered
Parenting, altered, potential
Personal identity disturbance
Poisoning, potential for
Post-trauma response
Powerlessness

Rape-trauma syndrome
Rape-trauma syndrome: compound reaction
Rape-trauma syndrome: silent reaction
Role performance, altered

Self-care deficit, bathing/hygiene
Self-care deficit, dressing/grooming
Self-care deficit, feeding
Self-care deficit, toileting
Self-esteem, disturbance
Self-esteem, chronic low
Self-esteem, situational low
Sensory/perceptual alterations (specify) (visual, auditory, kinesthetic, gustatory, tactile, olfactory)

Sexual dysfunction
Sexuality patterns, altered
Skin integrity, impaired
Skin integrity, impaired, potential
Sleep pattern disturbance
Social interaction, impaired
Social isolation
Spiritual distress (distress of the human spirit)
Suffocation, potential for
Swallowing, impaired

Thermoregulation, ineffective
Thought processes, altered
Tissue integrity, impaired
Tissue perfusion, altered (specify type) (renal, cerebral, cardiopulmonary, gastrointestinal, peripheral)
Trauma, potential for

Unilateral neglect
Urinary elimination, altered patterns
Urinary retention

Violence, potential for: self-directed or directed at others

Answers to Study Questions

Chapter 1	Chapter 5	Chapter 7	7. D	14. A
1. C	1. A	1. C	8. B	15. B
2. A	2. B	2. B	9. C	**Chapter 14**
3. D	3. C	3. D	10. D	1. D
4. D	4. A	4. B	**Chapter 11**	2. B
5. B	5. B	5. C	1. A	3. C
6. D	6. D	6. B	2. D	4. D
Chapter 2	7. C	7. B	3. D	5. A
1. C	8. B	8. B	4. C	6. C
2. D	**Chapter 6**	9. B	5. A	7. B
3. A	1. D	10. B	6. C	8. B
4. D	2. C	11. C	7. B	9. C
5. D	3. D	**Chapter 8**	8. C	10. A
6. C	4. D	1. A	9. D	**Chapter 15**
Chapter 3	5. D	2. A	10. A	1. D
1. A	6. D	3. C	**Chapter 12**	2. D
2. A	7. C	4. B	1. B	3. C
3. C	8. B	5. C	2. A	4. A
4. D	9. B	6. B	3. B	5. B
5. A	10. B	7. C	4. C	6. C
6. C	11. B	8. C	5. C	7. B
7. D	12. A	9. A	**Chapter 13**	**Chapter 16**
8. C	13. C	10. C	1. A	1. B
9. C	14. C	11. C	2. D	2. D
Chapter 4	15. A	12. D	3. B	3. A
1. B	16. B	13. D	4. A	4. C
2. C	17. D	14. A	5. A	5. A
3. D	18. A	**Chapter 9**	6. B	6. B
4. A	19. A	1. C	7. D	7. D
5. B	20. C	2. C	8. A	8. B
6. D	21. A	3. A	9. A	9. B
7. C	22. A	4. D	10. B	10. A
8. B	23. D	5. B	11. D	11. C
9. A	24. C	6. A	12. D	**Chapter 17**
10. D	25. C		13. A	1. B
11. A				2. D

824

3. A
4. C
5. B
6. D
7. C
8. A
9. B
10. C

Chapter 18
1. D
2. B
3. A
4. C
5. A
6. B
7. C
8. C

Chapter 19
1. A
2. C
3. C
4. D
5. B
6. B
7. A
8. D
9. A
10. D
11. A

Chapter 20
1. C
2. C
3. A
4. B
5. C
6. D
7. D
8. D
9. D
10. A
11. C
12. C
13. C
14. D
15. C

Chapter 21
1. B
2. D
3. C
4. C
5. A
6. C
7. B
8. D
9. C
10. A
11. D

Chapter 22
1. C
2. A
3. C
4. B
5. D
6. A
7. B
8. D
9. A
10. D
11. B
12. C
13. B
14. C
15. B

Chapter 23
1. B
2. C
3. B
4. A
5. C
6. A
7. C
8. B
9. C
10. A
11. D
12. C
13. D
14. C

Chapter 24
1. A
2. B
3. B
4. D
5. C
6. C
7. D
8. A
9. D
10. A
11. A

Chapter 25
1. C
2. C
3. D
4. D
5. B
6. C
7. B
8. C
9. D
10. B
11. D
12. D
13. A
14. B

15. C
16. D
17. A

Chapter 26
1. B
2. A
3. A
4. D
5. C
6. B
7. C
8. B
9. C
10. C

Chapter 27
1. D
2. D
3. C
4. C
5. A
6. A
7. C
8. B
9. D
10. C
11. B
12. A
13. A
14. B
15. B

Chapter 28
1. B
2. B
3. A
4. B
5. D
6. A
7. B
8. B
9. A
10. C
11. B
12. D
13. B
14. C

Chapter 29
1. D
2. D
3. C
4. C
5. A
6. A
7. C
8. D
9. C
10. B
11. A
12. B

Index

Propylthiouracil (PTU) for hyperthyroidism, 756
Prosobee, content of, 149
Prostate, 778
Protamine zinc, 773
Proteases, 669
Protective isolation, 220
Protein(s), 142
  digestion of, 669
  in infant formulas, 148
  metabolism of, and diabetes mellitus, 763
  physiologic functions of, 140
  sources of, 140
  synthesis of, thyroid hormones and, 744
Proteinuria, testing for, 706
Proternol; see Isoproterenol
Proteus
  and osteomyelitis, 500
  and urinary tract infections, 724
Prothrombin, 624
Protoporphyrins, 627
Proventil; see Albuteral sulfate
Providencia stuartii and burn wounds, 367
Proximodistal development, 15
Pruritus and atopic dermatitis, 353
Pseudomenstruation, 787
Pseudomonas
  and burn wounds, 367
  and cystic fibrosis, 548
  and meningitis, 417
  and osteomyelitis, 500
  and otitis externa, 461
  and urinary tract infections, 724
Psoas sign, 695
Psychosocial development of infants, 23-24; *see also* Developmental milestones
PTH; *see* Parathyroid hormone (PTH)
PTU; *see* Propylthiouracil (PTU)
Ptyalin, 669
Pubarche, premature, 794
Pubertal development
  in females, 783
  in males, 780
Pubescence, 35-36
  average age of milestones in American boys, 36
  average age of milestones in American girls, 35
Pubic hair
  development of
    in females, 783
    in males, 781
  growth of
    in boys, 36
    in girls, 35
Pubic lice, 801
Pulmonary artery banding, 590
Pulmonary ejection murmur, 583
Pulmonary function tests, 531
Pulmonary stenosis, 602
Pulmonary venous connection, total anomalous, 604-605
Pulse(s)
  apical, monitoring, in fluid and electrolytes alterations, 235
  assessment of, 129, 578
    in CPR, 240-241

Pulse(s)—cont'd
  normal rates of, 115
  techniques for taking, 115
Pulse pressure, assessment of, 581
Pulsus alternans, 581
  and pericarditis, 615
Puncture
  capillary, 221
  lumbar, restraining for, 217
  venous, 221
Punishment; *see* Discipline
Pupillary light reflex, 120, 121
Pupils, assessment of, 387, 449
Purinethol; *see* 6-Mercaptopurine
Purpura
  description of, 115
  idiopathic thrombocytopenic, 661-662
Pustules, 349
  and acne vulgaris, 364
  description of, 115
PV-IVH; *see* Periventricular-intraventricular hemorrhage (PV-IVH)
Pyelonephritis, 723, 724
Pyloric sphincter, 668
Pyloric stenosis, 689
  and dehydration, 232
Pyrogens, 217
Pyrvinium pamoate for oxyuriasis, 693
PZI; *see* Protamine zinc

Q

Questions in interviews, 94
Quinacrine for taeniasis, 693

R

Race, influence of, on child development, 14
Radiant warmers, overhead, 319
Radiation and increased body temperature, 217
Radiation therapy for brain tumors, 428, 431-432
Radiologic tests, 135
  for cardiovascular problems, 585
Rales, 127
Range-of-motion, assessment of, 133
Range-of-motion exercise, 496
Ranitidine for Curling's ulcer, 370
Rash(es)
  of chickenpox, 358
  diaper, 350
  of measles, 355
  rheumatoid, 505
  of rubella, 355
  of scarlet fever, 355
  skin, assessment of, 117
Rashkind septostomy, 604
RDAs; *see* Recommended Dietary Allowances (RDAs)
R-DPQ; *see* Denver Prescreening Questionnaire, Revised (R-DPQ)
Reach and grasp skills, 336
Reassessment, 106
Rebound tenderness, 130
Recommended Dietary Allowances (RDAs), 139
Recreation and adolescents, 90-91

Rectal swab, 670
Rectum, 668
  physical assessment of, 131-132
Rectus femoris muscle for injections in thigh, 209
Red blood cells, examination of, in urine, 707; *see also* Erythrocytes
Red cell infusion, packed, 629
Red measles; *see* Rubeola
Red reflex, 121-122
Reed-Sternberg cell, 662
Reflex(es); *see also* specific reflexes
  assessment of, 388
  cremasteric, 131, 391, 786
  deep tendon, assessment of, 134
  extrusive, 72
  infantile, 391
  of newborn, 23
  primary, assessment of, 133-134
  red, 121-122
Reflex irritability and Apgar scoring, 303
Reflex movement, 481
Refraction of light, 444-445
Refractive errors, 467-469
Regional enteritis, 698-699
Regionalization of perinatal care, 323-325
Regression
  of hospitalized school-age children, 190
  of hospitalized toddler, 187-188
Rehabilitation
  for musculoskeletal problems 496
  for spinal cord injury, 440
Reinforced coughing, 212
Rejection of chronically ill children, 274
Related factors, 97
Religion
  and bereavement, 283
  and death, 281-282
  role of, in nursing care, 41
Renal biopsy, 709-710
Renal buffering, 227
Renal failure
  acute, 732-733
    as complication of shock, 245
    nursing care plan for, 734-736
  chronic, 733
Renal problems; *see also* Urinary problems
  in adolescent, 731-737
  in preschooler and school-age child, 728-731
  in toddler, 715-728
Renal scan, 709
Renal system
  in acid-base balance, 227
  diagnostic tests for, 704
  functional tests for, 707-709
Renal trauma, 730
Renin, 703
Replacement therapy, deficit, 233
Reproductive problems
  in adolescent, 796-805
  in newborn and infant, 789-790
  nursing diagnoses related to, 788
  in school-age child, 794-796
  in toddler and preschooler, 791-794
Reproductive system
  anatomy and physiology of, 777-784

Urine
average 24-hour outputs of, 710
collection of, 221-222, 223
dipstick tests and, 706
microscopic examination of, 707
normal values of, 221
normal volumes of, in different age groups, 234
pH of, 706
production of, 702-703
specific gravity of, 706
sugar in, testing for, 706
Urine concentration test, 704, 708
Urine specimens, 703
collection of, 705-706
12- or 24-hour, 707
Urticaria, 348
and drug eruption, 363
Uterine bleeding, dysfunctional, 797
Uterus, 778
UTI; see Urinary tract infections (UTIs)
Uvula, assessment of, 125

V

Vaccine for rubella, 359
Vaccinia, isolation for, 219
Vagina, 778
Vaginal orifice, 778
examination of, 787
Vaginitis, nonspecific, 801
Vagus nerve
assessment of, 388
function of, 389-390
testing, 389
Valium for meningitis, 420; see also Diazepam
Vanceril; see Beclomethasone dipropionate
Varicella, 357-359
isolation for, 219
and leukemia, 659
Varicella-zoster virus, 357
Vas deferens, 777, 778
VASC auditory screening method, 454
Vasogenic shock, 244
Vasopressin, 743, 744
lysine, for diabetes insipidus, 751
for subdural hematoma, 412
Vastus lateralis muscle for injections in thigh, 208
VCUG; see Voiding cystourethrogram (VCUG)
Vectorcardiogram, 584
Vegetables
average-size servings per age, 156
recommended servings of, 142
Vegetarianism, 142-143
Velopharyngeal flap operation, 681
Vena cava, inferior and superior, 576
Venereal disease and partial emancipation, 164-165; see also Sexually transmitted diseases
Venipuncture
femoral, restraining for, 217
jugular, restraining for, 216
Venous hum, 583
Venous puncture, 221
Ventilation, 528

Ventilatory support for high-risk neonate, 320-321
Ventolin; see Albuterol sulfate
Ventral suspension in neurological assessment of newborn, 21
Ventricular fibrillation, 582
Ventricular septal defect (VSD), 589-590
murmur of, 583
and transposition of great vessels, 604
Ventricular tachycardia, 582
Ventricular tap, 395
Ventriculogram, 394
Ventriculoperitoneal shunt, 404
VEPs; see Visual evoked potentials (VEPs)
Vernal conjunctivitis, 449
Vesicles, 348
description of, 115
Vesicopustules, 349
Vesicostomy, cutaneous, 730
Vesicoureteral reflux, 724
Vessels, great, transposition of, 603-604
Vestibular function test, 123-124
Vestibular stimulation
of high-risk neonates, 326
of mentally retarded infant, 335
Viar-A; see Vidarabine
Vibration as chest physical therapy, 212, 213
Vidarabine for herpes encephalitis, 424
Vinblastine for Hodgkin's disease, 663
Vincristine
for Hodgkin's disease, 663
for leukemia, 653, 656, 657, 658
for medulloblastoma, 419
for osteogenic and Ewing sarcoma, 515
for Wilms' tumor, 711
Vineland Social Maturity Scale, 332
Violence
and child care, 7
in family, 248
potential for, related to child abuse, 256
on television, and school-age child, 85
Viral pharyngitis, 565
Viral respiratory infections, 566, 567-568
Virus(es)
Epstein-Barr, 664
herpes simplex, type 2, 800
human immunodeficiency, 629
and pneumonia, 545
respiratory syncytial, 541-542
and bronchiolitis, 538
Vision; see also Eye(s)
assessment of, 448-449
screening of, 122
Vistaril; see Hydroxyzine hydrochloride
Visual acuity, diagnostic tests for, 452-453
Visual evoked potentials (VEPs), 452
Visual fields, assessment of
in child, 387
in infant, 388
Visual impairment; see also Blindness
child with, nursing management of, 455
mental retardation and, 339
Visual stimulation
of high-risk neonates, 326
of infants, 71, 72, 73, 74, 75

Visual stimulation—cont'd
of mentally retarded infant, 335
of newborns, 70
Vital capacity (VC), 531
Vital signs
of children and adolescents, 23
monitoring, in fluid and electrolyte alterations, 235-236
normal, 115-116
technique for taking
in older infant, 112
in young infant, 111
Vitamin(s), 143
fat-soluble, 144
in infant formulas, 148
metabolism of, thyroid hormones and, 744
water-soluble, 144-145
Vitamin A
functions and sources of, 144
physiologic functions of, 140
sources of, 140
Vitamin A-acid for acne vulgaris, 365
Vitamin B; see Thiamin
Vitamin B_2; see Riboflavin
Vitamin C
functions and sources of, 144
physiologic functions of, 140
sources of, 140, 146
Vitamin D
functions and sources of, 144
for hypoparathyroidism, 758
Vitamin E, 144
Vitamin K
functions and sources of, 144
in hemorrhagic disease of newborn, 316
VM-26; see Tenoposide
Vocal fremitus, 126-127
Voided specimens, clean, 221-222
Voiding cystourethrogram (VCUG), 704, 708-709
Volkmann's ischemic contracture, 493
Vomiting
assessment of, in fluid and electrolyte alterations, 234
and dehydration, 230, 231
protracted, 232
VP-16; see Etoposide
VSD; see Ventricular septal defect (VSD)
Vulva, 778
Vulvovaginitis, 794-795

W

Walking, assessment of, 132
Walking reflex, 133
Warmers, overhead radiant, 319
Wasp stings, 361
Water
distribution body, internal exchange of, 225
distribution in body, factors influencing, 225
importance of, to human body, 224
as nutrient, 146-147
in replacement therapy, 233
and sodium balance, 702
Water deprivation test, 746

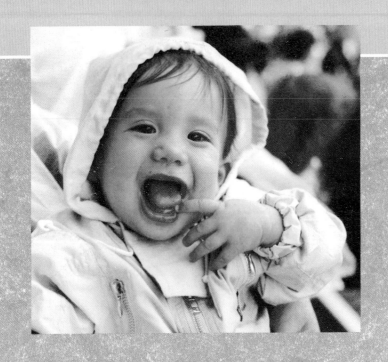
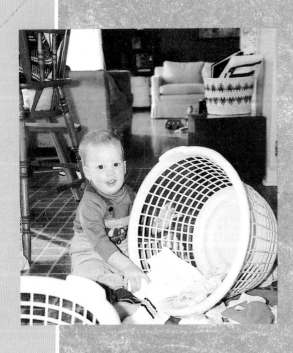
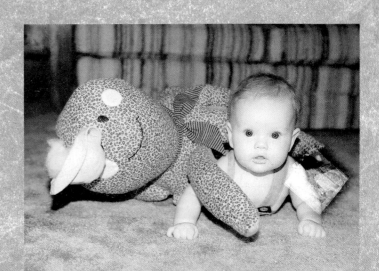